THE JOHNS HOPKINS MANUAL OF GYNECOLOGY AND OBSTETRICS

Sixth Edition

T0200186

THE JOHNS HOPKINS MANUAL OF GYNECOLOGY AND OBSTETRICS

Sixth Edition

Betty Chou, MD
Residency Program Director
Assistant Professor
Department of Gynecology and Obstetrics
Johns Hopkins University School of Medicine
Baltimore, Maryland

Jessica L. Bienstock, MD, MPH
Associate Dean for Graduate Medical Education and
Designated Institutional Official
Vice Chair for Education
Department of Gynecology and Obstetrics
Professor, Maternal Fetal Medicine
Johns Hopkins University School of Medicine
Baltimore, Maryland

Andrew J. Satin, MD
The Dr. Dorothy Edwards Professor and
Director (Chair) of Gynecology and Obstetrics
Obstetrician/Gynecologist-in-Chief
Johns Hopkins Medicine
Baltimore, Maryland

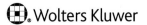

Philadelphia • Baltimore • New York • London
Buenos Aires • Hong Kong • Sydney • Tokyo

Acquisitions Editor: Chris Teja
Development Editor: Robyn Alvarez/Thomas Celona
Editorial Coordinator: Julie Kostelnik
Marketing Manager: Phyllis Hitner
Production Project Manager: David Saltzberg
Design Coordinator: Stephen Druding
Manufacturing Coordinator: Beth Welsh
Prepress Vendor: Absolute Service, Inc.

Sixth edition

Copyright © 2021 Wolters Kluwer

Copyright © 2015 Wolters Kluwer
Copyright © 2011 Lippincott Williams & Wilkins, a Wolters Kluwer business
Copyright © 2007, 2002 by Lippincott Williams & Wilkins

9 8 7 6 5 4 3 2

Printed in the United States of America

Library of Congress Cataloging-in-Publication Data
Library of Congress Control Number: 2020932847

shop.lww.com

MPP1121

Dedication

We have dedicated previous editions to our mentors, mentees, and loved ones who energize and inspire us. We would be remiss not to recognize those groups again. We are honored to continue the tradition of this manual, to work with dedicated colleagues at Johns Hopkins and beyond, all in an effort to advance the health of women and families.

Andrew J. Satin, MD
Jessica Bienstock, MD, MPH
Betty Chou, MD

Preface

The history of the Department of Gynecology and Obstetrics extends over 130 years. We are very proud of our historic tradition of leadership in gynecology, obstetrics, and our subspecialties, dating back to Drs. Howard Kelly, J.W. Williams, Richard TeLinde, Nicholson Eastman, Howard and Georgeanna Jones, and so many others who have come before us. Our proud tradition inspires us today to advance our tripartite mission of clinical care, research, and education. In an era of economic and market challenges to academic medicine, we remain steadfast to ensuring advances in all arms of our tripartite mission. Now in its sixth edition, this manual continues to be created by the cooperative efforts of a resident or fellow, faculty preceptor, and a senior faculty editor at Johns Hopkins. It draws its strength from the collaboration of experienced faculty and insightful practical input from rising stars in our field. In using this edition, we hope you will appreciate the camaraderie in which the manual was created. This manual is truly a team effort. Over the years, this book has been a trusted companion carried in the lab coats of residents, medical students, and busy clinicians.

This edition contains several new chapters addressing contemporary topics affecting our patients. Substance abuse, specifically opioid use, in pregnancy has escalated dramatically in recent years. The rise of fetal therapy programs including management options for twin-to-twin transfusion led us to expand content on multifetal gestation. The recognition of the role of genetics prompted a new chapter on genetic and hereditary syndromes. In addition to new chapters in obstetrics addressing substance abuse and multifetal gestation we added chapters on psychiatric disorders, dermatologic disease, and neoplastic disease in pregnancy. New gynecologic chapters focus on organ prolapse, incontinence, and benign vulvar disease. Emphasis on safety sciences and value-based care is pervasive in modern medicine and is now incorporated throughout the practice of obstetricians and gynecologists. We dedicate a new chapter in this edition of the manual to this most important topic. As much as things change, we hope and trust that the content, readability, portability, format, and size continue to have great appeal for practicing clinicians and learners.

Andrew J. Satin, MD
Jessica Bienstock, MD, MPH
Betty Chou, MD

Contributors

All chapter first authors are current or former residents/clinical fellows of the Johns Hopkins Department of Gynecology and Obstetrics. All chapter senior authors are current or former faculty of the Johns Hopkins University School of Medicine.

Crystal Aguh, MD
Director, Ethnic Skin Fellowship
Assistant Professor
Johns Hopkins University School of Medicine
Baltimore, Maryland

Abimbola Aina-Mumuney, MD
Assistant Professor
Division of Maternal Fetal Medicine
Department of Gynecology and Obstetrics
Johns Hopkins University School of Medicine
Baltimore, Maryland

Steve C. Amaefuna, MD
Resident Physician
Department of Gynecology and Obstetrics
Johns Hopkins University School of Medicine
Baltimore, Maryland

Jean R. Anderson, MD
Professor
Department of Gynecology and Obstetrics
Johns Hopkins University School of Medicine
Baltimore, Maryland

Ana M. Angarita, MD
Resident Physician
Department of Gynecology and Obstetrics
Johns Hopkins University School of Medicine
Baltimore, Maryland

Maria Facadio Antero, MD
Clinical Fellow, Female Pelvic Medicine and
  Reconstructive Surgery
Department of Gynecology and Obstetrics
Johns Hopkins University School of Medicine
Baltimore, Maryland

Cynthia H. Argani, MD
Assistant Professor
Department of Gynecology and Obstetrics
Johns Hopkins University School of Medicine
Baltimore, Maryland

Deborah K. Armstrong, MD
Professor, Department of Oncology
Professor, Department of Gynecology and
  Obstetrics
Johns Hopkins University School of Medicine
Baltimore, Maryland

Ahmet Baschat, MD
Professor
Director, Johns Hopkins Center for Fetal
  Therapy
Department of Gynecology and Obstetrics
Johns Hopkins University School of Medicine
Baltimore, Maryland

Anna L. Beavis, MD, MPH
Assistant Professor
Kelly Gynecologic Oncology Service
Department of Gynecology and Obstetrics
Johns Hopkins University School of Medicine
Baltimore, Maryland

Jessica L. Bienstock, MD, MPH
Associate Dean for Graduate Medical
  Education and Designated Institutional
  Official
Vice Chair for Education
Department of Gynecology and Obstetrics
Professor, Maternal Fetal Medicine
Johns Hopkins University School of Medicine
Baltimore, Maryland

Juliet C. Bishop, MD
Clinical Fellow, Maternal Fetal Medicine/
  Genetics
Department of Gynecology and Obstetrics
Johns Hopkins University School of Medicine
Baltimore, Maryland

Mostafa A. Borahay, MD, MPH
Associate Professor
Department of Gynecology and Obstetrics
Johns Hopkins University School of Medicine
Baltimore, Maryland

Carla Bossano, MD
Assistant Professor
Department of Gynecology and Obstetrics
Johns Hopkins University School of Medicine
Baltimore, Maryland

Irina Burd, MD, PhD
Associate Professor
Director, Maternal Fetal Medicine
  Fellowship
Department of Gynecology and Obstetrics
Johns Hopkins University School of Medicine
Baltimore, Maryland

Kamaria C. Cayton Vaught, MD
Clinical Fellow, Reproductive Endocrinology,
  Infertility, and Genetics
Department of Gynecology and Obstetrics
Johns Hopkins University School of Medicine
Baltimore, Maryland

Danielle B. Chau, MD
Resident Physician
Department of Gynecology and Obstetrics
Johns Hopkins University School of Medicine
Baltimore, Maryland

Katherine F. Chaves, MD
Resident Physician
Department of Gynecology and Obstetrics
Johns Hopkins University School of Medicine
Baltimore, Maryland

Chi Chiung Grace Chen, MD, MHS
Associate Professor
Department of Gynecology and Obstetrics
Johns Hopkins University School of Medicine
Baltimore, Maryland

Mindy S. Christianson, MD
Assistant Professor
Medical Director, Johns Hopkins Fertility
  Center
Department of Gynecology and Obstetrics
Johns Hopkins University School of Medicine
Baltimore, Maryland

Jensara Clay, MD
Assistant Professor
Department of Gynecology and Obstetrics
Johns Hopkins University School of Medicine
Baltimore, Maryland

Jenell S. Coleman, MD, MPH
Associate Professor
Division Director, Gynecologic Specialties
Medical Director, JHOC Women's Health
  Center
Department of Gynecology and Obstetrics
Johns Hopkins University School of Medicine
Baltimore, Maryland

Chantel I. Cross, MD
Assistant Professor
Department of Gynecology and Obstetrics
Johns Hopkins University School of Medicine
Baltimore, Maryland

Kristin Darwin, MD
Resident Physician
Department of Gynecology and Obstetrics
Johns Hopkins University School of Medicine
Baltimore, Maryland

Samantha de los Reyes, MD
Clinical Fellow, Maternal Fetal Medicine
Department of Gynecology and Obstetrics
University of Chicago
Chicago, Illinois

Rita W. Driggers, MD
Associate Professor
Department of Gynecology and Obstetrics
Johns Hopkins University School of Medicine
Baltimore, Maryland

Jill Edwardson, MD, MPH
Assistant Professor
Division of Family Planning
Department of Gynecology and Obstetrics
Johns Hopkins University School of Medicine
Baltimore, Maryland

Cybill R. Esguerra, MD
Assistant Professor
Department of Gynecology and Obstetrics
Johns Hopkins University School of Medicine
Baltimore, Maryland

Amanda Nickles Fader, MD
Associate Professor
Chief, Vice Chair of Gynecology Surgery
  Operations
Director, Center for Rare Gynecologic
  Cancers
Kelly Gynecologic Oncology Service
Johns Hopkins University School of Medicine
Baltimore, Maryland

Tola Fashokun, MD
Medical Student Instructor
Department of Obstetrics and Gynecology
Johns Hopkins University School of Medicine
Baltimore, Maryland

Jerome J. Federspiel, MD, PhD
Clinical Fellow, Maternal Fetal Medicine
Department of Obstetrics and Gynecology
Duke University
Durham, North Carolina

Braxton Forde, MD
Clinical Fellow, Maternal Fetal Medicine
Department of Obstetrics and Gynecology
University of Cincinnati Medical Center
Cincinnati, Ohio

Anja Frost, MD
Resident Physician
Department of Gynecology and Obstetrics
Johns Hopkins University School of Medicine
Baltimore, Maryland

Timothee Fruhauf, MD, MPH
Resident Physician
Department of Gynecology and Obstetrics
Johns Hopkins University School of Medicine
Baltimore, Maryland

Stéphanie Gaillard, MD, PhD
Assistant Professor
Department of Oncology and Gynecology/
  Obstetrics
Johns Hopkins University School of Medicine
Baltimore, Maryland

Nicole R. Gavin, MD
Clinical Fellow, Maternal Fetal Medicine
Department of Gynecology and Obstetrics
Johns Hopkins University School of Medicine
Baltimore, Maryland

Megan E. Gornet, MD
Resident Physician
Department of Gynecology and Obstetrics
Johns Hopkins University School of Medicine
Baltimore, Maryland

Ernest M. Graham, MD
Professor
Department of Gynecology and Obstetrics
Johns Hopkins University School of Medicine
Baltimore, Maryland

Marielle S. Gross, MD, MBE
Hecht-Levi Postdoctoral Fellow
Berman Institute of Bioethics
Johns Hopkins University Bloomberg School
  of Public Health
Baltimore, Maryland

Marlena Simpson Halstead, MD
Physician
Complete Care for Women
Department of Obstetrics and Gynecology
Chippenham Hospital
Richmond, Virginia

Esther S. Han, MD, MPH
Clinical Fellow, Minimally Invasive
  Gynecologic Surgery
Columbia University Medical Center
New York-Presbyterian Hospital
New York, New York

Katerina Hoyt, MD
Resident Physician
Department of Gynecology and Obstetrics
Johns Hopkins University School of Medicine
Baltimore, Maryland

Nancy A. Hueppchen, MD, MSc
Associate Professor
Associate Dean, Undergraduate Medical
* Education*
Division of Maternal-Fetal Medicine
Department of Gynecology and Obstetrics
Johns Hopkins University School of Medicine
Baltimore, Maryland

Tochi Ibekwe, MD
Instructor
Department of Gynecology and Obstetrics
Johns Hopkins University School of Medicine
Baltimore, Maryland

Angie C. Jelin, MD
Assistant Professor, Maternal Fetal Medicine/
* Genetics*
Department of Gynecology and Obstetrics
Johns Hopkins University School of Medicine
Baltimore, Maryland

Clark T. Johnson, MD, MPH
Assistant Professor
Department of Gynecology and Obstetrics
Johns Hopkins University School of Medicine
Baltimore, Maryland

Tiffany Nicole Jones, MD, MS
Resident Physician
Department of Gynecology and Obstetrics
Johns Hopkins University School of Medicine
Baltimore, Maryland

Svena D. Julien, MD
Assistant Professor
Division of Maternal Fetal Medicine
Department of Gynecology and Obstetrics
Johns Hopkins University School of Medicine
Baltimore, Maryland

Chavi Kahn, MD, MPH
Physician
Planned Parenthood of Maryland
Baltimore, Maryland

Edward K. Kim, MD, MPH
Resident Physician
Department of Gynecology and Obstetrics
Johns Hopkins University School of Medicine
Baltimore, Maryland

Benjamin K. Kogutt, MD
Clinical Fellow, Maternal Fetal Medicine
Department of Gynecology and Obstetrics
Johns Hopkins University School of Medicine
Baltimore, Maryland

Jaden R. Kohn, MD, MPH
Resident Physician
Department of Gynecology and Obstetrics
Johns Hopkins Hospital
Baltimore, Maryland

Lauren M. Kucirka, MD, PhD
Resident Physician
Department of Gynecology and Obstetrics
Johns Hopkins University School of Medicine
Baltimore, Maryland

Megan E. Lander, MD
Resident Physician
Department of Gynecology and Obstetrics
Johns Hopkins University School of Medicine
Baltimore, Maryland

Shari M. Lawson, MD, MBA
Assistant Professor
Division Director, Generalist Obstetrics and
* Gynecology*
Department of Gynecology and Obstetrics
Johns Hopkins University School of Medicine
Baltimore, Maryland

Jessica K. Lee, MD, MPH
Assistant Professor
Department of Obstetrics, Gynecology and
* Reproductive Sciences*
University of Maryland School of Medicine
Baltimore, Maryland

Judy M. Lee, MD, MPH, MBA
Adjunct Assistant Professor, Division of
  Gynecologic Specialties
Department of Gynecology and Obstetrics
Johns Hopkins University School of Medicine
Baltimore, Maryland

Kristen Ann Lee, MD
Resident Physician
Department of Gynecology and Obstetrics
Johns Hopkins University School of Medicine
Baltimore, Maryland

Kimberly Levinson, MD, MPH
Assistant Professor
Department of Gynecology and Obstetrics
Johns Hopkins University School of Medicine
Baltimore, Maryland

Melissa H. Lippitt, MD, MPH
Clinical Fellow, Gynecology Oncology
Department of Gynecology and Obstetrics
Johns Hopkins University School of Medicine
Baltimore, Maryland

David A. Lovejoy, MD
Associate Professor
Department of Obstetrics and Gynecology
Mercer University School of Medicine
Macon, Georgia

Jacqueline Y. Maher, MD
Assistant Research Physician and Staff
  Clinician
Division of Pediatric and Adolescent
  Gynecology
Division of Reproductive Endocrinology and
  Infertility
Eunice Kennedy Shriver *National Institute*
  of Child Health and Human Development
  (NICHD)
Bethesda, MD

Amanda C. Mahle, MD, PhD
Resident Physician
Department of Gynecology and Obstetrics
Johns Hopkins University School of Medicine
Baltimore, Maryland

Morgan Mandigo, MD, MSc
Obstetrician/Gynecologist
York Hospital
York, Maine

Melissa Pritchard McHale, MD
Resident Physician
Department of Gynecology and Obstetrics
Johns Hopkins University School of Medicine
Baltimore, Maryland

Meghan McMahon, MD
Resident Physician
Department of Gynecology and Obstetrics
Johns Hopkins Hospital
Baltimore, Maryland

Lorraine A. Milio, MD
Assistant Professor
Department of Gynecology and Obstetrics
Johns Hopkins University School of Medicine
Baltimore, Maryland

Christina N. Cordeiro Mitchell, MD
Clinical Fellow, Reproductive,
  Endocrinology, and Infertility
Department of Gynecology and Obstetrics
Johns Hopkins University School of Medicine
Baltimore, Maryland

Bernard D. Morris III, MD
Resident Physician
Department of Gynecology and Obstetrics
Johns Hopkins University School of Medicine
Baltimore, Maryland

Chailee Faythe Moss, MD
Assistant Professor
Department of Gynecology and Obstetrics
Johns Hopkins University School of Medicine
Baltimore, Maryland

Reneé Franklin Moss, MD
Resident Physician
Department of Gynecology and Obstetrics
Johns Hopkins University School of Medicine
Baltimore, Maryland

Lea A. Moukarzel, MD
Clinical Fellow, Gynecology Oncology
Department of Surgery
Memorial Sloan Kettering Cancer Center
New York, New York

Jamie Murphy, MD
Associate Professor
Director of Obstetrics, Gynecology and Fetal
  Anesthesiology Division
Department of Anesthesiology and Critical
  Care Medicine
Johns Hopkins University School of Medicine
Baltimore, Maryland

Emily Myer, MD
Urogynecologist
Department of Obstetrics and Gynecology
Minnesota Women's Care
Woodbury, Minnesota

Shriddha Nayak, MD
Assistant Professor
Department of Gynecology and Obstetrics
Johns Hopkins University School of Medicine
Baltimore, Maryland

Victoire Ndong, MD
Resident Physician
Department of Gynecology and Obstetrics
Johns Hopkins University School of Medicine
Baltimore, Maryland

Donna Maria Neale, MD
Assistant Professor
Department of Gynecology and Obstetrics
Johns Hopkins University School of Medicine
Baltimore, Maryland

Christopher M. Novak, MD
Assistant Professor
Department of Gynecology and Obstetrics
Johns Hopkins University School of Medicine
Baltimore, Maryland

Elizabeth Oler, MD
Physician and Surgeon
Department of Obstetrics and Gynecology
Evergreen Women's Health
Roseburg, Oregon

Lauren M. Osborne, MD
Assistant Professor
Departments of Psychiatry and Behavioral
  Sciences
Department of Gynecology and Obstetrics
Johns Hopkins University School of Medicine
Baltimore, Maryland

Yangshu Linda Pan, MD
Resident Physician
Department of Gynecology and Obstetrics
Johns Hopkins Hospital
Baltimore, Maryland

Prerna Raj Pandya, MD, MS
Clinical Fellow, Female Pelvic Medicine and
  Reconstructive Surgery
Department of Gynecology and Obstetrics
Johns Hopkins University School of Medicine
Baltimore, Maryland

Silka Patel, MD, MPH
Assistant Professor
Department of Gynecology and Obstetrics
Johns Hopkins University School of Medicine
Baltimore, Maryland

Kristin Patzkowsky, MD
Assistant Professor
Department of Gynecology and Obstetrics
Johns Hopkins University School of Medicine
Baltimore, Maryland

Jennifer A. Robinson, MD, MPH,
  PhD
Assistant Professor
Department of Gynecology and Obstetrics
Johns Hopkins University School of Medicine
Baltimore, Maryland

Linda C. Rogers, CRNP
Nurse Practitioner
Johns Hopkins Bayview Medical Center
Baltimore, Maryland

Isa Ryan, MD
Resident Physician
Department of Gynecology and Obstetrics
Johns Hopkins University School of Medicine
Baltimore, Maryland

Brittany L. Schuh, MD
Resident Physician
Department of Gynecology and Obstetrics
Johns Hopkins University School of Medicine
Baltimore, Maryland

Marla Scott, MD
Clinical Fellow, Gynecology Oncology
Cedars-Sinai Medical Center
Los Angeles, California

Rachel Chan Seay, MD
Assistant Professor
Department of Gynecology and Obstetrics
Johns Hopkins University School of Medicine
Baltimore, Maryland

Angela K. Shaddeau, MD, MS
Clinical Fellow, Maternal Fetal Medicine
Department of Gynecology and Obstetrics
Johns Hopkins University School of Medicine
Baltimore, Maryland

Jeanne S. Sheffield, MD
Professor
Division Director, Maternal Fetal Medicine
Department of Gynecology and Obstetrics
Johns Hopkins University School of Medicine
Baltimore, Maryland

Wen Shen, MD, MPH
Assistant Professor
Department of Gynecology and Obstetrics
Johns Hopkins University School of Medicine
Baltimore, Maryland

Khara M. Simpson, MD
Assistant Professor
Department of Gynecology and Obstetrics
Johns Hopkins University School of Medicine
Baltimore, Maryland

Anna Jo Smith, MD, MPH, MSc
Resident Physician
Department of Gynecology and Obstetrics
Johns Hopkins University School of Medicine
Baltimore, Maryland

Malorie Snider, MD
Attending Physician
Department of Obstetrics and Gynecology
Tanner Clinic
Layton, Utah

Rebecca Stone, MD, MS
Associate Professor
Division Director, Kelly Gynecologic
  Oncology Service
Department of Gynecology and Obstetrics
Johns Hopkins University School of Medicine
Baltimore, Maryland

Carolyn Sufrin, MD, PhD
Assistant Professor
Division of Family Planning
Department of Gynecology and Obstetrics
Johns Hopkins University School of Medicine
Baltimore, Maryland

Stacy Sun, MD, MPH
Clinical Fellow, Family Planning
Department of Gynecology and Obstetrics
Johns Hopkins University School of Medicine
Baltimore, Maryland

Sunitha Suresh, MD
Clinical Fellow, Maternal Fetal Medicine
Department of Obstetrics and Gynecology
University of Chicago
Chicago, Illinois

Edward J. Tanner III, MD
Associate Professor
Department of Obstetrics and Gynecology
Northwestern University
Chicago, Illinois

Lauren Thomaier, MD
Clinical Fellow, Gynecology Oncology
Department of Obstetrics, Gynecology and Women's Health
University of Minnesota
Minneapolis, Minnesota

Orlene Thomas, MD
Assistant Professor
Department of Gynecology and Obstetrics
Johns Hopkins University School of Medicine
Baltimore, Maryland

Julia Timofeev, MD
Assistant Professor
Division of Maternal Fetal Medicine
Department of Gynecology and Obstetrics
Johns Hopkins University School of Medicine
Baltimore, Maryland

Connie L. Trimble, MD
Professor
Departments of Gynecology and Obstetrics, Oncology, and Pathology
Johns Hopkins University School of Medicine
Baltimore, Maryland

Sandy R. Truong, MD
Resident Physician
Department of Gynecology and Obstetrics
Johns Hopkins University School of Medicine
Baltimore, Maryland

Katelyn A. Uribe, MD
Resident Physician
Department of Gynecology and Obstetrics
Johns Hopkins University School of Medicine
Baltimore, Maryland

Arthur Jason Vaught, MD
Assistant Professor
Department of Gynecology and Obstetrics
Johns Hopkins University School of Medicine
Baltimore, Maryland

Karen C. Wang, MD
Assistant Professor
Department of Gynecology and Obstetrics
Johns Hopkins Hospital
Baltimore, Maryland

Stephanie L. Wethington, MD, MSc
Assistant Professor, Gynecology Oncology
Department of Gynecology and Obstetrics
Johns Hopkins University School of Medicine
Baltimore, Maryland

MaryAnn Wilbur, MD, MPH, MHS
Instructor
Department of Obstetrics and Gynecology
Harvard Medical School
Boston, Massachusetts

Tenisha Wilson, MD, PhD
Resident Physician
Department of Gynecology and Obstetrics
Johns Hopkins University School of Medicine
Baltimore, Maryland

Harold Wu, MD
Clinical Fellow, Minimally Invasive Gynecology
Department of Gynecology and Obstetrics
Johns Hopkins University School of Medicine
Baltimore, Maryland

Camilla Yu, MD
Resident Physician
Department of Gynecology and Obstetrics
Johns Hopkins University School of Medicine
Baltimore, Maryland

Howard A. Zacur, MD, PhD
Theodore and Ingrid Baramki Professor of Reproductive Endocrinology
Fellowship Director for Reproductive Endocrinology and Infertility
Division of Reproductive Endocrinology and Infertility
Department of Gynecology and Obstetrics
Johns Hopkins University School of Medicine
Baltimore, Maryland

Contents

Obstetrics

1 Prepregnancy Counseling and Prenatal Care

Marlena Simpson Halstead and Rachel Chan Seay

PREPREGNANCY CARE AND COUNSELING

- Prepregnancy care is an important time during the women's health continuum that can reduce maternal-fetal morbidity and mortality. It is an opportunity prior to conception to optimize health, identify and modify risk factors, and provide education about considerations and behaviors that could affect a future pregnancy. Preconception counseling is becoming ever more important as more women are diagnosed with chronic conditions such as hypertension, diabetes mellitus, obesity, autoimmune diseases, and psychiatric illness. Preconception counseling should be implemented into the routine medical care of all reproductive-aged women. Any encounter with nonpregnant women with reproductive potential is an opportunity to improve reproductive health and impact future obstetric outcomes.
- A thorough review of medical, surgical, psychiatric, gynecologic, and obstetric health can expose potential complications in a planned pregnancy or factors contributing to infertility.
  - A full **obstetric history** should be taken during prepregnancy care and reviewed at the initial prenatal visit. Family planning and pregnancy spacing needs should be discussed, and women should be advised about the risks of interpregnancy intervals shorter than 6 months. Prior pregnancy complications should be discussed as well as the risk of recurrence and possible interventions that might decrease that risk.
- Prepregnancy care should include a review of **age-appropriate cancer screening**. If there is a history of inconsistent or outdated testing, this evaluation should be completed. Discussion about appropriate pregnancy timing should be considered to avoid delayed cancer diagnosis or treatment.
- Consultation with maternal-fetal medicine or reproductive endocrinology and infertility may be considered in women with a history of poor obstetric outcomes or chronic medical conditions.

1

Health Optimization and Medical Assessment

Approximately half of pregnancies are unintended or unplanned, so it is important to counsel all women with reproductive potential about wellness and healthy habits. In turn, a large portion of women consciously attempt pregnancy and actively seek counseling about health optimization, management of chronic illness, risk identification, and behavior modification prior to conception.

- Preconception care should include a thorough assessment of an individual's medical problems and risk assessment (Table 1-1). Many chronic medical conditions have implications for fertility and pregnancy, and the goal of prepregnancy care is to identify and optimally manage these conditions prior to pregnancy. Referral to specialists, including maternal-fetal medicine, may be appropriate, both for health optimization and for discussion of potential effects of a pregnancy on the chronic medical condition. While there are many medical conditions that should be optimized before conception, we discuss three common conditions here:
  - **Diabetes mellitus.** See chapter 11. Preconception counseling should include a review of current management in women with a prior diagnosis or a review of risk factors and recommendations to obtain diagnostic testing when applicable. Poorly controlled diabetes is associated with a risk of major fetal malformations. Pregestational diabetes mellitus is also associated with spontaneous abortion, preterm birth, and accelerated or excessive fetal growth.
  - **Chronic hypertension.** See chapter 12. The assessment of chronic hypertension should include the duration of illness, current medication regimen, and its

Table 1-1	Preconception Risk Assessment: Laboratory Testing[a]
Recommended for All Women	**Recommended Screening for Some Women**
Hemoglobin level or hematocrit	Tuberculosis
Rh factor	Hepatitis C
Offer genetic screening for cystic fibrosis, spinal muscular atrophy.	Gonorrhea and chlamydia
Urine dipstick	HIV
Age-appropriate cervical cancer screening (Pap smear ± HPV co-testing)	Syphilis
	Varicella IgG
	Toxoplasmosis IgG
Hepatitis B surface antigen	CMV IgG
Rubella IgG	Parvovirus B19 IgG
Illicit drug screen	Consider genetic carrier screening for hemoglobinopathies, Tay-Sachs disease, Canavan disease, or other genetic diseases.
	Lead level

Abbreviations: CMV, cytomegalovirus; HIV, human immunodeficiency virus; HPV, human papillomavirus; IgG, immunoglobulin G.

[a]Adapted from U.S. Department of Health and Human Services. *Caring for Our Future: The Content of Prenatal Care. A Report of the Public Health Service Expert Panel.* Washington, DC: U.S. Department of Health and Human Services; 1989.

degree of successful control. Further investigation into secondary causes of hypertension and other systemic sequelae may be needed, such as an assessment of baseline renal function or testing for ventricular hypertrophy. Recommendations should be made to alter current medication regimens to avoid angiotensin-converting enzyme inhibitors and angiotensin receptor blockers, as these agents are contraindicated in pregnancy. Preconception counseling should include a discussion about the risk of adverse outcomes during the pregnancy, including superimposed heart failure, stroke, worsening underlying renal disease, preeclampsia, placental abruption, fetal growth restriction, and preterm delivery.

- **Obesity.** The incidence of obesity in reproductive-aged women is increasing. Obesity is associated with problems including but not limited to infertility, recurrent pregnancy loss, preterm delivery, pregnancy-induced hypertension, gestational diabetes, stillbirth, and higher rates of cesarean delivery.
  - Optimal control and management obesity ideally occurs prior to conception. Improvement in medical comorbidities has been demonstrated in women with even modest weight loss prior to pregnancy. This weight loss can be achieved by medical or surgical means. Medications used for weight loss are not recommended during conception or pregnancy. Motivational interviewing to support healthy diet and physical activity has been used within the clinical setting to promote weight loss in this population.
  - The number of bariatric surgical procedures performed annually is increasing, and the majority of these patients are reproductive-aged females. Higher fertility rates are seen following surgery as a result of the rapid weight loss and restoration of predictable ovulation. Women should be counseled regarding contraceptive options with the recommendation to avoid pregnancy for 12 to 24 months following bariatric surgery.

Substance Use Assessment

All patients should routinely be asked about their use of nicotine products, alcohol, and prescription as well as illicit substances. The preconception interview allows timely education about drug use and effects on pregnancy, informed decision making about the risks of using these substances at the time of conception and throughout pregnancy, and the introduction of interventions for women who need treatment (see chapter 19).

- **Nicotine products.** Tobacco use remains the single largest preventable cause of disease and premature death in the United States. Screening for tobacco use and providing cessation counseling are some of the most effective preventive health actions provided by health care providers.
  - Tobacco use can negatively impact fertility and a future pregnancy by increasing rates of miscarriage, ectopic pregnancy, preterm birth, placental abruption, intrauterine growth restriction, low infant birth weight, and perinatal mortality. Tobacco exposure can continue to negatively impact the neonate, as children of smokers have increased risk of asthma, infantile colic, and childhood obesity.
  - Tobacco cessation should be recommended prior to conception and readdressed throughout the pregnancy and postpartum period. *Nicotine replacement therapy* with either gum or transdermal patch can be considered for women attempting to stop smoking. These forms of replacement reduce fetal exposure to toxic chemicals like carbon monoxide. In general, emphasis on offering techniques to stop smoking rather than mandating cessation alone has been found to be a more successful strategy in counseling cessation.

- **Alcohol.** Alcohol is a well-established teratogen. There is no known safe amount of alcohol use during pregnancy or while trying to get pregnant. Ethanol freely traverses the maternal-fetal placental barrier and the fetal blood-brain barrier. Although the threshold for adverse events is not currently known, a dose-related relationship between alcohol and the consequences in pregnancy has been established. The US Surgeon General advises woman who are pregnant or planning pregnancy to abstain from drinking alcohol.
  - *Fetal alcohol spectrum disorder* refers to a range of effects that can occur when a fetus is exposed to alcohol during pregnancy, including disturbances in intellect, learning abilities, behavior, growth, vision, and hearing. Alcohol can alter cardiac development, presenting as atrial or ventricular septal defects or conotruncal heart defects. Children born to women who abuse alcohol are at higher risk for skeletal, renal, and ocular defects than those not exposed to alcohol during pregnancy. Fetal alcohol syndrome represents the most severe form of the fetal alcohol spectrum disorder and is characterized by neurodevelopmental and central nervous system disturbances, growth deficiencies, and characteristic abnormal facial features. This group of conditions is preventable.
  - All women should be screened annually for alcohol dependence and abuse, and all pregnant women should be screened as early as possible in pregnancy. American College of Obstetricians and Gynecologists (ACOG) recommends the use of short validated screening tools, such as the T-ACE tool (Table 1-2). Identifying at-risk behavior allows for early intervention and timely referral for treatment.
- **Marijuana.** Marijuana is the most commonly used illicit substance during pregnancy, and marijuana use is increasing with marijuana legalization. The receptor on which marijuana acts has been found in the central nervous system of fetuses as early as 14 weeks' gestation. Animal models have suggested that tetrahydrocannabinol is able to cross the placenta, and there is some evidence in human research that it is also present in breast milk. Emerging evidence suggests that prenatal exposure to marijuana may result in impaired cognition and possibly an increased susceptibility to other illicit or abused substances. Marijuana use in pregnancy may be associated with an increased risk of stillbirth, preterm delivery, and lower birth weights. In addition to potential physiologic effects, patients should also be informed of the potential ramifications of a positive toxicology screen result in pregnancy.

Table 1-2	T-ACE Screening Tool for Alcohol Misuse[a]
Tolerance	How many drinks does it take to make you feel high?
Annoyed	Have people annoyed you by criticizing your drinking?
Cut down	Have you ever felt you ought to cut down on your drinking?
Eye-opener	Have you ever had a drink first thing in the morning to steady your nerves or get rid of a hangover?

[a]Positive score is 2 or more points. Two points are assigned if more than two drinks for the Tolerance question. One point is assigned if person responds "yes" to the Annoyed, Cut down, or Eye-opener question.

- **Opioids.** The prevalence of opioid use in pregnancy has increased dramatically in recent years. Opioid use disorder is a chronic disease that can be managed successfully when identified. Several validated screening tools exist, and ACOG recommends early universal screening in pregnancy for opioid use disorder.
  - Opioids can be ingested orally, intravenously, or by inhalation. They can be swallowed, chewed, or placed as suppositories. All opioid substances may result in overdose, causing respiratory depression or death. Additionally, injected opioids carry the risk of blood-borne diseases such as human immunodeficiency virus (HIV) and hepatitis, and additional vaccination and testing should be considered. Opioid use disorder is also associated with concomitant psychiatric disorders such as depression, anxiety, and posttraumatic stress disorder. Thus, mental health screening is particularly important in these patients.
  - The literature is inconsistent regarding the risk of congenital anomalies following prenatal opioid exposure. Chronic use during pregnancy is associated with an increased risk of fetal growth restriction, preterm birth, stillbirth, and placental abruption. *Neonatal abstinence syndrome* is the drug withdrawal pattern that may develop in neonates exposed to chronic maternal opioid use in utero. It may last days to weeks and is characterized by poor feeding, poor sleep, hypertonicity, sneezing, high-pitched cry, diarrhea, tremors, or seizure.
- **Cocaine.** Many of the adverse effects of cocaine are related to vasoconstriction or hypertensive events. Cocaine use is associated with cardiac ischemia, cerebral infarction or hemorrhage, and malignant hypertension and may lead to sudden cardiac death. Cocaine use in pregnancy is associated with spontaneous abortion, stillbirth, placental abruption, preterm labor, preterm rupture of membranes, and fetal growth restriction. Fetuses exposed to cocaine in utero have an increased risk of behavioral abnormalities, cognitive impairment, and impaired motor function.
- **Amphetamine.** Data are limited when looking specifically at methamphetamine use in pregnancy. Women who use methamphetamine frequently use other illicit drugs as well which can confound outcomes. As trends demonstrate an increase in use within the United States, it is important to be aware of this compound and its effects. Methamphetamine can be ingested orally, intravenously, or rectally as well as by inhalation or nasal insufflation. Intrauterine exposure has been consistently associated with infants who are small for gestational age and may increase the risk of early childhood neurodevelopmental abnormalities. At present, teratogenicity has not been demonstrated.

Psychiatric Health

Psychiatric illness during pregnancy is associated with a higher risk of postpartum psychiatric illness, less or inconsistent prenatal care, and poor maternal and infant outcomes. In addition, antidepressants and antipsychotic medications have been associated with decreased ovulation and infertility. Evaluation for psychiatric illness and optimization of a medical regimen should be encouraged prior to pregnancy (see chapter 18).

Review of Medications

All prescription medications, over-the-counter drugs, and dietary supplements should be reviewed. Male partners should also be screened for the use of androgens, which is associated with male factor infertility. If attempting pregnancy, it is important to review the safety of all current medications prior to conception. Secondary to the oversimplification of safety profiles, the historic categories for medications in pregnancy have been replaced with descriptions that are felt to be more comprehensive. Assistance in answering questions about reproductive toxicology is available through the online database REPROTOX (http://www.reprotox.org). Potentially teratogenic medications should be adjusted in collaboration with the prescribing health care providers. Both the maternal and fetal risk of continuing or discontinuing medication should be considered. In some cases, discontinuation of a medication may be associated with a greater risk for maternal well-being when compared to potential medication-related risks to the fetus.

Infectious Disease Screening

It is important to clarify a history of infectious diseases and assess past and current risk of exposure and need for screening. A woman should be screened based on age and risk factors for gonorrhea, chlamydia, syphilis, HIV, hepatitis, tuberculosis, toxoplasmosis, and Zika virus as appropriate. A history of herpes simplex virus, particularly genital involvement, should be assessed. Listeria infection is associated with obstetric and neonatal complications, and dietary recommendations should be reviewed.

Immunizations

Both prepregnancy and prenatal counseling should include a review of immunization status and recommendations for appropriate vaccination.

- **Influenza.** This vaccine is recommended annually during the flu season for all pregnant women regardless of gestational age. Patients with conditions that make them more susceptible to the illness, such as cardiopulmonary disorders, immunosuppression, and diabetes mellitus, should be especially urged to comply with this recommendation.
- **Tetanus, diphtheria, and pertussis.** The Centers for Disease Control and Prevention recommends administering the tetanus, diphtheria, and pertussis vaccine during each pregnancy between 27 and 36 weeks, preferably during the earlier part of this time period.
- **Hepatitis B.** Administration of the hepatitis B virus (HBV) vaccine or hepatitis B immune globulin is safe in pregnancy. Women at high risk for HBV who should receive the vaccine during pregnancy include those with a history of intravenous drug use, those at risk from sexual exposure (multiple sex partners, partners of hepatitis B surface antigen–positive persons, receiving treatment for another sexually transmitted disease) or occupational exposure, those who reside in places where adults have high risk for hepatitis B infection (dialysis unit, nursing institutions), and those who are recipients of clotting factor concentrates.
- **Pneumococcal vaccine.** This vaccine is indicated for pregnant women at high risk for this infection, such as women with heart disease, HIV infection, lung disease, sickle cell disease, and diabetes.
- Live vaccines should be administered either prior to or after pregnancy.
  - The measles, mumps, and rubella vaccine contains live attenuated antigens. This vaccine should be administered outside of pregnancy and optimally more than 4 weeks prior to conception.
  - The varicella vaccine is a live attenuated vaccine and should be administered outside of pregnancy to those without a clinical history of the chicken pox or verified immunity.
  - The human papillomavirus vaccination is not currently recommended during pregnancy.

Social Assessment

- **Violence, intimate partner violence, and reproductive coercion.** Women of all ages may experience violence, but those of reproductive age are at highest risk. Screening for violence and intimate partner violence is a core part of women's preventive health and should routinely be included in prepregnancy and prenatal care. In addition to maternal trauma, physical abuse during pregnancy has been associated with fetal injury, stillbirth, antepartum hemorrhage, placental abruption, and preterm labor. All patients should be screened early and often, and patients should be made aware that all patients are screened. Legal and community resources should be provided to women who disclose abuse or reproductive coercion (see chapter 37).
- **Housing and food security.** Patients should be asked about social support and screened for housing and food security. Referral to social work and appropriate assistance programs should be incorporated into care as needed.
- **Insurance coverage and financial difficulties.** Many women do not know the eligibility requirements or extent of maternity coverage provided by their insurance carrier or may lack medical insurance coverage altogether. Referral for medical assistance programs should be part of preconception planning as needed.

Family History

- The preconception evaluation should include a thorough family history of the patient and her partner, including genetic disorders; congenital or chromosomal anomalies; mental disorders; consanguinity; and breast, ovarian, uterine, and colon cancer. Ethnic background of a couple may help guide recommendations for carrier screening. Referral to a genetics counselor may be considered.
- Early identification of carrier status can help guide reproductive goals and plans for attempting pregnancy; performing testing before, during, and after pregnancy; or using assistive technologies to achieve pregnancy.

Maternal Age

- Women who will be 35 years or older at the time of delivery are considered to be of advanced maternal age and are at increased risk for fetal aneuploidy, infertility, stillbirth, and other pregnancy-associated diseases such as hypertension and diabetes. Patients should be counseled on their options for aneuploidy screening and diagnostic testing.

Nutritional Assessment

- **Folic acid.** All women of reproductive age should take folic acid supplementation. Adequate folic acid intake decreases the risk for defects related to complete closure of the neural tube (NTDs). Average-risk women should consume 400 μg daily. Most prenatal multivitamins contain sufficient folic acid for average-risk women. Women who take antiepileptic medications or have had a prior pregnancy affected by an NTD are at higher risk and should consume higher levels (4 mg daily) of folic acid.
- Excessive use of supplements containing vitamin A should be avoided. At dosages of more than 20,000 IU daily, vitamin A carries a risk of teratogenic effects.
- **Eating habits and disorders.** Patterns in eating (eg, fasting, caloric restriction, use of nutritional supplements) should be discussed. Women at risk of eating disorders should be counseled, and multimodal treatment teams should ideally be established prior to pregnancy and include a nutritionist and a mental health provider.

ROUTINE PRENATAL CARE

Prenatal care is an ongoing process of health optimization for the woman and her fetus and requires continual assessment of medical and social determinants of health. Prenatal care is associated with improved reproductive outcomes including decreases in preterm birth, fetal growth restriction, and neonatal death. See Table 1-3 for recommendations for routine prenatal tests.

Pregnancy Dating

It is important to establish the correct gestational dating of a pregnancy as soon as possible during prenatal care. This can influence interpretation of antenatal testing and determine optimal delivery timing. Assuming that ovulation and conception occurred on the 14th day of a 28-day cycle, the average length of a human pregnancy is 280 days, counting from the first day of the last menstrual period (LMP). As soon

Table 1-3	Routine Prenatal Care
Timing	Exams and Tests
Initial obstetric visit	History and physical exam
	Blood/Rh type, antibody screen, CBC, rubella, Hgb electrophoresis (if at risk for hemoglobinopathy), urine culture, urine toxicology[a]
	Infection screening for syphilis[a], HBV, HIV[a], chlamydia, and gonorrhea. Consider HCV screening in pregnancy women at increased risk.
	Cervical cancer screening as needed
	Sonogram to confirm gestational age, viability, and number of fetuses
	Offer genetic testing for CF, SMA, or other carrier screening tests based on personal or family history.
11-14 wk gestation	Aneuploidy screening option: first trimester screen
16-20 wk gestation	Offer MSAFP.
	Aneuploidy screening option: quadruple ("quad") screen
18-22 wk gestation	Ultrasound evaluation of fetal anatomy and placental location
24-28 wk gestation	Blood/Rh type, antibody screen, CBC, GDM screening
	Infection screening: syphilis[a], HIV[a]
36 wk gestation	Group B streptococcus rectovaginal culture
	Consider repeat screening for gonorrhea/chlamydia.
	Verify fetal presentation.

Abbreviations: CBC, complete blood count; CF, cystic fibrosis; GDM, gestational diabetes mellitus; HBV, hepatitis B virus, HCV, hepatitis C virus; Hgb, hemoglobin; HIV, human immunodeficiency virus; MSAFP, maternal serum α-fetoprotein; SMA, spinal muscular atrophy.
[a]State-mandated testing may vary by location.

Table 1-4	Accuracy of Pregnancy Dating by Ultrasonography According to Gestational Age[a]		
Gestational Age (wk)	**Ultrasonographic Measurements**		**Accuracy**
<8 6/7	CRL		±5 d
9–13 6/7	CRL		±7 d
14–15 6/7	BPD, HC, FL, AC		±7 d
16–21 6/7	BPD, HC, FL, AC		±10 d
22–27 6/7	BPD, HC, FL, AC		±14 d
>28	BPD, HC, FL, AC		±21 d

Abbreviations: AC, abdominal circumference; BPD, biparietal diameter; CRL, crown-rump length; FL, femur length; HC, head circumference.
[a]Adapted with permission from American College of Obstetricians and Gynecologists Committee on Obstetric Practice. ACOG Committee Opinion No. 700: methods for estimating the due date. *Obstet Gynecol.* 2017;129(5):e150-e154. (Reaffirmed 2019). Copyright © 2017 by The American College of Obstetricians and Gynecologists.

as data from the LMP and first ultrasound are obtained, an estimated date of delivery (EDD) should be established and clearly communicated with the patient.

- Pregnancies resulting from assisted reproductive technology should use the assisted reproductive technology–guided gestational age for establishing the EDD.
- **Naegele's rule.** To estimate the date of delivery, determine the first day of the LMP, add 7 days, then add 1 year, and then subtract 3 months.
- **Ultrasonographic dating.** If EDD by ultrasound measurements falls within the range of accuracy, the LMP is used to establish the EDD as confirmed by ultrasound (Table 1-4).

Nutrition, Weight Gain, and Exercise

- **Nutrition.** A pregnant woman requires approximately 15% more calories than she does when not pregnant, that is, typically an additional 300 to 500 kcal/d.
- **Iron.** Consumption of iron-rich foods is encouraged throughout pregnancy. The National Academy of Sciences recommends adding 27-mg iron supplementation (typically present in prenatal vitamins) to the average diet. Additional supplementation may be required.
- **Weight gain.** Recommendations regarding total weight gain in pregnancy aim to optimize maternal and fetal outcomes. These recommendations are based on prepregnancy body mass index (BMI) and were established by the Institute of Medicine (Table 1-5).
- Obesity (BMI > 30 kg/m^2) is associated with an increased risk for poor pregnancy outcomes including miscarriage, stillbirth, fetal anomalies, preterm delivery, gestational diabetes and hypertension, preeclampsia, thromboembolic event, cesarean delivery, and shoulder dystocia. Women with a history of gastric bypass surgery should be evaluated for nutritional deficiencies (eg, protein, iron, vitamin B_{12}, folate, vitamin D, calcium). Weight loss counseling and referral to a nutritionist should be offered.
- **Physical exercise.** The US Department of Health and Human Services recommends that women participate in at least 150 minutes of moderate physical activity per week

Table 1-5	Recommended Range of Total Weight Gain in Pregnancy		
Prepregnancy Weight Category	*Prepregnancy Body Mass Index (kg/m²)*	Singleton	Twin Gestation
Underweight	<18.5	28-40 lb	No recommendation
Normal weight	18.5-24.9	25-35 lb	37-54 lb
Overweight	25-29.9	15-25 lb	31-50 lb
Obese (all classes)	30 and greater	11-20 lb	25-42 lb

during pregnancy and the postpartum period. This should be continued as tolerated during the pregnancy. Absolute contraindications to aerobic exercise during pregnancy include severe cardiac or pulmonary disease, cervical insufficiency or cerclage, multiple gestation at risk of premature labor, persistent second- or third-trimester bleeding, placenta previa, ruptured membranes, pregnancy-induced hypertension, and severe anemia. Relative contraindications to aerobic exercise during pregnancy include poor health status prior to pregnancy, anemia, unevaluated maternal cardiac arrhythmia, lung disease, poorly controlled type 1 diabetes, extremes of maternal weight, orthopedic or neurologic limitations, poorly controlled thyroid disease, and fetal growth abnormalities. Contact sports and activities with increased risk of falling or involving extremes in temperature should be avoided.

Immunizations

- See "Immunizations" under "Prepregnancy Care and Counseling" section.

Genetic Screening

- All pregnant women should be offered testing to assess risk of fetal aneuploidy. Fetal aneuploidy refers to conditions associated with an abnormal number of chromosomes. Whereas chromosomal abnormalities occur in approximately 1 in 150 live births, the prevalence is greater as aneuploidy accounts for a large proportion of early pregnancy loss.
- Risk factors to consider for referral to genetic counseling (Table 1-6) include family history, maternal age, ethnicity, drug and environmental exposures, and obstetric and medical history.
- Providing access to prenatal genetic counseling and screening allows providers to provide adequate prenatal interventions if needed, optimize neonatal outcomes by organizing appropriate resources following delivery, and provide relative reassurance to parents when testing is normal.
- ACOG recommends providing universal carrier screening for cystic fibrosis and spinal muscular atrophy to women who are considering pregnancy or are currently pregnant. Case-specific carrier screening can be offered for Tay-Sachs disease, fragile X syndrome, and certain hemoglobinopathies.
- **Down syndrome (trisomy 21)** is the most common condition associated with an abnormal chromosome number found in live born children that is not related

Table 1-6	Reasons to Consider Referral for Genetic Counseling

Mother age 35 or older at estimated date of delivery
Fetal anomalies detected via ultrasonography
Abnormal first trimester serum/nuchal translucency screening
Abnormal triple/quad screening or abnormal α-fetoprotein test results
Parental exposure to teratogens (includes certain drugs, radiation)
Family history of genetic disease (includes chromosome, single gene, and
    multifactorial disorders)
Personal or family history of birth defects or mental retardation
Certain parental medical conditions (eg, cancer, congenital heart disease)
Membership in ethnic group in which certain genetic disorders are frequent
    when appropriate screening for or prenatal diagnosis of the disease is
    available (eg, sickle cell anemia, Tay-Sachs disease, Canavan disease,
    thalassemia)
Consanguinity
Infertility
Recurrent pregnancy loss
Stillbirth or neonatal death
Infant, child, or adult with dysmorphic features, developmental and/or growth
    delay, ambiguous genitalia, or abnormal sexual development

to a sex chromosome disorder. All cases are identified by the presence of an extra chromosome 21, which can result from nondisjunction, translocations, or mosaicism. Down syndrome can vary in presentation and is associated with hypotonia, characteristic facial features, congenital heart defects, intellectual disability, and intestinal atresia (see chapter 9).

- **Patau syndrome (trisomy 13) and Edward syndrome (trisomy 18)** are more severe disorders associated with multiorgan birth defects and intellectual disability. The majority of cases die in utero or within the first year of life.

Screening Tests

See Table 1-7 for a summary of the common prenatal genetic screening tests.

First Trimester Screening

- First trimester screening is performed between 10 0/7 weeks' and 13 6/7 weeks' gestation. The test includes nuchal translucency, maternal age, and two maternal serum markers: free β-human chorionic gonadotrophin (hCG) and pregnancy-associated plasma protein-A.
- Factors required for accurate risk calculation include a history of prior birth with aneuploidy, race, number of fetuses, and current maternal weight.
- The detection rate for trisomy 21 is approximately 82% to 87% with a 5% false-positive rate, which is improved by adding an ultrasound assessment of the fetal nasal bone (about 95%). Detection rate for trisomy 18 is about 95%.
- First trimester screening does not include assessment of risk for NTDs.

Table 1-7   Summary of Prenatal Genetic Screening Tests[a]

Test	Components	Testing Time Frame	Comments	Detection Rate for Trisomy 21
First trimester screen	Maternal age Maternal serum: • hCG • PAPP-A Fetal ultrasound: • Nuchal translucency • ± Nasal bone	10-13 6/7 wk	Provides risk for trisomy 21 and 13/18; improved detection when fetal nasal bone is assessed	82%-87% 95% (including nasal bone assessment)
Quad screen	Maternal serum: • hCG • MSAFP • uE3 • DIA	15-22 6/7 wk	Provides risk for trisomy 21, 18, and open NTDs	81%
Combined screening (integrated)	Fetal nuchal translucency Maternal serum: • PAPP-A • hCG • MSAFP • uE3 • DIA	First and second trimester (as noted above)	Detection rate for trisomy 21 equivalent to first trimester screen when nasal bone is included	94%-96%
Combined screening (sequential)	Patient given results of first trimester screen and then decide whether to undergo invasive testing (if positive) or quad screen (if negative).	First and second trimester (as noted above)	Allows patients to decide the extent of testing they wish to pursue	95%
MSAFP	MSAFP	Second trimester	Provides risk for open NTDs	NA
Cell-free fetal DNA analysis	Maternal blood draw with analysis of fetal DNA	10 wk and later	Only recommended for patients at higher risk of aneuploidy	>98%

Abbreviations: β-hCG, β-human chorionic gonadotropin; DIA, dimeric inhibin A; MSAFP, maternal serum α-fetoprotein; NTDs, neural tube defects; PAPP-A, pregnancy-associated plasma protein-A; uE3, unconjugated estriol.
[a]Data from American College of Obstetricians and Gynecologists Committee on Practice Bulletins—Obstetrics, Committee on Genetics, Society for Maternal-Fetal Medicine. ACOG Practice Bulletin No. 163: screening for fetal aneuploidy. *Obstet Gynecol.* 2016;127:e123-e137.

Second Trimester Screening

- The quad screen is typically performed between 15 0/7 weeks' and 22 6/7 weeks' gestation and can establish risk for trisomy 18 and 21 and NTDs.
- Four maternal serum markers are evaluated: hCG, maternal serum α-fetoprotein (MSAFP), unconjugated estriol (uE3), and dimeric inhibin A (DIA). Maternal age is also noted during the evaluation.
- Trisomy 21 is detected at a rate of 75% for women younger than 35 years and 90% for those older than 35 years.
- Elevated α-fetoprotein is associated with defects of the abdominal wall or NTDs.

Combined Screening

- Combined screening uses combined first and second trimester screening to adjust a woman's age-related risk for fetal aneuploidy.
- **Integrated screening** uses nuchal translucency and pregnancy-associated plasma protein-A from the first trimester screening as well as hCG, MSAFP, uE3, and DIA from the second trimester screening. Results are reported only after *both* screening tests are completed. The detection rate for this method is 94% to 96% with 5% false positives; this is equivalent to first trimester screening when nasal bone is included in the risk assessment.
- **Sequential screening** involves giving the patient the first trimester screen results. If at high risk, patients are given the option for invasive testing, whereas those at low risk can still undergo second trimester screening to achieve a higher detection rate.

Cell-Free Fetal DNA Screening

- Fragments of fetal DNA can be isolated from maternal blood to determine the risk for several fetal conditions. This test can be performed between 10 weeks' gestation and term and detects >98% of trisomy 21 pregnancies. The false-positive rate is <0.5%, although this rate is higher in women at low risk of Down syndrome. The rate of detection is lower for trisomy 13 and 18. Women with no reportable result are also at increased risk of fetal aneuploidy.

Screening for Neural Tube Defects

- NTDs are the second most common type of congenital abnormality, after cardiac anomalies. This group of disorders is characterized by failure of the neural tube to close or be sealed by normal musculoskeletal coverings during embryogenesis. Incomplete neural tube closure can result in a range of disorders including meningocele, myelomeningocele, or anencephaly. Depending on the severity, some defects may have potential for surgical correction. The NTDs can be isolated defects or associated with syndromes and are associated with certain environmental disorders, maternal diseases, and ethnicities. Primary prevention of NTDs is recommended with folic acid supplementation (see chapter 9).
- Screening for NTDs should be offered to all pregnant women either with second trimester MSAFP and/or targeted fetal anatomy ultrasound.
- The MSAFP is a glycoprotein secreted by the fetal liver and yolk sac. Although not diagnostic, abnormally elevated levels of MSAFP (greater than 2.5 multiples of the median) are suspicious for open NTDs. Elevated MSAFP can also be detected in pregnancies complicated by abdominal wall defects, cystic hygroma, teratomas, fetal demise, multiple gestation, or incorrect pregnancy dating, whereas abnormally low levels of α-fetoprotein may be associated with fetal aneuploidy. Diagnostic ultrasonography should be performed in cases with abnormal MSAFP.

Ultrasonographic Screening

- Ultrasound evaluation of fetal anatomy and placental location should be performed between 18 and 22 weeks' gestation. Midtrimester ultrasonography seeks to identify major structural abnormalities (eg, enlarged nuchal translucency, cystic hygroma, cardiac malformations) and ultrasonographic "soft markers" of aneuploidy (eg, thickened nuchal fold, pyelectasis, echogenic bowel, short femur length). However, the sensitivity of ultrasound is widely variable depending on ultrasonographer experience, machine quality, number of fetuses, and maternal BMI. Women with high a priori risk of fetal aneuploidy should be offered diagnostic testing even when fetal anatomy is thought to appear normal on ultrasound evaluation.

Diagnostic Testing

- Prenatal diagnostic testing is most commonly done to evaluate for fetal chromosomal abnormalities. Fetal cells obtained by either chorionic villus sampling (CVS) or amniocentesis can then be evaluated using traditional karyotype, fluorescence in situ hybridization, or chromosomal microarray analysis. Unsensitized Rh-negative women undergoing prenatal diagnostic testing should receive Rho(D) immune globulin.
- In **chorionic villus sampling**, placental tissue is retrieved via transcervical or transabdominal aspiration.
  - This procedure is most commonly performed between 10 and 13 weeks of gestation, although the transabdominal approach may be offered throughout the second and third trimesters. There is no significant difference in the risks of the two approaches.
  - The CVS can be performed at an earlier gestational age than amniocentesis, allowing earlier diagnosis and thus earlier option for pregnancy termination.
  - The risk of CVS-related pregnancy loss is approximately 1:455 (0.22%).
  - In 1991, reports of limb defects after CVS were first reported. The risk of this outcome is decreased when the procedure is performed after 10 weeks' gestation.
  - Other risks of CVS include vaginal spotting, which is more frequent with the transcervical approach. Amniotic fluid leak or infection after CVS is very rare.
  - Unsensitized Rh-negative women undergoing CVS should receive Rh immunoglobulin.
- **Amniocentesis** is the transabdominal aspiration of 20 to 30 mL of amniotic fluid. Amniotic fluid contains fetal cells shed from the fetal gastrointestinal tract, skin, and bladder.
  - This procedure is typically performed between 15 and 20 weeks' gestation but can also be performed at more advanced gestational ages.
  - Placental puncture should be avoided because fetal blood can contaminate the specimen and lead to false-positive results.
  - Although accurate data are difficult to obtain, the rate of procedure-related pregnancy loss attributable to prenatal diagnostic procedures is estimated to be 0.1% to 0.3% when performed by experienced health care providers, and overall, the pregnancy loss rate for amniocentesis is very low. Other complications, including vaginal bleeding, leakage of amniotic fluid, and fetal trauma, occur infrequently, approximately 1% to 2% of all cases.

SUGGESTED READINGS

American College of Obstetricians and Gynecologists Committee on Gynecologic Practice. ACOG Committee Opinion No. 762: prepregnancy counseling. *Obstet Gynecol.* 2019;133: e78-e89.

American College of Obstetricians and Gynecologists Committee on Obstetric Practice. ACOG Committee Opinion No. 650: physical activity and exercise during pregnancy and the postpartum period. *Obstet Gynecol.* 2015;126:e135-e142. (Reaffirmed 2019)

American College of Obstetricians and Gynecologists Committee on Obstetric Practice. ACOG Committee Opinion No. 721: smoking cessation during pregnancy. *Obstet Gynecol.* 2017;130:e200-e204.

American College of Obstetricians and Gynecologists Committee on Practice Bulletins— Obstetrics. ACOG Practice Bulletin No. 156: obesity in pregnancy. *Obstet Gynecol.* 2015;126:e112-e126. (Reaffirmed 2018)

American College of Obstetricians and Gynecologists Committee on Practice Bulletins— Obstetrics. ACOG Practice Bulletin No. 162: prenatal diagnostic testing for genetic disorders. *Obstet Gynecol.* 2016;127:e108-e122. (Reaffirmed 2018)

American College of Obstetricians and Gynecologists Committee on Practice Bulletins— Obstetrics. ACOG Practice Bulletin No. 163: screening for fetal aneuploidy. *Obstet Gynecol.* 2016;127:e123-e137. (Reaffirmed 2018)

American College of Obstetricians and Gynecologists Immunization, Infectious Disease, and Public Health Preparedness Expert Work Group. ACOG Committee Opinion No. 741: maternal immunization. *Obstet Gynecol.* 2018;131:e214-e217. (Reaffirmed 2019)

Normal Labor and Delivery, Operative Delivery, and Malpresentations

Samantha de los Reyes and Orlene Thomas

Labor is defined as repetitive uterine contractions of sufficient frequency, intensity, and duration to cause progressive cervical effacement and dilation.

STAGES AND PHASES OF LABOR

- The **first stage of labor** begins with the onset of labor and ends with full cervical dilation. It is divided into latent and active phases.
  - The **latent phase** begins with regular contractions and ends when there is an increase in the rate of cervical dilation.
  - The **active phase** is characterized by an increased rate of cervical dilation and descent of the presenting fetal part, which may not occur until after 6 cm

of dilation. It ends with complete cervical dilation and is further subdivided into the following:

- **Acceleration phase:** A gradual increase in the rate of dilation initiates the active phase and marks a change to rapid dilation.
- **Phase of maximum slope:** the period of active labor with the greatest rate of cervical dilation
- **Deceleration phase:** the terminal portion of the active phase in which the rate of dilation may slow until full cervical dilation

- The **second stage of labor** is the interval between full cervical dilation and delivery of the neonate.
- The **third stage of labor** is the interval between delivery of the neonate and delivery of the placenta.
- The **fourth stage of labor**, or puerperium, follows delivery and concludes with resolution of the physiologic changes of pregnancy, usually by 6 weeks postpartum. During this time, the reproductive tract returns to its nonpregnant state, and ovulation may resume.

MECHANISM OF LABOR

The **cardinal movements of labor** refer to the changes in position of the fetal head during its descent through the birth canal in vertex presentation:

- **Descent (lightening):** movement of the fetal head through the pelvis toward the pelvic floor. The highest rate of descent occurs during the deceleration phase of the first stage and during the second stage of labor.
- **Engagement:** the descent of the widest diameter of the presenting fetal part below the plane of the pelvic inlet. The widest diameter in cephalic presentation is the biparietal diameter. In breech presentation, the bitrochanteric diameter determines the station.
- **Flexion:** a passive movement that permits the smallest diameter of the fetal head (suboccipitobregmatic diameter) to pass through the maternal pelvis
- **Internal rotation:** The fetal occiput rotates from its original position (usually transverse) toward the symphysis pubis (occiput anterior) or, less commonly, toward the hollow of the sacrum (occiput posterior).
- **Extension:** The fetal head is delivered by extension from the flexed position as it travels beneath the symphysis pubis.
- **External rotation:** The fetal head turns to realign with the long axis of the spine, allowing the shoulders to align in the anterior-posterior axis.
- **Expulsion:** The anterior shoulder descends to the level of the symphysis pubis. After the shoulder is delivered under the symphysis pubis, the remainder of the fetus is delivered.

MANAGEMENT OF NORMAL LABOR AND DELIVERY

Initial Assessment

History

- Age, parity (full-term deliveries [≥37 wk], preterm deliveries [≥20 to <37 wk], abortions [<20 wk], and living children), estimated gestational age (GA)
- Labor-related symptoms including (1) onset, strength, and frequency of contractions; (2) leakage of fluid; (3) vaginal bleeding; and (4) fetal movement

- Maternal drug allergies
- Medications
- Last oral intake
- Review of prenatal labs and imaging studies including fetal ultrasounds
- Past medical and surgical history, gynecologic history including abnormal Pap smears and sexually transmitted infections, obstetric history including birth weight and method of delivery of previous children, social history including tobacco/alcohol/illicit drug use

Physical Exam

- Maternal vital signs (pulse, blood pressure, respiratory rate, and temperature)
- Confirmation of GA, where appropriate, and confirmation of viability at ≥ approximately 24 weeks
- Assessment of fetal well-being (fetal heart rate [FHR])
- Frequency and intensity of contractions
- Fetal presentation
- Estimated fetal weight (may be performed via **Leopold maneuvers**, below)
  - Step 1: Palpate the fundus to ascertain a fetal pole and obtain fundal height.
  - Step 2: Palpate the lateral walls of the uterus to determine fetal lie (vertical vs transverse) and the location of fetal spine and extremities.
  - Step 3: Grasp and palpate the upper and lower poles to determine presentation, to assess mobility and fetal weight, and to estimate the amniotic fluid volume.
  - Step 4: Palpate the presenting part from lateral to medial to assess engagement in the maternal pelvis, the location of the fetal brow, and the degree of flexion.
- **Speculum exam**
  - Vulvar, vaginal, and cervical inspection (especially noting lesions or scars)
  - Evaluate for **ruptured membranes:** vaginal pooling of fluid in the posterior fornix, nitrazine test, and ferning seen on microscopic slide.
  - Wet mount, gonorrhea/chlamydia screening, group B *Streptococcus* culture, if indicated
- **Digital exam**—defer if estimated GA is <34 weeks with ruptured membranes. This exam can provide the following data:
  - **Cervical dilatation** is the estimated diameter of the internal os in centimeters. Ten centimeters corresponds to complete dilation.
  - **Cervical effacement** is the length of the cervix, expressed as the percentage change from full length, approximately 4 cm. (Zero percent or "long" means not shortened at all, whereas 100% means only a paper-thin rim of cervix is detected).
  - **Fetal station** describes the distance in centimeters between the presenting *bony* part and the plane of the ischial spines. Station 0 defines the level of the ischial spines. Below the spines is +1 cm to +5 at the perineum. Station above the spines is −1 cm to −5 at the level of the pelvic inlet.
  - **Clinical pelvimetry:** evaluation of the maternal pelvis by vaginal exam
    - **Diagonal conjugate:** the distance between the sacral promontory and the posterior edge of the pubic symphysis. A distance of at least 11.5 cm suggests a sufficiently adequate pelvic inlet for an average-weight fetus.
    - **Transverse diameter:** the distance between the ischial tuberosities, which can be approximated by placing a closed fist of known width at the perineum. An intertuberous diameter of at least 8.5 cm suggests an adequate pelvic outlet.
- The **pelvic type** can be classified into four types based on general shape and bony characteristics. Gynecoid and anthropoid types are most amenable to a successful vaginal birth.

Standard Admission Procedures

- Standard admission labs include urine testing (for protein and glucose), complete blood count, and a type and screen.
- For patients without prenatal care, hepatitis B surface antigen, human immunodeficiency virus, ABO blood group and antibody screen, urine culture and toxicology, rubella immunoglobulin G, complete blood count, and syphilis screening should be sent.
- Intravenous access (heplock or continuous infusion) is recommended.
- Informed consent for management of labor and delivery, contraception (if desired) and for administration of blood products, should they become necessary, should be obtained.

Management of Labor

- The quality and frequency of uterine contractions should be assessed regularly by palpation, tocodynamometer, or intrauterine pressure catheter (if indicated).
- The FHR should be assessed by intermittent auscultation, continuous electronic fetal monitoring, or fetal scalp electrode (FSE) (if indicated).
- Cervical examinations should be kept to the minimum required to detect abnormalities in the progression of labor.
- The lithotomy position is the most frequently assumed position for vaginal delivery in the United States, although birthing positions are highly cultural and alternative birthing positions, such as the lateral or Sims position or the partial sitting or squatting positions, are preferred by some patients, physicians, and midwives.

Induction of Labor

- **Indications:** Induction of labor is indicated when the benefits of delivery (for the mother or fetus) outweigh the benefits of continued pregnancy. The favorability of the cervix at the time of induction is related to the success of labor induction. When the Bishop score (Table 2-1) exceeds 8, the likelihood of vaginal delivery after induction is similar to that with spontaneous labor. Induction with a lower Bishop score has been associated with a higher rate of failure, prolonged labor, and

Table 2-1	Components of the Bishop Score[a]			
		Rating		
Factor	0	1	2	3
Dilation	Closed	1-2 cm	3-4 cm	5+ cm
Effacement	0%-30%	40%-50%	60%-70%	80%+
Station	−3	−2	−1, 0	>+1
Consistency	Firm	Medium	Soft	—
Position	Posterior	Midposition	Anterior	—

[a]Adapted with permission from Bishop EH. Pelvic scoring for elective induction. *Obstet Gynecol.* 1964;24:267.

| Table 2-2 | Induction of Labor: Indications and Contraindications[a] |

Indications	Contraindications
• Abruptio placentae, chorioamnionitis, gestational hypertension	• Vasa previa or complete placenta previa
• Premature rupture of membranes, postterm pregnancy, preeclampsia, eclampsia	• Transverse fetal lie
	• Infection—active genital HSV, high viral load HIV
• Maternal medical conditions (eg, diabetes mellitus, renal disease, chronic pulmonary disease, chronic hypertension)	• Pelvic structural deformities
	• Umbilical cord prolapse
• Fetal compromise (eg, severe fetal growth restriction, isoimmunization)	• Advanced cervical cancer
• Fetal demise	
• Elective inductions for gestational age >39 wk	

Abbreviations: HIV, human immunodeficiency virus; HSV, herpes simplex virus.

[a]Adapted with permission from American College of Obstetricians and Gynecologists Committee on Practice Bulletins—Obstetrics. ACOG Practice Bulletin No. 107: induction of labor. *Obstet Gynecol.* 2009;114(2):386-397. (Reaffirmed 2019). Copyright © 2009 by The American College of Obstetricians and Gynecologists.

cesarean delivery. Induction should not be initiated if vaginal delivery is contraindicated (Table 2-2).
- **Cervical ripening** may be used to soften the cervix before induction if the Bishop score is low. Cervical ripening can be achieved using pharmacologic and mechanical methods.
- **Pharmacologic methods of induction of labor and cervical ripening**
- **Low-dose oxytocin** may be used with or without mechanical dilators.
- **Prostaglandin E_2** is superior to placebo in promoting cervical effacement and dilation and may enhance sensitivity to oxytocin.
  - **Prepidil** gel contains 0.5 mg of dinoprostone in a 2.5-mL syringe; the gel is injected into the cervical canal every 6 hours for up to 3 doses in a 24-hour period.
  - **Cervidil** is a vaginal insert containing 10 mg of dinoprostone. It provides a lower rate of release (0.3 mg/h) than the gel but has the advantage that it can be removed if uterine tachysystole occurs (>5 contractions in 10 min).
- **Prostaglandin E_1** is also effective in stimulating cervical ripening.
  - **Misoprostol** is administered as 25 to 50 mg every 3 to 6 hours intravaginally, orally, or buccally. The use of misoprostol for cervical ripening is off-label.
- **Side effects:** Any pharmacologic induction method includes a risk of uterine tachysystole. If oxytocin is being used, it can be titrated down or turned off with quick effect due to its short half-life. If Cervidil is being used, the insert can be removed. If indicated, a β-adrenergic agonist (eg, terbutaline sulfate) can be administered. Maternal systemic effects of prostaglandins may include fever, vomiting, and diarrhea.
- **Contraindications:** Cervical ripening agents should be used with caution in patients with a history of uterine scar or prior cesarean delivery. Caution should

be exercised when using prostaglandin E_2 in patients with glaucoma or severe hepatic or renal impairment.

- **Mechanical methods of labor induction and cervical ripening**
  - **Membrane stripping (sweeping):** increases levels of phospholipase A2 and prostaglandins and increases likelihood of spontaneous labor within 48 hours
  - **Amniotomy** (artificial rupture of membranes): The risk of umbilical cord prolapse can be reduced by performing the amniotomy while the fetal presenting part is well applied to the cervix.
  - **Balloon catheters placed transcervically:** a single-balloon device such as a 24-French Foley catheter with inflation volumes of 30 to 80 mL inserted into the extraamniotic space. Other options are to use larger volume bulb catheters or a double-balloon device.
    - Recent evidence suggests that use of a mechanical method of induction with concurrent use of a pharmacologic agent results in a faster median time to delivery than single-agent alone.
- Osmotic dilators (laminaria)

Oxytocin Administration

- **Indications:** Oxytocin is used for both induction and augmentation of labor. Augmentation should be considered for protracted or arrest disorders of labor or the presence of a hypotonic uterine contraction pattern. A range of options regarding the dosing of oxytocin exist. A reasonable starting dosage is 0.5 to 4 mIU/min, with incremental increases of 1 to 2 mIU/min every 20 to 30 minutes. Cervical dilation of at least 1 cm/h in the active phase indicates that oxytocin dosing is adequate. If an intrauterine pressure catheter is in place, 180 MVU per 10-minute period are considered adequate. However, some practitioners use a threshold of 250 to 275 MVU with increased success of induction and minimal adverse consequences.
- **Complications:** Adverse effects of oxytocin are primarily dose related. The most common complication is uterine tachysystole (greater than 5 contractions in 10 min), which may result in uteroplacental hypoperfusion and nonreassuring fetal heart tracings (FHTs). Uterine tachysystole is usually reversible when the oxytocin infusion is decreased or discontinued. If necessary, a β-adrenergic agent may be administered. Rapid infusion of oxytocin can result in hypotension. Prolonged infusion can result in water intoxication and hyponatremia because oxytocin structurally resembles antidiuretic hormone; prolonged use also increases the risk of postpartum uterine atony and hemorrhage.

Labor Progress Assessment: Historical and Contemporary

- Dr. Emanuel Friedman's historic studies on normal labor resulted in widely used guidelines for normal labor progress.
  - **Latent phase prolongation** is somewhat controversial, as measurement of this phase is difficult and inexact. Generally speaking, without induction, this phase is considered prolonged if it exceeds 20 hours in a nulliparous patient and 14 hours in a multiparous patient.
  - The **active phase** is considered protracted if the rate of cervical change is <1.2 cm/h for the nulliparous patient and <1.5 cm/h in the multiparous patient. **Arrest of dilation** occurs when there is no apparent cervical change over a 2-hour period despite adequate contractions (180–250 MVU).

- The **second stage of labor** is considered protracted after 2 hours of pushing in nulliparous patients or 1 hour in parous patients. An additional hour may be allowed if epidural anesthesia is used. Arrest of descent occurs when there is no apparent descent of the presenting part over a 1-hour period of pushing during the second stage.
- The **third stage of labor** averages 10 minutes and is considered prolonged if it lasts longer than 30 minutes.
- More recently, data from the **Consortium on Safe Labor** suggest a revision of the definitions of normal and protracted labor to reflect a more contemporary obstetric population.
  - The evidence from this large retrospective study suggests a slower rate of cervical change than Friedman's work.
    - **For nulliparous women:** 0.5 to 0.7 cm/h
    - **For multiparous women:** 0.5 to 1.3 cm/h
- First-stage arrest
  - From 4 to 6 cm, nulliparous and multiparous women dilated at approximately the same rate but still at a slower rate than described by Friedman. From 6 cm and beyond, multiparous women dilated at a faster rate.
  - The active phase **did not start** until 6 cm.
- The Consortium on Safe Labor did not specifically address duration for diagnosis of arrest of labor but recommend diagnosis of arrest of labor to be reserved beyond 6 cm of dilation. Generally, if a patient remains at ≥ 6 cm for more than 4 hours in the setting of an adequate contraction pattern or for more than 6 hours without an adequate contraction pattern, she is said to have active phase arrest of labor.
- Second-stage arrest: no progress (descent or rotation) when pushing for over 3 hours in nulliparous women and over 2 hours in multiparous women. An additional hour is allowed if epidural anesthesia is used.
- **Abnormal labor** may be due to the following:
  - Power: inadequate uterine contractions or maternal expulsive effort
  - Passenger: size of fetus or abnormal proportions, presentation, or position
  - Passage: small pelvis or obstructed birth canal
- **Risk factors** for abnormal labor could be any medical condition or clinical situation that affects the categories above.
  - Risks for an abnormal first stage of labor: increased maternal age, diabetes, hypertension, premature rupture of membranes, macrosomia (usually defined as ≥ 4000 g or ≥ 4500 g), epidural anesthesia, chorioamnionitis, a history of previous complications like perinatal death, and amniotic fluid abnormalities
  - Risks for an abnormal second stage of labor: a prolonged first stage, occiput posterior position, epidural anesthesia, nulliparity, short maternal stature, increased birth weight, and high station at complete cervical dilation

Interventions for Abnormal Labor

- **Amniotomy:** Artificial rupture of membranes may enhance progress for a patient who is in active labor. It may increase the risk of chorioamnionitis, although the evidence has not demonstrated a significant increase in the risk.
- **Augmentation of labor via oxytocin:** Oxytocin has been shown to decrease the time of active labor in nulliparous women. In addition, some studies have shown that it decreases the rate of cesarean delivery for failure to progress.

- **Uterine contraction monitoring:** Placement of an intrauterine pressure catheter provides information about the frequency and strength of contractions and may be useful for titrating oxytocin to maximize the chance for successful vaginal delivery.

FETAL HEART RATE EVALUATION

The three-tiered guidelines for FHR or FHT interpretation are given in Table 2-3.

- **Baseline rate:** lasts for at least 2 minutes during a 10-minute section rounded to the nearest 5 beats/min.
- **Normal rate:** 110 to 160 beats/min
- **Bradycardia:** A baseline FHR <110 beats/min. Causes of bradycardia include fetal head compression, hypoxemia, and maternal hypothermia. The clinical picture is as important as the heart rate in interpreting fetal bradycardia.
- **Tachycardia:** A baseline FHR >160 beats/min. The most common cause is maternal fever or infection. Other less common causes of fetal tachycardia include fetal arrhythmias or maternal administration of parasympatholytic or sympathomimetic drugs.
- **Variability:** fluctuations in the FHR. It is most reliable when measured with an FSE.
  - **Absent:** absent variability
  - **Minimal:** detectable variability of <5 beats/min
  - **Moderate:** variability of 6 to 25 beats/min
  - **Marked:** variability of >25 beats/min
- **Accelerations:** For GA >32 weeks, an acceleration is an increase in FHR of at least 15 beats/min that lasts for at least 15 seconds. For GA <32 weeks, an acceleration is an increase in FHR >10 beats/min for 10 seconds.
- An FHT is **reactive** if it shows two accelerations within 10 minutes.
- A **sinusoidal** FHT is a persistent smooth undulating pattern with a frequency of 3 to 5 cycles/min. It is concerning and requires immediate evaluation. Fetal anemia; analgesic drugs such as morphine, meperidine, alphaprodine, and butorphanol; and chronic fetal distress should be considered.
- **Decelerations:** a decrease in FHR below the baseline. In some instances, the pattern of deceleration of the FHR can be used to identify the cause.
  - **Variable decelerations** may start before, during, or after the uterine contraction starts (hence, the designation "variable"). They usually show an abrupt onset to nadir in <30 seconds and return, which gives them a characteristic V shape. The decrease is >15 beats/min lasting >15 seconds but <2 minutes. Variable decelerations are commonly caused by umbilical cord compression.
  - **Early decelerations** are shallow and symmetric and reach their nadir at the peak of the contraction. They are caused by vagus nerve–mediated response to fetal head compression.
  - **Late decelerations** are U-shaped decelerations of gradual onset to nadir in >30 seconds and gradual return, reach their nadir after the peak of the contraction, and do not return to the baseline until after the contraction is over. They may result from uteroplacental insufficiency and relative fetal hypoxia. Recurrent late decelerations can be an ominous sign.
  - **Prolonged deceleration:** a deceleration that lasts longer than 2 minutes but <10 minutes
  - **Recurrent decelerations:** occur with >50% of uterine contractions in any 20-minute span
  - **Intermittent decelerations:** occur with <50% of uterine contractions in any 20-minute span.

| Table 2-3 | Fetal Heart Tracing Interpretation, Categories, and Criteria[a] |

Category	Description
Category I	All of the following: • Baseline rate: 110-160 beats/min • Baseline FHR variability: moderate • Late or variable decelerations: absent • Early decelerations: present or absent • Accelerations: present or absent
Category II	All FHR tracings not categorized as category I or category III. Category II tracings may represent an appreciable fraction of those encountered in clinical care. Examples of category II FHR tracings include any of the following: Baseline rate • Bradycardia not accompanied by absent baseline variability • Tachycardia Baseline FHR variability • Minimal baseline variability • Absent baseline variability with no recurrent decelerations • Marked baseline variability Accelerations • Absence of induced accelerations after fetal stimulation • Periodic or episodic decelerations • Recurrent variable decelerations accompanied by minimal or moderate baseline variability • Prolonged deceleration more than 2 min but less than 10 min • Recurrent late decelerations with moderate baseline variability • Variable decelerations with other characteristics such as slow return to baseline, overshoots, or "shoulders"

Category III	Either
	• Absent baseline FHR variability and any of the following:
	  • Recurrent late decelerations
	  • Recurrent variable decelerations
	  • Bradycardia
	Or
	• Sinusoidal pattern

Abbreviation: FHR, fetal heart rate.
[a]Reprinted with permission from Macones GA, Hankins GD, Spong CY, et al. The 2008 National Institute of Child Health and Human Development workshop report on electronic fetal monitoring: update on definitions, interpretation, and research guidelines. *Obstet Gynecol.* 2008;112(3):661-666. Copyright © 2008 by The American College of Obstetricians and Gynecologists.

Overall Assessment

- **Category I FHT** must have a baseline FHR between 110 and 160 beats/min and moderate variability, and accelerations may be present or absent, with no late or variable decelerations.
- **Category II FHT** are those that cannot be classified as category I or III.

- **Category III FHT** have concerning findings such as absent variability with recurrent variable or late decelerations, bradycardia, or sinusoidal pattern. Consideration for delivery should be given.

Management of Nonreassuring Fetal Heart Rate Patterns

- Nonreassuring FHR patterns do not necessarily predict adverse events, and although electronic fetal heart monitoring has resulted in increased cesarean deliveries, there has not been a decrease in long-term adverse neurologic outcomes such as cerebral palsy. Nevertheless, the known relationships between fetal hypoxemia/acidemia and abnormal heart rate patterns make FHT interpretation a critical part of labor management.

Noninvasive Management

- **Oxygen:** Maternal supplemental oxygen often results in improved fetal oxygenation, assuming adequate placental exchange and circulation.
- **Maternal position:** Left lateral positioning releases vena cava compression by the gravid uterus, promoting increased venous return, increased cardiac output, increased BP, and improved uterine blood flow.
- **Discontinue oxytocin** until the FHR and uterine activity become normal.
- **Vibroacoustic stimulation** or **fetal scalp stimulation:** Fetal stimuli may be used to induce accelerations when the FHR lacks variability for a long period of time. Heart rate acceleration in response to these stimuli indicates the absence of acidosis and correlates with a mean pH value of about 7.30. Conversely, a 50% chance of acidosis exists in a fetus that fails to respond to vibroacoustic stimulation in the setting of a nonreassuring heart rate pattern.

Invasive Management

- **Amniotomy:** If the FHR cannot be monitored adequately externally, an amniotomy should be performed to place internal monitors, unless these are contraindicated by the clinical situation.
- **Fetal scalp electrode:** Direct application of an FSE records the fetal electrocardiogram waveform and may allow closer evaluation of the FHR. An FSE may be contraindicated in cases of fetal coagulopathy or maternal infections such as human immunodeficiency virus or hepatitis B or C.
- **Intrauterine pressure catheter and amnioinfusion:** A catheter is inserted into the chorioamnionic sac and attached to a pressure gauge. Pressure readings provide quantitative data on the strength and duration of contractions. Amnioinfusion of room temperature normal saline can be used to replace amniotic fluid volume to relieve recurrent variable decelerations in patients with oligohydramnios. Care should be used to avoid overdistention of the uterus.
- **Tocolytic agents:** β-Adrenergic agonists (eg, terbutaline, 0.25 mg subcutaneously or 0.125-0.25 mg intravenously) can be administered to decrease uterine activity in the presence of uterine tachysystole. Potential side effects of β-adrenergic agonists include elevated serum glucose levels and increased maternal and FHRs.
- **Management of maternal hypotension:** Maternal hypotension, as a complication of the sympathetic blockade associated with epidural anesthesia or from compression of the vena cava, can lead to decreased placental perfusion and FHR decelerations. Intravenous fluid bolus, left uterine displacement, and ephedrine or phenylephrine administration may be appropriate.

ASSISTED SPONTANEOUS VAGINAL DELIVERY

The goals of assisted spontaneous vaginal delivery are reduction of maternal trauma, prevention of fetal injury, and initial support of the newborn.

- **Episiotomy** is an incision into the perineal body to enlarge the outlet area and facilitate delivery and is no longer routinely performed. Episiotomy may occasionally be necessary in cases of vaginal soft tissue dystocia or as an accompaniment to forceps- or vacuum-assisted vaginal delivery. Recent evidence demonstrates restrictive episiotomy practices were associated with a lower risk of perineal trauma and complications and are thus recommended over routine episiotomy.
  - **Median or midline episiotomy:** more commonly performed in the United States. Starts within 3 mm of the midline of the posterior fourchette. The incision should extend inferiorly between 0 and 25 degrees of the sagittal plane. These are associated with an increased risk of extension to a third- or fourth-degree laceration.
  - **Mediolateral episiotomy:** more commonly performed in Europe. Starts within 3 mm of the midline of the posterior fourchette. The incision should be directed at an angle of at least 60 degrees from the midline toward the ischial tuberosities.
- **Delivery of the head:** The goal is to prevent excessively rapid delivery by controlling the expulsion of the head. If extension of the head does not occur easily, a modified Ritgen maneuver can be performed by palpating the fetal chin through the perineum and applying pressure upward. After delivery of the head, external rotation is possible, which brings the occiput in line with the fetal spine. If a nuchal cord is present, it is reduced over the head or double-clamped and cut.
- **Delivery of the shoulders and body:** The fetus is directed posteriorly with gentle downward pressure until the anterior shoulder has passed beneath the symphysis pubis. The fetus is then directed anteriorly until the posterior shoulder passes the perineum. After the shoulders are delivered, the fetus is grasped with one hand supporting the head and neck, and the other hand along the spine.

OPERATIVE VAGINAL DELIVERY

Operative vaginal delivery can be an effective alternative to cesarean section for women in the second stage of labor who meet specific criteria.

Forceps Delivery

- Classification is by station of the fetal head at the time that the forceps are applied.
  - **Midforceps:** Head is engaged but higher than +2 station.
  - **Low forceps:** Station is +2 or lower.
  - **Outlet forceps:** Scalp is visible without separating the labia, skull has reached pelvic floor, head is at or on perineum, and the occiput is either directly anterior-posterior in alignment or does not require more than 45 degrees of rotation.
- **Application:**
  - Sagittal suture should be perpendicular to the plane of the shanks of the forceps.
  - The posterior fontanelle should be halfway between the blades and one fingerbreadth above the plane of the shanks.
  - If using fenestrated blades, equal amounts of fenestration should be palpable on each blade.

- **Indication:** None are absolute but include the following:
  - Prolonged second stage of labor
  - Maternal exhaustion
  - Inadequate maternal expulsive effort
  - Concern for fetal compromise
  - A maternal condition requiring a shortened/passive second stage
- **Prerequisites:** Before operative vaginal delivery with forceps is attempted, the following criteria should be met:
  - The fetal head must be engaged in the pelvis.
  - The cervix must be fully dilated and membranes ruptured.
  - The bladder should be empty.
  - The exact station and position of the fetal head should be known.
  - Maternal pelvis must be adequate.
  - If time permits, the patient should be given adequate anesthesia.
  - If forceps delivery is done for nonreassuring fetal status, someone who is able to perform neonatal resuscitation should be available.
  - The operator should have knowledge about, and experience with, the appropriate instrument, its proper application, and the possible complications.
- **Maternal complications:** uterine, cervical, or vaginal lacerations, extension of an episiotomy, bladder or urethral injuries, and hematomas
- **Fetal complications:** cephalohematoma, bruising, lacerations, facial nerve injury, and, rarely, skull fracture and intracranial hemorrhage

Vacuum Delivery

- Indications, contraindications, and complications are largely the same as for forceps delivery.
- The suction cup is applied in the midline on the sagittal suture with the center of the cup about 3 cm anterior to the posterior fontanelle (the "flexion point").
- Maximum vacuum suction of 0.7 to 0.8 kg/cm^2 (500-600 mm Hg) is applied and then one hand maintains fetal flexion and supports the vacuum cup, whereas the other applies sustained traction to assist delivery of the fetal head, without rocking or twisting, only during contractions.
- Vacuum pressure can be released between contractions and should not be maintained for longer than 30 minutes.
- Vacuum use should be avoided in fetuses <34 weeks' GA, weight <2500 g or concern for fetal blood disorders.

OBSTETRIC LACERATIONS

Obstetric lacerations are commonly encountered after a vaginal delivery. The use of operative vaginal delivery is a known risk factor for third- and fourth-degree perineal lacerations.

- **First-degree laceration:** superficial laceration of the vaginal mucosa
- **Second-degree laceration:** first-degree laceration that involves the vaginal mucosa and perineal body and may extend into the transverse perineal muscles
- **Third-degree laceration:** second-degree laceration that extends into the muscle of the perineum and may involve the transverse perineal muscles and external anal sphincter; does not involve the rectal mucosa
- **Fourth-degree laceration:** third-degree laceration that involves the rectal mucosa

SHOULDER DYSTOCIA

Shoulder dystocia occurs in 0.2% to 3.0% of all vaginal deliveries and is defined as an impaction of the fetal shoulder after delivery of the head. It is associated with increased fetal morbidity and mortality secondary to brachial plexus injuries and fetal asphyxia. The diagnosis should be considered when the application of gentle, downward pressure of the fetal head fails to accomplish delivery.

- **Macrosomia** is associated with shoulder dystocia. With infants weighing >4500 g, the risk of shoulder dystocia has been reported to be 9% to 14%. When maternal diabetes is factored in with weight >4500 g, the incidence is as high as 20% to 50%.
- Other **risk factors** include maternal obesity, previous macrosomic infant, diabetes mellitus, and gestational diabetes. However, it should be noted that most cases occur in nondiabetic women with normal-sized infants. Clinicians should be aware of the risk factors, but a level of caution should be extended to all patients.

Management

- Anticipation and preparation are important. Help should be available as extra hands may be needed during the delivery. A pediatrician should be notified. If available, an anesthesiologist should also be informed.
- The time should be marked when the dystocia is called, if Pitocin has been used, it should be discontinued, and the total time until delivery recorded in the notes. Once the shoulder dystocia is identified, no significant downward pressure should be applied to the head until the shoulders are delivered. Fundal pressure should *never* be applied as it only exacerbates the shoulder impaction.
- **McRoberts maneuver** is performed by hyperflexion and abduction of the maternal hips, flattening the lumbar spine, and rotating the pelvis to increase the anterior-posterior outlet diameter.
- **Suprapubic pressure** is applied in a vector chosen to anteriorly rotate the anterior fetal shoulder and dislodge the shoulder from the symphysis.
- Other measures in combination are chosen for the specific clinical situations based on clinician experience. There is no "right order" in which the maneuvers described below should be performed, and maneuvers can and should be used more than once, as needed.
  - **Delivery of the posterior arm:** By grasping the posterior hand, the posterior arm can be flexed and swept across the fetal chest, delivered first, thereby creating more room for the anterior shoulder. If the entire posterior arm cannot be delivered, an attempt at delivering the posterior shoulder by gentle upward traction on the fetal head can be performed.
  - **Episiotomy:** Incision of the perineum provides additional room and should be considered if it might facilitate delivery or additional maneuvering.
  - **Rubin maneuver:** The anterior fetal shoulder is rotated obliquely with a vaginal hand. This maneuver may also be performed in a posterior manner.
  - **Wood corkscrew:** The posterior shoulder is rotated over 180 degrees with a vaginal hand to assist delivery of the shoulders.
  - **Gaskin maneuver:** Facilitated in a patient without regional anesthesia, she is turned over on "all fours," inverting the anterior and posterior shoulders.

- Delivery that does not occur following the above maneuvers may require some of the more invasive and traumatic procedures noted below for the sake of fetal viability.
  - **Management of neonatal clavicular fracture:** Palpate the clavicles and apply outward pressure with the thumb to avoid lung or subclavian artery injury.
  - In extreme cases, the **Zavanelli maneuver** (in which the fetal head is flexed and pushed back up into the uterus as preparations for emergent cesarean section are made) or **symphysiotomy** (performed by laterally displacing the urethra using the index and middle fingers placed against the posterior aspect of the symphysis and incising the cartilaginous portion of the symphysis) could be performed.

CESAREAN SECTION

- **Fetal indications** for cesarean delivery include the following:
  - Nonreassuring FHT
  - Nonvertex presentation (malpresentation)
  - Fetal anomalies, such as hydrocephalus, that would make successful vaginal delivery unlikely
  - Umbilical cord prolapse
  - Conjoined twins
- **Maternal indications** for cesarean delivery include the following:
  - Obstruction of the lower genital tract (eg, large condyloma)
  - Previous cesarean section (if vaginal birth after cesarean [VBAC] is declined or not appropriate)
  - Previous uterine surgery involving the contractile portion of the uterus (ie, classical cesarean, transmural myomectomy)
  - History of severe pelvic floor injury from a prior vaginal delivery
  - Abdominal cerclage
- **Maternal and fetal indications** include the following:
  - Some cases of abruptio placentae
  - Active maternal genital herpes simplex virus infection
  - Labor dystocia or cephalopelvic disproportion
  - Placenta previa or known vasa previa
  - Failed operative vaginal delivery
- The patient should be counseled regarding standard **risks of surgery**, such as pain, bleeding that may require transfusion, infection, damage to nearby organs, and a small but increased risk of death when compared to vaginal delivery.

VAGINAL BIRTH AFTER CESAREAN SECTION

- Provided there are no contraindications to vaginal delivery, a patient may be counseled and offered a trial of labor after previous cesarean delivery (TOLAC). An online prediction model created by the Maternal-Fetal Medicine Units Network has been developed that calculates a percentage for a successful VBAC based on the presence or absence of six variables known to contribute to VBAC success rates. Success rates of VBAC are higher for patients with nonrecurring conditions, such as malpresentation or fetal intolerance of labor (60% to 85%) than for those with a prior diagnosis of dystocia (15% to 30%). Patients should be counseled regarding the risk of uterine rupture (0.5% to 3.7%), failed trial of labor, and need for cesarean delivery. A patient with a history of two prior cesarean sections may consider a TOLAC, depending on prior indications. The likelihood of a successful VBAC for patients with two prior cesarean sections is the same as for women with one prior cesarean section. The risk of uterine rupture with two prior cesarean sections is 1.6%.

- **Contraindications** include previous classical or inverted T-shaped uterine incision, transfundal uterine surgery, history of uterine rupture, contracted pelvis, and medical or obstetric contraindications to vaginal delivery.
- Epidural anesthesia and oxytocin may be used with TOLAC. The use of prostaglandins is contraindicated. The delivery hospital must have facilities and staffing for emergency cesarean delivery. Blood products should be readily available. The most common sign of uterine rupture is a nonreassuring FHR pattern with variable decelerations evolving into late decelerations, bradycardia, and undetectable FHR. Other findings include uterine or abdominal pain, loss of station of the presenting part, vaginal bleeding, and hypovolemia (see chapter 3).

MALPRESENTATIONS

Normal presentation is defined by longitudinal lie, cephalic presentation, and flexion of the fetal neck. All other presentations are malpresentations. Occurring in approximately 5% of all deliveries, malpresentations may lead to abnormalities of labor and increased risk for mother or fetus.

- **Risk factors** for malpresentation are conditions that decrease the polarity of the uterus, increase or decrease fetal mobility, or block the presenting part from the pelvis.
  - **Maternal factors** include grand multiparity, pelvic tumors, uterine fibroids, pelvic contracture, and uterine malformations.
  - **Fetal factors** include prematurity, multiple gestation, polyhydramnios or oligohydramnios, macrosomia, placenta previa, hydrocephaly, aneuploidy, anencephaly, and myotonic dystrophy.

Breech Presentation

- **Breech** presentation occurs when the cephalic pole is in the uterine fundus. Major congenital anomalies occur in 6.3% of term breech presentation infants compared to 2.4% of vertex presenting infants.
  - The incidence of breech presentation is 25% of pregnancies at <28 weeks' gestation, 7% of pregnancies at 32 weeks' gestation, and 3% to 4% of term pregnancies in labor.
  - The three types of breech presentation are the following:
    - **Frank breech** (48% to 73%) occurs when both hips are flexed and both knees are extended.
    - **Complete breech** (5% to 12%) occurs when the fetus is flexed at the hips and flexed at the knees.
    - **Incomplete, or footling breech** (12% to 38%), occurs when the fetus has one or both hips extended.
- **Risks** of breech presentation include cord prolapse (15% in footling breech, 5% in complete breech, and 0.5% in frank breech), head entrapment, and spinal cord injury (with neck hyperextension).

- Fetuses in a complete or frank breech presentation may occasionally be considered for vaginal delivery with appropriate selection and counseling.
- Cesarean delivery poses risk of increased maternal morbidity and mortality.
- Vaginal breech delivery poses increased risk of fetal asphyxia, cord prolapse, birth trauma, spinal cord injury, and mortality. Planned vaginal breech delivery is not routinely offered but with careful selection and evaluation may be permitted.
- A **trial of labor** may be attempted if
  - The breech is frank or complete.
  - The estimated fetal weight is <3800 g.
  - Pelvimetry suggests an adequate pelvis.
  - The fetal head is flexed.
  - Anesthesia is immediately available.
  - The fetus is continuously monitored.
  - A pediatrician is available.
  - An obstetrician is available who is experienced with vaginal breech delivery.
- In breech presentation, the fetus usually emerges in the sacrum transverse or oblique position. As crowning occurs (the bitrochanteric diameter passes under the symphysis), an episiotomy can be considered. When the umbilicus appears, place fingers medial to each thigh and press out laterally to deliver the legs (Pinard maneuver). The fetus should then be rotated to the sacrum anterior position, and the trunk can be wrapped in a towel to allow for application of downward traction. When the infant's scapulae appear, the arms can be delivered. The fetus is rotated so that the shoulder is anterior, the humerus followed down, and each arm rotated across the chest and out (Lovset maneuver). To deliver the *right* arm, the fetus is turned in a *counterclockwise* direction; to deliver the *left* arm, the fetus is turned in a *clockwise* direction. If the head does not deliver spontaneously, the head may be flexed by placing downward traction and pressure on the maxillary ridge (Mauriceau-Smellie-Veit maneuver). Direct vertical suprapubic pressure may also be applied. Piper forceps may be used to assist in delivery of the head.
- For delivery of a **breech second twin**, ultrasonography should be available in the delivery room. The operator reaches into the uterus and grasps both feet, trying to keep the membranes intact. The feet are brought down to the introitus and then amniotomy is performed. The body is delivered to the scapula by applying gentle traction on the feet. The remainder of the delivery is the same as that described earlier for a singleton breech.
- **Head entrapment** during breech vaginal delivery may be managed by one or more of the following procedures:
  - **Application of Piper forceps**
    - If the cervix has contracted around the fetal neck, **Dührssen incisions** are made in the cervix at the 2, 6, and 10 o'clock positions. Up to three incisions may be needed to facilitate delivery of the fetal head through the cervix. The 3- and 9-o'clock positions should be avoided due to the risk of dividing the cervical vessels with resultant hemorrhage.
    - Relaxation agents (nitric oxide or nitroglycerine) may release the entrapped head, enabling proper head flexion and vaginal delivery.
    - Cephalocentesis can be performed if the fetus is not viable. The procedure is performed by perforating the base of the skull and suctioning the cranial contents.

External Cephalic Version

- **Indication** is persistent breech (or other nonvertex) presentation at term. The version is performed to avoid malpresentation in labor.
- **Risks** include compromised umbilical blood flow, placental separation, fetal distress, fetal injury, premature rupture of membranes, and fetomaternal bleeding (overall incidence is 0% to 1.4%). The most common "risk" is failed version.
- **Success rate** for external cephalic version ranges from 35% to 86%, but in 2% of cases, the fetus reverts back to breech presentation.
- **Technique:** Prerequisites include a GA of at least 36 weeks, reactive nonstress test, and informed consent. Version is generally accomplished by applying a liberal amount of lubrication to the maternal abdomen, then transabdominally grasping the fetal head and fetal breech, and manipulating the fetus through a forward or backward roll. Ultrasonographic guidance is an important adjunct to confirm position and monitor FHR. Tocolysis and spinal or epidural anesthesia may improve success rates. After the procedure, the patient should be monitored continuously until the FHR is reactive, no decelerations are present, and no evidence of regular contractions exists. Rh-negative patients should receive $Rh_o(D)$ immune globulin after the procedure because of the potential for fetomaternal bleeding.
- **Factors associated with failure** include obesity, oligohydramnios, deep engagement of the presenting part, a partial uterine septum, and fetal back posterior. Nulliparity and an anterior placenta may also reduce the likelihood of success.
- **Contraindications** to external cephalic version include conditions in which labor or vaginal delivery would be contraindicated. Version is not generally recommended in cases of ruptured membranes, third-trimester bleeding, oligohydramnios, multiple gestations, or after labor has begun.

Abnormal Lie

- Lie refers to the alignment of the fetal spine in relation to the maternal spine. Longitudinal lie is normal, whereas oblique and transverse lies are abnormal. Abnormal lie is associated with multiparity, prematurity, pelvic contraction, and disorders of the placenta.
- **Incidence** of abnormal lie is 1 in 300 term pregnancies. At 32 weeks' gestation the incidence is <2%.
- **Risk:** The greatest risk of abnormal lie is cord prolapse because the fetal parts do not fill the pelvic inlet.
- **Management:** If abnormal lie persists beyond 35 to 38 weeks, external version may be attempted. An ultrasonographic examination should be performed to rule out major anomalies and abnormal placentation. If an abnormal lie persists, mode of delivery should be cesarean section. An intraoperative cephalic version may be attempted. A vertical uterine incision may be prudent in cases with back down transverse or oblique lie with ruptured membranes or poorly developed lower uterine segment.
- **Abnormal attitude and deflexion:** Full flexion of the fetal neck is considered normal. Abnormalities range from partial deflexion to full extension:
  - **Face presentation** results from extension of the fetal neck. The chin is the presenting part.
    - **Incidence** is between 0.14% and 0.54%. In 60% of cases, face presentation is associated with a fetal malformation. Anencephaly accounts for 33% of all cases.
    - **Diagnosis:** Face presentation may be diagnosed by vaginal examination, ultrasonography, or palpation of the cephalic prominence and the fetal back on the same side of the maternal abdomen when performing Leopold maneuvers.

- o **Risk:** Perinatal mortality ranges from 0.6% to 5.0%.
- o **Management:** The fetus must be mentum (chin) anterior for a vaginal delivery to allow for flexion of the fetal head and successful vaginal delivery. Mentum posterior should be managed by cesarean delivery.
- **Brow presentation** results from partial deflexion of the fetal neck.
- o **Incidence** is 1 in 670 to 1 in 3433 pregnancies. Causes of brow presentation are similar to those of face presentation.
- o **Risks:** Perinatal mortality ranges from 1.28% to 8.00%.
- o **Management:** The majority of cases spontaneously convert to a flexed attitude. A vaginal delivery of a persistent brow presentation can be considered if the maternal pelvis is large, the fetus is small, and labor progresses adequately.
- **Compound presentation** occurs when an extremity prolapses beside the presenting part.
  - **Incidence** is 1 in 377 to 1 in 1213 pregnancies and is associated with prematurity.
  - **Risks:** Fetal risks are cord prolapse in 10% to 20% of cases and birth trauma including neurologic and musculoskeletal damage to the involved extremity.
  - **Management:** The prolapsing extremity should not be manipulated. Continuous fetal monitoring is recommended because compound presentation can be associated with occult cord prolapse. Spontaneous vaginal delivery occurs in 75% of vertex/upper extremity presentations. Cesarean section is indicated in cases of nonreassuring FHT, cord prolapse, and failure of labor to progress.

SUGGESTED READINGS

American College of Obstetricians and Gynecologists Committee on Practice Bulletins—Obstetrics. ACOG Practice Bulletin No. 107: induction of labor. *Obstet Gynecol.* 2009; 114(2, pt 1):386-397. (Reaffirmed 2019)

American College of Obstetricians and Gynecologists Committee on Practice Bulletins—Obstetrics. ACOG Practice Bulletin No. 154: operative vaginal delivery. *Obstet Gynecol.* 2015;126(5):e56-e65. (Reaffirmed 2018)

American College of Obstetricians and Gynecologists Committee on Practice Bulletins—Obstetrics. ACOG Practice Bulletin No. 173: fetal macrosomia. *Obstet Gynecol.* 2016; 128(5):e195-e209. (Reaffirmed 2018)

American College of Obstetricians and Gynecologists Committee on Practice Bulletins—Obstetrics. ACOG Practice Bulletin No. 178: shoulder dystocia. *Obstet Gynecol.* 2017; 129:e123-e133. (Reaffirmed 2019)

American College of Obstetricians and Gynecologists Committee on Practice Bulletins—Obstetrics. ACOG Practice Bulletin No. 198: prevention and management of obstetric lacerations at vaginal delivery. *Obstet Gynecol.* 2018;132:e87-e102.

American College of Obstetricians and Gynecologists Committee on Practice Bulletins—Obstetrics. ACOG Practice Bulletin No. 205: vaginal birth after cesarean delivery. *Obstet Gynecol.* 2019;133:e110-e127.

American College of Obstetricians and Gynecologists, Society for Maternal-Fetal Medicine. Obstetric Care Consensus No. 1: safe prevention of the primary cesarean delivery. *Obstet Gynecol.* 2014;123(3):693-711.

Cunningham FG, Leveno KJ, Bloom SL, et al, eds. Delivery. In: *Williams Obstetrics.* 25th ed. New York, NY: McGraw-Hill; 2018:516-605.

Cunningham FG, Leveno KJ, Bloom SL, et al, eds. Labor. In: *Williams Obstetrics.* 25th ed. New York, NY: McGraw-Hill; 2018:400-515.

Complications of Labor and Delivery

Benjamin K. Kogutt and Clark T. Johnson

UTERINE DEHISCENCE OR RUPTURE

- **Dehiscence** is defined as lower uterine scar separation that does not breach the serosa; it rarely causes significant bleeding. **Rupture** is defined as complete separation of the uterine wall and may lead to fetal distress and significant maternal hemorrhage.
- **Incidence.** Uterine rupture occurs in 0.2% to 1.8% of patients with one or more previous low-segment transverse cesarean deliveries and in 4% to 9% of patients with a prior uterine active segment incision (classical cesarean, T incision, other disruption of the myometrium such as a myomectomy). One-third of prior classical cesarean scar ruptures occur before the onset of labor.
- **Etiology.** Significant risk factors include the following:
  - Prior cesarean delivery
  - Prior uterine perforation
  - Previous resection of cornual ectopic pregnancy
  - Prostaglandin induction of labor with history of prior cesarean
  - Collagen disorders
  - Abdominal myomectomies in which the endometrial cavity was invaded
- **Diagnosis and management**
  - Fetal bradycardia is clinically manifested in 33% to 70% of cases. Fetal distress may be the initial presentation in catastrophic uterine rupture. In more subtle cases, the initial presentation may be a simple rise in fetal station or change in the position for fetal heart monitor placement. Maternal signs and symptoms include hypotension, uterine tenderness, a change in uterine shape, or constant abdominal pain.
  - When uterine rupture is suspected, it is important to proceed emergently to laparotomy with delivery of the infant and repair of the uterine rupture. Rates of recurrent rupture in subsequent pregnancies carried to term approach 22%. Recommendations are for early delivery via cesarean delivery by 36 weeks for patients who have experienced a prior uterine rupture.

UMBILICAL CORD PROLAPSE

- **Umbilical cord prolapse** occurs when the umbilical cord slips beyond the presenting fetal part and passes through the open cervical os (overt) or descends alongside the presenting part (occult). The fetal blood supply is effectively compromised when the cord is compressed. The overall incidence is 1 to 6 per 1000 births. The incidence in breech deliveries is slightly higher than 1% and in footling breech or rupture of membranes with transverse lie may be as high as 10% to 15%.
- **Etiology.** Risk factors include ruptured membranes, unengaged fetal presenting part (including disengagement), malpresentation (breech, transverse, oblique), prematurity, multiple gestation (second twin), multiparity, and polyhydramnios.

- **Diagnosis.** Cord prolapse usually causes severe prolonged fetal bradycardia or persistent moderate to severe variable decelerations. Vaginal exam may confirm overt prolapse; the cord will be palpable.
- **Management**
  - If the cord is felt on vaginal examination, elevate the presenting part to relieve pressure off of the cord, call for help, and move to the operating room for emergent cesarean delivery.
  - Appropriate anesthesia should be administered in the operating room and the viability of the fetus confirmed before proceeding with cesarean delivery.
  - Placing the patient in Trendelenburg or knee-chest position may relieve cord compression with prolapse, but the vaginal hand should continue to elevate the presenting part. This should not delay transportation to the operating room.
  - The interval between cord prolapse and delivery is the major predictor of newborn status. If delivered expeditiously, the neonatal outcomes are generally favorable. A cord gas should be obtained at the delivery to assess the degree of hypoxia.

EMBOLIC DISEASE

Amniotic Fluid Embolism

- **Amniotic fluid embolism (AFE)** is a rare complication. Fetal fluid, tissue, or debris enters the maternal circulation via the placental bed and triggers acute anaphylaxis.
- **Incidence**
  - Approximately 1 in 20 000 singleton pregnancies is complicated by AFE.
  - Mortality is around 25% in the United States, much lower than the typically reported 60% to 80%. AFE accounts for 10% of maternal deaths in the United States. Severe neurologic deficits occur in a high percentage of survivors. Neonatal survival is reported at 70%.
- **Etiology and diagnosis**
  - The term *embolism* is a misnomer because the clinical findings are probably a result of anaphylactic shock rather than pulmonary embolism (PE). Amniotic fluid has been shown to cause vasospasm of the pulmonary vasculature in animal models.
  - Risk factors include induced labor, advanced maternal age, multiparity, uterine rupture, abdominal trauma, placental abruption, diabetes, cervical lacerations, and operative delivery.
  - AFE is primarily a clinical diagnosis of exclusion, made when a woman acutely presents with profound hypoxia, shock, and cardiovascular collapse during or immediately after labor. Cyanosis, hemorrhage, coma, and disseminated intravascular coagulation (DIC) rapidly ensue.
  - The differential diagnosis includes other acute events such as PE, hemorrhage, drug reaction, anaphylaxis, sepsis, and myocardial infarction.
  - Useful laboratory data include arterial blood gas, serum electrolytes, calcium and magnesium levels, coagulation profile, and complete blood count.
  - Definitive diagnosis is made only at autopsy, when amniotic fluid debris (eg, fetal squamous cells or hair) are found in the maternal pulmonary vasculature. These debris may be present in the maternal circulation of women without AFE, however, so this finding is not pathognomonic.

- **Management**
  - Approximately 65% of AFE occurs before delivery. Emergent delivery is required for both fetal and maternal benefits.
  - The patient should be intubated and aggressively resuscitated.
  - Administer intravenous (IV) fluids, inotropic agents, and vasopressors to maintain adequate blood pressure. Packed red blood cells (PRBCs) and fresh frozen plasma (FFP) should be available because there is a high risk for DIC. Factor VII has been used in cases of severe DIC. Despite all efforts, significant maternal morbidity and mortality remain high.

Venous Thromboembolism

- **Pulmonary embolism** and **deep vein thrombosis (DVT)** both compose a single disease defined as venous thromboembolism (VTE). The VTE can manifest as isolated lower extremity DVT or a clot can break off from the lower extremities and travel to the lungs and present as a PE.
- **Incidence.** Pregnancy and the postpartum period are known risk factors for the development of VTE, with the potential risk for PE. The incidence of VTE is estimated at 0.76 to 1.72 per 1000 pregnancies (4 times as great as in the nonpregnant population). In the United States, PE is the sixth leading cause of maternal mortality and occurs in the postpartum period 43% to 60% of the time.
- **Etiology and risk factors.** Pregnancy alone is a risk factor for the development of VTE. Risk is highest in the postpartum period. Additional risk factors include thrombophilias, multiple gestation, varicose veins, inflammatory bowel disease, urinary tract infection, diabetes, body mass index $>30 \text{ kg/m}^2$, increased maternal age >35 years. The DVT is most likely to occur in the left leg (70%-90% of cases), possibly due to compression of the left iliac vein by being crossed by the right iliac artery.
- **Evaluation.** Clinical signs or symptoms for PE are nonspecific, challenging diagnosis in pregnancy. Complicating the nonspecific nature of the presentation of PE is the overlap between many physiologic changes in pregnancy and those symptoms that can be associated with a PE (VTE is confirmed in $<10\%$ of suspected cases versus 25% of suspected cases in nonpregnant patients). The four most common presenting symptoms of PE are dyspnea, pleuritic chest pain, cough, and sweating.
- **Diagnosis.** A high index of suspicion and low threshold for obtaining objective testing are the key to prompt and successful diagnosis of PE. See chapter 20 for further discussion regarding evaluation for PE, including imaging modalities.
- **Management.** When high suspicion for PE exists, empiric anticoagulation therapy is indicated prior to diagnostic evaluation and can be discontinued if and once VTE is excluded. Once anticoagulation therapy is indicated, it should be initiated with one of the following medications: subcutaneous low-molecular-weight heparin, subcutaneous unfractionated heparin, or IV unfractionated heparin. Meanwhile, supportive care with respiratory support as needed should be provided (see chapter 20).

Postpartum Hemorrhage

- **Postpartum hemorrhage (PPH) is defined as the following:**
  - Estimated blood loss (EBL) of >1000 mL for a vaginal or cesarean delivery
  - Any bleeding within 24 hours after birth sufficient to cause symptoms

- **Incidence.** PPH is a leading cause of maternal death, accounting for at least 25% of maternal deaths worldwide. It is the second leading cause of pregnancy-related death in the United States, accounting for slightly more than 10% of maternal mortality.
- **Etiology and management** (Table 3-1)
  - Patients often tolerate loss of up to 20% of blood volume before symptoms of hypovolemia develop. Prompt, even anticipatory, action is crucial. Blood flow to the gravid uterus is 600 to 900 mL/min; patients can become unstable rapidly.

Table 3-1	Etiologies of Postpartum Hemorrhage[a]
Etiology	**Risk Factor(s)**
Abnormal placentation	Placenta previa in the setting of prior cesarean delivery
	Sonographic evidence of placenta accreta spectrum disorders
Birth canal injuries	Episiotomy and lacerations
	Rapid labor and cervical dilation
	Cesarean delivery or hysterectomy
Uterine rupture	History of uterine scar
	High parity
	Uterine hyperstimulation
	Obstructed labor
	Intrauterine manipulation
	Midforceps rotation
	Breech extraction
Uterine atony	Uterine overdistension: large fetus, multiple gestation, polyhydramnios, retained clot
	Induction of labor
	Halogenated anesthetic agents
	Labor abnormalities: rapid labor, prolonged labor, augmented labor, chorioamnionitis
	History of uterine atony
Coagulation disorders	Massive transfusion
	Placental abruption
	Sepsis
	Severe preeclampsia
	Acute fatty liver of pregnancy
	Anticoagulation
	Coagulopathies
	Amniotic fluid embolism

[a]Adapted with permission from American College of Obstetricians and Gynecologists Committee on Practice Bulletins—Obstetrics. ACOG Practice Bulletin No. 183: postpartum hemorrhage. *Obstet Gynecol.* 2017;130(4):e168-e186. Copyright © 2017 by The American College of Obstetricians and Gynecologists.

- Establish large bore IV access. Initiate IV fluid resuscitation. Administer supplemental oxygen, and order crossmatched blood. After these initial steps, examine the patient to determine the underlying cause and address the problem expeditiously.
- Blood transfusion should be considered after 1 to 2 L EBL and may be initiated earlier if bleeding is expected to continue, the patient's starting hemoglobin was low, or the patient is symptomatic.
- Coagulation factors (FFP and cryoprecipitate) and platelets should be repleted with massive blood loss. Historically, 1 unit of FFP was given for every 4 to 6 units of PRBCs to reduce dilutional and citrate coagulopathy as every 500 mL of red cells is expected to dilute coagulation factors by 10%. Additionally, platelets were transfused when the platelet count dropped below 50 000/mL or after 6 to 10 units of red cell transfusion. More recent evidence suggests better outcomes with a protocol of 1:1:1 repletion of PRBC, FFP, and platelets when bleeding is ongoing or massive (>8 units of PRBC) transfusion is needed. In the operative setting, direct manual aortic compression can decrease pulse pressure and slow active bleeding to allow hemodynamic stabilization before proceeding with definitive management.
- Factor VII infusion may be considered in extreme cases of hemorrhage with DIC.
- Tranexamic acid administration should be considered for all cases of hemorrhage with an EBL greater than 1 L, with redosing permissible 1 hour after the initial dose if continued bleeding is a concern.

Uterine Atony

- **Uterine atony** (postpartum uterine contraction inadequate for hemostasis) is the most common cause of PPH.
- Normally, uterine contraction after delivery compresses placental bed spiral arterioles, thereby reducing blood loss. Atony permits continuous brisk bleeding.
- Risk factors include uterine overdistention (as with fetal macrosomia, polyhydramnios, or multiple gestation); prolonged, augmented, or precipitous labor; chorioamnionitis; grand multiparity; and use of tocolytic agents.
- Initial management is oxytocin administration and bimanual massage of the uterus to stimulate contraction and evacuation of clot from the lower uterine segment to remove a distending mass. This is sufficient in most cases.
- Procontractile agents can be administered if atony persists (Table 3-2). Additional oxytocin, methylergonovine, and prostaglandins are appropriate. Rectal misoprostol (800-1000 µg) is often used to stimulate sustained uterine contraction.
- Selective **uterine arterial embolization** may also be considered for continued postpartum atony if the patient is stable for transport to a fluoroscopy suite.
- When these more conservative interventions are unsuccessful, **surgical exploration** through a vertical midline incision should be considered. Depending on the patient's desire for future childbearing, the extent of hemorrhage, and the experience of the surgeon, several approaches may be used:
  - **Uterine compressive sutures** can be effective for uterine atony. The B-Lynch suture was the original technique described (Figure 3-1). Since then, multiple compressive sutures have been proposed including combinations of vertical and horizontal sutures to transfix the anterior and posterior uterine walls. All have similar efficacy in achieving hemostasis.

Table 3-2 Management of Postpartum Hemorrhage With Uterotonic Agents[a]

Agent	Dose	Comments and Contraindications
Oxytocin (Pitocin)	10-40 U/L IV at 120 mL/h or 10 U IM	Do not give undiluted IV bolus. Antidiuretic effect with prolonged infusion or high dose; can cause volume overload
Methylergonovine maleate (Methergine)	0.2 mg IM every 2-4 h or 0.2 mg orally every 6 h. Do not start orally until 4 h after last parenteral dose.	Avoid in patients with hypertension, preeclampsia, or Raynaud phenomenon. May cause nausea and vomiting
15-Methyl prostaglandin $F_2\alpha$ (Hemabate)	0.25 mg IM (skeletal or myometrium) every 15-90 min to a maximum of 8 doses	Avoid in patients with asthma. Renal, hepatic, and cardiac diseases are relative contraindications. May cause nausea/vomiting, tachycardia, diarrhea, pyrexia
Prostaglandin E_1 analog (misoprostol [Cytotec])	800-1000 μg orally, sublingually, or rectally; once	May cause nausea, vomiting, diarrhea, fever, shivering, headache

Abbreviations: IM, intramuscular; IV, intravenous.
[a]Adapted with permission from American College of Obstetricians and Gynecologists Committee on Practice Bulletins—Obstetrics. ACOG Practice Bulletin No. 183: postpartum hemorrhage. *Obstet Gynecol.* 2017;130(4):e168-e186. Copyright © 2017 by The American College of Obstetricians and Gynecologists.

- **O'Leary bilateral uterine artery ligation** effectively reduces blood loss (Figure 3-2). After identifying the ureter, ascending branches of the uterine arteries are ligated at the level of the vesicouterine peritoneal reflection. The suture is placed through the lateral lower uterine segment, close to the cervix, and then passed through an avascular area of the broad ligament lateral to the uterine vessels. Utero-ovarian vessels (near the cornua) and infundibulopelvic vessels may also be ligated if needed.
- **Hysterectomy** is the definitive procedure for intractable uterine bleeding and should not be delayed when needed. Delay to hysterectomy is associated with increased mortality. Intensive care monitoring may be required after peripartum hysterectomy due to massive blood loss, large postoperative fluid shifts, and potential need for ventilatory support.

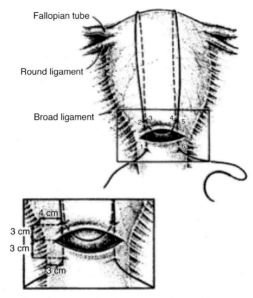

Figure 3-1. B-Lynch suture. Reprinted with permission from Dildy GA III. Postpartum hemorrhage: new management options. *Clin Obstet Gynecol.* 2002;45(2):330-344.

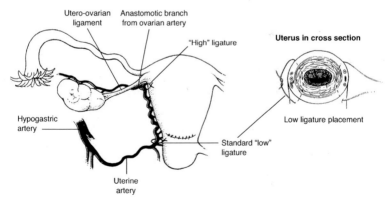

Figure 3-2. O'Leary uterine artery ligation. From Rock JA, Jones HW, eds. *TeLinde's Operative Gynecology.* 10th ed. Philadelphia, PA: Lippincott Williams & Wilkins; 2008. With permission from *Contemp Obstet Gynecol.* 1984;24:70, and *Surgical Obstetrics.* Philadelphia, PA: WB Saunders; 1992:272.

Lacerations and Hematomas

- **Uterine**, **vaginal**, or **cervical laceration** should be suspected if the uterine fundus is well contracted but bleeding persists, particularly if operative delivery or episiotomy was performed. Adequate visualization (light and exposure) is mandatory to investigate a laceration. Adequate analgesia is also valuable.
- The cervix, entire vagina, and perineum should be evaluated systematically. Moving to the operating room often facilitates this process with adequate exposure and instrumentation.
- Occult bleeding in **vulvar** and **vaginal hematomas** is identified mainly by hypotension and pelvic pain. Stable hematomas may be managed conservatively, but expanding hematomas should be evacuated by performing a generous incision, copiously irrigating, and ligating the bleeding vessels. Layered closure is recommended to assist hemostasis and eliminate dead space. Vaginal packing (for 12-18 h) may be helpful. Broad-spectrum antibiotics should be administered. Arterial embolization may be helpful if the bleeding is unable to be managed surgically.
- **Retroperitoneal hematoma** is potentially life-threatening due to the volume of blood that can develop in that space. Definitive diagnosis is made via computed tomography (CT) with IV contrast. It may present as hypotension, cardiovascular shock, or flank pain. Stable retroperitoneal bleeding can be managed conservatively. The pressure from the expanding hematoma will tamponade vessels and stop blood loss. Continued expansion necessitates surgical exploration or interventional radiology embolization.

Retained Products of Conception

- Retained products of conception can cause PPH.
- Risk factors include accessory placental lobes, abnormal placentation, *placenta accreta*, chorioamnionitis, and very preterm delivery.
- If retained products are suspected, blunt curettage may be performed. Using large "banjo" curettes with a broad tip under ultrasound guidance may reduce the risk of uterine perforation.

Placenta Accreta Spectrum Disorders

- In *placenta accreta*, the normal plane of separation between uterus and placenta is absent. If the third stage of labor lasts longer than 30 minutes, abnormal placentation should be considered. Manual extraction and uterine exploration are performed. Blunt curettage may be required. It may be impossible to remove the entire placenta without damaging the uterus. If bleeding is controlled with uterotonic agents, conservative management may be sufficient.
- Balloon catheter (Bakri balloon), with instillation of up to 500 mL of saline, can be placed in the uterus and inflated to tamponade bleeding from abnormal placentation. It may provide complete hemostasis or simply give time to stabilize the patient and arrange additional care, such as uterine artery embolization. The balloon catheter may be left in place for 12 to 24 hours.
- Laparotomy and peripartum hysterectomy are the definitive procedures for bleeding due to *placenta accreta*.

Coagulopathy

- **Coagulopathy** can cause or contribute to PPH.
- Risk factors include severe preeclampsia, abruptio placentae, idiopathic/autoimmune thrombocytopenia, AFE, DIC, intrauterine fetal demise, and hereditary coagulopathies (eg, von Willebrand disease).

• If bleeding is due to coagulopathy, surgical treatment will only increase the hemorrhage. Replete coagulation factors and platelets as needed.

UTERINE INVERSION

• In **uterine inversion**, the uterus is turned inside out, with the fundus protruding through the cervical os into or out of the vagina. It is classified as *incomplete* if the corpus travels partially through the cervix, *complete* if the corpus travels entirely through the cervix, and *prolapsed* if the corpus travels beyond the vaginal introitus.
• **Incidence.** Occurs in approximately 1 in 2500 deliveries, usually with a fundal placenta
• **Etiology and management**
  • Risk factors include multiparity, long labor, short umbilical cord, abnormal placentation (ie, accreta), connective tissue disorders, and excessive traction on the cord.
  • Establishment of additional IV access with aggressive fluid resuscitation, anticipating massive PPH. Uterotonics including oxytocin should be discontinued.
  • An attempt to replace the uterus manually should be made.
  • In the *Johnson maneuver*, the inverted fundus is grasped and replaced cephalad through the cervix into the normal position. Leaving the placenta in place may reduce blood loss; it can be removed manually after normal anatomy is restored. However, if the placenta prevents replacement of the uterus, it should be removed quickly before attempting to push the fundus into place.
  • If the maneuver is unsuccessful or a contracted ring of uterine tissue prevents access, uterine-relaxing agents can be administered. The preferred agent is nitroglycerin (up to three doses of 50-100 mg IV or sublingual spray); it has a rapid onset of about 30 seconds and a short half-life. Other uterine relaxants such as terbutaline sulfate or halogenated general anesthetics (eg, halothane, isoflurane) can also be used.
  • Uterotonics should be implemented as soon as normal uterine anatomy is restored.
  • Laparotomy is indicated if manual restoration fails. Vaginal elevation, sequential upward traction from the round ligaments with an atraumatic instrument (Huntington procedure) or a posterior vertical incision on the lower uterine segment and cervical ring (Haultain procedure) can all facilitate replacement of the fundus.

CHORIOAMNIONITIS

• **Chorioamnionitis** is infection/inflammation of the placenta, chorion, and amnion.
• **Incidence.** Occurs in 1% to 2% of term and 5% to 10% of preterm deliveries
• **Etiology and diagnosis**
  • Risk factors include nulliparity, prolonged labor, prolonged ruptured membranes, use of internal monitors, maternal bacterial vaginosis, untreated infection, and multiple vaginal examinations.
  • Chorioamnionitis is an ascending polymicrobial infection. The most common pathogens are *Ureaplasma urealyticum, Mycoplasma hominis, Bacteroides bivius, Gardnerella vaginalis*, group B streptococci, and *Escherichia coli*.

- The diagnosis is clinical. Signs and symptoms include maternal fever 38.0°C or higher without other obvious infection, maternal or fetal tachycardia, uterine tenderness, foul-smelling amniotic fluid or frankly purulent discharge, and leukocytosis (typically >15 000 with a left shift).
- If the diagnosis is uncertain and the clinical situation warrants, amniocentesis may be performed. Positive amniotic fluid culture gives definitive diagnosis. An amniotic fluid white blood cell count >30 cells/μL, glucose level <15 mg/dL, interleukin-6 $\geq$11.2 ng/mL, or a positive Gram stain also suggest infection.
- **Management**
  - Definitive treatment is delivery and evacuation of the uterine contents. Antibiotics are administered during labor for fetal benefit. When the diagnosis of chorioamnionitis is made, delivery is indicated. Often, a rapidly progressing preterm delivery will ensue without assistance. Vaginal delivery should be considered unless contraindicated.
  - Acceptable antibiotic regimens include the following:
    - Ampicillin (2 g IV every 6 h) plus gentamicin sulfate (2 mg/kg IV to load and then 1.5 mg/kg IV every 8 h) until delivery. If cesarean delivery is performed, clindamycin or metronidazole may be added for anaerobic coverage postpartum.
    - For nonanaphylactic penicillin allergy, substitute cefazolin (1 g IV every 8 h) for ampicillin.
    - For severe penicillin allergy, substitute clindamycin (900 mg IV every 8 h) or vancomycin (500 mg every 6 h) for ampicillin.
    - Single-drug regimens have also been used: ampicillin/sulbactam (Unasyn; 3 g IV every 6 h), piperacillin/tazobactam (Zosyn; 3.375 g IV every 6 h), and ticarcillin/clavulanate (Timentin; 3.1 g every 6 h).
    - No data suggest that one regimen is better than another.
  - At delivery, the pediatrician should be notified because the neonate may be affected.
  - The placenta should be sent to pathology for histologic examination. Membrane culture can be obtained by carefully peeling the amnion and chorion apart and swabbing between the layers. Cord blood may also be sent for culture.
  - Unless the patient remains febrile, maternal antibiotics are not indicated beyond one dose after vaginal delivery.
  - After cesarean delivery with chorioamnionitis, broad coverage should be continued for at least one additional dose of antibiotics (8 h). It may be reasonable to continue antibiotics for as long as 48 hours after the last recorded temperature of 38.0°C or higher. Gentamicin and clindamycin is the typical regimen, but ampicillin can be added to achieve broader coverage (especially for enterococcus).

POSTPARTUM ENDOMYOMETRITIS

- **Postpartum endomyometritis** is infection of the endometrium, myometrium, and parametrial tissues.
- **Incidence.** About 5% of vaginal deliveries and 10% of cesarean deliveries are affected by postpartum uterine infection. Rates are significantly higher in women of lower socioeconomic status.

- **Etiology and diagnosis**
  - Risk factors include cesarean delivery, maternal diabetes mellitus, manual removal of the placenta, and all of the risks for chorioamnionitis.
  - Endomyometritis, like chorioamnionitis, is an ascending polymicrobial infection often caused by normal vaginal flora.
  - It may develop immediately to several days after delivery.
  - Diagnosis is clinical: fever 38.0°C or greater on two separate occasions >2 to 4 hours apart or a single temperature >39.0°C, uterine tenderness, tachycardia, purulent vaginal discharge, and associated findings such as dynamic ileus, pelvic peritonitis, pelvic abscess, and bowel obstruction.
  - Endometrial cultures are unnecessary; they are typically contaminated by normal flora and yield results much later than clinically required. Blood culture is indicated only for the most severe cases with concern for sepsis.
- **Management.** Acceptable broad-spectrum antibiotic regimens include the following:
  - Therapy with gentamicin and clindamycin ± ampicillin until 24 to 48 hours afebrile
  - Alternate single-agent therapies include ertapenem, ceftriaxone, cefotetan, Unasyn, Zosyn, or Timentin. The aim is broad polymicrobial coverage.
  - Gentamicin is administered every 8 hours before delivery. For postpartum treatment, however, several studies show 5 to 7 mg/kg daily dosing is safe, efficacious, and cost-effective. Drug levels are not monitored for daily dosing.
- Endomyometritis typically resolves with 48 hours of antibiotic treatment. Oral antibiotics are not required after completion of IV course.
- If fever persists or patient develops sepsis, additional workup should be considered. This may include urine and blood cultures; chest and abdominal radiographs; pelvic examination; and pelvic/abdominal ultrasound, CT, or magnetic resonance imaging.
- Infections with clostridia, group A streptococci, and staphylococci should be suspected in patients presenting with sepsis. Group A streptococcal septicemia is the leading cause of peripartum sepsis worldwide but is relatively rare in the United States (for management, see chapter 8). Toxic shock syndrome may be suspected when there is high fever, desquamation, diffuse macular rash, or multisystem organ failure. In rare cases, postpartum hysterectomy has been reported for uterine myonecrosis.

SEPTIC PELVIC THROMBOPHLEBITIS

- **Septic pelvic thrombophlebitis (SPT)** exists in two forms: **ovarian vein thrombosis/thrombophlebitis** and **deep pelvic septic thrombophlebitis**. The SPT occurs in 1 in 2000 to 1 in 3000 deliveries, most commonly after cesarean delivery.
- **Diagnosis and etiology**
  - The SPT should be considered in patients with persistent spiking fevers despite 3 days of antibiotic treatment for endometritis. The patient usually appears well between febrile episodes, and pain is minimal.
  - Thrombi form in the deep pelvic veins as a result of pregnancy-induced hypercoagulability and venous congestion. These may become infected, releasing septic emboli that travel to the lungs. Less than 2% of cases have pulmonary emboli by imaging. When other causes of postpartum fever have been excluded,

pelvic ultrasound and pelvic/abdominal CT or magnetic resonance imaging help diagnose abscess or large thrombus. A negative result, however, does not rule out SPT, which is largely a diagnosis of exclusion. Blood cultures are typically negative.

- **Management**
  - Because SPT is often a diagnosis of exclusion in patients with persistent fever, most are already being treated with broad-spectrum antibiotics, which also cover the typical pathogens of endomyometritis. Once the diagnosis is suspected, anticoagulation with heparin or enoxaparin is initiated.
  - Heparin theoretically terminates embolic showers that may cause the spiking fever. Therapeutic IV heparin infusion may be initiated with a 5000-unit heparin bolus and then a continuous infusion (usually 16-18 mm/kg/h) with an activated partial thromboplastin time ratio goal of 1.5 to 2.0 times normal. Low-molecular-weight heparin at a dose of 1 mg/kg every 12 hours is also acceptable.
  - Antibiotics may be continued until the patient is 24 to 48 hours afebrile. The duration of anticoagulation is somewhat controversial, with recommendations ranging from 24 hours to 2 weeks after the last fever. If imaging clearly detects a deep vein or pulmonary thrombus, 6 months of anticoagulation with warfarin or enoxaparin are indicated.

SUGGESTED READINGS

American College of Obstetricians and Gynecologists Committee on Practice Bulletins—Obstetrics. ACOG Practice Bulletin No. 183: postpartum hemorrhage. *Obstet Gynecol.* 2017;130:e168-e186.

Chandraharan E, Krishna A. Diagnosis and management of postpartum haemorrhage. *BMJ.* 2017;358:j3875.

Kogutt BK, Vaught AJ. Postpartum hemorrhage: blood product management and massive transfusion. *Semin Perinatol.* 2019;43(1):44-50. doi:10.1053/j.semperi.2018.11.008.

Mackeen AD, Packard RE, Ota E, Speer L. Antibiotic regimens for postpartum endometritis. *Cochrane Database Syst Rev.* 2015;(2):CD001067.

Pacheco LD, Saade G, Hankins GDV, Clark SL; for Society for Maternal-Fetal Medicine. Amniotic fluid embolism: diagnosis and management. *Am J Obstet Gynecol.* 2016;215(2): B16-B24.

Weeks A. The prevention and treatment of postpartum haemorrhage: what do we know, and where do we go to next? *BJOG.* 2015;122(2):202-210.

Fetal Assessment
Nicole R. Gavin and Ahmet Baschat

BACKGROUND

Antenatal fetal surveillance is performed using various modalities that allow care providers to closely monitor fetuses at risk for deterioration of well-being. The majority of surveillance tests detect signs of fetal compromise related to uteroplacental insufficiency in order to circumvent fetal hypoxemia, acidemia, and death. Performed serially at regular intervals, antenatal fetal testing is used to assess ongoing fetal well-being, guide antenatal management, and determine possible need for imminent delivery or other acute obstetric management. It is therefore important that providers of obstetrical care be well versed in the different modalities of fetal testing, including their limitations and implications.

METHODS OF FETAL ASSESSMENT

There are numerous methods of assessing fetal well-being, and no single test is superior to another method, although some surveillance tests perform better for specific fetal conditions. Each test has its own individual merits (as well as limitations), and tests are often used in combination to create an overall picture of the fetal state and help identify fetal compromise (Table 4-1).

Fetal Movement

- **Maternal assessment of fetal movement (kick counts)**
  - Least expensive and least invasive fetal assessment test.
  - Requires neither equipment nor hospital setting.
- **Purpose:** Kick counts can be used for routine screening and reassurance in low-risk pregnancies when a patient perceives decreased fetal movement or as a complement to other disease-specific surveillance modalities. It can also be used as a method of surveillance in some higher risk pregnancies, for example, in women with a prior history of stillbirth.
- **Method of testing:** The patient counts the number of fetal movements in a finite period. While performing this test, the woman should lie on her left side to improve blood flow to the uterus and placenta and eat prior to starting the test, to stimulate the fetus. Multiple testing strategies have been described, all with equal efficacy.
  - To perform the Cardiff technique, the patient counts fetal movements when she first gets up in the morning and records the time required for the fetus to move 10 times. Lack of 10 movements over 3 hours should prompt the patient to call her physician for further fetal testing.
  - Using the Sadovsky technique, the patient counts fetal movements over the course of 1 hour. To be considered "reassuring," 4 or more fetal movements should be felt over the course of the hour. However, a second hour of monitoring

Table 4-1 Summary of Antenatal Testing[a]

	Components	Results	False-Negative Rate	False-Positive Rate
NST	• Continuous FHR monitoring	**Reactive:** ≥2 accelerations within 20 min (may be extended to 40 min) **Nonreactive:** <2 accelerations in 40 min	0.2%–0.65%	55%-90%
CST/OCT	• Continuous FHR monitoring • At least three contractions of ≥40 s duration within 10 min	**Negative:** no late or significant variable decelerations **Positive:** late decelerations following ≥50% of contractions **Equivocal:** intermittent decelerations	0.04%	35%-65%
BPP	Five components within 30 min: • NST • Episode of fetal breathing movements lasting ≥30 s • ≥3 discrete body or limb movements • ≥1 episode of extremity extension with return to flexion • Maximum vertical AF pocket >2 cm or AFI >5 cm	**Normal:** ≥8/10 or 8/8 excluding NST **Equivocal:** 6/10 **Abnormal:** ≤4/10	0.07%–0.08%	40%-50%
Modified BPP	• NST • AFI	**Normal:** reactive NST and AFI >5 cm **Abnormal:** nonreactive NST and/or AFI ≤5 cm	0.08%	60%

Abbreviations: AF, amniotic fluid; AFI, amniotic fluid index; BPP, biophysical profile; CST, contraction stress test; FHR, fetal heart rate; NST, nonstress test; OCT, oxytocin challenge test.

[a]Adapted with permission from Signore C, Freeman RK, Spong CY. Antenatal testing-a reevaluation: executive summary of a Eunice Kennedy Shriver National Institute of Child Health and Human Development workshop. *Obstet Gynecol.* 2009;113(3):687-701. Copyright © 2009 by The American College of Obstetricians and Gynecologists.

to attain 4 movements is permissible. If 4 fetal movements have not been felt after 2 hours, the patient should contact her doctor for further recommendations.

- **Management after abnormal results:** After the observation of decreased fetal movement, the follow-up test to evaluate fetal well-being is a nonstress test (NST).

Fetal Heart Rate Monitoring

- **Nonstress test**
  - In the absence of acidosis or neurologic impairment, the fetal heart rate normally rises temporarily and randomly during fetal movement. These increases in heart rate or accelerations are documented using cardiotocography.
  - **Method of testing:** The NST is a noninvasive assessment that records the fetal heart rate simultaneously with uterine activity. The fetal heart rate is monitored with an external cardiotachometer, which uses ultrasound to evaluate fetal heart motion, giving an average of fetal heart beats. Uterine activity is monitored with an external tocodynamometer.
  - **Criteria for test results:** A "reactive" NST demonstrates at least two accelerations of the fetal heart rate over a 20-minute period.
    - Prior to 32 weeks' gestation, accelerations must be 10 seconds in duration and reach a peak 10 beats above the baseline to qualify as "reactive."
    - As the sympathetic and parasympathetic nervous systems mature, more stringent criteria are applied. In a fetus 32 weeks' gestation or greater, each of the 2 accelerations must be 15 seconds in duration and must reach a peak of 15 beats above the baseline level (Figure 4-1).
    - If the fetal heart rate is "nonreactive" after 20 minutes, the fetal heart rate should be observed for an additional 20 minutes to account for the possibility that the fetus may have been in quiet sleep during the initial observation period.
    - There are many other factors that can influence the fetal heart rate tracing (see below). Specifically, the development of fetal behavioral states results in a gradual increase of nonreactive heart rate tracings from 32 weeks onward.

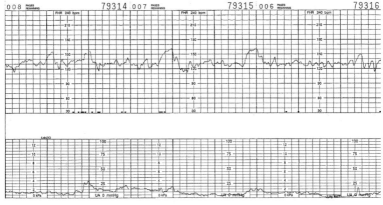

Figure 4-1. Reactive nonstress test. Fetal monitor strip records fetal heart rate **(top)** and uterine contractile activity **(bottom)**. Several accelerations are evident.

These often coincide with periods of fetal quiescence and therefore may require additional testing to distinguish this physiologic state from compromise.

- **Strengths and limitations:** A "reactive" NST is highly predictive of a low risk of fetal mortality. The stillbirth rate in the week following a reactive NST is 1.9/1000, depending on the indication for fetal testing. The negative predictive value of an NST is >90%. The positive predictive value is only 50% to 70%. Therefore, the NST is better suited to rule out rather than predict fetal compromise. Given the high false-positive rate, a "nonreactive" NST should be followed by more extensive testing such as biophysical profile (BPP), vibroacoustic stimulation (VAS), or contraction stress test (CST). The VAS test is specifically designed to induce fetal heart rate accelerations by an acoustic stimulus that "awakens" the fetus from a resting state.

- **Contraction stress test or oxytocin challenge test**
  - **Purpose:** The CST is designed to assess fetal response to the stress of induced uterine contractions causing transient uteroplacental insufficiency.
  - **Method of testing:** The mother is placed in the left lateral tilt position and external monitors are applied. If three contractions of 40 seconds duration or greater are noted, a "spontaneous" CST can be performed without stimulation. In the absence of spontaneous contractions, uterine activity can be induced either by nipple stimulation or with a dilute solution of oxytocin until three contractions occur in a 10-minute period.

- **Criteria for test results:** A "positive" CST demonstrates late decelerations with more than 50% of contractions (Figure 4-2). Late decelerations reach their nadir after the peak of the contraction. A "negative" CST demonstrates no late decelerations. A CST with intermittent late decelerations is considered equivocal, and further evaluation of the pregnancy is warranted. An "inadequate" or "unsatisfactory" CST is one in which adequate contractions are not achieved. If hyperstimulation occurs, an abnormal fetal response may be the result of the testing technique alone and should be repeated or another form of testing should be done.

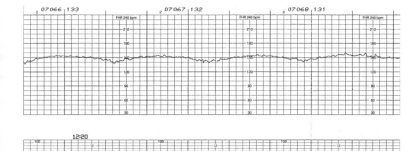

Figure 4-2. Fetal heart tracing with late decelerations. Following each contraction (**bottom tracing**) is a slight depression of the fetal heart rate (**top tracing**), suggesting uteroplacental insufficiency. Original fetal monitor strip courtesy of Janice Henderson, MD, Division of Maternal Fetal Medicine, Department of Gynecology and Obstetrics, Johns Hopkins Hospital.

- **Strengths and limitations:** The CST is one of the most labor-intensive methods of fetal surveillance but has the highest specificity for detecting the compromised fetus. It has a negative predictive value of >99%. Relative contraindications to CST include preterm labor, preterm premature rupture of membranes, placenta previa, and high risk for uterine rupture. Previous low transverse cesarean delivery is not a contraindication.

Fetal Heart Monitoring With Ultrasonography

- **Biophysical profile**
  - **Purpose:** The BPP uses ultrasound observations in conjunction with the NST to help predict acute and chronic tissue hypoxia. It has excellent negative predictive value for fetal mortality in the 72 to 96 hours after the test. It has been shown to reduce perinatal morbidity and mortality.
  - **Method of testing:** The BPP has five components: fetal breathing, fetal movement, fetal tone, amniotic fluid assessment determined by ultrasound, and the NST. Two points are awarded for each observed parameter. No points are awarded for a nonreactive NST or the absence of any parameter. Therefore, only even number scores are possible with a maximum score of 10. The specific criteria of these components are listed in Table 4-2. All of the sonographic criteria must be observed within a 30-minute period.
  - **Criteria for test results:** The BPP is reported as normal, equivocal, or abnormal. A score of 8 or 10 is normal, and routine surveillance and expectant obstetric management may continue. A score of 8 with a maximum vertical pocket <2 cm or score of 6 is equivocal, and the BPP should be repeated in 6 to 24 hours, especially in fetuses over 32 weeks' gestation. If the score does not improve, delivery should be considered, depending on gestational age and individual circumstances. A score of 6 with maximum vertical pocket <2 cm or

Table 4-2	Biophysical Profile	
Biophysical Variable	Normal (Score = 2)	Abnormal (Score = 0)
Fetal breathing movements	One episode of fetal breathing 30 s	Less than 30 s of fetal breathing; absent breathing
Fetal movements	Three discrete body/limb movements	Two or fewer body/limb movements
Fetal tone	One episode of active extension, with return to flexion of fetal limbs or trunk	Extended position with no or slow return to flexion; absent movement
Nonstress test	Reactive	Nonreactive
Amniotic fluid volume	One pocket of fluid at least 2 cm in two perpendicular planes	No amniotic fluid or pocket <2 cm in size

a score of 4 or below is abnormal, and delivery should be considered, again depending on gestational age and clinical context. Regardless of the composite score, oligohydramnios (as defined by amniotic fluid volume with the deepest pocket <2 cm) warrants further evaluation. It is important to consider that fetal breathing can be reduced in preterm fetuses <34 weeks' gestation, and this may affect interpretation.

- **Modified BPP**
  - **Purpose:** This test combines the **NST and amniotic fluid volume**, which are often used together to assess fetal well-being in the third trimester. In general, the amniotic fluid volume reflects fetal perfusion and, if decreased, raises suspicion for uteroplacental insufficiency.
  - **Criteria for test results:** A normal test includes a reactive NST and an amniotic fluid volume with a deepest vertical pocket >2 cm. An abnormal test lacks one or both of these findings and should be further evaluated.
  - **Strengths and limitations of the BPP:** A normal BPP is highly predictive of normal fetal status, whereas an abnormal BPP strongly predicts prelabor acidemia with a fetal pH <7.20. A disadvantage of the BPP is that it has limited ability to predict impending fetal deterioration. The stillbirth rate within a week of a normal BPP is 0.9/1000 with fetomaternal hemorrhage, acute obstetric events, and deteriorating placental function as the primary contributors to fetal demise.

Fetal Blood Flow/Velocity and Dopplers

- **Purpose:** Doppler velocimetry is a noninvasive method of assessing fetal vascular impedance, or absolute blood flow velocity in several vascular beds. The purpose of Doppler surveillance is to evaluate the severity of placental dysfunction or the degree of fetal cardiovascular compromise in a variety of fetal conditions. The primary vessels used in fetal surveillance are the umbilical artery, the middle cerebral artery (MCA), and the ductus venosus (DV).
- **Umbilical artery Doppler velocimetry**
  - **Method of umbilical artery Doppler testing:** Umbilical artery blood flow is measured in a free-floating loop of umbilical cord. The waveform pattern is recorded and analyzed (Figure 4-3), most commonly with the systolic/diastolic (S/D) ratio, whereas the pulsatility index (PI) provides the most consistent measurement. A reduction in diastolic flow is associated with placental insufficiency and produces an increase of the Doppler indices above the gestational age-specific reference range (S/D and PI). A significant reduction leading to absence or reversal of end-diastolic velocity is observed with significant placental dysfunction. Abnormal umbilical artery Doppler is associated with intrauterine growth restriction (IUGR), fetal hypoxia, fetal acidosis, and therefore with higher rates of perinatal morbidity and mortality.
  - **Strengths and limitations:** Abnormal umbilical artery blood flow patterns are reported to precede abnormal fetal heart rate patterns by a median of 7 days. For this reason, it is used in conjunction with other tests for pregnancies complicated by IUGR, preeclampsia, or chronic hypertension. Umbilical artery Doppler is particularly useful in conditions that are associated with abnormal perfusion of the placental circulation as observed in IUGR. Mildly abnormal placental dysfunction that affects fetal oxygenation is not necessarily detected by umbilical artery Doppler.

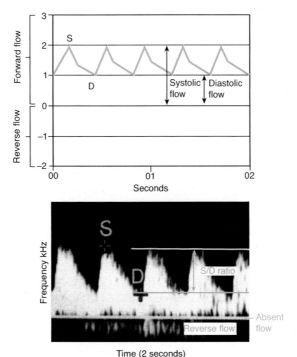

Figure 4-3. Evaluation of umbilical artery flow by Doppler velocimetry. **Top panel** illustrates the findings for a normal umbilical artery. **Bottom image** is a typical normal Doppler recording. Ratio of flow during systole and diastole (S/D ratio) reflects placental bed resistance. D, diastole; S, systole. Adapted from Druzin ML, Gabbe SG, Reed KL. Antepartum fetal evaluation. In: Gabbe SG, Niebyl JR, Simpson JL, eds. *Obstetrics: Normal and Problem Pregnancies.* 4th ed. New York, NY: Churchill Livingstone; 2001:334 and MacDonald MG, Mullet MD, Seshia MMK, eds. *Avery's Neonatology: Pathophysiology & Management of the Newborn.* 6th ed. Philadelphia, PA: Lippincott Williams & Wilkins; 2005.

- **Indications for use**: Umbilical artery Doppler velocimetry should not be used as a screening tool in the general population. It has been shown to be useful in pregnancies complicated by IUGR, hypertension, or preeclampsia.
- **Middle cerebral artery Doppler velocimetry**
  - The MCA blood flow is measured in the fetal brain and the waveform is analyzed using the S/D ratio but more consistently with the PI. In addition, the peak systolic velocity can also be recorded. A significant increase in diastolic flow leads to reduction of the Doppler index and may be observed with significant fetal hypoxemia and placental dysfunction (this is called "brain sparing"). An increase in the peak systolic velocity is observed when there is fetal anemia.
  - **Strengths and limitations:** Abnormal MCA Doppler can detect placental dysfunction that is below the detection threshold of umbilical artery Doppler, as

is frequently observed with term IUGR. In the term IUGR fetus with normal umbilical artery Doppler, new-onset brain sparing (as seen by abnormal MCA Doppler testing) is associated with stillbirth within 1 week. The middle cerebral peak systolic velocity has become the primary surveillance tool for fetuses at risk for fetal anemia (Rh isoimmunization, fetomaternal hemorrhage) because it predicts severe fetal anemia with a high sensitivity.

- **Indications for use:** The MCA Doppler should not be used as a screening tool because its ability to predict fetal compromise is limited to specific fetal conditions. It has been shown to be useful in pregnancies complicated by IUGR, hypertension, preeclampsia, or fetal anemia.

- **Ductus venosus Doppler velocimetry**
  - The DV is responsible for delivering oxygenated blood directly to the heart and as a venous vessel possesses a triphasic waveform (systole, diastole, atrial systole). A significant decrease in forward flow during atrial systolic flow leads to an increase in the Doppler index and may be observed with progression to acidemia in fetuses with severe IUGR. Loss or reversal of atrial systolic forward flow in this setting is associated with an increased risk for stillbirth within 1 week. Therefore, delivery is recommended when this occurs even in the preterm IUGR fetus presenting from 26 weeks onwards.
  - **Strengths and limitations:** Abnormal DV Doppler is useful to detect advancing deterioration in IUGR fetuses that requires delivery. In early-onset IUGR, DV Doppler becomes abnormal after the umbilical or MCA abnormalities have already occurred. A randomized trial has established that waiting for DV Doppler abnormality gains significant gestational age and is associated with improved composite outcome in IUGR.
  - **Indications for use:** The DV is a disease-specific surveillance tool used in early-onset IUGR presenting before 32 weeks' gestation. A DV Doppler should not be used as a screening tool because its ability to predict fetal acidemia and compromise is limited to IUGR. A DV Doppler may not always reflect compromise and therefore concurrent monitoring with fetal heart rate and/or BPP is recommended as a safety net. Of note, in the above-mentioned randomized trial, fetal heart rate triggered delivery in the majority of cases, rather than Dopplers.

CONFOUNDING FACTORS IN FETAL ASSESSMENT

- **Sleep cycles:** The fetus may have sleep cycles 20 to 80 minutes in duration. During these periods, the long-term variability of the fetal heart rate is decreased and the tracing is likely to be nonreactive. To rule out sleep cycle as a cause for a nonreactive NST, prolonged monitoring (longer than 80 minutes at times) or VAS may be required.
- **Medications:** Certain maternal medications cross the placenta and can have an effect on the fetal heart rate, movement, and amniotic fluid volume. There are a number of medications administered in the management of labor and complications of labor that can have an influence on the tests for fetal well-being. Glucocorticosteroids given for the purpose of enhancing fetal maturity have been shown to influence BPP scores by decreasing the amniotic fluid index, decreasing fetal movement, and decreasing breathing motion. Magnesium sulfate can decrease the fetal heart rate variability. Other medications, such as narcotics,

sedatives, and β-blockers have been shown to decrease fetal heart rate variability and reactivity.

- **Maternal smoking and illicit drugs:** The maternal use of illicit drugs and smoking results in a transient decrease in fetal heart rate variability.
- **Maternal hypoglycemia:** Maternal hypoglycemia may reduce fetal heart rate variability as well as fetal movement and breathing.

INDICATIONS FOR FETAL TESTING

- **Maternal conditions and complications of pregnancy:** There are numerous maternal medical conditions, complications of pregnancy, and fetal conditions that confer increased risk of adverse fetal outcomes. Therefore, antenatal fetal surveillance is recommended in these high-risk pregnancies in an attempt to decrease fetal morbidity and mortality. Tables 4-3 and 4-4 outline some of the maternal and fetal indications for antenatal fetal surveillance, the methods of testing to be employed for fetal assessment, the gestational age to begin testing, and the frequency of monitoring.
- **Commencement and frequency of testing:** Each maternal and fetal indication for fetal surveillance has its own recommendations for the commencement and frequency of testing based on the underlying etiology of disease and the perceived risk to the fetus.

Table 4-3	Recommendations for Antenatal Fetal Assessment: Maternal/Pregnancy Conditions[a]
Maternal Conditions	**Pregnancy-Related Conditions**
• Pregestational diabetes	• Gestational hypertension
• Hypertension	• Preeclampsia
• Systemic lupus erythematosus	• Decreased fetal movement
• Chronic renal disease	• Gestational diabetes (poorly controlled or medically treated)
• Antiphospholipid syndrome	• Oligohydramnios
• Hyperthyroidism (poorly controlled)	• Preterm premature rupture of membranes
• Hemoglobinopathies (sickle cell, sickle cell–hemoglobin C, or sickle cell–thalassemia disease)	• Fetal growth restriction
• Cyanotic heart disease	• Chronic abruption
	• Late-term or postterm pregnancy
	• Isoimmunization
	• Previous fetal demise
	• Monochorionic multiple gestation (with significant growth discrepancy)
	• Cholestasis of pregnancy

Table 4-4	Recommendations for Antenatal Fetal Testing: Fetal Conditions		

Indication	Recommended Tests	Suggested Gestational Age for Commencement	Frequency of Testing
Intrauterine growth restriction	Umbilical Dopplers NST AFI BPP	Time of diagnosis	Weekly or twice weekly Weekly to daily Weekly Weekly to daily
Isoimmunization	MCA Doppler for fetal anemia	16-18 wk	Weekly
Preterm premature rupture of membranes (PPROM)	NST BPP	At time of PPROM	Daily to twice a week
History of prior stillbirth	Kick counts NST, AFI, BPP	26-28 wk 32 wk or 1-2 wk prior to GA of previous stillbirth	Daily Weekly to twice a week

Abbreviations: AFI, amniotic fluid index; BPP, biophysical profile; GA, gestational age; MCA, middle cerebral artery; NST, nonstress test.

SUGGESTED READINGS

American College of Obstetricians and Gynecologists Committee on Practice Bulletins—Obstetrics. ACOG Practice Bulletin No. 145: antepartum fetal surveillance. *Obstet Gynecol.* 2014;124:182-192. (Reaffirmed 2019)

American College of Obstetricians and Gynecologists Committee on Practice Bulletins—Obstetrics. ACOG Practice Bulletin No. 204: fetal growth restriction. *Obstet Gynecol.* 2019;133:e97-e109.

Baschat AA. Planning management and delivery of the growth-restricted fetus. *Best Pract Res Clin Obstet Gynaecol.* 2018;49:53-65.

Devoe LD. Antenatal fetal assessment: contraction stress test, nonstress test, vibroacoustic stimulation, amniotic fluid volume, biophysical profile, and modified biophysical profile—an overview. *Semin Perinatol.* 2008;32:247-252.

Lees CC, Marlow N, van Wassenaer-Leemhuis A, et al. 2 Year neurodevelopmental and intermediate perinatal outcomes in infants with very preterm fetal growth restriction (TRUFFLE): a randomised trial. *Lancet.* 2015;385:2162-2172.

Nageotte M. Antenatal testing: diabetes mellitus. *Semin Perinatol.* 2008;32:269-270.

Turan S, Miller J, Baschat A. Integrated testing and management in fetal growth restriction. *Semin Perinatol.* 2008;32:194-200.

Prenatal Complications
Jerome J. Federspiel and Jeanne S. Sheffield

NAUSEA AND VOMITING OF PREGNANCY

- Nausea and vomiting are common symptoms in pregnancy, with an incidence of nausea from 50% to 80% and vomiting of 50%. **Hyperemesis gravidarum** is much less common, complicating approximately 1% of pregnancies. There is no universally accepted definition of hyperemesis gravidarum, but diagnostic criteria include a combination of the following: exclusion of alternative etiologies for nausea and vomiting (Table 5-1), acute starvation (eg, ketonuria), and weight loss (eg, 5% from pregravid weight) and may also include electrolyte, thyroid, and hepatic function testing abnormalities. Hyperemesis gravidarum, which peaks around 9 weeks, is generally viewed as a severe manifestation of nausea and vomiting of pregnancy, rather than a separate disorder (see chapter 15).

- The etiology of nausea and vomiting of pregnancy is poorly understood. Increased levels of human chorionic gonadotropin (such as is produced by multiple gestations and molar pregnancy) and estradiol are associated with worsened symptoms, although the exact mechanism is unclear. Theories that nausea and vomiting of pregnancy are driven by a psychological predisposition to the condition are less helpful in understanding and managing the condition. Other risk factors include history of motion sickness, migraine headaches, family or personal history of the condition, and female fetus.

- Serious complications of nausea and vomiting in pregnancy (such as Boerhaave syndrome or Wernicke encephalopathy) are rare in modern obstetric practice, but the disorder remains the second most common reason for antepartum hospitalization (after preterm labor) in the United States and has a considerable impact on maternal quality of life. Mild to moderate nausea and vomiting in pregnancy has not been associated with fetal or neonatal impacts. Severe nausea and vomiting and hyperemesis may be associated with higher rates of low birthweight and preterm birth, but there has been no association between hyperemesis and either perinatal or neonatal mortality in large cohorts.

- **Management:** Preventative efforts include recommending patients start prenatal vitamins at least 1 month prior to conception, and for women with a history of hyperemesis, starting antiemetic treatment prior to onset of symptoms. For management of nausea and vomiting once it manifests, current American College of Obstetrics and Gynecologists (ACOG) guidance recommends nonpharmacologic therapies as first-line management, starting with transition from prenatal vitamins to only folic acid supplementation, ginger capsules, and consideration of P6 acupressure wrist bands. See Table 5-2. Counseling regarding small frequent meals and avoidance of foods that trigger symptoms are reasonable, albeit non–evidence-based interventions. In the event nonpharmacologic management is unsuccessful, ACOG recommends products containing a combination of vitamin B_6 (pyridoxine) and doxylamine as the first-line pharmacotherapeutic option. For patients with persistent symptoms, escalation to a sedating antihistamine (eg, dimenhydrinate or

Table 5-1 Differential Diagnosis of Nausea and Vomiting of Pregnancy[a]

Gastrointestinal conditions	Gastroenteritis
	Gastroparesis
	Achalasia
	Biliary tract disease
	Hepatitis
	Intestinal obstruction
	Peptic ulcer disease
	Pancreatitis
	Appendicitis
Conditions of the genitourinary tract	Pyelonephritis
	Uremia
	Ovarian torsion
	Kidney stones
	Degenerating uterine leiomyoma
Metabolic conditions	Diabetic ketoacidosis
	Porphyria
	Addison disease
	Hyperthyroidism
	Hyperparathyroidism
Neurologic disorders	Pseudotumor cerebri
	Vestibular lesions
	Migraine headaches
	Tumors of the central nervous system
	Lymphocytic hypophysitis
Miscellaneous conditions	Drug toxicity or intolerance
	Psychological condition
Pregnancy-related conditions	Acute fatty liver of pregnancy
	Preeclampsia
	"Morning sickness"
	Hyperemesis gravidarum

[a]Adapted from Goodwin TM. Hyperemesis gravidarum. *Obstet Gynecol Clin North Am.* 2008;35(3): 401-417, viii. Copyright © 2008 Elsevier. With permission.

diphenhydramine) or phenothiazine derivative (eg, prochlorperazine or promethazine) is suggested. Further escalation in the absence of dehydration could include metoclopramide, ondansetron, promethazine, or trimethobenzamide. In escalating therapy, it is important to consider that combinations of dopamine antagonists and phenothiazines increase the risk of extrapyramidal side effects and neuroleptic malignant syndrome, whereas combinations of ondansetron and phenothiazines may lead to excessive QTc prolongation.

- For patients who present with dehydration or who cannot tolerate oral rehydration, current ACOG guidance recommends the use of parenteral hydration as

Table 5-2 Treatment of Nausea and Vomiting in Pregnancy[a]

Step of Treatment[b]	Treatment
1	Nonpharmacologic options: • Transition from prenatal vitamins to folic acid only • Ginger capsules, 250-mg tablets 4 times orally daily • P6 acupressure wrist bands
2	Add one of the following medications: • Vitamin B_6 (pyridoxine) 10-25 mg and/or doxylamine 12.5 mg orally 3-4 times a day • Vitamin B_6 10 mg/doxylamine 10 mg (Diclegis), two tablets orally at bedtime initially, up to four tablets a day (add one tablet in the morning and one tablet midafternoon) • Vitamin B_6 20 mg/doxylamine 20 mg (Bonjesta), one tablet orally at bedtime initially, up to two tablets per day (add one tablet in the morning)
3	Add any of the following: • Diphenhydramine 25-50 mg every 4-6 h orally • Prochlorperazine 25-50 mg every 12 h rectally • Promethazine 12.5-25 mg every 4-6 h orally or rectally • Dimenhydrinate 25-50 mg every 4-6 h orally (not to exceed 200 mg/d if taken with doxylamine)
4A (no dehydration)	Add any of the following: • Metoclopramide 5-10 mg every 6-8 h orally or IM • Ondansetron 4 mg every 8 h orally • Promethazine 12.5-25 mg every 4-6 h orally, rectally, or IM • Trimethobenzamide 200 mg every 6-8 h IM
4B (with dehydration)	Add intravenous fluid replacement AND any of the following: • Metoclopramide 5-10 mg every 8 h IV • Ondansetron 8 mg every 12 h IV • Promethazine 12.5-25 mg every 4-6 h IV • Dimenhydrinate 50 mg every 4-6 h IV
5 (with dehydration)	Continue intravenous fluid replacement AND add either of the following: • Chlorpromazine 25-50 mg every 4-6 h IV or IM • Chlorpromazine 10-25 mg every 4-6 h orally • Methylprednisolone 16 mg every 8 h for 3 days, orally or IV; taper over 2 wk to lowest effective dose; limit use to 6 wk

Abbreviations: IM, intramuscularly; IV, intravenously.
[a]Data from American College of Obstetricians and Gynecologists Committee on Practice Bulletins—Obstetrics. ACOG Practice Bulletin Number 189: nausea and vomiting of pregnancy. *Obstet Gynecol* 2018;131(1):e15-e30.
[b]If no improvement, move to the next step for management.

first-line therapy. Patients who require intravenous (IV) hydration, or who have been vomiting for more than 3 weeks, should receive 100 mg of thiamine with her first bag of IV fluids, and an additional 100 mg daily for the next 2 to 3 days to prevent Wernicke encephalopathy. Dextrose-containing fluids should be deferred until the first dose of thiamine is delivered. For patients whose vomiting is refractory to these management efforts, a corticosteroid is a further management option, which has been shown to reduce the risk of readmission. However, corticosteroids have been shown to increase the risk of oral cleft defects when given before 10 weeks of gestation, and given the potential risks of prolonged steroid use for both fetus and mother, should be limited to 6 weeks of therapy during pregnancy per ACOG guidelines as a last-resort therapy.

- While management of the patient's symptoms is in progress, it is important to also manage her nutritional status. For patients whose symptoms preclude oral intake or who cannot maintain weight despite pharmacotherapy, enteral feeding using a nasogastric or nasoduodenal tube should be first-line management. Prolonged use of central catheters, even peripherally inserted central catheters, are associated with significant morbidity in pregnancy, and for this reason, the use of total parenteral nutrition should be reserved for those patients who are not able to tolerate enteral feeding despite maximum pharmacologic management of nausea and vomiting.

- Gestational transient thyrotoxicosis is a common complication of nausea and vomiting of pregnancy. Abnormal thyroid function studies diagnosed in the setting of nausea and vomiting of pregnancy should not automatically be treated with antithyroid medication because the thyroid function abnormalities will resolve as the symptoms improve.

CERVICAL INSUFFICIENCY

- **Cervical insufficiency (CI)**, or cervical incompetence, occurs in 1 in 100 to 1 in 2000 gestations. Risk factors include prior cervical laceration, history of cervical conization, multiple terminations with mechanical cervical dilation, intrauterine diethylstilbestrol exposure, and congenital cervical anomaly.

- The epidemiology is as imprecise as the various, sometimes controversial, criteria used to diagnose CI. One reasonable definition is painless cervical dilation during the second trimester in the absence of infection, placental abruption, uterine contractions, or uterine anomaly. Because CI is a diagnosis of exclusion, alternate diagnoses must be rigorously sought. Admittedly, diagnosis of CI and selection of patients for cervical cerclage can be difficult. Progesterone supplementation, pessary placement, and cervical cerclage have been suggested to prevent pregnancy loss from CI, but the evidence for their effectiveness is mixed. See chapter 6.

- Patients may qualify for
  - **History-indicated cerclage:** history of one or more prior second-trimester pregnancy losses in setting of painless dilation and absence of labor or abruption and typically placed at 12 to 14 weeks' gestation
  - **Ultrasound-indicated cerclage:** cervical length less than 25 mm with a history of at least one preterm delivery, as assessed by serial ultrasounds from 16 to 24 weeks' gestation
  - **Rescue cerclage:** patient with cervical dilation not suspected to be due to labor or abruption (see chapter 6, Table 6-1)

- Vaginal cerclage may be performed by either using the McDonald or Shiradkor techniques. Permanent suture, either Prolene (polypropylene) or Mersiline (polyester fiber), is commonly employed. Prophylactic antibiotics and postoperative tocolytics have not been proven to affect outcome, except possibly in the case of rescue cerclage where such use is associated with a higher percentage of patients with pregnancies prolonged by at least 28 days.
  - The risk of iatrogenic pregnancy loss ranges from 1% to 20% for elective cases. Rescue cerclage for CI/bulging membranes is associated with >50% risk of complications.
  - An abdominal cerclage is placed at laparotomy or using minimally invasive (laparoscopic or robotic methods) techniques for women who have minimal to no residual cervical length (often due to large cone biopsies or trachelectomy) or who had prior pregnancy losses with a vaginal cerclage in situ. Subsequent cesarean delivery is necessary in the setting of an abdominal cerclage.
- Progesterone supplementation, in the form of 17-hydroxyprogesterone caproate, is commonly prescribed to patients with a history of preterm delivery, whether caused by CI or not. Evidence has not proven an incremental benefit to this treatment when added to cerclage. Vaginal progesterone may be employed for treatment of patients with cervical shortening in the absence of history of preterm birth.
- Vaginal pessaries are designed to transfer the weight of uterine contents away from the cervix, and by changing the axis of the cervical canal. The best studied pessaries for CI are the Arabin design. In meta-analyses of randomized controlled trials among singleton pregnancies with pessaries placed for cervical shortening without history of preterm delivery, pessaries were not shown to provide a significant benefit. Data from twin gestations, an area in which cerclage has been shown to be ineffective, have been more promising. Further research is needed to understand the optimal use of pessaries in current obstetric practice; currently, their use may be considered reasonable for twin gestations and for cervical shortening in singleton gestations for patients without history of preterm delivery.

AMNIOTIC FLUID DISORDERS

- **Amniotic fluid volume (AFV)** represents the balance between production and removal of fetal fluids. In early gestation, fluid is produced from the fetal surface of the placenta, from transfer across the amnion, and from embryonic surface secretions. In mid to late gestation, fluid is produced by fetal urination and alveolar transudate. Fluid is removed by fetal swallowing and absorption at the amnion-chorion interface.
- Ultrasound is used to estimate AFV.

Polyhydramnios

- **Polyhydramnios** is the pathologic accumulation of amniotic fluid more than the 95th percentile for gestational age, the deepest vertical pocket of >8 cm, or an amniotic fluid index (AFI) >24 cm at term. The incidence of polyhydramnios in the general population is about 1%.
- Mildly increased AFV is usually clinically insignificant. Markedly increased AFV is associated with increased perinatal morbidity due to preterm labor, cord prolapse upon membrane rupture, underlying comorbidities, and congenital malformations.

Abruptio placentae is associated with polyhydramnios and rupture of membranes due to rapid decompression of the overdistended uterus. Increased maternal morbidity also results from postpartum hemorrhage due to uterine overdistention leading to atony. If polyhydramnios is severe, uterine distention can cause venous and ureteral compression causing severe lower extremity edema and hydronephrosis. The most common **etiology** of polyhydramnios is idiopathic; however, in severe cases, a cause is more likely to be associated with a detectable fetal anomaly. Specific causes include the following:

- **Fetal structural malformations.** In cases of acrania or anencephaly, polyhydramnios occurs from an impaired swallowing mechanism, low antidiuretic hormone causing polyuria, and possibly transudation across the exposed fetal meninges. Gastrointestinal tract anomalies may also lead to polyhydramnios by either direct physical obstruction or decreased absorption. Ventral wall defects increase AFV from transudation across the peritoneal surface or bowel wall.
- **Chromosomal and genetic abnormalities.** As many as 35% of fetuses with polyhydramnios have chromosomal abnormalities. The most common are trisomy 13, 18, and 21.
- **Neuromuscular disorders.** Impaired fetal swallowing can increase AFV.
- **Diabetes mellitus.** Maternal diabetes mellitus is a common cause of polyhydramnios, especially with poor glycemic control or associated fetal malformations. Fetal hyperglycemia can increase fluid transudation across the placental interface and cause fetal polyuria.
- **Alloimmunization.** *Hydrops fetalis* can increase AFV.
- **Congenital infections.** In the absence of other factors, polyhydramnios may warrant screening for congenital infections, such as toxoplasmosis, cytomegalovirus, and syphilis. These are, however, rare causes of polyhydramnios.
- **Twin-to-twin transfusion syndrome.** The recipient twin develops polyhydramnios and occasionally *hydrops fetalis*, whereas the donor twin develops growth restriction and oligohydramnios.
- **Treatment.** Mild to moderate polyhydramnios can be managed expectantly until the onset of labor or spontaneous rupture of membranes. Current Society for Maternal and Fetal Medicine guidance does not require antenatal testing for patients with mild polyhydramnios in the absence of other indications for testing. If the patient develops significant dyspnea, abdominal pain, or difficulty ambulating, treatment becomes necessary.
  - **Amnioreduction** can alleviate significant maternal symptoms. Amniocentesis is performed, and fluid is removed. Frequent removal of smaller volumes (total 1500 to 2000 mL or until the AFI is <8 cm) will result in a lower risk of preterm labor compared with removal of larger volumes. Amnioreduction is repeated as needed. Antibiotic prophylaxis is unnecessary. Because of the risks inherent in this invasive procedure, amnioreduction is reserved for patients with severe maternal discomfort or dyspnea with severe polyhydramnios.
  - **Pharmacologic treatment** with indomethacin reduces fetal urine production. Fetal renal blood flow and glomerular filtration rate are sensitive to prostaglandins. Indomethacin (25 mg PO every 6 h) can decrease fetal renal blood flow and urination. Premature closure of the fetal ductus arteriosus is a potential complication of indomethacin that requires close AFV and ductus diameter monitoring. Discontinue therapy if there is any suggestion of ductus closure. The risk of complications is low if the total daily dose of indomethacin is <200 mg, the

treatment is limited to pregnancies <32 weeks, and the duration of therapy is <48 h; however, given the significant risks of adverse neonatal outcomes associated with indomethacin use in use pregnancy, contemporary guidance from the Society for Maternal and Fetal Medicine discourages its use.

- Delivery planning and intrapartum management can be individualized, but in general, deliveries for polyhydramnios should be deferred until 39 weeks, barring another obstetric indication to earlier delivery. During the intrapartum course, patients with polyhydramnios are at increased risk for unstable lie, cord prolapse, dysfunctional labor, and postpartum hemorrhage, and these risks should be monitored closely.

Oligohydramnios

- **Oligohydramnios** has multiple definitions, including AFI of less than 5 cm, maximum vertical pocket less than 2 cm, or AFI less than the 5th percentile for gestational age. Maximum vertical pocket may be a superior option to AFI because AFI measurement has a higher rate of false positives for oligohydramnios and thus increases induction and cesarean delivery rates without evidence of improvement in neonatal outcomes.
- It is associated with increased perinatal morbidity and mortality at any gestational age, but the risks are particularly high during the second trimester when perinatal mortality approaches 80% to 90%. Pulmonary hypoplasia can result from insufficient fluid filling the terminal air sacs. Prolonged oligohydramnios in the second and third trimester leads to cranial, facial, or skeletal abnormalities in 10% to 15% of cases. Cord compression leads to an increased incidence of fetal heart rate decelerations in labor.
- The **etiology** of oligohydramnios includes ruptured membranes, fetal urinary tract malformations, postterm pregnancy, placental insufficiency, and medications reducing fetal urine production. Rupture of membranes must be considered at any gestational age. Renal agenesis or urinary tract obstruction often becomes apparent during the second trimester of pregnancy, when fetal urine flow begins to contribute significantly to AFV. Placental insufficiency can cause both oligohydramnios and intrauterine growth restriction (IUGR). The cause of oligohydramnios in postterm pregnancies may be deteriorating placental function.
- **Ultrasound** is used to diagnose oligohydramnios. Rupture of membranes should be evaluated.
- **Treatment** for oligohydramnios is limited. Maternal intravascular fluid status appears to be closely tied to that of the fetus; maternal hydration (IV or oral) may improve the AFV depending on the etiology of oligohydramnios. In cases of obstructive genitourinary defects, in utero surgical diversion has produced some promising results. For optimal benefit, urinary diversion must be performed before renal dysplasia develops and early enough in gestation to permit normal lung development. Amnioinfusion has been proposed as a temporizing measure, particularly for patients with bilateral renal agenesis, but its use is currently limited to research protocols. Oligohydramnios is managed with frequent fetal surveillance (twice-weekly nonstress testing) starting around 32 weeks' gestation or at time of diagnosis if later. If fetal testing is reassuring, delivery is advised at 36 to 37 6/7 weeks' gestation if deepest vertical pocket is <2 cm. Oligohydramnios is not a contraindication to labor.

FETAL GROWTH RESTRICTION

- **Intrauterine growth restriction** is suggested when the estimated fetal weight falls below the 10th percentile for gestational age. Approximately 70% of so-called IUGR is merely constitutional, although an underlying etiology may be difficult to elucidate in the antepartum period. The incidence of pathologic IUGR is between 4% and 8% of gestations in developed countries and between 6% and 30% in developing countries. Fetuses with IUGR have a 2- to 6-fold increase in perinatal morbidity and mortality. The degree of symmetry present in IUGR may suggest an etiology. In symmetrical IUGR, the fetus is proportionally small, whereas in asymmetrical IUGR, abdominal growth lags behind head circumference. Symmetrical growth restriction implies an early insult such as chemical exposure, infection, or aneuploidy. Asymmetrical growth is more associated with a late pregnancy insult such as placental insufficiency.

- The **etiology** of IUGR includes both maternal and fetal causes:
  - **Constitutionally small mothers and inadequate weight gain.** Women who weigh <100 lb at conception have double the risk for a small-for-gestational age newborn. Inadequate or arrested weight gain after 28 weeks of pregnancy is also associated with IUGR.
  - **Chronic maternal disease.** Multiple medical conditions of the mother, including chronic hypertension, cyanotic heart disease, pregestational diabetes, malnutrition, and collagen vascular disease, can cause growth restriction. Preeclampsia and smoking are associated with IUGR.
  - **Fetal infection.** Viral causes including rubella, cytomegalovirus, hepatitis A, parvovirus B19, varicella, and influenza are among the best known infectious antecedents of IUGR. In addition, bacterial (listeriosis), protozoal (toxoplasmosis), and spirochetal (syphilis) infections may be causative.
  - **Chromosomal abnormalities.** Chromosomal abnormalities, such as trisomy 13 and 18 and Turner syndrome, are often associated with IUGR. Trisomy 21 usually does not cause significant growth restriction.
  - **Teratogen exposure.** Any teratogen can produce fetal growth restriction. Anticonvulsants, tobacco, illicit drugs, and alcohol can impair fetal growth.
  - **Placental abnormalities.** Placental abnormalities that lead to decreased blood flow to the fetus can cause growth restriction.
  - **Multiple gestation** is complicated by growth impairment of at least one fetus in 12% to 47% of cases.

- **Diagnosis** is made by sonographic assessment. Gestational age must be established with certainty, preferably in the first trimester, to assess fetal growth accurately. A lag in fundal height of more than 2 cm from gestational age after 20 weeks should prompt sonographic evaluation.

- **Management** generally depends on gestational age. In general, growth restriction diagnosed in the second trimester, or in the setting of a structural defect, prompts offering amniocentesis or fetal blood sampling for karyotype and viral studies. Even when termination is not considered, the information gained from these tests may be important for parents, obstetricians, and pediatricians planning the delivery and newborn care. Other management includes the following:
  - **IUGR at or near term:** Fetal assessment includes serial fetal growth ultrasounds every 3 to 4 weeks, nonstress testing or biophysical profiles, Doppler studies, and assessment of AFV. For uncomplicated growth restriction in singleton gestation, ACOG recommends induction at 38 to 39 6/7 weeks. The ACOG recommends individualizing delivery timing between 32 and 37 6/7 weeks' gestation with

growth restriction complicated by oligohydramnios, abdominal Doppler studies, or maternal comorbidities such as preeclampsia or chronic hypertension.

- **IUGR remote from term:** Attempt conservative management and fetal testing as discussed in IUGR at or near term. Ensure adequate nutrition and initiate fetal surveillance. Umbilical artery Doppler velocimetry showing elevated systolic-to-diastolic ratio or absent or reversed end-diastolic flow suggests fetal compromise (see chapter 4) and should prompt escalating surveillance or delivery.

- The decision to **deliver** an IUGR infant remote from term, particularly before 32 weeks' gestation, weighs the risk of preterm birth against continued exposure to the intrauterine environment. Contemporary management combines information from nonstress testing, biophysical profiles, and umbilical artery Dopplers. In pregnancies prior to 32 weeks' gestation, the addition of Doppler information from the ductus venosus can be employed to better identify those pregnancies that can be prolonged, although use of this parameter is not yet incorporated into contemporary guidance. In general, vaginal delivery is not contraindicated, but there is an increased risk of fetal intolerance of labor. Growth-restricted newborns are susceptible to hypothermia and other metabolic abnormalities, such as hypoglycemia. Some data show that fetal growth restriction has long-term negative effects on cognitive function, independent of other variables.

POSTTERM AND LATE-TERM PREGNANCY

- **Postterm pregnancy** is defined as 42 *completed* weeks of gestation from the last menstrual period. **Late-term pregnancy** is defined as reaching between 41 0/7 and 41 6/7 weeks of gestation. In the United States, the overall incidence of postterm pregnancy is 5.5%. Postterm and late-term pregnancies are associated with an increased risk of perinatal morbidity and mortality.

- **Diagnosis** of postterm pregnancy is based on accurate estimation of gestational age. The **etiology** is most commonly incorrect dating, but risk factors for postterm pregnancy include primiparity, previous postterm pregnancy, placental sulfatase deficiency, fetal anencephaly, family history, and fetal male sex.

- **Complications** of postterm pregnancy include the following:
  - **Postmaturity syndrome** involves exhibiting subcutaneous wasting, intrauterine growth failure, meconium staining, oligohydramnios, absent *vernix caseosa* and lanugo hair, and peeling newborn skin. Such findings are described in only 10% to 20% of true postterm newborns.
  - **Macrosomia** is more common in postterm pregnancies. Twice as many postterm fetuses weigh more than 4000 g compared to term infants. This increase in macrosomia likely contributes to the increased risks of cesarean delivery, operative vaginal delivery, and shoulder dystocia in postterm pregnancies.
  - **Oligohydramnios** is more common in postterm pregnancies, probably due to decreasing uteroplacental function. Low AFV is associated with increased intrapartum fetal intolerance of labor and cesarean delivery.
  - **Meconium-stained amniotic fluid** and meconium aspiration syndrome increase in postterm gestation.

- **Delivery timing may be targeted to the late term or post-term period.** Current ACOG guidance recommends induction between 42 0/7 and 42 6/7 weeks, with management of singleton pregnancy continuing beyond 41 weeks' gestation consistent of either biophysical profile or nonstress testing plus amniotic fluid assessments.

Based on data from a systematic review that induction at 41 weeks was associated with fewer perinatal deaths and cesarean deliveries, ACOG concludes that induction "can be considered" at this gestational age.

INTRAUTERINE FETAL DEMISE

- Intrauterine fetal demise (IUFD), also called fetal demise in utero, is the antenatal diagnosis of a stillborn infant after 20 weeks' gestation. Approximately 50% of perinatal deaths are stillbirths. Of all fetal deaths in the United States, over two-thirds occur before 32 weeks' gestation, 20% occur between 36 and 40 weeks' gestation, and approximately 10% occur beyond 41 weeks' gestation.
- The IUFD is suspected with any maternal report of more than a few hours of absent fetal movement. Definitive diagnosis is by absent fetal cardiac activity on real-time ultrasonography.
- Fetal deaths can be categorized by occurrence during the antepartum period or during labor (intrapartum stillbirth). The antepartum fetal death rate in an unmonitored population is approximately 8 in 1000 and represents 86% of fetal deaths.
- The etiology of antepartum fetal death can be divided into broad categories: chronic hypoxia of diverse origin (30%), congenital malformation or chromosomal anomaly (20%), complications of pregnancy such as Rh alloimmunization (<1%), abruptio placentae (20%-25%), fetal infection (<5%), and idiopathic/unexplained (25% or more).
- Both expectant and active **management** are acceptable after fetal demise. Spontaneous labor occurs within 2 to 3 weeks in 80% of cases. In cases of prolonged demise, active management should be offered due to emotional burden and the risk of chorioamnionitis and rarely DIC. For patients with IUFD occurring at 24 weeks of gestation or earlier, either pregnancy induction or dilation and evacuation (D&E) are reasonable options; this age threshold may be higher or lower depending on local expertise and comfort with evacuation procedures. The D&E provides greater maternal safety and faster pregnancy resolution than does induction, whereas induction provides the opportunity to labor and to deliver an intact fetus, which also facilitates inspection and autopsy. If induction is chosen, third-trimester IUFD are managed in the same manner as a usual induction of labor. In the case of second trimester IUFD, induction with a combination of mifepristone and high-dose misoprostol, misoprostol alone, or high-dose oxytocin may be employed.
- Patients should be offered diagnostic evaluation for IUFD. The ACOG recommends fetal and placental inspection and offering the patient autopsy and cytogenetics. A comprehensive maternal and family history may identify an etiology for demise. Laboratory studies should include complete blood counts, fetal-maternal hemorrhage screens, human parvovirus serology, syphilis, lupus anticoagulant, anticardiolipin, and thyroid-stimulating hormone studies, with additional workup based on the patient's clinical history.

SUGGESTED READINGS

American College of Obstetricians and Gynecologists Committee on Practice Bulletins—Obstetrics. ACOG Practice Bulletin No. 102: management of stillbirth. *Obstet Gynecol.* 2009;113:748-761. (Reaffirmed 2019)

American College of Obstetricians and Gynecologists Committee on Practice Bulletins—Obstetrics. ACOG Practice Bulletin No. 142: cerclage for the management of cervical insufficiency. *Obstet Gynecol.* 2014;123:372-379. (Reaffirmed 2019)

American College of Obstetricians and Gynecologists Committee on Practice Bulletins—Obstetrics. ACOG Practice Bulletin No. 146: management of late-term and postterm pregnancies. *Obstet Gynecol.* 2014;124(2, pt 1):390-396. (Reaffirmed 2019)

American College of Obstetricians and Gynecologists Committee on Practice Bulletins—Obstetrics. ACOG Practice Bulletin No. 189: nausea and vomiting of pregnancy. *Obstet Gynecol.* 2018;131(1):e15-e30.

American College of Obstetricians and Gynecologists Committee on Practice Bulletins—Obstetrics, American Institute of Ultrasound in Medicine. ACOG Practice Bulletin No. 175: ultrasound in pregnancy. *Obstet Gynecol.* 2016;128:e241-e256. (Reaffirmed 2018)

American College of Obstetricians and Gynecologists Committee on Practice Bulletins—Obstetrics, Society for Maternal-Fetal Medicine. ACOG Practice Bulletin No. 204: fetal growth restriction. *Obstet Gynecol.* 2019;133:e97-e109.

Goya M, de la Calle M, Pratcoronoa L, et al. Cervical pessary to prevent preterm birth in women with twin gestation and sonographic short cervix: a multicenter randomized controlled trial (PECEP-Twins). *Am J Obstet Gynecol.* 2016;214(2):145-152.

Lees C, Marlow N, Arabin B, et al. Perinatal morbidity and mortality in early-onset fetal growth restriction: cohort outcomes of the Trial of Randomized Umbilical and Fetal Flow in Europe (TRUFFLE). *Ultrasound Obstet Gynecol.* 2013;42(4):400-408.

Nabhan AF, Abdelmoula YA. Amniotic fluid index versus single deepest vertical pocket as a screening test for preventing adverse pregnancy outcome. *Cochrane Database Syst Rev.* 2008;(3):CD006593.

Preterm Labor and Preterm Prelabor Rupture of Membranes

6

Kristin Darwin and Clark T. Johnson

PRETERM LABOR

Definitions

- Preterm labor (PTL) include the following:
  - Regular uterine contractions with cervical change (dilation, effacement, or both) before 37 weeks' gestation
  - Initial presentation with regular contractions and cervical dilation of 2 cm or more
- Preterm birth (PTB) is delivery between 20 0/7 and 36 6/7 weeks' gestation.
- Late PTB is delivery between 34 0/7 and 36 6/7 weeks' gestation.

Incidence and Significance

- In 2015, 9.6% of the approximately four million deliveries in the United States were PTBs, which is the leading cause of neonatal morbidity (Figure 6-1). PTL accounts for 40% to 50% of PTB. Other causes of PTB include preterm prelabor (premature) rupture of membranes (PPROM), placental abruption, and indicated preterm deliveries.

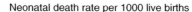

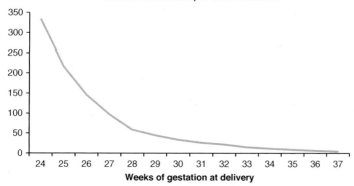

Figure 6-1. Mortality based on gestational age at delivery, 2007-2016. Adapted from United States Department of Health and Human Services, Centers for Disease Control and Prevention, National Center for Health Statistics, Division of Vital Statistics. Linked Birth/Infant Death Records 2007-2016, as compiled from data provided by the 57 vital statistics jurisdictions through the Vital Statistics Cooperative Program, on CDC WONDER Online Database.

- It is difficult to identify which women who present with PTL will give birth preterm. Approximately 50% of patients admitted to the hospital with a diagnosis of PTL give birth after 37 weeks.
- Short-term neonatal morbidity associated with PTB includes respiratory distress syndrome, hypothermia, hypoglycemia, jaundice, intraventricular hemorrhage, necrotizing enterocolitis, bronchopulmonary dysplasia, sepsis, and patent ductus arteriosus.
- Long-term morbidity includes cerebral palsy, intellectual disability, and retinopathy of prematurity.

Risk Factors

- Causes of PTL are often multifactorial. Additionally, PTL is not the only cause of PTB. There are no tools with which clinicians can accurately predict occurrence of PTL. However, there are known maternal and pregnancy risk factors for PTL, which include the following:
  - Previous PTB: most strongly associated with PTL, recurrence risk 17% to 30%
  - Infection:
    - Systemic or local infections including urinary tract infections, pyelonephritis, bacterial vaginosis, sexually transmitted infections, pneumonia, appendicitis, periodontal disease
    - Chorioamnionitis affects 25% of preterm deliveries. Release of cytokines from endothelial cells, including interleukin-1, interleukin-6, and tumor necrosis factor-α stimulates a cascade of prostaglandin production that stimulates contractions.
  - Uterine overdistension: multiple gestation, polyhydramnios
  - Short cervix (see "Steps to Minimize Risk of Preterm Labor and Delivery")
  - History of cervical surgical manipulation: loop electrosurgical excision procedure or cold knife cone.

- Uterine malformations: bicornate uterus, leiomyomata, uterine didelphys
- Second- or third-trimester bleeding; placenta previa or placental abruption
- Social characteristics and health behaviors associated with PTL include African American race, maternal age <18 or >35 years, low socioeconomic status, anxiety, depression, stressful life events, tobacco use, and alcohol or drug abuse.

Steps to Minimize Risk of Preterm Labor and Delivery

- Any discussion regarding interventions to minimize risk of PTL must contain the caveat that the most significant risk factor for PTL, which is prior PTB, is not modifiable.
- **Education** of patients regarding signs and symptoms of PTL and clear directions regarding when to call providers with questions and/or present for evaluation
- **Treat infections** during pregnancy, such as urinary tract and lower genital infections (see chapter 8).
  - Chorioamnionitis is an indication for delivery, regardless of gestational age.
  - Treatment of infection may not alleviate risks as mechanism of influence may be from associated inflammation rather than the infection itself.
    - o Bacterial vaginosis: Bacterial vaginosis is present in approximately 20% of women during pregnancy. It represents an overgrowth of normal vaginal flora rather than pathogenic infection. Routine screening is not recommended, and diagnosis is reserved to diagnose and treat symptomatic individuals. The presence of bacterial vaginosis is associated with increased risk of PTB, but causal relationship has not been established, and treatment has not been shown to reduce this risk. Treatment with metronidazole 500 mg orally twice a day for 7 days, 250 mg orally thrice a day for 7 days, or 2% clindamycin cream per vagina nightly for 7 days is effective at eradicating discharge symptoms but does NOT reduce risk of PTB. Recurrence can occur.
    - o Among women with intact membranes, empiric broad-spectrum antibiotics have not been shown to reduce risk of PTL and delivery, are associated with increased neonatal morbidity, and are not recommended for routine use.
- **Progesterone therapy**
  - Intramuscular (IM) progesterone therapy was previously universally recommended for singleton pregnancies in women with a prior PTB to reduce the risk of recurrent PTB, although more recently, its benefit has been called into question based on large-scale evaluation. Further study is needed to demonstrate definitive benefit of this therapy, and evolution of its recommended use is likely in the near future at time of this publication.
    - o There have not been long-term neonatal risks associated with progesterone use, but study in this regard is limited and ongoing.
    - o Women at highest risk of PTB would seem most likely to benefit based on clinical study to date (eg, very PTB history or multiple prior PTBs), although definitive benefit remains unclear.
  - Use of IM progesterone therapy should be individualized, considering the uncertain benefits and potential risks of using a limited studied medication in pregnancy. An algorithm for progesterone therapy, if employed, is shown in Figure 6-2.

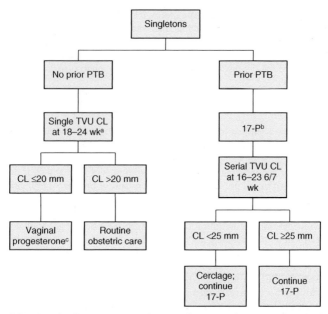

Figure 6-2. Algorithm for consideration of the use of progestins for reducing the risk of preterm birth (PTB). [a]If transvaginal ultrasound (TVU) cervical length (CL) screening is performed. [b]17-α hydroxyprogesterone caproate (17-P) 250 mg intramuscularly every week from 16-20 to 36 weeks, if selected weighing the risk and benefits of research to late discussed on the prior page. [c]For example, daily 200-mg suppository or 90-mg gel from time of diagnosis of short CL to 36 weeks. Reprinted from Society for Maternal-Fetal Medicine. Progesterone and preterm birth prevention: translating clinical trials data into clinical practice. *Am J Obstet Gynecol.* 2012;206(5):376-386. Copyright © 2012 Elsevier. With permission.

- Singleton pregnancy with prior spontaneous PTB, if IM progesterone is employed (considering the risks and benefits as outlined on previous page).
  - 17-α hydroxyprogesterone caproate (Makena) or 17-P: 250 mg IM weekly
    - Begin between 16 and 20 weeks until 36 weeks.
    - If initiated, suggested to start at <21 weeks but also has shown benefit up to initiation at 27 weeks.
    - There is mixed data regarding vaginal progesterone's effectiveness at preventing PTB patients with prior PTB. However, initiation of vaginal progesterone may be reasonable in certain clinical circumstances or when IM 17-P is unavailable.
- Singleton pregnancy with no prior history of PTB *BUT* cervical length ≤20 mm at ≤24 weeks
  - Vaginal progesterone: 90 mg gel or 200 mg suppository daily
    - Begin from diagnosis of short cervical length until 36 weeks
    - In women with singleton pregnancies and risks associated with cervical insufficiency or PTL, consider following with serial transvaginal ultrasound in second trimester between 16 and 24 weeks' gestation.
- Progesterone has not been shown to be effective in singleton pregnancies, without history of prior PTB and normal or unknown cervical length, multifetal gestation, or in symptomatic (active) PTL or PPROM.

- **Cerclage**
  - Cervical insufficiency is the inability of the cervix to retain a pregnancy in the absence of signs or symptoms of PTL (see chapter 5).
  - Clinical requirements and considerations of history-indicated, physical examination–indicated, and ultrasound-indicated cerclage as defined by American College of Obstetricians and Gynecologists are outlined in Table 6-1.
  - There is no current evidence to support cerclage in multifetal gestation.

Table 6-1 Indications for Cerclage[a]

Indication Type	History-Indicated ("Prophylactic")	Physical Examination–Indicated ("Emergency" or "Rescue")	Ultrasound-Indicated
Clinical requirements	• History of one or more second-trimester pregnancy losses related to painless cervical dilation[b] • Prior cerclage due to painless cervical dilation in second trimester	• Painless cervical dilation in second trimester without evidence of preterm labor or placental abruption[c,d]	• Cervical length <25 mm in patient with history of PTB less than 34 wk gestation and current singleton pregnancy before 24 wk of gestation[e,f]
Timing and placement considerations	• Place at 13-14 wk gestation	• Place at time of diagnosis • Must rule out PTL and intraamniotic infection	• Place at time of diagnosis • If patient on 17-P, continue weekly therapy until 36 wk.

Abbreviations: PTB, preterm birth; PTL, preterm labor; 17-P, 17-α hydroxyprogesterone caproate.

[a]Adapted with permission from American College of Obstetricians and Gynecologists Committee on Practice Bulletins—Obstetrics. ACOG Practice Bulletin No. 142: cerclage for the management of cervical insufficiency. *Obstet Gynecol.* 2014;123(2 Pt 1):372-379. (Reaffirmed 2019). Copyright © 2014 by The American College of Obstetricians and Gynecologists.

[b]Data is mixed regarding benefit of cerclage in this population.

[c]May consider indomethacin and antibiotics for placement: cefazolin 1-2 g preoperatively and every 8 h × 2 (clindamycin 600 mg if penicillin allergy); indomethacin 50 mg postprocedure and every 8 h × 2.

[d]Possible benefit of cerclage in this population; however, no randomized control trials have been performed that demonstrate clear benefit.

[e]Meta-analysis has shown cerclage is beneficial in this population.

[f]Cerclage for shortened cervical length on ultrasound is not clearly indicated in women without history of PTB (see "Progesterone Therapy").

- Transvaginal cervical cerclage removal is indicated at 36 to 37 weeks' gestation and removal is not an indication for delivery.
- Patients who will undergo cesarean delivery at 39 weeks may keep cerclage in place until that time with removal at the time of surgery. However, clinician must weigh risks of cervical trauma if preterm or early term contractions occur and counsel patients regarding signs of labor.
- **Abdominal cerclage** may be considered in patients with previous failed transvaginal cervical cerclage (ie, previous placement in pregnancy that ultimately resulted in second trimester pregnancy loss).
  - Performed in late first trimester and early second trimester or in nonpregnant patient.
  - May be kept in place between pregnancies with planned cesarean deliveries
- **Pessary** may be considered as an alternative to cerclage, although data are mixed regarding effectiveness.
  - Counseling should include that pessaries are typically well tolerated, are associated with increased vaginal discharge, do not have to be removed for cleaning, and do not increase risk of infection.
  - When placing a pessary, insert the pessary so the smallest diameter is upward toward the cervix. Confirmation of the patients ability to void following placement is recommended.

Evaluation

For the patient presenting with signs and symptoms of PTL:
- **Establish best dating:** use last menstrual period, fundal height, ultrasound data, and available prenatal records.
- Collect history regarding prior PTB; duration and quality of PTL symptoms; precipitating factors such as abdominal trauma; and presence of other associated symptoms including leakage of fluid, abdominal pain, subjective fevers.
- **Obtain vital signs.**
  - Temperature >38°C or fetal or maternal tachycardia may indicate underlying infection.
  - Hypotension with fetal or maternal tachycardia may suggest placental abruption.
- **Physical examination**
  - Fundal tenderness may suggest chorioamnionitis or placental abruption.
  - Costovertebral angle tenderness may suggest pyelonephritis.
  - Initiate continuous fetal heart monitoring and tocodynamometry. Nonreassuring fetal heart tracing may indicate chorioamnionitis, abruption, or cord compression.
  - **Sterile speculum examination**
    - Inspect visually for bleeding, amniotic fluid pooling, advanced dilation, bulging membranes, and purulent cervical discharge.
    - Consider collecting **fetal fibronectin (fFN)** swab.
      - The fFN is an optional adjunct and may assist in risk stratification of patient with preterm contractions. The fFN is a component of the extracellular membranes of the amniotic sac and is typically not present between 22 and 34 weeks' gestation.
      - Should be first test performed during exam: Insert speculum without gel and collect sample from posterior fornix (rotate swab across posterior fornix for approximately 10 s); may collect from 24 to 34 weeks' gestation
      - Valid if cerclage in place

- Invalid with vaginal bleeding, ruptured membranes, cervical dilation >3 cm, or history of cervical manipulation (eg, intercourse or vaginal examination) within 24 hours
- Negative predictive value is approximately 99.5% for delivery within 7 days and 99.2% for delivery within 14 days.
- Positive predictive value for delivery within 7 days is as low as 14%; thus, a positive result provides little clinical insight.
- May consider obtaining a **cervical length** in order to aid in risk stratification of patient in certain clinical circumstances
- **Membrane status** (intact or ruptured) alters management and should be determined during early evaluation.
  - Pooling: If pooling not apparent, have the patient cough or Valsalva to see whether apparent amniotic fluid accumulates in the vagina.
  - Nitrazine: Normal vaginal pH is <4.5, with amniotic fluid pH usually 7.0 to 7.5. Vaginal pH >6.5 or blue on nitrazine paper is consistent with rupture of membranes. However, be cognizant that false-positive tests can be observed with blood, semen, *Trichomonas* or other infection, cervical mucus, or urine contamination.
  - Ferning: The presence of ferning of vaginal fluid on a slide can indicate rupture of membranes. Ferning may be falsely absent (falsely negative) in presence of blood. Avoid swabbing cervical mucus because it can result in a false positive.
  - Amniotic fluid index <5th percentile for gestational age, maximum vertical pocket <2 cm, or change in amniotic fluid index measurement from previous and recently documented measurement is suspicious for rupture of membranes but is not diagnostic.
  - If assessment for rupture of membranes is negative but clinical suspicion remains high, consider repeating examination after multiple hours and have patient lay supine between exams. Alternatively, amniocentesis with indigo carmine injection can confirm the presence of ruptured membranes and may be helpful in certain clinical circumstances
- Obtain **Group B *Streptococcus* (GBS) anovaginal culture** because the result of culture will determine need for prophylactic antibiotics in labor.
- Obtain cervical or vaginal cultures for gonorrhea and chlamydia.
- Evaluate wet mount for bacterial vaginosis, *Trichomonas*, and yeast.
- **AFTER ascertaining intact membranes, digital examination** is performed to assess cervical dilation, effacement, and station.
- Obtain **laboratory studies** including complete blood count, urinalysis with microscopic evaluation, and cultures obtained in the sterile speculum examination. Obtain cultures before administration of antibiotics.
- Perform an **ultrasound** to assess for multiple gestation, fetal presentation, estimated fetal weight (EFW), placental location, amniotic fluid index (per above), and fetal or uterine anomalies.

Management

- **Goals** of management:
  - Ultimate goal in managing PTL is to optimize outcomes with administration of corticosteroids and use of magnesium sulfate for fetal neuroprotection.
  - These intervention and management recommendations must be tailored to each patient and pregnancy; risks or prolonging pregnancy to mother must be

weighed against risk of prematurity to fetus and fetal morbidity associated with worsening clinical status of mother.

- **Oral or intravenous (IV) hydration** can be used as an initial approach to preterm contractions due to dehydration.
  - Randomized trials have shown that hydration does not reduce the incidence of PTB.
  - Clinical judgment will guide initial treatment and consideration for admission.
- Bed rest is not clinically indicated for patients hospitalized with PTL, and there are no data to support its use. There are significant risks of bed rest including increased risk of venous thromboembolism. In the setting of concomitant ruptured membranes, cervical dilation, and fetal malpresentation, bed rest may help avoid umbilical cord prolapse. There is limited evidence that associates prolonged standing, strenuous activity, or sexual activity with PTL.
- Thromboembolic prophylaxis should be considered and a physical therapy consult obtained for all patients with activity limitations.
- **Antenatal corticosteroids**
  - Administration of corticosteroids is the most beneficial intervention to improve neonatal outcomes. **Preterm infants between 24 0/7 and 33 6/7 weeks' gestation who receive antenatal corticosteroids have lower risk of respiratory distress syndrome, intracranial hemorrhage, necrotizing enterocolitis, and death.** Late preterm infants between 34 0/7 and 36 6/7 weeks who receive their first course of corticosteroids during that time have decreased respiratory morbidity.
    - Treatment benefit is seen >24 hours after administration; still administer if delivery anticipated sooner than 24 hours.
    - Greatest benefit of steroid administration is 2 to 7 days after administration.
    - Maternal side effects include (1) transient hyperglycemia of mother, beginning approximately 12 hours after first administration, with effect peaking around 2 to 3 days, and lasting up to 5 days and (2) leukocytosis within first 24 hours that generally resolves in approximately 3 days. Exercise caution when interpreting lab values during this time period.
    - Poorly controlled diabetes mellitus is not a contraindication for corticosteroid administration prior to 34 weeks of gestation. Inpatient observation and glucose management may be considered for the patient who receives betamethasone and has poorly controlled gestational diabetes mellitus or pregestational diabetes in order to avoid morbidity associated with hyperglycemia.
  - **Recommendations for administration**
    - Administer a single course of corticosteroids if fetus is between 24 0/7 and 33 6/7 weeks and preterm delivery in next 7 days is likely. A provider may consider administration beginning at 23 weeks' gestation depending on clinical circumstances and patient preferences. In the event of PTL and periviability with possible delivery within the next 7 days, a discussion with the patient regarding fetal prognosis and patient's preferences for intervention and resuscitation should be carried out before corticosteroid, tocolytic, or magnesium administration.
    - **Dosing**
      - Betamethasone 12 mg IM every 24 hours for 2 doses
      - Dexamethasone 6 mg IM every 12 hours for 4 doses

- A **single rescue course** of steroids may be administered 7 to 14 days after initial steroid course if patient did not deliver, is deemed clinically at risk for delivery within next 7 days, and is still <34 weeks' gestation.
  - There is no data supporting or refuting use of rescue course of steroids in the event of PPROM.
  - Rescue steroids have not been studied and are not indicated in the late preterm period (34-37 wk).
- Serial courses of additional doses are not indicated and are associated with growth restriction and neonatal morbidity.
- **Late preterm steroids** (between 34 0/7 and 36 6/7 wk gestation) may be administered if patient has not previously received corticosteroids and may deliver in next 7 days.
  - Administration of late preterm steroids reduces the need for respiratory support in first 72 hours, respiratory distress syndrome, transient tachypnea, bronchopulmonary dysplasia, and need for surfactant.
  - Tocolysis should not be performed in order to delay delivery to facilitate administration of late preterm steroids and indicated late preterm deliveries should not be delayed for administration.
- **Magnesium** should be considered prior to 32 weeks' gestation for fetal neuroprotection when patient is thought to be at risk for delivery between next 30 minutes to 24 hours. Risk of moderate to severe cerebral palsy of fetus is decreased by approximately 40%. The number needed to treat to prevent one case of cerebral palsy is 1:63.
  - There are multiple regimens for magnesium sulfate for neuroprotection that were included in the meta-analysis that demonstrated this benefit.
    - 4-g bolus over 30 minutes × 1
    - 1 g/h for 24 hours
    - 2 g/h for 12 hours
  - It is generally accepted to use any of these proposed regimens.
  - Consider restarting magnesium infusions that have been discontinued for the fetus <32 weeks' gestation if delivery is thought to be imminent.
- The **GBS prophylaxis** is continued until cervical exam is stable and risk for progression to PTB is lower.
  - Prophylactic antibiotics for GBS are not indicated outside of concern for active PTL.
  - Prolonged risk of empiric antibiotics in the case of intact membranes may increase neonatal risk of sepsis.
- **Tocolysis**
  - The goal of tocolysis is to prolong pregnancy to administer steroids and magnesium sulfate for neuroprotection. Also may consider tocolysis in order to facilitate maternal transport. There is no data to suggest that tocolysis for longer than 48 hours improves fetal or maternal outcomes.
  - Tocolytic agents include nifedipine and indomethacin, both of which have been shown to increase likelihood of completion of betamethasone administration. Terbutaline is a tocolytic but has not demonstrated efficacy in this regard. Magnesium has been historically used for tocolytic benefit but has been shown ineffective in this regard (Table 6-2). After 32 weeks, nifedipine, rather than indomethacin, is used for tocolysis in the absence of maternal contraindications.
    - **Indomethacin is contraindicated after 32 weeks or in the setting of oligohydramnios.**

Table 6-2 Indomethacin and Nifedipine Tocolytic Overview

Drug	Mechanism of Action	Dosing Regimen	Contraindications	Side Effects	Notes
Indomethacin	Prostaglandin synthetase inhibitor: prevents production of prostaglandin $F_{2\alpha}$, which normally stimulates uterine contractions	Loading dose: 50-100 mg orally or per rectum Maintenance dose: 35-50 mg orally or per rectum every 4 h for 72 h	Peptic ulcer disease Renal disease Hepatic dysfunction Coagulopathy Oligohydramnios	Oligohydramnios Nausea GERD/gastritis Emesis Platelet dysfunction (rare)	First-line agent in gestations <32 wk Avoid at >32 wk gestation (associated with premature closure of fetal ductus arteriosus). Avoid using for >72 h (associated with oligohydramnios).
Nifedipine	Calcium channel blocker: inhibits myometrial calcium entry	10-20 mg orally every 6 h	Hypotension Congestive heart failure Aortic stenosis	Hypotension Flushing Light-headedness Dizziness Nausea	First-line agent

Abbreviation: GERD, gastroesophageal reflux disease.

- o **Nifedipine is contraindicated in the setting of hypotension.** There is a theoretical risk of pulmonary edema with concurrent use of magnesium and nifedipine, although this interaction has not been supported in large-scale studies to date and is not considered a contraindication to combination therapy if indicated.
- o Magnesium is not routinely an evidence-based tocolytic but is frequently used in this population for neuroprotective benefit until 32 weeks of gestation.
- o Terbutaline is a β-sympathomimetic agent administered in 0.25-mg subcutaneous dose that causes smooth muscle relaxation in the acute setting. It has not been shown to prolong pregnancy for steroid or magnesium administration.
- Contraindications to tocolysis include intrauterine fetal demise, lethal fetal anomaly, nonreassuring fetal status, preeclampsia with severe features or eclampsia, maternal bleeding with hemodynamic instability, chorioamnionitis, and agent-specific maternal contraindications to tocolysis.
- Special considerations
  - o Tocolysis may be considered in PPROM in the absence of signs of maternal infection in order to facilitate administration of steroids or for maternal transport.
  - o Tocolysis is generally **not** indicated:
    - o Before neonatal viability. Tocolysis may be considered in the previable or periviable neonate when a known precipitant of PTL (such as abdominal surgery) has occurred. It may also be considered in periviable period based on family's wishes regarding resuscitation.
    - o In presence of preterm contractions without cervical change
- **Fetal monitoring**
  - No optimal schedule has been established.
  - Maintain external fetal monitoring and tocodynamometry until active PTL has resolved.
  - Once PTL has subsided, patient does not need to undergo continuous monitoring for this indication.

Route of Delivery Varies by Gestational Age

- If <26 weeks or EFW <750 g, vaginal delivery is appropriate depending on clinical circumstances.
  - **Breech delivery may be considered depending on clinical circumstances**
  - There is limited data to suggest cesarean delivery improves neonatal outcomes at this early gestation in part because of generally poor neonatal outcomes regardless of delivery method.
- A frank discussion of the risks and benefits of cesarean delivery for fetal intolerance of labor or otherwise should take place, given the increased maternal morbidity and poor neonatal prognosis. The risks and future implications of classical cesarean delivery should be discussed. Document your discussion carefully in the chart, and revisit the issue as gestation progresses.
- If the fetus is malpresenting and is either >26 weeks or EFW is >800 g, cesarean delivery should be considered to minimize neonatal morbidity.
- Disproportionate head-to-body ratio after this gestational age contributes to an increased risk of fetal head entrapment and associated morbidity.
- Preterm gestation alone is not an indication for cesarean delivery in cephalic presenting fetuses.

PRETERM PRELABOR RUPTURE OF MEMBRANES

Definitions

- **Preterm prelabor (or premature) rupture of membranes** is spontaneous rupture of amnion and chorion membranes before the onset of labor at a gestational age <37 weeks.
- **Prelabor (or premature) rupture of membranes (PROM)** occurs after 37 weeks' gestation. The **latency period** is the time from PPROM or PROM to onset of labor.

Incidence and Significance

- PROM occurs in approximately 8% of term pregnancies.
- PPROM occurs in approximately 3% of pregnancies and accounts for approximately 30% of PTB.
  - After PPROM, approximately 50% of patients deliver within 24 to 48 hours. Of the remaining 50%, around half deliver within 1 week.
  - There is a 1% to 2% risk of fetal demise after PPROM secondary to risks of infection and umbilical cord accident.
  - Placental abruption occurs in 2% to 5% of pregnancies with PPROM.

Etiology

- Like PTL, in many cases, risk factors of PPROM are difficult to predict and the cause of PPROM is often likely multifactorial. Risk factors include intrauterine infection, prior history of PPROM, trauma, amniocentesis, and polyhydramnios.
  - History of PPROM is a risk factor for PTL and PPROM in future pregnancies.
  - Intrauterine infection complicates approximately 15% to 25% of pregnancies with PPROM with postpartum infection in 15% to 20%. Risks of infection are increased with earlier gestational age.

Evaluation

- Similar to PTL (see pages 70-71). Make careful note of the circumstances, character, and timing of rupture of membranes and consistency of fluid.
- **ONLY a sterile speculum examination should be performed**. Assess for pooling, ferning, and fluid pH using nitrazine paper. Inspect for cord prolapse, cervical dilation (visually), and collect swabs as outlined pages 70-71. **Avoid digital cervical exam unless delivery is thought to be imminent.** Digital examination decreases the latency period and increases the risk of neonatal sepsis.
- In the event of equivocal or negative tests but high clinical suspicion, the following adjunctive methods may be of benefit:
  - Assess amniotic fluid index, which can aid in evaluation but is not diagnostic.
  - Fetal fibronectin is sensitive but not specific; therefore, a negative test suggests intact membranes.
  - May consider commercially available tests, such as AmniSure.
  - Retest several hours after prolonged recumbency.

Management

- Goals of management:
  - Screen for underlying chorioamnionitis or nonreassuring fetal status. Move toward delivery if these conditions are identified. Otherwise, depending on gestational age, prolonging the latent period is the goal.

- Interval development of clinical chorioamnionitis or placental abruption compromising fetal status indicate prompt mobilization for delivery to minimize fetal morbidity and fetal demise in utero.
- Administer **antenatal corticosteroids** per guidelines pages 72-73. No evidence to suggest that corticosteroids are associated with increased maternal or neonatal infection risk.
- There is no evidence to support strict bed rest for women with PPROM, although limited activity may be considered where there is a risk for potential cord prolapse as with unstable lies.
- **Before 34 to 35 weeks' gestation** in the absence of chorioamnionitis: Initiate latency antibiotics, which have been shown to prolong pregnancy and therefore decrease neonatal morbidity.
  - Standard latency regimen is IV ampicillin 2 g and erythromycin 250 mg IV every 6 hours for 48 hours.
  - This is followed by oral amoxicillin 250 mg orally every 8 hours and erythromycin 333 mg every 8 hours or 250 mg erythromycin every 6 hours for 5 additional days.
  - In the absence of evidence of infection or nonreassuring fetal status, continue expectant management.
- Once the patient and fetus are stable, daily nonstress test should be performed with additional testing as clinically indicated. Changes in fetal heart rate monitoring or contractions may indicate occult infection.
- When an inpatient with PPROM begins to endorse regular contractions, advise immediate evaluation. Regular contractions and new leukocytosis (in the absence of recent betamethasone administration) may indicate early signs of infection even in the absence of fever. Begin magnesium for neuroprotection (if <32 weeks) and penicillin for GBS unknown or GBS-positive status as indicated.
- **After 34 to 35 weeks' gestation**, move toward delivery (induction or cesarean delivery for standard obstetric indications).
- Tocolysis is generally contraindicated in PPROM except for extreme prematurity to allow corticosteroid administration. If chorioamnionitis or significant placental abruption is suspected, tocolysis is contraindicated.
- Continue inpatient management until delivery.

SUGGESTED READINGS

American College of Obstetricians and Gynecologists Committee on Obstetric Practice, Society for Maternal-Fetal Medicine. ACOG Committee Opinion No. 455: magnesium sulfate before anticipated preterm birth for neuroprotection. *Obstet Gynecol*. 2010;115(3):669-671. (Reaffirmed 2018)

American College of Obstetricians and Gynecologists Committee on Practice Bulletins—Obstetrics. ACOG Practice Bulletin No. 171: management of preterm labor. *Obstet Gynecol*. 2016;128(4):e155-e164. (Reaffirmed 2018)

American College of Obstetricians and Gynecologists Committee on Practice Bulletins—Obstetrics. ACOG Practice Bulletin No. 188: prelabor rupture of membranes. *Obstet Gynecol*. 2018;131:e1-e14.

Blackwell SC, Gyamfi-Bannerman C, Biggio JR Jr, et al. 17-OHPC to prevent recurrent preterm birth in singleton gestations (PROLONG study): a multicenter, international, randomized double-blind trial [published online ahead of print October 25, 2019]. *Am J Perinatol*. doi:10.1055/s-0039-3400227.

Crowther CA, McKinlay CJ, Middleton P, Harding JE. Repeat doses of prenatal corticosteroids for women at risk of preterm birth for improving neonatal health outcomes. *Cochrane Database Syst Rev*. 2015;(7):CD003935.

Gyamfi-Bannerman C, Thom EA, Blackwell SC, et al. Antenatal betamethasone for women at risk for late preterm delivery. *N Engl J Med.* 2016;374(14):1311-1320.

Meis PJ, Klebanoff M, Thom E, et al. Prevention of recurrent preterm delivery by 17 alpha-hydroxyprogesterone caproate. *N Engl J Med.* 2003;348(24):2379-2385.

Mercer BM, Miodovnik M, Thurnau GR, et al. Antibiotic therapy for reduction of infant morbidity after preterm premature rupture of the membranes. A randomized controlled trial. National Institute of Child Health and Human Development Maternal-Fetal Medicine Units Network. *JAMA.* 1997;278(12):989-995.

Roberts D, Brown J, Medley N, Dalziel SR. Antenatal corticosteroids for accelerating fetal lung maturation for women at risk of preterm birth. *Cochrane Database Syst Rev.* 2017;(3):CD004454.

Shepherd E, Salam RA, Middleton P, et al. Antenatal and intrapartum interventions for preventing cerebral palsy: an overview of Cochrane systematic reviews. *Cochrane Database Syst Rev.* 2017;(8):CD012077.

7 Third-Trimester Bleeding

Isa Ryan and Shari M. Lawson

Third-trimester bleeding ranging from spotting to massive hemorrhage, occurs in 2% to 6% of all pregnancies. The differential diagnosis includes the following:

* Bloody show from labor
* Abruptio placentae (AP)
* Placenta previa (PP)
* Vasa previa (VP)
* Cervicitis
* Postcoital bleeding
* Trauma
* Uterine rupture (see chapter 3)
* Carcinoma

Third-trimester bleeding should be carefully evaluated, diagnosed, and managed. See Table 7-1. The AP, PP, and VP can lead to significant maternal and fetal morbidity and mortality.

ABRUPTIO PLACENTAE

The AP is the premature separation of the normally implanted placenta from the uterine wall due to maternal/uterine bleeding into the *decidua basalis*. See chapter 3.

Epidemiology

* One third of all antepartum bleeding is due to AP, with an incidence of 1 in 75 to 1 in 225 births. The incidence increases with maternal age.

Table 7-1	Important Steps in the Diagnosis and Management of Third-Trimester Vaginal Bleeding

- Assess maternal hemodynamic status through vital signs and laboratory studies. Ensure the patient has appropriate IV access and order fluid resuscitation when indicated. If bleeding is substantial, obtain a type and cross.
- Assess fetal status through continuous external fetal monitoring.
- Obtain history from patient, including the duration/severity of bleeding, whether or not the bleeding is painful, and whether there has been any trauma. Be sure to rule out other sources of bleeding, such as rectal bleeding.
- Use ultrasound to assess the location and appearance of the placenta.
- Once previa is ruled out through imaging, a pelvic exam should be performed and the patient's cervix should be assessed.
- Formulate a plan for management and/or delivery, taking into account the patient's gestational age and hemodynamic status.
- Consider administering medications, when appropriate, including betamethasone, Rho(D) immunoglobulin, and/or magnesium sulfate for neuroprotection.

Abbreviation: IV, intravenous.

- The AP recurs in 5% to 17% of pregnancies after one prior episode and up to 25% after two prior episodes.
- There is a 7% incidence of stillbirth in future pregnancies after AP leading to fetal death.

Etiology

- Vaginal bleeding does not correlate with abruption size and may vary from scant to massive.
- An AP without vaginal bleeding can result in delayed diagnosis and consumptive coagulopathy.
- Blood in the *basalis* layer stimulates forceful, classically tetanic, uterine contractions leading to ischemic abdominal pain.
- An AP is associated with maternal hypertension, advanced maternal age, multiparity, cocaine use, tobacco use, chorioamnionitis, preterm premature rupture of membranes, coagulopathy, and trauma. Many cases are idiopathic.
  - Patients with chronic hypertension, superimposed preeclampsia, or severe preeclampsia have 5-fold increased risk of severe abruption compared to normotensive women. Antihypertensive medications do not reduce the risk.
  - Cigarette smoking increases the risk of stillbirth from AP by 2.5-fold. The risk increases by 40% for each pack per day smoked.
- Rapid changes in intrauterine volume can lead to abruption, such as rupture of membranes, therapeutic amnioreduction for polyhydramnios, or during delivery of multiple gestations.
- Abruption occurs more frequently when the placenta implants on abnormal uterine surfaces as with submucosal myomas or uterine anomalies.
- Hyperhomocysteinemia, factor V Leiden, and prothrombin 20210 mutations (thrombophilias) are associated with an increased risk of abruption.

Complications

- Massive maternal blood loss may lead to **hemorrhagic shock**. See chapter 61.
- Maternal **disseminated intravascular coagulation** can occur and is found in 10% to 20% of AP with stillbirth.
- Extravasation of blood directly into the uterine muscle (Couvelaire uterus) can lead to **uterine atony** and massive postpartum hemorrhage.
- **Fetal hypoxia** may occur, leading to acute fetal distress, hypoxic-ischemic encephalopathy, premature delivery, and fetal death. Milder chronic abruption may lead to growth restriction, major malformations, or anemia.

Diagnosis

History and physical examination

- Classically presents late in pregnancy with vaginal bleeding and acute severe abdominal pain. Even slight clinical suspicion should prompt rapid investigation and close monitoring.
- Maternal vital signs, fetal heart rate assessment, and uterine tone should be evaluated immediately.
- Defer digital cervical exam until PP and VP have been ruled out.
- Mark or record the fundal height to follow expansion of concealed hemorrhage. Blood may be sequestered between the uterus and placenta when the placental margins remain adherent. Membranes or the fetus itself may obstruct the cervical os and prevent accurate assessment of blood loss.
- Ultrasound is insensitive in diagnosing AP, but large abruptions may be seen as hypoechoic areas underlying the placenta.
- Perform a speculum exam to evaluate for vaginal or cervical lacerations and the amount of bleeding.

Laboratory tests

- **Complete blood cell count** with hematocrit and platelets ($<$100 000/mL suggests severe abruption.)
- Blood **type and screen** (Crossmatch should be strongly considered.)
- **Prothrombin/activated partial thromboplastin time**
- **Fibrinogen** ($<$200 mg/dL suggests severe abruption.)
- **Fibrin split-products**
- Consider holding a **whole blood** specimen at the bedside while lab work is pending. If a clot does not form within 6 minutes or forms and lyses within 30 minutes, disseminated intravascular coagulation may be present.
- Consider a thromboelastogram.
- The **Kleihauer-Betke test** for fetal hemoglobin in the maternal circulation is not valuable in diagnosing AP.

Management

- **Large-bore intravenous** access should be obtained.
- **Fluid resuscitation** should be initiated and a **Foley catheter** placed to monitor urine output (more than 0.5 mL/kg/h or at least 30 mL/h should be observed).
- Close monitoring of **maternal vital signs** and continuous **fetal monitoring** should be maintained.

- **Rho(D) immunoglobulin** should be administered to Rh-negative individuals.
- Further management depends on the gestational age and hemodynamic status of both mother and fetus.

Term Gestation, Hemodynamically Stable

- Plan for vaginal delivery via induction of labor, with cesarean delivery for usual indications.
- Follow serial hematocrit and coagulation studies.
- Consider fetal scalp electrode for accurate and continuous fetal monitoring and intrauterine pressure catheter to assess resting uterine tone.

Preterm and Term Gestations, Hemodynamic Instability

- Aggressively fluid resuscitate.
- Transfuse packed red blood cells, fresh frozen plasma, and platelets as needed. Maintain fibrinogen level >150 mg/dL, hematocrit more than 25%, and platelets over 60 000/mL.
- Once the mother is stabilized, proceed to urgent cesarean delivery, unless vaginal delivery is imminent.

Preterm Gestation, Hemodynamically Stable

- Eighty-two percent of patients with evidence of AP at <20 weeks' gestation will progress to term. Only 27% of patients who present after 20 weeks' gestation, however, will have a term delivery.
- In the absence of labor, preterm AP should be followed closely with serial ultrasound evaluation of fetal growth from 24 weeks and regular antepartum testing. Steroids should be given to promote fetal lung maturity. If maternal instability or fetal distress arises, delivery should be performed as described in the section on hemodynamic instability. Otherwise, labor can be induced at term.
- For preterm AP with labor, completely stable hemodynamics, and reassuring fetal signs, tocolysis may be used in selected rare cases, giving time to administer a course of corticosteroids. Indomethacin is avoided because of its effect on platelet function. If maternal or fetal compromise arises, delivery should be performed after appropriate resuscitation.

PLACENTA PREVIA

The **PP** is the presence of placental tissue over or immediately adjacent to the internal cervical os. It is classified based on the placental location relative to the cervical os (Figure 7-1):
- **Complete** or **total previa:** Placenta covers the entire cervical os.
- **Partial previa:** The edge of the placenta covers part, but not all, of the internal os.
- **Marginal previa:** The edge of the placenta lies adjacent to the internal os.

Epidemiology

- In general, the incidence of PP is approximately 1 in 300 pregnancies over 20 weeks' gestational age. The frequency varies with parity, however, giving an incidence of 0.2% in nulliparas and as high as 5% in grand multiparas.
- The placenta covers the cervical os in 5% of pregnancies in the second trimester. Usually, the placenta will migrate away from the cervical os as the uterus grows with gestational age and the upper third of the cervix develops into the lower uterine segment.

Placenta previa

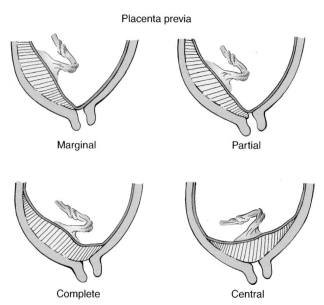

Figure 7-1. Three types of placenta previa: marginal, partial, complete. Central previa refers to a complete previa where the central portion the placenta is located over the cervical os. Reprinted with permission from Kay HH. Placenta previa and abruption. In: Gibbs RS, Karlan BY, Haney AF, Nygaard I, eds. *Danforth's Obstetrics and Gynecology*. 10th ed. Baltimore, MD: Lippincott Williams & Wilkins; 2008:386, Figure 21-1.

Etiology

- The most important risk factor for PP is a **previous cesarean delivery**. The PP occurs in 1% of pregnancies after a single cesarean delivery. The incidence after four or more cesarean deliveries increases to 10%, a 40-fold increased risk compared with no cesarean delivery. Anterior PP in these patients should be carefully evaluated for coexistent accreta.
- Other risk factors for PP include increasing maternal age (especially over the age of 40), multiparity, smoking, residing at higher elevations, male fetus, multiple gestation, and previous uterine curettage.

Complications

- Bleeding occurs with the development of the lower uterine segment in the third trimester in preparation for labor. The placenta separates, and the thinned lower segment cannot contract sufficiently to stop blood flow from the exposed uterine vessels. Cervical exams or intercourse may also cause separation of the placenta from the lower uterine segment. Bleeding can range from spotting to massive hemorrhage.
- The PP increases the risk for other abnormalities of placentation:
  - **Placenta accreta:** The placenta adheres directly to the uterus without the usual intervening *decidua basalis*. The incidence in patients with previa who have not

had previous uterine surgery is approximately 4%, increasing to as many as 25% of patients who have had a previous cesarean delivery or uterine surgery.

- **Placenta increta:** The placenta invades the myometrium but does not cross the serosa.
- **Placenta percreta:** The placenta penetrates the entire uterine wall, potentially growing into bladder or bowel.
- The PP is associated with double the rate of fetal congenital malformations, including anomalies of the central nervous system, digestive system, cardiovascular system, and respiratory system. No specific syndrome has been identified.
- The PP is also associated with fetal malpresentation, preterm premature rupture of membranes, intrauterine growth restriction, velamentous cord insertion, and VP.

Diagnosis

History and Physical Exam

- Seventy percent to 80% of PP presents with the acute onset of **painless vaginal bleeding** with bright, red blood.
- The first bleeding episode is usually around 34 weeks. About one-third of patients develop bleeding before 30 weeks, whereas another one-third present after 36 weeks and 10% go to term. The number of bleeding episodes is unrelated to the degree of PP or the prognosis for fetal survival.
- A thorough medical, obstetric, and surgical history should be obtained along with documentation of previous ultrasound examinations. Other causes of vaginal bleeding must also be ruled out, such as placental abruption.
- Maternal vital signs, abdominal exam, uterine tone, and fetal heart rate monitoring should be assessed.
- Vaginal **sonography** is the gold standard for diagnosis of previa. The diagnosis may be missed by a transabdominal scan, especially if the placenta lies in the posterior portion of the lower uterine segment where it is poorly visualized. Having the patient empty her bladder may help in identifying anterior PP. Trendelenburg position may be useful in diagnosing posterior PP.
- If PP is present or suspected, **digital examination is contraindicated**. A gentle speculum exam can be used to evaluate the presence and quantity of vaginal bleeding, but in most cases, this can be assessed adequately by inspecting the perineum and thereby avoid exacerbating the hemorrhage.

Laboratory Studies

- **Complete blood cell count**
- **Type and crossmatch**
- **Prothrombin time** and **activated thromboplastin time**
- **Kleihauer-Betke test** to assess for fetomaternal hemorrhage in Rh-negative unsensitized patients; not useful for the diagnosis of PP

Management

- Of note, many previas diagnosed on ultrasound in the early second trimester will resolve.
- In general, patients diagnosed with PP but *without* bleeding in the third trimester should have ultrasound confirmation of persistent previa. They should maintain

strict pelvic rest (ie, nothing in the vagina, including intercourse or pelvic exams) and avoid strenuous activity or exercise. They should receive advice about when to seek medical attention and be scheduled for fetal growth **ultrasounds** every 3 to 4 weeks.

- In general, patients with PP who *are* bleeding should be hospitalized for hemodynamic stabilization and close **maternal and fetal monitoring**. **Laboratory studies** should be ordered as described. **Steroids** are administered to promote lung maturity for gestations between 24 and 36 weeks, and **Rho(D) immunoglobulin** should be administered to Rh-negative mothers.

- Management of placenta accreta, or its variants, can be challenging. In patients with PP and a prior history of cesarean delivery, cesarean hysterectomy may be required if bleeding cannot be controlled after delivery. In cases where uterine preservation is highly desired and no bladder invasion has occurred, bleeding might be successfully controlled with selective arterial embolization or packing of the lower uterine segment, with removal of the pack through the vagina in 24 hours. The Bakri balloon catheter has also been used to help control bleeding from the placental bed.

- Specific management of PP is based on gestational age and assessment of the maternal and fetal status.

Term Gestation, Hemodynamically Stable

- Patients with **complete previa** at term require cesarean delivery. This is generally performed at 36 to 37 6/7 weeks.

- Patients with **partial** or **marginal previa** at term may deliver vaginally, with thorough consent regarding risks for blood loss and need for transfusion. The staff and facilities for immediate emergent cesarean delivery must be available. If maternal or fetal stability is compromised at any point in labor, urgent cesarean delivery is performed.

Preterm and Term Gestation, Hemodynamic Instability

- Stabilize the mother with fluid resuscitation and blood products.

- Cesarean delivery is indicated for nonreassuring fetal heart monitoring, life-threatening maternal hemorrhage, or bleeding after 34 weeks.

- If the mother is stable and intrauterine fetal loss occurs or the fetus is <24 weeks' gestational age, vaginal delivery can be considered.

Preterm Gestation, Hemodynamically Stable

- Patients at 24 to 37 weeks' gestation with PP *in the absence of labor can be* managed expectantly until 36 to 37 6/7 weeks.

- In general, once a patient has been hospitalized for three separate episodes of bleeding, she should remain in the hospital until delivery. For each bleeding episode, the following are recommended:
  - Hospitalization on bed rest with bathroom privileges until stabilized
  - Periodic assessment of maternal hematocrit and maintenance of an active type and screen
  - Red blood cell transfusion as needed to maintain hematocrit above 30% for slight but continuous bleeding
  - Corticosteroids and RhoGAM as indicated
  - Fetal testing and growth ultrasounds to assess for intrauterine growth restriction

- Tocolysis is not warranted unless to administer a course of steroids in an otherwise stable patient.
- After initial hospital management, outpatient care may be considered if bleeding stops for greater than 48 hours, no other complications exist, and the following criteria are met:
  - The patient can maintain strict pelvic rest at home and is adherent to medical care.
  - There is a responsible adult present at all times who can assist in an emergency.
  - The patient lives near the hospital with dependable transportation.
- For preterm gestations with PP *and contractions*, it can be difficult to diagnose labor. Cervical exams are contraindicated, and 20% of patients with PP show some uterine activity. If the patient and fetus are stable, tocolytics may be considered to prolong pregnancy. Indomethacin should be avoided.

LOW-LYING PLACENTA

A placenta that ends within 2 cm of the internal cervical os but that is not abutting the internal os is known as a low-lying placenta. Patients with a low-lying placenta are at increased risk for antepartum hemorrhage and cesarean delivery, although descent of the fetal head in labor often tamponades any intrapartum bleeding that may occur.

- A vaginal delivery is successful in 43% of patients with a placenta that is within 10 mm of the internal cervical os.
  - Patients with a placenta within 10 mm of the internal cervical os may be allowed to labor but should be counseled about the increased risk for cesarean delivery and bleeding.
  - Excellent intravenous access and blood type and screen are necessary for these patients.
- Patients whose placental end is 11 to 20 mm from the internal cervical os have an 85% rate of successful vaginal delivery, similar to that of patients whose placenta ends >20 mm from the internal cervical os.

VASA PREVIA

A **VP** occurs when the umbilical cord inserts into the membranes, instead of the central placental disc and the vessels traverse the membranes near the internal os in advance of the fetal presenting part. This puts the vessels at risk for rupture, causing fetal hemorrhage. Velamentous cord insertion also increases the risk of VP and is much more common in multiple gestations.

Epidemiology

- The incidence of VP is estimated to be approximately 1 in 5000 pregnancies.
- Fetal mortality may be as high as 60% with intact membranes and 75% when membranes rupture.

Etiology

- The cause of VP is unknown. Because of the association between velamentous cord insertion, multiple gestations, and VP, one theory suggests that it develops due to trophoblastic growth and placental migration toward the more vascular uterine fundus. The initial cord insertion at the center of the placenta becomes more peripheral as one portion of the placenta actively grows and another portion does not. In vitro fertilization may also be a risk factor.

Complications

- Even small amounts of fetal hemorrhage can result in morbidity and possible death, due to the small total fetal blood volume.
- Rupture of the membranes can result in rapid exsanguination of the fetus.

History

- The patient usually presents with acute onset vaginal bleeding after rupture of membranes.
- The bleeding is associated with an acute change in fetal heart pattern. Typically, fetal tachycardia occurs, followed by bradycardia with intermittent accelerations. Short-term variability is often maintained. Occasionally, a sinusoidal pattern may be seen.

Diagnosis

- **Transvaginal ultrasound**, in combination with color Doppler ultrasonography, is the most effective tool in antenatal diagnosis.
- In one study, there was a 97% survival rate in cases diagnosed antenatally compared to a 44% survival rate in those without prenatal diagnosis.

Management

- Third-trimester bleeding caused by VP is often accompanied by acute and severe fetal distress. **Emergency cesarean delivery** is indicated.
- If VP is diagnosed antenatally, **planned cesarean delivery** should be scheduled at 34 to 37 weeks under controlled circumstances and before the onset of labor, to reduce fetal mortality.

SUGGESTED READINGS

Gyamfi-Bannerman C. Society for Maternal-Fetal Medicine (SMFM) Consult Series #44: management of bleeding in the late preterm period. *Am J Obstet Gynecol.* 2018;218(1):B2-B8.

Hill JS, Devenie G, Powell M. Point-of-care testing of coagulation and fibrinolytic status during postpartum haemorrhage: developing a thrombelastography®-guided transfusion algorithm. *Anaesth Intensive Care.* 2012;40:1007-1015.

Jansen C, de Mooij YM, Blomaard CM, et al. Vaginal delivery in women with a low-lying placenta: a systematic review and meta-analysis. *BJOG.* 2019;126:1118-1126.

McCormack RA, Doherty DA, Magann EF, Hutchinson M, Newnham JP. Antepartum bleeding of unknown origin in the second half of pregnancy and pregnancy outcomes. *BJOG.* 2008;115(11):1451-1457.

Silver RM. Abnormal placentation: placenta previa, vasa previa, and placenta accreta. *Obstet Gynecol.* 2015;126(3):654-668.

Silver RM, Branch DW. Placenta accreta spectrum. *N Engl J Med.* 2018;378:1529-1536.

Perinatal Infections
Edward K. Kim and Jeanne S. Sheffield

Perinatal infections encompass a range of viruses, parasites, and bacteria that can be transmitted during pregnancy from mother to fetus. Asymptomatic or undiagnosed maternal disease can result in significant fetal and neonatal morbidity and mortality. For this reason, it is important to understand the clinical manifestations, diagnostic criteria, and management of these perinatal infections. This chapter focuses on infectious diseases that are prevalent or of particular clinical significance among pregnant women in the United States.

VIRAL INFECTIONS

Human Immunodeficiency Virus

- **Epidemiology**
  - Approximately 2 million infants are born to human immunodeficiency virus (HIV)-infected women annually in the world. In addition, mother-to-child transmission (MTCT) makes up about 90% of HIV infections among children worldwide.
  - Antiretroviral (ARV) use during pregnancy, intrapartum, and postpartum during breastfeeding has decreased this type of transmission by 50% worldwide since 2010.
- **Diagnosis**
  - The American College of Obstetricians and Gynecologists (ACOG) and Centers for Disease Control and Prevention (CDC) recommend HIV testing in the following settings:
    - All pregnant women as a routine part of antenatal care
    - Repeat testing in the third trimester for women in areas of high HIV prevalence, for those known to be at risk, and for those who declined earlier testing.
    - Screen on presentation to labor and delivery for any pregnant woman of unknown HIV status or any pregnant woman who tested negative in early pregnancy but is at high risk for infection (sexually transmitted infection diagnosis, illicit drug use, transactional sex, multiple partners, HIV-positive partner, signs/symptoms of HIV, or living in an area with high HIV incidence/prevalence) and was not tested in the third trimester.
  - The most commonly used HIV screening test is a laboratory serum enzyme-linked immunosorbent assay. A positive or indeterminate test is followed by a confirmatory test (Western blot most common).
  - Rapid HIV antibody assays are available. The sensitivity and specificity of these tests are comparable to the enzyme-linked immunosorbent assay HIV test. A positive result with a rapid HIV test must be confirmed by the Western blot test.

- **Management**
  - Prenatal
    - Accurate determination of gestational age based on ultrasound
    - Tests to obtain include the following:
      - HIV viral load and CD4 count
      - HIV drug resistance testing
      - Baseline complete blood count and comprehensive metabolic panel to allow for later assessment of ARV toxicity (bone marrow suppression, renal and hepatotoxicity)
      - Hepatitis B and C
      - Tuberculosis testing
      - Other sexually transmitted infections
      - Toxoplasma serology
      - Cytomegalovirus (CMV) serology
    - Immunizations recommended in addition to routine prenatal immunization include pneumococcal vaccines and hepatitis A and B vaccines.
    - The MTCT risk reduction: All pregnant HIV-infected women, regardless of CD4 count or viral load, should receive combination antiretroviral therapy (ART). For ARV use and preventive measures, refer to "'Prevention' under 'Viral Infections.'"
  - Antepartum
    - Women on ARV should undergo fetal anatomy ultrasound in the second trimester. Although the current data suggest no increase in overall birth defects with exposure to ARV, there is only a limited amount of data on newer ARTs.
    - Due to a possible association of low birth weight with some ARV medications, fundal height measurements in conjunction with growth ultrasounds are recommended to assess fetal growth.
  - Intrapartum
    - Medication
      - The ARV regimen should be continued intrapartum.
      - Intravenous (IV) zidovudine should be administered to women with an HIV viral load >1000 copies/mL or unknown viral load near delivery, regardless of antepartum regimen or mode of delivery.
      - Women on ARV and with HIV viral load up to 999 copies/mL near delivery should continue their ART regimen and consider IV zidovudine on a case-by-case basis.
      - The IV zidovudine should be started immediately in women presenting in labor with a positive rapid HIV test; CD4 T lymphocyte and HIV-1 RNA viral load should accompany confirmatory HIV antibody testing.
    - Instrumentation: In general, amniotomy (in setting of detectable HIV viral load), fetal scalp electrodes, operative vaginal delivery, and episiotomy should be avoided if possible.
    - Delivery route: A scheduled cesarean delivery at 38 weeks is recommended for women with an HIV viral load >1000 copies/mL near delivery. When cesarean delivery is planned, IV zidovudine should be administered for at least 3 hours prior to the cesarean delivery to ensure therapeutic blood levels (2 mg/kg IV load for 1 h followed by 1 mg/kg IV infusion for 2 h).
  - Postpartum
    - Maternal: Continuation of ARV treatment in the postpartum period should involve the patient and her primary HIV care provider.

- o Neonatal: Infants should receive zidovudine starting 6 to 12 hours after birth and continuing for 6 weeks. Neonates may require a more expanded regimen depending on the maternal HIV status at delivery. Refer to a pediatric ID specialist for evaluation.
- o Breastfeeding: Adherence to ARV significantly reduces risk of MTCT via breastfeeding. However, recommendations differ depending on the setting.
  - o In resource-rich countries such as in the United States, formula feeding is recommended for infants born to HIV-positive mothers. If the woman chooses to breastfeed, harm reduction measures such as continuing ART, exclusively breastfeeding for 6 months, and slow weaning should be discussed.
  - o In developing countries, formula feeding may pose a challenge in terms of access to quality-controlled formula and clean water. In this setting, breastfeeding is recommended, especially for mothers who are adherent to ARV.

- **Prevention**
  - Pregnancy intentions and information on effective contraception should be discussed on a routine basis with women of childbearing age. Current data suggest that over 50% of pregnancies in HIV-positive women are unintended. In HIV-positive adolescents, the rate of unintended pregnancy is as high as 83%.
  - All pregnant women with HIV should have potentially modifiable behaviors addressed, such as cigarette smoking, drug use, and high-risk sexual practices.
  - In pregnancies complicated by HIV, the major goals are to optimize maternal health and to reduce the risk of perinatal transmission. Ideally, a treatment plan will be made during preconception counseling that excludes drugs with teratogenic potential. Women on ARV should be encouraged to achieve an undetectable HIV-1 RNA viral load prior to conception to decrease the risk of MTCT.
  - Women who meet criteria to initiate ARV for maternal viral status should do so prior to pregnancy. In most cases, women already on ART at presentation for obstetric care should continue their current regimens if virally suppressed.
  - Women who are not on ARV or who have a new diagnosis should have their initial labs (eg, HIV viral load and resistance testing) reviewed prior to initiating therapy. If the patient is experiencing significant nausea and vomiting, do not start the medications until this is controlled. Intermittent use of medications is associated with antiviral resistance developing. Efavirenz and dolutegravir should not be initiated in women who may become pregnant or during the first trimester of pregnancy due to potential teratogenic effects.
  - The ART regimens should contain three to four drugs from at least two different classes: nucleoside/nucleotide reverse transcriptase inhibitor, nonnucleoside reverse transcriptase inhibitor, protease inhibitor, entry inhibitor, and integrase inhibitor.

Cytomegalovirus

- **Epidemiology. Cytomegalovirus** is the most common congenital viral infection, with intrauterine infection occurring in 0.2% to 2.5% of live births. The CMV is a ubiquitous DNA herpes virus with approximately 50% of the US population having antibodies to CMV. Transmission occurs through direct contact with infected saliva, semen, cervical and vaginal secretions, urine, breast milk, or blood products.

Vertical transmission can occur transplacentally, during delivery, or postpartum. An estimated 40 000 infants are born with CMV infection in the United States annually.

- **Clinical manifestations**
  - **Maternal infection.** In immunocompetent adults, CMV infection is typically silent. Symptoms, however, can be flu-like, including fever, malaise, swollen glands, and rarely hepatitis. After the primary infection, the virus becomes dormant, with periodic episodes of reactivation and viral shedding.
  - **Congenital (fetal) infection.** Most fetal infections are due to recurrent maternal infection and lead to congenital abnormalities in approximately 1.4% of cases. Previously acquired maternal immunity confers protection from clinically apparent disease by maternal antibodies. Mothers determined to be seronegative for CMV before conception or early in gestation have a 1% to 4% risk of acquiring the infection during pregnancy and 30% rate of fetal transmission after seroconversion.
  - Approximately 90% of infants with congenital CMV infection will be asymptomatic at birth. Ten percent to 15% of these may later develop symptoms including developmental delay, hearing loss, and visual and dental defects.
  - Unlike recurrent infection, primary maternal infection during pregnancy can often lead to serious neonatal sequelae with neonatal mortality of approximately 5% but as high as 30% in some investigations. Approximately 5% to 20% of newborns of mothers with primary CMV infection are overtly symptomatic at birth. Infection in the first trimester leads to higher risk of sequelae than in the third trimester.
  - The most common clinical findings at birth include the presence of petechiae, hepatosplenomegaly or jaundice, and chorioretinitis. These symptoms constitute fulminant cytomegalic inclusion disease. Infants show signs of respiratory distress, lethargy, and seizures. Long-term sequelae include mental retardation, motor disabilities, and hearing and visual loss.
- **Diagnosis**
  - **Maternal CMV screening** is not routine. Testing may be indicated as part of the workup for mononucleosis-like symptoms. Presence of CMV immunoglobulin M (IgM) is not helpful for timing the onset of infection because it is present in only 75% to 90% of women with acute infection, can remain positive following acute infection, and may represent reactivation or reinfection with a different strain. High anti-CMV immunoglobulin G (IgG) avidity (>65%) suggests that the primary infection occurred more than 6 months in the past; low avidity anti-CMV IgG (<30%) suggests a recent primary infection.
  - Fetal ultrasound may demonstrate microcephaly, ventriculomegaly, intracranial calcifications, oligohydramnios, and intrauterine growth restriction. Amniocentesis and cordocentesis for polymerase chain reaction (PCR) DNA testing have also been used to diagnose intrauterine infection.
- **Management.** There is no effective in utero therapy for CMV. Because it is difficult to predict the severity of sequelae, counseling patients appropriately about the option of pregnancy termination is problematic. Use of antiviral drugs in immunocompetent individuals is not indicated. Most infected fetuses do not suffer serious problems. The benefits of breastfeeding outweigh the risk of infection transmission by breastfeeding and may be encouraged.

• **Prevention.** The CMV transmission requires close personal contact or contact with contaminated bodily fluids. Preventive measures include transfusing only CMV-negative blood products, safe sex practices, and frequent handwashing.

Varicella Zoster Virus

• **Epidemiology**
  • Primary varicella infection, "chickenpox," is estimated to affect only 1 to 5 of every 10 000 pregnancies. Fewer than 2% of cases occur in adults, but this group represents 25% of mortality from varicella zoster virus (VZV). Herpes zoster, "shingles," is due to reactivation of latent VZV but is not associated with an increased risk for congenital varicella syndrome.
  • The major mode of transmission is respiratory, although direct contact with vesicular or pustular lesions may result in disease. In the past, nearly all persons were infected before adulthood, 90% before age 14 years. Since use of the varicella vaccine, most people in the United States have vaccine-induced immunity.
  • Varicella outbreaks occur most frequently during the winter and spring. The incubation period is 10 to 21 days. Infectivity is greatest 24 to 48 hours before the onset of rash and lasts 3 to 4 days into the rash. The virus is rarely isolated after the lesions have crusted over.
• **Clinical manifestations**
  • **Maternal.** The characteristic pruritic rash starts as macules, evolves into papules, and then vesicles. Primary varicella infection tends to be more severe in adults than in children and can be especially severe in pregnancy. A particularly morbid complication of VZV in pregnancy is varicella pneumonia. Maternal mortality with varicella pneumonia may reach 40% in the absence of antiviral therapy (3%-14% with antiviral therapy). In contrast, herpes zoster infection (reactivation of varicella) is more common in older and immunocompromised patients and poses little risk to the fetus.
  • **Congenital.** Fetal infection with varicella zoster can occur in utero, intrapartum, or postpartum. Intrauterine infection infrequently causes congenital abnormalities including cutaneous scars, limb-reduction anomalies, malformed digits, muscle atrophy, growth restriction, cataracts, chorioretinitis, microphthalmia, cortical atrophy, microcephaly, and psychomotor retardation.
    ○ The risk of congenital malformation after fetal exposure to primary maternal varicella before 20 weeks' gestation is estimated to be <2% and is <0.4% before 12 weeks.
    ○ Infection after 20 weeks' gestation may lead to postnatal disease with symptoms ranging from typical varicella with a benign course to fatal disseminated infection or shingles appearing months to years after birth. If maternal infection occurs within 5 days of delivery, hematogenous transplacental viral transfer may cause significant neonatal morbidity with mortality rates as high as 25%. Sufficient transplacental antibody transfer to confer fetal immunity requires at least 5 days after the onset of the maternal rash. Women who develop chickenpox, especially near term, should be observed. Neonatal therapy with immunoglobulin is also important when a mother develops signs of chickenpox within 3 days postpartum. Herpes zoster infection during pregnancy is not associated with fetal sequelae due to maternal antibody transfer.

- **Diagnosis**
  - **Clinical.** The diagnosis of acute varicella zoster in the mother usually can be established by the characteristic cutaneous manifestations described as chickenpox. The generalized vesicular rash usually appears on the head and ears and then spreads to the face, trunk, and extremities. Mucous membrane involvement is common. Vesicles and pustules evolve into crusted lesions, which then heal and may scar. Herpes zoster, or shingles, demonstrates a unilateral vesicular eruption in a dermatomal distribution.
  - **Laboratory.** Confirmation of the diagnosis may be obtained by examining scrapings of vesicular lesions that will reveal multinucleated giant cells. For rapid diagnosis, varicella zoster antigen may be demonstrated in exfoliated cells from lesions by immunofluorescent antibody staining.
  - **Ultrasonography.** Detailed ultrasonographic examination is the best means for assessing a fetus for major limb abnormalities or growth disturbances associated with varicella infection. Ultrasound findings in combination with PCR testing of amniotic fluid can estimate the risk of intrauterine infection and congenital syndrome.
- **Management**
  - **Varicella exposure during pregnancy.** An IgG titer should be obtained within 24 to 48 hours of exposure to a person with noncrusted lesions. The presence of IgG reflects prior immunity, whereas absence of varicella IgG indicates susceptibility.
  - **Varicella zoster immune globulin (VariZIG)** may be administered to susceptible women (ie, women without detectable varicella IgG) within 10 days of exposure (best if within 96 h) to reduce the severity of maternal infection. The VariZIG is administered intramuscularly (IM) at a dose of 125 U/10 kg to a maximum of 625 U. Maternal administration of VariZIG, however, does not ameliorate or prevent fetal infection.
  - Usually, the disease course is similar in pregnant and nonpregnant patients. Supportive care with fluids and analgesics should be administered. In addition, oral acyclovir, when started within 72 hours of symptom onset, has been shown to be associated with faster healing of lesions, a shorter febrile time, and less progression to pneumonia. It has low rates of teratogenicity, and its use is recommended by ACOG.
  - **Varicella pneumonia** is a medical emergency with significant risk for mortality. Patients should be admitted to the hospital for treatment with IV acyclovir. Acyclovir administered to pregnant women with varicella pneumonia during the second or third trimester decreases maternal morbidity and mortality. The dosage of acyclovir is 10 to 15 mg/kg IV every 8 hours for 7 days or 800 mg by mouth 5 times per day. Tocolytics are generally avoided in women with varicella pneumonia. Delivery should be performed for obstetric indications.
- **Prevention.** Preconception counseling plays an important role in prevention of VZV. An attenuated live vaccine was approved by the FDA in 1995. Two doses are recommended for all children, adolescents, and adults without history of varicella infection. The seroconversion rate after vaccination is approximately 82% in adults and 91% for children. Use of the vaccine during pregnancy is not recommended, but it is appropriate for breastfeeding mothers.

Parvovirus B19

- **Epidemiology**
  - Parvovirus B19 is a single-stranded DNA virus passed primarily by respiratory secretions. Also known as erythema infectiosum or fifth disease, it commonly occurs in school-aged children. By adulthood, 30% to 60% of women have acquired immunity (IgG) to the virus. Outbreaks usually occur in the midwinter to spring months. Prevalence in pregnancy is approximately 3.3% and is highest among teachers, day care workers, and stay-at-home parents.
- **Clinical manifestations**
  - **Maternal.** Adults may present with typical clinical features: a red, macular rash and facial erythroderma, which gives a characteristic "slapped cheek" appearance (more common in children). The rash may also cover the trunk and extremities. Infected adults often have acute joint swelling, usually with symmetric involvement of peripheral joints. The arthritis may be severe and chronic. Patients may also present with constitutional symptoms of fever, malaise, myalgia, and headaches. Some adults have a completely asymptomatic infection. Parvovirus B19 preferentially effects rapidly dividing cells and is cytotoxic to erythroid progenitor cells. It may cause aplastic crisis in patients with chronic anemia (eg, sickle cell disease or thalassemia).
  - **Congenital.** Approximately one-third of maternal infections are associated with fetal infection via transplacental transfer of the virus. Infection of fetal red blood cell precursors can result in fetal anemia, which, if severe, leads to nonimmune hydrops fetalis. Hydrops can lead to rapid fetal death or can resolve spontaneously. In cases of mild to moderate hydrops, approximately one-third resolve; this number decreases in cases of severe hydrops. The likelihood of severe fetal disease is increased if maternal infection occurs during the first 18 weeks of pregnancy, but the risk of hydrops fetalis persists even when infection occurs in the late third trimester. The overall risk of fetal death after maternal infection before 20 weeks is 6% to 11% and after 20 weeks' gestation is <1%. Parvovirus B19 infection has not been directly associated with specific congenital abnormalities.
- **Diagnosis**
  - The illness may be suspected if a regional outbreak is ongoing or if family members are affected. Children are the most common vectors for parvovirus B19 transmission.
  - A pregnant woman who has been exposed to fifth disease and presents with clinical symptoms or who has a known history of chronic hemolytic anemia and presents with an aplastic crisis should be evaluated with parvovirus B19 immunoglobulin titers. Parvovirus B19 IgM appears 3 days after the onset of illness, peaks in 30 to 60 days, and may persist for 3 to 4 months. Parvovirus B19 IgG is usually detected by the seventh day of illness and persists for years. The PCR of amniotic fluid can be used to detect fetal infection in a woman who was recently exposed or has ultrasound findings of fetal hydrops.
- **Management**
  - No specific antiviral therapy exists for parvovirus B19 infection. The IV gamma globulin may be administered on an empiric basis to immunocompromised patients with known exposure to parvovirus B19 and should be used for treatment of women in aplastic crisis with viremia.

- Parvovirus B19 can infect the fetal bone marrow, which may lead to severe fetal anemia. Therefore, when maternal infection is confirmed, serial screening sonograms should be performed to assess for fetal signs such as hydrops. Hydrops fetalis usually develops within 6 weeks but can develop as late as 10 weeks after maternal infection. Fetal middle cerebral artery (MCA) Doppler evaluation should be performed every 1 to 2 weeks to screen for fetal anemia.
- If severe anemia is suspected based on ultrasound findings, fetal hemoglobin levels may be determined with percutaneous umbilical vein sampling. Intrauterine blood transfusion can be used to correct fetal anemia and hydrops. Single or serial intrauterine transfusions may be undertaken.
- **Prevention.** Conscientious handwashing and avoiding known infected contacts are advised.

Rubella (German Measles)

- **Epidemiology.** Despite widespread immunization programs in the United States, the CDC reports 10% to 20% of adults remain susceptible to rubella. The annual number of reported cases in the United States, however, remains extremely low, with fewer than 10 cases of rubella occurring annually. The disease remains endemic in many areas of the world, and positive rubella antibodies in individuals from these areas can represent active infection.
- **Clinical manifestations**
  - The disease is communicable for 1 week before and for 4 days after the onset of the rash, with the most contagious period occurring a few days before the onset of the maculopapular rash. The incubation period ranges from 14 to 21 days. Transmission results from direct contact with the nasopharyngeal secretions of an infected person.
  - **Maternal.** Rubella usually presents as a maculopapular rash that persists for 3 days, generalized lymphadenopathy (especially postauricular and occipital), which may precede the rash, transient arthritis, malaise, and headache. Rubella typically follows the same mild course in pregnancy and may be asymptomatic. The majority of women with affected infants report no history of a rash during their pregnancies.
  - **Congenital.** Maternal viremia leads to fetal infection in 25% to 90% of cases. Fetal sequelae are dependent on gestational age, with 90% of first trimester exposures resulting in clinical signs, 54% at 13 to 14 weeks, and 25% by the end of the second trimester. Congenital rubella syndrome involves multiple organs. The most common manifestations are sensorineural hearing loss, developmental delay, growth retardation, and cardiac and ophthalmic defects. Additionally, as many as one-third of asymptomatic exposed infants may develop late manifestations, including diabetes mellitus, thyroid disorders, and precocious puberty. The extended rubella syndrome (progressive panencephalitis and type 1 diabetes mellitus) may develop as late as the second or third decade of life.
- **Diagnosis**
  - Infection is confirmed by serology. Specimens should be obtained as soon as possible after exposure, 2 weeks later, and if necessary, 4 weeks after exposure. Serum specimens from both acute and convalescent phases should be tested; a 4-fold or greater increase in titer or seroconversion indicates

acute infection. If the patient is IgG-seropositive on the first titer (performed within the first few days after exposure), there is no risk to the fetus. Primary rubella confers lifelong immunity. Reinfection with rubella is usually sub-clinical, rarely associated with viremia, and infrequently results in a congen-itally infected infant.

- Prenatal diagnosis is made by identification of rubella-specific IgM antibody in fetal blood samples obtained at 22 weeks' gestation or later. An IgM does not cross the placenta, and therefore, its presence indicates fetal infection.
- **Management.** If a pregnant woman is exposed to rubella, serologic evaluation is recommended. If primary rubella is diagnosed, the mother should be informed about the implications of the infection for the fetus including the high rate of fetal infection and the option for termination discussed. Women electing to continue the pregnancy may be given immune globulin, which may modify clinical rubella in the mother. Immune globulin, however, does not prevent infection or viremia and affords no protection to the fetus.
- **Prevention.** Pregnant women should have a rubella IgG performed as part of rou-tine prenatal care. A clinical history of rubella is unreliable. If the patient is non-immune, she should receive rubella vaccine after delivery. The rubella vaccine is a live attenuated virus and should be avoided in pregnancy due to the theoretic risk of teratogenicity. The CDC maintains a registry to monitor fetal effects of vacci-nation, and there have been no reported cases of congenital rubella syndrome after vaccination. Nonetheless, the CDC recommends contraception for 28 days after vaccination.

Influenza

- **Epidemiology.** In recent years, the number of cases of influenza has increased in the general population. The pattern of outbreaks is determined by the changing antigenic properties of the virus and their effect on the transmissibility and infectiv-ity of the virus. During pregnancy, physiologic changes make women more likely to become infected with influenza and more likely to have severe infection with significant morbidity and mortality.
- **Clinical manifestations**
  - **Maternal:** Clinical manifestations of influenza in pregnancy are similar to the general population. The symptoms include fever, cough, rhinorrhea, sore throat, myalgia, and headaches. During the pandemics of 1918, 1957, and 2009, preg-nant women were noted to have a disproportionate risk of mortality compared to the general population.
  - **Fetal:** There is some evidence that pandemic influenza infection may increase the risk of spontaneous abortion, preterm delivery, and low-birth-weight fetuses. However, this is not well studied.
- **Management/prevention.** Antiviral therapies have not been well studied but can be used for postexposure chemoprophylaxis and treatment of influenza. Oseltami-vir (75 mg twice daily for 5 d [treatment] and once daily for 10 d [chemopro-phylaxis]) and zanamivir are currently used. The CDC maintains a Web site with up-to-date treatment recommendations: https://www.cdc.gov/flu/treatment/index .html. Treatment is otherwise supportive with antipyretics and fluids. The CDC and ACOG recommend use of an inactivated influenza vaccine at any point during pregnancy.

Viral Hepatitis

Hepatitis A

- **Epidemiology.** An estimated 200 000 cases of hepatitis A virus (HAV) infection occur annually in the United States and affect approximately 1 in 1000 pregnancies. The HAV is transmitted primarily through fecal–oral contamination and typically is not excreted in urine or other bodily fluids. Obstetric patients at highest risk for developing HAV infection are those who have emigrated from or traveled to countries where the virus is endemic (eg, Southeast Asia, Africa, Central America, Mexico, and the Middle East).
- **Clinical manifestations**
  - **Maternal.** Symptoms of HAV infection include malaise, fatigue, anorexia, nausea, and abdominal pain, typically right upper quadrant or epigastric. Physical findings include jaundice, upper abdominal tenderness, and hepatomegaly.
  - **Congenital.** Perinatal transmission of HAV has not been documented.
- **Diagnosis.** A complete travel history suggests the diagnosis in a jaundiced patient. Laboratory studies may reveal transaminitis (elevated alanine aminotransferase and aspartate aminotransferase) and hyperbilirubinemia. Abnormal coagulation studies and hyperammonemia may suggest more significant liver injury. The presence of IgM antibody to HAV confirms the diagnosis. The IgG antibody will persist in patients with a history of exposure.
- **Management**
  - Individuals with close personal or sexual contact with an affected individual may receive HAV immune globulin in a single IM dose.
  - Treatment of HAV is supportive. There is no antiviral therapy. Activity level should be decreased, and upper abdominal trauma should be avoided. Patients with hepatitis-induced encephalopathy or coagulopathy and debilitated patients should be hospitalized.
- **Prevention.** The HAV vaccine, an inactivated vaccine, may be used in pregnancy. The vaccine is recommended for individuals traveling to endemic areas and is administered in two injections, 4 to 6 months apart.

Hepatitis B

- **Epidemiology**
  - In North America, hepatitis B virus (HBV) transmission occurs most commonly via parenteral exposure or sexual contact. Approximately 43 000 persons in the United States are newly diagnosed each year, with an estimated 2.2 million chronic carriers. Acute HBV occurs in 1 to 2 per 1000 pregnancies and chronic HBV in 5 to 15 per 1000 pregnancies. The MTCT is an important cause of chronic HBV infection worldwide. Transmission can occur prenatally, during delivery, or postpartum and is highest in women who are HBV envelope antigen (HBeAg) positive. The vertical transmission rate in these women is as high as 90% in the puerperium if prophylaxis is not given to their neonates.
  - **Natural history.** The HBV contains three principal antigens: HBV surface antigen (HBsAg), HBV core antigen, and HBeAg. The HBsAg is detectable in serum during acute and chronic infection. HBV core antigen compromises the central nucleocapsid of the virus; it is found only in hepatocytes during active viral replication and is not detected in serum. The HBeAg is a secretory product that is processed from the precore protein; it is a marker of active HBV replication

and increased infectivity. The presence of HBeAg is usually associated with high levels of HBV DNA in serum and higher rates of HBV transmission. Circulating antibodies against these viral antigens develop in response to infection.

- **Clinical manifestations**
  - **Maternal.** The clinical manifestations of HBV during pregnancy are similar to those for the nonpregnant patient. The HBV infection presents with nonhepatic prodromal symptoms, including rash, arthralgia, myalgia, and occasionally frank arthritis. Jaundice occurs in a minority of patients. In adults, around 90% to 95% acute infections resolve completely, and the patient develops protective levels of antibody. The remaining 5% to 10% of patients become chronically infected. These patients are clinically asymptomatic and usually have normal liver function tests. They nonetheless have detectable levels of HBsAg. The incidence of cirrhosis in a chronic HBV carrier is 8% to 20%. Acute hepatitis B carries a 1% risk of maternal mortality.
  - **Congenital.** Maternal-fetal transmission can occur at any time during pregnancy but most commonly occurs at the time of delivery. In women who are seropositive for both HBsAg and HBeAg (indicating active replication), the vertical transmission rate approaches 90%. However, in a woman who is HBsAg positive and hepatitis B core antibody positive with an undetectable hepatitis B viral load (carrier state), the risk of transmission drops to 10% to 30%. The frequency of vertical transmission is also affected by the timing of maternal infection. When maternal infection occurs in the first trimester, 10% of neonates are seropositive; when it occurs in the third trimester, 80% to 90% of neonates are infected. Whether infection occurs in utero or intrapartum, the presence of HBeAg in the neonates carries an 85% to 90% likelihood of progression to chronic HBV infection and the associated hepatic sequelae. Prophylactic administration of hepatitis B immunoglobulin to infants after birth reduces transmission to 5% to 10%, and antiviral medications now reduce that risk even further.
- **Diagnosis**
  - Diagnosis is confirmed by serology. The HBV viral load should also be performed.
  - The HBsAg appears in the serum 1 to 10 weeks after an acute exposure prior to the onset of clinical symptoms and then becomes undetectable after 4 to 6 months in patients who eventually recover. Persistence of HBsAg for >6 months implies chronic infection.
  - The disappearance of HBsAg is followed by the appearance of anti-HBs. In most patients, anti-HBs persist for life, conferring long-term immunity.
  - The HBeAg is detected during active viral replication.
- **Management**
  - Patients with acute hepatitis B infection may require hospitalization and supportive care. The disease is generally self-limited, and symptoms resolve within 1 to 2 weeks.
  - Current CDC recommendations include universal screening of all pregnant women for HBV at the first prenatal visit.
  - Women exposed to HBV should receive passive immunization with HBV immune globulin (HBIG) and receive recombinant HBV vaccine. The HBIG is 75% effective in preventing maternal HBV infection.
  - The HBIG should be administered to the neonate of an infected mother within the first 12 hours of life. The HBIG is followed immediately by the standard

three-dose HBV immunization series. The combination of HBIG and HBV vaccine prevents vertical transmission in 85% to 90% of cases.

- The use of antiviral therapy (tenofovir, telbivudine, or lamivudine) starting at 28 to 32 weeks' gestation to decrease MTCT is now recommended for women with a hepatitis B viral load $>2 \times 10^5$ IU/mL.
- Invasive intrapartum fetal monitoring (fetal scalp electrodes or fetal scalp blood sampling) should be avoided if maternal infection is known to help minimize vertical transmission risk.
- **Prevention.** Vaccination for hepatitis B is recommended for all women of reproductive age who were not immunized in childhood, preferably during preconception or routine gynecologic care, but is also safe to use during pregnancy.

Hepatitis C

- **Epidemiology.** Transmission of the hepatitis C virus (HCV) is similar to that of HBV but occurs via percutaneous blood contamination and rarely through sexual contact. An increased incidence of HCV is noted among IV drug abusers and recipients of blood products. Mass screening of the blood supply for HCV has markedly decreased the risk of HCV infection to <1 per 1 million screened units of blood.
- **Clinical manifestations**
  - **Maternal.** Acute HCV infection presents after an incubation period of 30 to 60 days. Asymptomatic infection occurs in 75% of patients, and at least 50% of infected individuals progress to chronic infection, regardless of the mode of acquisition or severity of initial infection. Of these patients, approximately 20% subsequently develop chronic active hepatitis or cirrhosis. Concomitant infection with HIV may accelerate the progression and severity of hepatic injury. Unlike HBV antibodies, antibodies to HCV are not protective. The HCV causes acute hepatitis in pregnancy but may go undetected if liver function tests and HCV antibody tests are not performed.
  - **Congenital.** Vertical transmission is proportional to the maternal serum HCV viral RNA titer. Transmission is approximately 2% in women with HCV viremia and is approximately 15% to 19% in the setting of maternal coinfection with HIV. Higher HCV RNA levels in pregnancy are associated with vertical transmission. Currently, there is no method or technique to prevent prenatal transmission. If transmission occurs transplacentally, the neonate is at increased risk for acute hepatitis and probable chronic hepatitis or carrier status. To date, no teratogenic syndromes associated with HCV have been described.
- **Diagnosis.** Anti–hepatitis C antibody is detected in serum but may take up to 1 year from exposure to test positive. The HCV viral RNA can be detected by PCR assay of serum soon after infection and in chronic disease and can be used to quantify active viral replication.
- **Management.** Because there is no prophylaxis for transmission, primary prevention of maternal infection is the mainstay of management. Treatment (both alpha interferon and direct-acting antiviral therapy) in pregnant women has not been well studied. During labor, invasive procedures such as a fetal scalp electrode or fetal scalp blood sampling should be avoided. According to CDC guidelines, maternal infection with hepatitis C is not an absolute contraindication to breastfeeding.

Herpes Simplex Virus 1 and 2

- **Epidemiology**
  - Type 1 herpes simplex virus (HSV) is responsible for most nongenital herpetic infections and up to 50% of genital lesions. Type 2 HSV is usually recovered from the genital tract. Approximately 1 in 7500 live-born infants contract HSV perinatally. Whether pregnancy alters the rate of recurrence or frequency of cervical shedding of virus is debated. The incidence of asymptomatic shedding in pregnancy is highest in the first year after a primary infection and 0.5% after a recurrent episode.
  - Primary maternal infection with HSV results from direct contact with mucous membranes or skin infected with the virus, commonly through sexual contact.
  - Fetal infection with HSV can occur transplacentally, as an ascending infection from the cervix, or most commonly through direct contact with infectious maternal genital lesions during delivery.
- **Clinical manifestations**
  - **Maternal.** Primary infections range from mild or asymptomatic to severe. Vesicles may appear on the cervix, vagina, or vulva 2 to 10 days after exposure. Swelling, erythema, pain, and regional lymphadenopathy are common. The lesions can persist for 1 to 3 weeks with concomitant viral shedding. Reactivation occurs in 50% of patients within 6 months of the initial outbreak and subsequently at irregular intervals. Symptoms of recurrent outbreaks are generally milder, with viral shedding lasting less than a week. In pregnancy, primary outbreaks may increase the incidence of preterm labor in the latter half of pregnancy.
  - **Congenital.** The highest rate of congenital infection occurs in women with a primary infection. Infection is usually the result of primary maternal infection. The most common form of transmission is direct contact with vaginal secretions during delivery. Viral shedding during labor is the strongest predictor of transmission. Overall, congenital infections are very rare, and few are asymptomatic. The majority ultimately produce disseminated or CNS disease. Localized infection is usually associated with a good outcome, but infants with disseminated infection have a mortality rate of 60%, even with treatment. At least half of infants surviving disseminated infection develop serious neurologic and ophthalmic sequelae.
  - **Diagnosis.** When HSV is suspected, a swab specimen may be obtained from the lesion for culture and immunofluorescent or PCR studies. Seven to 10 days must be allowed for isolation of the virus via tissue culture, but the sensitivity is 95% and specificity is also high. Serology is of limited value in diagnosis because a single antibody titer is not predictive of viral shedding and IgG will be positive indefinitely after the primary outbreak. Smears of scrapings from the bases of vesicles may be stained using the Tzanck or Papanicolaou technique. The PCR for HSV DNA is sensitive and rapid.
  - **Management.** Patients with a history of genital herpes should undergo a careful perineal examination at the time of delivery. Vaginal delivery is permitted if no signs or symptoms of HSV are present. Active genital HSV in patients in labor or with ruptured membranes at or near term is an indication for cesarean delivery, regardless of the duration of rupture. Evidence shows that HSV recurrences in the regions of the buttocks, thighs, and anus are associated with low rates of cervical virus shedding. Lesions in these areas should not preclude a vaginal delivery; however, it is recommended that the lesion(s) be covered for delivery. Acyclovir may

be used to treat HSV infection in pregnancy; however, valacyclovir hydrochloride (Valtrex) is more easily tolerated due to a twice-daily dosing schedule. Third trimester suppression with valacyclovir, 500 mg orally daily or twice daily, should be considered in women with frequent outbreaks during their pregnancies.

- **Prevention.** Barrier contraception can be recommended to avoid primary maternal infection as part of routine safe sex counseling.

BACTERIAL INFECTIONS

Group A Streptococcus (Bacteremia)

- **Epidemiology.** Women in the peripartum period have a 20-fold increased risk of bacteremia from group A *Streptococcus* (GAS) infection than nonpregnant women. Most cases are community acquired via upper respiratory tract infection unlike group B *Streptococcus* (GBS) that colonizes the genital tract. This can lead to hematogenous seeding of the placenta and uterus. In the postpartum period, exposed mucosal membranes in the reproductive tract and/or open wounds (laceration, episiotomy, surgical incision for cesarean delivery) may be responsible for increased vulnerability to GAS infection.
- **Clinical manifestations**
  - **Maternal.** The GAS bacteremia presents with fever, abdominal pain, respiratory distress, and renal dysfunction with or without a systemic inflammatory response syndrome such as tachycardia, hypotension, and leukocytosis. The GAS bacteremia can also cause streptococcal toxic shock syndrome or necrotizing fasciitis. These can manifest in the reproductive tract as well as respiratory tract and breast.
- **Diagnosis**
  - Rapid diagnosis is critical because maternal mortality rate for GAS bacteremia approaches 60%.
  - Diagnosis can be difficult due to the relatively low prevalence of GAS infection and nonspecific nature of presenting symptoms. Thus, onset of signs and symptoms of septic shock in a woman in the peripartum period should raise concern for GAS bacteremia.
  - Blood and urine cultures should be obtained. Postpartum women should have endometrial culture obtained.
  - Imaging studies such as computed tomography, magnetic resonance imaging, and ultrasound may be useful but should not delay treatment.
- **Management**
  - Treatment involves fluid resuscitation, prompt initiation of antibiotics, and source control.
  - The typical antibiotic regimen is penicillin G 4 million U IV every 4 hours and clindamycin 900 mg IV every 8 hours. Vancomycin may be used for women with penicillin allergy. Typical duration is 14 days of parenteral antibiotics. Sensitivity testing should be obtained to help tailor antibiotic coverage.
- **Prevention**
  - Antibiotic prophylaxis in the setting of cesarean delivery, prolonged premature rupture of membranes, and observation of hygiene and infection control among health care providers can help prevent GAS infections.
  - Unlike GBS infection, the role of screening in pregnancy is unclear.

Group B Streptococcus

- **Epidemiology.** The GBS (*Streptococcus agalactiae*), a gram-positive bacteria, can be isolated from the vagina and/or rectum in approximately 10% to 30% of pregnant women in the United States. The gastrointestinal tract is the reservoir for the bacteria and is the source of any vaginal and urinary colonization or infection. Neonatal colonization may occur as a result of ascending infection from the maternal genital tract or during passage of the fetus through the birth canal during a vaginal delivery. The vertical transmission rate may be as high as 72%, but invasive disease in term neonates is rare. In preterm infants, however, invasive disease is more common and is accompanied by significant morbidity and mortality.
- **Clinical manifestations**
  - **Maternal.** The GBS is a common urinary pathogen in pregnant women. The GBS is isolated in 5% to 29% of cases of asymptomatic bacteriuria and in 1% to 5% of cases of acute cystitis during pregnancy. When inadequately treated, both asymptomatic bacteriuria and acute cystitis can progress to pyelonephritis, necessitating hospitalization. Maternal GBS infection has also been associated with premature rupture of membranes, preterm labor, chorioamnionitis, bacteremia, puerperal endometritis, and postoperative wound infections after cesarean delivery.
  - **Congenital.** Neonatal colonization with GBS results from contamination from the mother's genital tract in 75% of cases. One percent to 2% of colonized infants will develop early-onset GBS infection (infection occurring within the first 7 d of life), with a case fatality of 11% to 50%. Preterm and/or low-birth-weight infants are at higher risk than term neonates. Maternal risk factors that predispose a neonate to early-onset GBS infection include preterm delivery, prolonged rupture of membranes (>18 h), intrapartum temperature of at least 38°C or 100.4°F, or a prior infant who had GBS infection.
    - Late-onset GBS infection, which occurs 7 days or more after birth, affects 0.5 to 1.8 per 1000 live births. It may result from maternal-neonatal transmission, nosocomial, or community contacts. Mortality for late-onset disease is approximately 10%.
    - Meningitis is common in infected neonates, but infants may also present with bacteremia without localizing symptoms. Other clinical syndromes include pneumonia, osteomyelitis, cellulitis, and sepsis. Neurologic sequelae develop in 15% to 30% of meningitis survivors.
- **Diagnosis.** Group B streptococcal colonization can be detected by anovaginal culture or nucleic acid amplification testing. A single swab is used to obtain a sample of the lower third of the vagina and anus/rectum. The predominant limitation of culture is time. Results are not available for 24 to 48 hours, making management difficult if delivery is imminent. Rapid-diagnostic tests are available that detect specific polysaccharide antigens. They are easy to perform, generally less expensive than a culture, and produce results within a short period of time (usually 1 h). The tests are highly sensitive in patients who are heavily colonized with GBS; however, their lower sensitivity and higher false-negative rate compared with those of cultures prevent their widespread clinical application in obstetrics.
- **Management**
  - Treatment of uncomplicated GBS lower urinary tract infection is with amoxicillin or penicillin. Hospitalization is required for cases of pyelonephritis, and patients should be treated with an appropriate regimen until afebrile and

asymptomatic for 24 to 48 hours. She may then be discharged to complete a total of 10 days of antibiotics.

- The ACOG recommends universal screening for GBS between 36 0/7 and 37 6/7 weeks' gestation with a swab of the lower vagina and rectum. Women with a positive screen, a previous infant with GBS invasive infection, urine colonization or infection with GBS during the current pregnancy, labor before 37 weeks with unknown GBS status, rupture of membranes >18 hours at term with unknown GBS status, or signs of chorioamnionitis should receive intrapartum antibiotics. Treatment is typically with penicillin 5 million U IV loading dose followed by 2.5 million U IV every 4 hours. Prophylaxis is most effective if started at least 4 hours before delivery. For patients with a penicillin allergy, cephalosporins can be used if the allergy is mild (rash) but should be avoided for more severe allergies (anaphylaxis). Genital culture results should be evaluated for sensitivity to clindamycin, where resistance precludes effectiveness of clindamycin. If culture results demonstrate resistance or if sensitivities are unknown and the patient has a severe penicillin allergy, vancomycin should be administered.

Listeria

- **Epidemiology**
  - In the United States, it is estimated that approximately 1600 cases of listeriosis occur annually. Listeriosis is notable for having one of the highest mortality rates among foodborne infections, and it accounts for approximately 19% of all foodborne infection–related deaths.
  - *Listeria* gastroenteritis has an incubation period around 24 hours and occurs as a result of consumption of contaminated food. Symptoms usually are self-limited and last for a few days.
  - Invasive *Listeria* may have an incubation period ranging from 1 to 4 weeks.
  - Pregnant women are especially vulnerable to *Listeria* infection. In fact, pregnant women make up approximately 33% of all reported cases.
- **Clinical manifestations**
  - **Maternal.** Listeriosis in pregnancy occurs most frequently in the third trimester. Presenting symptoms range from fever, myalgia, fatigue, malaise, chills, and back pain. Most infections are mild and self-limited. *Listeria* can also cause invasive disease that involves the central nervous system (CNS) or bacteremia. The CNS manifestation is usually in the form of meningoencephalitis. Symptoms can range from fever and acute mental status changes to coma. Listeria bacteremia is seen mostly in elderly or immunocompromised individuals but can occur in pregnant women.
  - **Congenital.** Fetal effects become less common with increasing gestational age. Fetal and neonatal effects include miscarriage, fetal death, and preterm delivery. Granulomatosis infantiseptica follows a severe in utero infection. Newborns with this condition may have granulomas and abscesses in multiple organs or skin lesions. Most of these newborns die soon after delivery. Placental pathology can help confirm this diagnosis.
- **Diagnosis**
  - Diagnosis is established by culture showing *Listeria*.
  - Symptomatic pregnant women who have consumed foods contaminated with *Listeria* should have blood and stool cultures performed.

- **Management**
  - Pregnant women who have consumed foods contaminated with *Listeria* but otherwise do not have symptoms that suggest listeriosis can be managed expectantly.
  - Gastroenteritis: Oral amoxicillin or ampicillin can be initiated. If cultures are negative, treatment may be discontinued.
  - Invasive listeriosis: IV ampicillin and gentamicin for 14 to 21 days
- **Prevention**
  - Because listeriosis is typically foodborne, avoiding certain foods is advisable per the CDC.
    - Avoid nonpasteurized dairy products.
    - Avoid raw or lightly cooked alfalfa, clover, radish, and mung bean sprouts.
    - Avoid luncheon meats, deli meats, hotdogs, or dry sausages unless cooked.
    - Avoid uncooked smoked seafood unless canned or shelf-stable.
  - More recommendations can be found at https://www.foodsafety.gov/.

Lyme disease

- Recent studies do not support a link between Lyme disease in pregnancy and negative fetal outcomes. If adequately treated, Lyme disease in pregnancy does not seem to affect the fetus.
- The standard antibiotic choice for Lyme disease in pregnancy is a β-lactam antibiotic such as amoxicillin or cefuroxime. Typical dosage is amoxicillin 500 mg orally 3 times a day for 14 days or cefuroxime 500 mg orally twice daily for 14 days.

Syphilis

- **Epidemiology.** In the United States, the rate of primary and secondary syphilis infection in women has increased recently. The rate of congenital syphilis also has increased. In 2017, 918 cases of congenital syphilis were reported.
- **Clinical manifestations**
  - **Fetal.** *Treponema pallidum* can infect the placenta and be transmitted to the fetus during any phase of maternal infection. Syphilis infection can lead to miscarriage, restricted fetal growth, fetal death in utero, preterm delivery, and stillbirth. The rate of congenital infection depends on the gestational age at diagnosis, treatment of maternal disease, and stage of maternal disease. Presence of spirochetes in the fetal circulation can lead to polyhydramnios, fetal anemia, hydrops fetalis, and hepatomegaly.
  - **Congenital.** Jaundice, hepatomegaly, rhinorrhea ("snuffles"), rash, generalized lymphadenopathy, long bone abnormalities
- **Diagnosis**
  - All pregnant women should be screened during initial prenatal visit. Pregnant women with high risk of infection should be rescreened in the third trimester and at presentation to labor and delivery.
  - Serologic testing is the most widely employed diagnostic tool, and it includes both nontreponemal and treponemal tests.
    - Nontreponemal tests: Venereal Disease Research Laboratory and rapid plasma reagin
    - Treponemal test: fluorescent treponemal antibody absorption, *Treponema pallidum* particle agglutination, microhemagglutination assay for *T pallidum* antibodies, enzyme immunoassays, and chemiluminescence immunoassays

- Ultrasound to evaluate for evidence of congenital syphilis
- Fetal anemia (measured by fetal MCA Doppler), hydrops fetalis, polyhydramnios, hepatomegaly, or placentomegaly
- **Management**
  - Penicillin is the treatment of choice in pregnancy. Thus, pregnant women with penicillin allergy must be desensitized and treated with penicillin. Desensitization can be done in an inpatient or outpatient setting depending on the reported severity of the allergy. Maternal treatment will also treat fetal infection.
    - Primary, secondary, or early latent. Benzathine penicillin G 2.4 million U IM in a single dose.
    - Late latent, tertiary, or unknown duration. Benzathine penicillin G 2.4 million U IM weekly for 3 weeks. If a dose is missed, the course must be restarted.
    - Postexposure prophylaxis. Pregnant women who had sexual contact with individuals with known infection should receive 1 dose of benzathine penicillin G 2.4 million U IM.
    - The Jarisch-Herxheimer (J-H) reaction is a possible complication of treatment of syphilis. It is thought to stem from an inflammatory response from lysed spirochetes. The J-H reaction begins within hours of beginning treatment and resolves within a day or two. Symptoms include fever, headache, myalgia, rash, and hypotension.
      - J-H reaction may lead to preterm contractions, preterm delivery, and nonreassuring fetal heart tracing.
      - Management is supportive care with IV fluids and antipyretics.
  - In fetuses with the above ultrasound findings of congenital syphilis infection, serial ultrasound is recommended to assess the effect of maternal treatment using MCA Doppler, amniotic fluid index, and size of placenta and fetal liver.

PROTOZOAN INFECTIONS

Toxoplasmosis

- **Epidemiology.** In the United States, the incidence of acute toxoplasmosis infection in pregnancy is estimated at 0.2% to 1.0%. Congenital toxoplasmosis occurs in 1 to 8 per 1000 live births. The infective agent is the oocyst, shed by the alimentary tract of cats. Transmission occurs primarily by eating undercooked or raw meat containing cysts, ingesting food or water contaminated by the oocyst of an infected cat, inhaling aerosolized oocysts from cat litter, or handling material contaminated by the feces of an infected cat. Approximately one-third of American women carry antibodies to *Toxoplasma gondii*.
- **Clinical manifestations**
  - **Maternal.** Up to 90% of acute toxoplasmosis infections are asymptomatic. A mononucleosis-like syndrome, including fatigue, malaise, cervical lymphadenopathy, sore throat, and atypical lymphocytosis, may occur. Placental infection and subsequent fetal infection occur during the spreading phase of the parasitemia.
  - **Congenital.** The rate of fetal transmission is approximately 15% in the first trimester, 30% in the second trimester, and 70% in the third trimester. Fetal morbidity and mortality rates are higher after early transmission, with 11% risk of perinatal death from infection in the first trimester, 4% in the second

trimester, and minimal to zero in the third trimester. Infected neonates often exhibit low birth weight, hepatosplenomegaly, icterus, and anemia. Sequelae such as vision loss and psychomotor and mental retardation are common. Hearing loss is demonstrated in 10% to 30% and developmental delay in 20% to 75%. Up to 90% of infants with congenital toxoplasmosis are asymptomatic at birth.

- **Diagnosis**
  - Screening for toxoplasmosis is not routine in the United States. Because most women with acute toxoplasmosis are asymptomatic, the diagnosis is not suspected until an affected infant is born. For women who do present with symptoms of acute infection, both IgM and IgG titers should be measured.
  - Negative IgM excludes acute or recent infection, unless the serum has been tested so early that an immune response has not yet been mounted. A positive test is more difficult to interpret because IgM may be elevated for more than a year after infection. Seroconversion of IgG on repeat testing may be useful.
  - The PCR testing for *Toxoplasma* DNA can be performed on amniotic fluid. This is the best method for confirming congenital infection.
  - Sonographic findings include bilateral dilated cerebral ventricles, intracranial and intrahepatic lesions, and placental hyperdensities. Occasionally, pericardial and pleural effusions are observed.
- **Management**
  - For women who elect to continue their pregnancies after a diagnosis of acute toxoplasmosis, therapy should be started immediately. There remains debate concerning the effectiveness of antibiotics, but the mainstay of treatment is spiramycin or pyrimethamine with sulfadiazine.
  - Spiramycin reduces the incidence but not necessarily the severity of fetal infection. It is recommended for the treatment of acute maternal infections diagnosed before the third trimester and should then be continued for the duration of the pregnancy. If amniotic fluid PCR results for *Toxoplasma* are negative, spiramycin is used; if results are positive, pyrimethamine and sulfadiazine should be used.
  - Pyrimethamine and sulfadiazine. Patients with documented *T gondii* infection of the fetus may be offered treatment with pyrimethamine 25 mg orally daily and sulfadiazine orally 1 g 4 times daily for 28 days. Folinic acid, 6 mg IM or orally, is administered 3 times per week to prevent toxicity. During the first trimester, pyrimethamine is not recommended due to teratogenic risk. Sulfadiazine is omitted from the regimen at term.
- **Prevention.** Pregnant women should eat only fully cooked meats, wash their hands after preparing meat for cooking, wash fruits and vegetables well, and avoid contact with cat litter boxes.

Malaria

- **Epidemiology.** Malaria is most prevalent in tropical regions of the world. In an endemic region such as sub-Saharan Africa, the median prevalence of maternal malaria is 28%. Pregnant women, compared to nonpregnant women, exhibit a higher prevalence of malaria infection. In addition, pregnant women infected with malaria are more likely to suffer more severe disease. However, not all malaria species have the same effect.
  - *Plasmodium falciparum* is associated with high levels of parasitemia, placental sequestration, and more severe fetal sequelae.

- *Plasmodium vivax* is associated with less severe fetal sequelae and is not as commonly sequestered in the placenta.
- *Plasmodium ovale* and *Plasmodium malariae* are not usually associated with severe disease in pregnancy.

- **Clinical manifestation**
  - **Maternal.** Most common symptoms are fever, chills, sweats, headache, myalgia, malaise, abdominal pain, nausea and vomiting, and diarrhea. Hypoglycemia can be seen in more severe disease. Pregnant women are more likely to experience severe symptoms and can sometimes exhibit severe respiratory distress, anemia, and hypoglycemia.
  - **Congenital.** *P falciparum* and *P vivax* have been associated with miscarriage, preterm delivery, low birth weight, fetal growth restriction, and congenital diseases. Congenital malarial infection manifests usually weeks after birth and includes fever, irritability, diarrhea, vomiting, and poor feeding.
- **Diagnosis**
  - Malaria should be on the differential diagnosis when encountering a pregnant woman with possible geographical exposure and fever.
  - The standard diagnostic tool is light microscopy showing parasites on Giemsa-stained blood smear. The limitation of this method is that it is operator dependent. Peripheral blood smear is also important in establishing the diagnosis. Molecular diagnostic tools such as PCR also may play a role in low-resource areas.
- **Management**
  - Treatment of malaria in pregnant women depends on species and chloroquine resistance.
  - The CDC guideline for treatment is available at https://www.cdc.gov/malaria/resources/pdf/treatmenttable.pdf.
  - During the acute phase of malaria infection, ultrasound imaging should be obtained to evaluate amniotic fluid volume, biophysical profile, and fetal size and growth. After a malaria infection episode, fetal growth surveillance with ultrasound should be performed.
- **Prevention**
  - Protect from mosquito bites by wearing protective clothing outdoors and using N,N-diethyl-meta-toluamide (DEET)-containing insect repellents.
  - Chemoprophylaxis should be administered to pregnant women who are traveling to areas where malaria is endemic. Chloroquine is the preferred agent. Mefloquine can be used for women traveling to areas where chloroquine resistance is present.

EMERGING INFECTIONS

West Nile

- **Epidemiology.** The MTCT can occur with West Nile virus but appears to be rare. Although the data is limited, the CDC recorded pregnancy outcome of 77 women infected with West Nile virus from 2003 to 2004 in the United States. Three of the 72 infants followed had symptomatic West Nile disease.
- **Clinical manifestation**
  - **Maternal.** Most infected individuals are asymptomatic. After an incubation period of 2 to 14 days, symptoms such as fatigue, weakness, myalgia, memory

impairment, and balance issues may manifest. A morbilliform or maculopapular rash may be present. It tends to appear at the time of defervescence. More worrisome manifestations of West Nile virus include meningitis, encephalitis, or paralysis. Ophthalmic manifestation includes chorioretinitis, vitreitis, and retinal hemorrhage.

- **Congenital.** Although there is some evidence that MTCT can occur with West Nile virus, there is no documented evidence of fetal abnormalities associated with maternal infection.
- **Diagnosis.** Pregnant women with meningitis, encephalitis, paralysis, or inexplicable fever in West Nile endemic areas should have testing for IgM antibody to West Nile virus. Cerebrospinal fluid should also be tested in the presence of neurologic or ophthalmic symptoms.
- **Management**
  - The mainstay of management is supportive. There is no clear evidence of invasive fetal testing.
  - Screening in asymptomatic pregnant women is not recommended.
- **Prevention.** Protect from mosquito bites by wearing protective clothing outdoors and using DEET-containing insect repellents.

Zika

- **Epidemiology**
  - Whereas Zika virus is primarily transmitted by mosquito bites, it can also be transmitted transplacentally and by sexual contact, blood transfusion, and organ transplantation.
  - Zika virus is currently endemic in Africa, Southeast Asia, and the Pacific Islands. As the outbreak pattern is dynamic, the most current geographical distribution of Zika virus may be viewed at the CDC's Web site on Zika: https://www.cdc .gov/zika/geo/index.html.
- **Clinical manifestation**
  - **Maternal.** Symptoms include fever, pruritic rash (erythematous maculopapular rash in the face, extremities, and trunk), joint pain, myalgia, and conjunctivitis. Guillain-Barré syndrome has also been associated with Zika virus infection.
  - **Congenital.** Congenital Zika syndrome may be identified in the fetuses/neonates of a subset of mothers infected with Zika virus. Microcephaly, other CNS abnormalities such as ventriculomegaly, intracranial calcifications, atrophy or hypoplasia of cerebral tissue, fetal growth restriction, miscarriage, stillbirth, and hydrops fetalis all have been documented.
- **Diagnosis**
  - All pregnant women should be screened for possible Zika virus exposure by inquiring about recent travel or sexual contact with a person who traveled to or lives in an area with ongoing Zika transmission.
  - Testing guidance has been updated frequently because more data are available regarding the current epidemic. The testing algorithms can be found at https://www .cdc.gov/pregnancy/zika/testing-follow-up/testing-and-diagnosis.html.
- **Management**
  - Management focuses on symptomatic support consisting of hydration and antipyretic.

- It is important to note that nonsteroidal anti-inflammatory drugs should be avoided until dengue infection has been ruled out, in order to reduce the risk of hemorrhage.
- **Prevention**
  - **Travel.** The current CDC recommendation is for pregnant women to avoid traveling to areas where Zika virus is ongoing. The most current travel advisory data can be found on the CDC's Web site: https://wwwnc.cdc.gov/travel/page /world-map-areas-with-zika.
  - **Mosquito bite prevention.** It is recommended that women in endemic areas wear clothes that provide coverage of arms and legs. In addition, they should wear DEET-containing insect repellents.
  - **Sexual.** It is recommended that women in endemic areas use barrier protection if sexually active. The World Health Organization also recommend that individuals who have travelled to endemic areas abstain from sex for at least 3 months before engaging in unprotected sex regardless of presence of symptoms.

SUGGESTED READINGS

American College of Obstetricians and Gynecologists Committee on Obstetric Practice. ACOG Committee Opinion No. 782: prevention of group B streptococcal early-onset disease in newborns. *Obstet Gynecol.* 2019;134:e19-e40.

American College of Obstetricians and Gynecologists Women's Health Care Physicians. ACOG Practice Bulletin No. 752: prenatal and perinatal human immunodeficiency virus testing–expanded recommendations (replaces Committee Opinion No. 635, June 2015). *Obstet Gynecol.* 2018;132:e138-e142.

Centers for Disease Control and Prevention. Sexually transmitted diseases treatment guidelines, 2015. *MMWR Morb Mortal Wkly Rep.* 2015;64(3):1-137.

Leddy MA, Gonik B, Schulkin J. Obstetrician-gynecologists and perinatal infections: a review of studies of the Collaborative Ambulatory Research Network (2005-2009). *Infect Dis Obstet Gynecol.* 2010;2010:583950.

Tan KR, Arguin PM. Malaria. Centers for Disease Control and Prevention Web site. https:// wwwnc.cdc.gov/travel/yellowbook/2018/infectious-diseases-related-to-travel/malaria. Accessed July 22, 2019.

US Department of Health and Human Services. Recommendations for the use of antiretroviral drugs in pregnant women with HIV infection and interventions to reduce perinatal HIV transmission in the United States. AIDSinfo Web site. https://aidsinfo.nih.gov/guidelines /html/3/perinatal/0. Accessed July 22, 2019.

Congenital Anomalies
Juliet C. Bishop and Angie C. Jelin

Congenital anomalies, also known as *birth defects*, are defined as structural or functional anomalies that exist at or before birth and are among the most common causes of neonatal morbidity and mortality. Birth defects can involve an isolated organ system or multiple organ systems; multiple anomalies may encompass a syndrome. Congenital anomalies can have medical, surgical, cosmetic, and/or social significance and may have long-term impact on the development and health of the affected individual.

EPIDEMIOLOGY

- According to the Centers for Disease Control and Prevention, major congenital anomalies occur in approximately 3% of live births and are the leading cause of infant deaths, accounting for 20% of all infant deaths.
- **Major anomalies** often require surgical repair or are life-threatening and are more common in spontaneous miscarriages.
- **Minor anomalies** are rarely medically significant and rarely require surgical intervention. Some minor anomalies can represent a part of the normal variation in the population and thus are more common than major anomalies. However, infants with multiple minor anomalies are at increased risk for having a syndrome.

ETIOLOGY

- Causes of congenital anomalies may be genetic, environmental, multifactorial, or idiopathic; hence, obtaining a thorough family history and screening all pregnant patients is important. Approximately 70% of all congenital anomalies are linked to a specific cause. See Table 9-1 for risk factors associated with congenital anomalies.
- **Genetic etiologies** include the following: aneuploidy disorders such as trisomy 21 (Down syndrome) or monosomy X (Turner syndrome), disorders caused by copy number variations such as deletion of chromosome 22q.11 (DiGeorge syndrome) or duplication of a chromosomal segment, and monogenic disorders such as Noonan syndrome and Smith-Lemli-Opitz syndrome. There are also anomalies that can be one of multiple findings in a specific syndrome or have a multifactorial etiology such as isolated congenital heart disease (CHD), cleft lip and palate, or arthrogryposis, which may result from interactions of several genes and environmental factors.
- **Nongenetic/environmental etiologies** include the following: certain medications such as tretinoin (Retin A) and warfarin (Coumadin), some illicit drugs, ethanol, maternal exposure to radiation, maternal nutritional deficiencies (folate), maternal medical conditions such as uncontrolled diabetes, maternal infections such as toxoplasmosis, syphilis, rubella, or Zika (see chapter 8), and maternal age.

Table 9-1	Factors Associated With Increased Risk for Congenital Anomalies

Advanced maternal age (maternal age ≥35 years at time of delivery)

Pregestational diabetes

Exposure to a known teratogen
  Infection (TORCH infections, varicella, CMV, Zika)
  Drugs/alcohol/chemicals
  Radiation/heat

History of having a child with birth defect

Personal or family history of a known genetic abnormality
  Aneuploidy
  Balanced translocation
  Deletion/duplication
  Gene mutation

Multiple gestation

Assisted reproductive technology

Abbreviations: CMV, cytomegalovirus; TORCH, toxoplasmosis, other (syphilis, varicella-zoster, parvovirus B19), rubella, cytomegalovirus, and herpes.

SCREENING AND MANAGEMENT

- Given the significant morbidity and mortality of congenital defects, all patients should be offered screening for fetal chromosomal abnormalities, preferably during the first trimester, and a level II anatomy ultrasound at 18 to 22 weeks. Detailed ultrasonography by an experienced technician can detect greater than 80% of fetal anomalies, allowing for a full range of management options: further workup (eg, karyotyping, microarray, and/or viral studies), expectant management, fetal monitoring and/or in utero therapy, and for those who desire it, pregnancy termination.

- Management should include counseling that takes into consideration the fetus, the mother, and the family. Treatment options and prognosis should be discussed. With a fetal congenital anomaly, multidisciplinary approach facilitates a unified plan of care. The obstetrician or maternal-fetal medicine (MFM) specialist can coordinate care with genetic counselors, neonatologists, and other pediatric specialists such as surgeons, cardiologists, urologists, and neurosurgeons. Social work and bereavement counseling can also be part of the care plan if indicated. The care plan must be timely, unbiased, and sensitive to the concerns and values of the patient and her family.

- **Ultrasonography** can be used to diagnose many major anomalies. The other clinical uses for ultrasound entail confirmation of gestational age, definition of placental location, determination of amniotic fluid volume, and evaluation of fetal growth.

- Optimal timing for the anatomic survey is between 18 and 22 weeks' gestation. At this gestational age, organogenesis is complete, bony ossification in the skull does not yet obscure sonography, and structures are large enough for accurate assessment but still small enough to visualize within a single ultrasound window. With a detected anomaly at this time, a patient can pursue a genetic workup and has a full set of options available to her at the time the anomaly is discovered. Detection of some anomalies is possible as early as 11 to 14 weeks; however, a screen for major fetal anomalies in the first trimester should not replace the more appropriate screening of fetal anatomy in the second trimester.

- The structures that are assessed in the level II anatomy screen include the following:
  - **Head.** The biparietal diameter and head circumference are measured, both in the same view at the level of the thalamus and cavum septum pellucidum. The intracranial contents including the ventricular structures, choroid plexus, midline falx, cavum septum pellucidum, cerebellum, and cisterna magna are evaluated. The profile, orbits, upper lip, and palate are also evaluated.
  - **Spine.** Sagittal, transverse, and/or coronal views are obtained at all levels (cervical, thoracic, lumbar, and sacral) to screen for neural tube defects (NTDs).
  - **Heart.** Four-chamber view and visualization of left and right ventricular outflow tracts are required. If an abnormality is suspected, fetal echocardiography should be performed.
  - **Abdomen.** The fetal stomach is evaluated for presence, size, and situs, and the umbilical cord is evaluated for insertion site and vessel number. The stomach and umbilical vein should be visualized in the same plane for the abdominal circumference measurement. Abdominal wall defects are ruled out by verifying normal cord insertion and the absence of bowel loops in the amniotic fluid. The kidneys, renal pelvises, and bladder are evaluated for location, structure, and evidence of obstruction.
  - **Limbs.** The four limbs should be imaged to their distal ends and the humerus and femur measured. The hands should be seen to open and close and the feet examined for normal positioning and appearance.
  - **Fetal sex.** Fetal genitalia should be evaluated for ambiguity because this may be relevant some medical conditions and/or genetic disorders.
- Several sonographic "soft markers" occur more frequently in fetuses with aneuploidy, specifically trisomy 21. These markers include increased nuchal translucency, renal pelvis dilation, echogenic intracardiac focus (EIF) (small bright spot within the fetal heart on ultrasound), echogenic bowel, and shortening of the long bones. Aneuploidy risk increases with an increased number of markers identified; previous studies have reported likelihood ratios for the individual markers.

CHROMOSOMAL ABNORMALITIES WITH ASSOCIATED CONGENITAL ANOMALIES

In many specific chromosomal syndromes, there are characteristic findings detected sonographically that assist in prenatal diagnosis (Table 9-2).

Trisomy 21 (Down Syndrome)

- Down syndrome is the most common aneuploidy among liveborn infants, with a frequency of 1:700 births. Down syndrome is a genetic disorder caused by the presence of all or part of a third copy of chromosome 21 instead of the usual two copies. Although women of any age can have a child with Down syndrome, the frequency of nondisjunction trisomy 21 increases with increasing maternal age.

Table 9-2 Common Aneuploidies With Associated Findings

Chromosomal Defect	Prenatal Ultrasound Findings	Neonatal Clinical Features[a]
Trisomy 21 (Down syndrome)	• Increased nuchal translucency • Absent nasal bone • Short femur/humerus • Clinodactyly • Sandal gap between first and second toes • Echogenic intracardiac focus • Cardiac anomalies • Echogenic bowel • Duodenal atresia • Renal pyelectasis	• Hypotonia • Flat facial profile • Upslanting palpebral fissures • Small ears • Excess dorsal nuchal skin • Single palmar crease • Hypoplasia of fifth finger middle phalanx
Trisomy 13 (Patau syndrome)	• Increased nuchal translucency • Holoprosencephaly/CNS anomalies • Facial anomalies (eye abnormalities, cleft lip/palate) • Cardiac anomalies • Renal anomalies (echogenic, enlarged kidneys, urinary tract dilation) • Gastrointestinal anomalies • Polydactyly/clenched hands • Fetal growth restriction	• Hypotonia • Hypotelorism/microphthalmia/coloboma • Microcephaly • Low-set ears • Brain/spinal cord, heart, kidney defects • Skin aplasia • Polydactyly/clenched hands/single palmar crease • Undescended testicles • Seizures • Severe intellectual disability
Trisomy 18 (Edwards syndrome)	• Increased nuchal translucency • Brain/CNS anomalies (choroid plexus cyst, posterior fossa abnormalities, holoprosencephaly, ventriculomegaly) • Facial anomalies (eye abnormalities, cleft lip/palate) • Cardiac anomalies • Single umbilical artery • Renal anomalies (horseshoe kidney) • Gastrointestinal anomalies (omphalocele, malrotation) • Musculoskeletal anomalies (clenched hands, rocker bottom feet, hemivertebrae) • Fetal growth restriction	• Prominent occiput, broad forehead • Short palpebral fissures • Small mouth • Rotated and malformed ears • Brain/spinal cord, heart, kidney defects • Clenched hands with second and fifth fingers overlapping third and fourth fingers • Imperforate anus • Severe intellectual disability

Table 9-2 Common Aneuploidies With Associated Findings *(Continued)*

Chromosomal Defect	Prenatal Ultrasound Findings	Neonatal Clinical Features[a]
Monosomy X (Turner syndrome)	• Cystic hygroma • Hydrops • Cardiac anomalies • Short femur/humerus • Horseshoe kidney	• Low hairline • Webbed neck • Short stature • Shield chest • Coarctation of the aorta • Wide-spaced hypoplastic nipples • Gonadal dysgenesis • Lymphedema
Triploidy	• Severe IUGR • Cystic placenta • Ventriculomegaly • Facial anomalies • Syndactyly • Cardiac anomalies • Renal anomalies	• Hypertelorism • Low nasal bridge • Cleft lip/palate • Low-set, malformed ears • Brain/spinal cord, heart, kidney defects • Short stature • Seizure • Intellectual disability

Abbreviations: CNS, central nervous system; IUGR, intrauterine grown restriction.
[a]In addition to corresponding prenatal ultrasound findings.

- Down syndrome can occur due to complete trisomy 21 in which all cells have three copies of chromosome 21 (94% of cases) or due to mosaic trisomy 21 in which only some cells in the body have an abnormal number of chromosome 21 (2%-3%). A third etiology of Down syndrome results from a mother who has a balanced translocation, in which an extra piece of chromosome 21 is attached to another chromosome and, when passed to the fetus, results in having three copies of chromosome 21.
- The finding of an EIF should prompt a search for other ultrasonographic markers of Down syndrome. The extent of the discussion with regard to associated Down syndrome risk is dependent on the preultrasound risk based on prior screening results. If Down syndrome is suspected, a fetal echocardiogram is recommended because these fetuses have a higher incidence of congenital heart defects. However, as an EIF is not a structural defect, it is not an indication for a fetal echocardiogram when found in isolation.
- Children with Down syndrome have some degree of intellectual disability, and in prenatal counseling, it is important to discuss that there is a spectrum of disease and the severity of disease cannot be predicted prenatally or by genetic testing.

Trisomy 13 and 18

- **Trisomy 13** (Patau syndrome) is usually due to meiotic primary nondisjunction giving rise to a 47,XX/47,XY, +13 genotype but can also be due to mosaic or partial trisomy 13. Trisomy 13 is characterized by severe, multiple anomalies and is invariably fatal; approximately 80% of newborns die in the first month of life, and 90% die by 1 year. Anomalies associated with trisomy 13 may include heart defects, holoprosencephaly, spinal cord abnormalities, microcephaly, microphthalmia or anophthalmia, cleft lip and/or cleft palate, polydactyly, rocker bottom feet, omphalocele, and hypotonia. The majority of prenatally diagnosed cases of trisomy 13 die in utero. Those who survive have severe intellectual disability and medical complications due to multiple anomalies.

- **Trisomy 18** (Edwards syndrome) is most commonly (>90%) due to meiotic primary nondisjunction giving rise to a 47,XX/47,XY, +18 genotype but can also be due to mosaic or partial trisomy 18. Life expectancy for these infants is usually very limited, with 50% of newborns dying within the first 2 weeks of life and only 5% to 10% surviving to or beyond 1 year of age. Anomalies associated with trisomy 18 may include growth restriction, microcephaly, micrognathia, heart defects, kidney defects, clenched fists with overlapping fingers, and rocker bottom feet. The majority of prenatally diagnosed cases of trisomy 18 die in utero. Those who survive have severe intellectual disability and medical complications due to multiple anomalies.

Turner Syndrome

- **Turner syndrome** (monosomy X) is usually 45,X genotype. Some individuals are mosaic, with both 45,X and 46,XX cell lines, with resultant variable characteristics. Most cases result in early miscarriage. These individuals can have normal intelligence or some degree of learning disability, short stature, and infertility. Anomalies associated with Turner syndrome include a thickened nuchal fold, lymphedema of the hands and feet, skeletal abnormalities, heart defects (coarctation of the aorta), and renal defects.

Triploidy

- **Triploidy** is a rare chromosomal abnormality in which there is one extra haploid set of chromosomes (ie, 69 chromosomes). Most cases are 69,XXY (60%) or 69,XXX (37%). Only 3% of cases are 69,XYY. Triploidy is uniformly fatal within the first few months of life, but most spontaneously abort early in pregnancy. Anomalies associated with triploidy include increased nuchal translucency thickness, placental abnormalities, growth restriction, craniofacial abnormalities, heart defects, NTDs, kidney defects, and limb defects.

COMMON SPECIFIC CONGENITAL ANOMALIES

- **Congenital heart disease** is the most common type of birth defect with a prevalence of approximately 1% and is the leading cause of neonatal death. Common congenital heart defects are described in Table 9-3. The etiology for the majority of these anomalies remains unknown, but there are some known etiologies for CHD, such as maternal diabetes or systemic lupus erythematosus, teratogen exposure, and certain genetic causes such as aneuploidy or 22q11 microdeletion (ie, DiGeorge syndrome). There is a long-established association between congenital heart defects and aneuploidy. The frequency of cytogenetic abnormalities with a congenital heart defect has been estimated to be 33% to 42% prenatally and 5% to 15% postnatally; the discrepancy in these rates is secondary to antenatal death occurring in

Table 9-3 Common Congenital Cardiac Defects

Cardiac Defect	Prevalence[a]	Findings
VSD	41.8	Abnormal communication between left and right ventricles, causing shunt
Atrial septal defect	13.1	Abnormal communication between left and right atria
Tetralogy of Fallot	4.7	VSD, overriding aorta, pulmonary artery stenosis, right ventricular hypertrophy
Coarctation of aorta	4.4	Narrowing of the aorta
Endocardial cushion defect/ atrioventricular septal defect	4.1	Missing "crux" of the heart in four-chamber view
Patent ductus arteriosus	2.9	Open ductus arteriosus, persistent connection between the pulmonary artery and the aorta
Hypoplastic left heart syndrome	2.3	Small left ventricle, aortic atresia, hypoplastic mitral valve
Transposition of great arteries	2.3	Aorta arises from right ventricle and pulmonary artery from left.
Total anomalous pulmonary venous return	0.8	Abnormal venous return of oxygenated blood from the lungs to right atrium instead of to the left atrium
Persistent truncus arteriosus	0.6	Single overriding arterial trunk

Abbreviation: VSD, ventricular septal defect.
[a]Per 10 000 live births.

fetuses with chromosomal abnormalities. The likelihood of a cardiac defect exceeds 50% for Down syndrome and is 90% for trisomies 13 and 18.

- **Prenatal diagnosis** of CHD has increased secondary to advances in ultrasound resolution and fetal echocardiography. A fetal echocardiogram is recommended for any abnormality detected in the standard heart views and for any fetus at high risk for a congenital heart defect (eg, diabetic mother, exposure to a teratogen in the first trimester, previous child with CHD). Some CHDs need a higher level of surveillance during the pregnancy to watch for signs of fetal heart failure in utero. Hydrops in utero is a poor prognostic sign.
- The functional consequences of cardiac anomalies are usually not evident until conversion from fetal to neonatal circulation after birth. Some common defects, such as ventriculoseptal defects and coarctation of the aorta, can be missed on prenatal ultrasounds and fetal echocardiograms.

- **Management** depends on the specific type of cardiac defect. Prenatal management entails offering genetic counseling secondary to the association of a chromosomal or genetic etiology for the CHD, the option of prenatal diagnosis with amniocentesis, and appropriate pediatric cardiology and pediatric cardiac surgery consultations. Most cardiac defects can be corrected surgically, although multiple procedures are usually required. Secondary to the complex nature of these cases, delivery at a tertiary care center is recommended.
- **Neural tube defects** are congenital structural abnormalities of the brain and spine and are the second most common form of structural congenital anomalies. The NTDs result from failure of neuropore closure during the third and fourth weeks after fertilization (fifth and sixth weeks of gestation). The main forms of NTD are anencephaly and spina bifida (Table 9-4). Spina bifida can be closed or open, and there are different types. The prevalence of NTDs is highly variable worldwide, reflecting differences in genetic and environmental predispositions. In the United States, they occur in approximately 5 per 10 000 births. The NTDs may occur as an isolated malformation, in combination with other malformations, as part of a genetic syndrome, or as a result of teratogenic exposure. The NTD risk factors include family history of NTD, poorly controlled diabetes, severe obesity, seizure medications, and poor nutritional status or low folate stores.
  - **Prevention** with preconception folate supplementation (0.4 mg/d) significantly lowers the incidence of NTDs. For women with a previously affected pregnancy, a higher dose of 4.0 mg of daily folate is recommended.
  - **Prenatal screening** by ultrasonography in the second trimester is recommended for all pregnant women with optimal examination between 18 and 22 weeks' gestation. Maternal serum α-fetoprotein (MSAFP) has been used as a primary

Table 9-4	Neural Tube Defects	
	Anencephaly	Spina Bifida
Ultrasound Findings	• Absent cranial vault • Absent telencephalon and encephalon • Polyhydramnios	• Vertebral splaying ± overlying soft tissue • Lemon sign • Banana sign
Associations	• Reported in trisomy 13 and 18 • Additional anomalies in 40%	• Arnold-Chiari type II malformation • Ventriculomegaly • Tethered spinal cord • Aneuploidy (4% in isolation, 14% with other anomalies)
Outcomes	• Fatal	• Severity depends on level of the lesion; worse with higher level defects • With lumbar/sacral: possible bowel, bladder, mobility, and neurologic dysfunction

prenatal screening method for NTDs since the 1980s. The MSAFP is elevated in 89% to 100% of pregnancies complicated by NTDs, and an abnormal value is defined as more than 2.5 times the normal. However, MSAFP can be elevated with multiple gestations, inaccurate dating, or in association with other fetal or placental conditions. It can also be normal in closed NTDs and thus has limited value in prenatal screening. With advances in ultrasonography, MSAFP is less important for detection of NTDs when high-quality, second-trimester fetal anomaly screen via ultrasonography can be obtained.

- **Prenatal diagnosis** can be made by ultrasound with confirmation by amniocentesis for α-fetoprotein and acetylcholinesterase levels. The prenatal ultrasound shows splaying of dorsal vertebral elements and a meningeal sac. Other intracranial findings are the "lemon sign" from scalloping of the frontal bones and the "banana sign" of the compressed cerebellum. Ventriculomegaly is also common along with Arnold Chiari II abnormalities. The NTD is associated with aneuploidy in 4% of isolated cases and in 14% of cases when other anomalies are present.

- **Management** of NTDs entails delivery at a tertiary care center where neonatology and neurosurgery are available. Delivery at term is preferred. The mode of delivery is determined on an individual basis, however; there have been no improved outcomes with cesarean delivery for these fetuses. In terms of when to repair this defect, the Management of Myelomeningocele Study (MOMS) trial compared prenatal versus postnatal closure and found that the children who had prenatal surgery had some improved outcomes but with an increased risk of preterm delivery and uterine dehiscence at delivery.

- **Hydrocephalus** is a pathologic dilatation of the brain's ventricular system due to an increase in intracranial cerebrospinal fluid volume with resultant increased pressure. The majority of cases are secondary to an obstruction at some level in the brain's ventricular system. In the fetus, this appears as **ventriculomegaly**, defined as dilation of the fetal cerebral ventricles and mild lateral ventriculomegaly (1.0-1.2 cm) and is a relatively common finding on second trimester ultrasound. Ventriculomegaly can be a normal variation or it can be secondary to various causes, some of which may result in or be associated with neurologic, motor, and/or cognitive impairment. Causes include structural abnormalities such as brain dysgenesis or atrophy, inability to resorb cerebrospinal fluid, fetal aneuploidy, genetic disorders such as X-linked hydrocephalus (*L1CAM* gene), genetic syndromes, or infections such as cytomegalovirus or toxoplasmosis. A less common cause of ventriculomegaly is cerebral hemorrhage. If this diagnosis is being considered, a workup for neonatal alloimmune thrombocytopenia should be offered (see chapter 20). In most cases of ventriculomegaly, the workup is negative and deemed idiopathic.

- **Prenatal diagnosis** of ventriculomegaly is made when enlarged ventricles are found on second-trimester ultrasound. The fetal biparietal diameter may or may not be increased with the finding of enlarged ventricles. The method for appropriately assessing ventricular size is by measuring the atrial diameter of the lateral ventricle with the fetal head in axial plane and at the level of the frontal horns and cavum septum pellucidum. If the mean diameter is greater than 10 mm, this indicates the presence of ventriculomegaly. After ventriculomegaly is detected, comprehensive sonographic examination for additional anomalies is important for diagnostic workup and appropriate patient counseling.

- **Management** of the pregnancy with enlarged ventricles includes a determination of the cause and follow-up ultrasounds to assess progression, stability, or resolution. Diagnostic studies may include amniocentesis for karyotype, DNA analysis for *L1CAM* mutations, viral studies, and fetal magnetic resonance imaging. A multidisciplinary team that includes perinatologists, genetic counselors, pediatric neurosurgeons, and neonatologists should be involved in the care of this pregnancy. Pregnancy termination may be considered in some cases. Fetuses with ventriculomegaly should be delivered at a tertiary care center where a pediatric neurosurgery team is available. **The timing and mode of delivery** should be based on standard obstetric indications. Because most cases have a normal head circumference, a vaginal delivery is reasonable. Significant head enlargement may preclude vaginal delivery and may be an indication for cesarean delivery and/or early delivery.
- **Prognosis** for ventriculomegaly depends on etiology, severity of ventriculomegaly, and the presence of associated abnormalities. The degree of ventricular dilation is not independently predictive of poor long-term outcome.
- **Congenital diaphragmatic hernia** (CDH) is a failure of the diaphragm to fuse properly during embryologic development, resulting in abdominal contents occupying the thoracic cavity. This creates a mass effect that can lead to underdevelopment of the lungs (pulmonary hypoplasia), potentially resulting in persistent pulmonary hypertension, with significant morbidity and mortality in the newborn. The CDH affects approximately 1 in 2500 newborns. Diaphragmatic hernias are most often unilateral, posterolateral, and left sided.
  - **Prenatal diagnosis** of CDH is accomplished in 60% to 90% of cases by ultrasonography or fetal magnetic resonance imaging. On ultrasound, abdominal contents (stomach, bowel, and/or liver) are seen in the thoracic cavity. Other signs seen on ultrasound are mediastinal shift, polyhydramnios, and abnormal cardiac axis. Associated structural anomalies are found in 40% of cases, and the most common anomalies are congenital heart defect, renal anomalies, central nervous system anomalies, and gastrointestinal anomalies. A detailed ultrasound and a fetal echocardiogram should be performed to assess for additional anomalies. Amniocentesis should be offered for karyotype and chromosomal microarray to evaluate for a chromosomal abnormality or genetic syndrome.
  - **Management** of the pregnancy may include expectant management with prenatal referral to a tertiary center with expertise in caring for infants with CDH, termination of pregnancy, or fetal intervention. A multidisciplinary team that involves MFM, neonatology, pediatric surgery, and genetic counselors can help the patient and her family determine a treatment plan. Delivery should be performed at tertiary center where pediatric extracorporeal membrane oxygenation is available.
  - **Prognosis** has significantly improved in recent years due to advances in techniques of ventilation and extracorporeal membrane oxygenation. Overall, survival now exceeds 80%.
- **Congenital pulmonary airway malformations (CPAM)** are rare developmental lung malformations characterized by an abnormal airway pattern and/or abnormal lung parenchyma that may lead to considerable morbidity and mortality. A CPAM is characterized by a malformation of pulmonary tissue that is cystic or hamartomatous with overgrowth of terminal bronchioles and reduction in the number of alveoli. Lesions can be macrocystic or microcystic. Two conditions included in this

group of disorders are **congenital cystic adenomatoid malformation (CCAM)** and **bronchopulmonary sequestration (BPS)**. These two abnormalities can exist in isolation or as a hybrid of the two lesions. The distinguishing feature is that CCAM typically has a pulmonary blood supply, whereas BPS has blood supply from anomalous systemic vessels.

- **Prenatal diagnosis** is possible for both lesions. In CCAM, prenatal ultrasound shows a lung mass that may be cystic or solid with its vascular supply from the pulmonary artery. A BPS is distinguished from a CCAM by the identification of a systemic (often aortic) feeding vessel on color Doppler sonography. It is often challenging to differentiate between the two in utero and lesions are often hybrid. Additional ultrasound findings with CPAM are pleural effusion, mediastinal shift, hydrops, and polyhydramnios.

- **Management** entails a detailed ultrasound examination and fetal echocardiogram to ensure there are no other anomalies. The incidence of associated chromosomal abnormalities is low; however, amniocentesis for fetal karyotype or microarray is offered, as chromosomal anomalies have been described. These fetuses should be delivered at tertiary care centers, and prenatal consultation with MFM, pediatric surgery, and neonatology is recommended. Pregnancies are serially monitored by an MFM specialist with ultrasound to watch for signs of progression or regression or an associated fetal complication such as hydrops. In the postnatal period, if these lesions persist, surgical excision is usually recommended.

- **Prognosis** is generally favorable for fetuses with CPAM in the absence of fetal hydrops, which is a predictor of poor outcome. The risk of hydrops is highest in fetuses with large lesions that may have mass effect on the vena cava and/or heart. Cases with hydrops and macrocystic lesions should be referred for possible drainage, whereas some evidence suggests those with microcystic lesions respond to maternal administration of betamethasone. In the absence of hydrops, the long-term outcome of infants with CPAM following resection is excellent.

- **Gastroschisis** and **omphalocele** are the two most common fetal abdominal wall defects that are detected in utero. Gastroschisis is an isolated abdominal wall defect where the herniated abdominal contents have no covering membrane. Omphalocele is a defect in the abdominal wall in which a membrane of peritoneum covers the herniated abdominal contents (Table 9-5).

- **Prenatal screening:** Both defects are associated with an elevated MSAFP.

- **Prenatal diagnosis** is usually made by ultrasound. Gastroschisis is not associated with an increased risk for aneuploidy. Omphalocele has a high incidence of associated malformations and chromosomal abnormalities. Amniocentesis for fetal karyotype and genetic testing should be offered in the case of omphalocele. Additionally, there is an increased incidence of congenital heart defects in cases of omphalocele, and fetal echocardiography is recommended.

- **Management** in pregnancy entails serial ultrasound assessments to follow the amount and type of abdominal contents that are herniated. A multidisciplinary team should be involved including MFM, genetic counseling, neonatology, and pediatric surgery. Delivery at a tertiary care center enables optimal care of the newborn. The mode of delivery can be vaginal in most cases, if standard obstetrical indications are met.

- **Prognosis** of infants with abdominal wall defects depends on whether there is the presence of other anomalies or an underlying chromosomal anomaly.

Table 9-5	Gastroschisis and Omphalocele	
	Gastroschisis	Omphalocele
Umbilical cord location	Umbilical cord inserts to left of the defect (with bowel herniation to the right)	Umbilical cord enters into the membrane-covered midline defect (with herniation of abdominal contents into base of cord)
Physical findings	• No covering membrane • Varies in size • Small bowel ± liver • Oligohydramnios > polyhydramnios	• Covered by membrane • Varies in size • Contains bowel loops ± liver
Additional anomalies	• Usually isolated • Increased risk for IUGR • Intestinal atresia in 10%-15%	• Additional structural anomalies common (25%-30%) • Cardiac defects • Gastrointestinal defects
Associated genetic abnormality	• No association with chromosomal abnormalities • Most are sporadic.	• 30%-40% with chromosomal abnormality • Association with Beckwith-Wiedemann and other syndromes

Abbreviation: IUGR, intrauterine growth restriction.

- **Congenital renal anomalies** can be diagnosed in the prenatal period and include renal agenesis, multicystic dysplastic kidney disease (MCKD), infantile polycystic kidney disease, and hydronephrosis secondary to ureteropelvic junction (UPJ) obstruction and outlet obstruction.
  - **Renal agenesis** can be unilateral or bilateral. Unilateral renal agenesis has a normal prognosis, and there is usually compensatory hypertrophy of the contralateral side. A portion of patients with unilateral renal agenesis have contralateral vesicoureteral reflux. Bilateral renal agenesis is rarely diagnosed prior to 18 weeks' gestation because the fetal kidneys do not contribute to the majority of amniotic fluid until after this gestation. On the prenatal ultrasound, the fetal kidneys and bladder are not visualized. This condition causes severe oligohydramnios or anhydramnios and is lethal secondary to severe pulmonary hypoplasia. Case reports have suggested the possibility of survival with serial amnioinfusions to preserve the fetal lungs. Surviving infants would still require dialysis and renal transplant. Current trials are in process to evaluate this fetal intervention.
  - **Multicystic dysplastic kidney disease** is a severe renal abnormality characterized by increased renal size and numerous large noncommunicating cysts alternating with areas of increased echogenicity on ultrasound. Because of the size of the kidney and the numerous cysts, this is usually detected by prenatal ultrasound. The MCKD is usually unilateral. In almost half of cases, the contralateral kidney has other malformations, the severity of which determines the overall prognosis. There is also an association with other nongenitourinary anomalies and some genetic syndromes. Amniocentesis should be offered during

a prenatal consultation. With unilateral MCKD, prenatal pediatric urology consultation is recommended. Bilateral multicystic dysplasia is associated with severe oligohydramnios and is fatal secondary to pulmonary hypoplasia.

- **Polycystic kidney disease** encompasses two inherited disorders with diffuse involvement of both kidneys. **Autosomal recessive polycystic kidney disease** is a single-gene disorder inherited in an autosomal recessive fashion. From the perspective of prenatal diagnosis and neonatal presentation, the recessive polycystic kidney disease is much more common. This disease is characterized by bilateral, enlarged, echogenic kidneys. Oligohydramnios can be present. The main cause of perinatal morbidity and mortality is pulmonary hypoplasia. Aggressive neonatal management has led to 1-year survival rates of 82% to 85% in autosomal recessive polycystic kidney disease. If infants survive the first month of life, they are predicted to live for many years. **Autosomal dominant polycystic kidney disease** rarely presents in the prenatal period; this disease usually has clinical findings in the third or fourth decade of life. Sonogram reveals enlarged kidneys with multiple cysts. Individuals with this form of polycystic kidney disease also have liver cysts, pancreatic cysts, and intracranial aneurysms. Renal ultrasound is recommended in both parents to evaluate for autosomal dominant polycystic kidney disease.

- **Urinary tract dilation** is diagnosed when the fetal renal pelvis is >0.4 cm at the time of an anatomy ultrasound. A follow-up ultrasound to evaluate for resolution or progression is recommended at 32 weeks' gestation. The most common etiology of pathologic fetal urinary tract dilation is **ureteropelvic junction obstruction**, which prevents urinary flow from the renal pelvis to the ureter. Most cases are unilateral; bilateral cases have a worse prognosis. Pregnancy management is generally unchanged in unilateral cases, but with bilateral UPJ obstruction, a fetal intervention of urinary shunting may be necessary. There is an overall increased incidence of chromosomal abnormalities with obstructive uropathy, thus amniocentesis for prenatal karyotype should be offered. A consultation with a pediatric urologist should be offered to the patient as well. With isolated UPJ obstruction, the prognosis is usually favorable.

- Bladder outlet obstructions have the potential to affect the entire urinary and pulmonary system. In males, the most common cause of bladder outlet obstruction is **posterior urethral valves**. In females, the most common cause is **urethral atresia**. The characteristic prenatal finding on ultrasound is a dilated bladder (megacystis) and bilateral hydroureteronephrosis. With posterior urethral valves, the bladder wall is thickened, and the urethra may have a characteristic keyhole appearance. There is an association with chromosomal abnormalities, thus amniocentesis and fetal karyotype should be offered in cases of bladder outlet obstruction. In utero interventions may be helpful in some cases, but there is often severe irreversible renal impairment. Pediatric urology consultation should be offered prenatally. Prognosis is determined by evaluation of amniotic fluid volume. The degree of oligohydramnios determines the extent of pulmonary hypoplasia, which is the most important determinant of prognosis for the fetus.

- **Musculoskeletal disorders** can be diagnosed prenatally. The most common skeletal dysplasia disorders that are diagnosed prenatally are **achondroplasia**, **thanatophoric dysplasia**, and **osteogenesis imperfecta** (Table 9-6). Ultrasound findings include shortened limbs, three to four standard deviations below the mean for gestational age as well as abnormalities in the skull, spine, and thorax. Options for further management of the pregnancy may depend on these ultrasound findings because type II osteogenesis imperfecta and thanatophoric dysplasia are lethal.

Table 9-6 Skeletal Dysplasias

Type of Dysplasia and Gene Mutation	Description	Outcome
Achondroplasia FGFR3	• Rhizomelic shortening of limbs • Frontal bossing • "Collar hoop" sign: rounded metaphyseal epiphyseal interface at the femur	• Normal intelligence • Joint problems • Craniocervical junction problems • Obstructive sleep apnea • Middle ear dysfunction • Kyphosis
Thanatophoric dysplasia FGFR3	• Very short extremities • Platyspondyly—flattened vertebral ossification centers • Small chest • Telephone receiver femur (type I) • Cloverleaf skull (type II)	Usually lethal
Osteogenesis imperfecta COL1A1 COL1A2 CRTAP/LEPRE1	• Bone fractures • Irregularity and angulation to long bones • Decreased skull ossification • Irregular shape of ribs	• Type II perinatal lethal • Variable features and disease severity based on the type of osteogenesis imperfecta

SUGGESTED READINGS

Agathoukleous M, Chaveeva P, Poon LCY, Kosinki P, Nicolaides KH. Meta-analysis of second-trimester markers for trisomy 21. *Ultrasound Obstet Gynecol.* 2013;41:247-261.

American College of Obstetricians and Gynecologists Committee on Practice Bulletins—Obstetrics. ACOG Practice Bulletin No. 162: prenatal diagnostic testing for genetic disorders. *Obstet Gynecol.* 2016;127:e108-e122. (Reaffirmed 2018)

American College of Obstetricians and Gynecologists Committee on Practice Bulletins—Obstetrics. ACOG Practice Bulletin No. 163: screening for fetal aneuploidy. *Obstet Gynecol.* 2016;127:e123-e137. (Reaffirmed 2018)

American College of Obstetricians and Gynecologists Committee on Practice Bulletins—Obstetrics, American Institute of Ultrasound in Medicine. ACOG Practice Bulletin No. 175: ultrasound in pregnancy. *Obstet Gynecol.* 2016;128:e241-e256. (Reaffirmed 2018)

Cunningham F, Leveno KJ, Bloom SL, et al, eds. Prenatal diagnosis. In: *Williams Obstetrics.* 24th ed. New York, NY: McGraw-Hill; 2013:283-305.

Driscoll DA, Simpson JL, Holzgreve W, Otaño L. Genetic screening and prenatal genetic diagnosis. In: Gabbe SG, Niebyl JR, Simpson JL, et al, eds. *Obstetrics: Normal and Problem Pregnancies.* 7th ed. Philadelphia, PA: Saunders; 2017:193-218.

Fox NS, Monteagudo A, Kuller JA, Craigo S, Norton ME; for Society for Maternal-Fetal Medicine. Mild fetal ventriculomegaly: diagnosis, evaluation, and management. *Am J Obstet Gynecol.* 2018;219:B2-B9.

10 Multifetal Gestation
Sunitha Suresh and Julia Timofeev

- The incidence of multifetal gestation has increased over the last several decades, now accounting for approximately 3% of all live births in the United States. Factors attributed to increasing multiple gestation rate include assisted reproductive technologies and increasing maternal age at birth. Other risk factors for multifetal gestation include race, family history, increasing parity, maternal weight and height, and possibly diet.
- Multiple gestation carries increased maternal and perinatal morbidity and mortality.
  - The majority of *perinatal* mortality and morbidity is associated with prematurity. In the United States, multifetal gestations account for nearly 25% of all very low-birth-weight (<1500 g) babies. The average duration of pregnancy is 35.3 weeks for twin gestation, 31.9 weeks for triplets, and 29.5 weeks for quadruplets. Perinatal mortality rate is higher for multifetal gestation, with infant mortality rates of 5/1000 live births for twin pregnancy, 20/1000 live births for triplet, and 47/1000 live births for quadruplets. Twin and higher order pregnancies have a higher rate of fetal growth restriction and congenital anomalies.
  - In terms of *maternal* mortality and morbidity, twin pregnancies are associated with higher risk of hypertension, preterm labor, preeclampsia, hemolysis, elevated liver enzymes, low platelets (HELLP), placental abruption, gestational diabetes, postpartum hemorrhage, acute fatty liver, preterm premature rupture of membranes (PPROM), and anemia.
- Maternal physiologic changes are exaggerated in multifetal gestation in comparison to singleton pregnancy. Levels of progesterone, estradiol, estriol, human placental lactogen, human chorionic gonadotropin, and α-fetoprotein are elevated. Maternal heart rate is increased by 4% and stroke volume increased by 15% in comparison to singletons. Maternal blood expansion is 50% to 60% as compared to 40% to 50% in singleton pregnancies; this expansion in plasma volume can lead to more significant dilutional anemia as well as an increased risk of pleural edema and other complications.

DIAGNOSIS

- Diagnosis of multiple gestation is confirmed by sonogram most accurately in the first trimester, when separate gestational sacs are easily seen to determine chorionicity: the "twin-peak" sign (also known as the "lambda sign") for dichorionic twins and the "T sign" for monochorionic diamniotic twins. Early determination of chorionicity is critical for guidance of further clinical care. Dichorionic chorionicity can be confirmed at later gestational age based on two placentas or differing fetal sex. Twin fetuses most commonly result from fertilization of two separate ova (dizygotic or fraternal twins). Monozygotic or identical twins arise when a single ovum divides after fertilization (Figure 10-1).

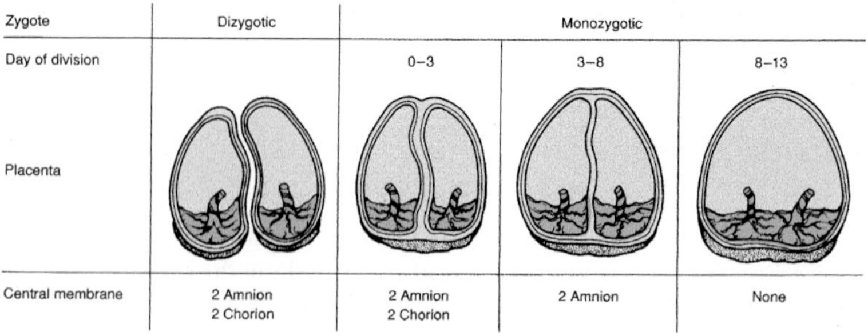

Zygote	Dizygotic	Monozygotic		
Day of division		0–3	3–8	8–13
Placenta				
Central membrane	2 Amnion 2 Chorion	2 Amnion 2 Chorion	2 Amnion	None

Figure 10-1. Types of placentation in dizygotic and monozygotic twinning. Reprinted with permission from Gibbs RS, Danforth DN. *Danforth's Obstetrics and Gynecology.* 10th ed. Philadelphia, PA: Wolters Kluwer Health/Lippincott Williams & Wilkins; 2008:222. Figure 14.1.

- **Dizygotic dichorionic/diamnionic twins** (70%-80% of all twins) result from the fertilization of two ova. Each fetus has its own placenta and a complete and separate amnion-chorion membrane. Before 8 weeks' gestation, separate gestational sacs surrounded by a thick echogenic ring is suggestive of dichorionicity.
- **Monozygotic twins** (20%-30% of all twins) result from cleavage of a single, fertilized conceptus. The timing of cleavage determines the placentation. This is more likely if separate echogenic rings are not visible before 8 weeks' gestation.
  - **Dichorionic/diamnionic monozygotic twins** (8% of all twins) result from cleavage in the first 3 days after fertilization. They will have separate amnions and chorions, just like dizygotic twins. They have the lowest perinatal mortality rate of all monozygotic twins.
  - **Monochorionic/diamnionic twins** (14%-20% of all twins) are produced by cleavage between days 4 and 8 after fertilization. They share a single placenta but have separate amniotic sacs. Two fetal poles with two yolk sacs suggest diamnionicity. The mortality rate for monochorionic/diamniotic twins is approximately 3 times higher than for dichorionic gestation.
  - **Monochorionic/monoamnionic twins** (<1% of cases) are produced by cleavage after the eighth day. The fetuses share a single placenta and a single amnionic sac because both amnion and chorion were formed before cleavage. Later cleavage is even more rare and results in conjoined fetuses. Two fetal poles with only one yolk sac suggest monoamnionic gestation. Monoamnionic gestations have historically been reported to have mortality up to 50% to 60%; however, more recent reports suggest mortality rate to be much lower.
- **Higher order multiples** have more frequent placental anomalies. Monochorionic and dichorionic placentation may both be present.

ANTEPARTUM MANAGEMENT

- **Diet, supplementation, weight gain recommendations:** Supplementation with 60 to 120 mg of elemental iron and 1 mg of folic acid is recommended due to increased risk for anemia related to iron deficiency/folate deficiency. Dietary intake for a woman with normal body mass index (BMI) should be approximately 300 kcal/day additional calories per fetus. Weight gain recommendations from the Institute of Medicine for twin gestations are 37 to 54 lb for a normal weight (BMI 18.5-24.9 mg/kg^2), 31 to 50 lb for overweight (BMI 25-29.9 mg/kg^2), and 25 to 42 lb for obese women (BMI >30 mg/kg^2). No recommendations are available for those who are underweight prepregnancy, and there is insufficient evidence to determine weight gain goals for higher order gestations.

- **Growth assessment:** Serial ultrasonography is used to assess fetal growth, typically every 3 to 4 weeks from 18 to 20 weeks' gestation. Serial ultrasonography can be every 2 to 3 weeks for monochorionic twins or if growth restriction/discordance is discovered. At 30 to 32 weeks, intrauterine growth of twins lags behind those of singletons. Growth is still determined typically based on singleton growth curves.
- **Aneuploidy screening:** Maternal serum screening tests are not as sensitive in multifetal gestations. Due to limitations of serum markers for the first trimester screen in multifetal gestations, the nuchal translucency can be used for aneuploidy screening. Chorionic villus sampling and amniocentesis can be done to definitively rule out aneuploidy and are associated with similar pregnancy loss rates in comparison to singleton gestations. There is a 1% risk of sampling error for chorionic villus sampling. Certain commercial laboratories offer noninvasive prenatal screening using cell-free DNA. Validation studies are limited by small number of patients, and this testing approach is not currently recommended by American College of Obstetricians and Gynecologists.
- **Antenatal testing:** Antenatal testing has not been validated for routine use; however, it is widely used in management of multiple gestations. Surveillance is indicated for significant growth restriction, growth discordance, and other routine obstetric indications such as oligohydramnios, decreased fetal movement, or maternal medical complications.

MATERNAL COMPLICATIONS

Medical complications associated with multifetal gestation include hyperemesis, hypertension, gestational diabetes, acute fatty liver, anemia, hemorrhage, increased risk of cesarean delivery and postpartum depression.

- Hyperemesis: The etiology is unclear but may be secondary to higher levels of human chorionic gonadotropin. Treatment for hyperemesis should be the same as with a singleton pregnancy.
- Hypertensive disorders of pregnancy and preeclampsia
  - Prevalence/etiology: Gestational hypertension and preeclampsia range from 10% to 20% in twins, 25% to 60% in triplets, and up to 90% in quadruplet pregnancies. This is thought to be in part secondary to the larger placental mass. Often, preeclampsia is more atypical in presentation in higher order multiple gestation, occurring earlier in pregnancy and is often more severe.
  - Management: Low-dose aspirin is recommended for preeclampsia prevention in multifetal gestation, starting in the first trimester between 12 weeks and 28 weeks, and ideally prior to 16 weeks. Delivery timing for indication of hypertensive disorders of pregnancy is the same as with singleton pregnancies.
- Gestational diabetes
  - Prevalence/etiology: There are no official guidelines regarding the timing of screening of gestational diabetes in multiple gestation; however, some experts suggest screening around 20 to 24 weeks given increased incidence of gestational diabetes with multifetal gestation.

- Management is the same as with a singleton pregnancy, with insulin often preferred as first-line treatment if dietary changes and exercise are not sufficient to achieve euglycemia.
- Acute fatty liver of pregnancy. Multiple gestation is a risk factor for acute fatty liver and should be considered in a differential when a woman with multiple gestation presents with hepatic dysfunction. Acute fatty liver is one of the imitators of HELLP syndrome. The typical onset is from 27 to 40 weeks' gestation. Symptoms may include malaise, anorexia, nausea, vomiting, and epigastric pain. Physical examination findings include jaundice, hypertension, proteinuria, and/or bleeding from coagulopathy. Typical lab findings include abnormal coagulation factors, elevated creatinine, and/or bilirubin. Maternal morbidity was previously reported as high as 70% but now is thought to be <10% secondary to higher supportive care. Perinatal morbidity and mortality are both increased. Treatment includes supportive care and delivery.

FETAL COMPLICATIONS

- Miscarriage and spontaneous reduction/vanishing twin: The overall miscarriage rate is higher in twin pregnancies (up to 7.3% per live birth) when compared to singleton pregnancies. One twin is lost before the second trimester in up to 10% to 40% of all twin pregnancies, with a higher rate in setting of assisted reproductive technologies. Miscarriage is higher in monochorionic twins than dichorionic gestations. Diagnosis of vanishing twin is important for serum maternal screening because serum markers are less precise if vanishing twin is diagnosed after 9 weeks, and testing ideally would be delayed by at least 4 weeks from demise of one twin. Maternal serum α-fetoprotein values can also be falsely elevated after the demise of one twin.
- Chromosomal abnormalities and congenital malformations: Incidence of congenital malformations is higher in comparison to singletons and also higher in monochorionic twins in comparison to dichorionic twins.
- Preterm birth
  - Prevalence: Preterm birth occurs in >50% of twin and 75% of triplet gestation.
  - Screening/prevention: Transvaginal cervical length assessment, routine digital examination, fetal fibronectin screening, and home monitoring have all been studied in asymptomatic women with multifetal gestations. None of these interventions has been shown to reduce the risk of spontaneous preterm delivery. Shortened cervix is associated with an increased risk of preterm delivery in singleton and multifetal gestations. For symptomatic women, positive predictive value of fetal fibronectin and cervical length is poor. Cerclage placement in women with multiple gestation complicated by short cervix has been observed to possibly double the rate of spontaneous preterm birth (studies are ongoing on potential benefit of cerclage placement in a subset of women with very short cervix of <15 mm). Bed rest was shown to have no benefit in prevention of preterm birth in a Cochrane review and is potentially dangerous because it results in deconditioning the mother and increasing the risk of thrombosis. There is no role for prophylactic or prolonged tocolytic use, and use of these agents has been associated with greater risk of maternal complications such as pulmonary edema. There is conflicting evidence regarding pessary placement for prevention of preterm delivery with a short cervix. There may be a benefit

for vaginal progesterone in the setting of a short cervix (less than 25 mm) and multiple gestation; however, prophylactic vaginal progesterone has not been shown to improve outcomes. Injectable 17-hydroxyprogesterone therapy has not been shown to be beneficial in reducing preterm delivery in multiple gestations.

- Management (steroids, PPROM, delayed delivery of second twin): Although there is no data specifically addressing antenatal steroid administration in multifetal gestations, corticosteroids are recommended to be administered to pregnant women between 24 0/7 and 33 6/7 weeks of gestation for those at risk of delivery within the next 7 days. Steroids may also be considered as early as 23 0/7 weeks' gestation. Whether multiple gestations benefit from administration of late preterm steroids is unknown. PPROM should be managed as in a singleton pregnancy. Median latency has been shown to be shorter with multifetal pregnancy than with a singleton. If delayed delivery of a second twin is attempted, the patient must be extensively counseled on significant risks associated with this approach, potential limited benefits (depending on gestational age and other considerations such as estimated fetal weight), and if elected, must be carefully monitored for infection, abruption, and other fetal and maternal complications (such as life-threatening infection).

- Growth discordance and fetal growth restriction: Growth discordance in monochorionic twins is usually attributed to abnormal placental vascular anastomoses and unequal sharing of placental mass, whereas in dizygotic pregnancies, it may be due to suboptimal implantation site of one of the placentas. Discordance is defined as a discrepancy of more than 20% in the estimated fetal weights and is calculated as a percentage of the larger twin's weight. Causes include twin-to-twin transfusion syndrome (TTTS), chromosomal or structural anomalies in either twin, discordant viral infection, and unequal division of the placental mass. When discordance exceeds 25%, the fetal and neonatal death rates increase 6.5-fold and 2.5-fold, respectively. Earlier discordance indicates a higher risk of fetal demise in the smaller twin.

- Complications of monochorionic gestation
  - Conjoined twins: This is a rare anomaly with an incidence of 1 in 50 000. Prognosis is poor given the presence of congenital anomalies. There is only an 18% overall survival rate.
  - Monochorionic-monoamniotic twins: These pregnancies are associated with increased risk of fetal death secondary to cord entanglement, anomalies, preterm birth, and TTTS. Due to unpredictability of cord entanglement, there is no clear prevention method. Typically, inpatient management with daily surveillance from 26 to 27 weeks has been shown to decrease stillbirth, with delivery around 32 to 34 weeks.
  - Monochorionic-diamniotic twins: These pregnancies are at higher risk for complications including TTTS, twin anemia polycythemia sequence (TAPS), and selective growth restriction. Delivery is recommended between 36 weeks and 37 6/7 weeks if the clinical course is otherwise uncomplicated.

- Special considerations
  - TTTS and management: TTTS occurs due to an imbalance in blood flow through arteriovenous communications in the placenta, leading to overperfusion of one twin and underperfusion of the second twin. The donor fetus typically demonstrates fetal growth restriction and oligohydramnios, and the recipient

fetus can be hyperperfused, hypertensive, and have polyhydramnios. The most important criterion is discrepancy in amniotic fluid with maximum vertical pocket <2 cm around donor and maximum vertical pocket >8 cm around the recipient. Management approaches include selective fetoscopic laser coagulation of placental anastomoses, serial reduction amniocentesis, amniotic septostomy, and delivery, depending on stage and gestational age at diagnosis. Fetoscopic laser coagulation of placental anastomoses is the primary treatment between 16 to 26 weeks, after which the other modalities may be considered.

- TAPS and management: TAPS can be diagnosed when the middle cerebral artery peak systolic velocity is greater than 1.5 multiples of the median in one fetus and less than 0.8 multiples of the median in the other fetus, but without any obvious amniotic fluid discrepancy. A TAPS can occur following laser treatment of TTTS in up to 13% of cases and can also be seen in approximately 5% of twin pregnancies never diagnosed with TTTS. Management depends on gestational age and can include preterm delivery, fetal transfusion, or repeat laser coagulation.

- Twin reversed arterial perfusion and management: Twin reversed arterial perfusion is specific to monochorionic twin gestations where one twin does not have a functioning heart. This results in a donor twin, or "pump" twin, who provides circulation for it and the recipient, the acardiac twin. Diagnosis is based on one normal appearing fetus and one abnormal appearing fetus. The pump twin may have polyhydramnios, cardiomegaly, and tricuspid regurgitation. Management is based on maximizing outcomes for the structurally normal pump twin, who is at risk for hydrops and may include prophylactic cord interruption at 16 to 18 weeks or delaying intervention until there are signs of cardiac decompensation.

- Fetal demise (of both fetuses) in the first trimester is generally considered a vanishing twin and does not carry significant risk to the remaining fetus. After the first trimester, risk of death/injury is more significant in monochorionic twin gestations because the remaining fetus may experience hypotension following the demise of the other twin, with risk of neurologic injury of up to 26% in the surviving twin. Death of a single fetus in utero increases the risk of demise and the risk of preterm birth for the co-twin, regardless of chorionicity.

DELIVERY

- Timing of delivery: The optimal time for delivery for multiple gestations is not well established. All twin fetuses should be delivered by 39 weeks' gestation, and uncomplicated dichorionic diamniotic twin gestations can undergo delivery after 38 weeks' gestation. Rate of stillbirth in multiple gestations at 39 weeks surpasses the risk of fetal death in singleton gestations greater than 42 weeks. For monochorionic twins, delivery should be considered at 36 to 37 weeks if otherwise uncomplicated. If fetal growth restriction, TAPS, or any other complications are present, delivery should be considered at 34 to 35 weeks. Although there are no high-quality studies to guide delivery of monochorionic/monoamniotic twin gestations, many experts consider delivery reasonable at 32 to 34 weeks' gestation.

- Mode of delivery: The optimal route of delivery for twins remains controversial and should be assessed on a case-by-case basis. Decisions about delivery must consider fetal presentations, gestational age, maternal or fetal complications, the experience of the obstetrician, and the availability of anesthesia and neonatal intensive care support. Monoamniotic monochorionic twin gestations are delivered via cesarean. Data from a large multicenter study found no benefit for planned cesarean for term twin pregnancy. There is no evidence regarding trial of labor after cesarean delivery for twin delivery, and these patients may be considered candidates. American College of Obstetricians and Gynecologists supports trial of labor after cesarean delivery for multiple gestation. In practice, twin deliveries are generally performed as a double set-up in the operating room.

- Vertex/vertex (43%) presentation can achieve a successful vaginal delivery in 70% to 80% of cases. Surveillance of twin B between deliveries is advised. Increasing interval time of delivery is associated with worse outcomes.
- Vertex/nonvertex (38%) presentation can achieve a vaginal delivery if estimated fetal weights are concordant. External cephalic version or internal podalic version and breech extraction of twin B may be attempted by an experienced operator. Vaginal delivery of twin B in nonvertex presentation may be considered for infants with an estimated weight between 1500 and 3500 g. Success rates are more than 96%. There is insufficient data to advocate a specific route of delivery for a second twin weighing <1500 g.
- Nonvertex presenting twins (19%) are typically delivered by cesarean for both fetuses.
- Locked twins is a rare condition occurring with breech/vertex twins, when the body of twin A delivers, but the chin "locks" behind the chin of twin B. Hypertonicity, monoamnionic twinning, or reduced amniotic fluid may contribute to interlocking fetal heads.
- Intrapartum/postpartum complications: Intrapartum complications including malpresentation, cord prolapse, cord entanglement, dysfunctional labor, fetal distress, and urgent cesarean delivery are more common for multiple gestations compared with singletons. The risk of uterine atony and postpartum hemorrhage is significantly increased.

SPECIAL CONSIDERATIONS

- Triplet/higher order gestation: There is no established ideal method of delivery for higher order multiples, with most being delivered via cesarean.
- Single anomalous fetus: Expectant management can lead to a 20% increase in risk of preterm delivery for the pregnancy overall.
- Selective reduction: For dichorionic gestation, ultrasound-guided intracardiac injection of potassium chloride is most commonly used for selective reduction. For monochorionic gestations, complete ablation of umbilical cord of anomalous fetus is suggested to avoid death/injury to the normal fetus. Cord ligation for a monochorionic twin can have up to a 10% failure rate and up to a 30% risk for PPROM.
- Multifetal pregnancy reduction can be considered for higher order multiple gestations. This is typically performed between 10 and 13 weeks' gestation. Reduction of triplets to twins has been shown to prolong gestation but has an increased risk of earlier miscarriage. Multifetal reduction also has been shown to possibly decrease risk of maternal complications, including preeclampsia. Typically, the fetuses are chosen based on technical considerations.

SUGGESTED READING

American College of Obstetricians and Gynecologists Committee on Practice Bulletins—Obstetrics. ACOG Practice Bulletin No. 169: multifetal gestations: twin, triplet, and higher-order multifetal pregnancies. *Obstet Gynecol.* 2016;128:e131-e146. (Reaffirmed 2019)

Hofmeyr GJ, Barrett JF, Crowther CA. Planned cesarean section for women with a twin pregnancy. *Cochrane Database Syst Rev.* 2015;(12):CD006553.

Jarde A, Lutsiv O, Park CK, et al. Preterm birth prevention in twin pregnancies with progesterone, pessary or cerclage: a systematic review and meta-analysis. *BJOG.* 2017;124(8): 1163-1173.

Kristiansen MK, Joensen BS, Ekelund CK, Petersen OB, Sandager P; and Danish Fetal Medicine Group. Perinatal outcome after first-trimester risk assessment in monochorionic and dichorionic twin pregnancies: a population-based register study. *BJOG.* 2015;122(10): 1362-1369.

Murray SR, Stock SJ, Cowan S, Cooper ES, Norman JE. Spontaneous preterm birth prevention in multiple pregnancy. *Obstet Gynaecol.* 2018;20(1):57-63.

Endocrine Disorders of Pregnancy

Tenisha Wilson and Svena D. Julien

DIABETES MELLITUS

Diabetes mellitus (DM) is the most common medical complication of pregnancy in the United States, affecting nearly 7% of all pregnancies. As the incidence of type 2 DM increases nationwide, cases of gestational diabetes mellitus (GDM) have also grown. In 86% of diabetic pregnancies, the cause is GDM.

- Diabetes in pregnancy is categorized as pregestational diabetes (diagnosed prior to pregnancy) or gestational diabetes (GDM) (carbohydrate intolerance developed during pregnancy). Pregestational diabetes is further classified as type 1 or type 2 (Table 11-1). One half percent to 1% of pregnancies are complicated by pregestational DM.

- Carbohydrate metabolism changes during pregnancy to provide adequate nutrition for both the mother and the fetus. In the fasting state, maternal serum glucose is lower in pregnancy than in the nonpregnant state (55-65 mg/dL), whereas free fatty acid, triglyceride, and plasma ketone concentrations are increased. A state of relative maternal starvation exists in pregnancy, during which glucose is spared for fetal consumption and alternate fuels are used by the mother.

- The GDM is similar to type 2 DM, in which increased pancreatic secretion of insulin cannot overcome decreased insulin sensitivity of maternal target tissues. Increased metabolism in pregnancy also increases insulin clearance. These changes are due to the effects of estrogen, progesterone, cortisol, prolactin, and human placental lactogen. The net result is maternal hyperglycemia.

Table 11-1	Comparison of Type 1 and Type 2 Diabetes Mellitus
Type 1	**Type 2**
Pathophysiology is absolute insulin deficiency.	Pathophysiology is tissue resistance to insulin.
Patients are at risk for severe hypoglycemia and DKA.	Patients may develop HONK. DKA is rare.
DKA can be encountered at relatively low blood glucose levels (<200 mg/dL).	HONK usually encountered at higher blood glucose levels (>500 mg/dL)
Increased risk for chronic microvascular disease at an early age	Lower incidence of microvascular disease during reproductive age range

Abbreviations: DKA, diabetic ketoacidosis; HON, hyperosmolar nonketotic coma.

Pregestational Diabetes Mellitus

Diagnosis

- The diagnosis of types 1 and 2 DM before pregnancy is by standard criteria: two abnormal fasting glucose levels ≥126 mg/dL or a random glucose level of ≥200 mg/dL.
- In a nonpregnant patient, screening includes one of the following:
  - Hemoglobin A1C ≥6.5%, confirmed on a repeat test
  - Fasting plasma glucose ≥126 mg/dL (7.0 mmol/L), with no caloric intake for at least 8 hours and confirmed on a repeat test
  - Two-hour plasma glucose ≥200 mg/dL (11.1 mmol/L) using an oral glucose tolerance test with a 75-g glucose load and confirmed on a repeat test
  - Random plasma glucose ≥200 mg/dL (11.1 mmol/L) with the presence of classic symptoms of hyperglycemia or hyperglycemic crisis
- Classic symptoms are polydipsia, polyuria, and polyphagia. Clinical signs include weight loss, hyperglycemia, persistent glucosuria, and ketoacidosis.

Fetal Complications

- Fetal and neonatal complications of DM in pregnancy are increased with both gestational and pregestational DM, but the incidence is much higher in pregestational DM and with poor glycemic control. Fetal glucose levels are similar to maternal blood glucose levels, and both fetal hyperglycemia and hypoglycemia have important effects.
- Spontaneous abortion ranges between 6% and 29% with pregestational DM and correlates with poor glucose control and an elevated hemoglobin A1C (HbA1C) around the time of conception. Type 1 and type 2 DM carry the same risk of pregnancy loss, but the main causes of fetal loss for type 1 DM are congenital anomalies and complications of prematurity, whereas for type 2 DM, they are in utero fetal demise, fetal hypoxia, and chorioamnionitis. The incidence of spontaneous abortion

in diabetics with excellent preconception glucose control (ie, HbA1C <6%) is the same as in the general population.

- Congenital malformations are the most common cause of perinatal mortality in pregestational diabetic pregnancies and correlate with maternal hyperglycemia and elevated HbA1C. Congenital anomalies account for 30% to 50% of perinatal mortality from diabetes, and 6% to 10% of infants of diabetic mothers have a major congenital anomaly (see chapter 9). However, there is no increase in congenital malformations when euglycemic and a normal HbA1C is present from conception through the first trimester.
  - The most common congenital malformations in diabetic pregnancies are in the cardiovascular and central nervous systems. Cardiac defects include transposition of the great vessels, ventricular and atrial septal defects, hypoplastic left ventricle, situs inversus, anomalies of the aorta, and complex cardiac anomalies. The rate of cardiac malformations is 5-fold higher in diabetics under poor glycemic control.
  - Sacral agenesis/caudal regression is highly suggestive of diabetic fetopathy. It is a rare malformation but diagnosed up to 400 times more frequently in diabetic pregnancies and is nearly pathognomonic for uncontrolled diabetes.
  - There is a 10-fold increase in the incidence of central nervous system malformations in infants of diabetic mothers, including anencephaly, holoprosencephaly, open spina bifida, microcephaly, encephalocele, and meningomyelocele.
  - Gastrointestinal system malformations, including tracheoesophageal fistula, bowel atresia, and imperforate anus, are also increased in diabetic gestations.
  - Genitourinary system anomalies including absent kidneys (leading to Potter syndrome), polycystic kidneys, and double ureter are more common in pregnancies complicated by diabetes.
- Polyhydramnios occurs in 3% to 32% of diabetic pregnancies, 30 times the rate for nondiabetic gestations. Diabetes alone is the leading known cause of polyhydramnios. Furthermore, diabetes-associated congenital anomalies of the central nervous and gastrointestinal systems can also lead to polyhydramnios. Mechanisms of polyhydramnios include increased fetal glycemic load resulting in polyuria, decreased fetal swallowing, and fetal gastrointestinal obstructions. Higher perinatal morbidity and mortality rates are associated with polyhydramnios, attributed in part to the higher incidence of both congenital anomalies and preterm delivery.
- Macrosomia is defined as an estimated fetal weight of 4500 g or more than the 90th percentile at any gestational age, depending on the authority. It occurs in 25% to 42% of hyperglycemic versus 8% to 14% of euglycemic pregnancies, and maternal diabetes is the most significant single risk factor. Diabetic macrosomia is characterized specifically by a large fetal abdominal circumference and decreased head to abdominal circumference ratio because fetal hyperinsulinemia leads to abnormal fat distribution. Macrosomic fetuses have an increased mortality rate and higher risk for hypertrophic cardiomyopathy, vascular thrombosis, neonatal hypoglycemia, and birth trauma. They are more likely to be delivered by cesarean and are at increased risk for shoulder dystocia during birth, which may result in fractured clavicles, facial paralysis, Erb palsy, Klumpke palsy, phrenic nerve injury, and intracranial hemorrhage.
- Intrauterine growth restriction (IUGR) may complicate pregnancy for pregestational diabetic women with microvascular disease. Placentas of diabetic pregnancies

can be compromised and may exhibit pathohistologic changes, including fibrinoid necrosis, abnormal villus maturation, and proliferative endarteritis of fetal stem arteries. There is wide variation, but these observations occur even with good glucose control, suggesting that irreversible placental abnormalities occur very early in gestation.

- Poorly controlled diabetes increases the risk of fetal demise in utero during the third trimester. Cord thrombosis and accelerated placental aging may be the cause.

Neonatal Complications

- Shoulder dystocia is increased 3-fold in diabetic gestations at any estimated fetal weight and is of even greater concern when macrosomia is also present. If shoulder dystocia occurs, infants of diabetic mothers are more likely to have brachial plexus injury than infants of women without DM. In macrosomic infants of diabetic mothers, vaginal delivery carries a 2% to 5% risk of brachial plexus injury.
- Twenty-five to 40% of infants of diabetic mothers develop neonatal hypoglycemia. The nadir of the serum glucose occurs at about 24 hours of life. Poor maternal glycemic control during late pregnancy and at delivery increases this risk. The pathogenesis is in utero stimulation of the fetal pancreas by maternal hyperglycemia leading to fetal islet β cell hyperplasia. When the maternal glucose source is eliminated, the continued overproduction of insulin may lead to newborn hypoglycemia with cyanosis, convulsions, tremor, apathy, diaphoresis, and a weak or high-pitched cry. Severe or prolonged hypoglycemia in the newborn is associated with neurologic sequelae and death. Standard of care includes testing neonatal blood glucose value within 1 hour of birth. Treatment should be instituted when the infant's blood glucose drops below 40 mg/dL.
- Neonatal hypocalcemia and hypomagnesemia are common in infants of diabetic mothers and correlate with the degree of glycemic control.
- Thirty-three percent of infants born to diabetic mothers have polycythemia (hematocrit higher than 65%). Chronic intrauterine hypoxia increases erythropoietin production, resulting in vigorous hematopoiesis. Alternatively, elevated glucose may lead to early increased red blood cell destruction, followed by increased erythrocyte production.
- Neonatal hyperbilirubinemia and neonatal jaundice occur more commonly in infants of diabetic mothers than in infants of nondiabetic patients of comparable gestational age. This may be related to delay in fetal liver maturation related to poor glycemic control.
- Neonatal respiratory distress syndrome may occur more frequently in diabetic pregnancies as a result of delayed fetal lung maturation. Fetal hyperinsulinemia may suppress production and secretion of surfactant required for normal lung function at birth.
- The risk of fetal cardiac septal hypertrophy and hypertrophic cardiomyopathy is increased in poorly controlled diabetic pregnancies (up to 10% have hypertrophic changes). As an isolated finding, cardiac septal hypertrophy is a benign neonatal condition. However, it increases the risk of morbidity and mortality in neonates with sepsis or congenital structural heart disease.

Maternal Complications

- **Diabetic ketoacidosis (DKA)** is a potentially life-threatening metabolic emergency for both mother and fetus. In pregnant patients, DKA can occur at lower blood glucose levels (ie, <200 mg/dL) and more rapidly than in nonpregnant diabetics. Although maternal death is rare with proper treatment, fetal mortality rates from 10% to 30% are reported. About half of DKA cases are due to medical illness, usually infection. Another 20% result from dietary or insulin noncompliance. In 30% of cases, *no precipitating cause is identified.* Antenatal steroids for fetal lung maturity and β-adrenergic tocolytics can precipitate or exacerbate hyperglycemia and DKA in pregestational diabetics.

- The pathophysiology of DKA is relative or absolute insulin deficiency. The resulting hyperglycemia and glucosuria lead to osmotic diuresis, promoting urinary potassium, sodium, and fluid loss. Insulin deficiency also increases lipolysis and hepatic oxidation of fatty acids, producing ketones and eventually causing metabolic acidosis.

- Diagnosis is by objective documentation of maternal hyperglycemia, acidemia, and serum ketosis. Signs and symptoms include abdominal pain, nausea and vomiting, polydipsia, polyuria, hypotension, rapid deep respiration, and impaired mental status (ranging from mild drowsiness to profound lethargy). Acidosis can be defined as a plasma bicarbonate level <15 mEq/L or arterial pH <7.3. In the presence of hyperglycemia, ketosis is presumed and can be verified by serum testing. Because pregnancy is a state of physiologic respiratory alkalosis, profound DKA may occur at a higher pH.

- In addition to hyperglycemia, severe **hypoglycemia**, requiring hospitalization, may occur in up to 45% of mothers with type 1 DM. Patients with poorer glycemic control can have blunted autonomic responses and milder symptoms, so they may present with more severe or prolonged episodes. Vomiting in early pregnancy also predisposes diabetics to low blood sugars. Severe hypoglycemia may be teratogenic in early gestation, but the effects on the developing fetus are not fully understood.

  - Symptoms include nausea, headache, diaphoresis, tremors, blurred or double vision, weakness, hunger, confusion, paresthesia, and stupor. Diagnosis is by careful history and review of symptoms and confirmed with a blood glucose measurement <60 mg/dL.

  - The Somogyi effect is rebound hyperglycemia after hypoglycemia, secondary to counter-regulatory hormone release. It usually occurs in the middle of the night but can happen after any hypoglycemic episode, manifesting as wide variations in blood glucose levels over a short period of time (eg, between 2:00 and 6:00 AM). Diagnosis is by checking additional blood glucose (ie, 3:00 AM) to identify unrecognized hypoglycemia. Treatment involves adding or modifying a nighttime snack or decreasing the overnight insulin dose in order to better match insulin needs with dietary intake.

- Rapid progression of **microvascular and atherosclerotic disease** can occur in pregnant diabetics. Any evidence of ischemic heart disease, heart failure, peripheral vascular disease, or cerebral ischemia should be evaluated carefully. A pregestational diabetic over age 30 should have a baseline electrocardiogram (ECG). Maternal echocardiogram and cardiology consultation may be warranted. Preconception counseling is useful for these patients. For the most severe maternal disease, termination in early pregnancy may be considered and offered.

- **Nephropathy** complicates 5% to 10% of diabetic pregnancies. In renal failure, with creatinine >1.5 mg/dL, there may be worsening failure with advancing pregnancy, but it is unclear if pregnancy actually hastens progression to end-stage disease. Diabetic nephropathy increases the risk for maternal hypertensive complications, preeclampsia, preterm birth, fetal growth restriction, and perinatal death. A new diagnosis of diabetic nephropathy is made in pregnancy if persistent proteinuria >300 mg/d in the absence of urinary tract infection is detected prior to 20 weeks' gestation. Creatinine clearance <50 mL/min is associated with increased incidence of severe preeclampsia and fetal loss. Intensive maternal and fetal surveillance throughout gestation is required in patients with renal disease.

- Diabetic **retinopathy** is the most common vascular manifestation of diabetes and a principal cause of adult-onset blindness in the United States. Proliferative retinopathy is believed to be a consequence of persistent hyperglycemia and is directly related to the duration of disease. Pregnancy does not change the long-term prognosis, but an ophthalmologic evaluation is recommended in preconception counseling or at the time of the pregnancy diagnosis. Progressive disease may be treated with laser treatment during pregnancy.

- The incidence of **chronic hypertension** is increased in patients with pregestational DM, especially those with nephropathy. **Preeclampsia** is 2 to 4 times more common in pregestational diabetics. The risk is increased with longer duration of disease, nephropathy or retinopathy, and chronic hypertension. Up to a third of women with long-standing diabetes (>20 years) will develop preeclampsia. The threshold for preeclampsia workup in these women should be very low (see chapter 12).

- **Preterm labor** and delivery may be 3 to 4 times higher in patients with DM. Worsening maternal medical status, poor glycemic control, noncompliance with diabetic management, and nonreassuring fetal status result in many iatrogenic preterm deliveries.

- Corticosteroids should be administered as indicated when there is an increased risk for preterm delivery before 37 weeks. Additional insulin or oral agents may be required for 5 to 7 days after steroid administration.

- Diabetics also have an increased risk for maternal adverse obstetric outcomes including third- and fourth-degree perineal lacerations and wound infection. Additionally, they are at increased risk for intrauterine fetal demise, particularly after 40 weeks' gestation.

Management of Pregestational Diabetes in Pregnancy

- Ideally, diabetic women desiring pregnancy should seek preconception counseling and attempt to achieve and maintain euglycemia before conception. The initial prenatal visit should include a detailed history and physical examination, an ophthalmologic examination, an ECG (for women older than age 30, smokers, or hypertensives), and 24-hour urine collection for protein and creatinine clearance. Echocardiography and cardiology consultation should be obtained for known or suspected cardiovascular disease. An HbA1C is helpful in evaluating recent (8-12 wk) glycemic control and in assessing risk for fetal malformations. An HbA1C >9.5% carries >20% risk of major fetal malformation. Strict glucose control (ie, HbA1C ≤6%) prior to and during organogenesis can reduce the risk of embryopathy to nondiabetic levels. Early nutrition consult and counseling may be beneficial.

- The recommended diet for pregnant diabetic women is 1800 to 2400 kcal daily, made up of 20% protein, 60% carbohydrates, and 20% fat. Carbohydrate counting, with 180 to 210 g of daily carbohydrates, is becoming more common and

Table 11-2	Goals for Glycemic Control in Pregnancy[a]
	Blood Glucose
Fasting	60-90 mg/dL (or 95b)
Premeal	<100 mg/dL
1 h postprandial	<140 mg/dL
2 h postprandial	<120 mg/dL
Bedtime	<120 mg/dL
2:00-6:00 AM	60-90 mg/dL

[a]Adapted from Metzger BE, Buchanan TA, Coustan DR, et al. Summary and recommendations of the Fifth International Workshop-Conference on Gestational Diabetes Mellitus. *Diabetes Care.* 2007;30(suppl 2):S251.
[b]From American College of Obstetricians and Gynecologists Committee on Practice Bulletins—Obstetrics. ACOG Practice Bulletin No. 190: gestational diabetes mellitus. *Obstet Gynecol.* 2018; 131:e49-e64.

replacing caloric guidelines. Three meals and three snacks are recommended for all diabetics in pregnancy. Nutrition consult should be part of preconception or early pregnancy planning.

- Goals for glycemic control are the same for GDM and pregestational DM (Table 11-2).
- Patients should start or continue intensive glucose monitoring early in pregnancy using a home glucometer. They should record fasting and 1-hour (or 2-h) postprandial blood glucose levels for each meal. The rationale for postprandial assessments (in contrast to premeal) is that postprandial glycemic control correlates most strongly with the risk for neonatal hypoglycemia, macrosomia, fetal death, and neonatal complications. Home monitoring records are reviewed every 1 to 2 weeks and therapy is optimized.
- Patients are usually continued on their normal prepregnancy insulin regimen while initial blood glucose monitoring is performed. The American Diabetes Association and American College of Obstetricians and Gynecologists (ACOG) recommend insulin for pregnant women with DM and for women with DM considering pregnancy. Patients taking oral hypoglycemic agent or a 70/30 (neutral protamine hagedorn [NPH]/regular) mixed insulin regimen may be switched to NPH and a rapid-acting insulin analog. Patients with type 1 DM usually require significant increases in insulin doses in the second half of pregnancy. Type 2 DM insulin dosing is frequently more than doubled in pregnancy.
- Insulin pumps provide a continuous subcutaneous infusion of insulin. Pump dosing must be managed carefully because the risk of severe hypoglycemia causing seizures and death is increased in pregnancy. Patients must be carefully selected; however, diabetic control may be improved in the correct patient population.
- For patients who opt for an oral agent, metformin may be administered. Metformin may be given at night and in the morning with breakfast. However, glycemic control is not as optimal with this agent, and postmeal elevations are often noted.

- A **DKA in pregnancy** needs aggressive management. Initial management consists of vigorous intravenous (IV) hydration followed by IV insulin drip and frequent blood sugar checks to titrate dosing. Potassium and bicarbonate supplementation may be necessary. Insulin cannot be given if potassium is less than 3.0 mEq/L because insulin drives potassium into the cells and can cause profound hypokalemia with resultant cardiac arrhythmias. Check electrolytes every 4 hours and blood sugar hourly until DKA is resolved. Evaluating for the underlying cause and pursuing treatment (eg, antibiotics for a urinary tract infection) is part of the management. See Table 11-3 for an algorithm for managing DKA.

Table 11-3	Initial Management of Diabetic Ketoacidosis[a]

IV Fluid Hydration
- 1-2 L of NS administered in the first hour
- 250-500 mL/h for the next 8 h depending on hydration state. If serum sodium is elevated, used half-NS.
- Change fluids to D5 half-NS when blood sugar decreases to 200 mg/dL.

Insulin Infusion (Regular Insulin)
- Loading dose of 0.1-0.2 U/kg
- IV infusion of 0.1 U/kg/h (Double the rate if glucose level does not decrease by 50-70 mg/dL in the first hour.)
- When blood sugar declines to 200 mg/dL, decrease infusion to 0.05-0.1 U/kg/h. Continue until urine ketones are cleared.
- Keep serum glucose between 100 and 150 mg/dL until resolution of diabetic ketoacidosis.
- When the patient is able to tolerate food, start the usual insulin regimen.

Potassium (K)
- If K is <3.3 mEq/L, hold insulin and give 20-30 mEq K/h until corrected.
- If K is between 3.3 and 5.3 mEq/L, give 20-30 mEq K in each liter of IV fluid to keep K between 4 and 5 mEq/L.
- If K is >5.3 mEq/L, do not give K and check serum K every 2 h.

Bicarbonate (HCO$_3$)
- pH >7: No HCO$_3$ is needed.
  Add one ampule HCO$_3$ (44 mEq) to 1 L of 0.45 NS, if pH is <7.1.
- pH is 6.9-7.0: Dilute HCO$_3$ (50 mmol) in 200 mL H$_2$O with 10 mEq KCL and infuse over 1 h. Repeat every 2 h until pH is 7.0. Monitor serum K.
- pH <6.9: Dilute HCO$_3$ (100 mmol) in 400 mL H$_2$O with 20 mEq KCL and infuse over 2 h. Repeat every 2 h until pH is 7.0. Monitor serum K.

Abbreviations: D5, 5% dextrose water; IV, intravenous; KCL, potassium chloride; NS, normal saline.
[a]Reprinted from Gabbe SG, Niebyl JR, Simpson JL, et al, eds. *Obstetrics: Normal and Problem Pregnancies.* 7th ed. New York, NY: Churchill Livingstone; 2016:885. Copyright © 2017 Elsevier. With permission.

Fetal Assessment for Pregestational Diabetes

Fetal assessment and monitoring for pregestational diabetes varies according to gestational age.

- **First trimester:** Obtain an early dating sonogram to confirm gestational age and document fetal viability. First trimester sonogram is also useful for aneuploidy screening. In addition, assessment of the fetal nuchal translucency allows identification of many fetuses at risk for congenital cardiac disease.

- **Second trimester:** Ultrasonography at 18 to 20 weeks is recommended for complete evaluation of the fetal anatomy. Fetal echocardiography is also recommended at 19 to 22 weeks for pregestational diabetics due to the increased risk for congenital heart disease.

- **Third trimester:** Twice weekly antenatal testing should be initiated for all pregestational diabetic pregnancies starting at 32 to 34 weeks' gestation. Patients with comorbidities or poor glycemic control may start assessment as early as 28 weeks. Serial ultrasonographic exams for fetal growth should be considered at 28 weeks and then, in conjunction with the fetal surveillance, at 4-week intervals. Umbilical artery Doppler velocimetry may be required to assess for IUGR in patients with microvascular disease (see chapter 4).

Labor and Delivery in Diabetic Pregnancies

- Timing of delivery (per ACOG recommendations):
  - Pregestational diabetes well controlled and uncomplicated: 39 0/7 to 39 6/7 weeks
  - Pregestational diabetes with vascular complications, poor glucose control, or prior stillbirth: 36 0/7 to 38 6/7 weeks
- Glucose control during labor and delivery should maintain euglycemia to improve neonatal outcomes. Continuous IV insulin and glucose infusions may be needed to optimize glycemic control. On admission, IV fluids are started along with serial glucose monitoring (every 1-2 h). The infusion fluids are adjusted to maintain blood glucose levels between 70 and 90 mg/dL. Short-acting insulin boluses may be required in addition to the IV drip.
- Route of delivery is determined by usual obstetric indications. If fetal macrosomia >4500 g is suspected, cesarean delivery is considered to decrease the risk of a shoulder dystocia or birth injury.

Postpartum Care for Diabetics

- For pregestational diabetics, blood glucose can be monitored with the patient's nonpregnant regimen. The insulin dose is typically one half the dose at the end of pregnancy, and oral hyperglycemic agents are significantly decreased. Blood glucose testing every 4 to 6 hours for 24 hours after cesarean delivery, with sliding scale insulin dosing, may be helpful until the patient can resume her normal routine. Keeping blood glucose values <180 mg/dL can help prevent wound breakdown, although overly strict glucose control leading to hypoglycemia should be avoided.

Gestational Diabetes

Screening and Diagnosis

- Universal screening for GDM with a laboratory-based test is standard in the United States. Testing is typically performed at 24 to 28 weeks, but if strong risk factors

Table 11-4	Gestational Diabetes Risk Assessment

Low Risk

Age younger than 25 years old

Not a member of an ethnic group with increased risk for type 2 DM
  (Hispanic, African, Native American, South or East Asian, or Pacific
  Islander ancestry)

BMI <25; normal weight at birth

No history of abnormal glucose tolerance

No history of poor obstetric outcomes

No first-degree relatives with DM

High Risk

Obesity

High-risk race or ethnicity for type 2 DM

Strong family history of type 2 diabetes

Previous history of GDM or impaired glucose metabolism

Previous baby with birth weight of 4000 g or more

History of hypertension, hypercholesterolism, or polycystic ovary syndrome

Abbreviations: BMI, body mass index; DM, diabetes mellitus; GDM, gestational diabetes mellitus.

such as obesity, family history, or a personal history of GDM are present, blood glucose screening may be performed at the first prenatal visit (Table 11-4). A normal early glucose screen needs to be repeated again at usual timing of 24 to 28 weeks' gestation.

- The two-step screening/diagnostic protocol is the most widely used.
  - In this screening, a **50-g oral glucose challenge** is consumed, followed by serum glucose measurement at 1 hour. No fasting or dietary preparation is required. A serum glucose ≥140 mg/dL identifies 80% of GDM, whereas decreasing the cutoff to ≥130 mg/dL identifies over 90% of GDM, but with more "false positives." A serum glucose ≥200 mg/dL is diagnostic of GDM without additional testing
  - If the screening test is positive, then a diagnostic **3-hour glucose tolerance test** (GTT) should be performed with 100 g oral glucose after at least 8 hours of fasting (Table 11-5). With abnormal fasting or any other two abnormal values, the diagnosis of DM is made. In patients at high risk for GDM with a normal GTT, a follow-up GTT can be performed at 32 to 34 weeks to identify later onset diabetes.
- An alternative to the two-step screening is the 2-hour GTT. In this protocol, a 75-g load is administered and GDM is diagnosed with a single abnormal value (fasting >92 mg/dL, 1-h value >180 mg/dL, or 2-h value >153 mg/dL).
- Classification of GDM depends on the management required to control blood glucose levels. In **type A1**, euglycemia is achieved with dietary changes alone. **Type A2** requires additional (ie, medical) therapy.

Table 11-5	Criteria for Diagnosis of Gestational Diabetes From Oral Glucose Tolerance Testing[a]	
Time Since 100-g Glucose Load (h)	Modified O'Sullivan Scale	Carpenter and Coustan Scale
Fasting	≥105 mg/dL	≥95 mg/dL
1	≥190 mg/dL	≥180 mg/dL
2	≥165 mg/dL	≥155 mg/dL
3	≥145 mg/dL	≥140 mg/dL

[a]Adapted from O'Sullivan JB, Mahan CM. Criteria for the oral glucose tolerance test in pregnancy. *Diabetes.* 1964;13:278-285 and Carpenter MW, Coustan DR. Criteria for screening tests for gestational diabetes. *Am J Obstet Gynecol.* 1982;144:768-773.

Fetal and Neonatal Complications

- Similar to pregestational diabetes, fetal and neonatal complications are increased in GDM, including **macrosomia**, **shoulder dystocia**, birth trauma, neonatal hypoglycemia, hyperbilirubinemia, and stillbirth.
- The GDM also has far-reaching health effects for the lifetime of the offspring because studies have demonstrated that fetal exposure to maternal diabetes contributes to obesity in childhood and adulthood as well as type II diabetes development.

Maternal Complications

- In the antepartum period, similar to women with pregestational diabetes, patients with GDM are at increased risk for developing **preeclampsia**. The risk is positively correlated with blood glucose control because the risk is increased to 9.8% in those with a fasting glucose <115 mg/dL and 18% in those with a fasting glucose >115 mg/dL.
- Women with GDM also have an **increased risk of cesarean delivery**. The risk is higher in patients requiring hypoglycemic agents compared to women with diet-controlled GDM, 25% versus 17%.
- Additionally, women with GDM have a **higher risk of developing diabetes**, primarily type II, within decades following pregnancy. This risk and rate of development are influenced by race. Although it is estimated that up to 70% of women with GDM will develop diabetes within 22-28 years after pregnancy, 60% of Latin American women with GDM are at risk for developing type II diabetes within 5 years of their pregnancy.

Gestational Diabetes Mellitus Management

- Management for GDM initially consists of **diet and exercise**:
  - Women with newly diagnosed GDM are started on a carbohydrate-controlled diet with three meals and three snacks daily. The recommended diet composition is 33% to 40% carbohydrates, 20% protein, and 40% fat.

- Moderate exercise can improve glycemic control in GDM. Patients are encouraged to maintain a consistent level of activity throughout pregnancy, provided there are no contraindications (eg, preterm labor).
- Women diagnosed with GDM should check their blood glucose levels 4 times daily, fasting and 1 or 2 hours postmeals. Goals for glycemic control are the same for pregestational diabetics (see Table 11-2).
- When diet and exercise fail to maintain glucose control, the introduction of pharmacologic treatment is recommended.
- **Insulin** is the preferred first-line pharmacologic therapy for GDM.
  - Insulin has traditionally been introduced to GDM management if fasting blood glucose levels are consistently ≥95 mg/dL, if 1-hour postprandial blood glucose levels are routinely ≥140 mg/dL, or if 2-hour postprandial blood glucose levels are consistently ≥120 mg/dL.
  - Different types of insulin may be combined to maintain euglycemia throughout the day and night (Figure 11-1). The NPH insulin is an intermediate-acting insulin usually given in the morning and at night, with peak activity at 5 to 7 hours. Rapid-acting insulin (eg, Humalog or Novolog) is typically administered with meals because its onset is 5 to 15 minutes and peak activity occurs at 1 to 3 hours.
  - If there are abnormally elevated glucose values at isolated and consistent specific times of the day, providers should focus their insulin regimen to correct the specifically timed hyperglycemia. For example, patients who only exhibit fasting hyperglycemia can be maintained on evening NPH insulin alone.
- Although insulin therapy is first line, an oral hypoglycemic agent can be a reasonable alternative for some women with GDM, particularly for women who decline insulin, cannot safely administer insulin, or cannot afford insulin.
  - **Metformin** is increasingly being used in the management of GDM. This agent is a biguanide, which helps control blood glucose by two main mechanisms: (1) inhibiting hepatic gluconeogenesis and glucose absorption and

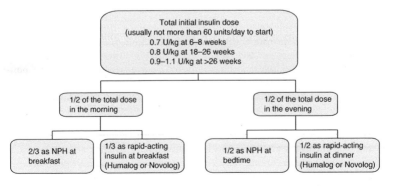

Figure 11-1. Calculation and dose distribution for initial insulin management in pregnancy. NPH, neutral protamine hagedorn. Adapted with permission from Gabbe SG, Graves CR. Management of diabetes mellitus complicating pregnancy. *Obstet Gynecol.* 2003;102(4):857-868. Copyright © 2003 by The American College of Obstetricians and Gynecologists.

(2) stimulating glucose uptake in peripheral tissue. Although metformin is an effective and convenient hypoglycemic agent for GDM, this medication, unlike insulin, crosses the placenta.

o **Glyburide** is a less commonly used oral hypoglycemic for GDM and is also believed to cross the placenta. It is a sulfonylurea that increases insulin secretion from the pancreas and insulin sensitivity of peripheral tissues.

o Given the lack of evidence that metformin or glyburide is superior to insulin and the absence of data on the long-term effects of oral hypoglycemics on offspring exposed to these agents in utero, insulin remains first-line for GDM management.

Fetal Assessment for Gestational Diabetes Mellitus

- Uncomplicated GDM well controlled with diet and exercise: no consensus regarding the need for antepartum fetal testing
- A GDM well controlled on medication: reasonable to consider twice weekly testing starting at 32 weeks. If other risk factors for poor pregnancy outcome are present, consider testing even earlier.

Labor and Delivery

- Timing of delivery (per ACOG recommendations):
  - Gestational diabetes well controlled with diet and exercise: 39 0/7 to 40 6/7 weeks
  - Gestational diabetes well controlled on medications: 39 0/7 to 39 6/7 weeks
  - Gestational diabetes poorly controlled: individualized decision
    - o Patients with poorly controlled GDM are at high risk for stillbirth. Therefore, delivery before 39 weeks may be appropriate. Delivery in the late preterm period, between 34 and 36 weeks 6 days of gestation, may also be a consideration for women who fail inpatient hospitalization methods to reduce blood glucose levels or have abnormal antepartum fetal testing.
- Given that macrosomia and shoulder dystocia are more common in patients with GDM, in addition to timing, method of delivery should also be a consideration. When the estimated fetal weight is ≥4500 g, women with GDM should receive counseling regarding the risks and benefits of a scheduled cesarean delivery.

Postpartum

- For GDM, no immediate postpartum testing is required. Most GDM diagnosed in the third trimester resolves rapidly after delivery. However, up to one third of affected women will have diabetes or impaired glucose metabolism at interval postpartum screening. Therefore, it is strongly recommended that these patients have a 4- to 12-week postpartum GTT. The preferred screening method, based on the Fifth International Workshop-Conference on Gestational Diabetes Mellitus recommendations, is the 75-g 2-hour fasting GTT (Table 11-6).
- Given that women with a history of GDM have a 7-fold increased risk of developing type 2 diabetes, GDM patients with normal postpartum screening test results should receive repeat testing every 1-3 years with their primary care physician.

THYROID DISORDERS

Thyroid disorders are common in women of reproductive age and are present in 3% to 4% of pregnancies. However, only 10% exhibit symptomatic disease.

Table 11-6	Postpartum Glucose Tolerance Test[a]		
	No DM	Impaired Glucose Tolerance	Overt DM
8 h fasting	<100 mg/dL	100-125 mg/dL	>126 mg/dL
2 h after 75-g glucose load	<140 mg/dL	140-199 mg/dL	>200 mg/dL

Abbreviation: DM, diabetes mellitus.

[a]Adapted from Metzger BE, Buchanan TA, Coustan DR, et al. Summary and recommendations of the Fifth International Workshop-Conference on Gestational Diabetes Mellitus. *Diabetes Care.* 2007;30(2):S251 and American Diabetes Association. Standards of Medical Care in Diabetes—2010. *Diabetes Care.* 2010;33(suppl 1):S11-S61.

Thyroid Hormones in Pregnancy

- Thyroid hormone levels are altered in pregnancy (Table 11-7).
- Total triiodothyronine (T_3) and thyroxine (T_4) increase due to human chorionic gonadotropin (hCG) stimulation of thyroid-stimulating hormone (TSH) receptors. In the first trimester, total serum T_4 can increase 2- to 3-fold and TSH may decrease, but hyperthyroid disease is not present because estrogen stimulates the liver to increase thyroxine-binding globulin, maintaining a constant proportion of

Table 11-7	Thyroid Function Test Results in Pregnancy Compared With Hyperthyroid and Hypothyroid Conditions		
Test	Normal Pregnancy	Hyperthyroidism	Hypothyroidism
Thyroid-stimulating hormone (TSH)	No change	Decreased	Increased
Thyroxine-binding globulin (TBG)	Increased	No change	No change
Total thyroxine (T_4)	Increased	Increased	Decreased
Free thyroxine (FT$_4$) or free T_4 index (FTI)	No change	Increased	Decreased
Total triiodothyronine (T_3)	Increased	Increased or no change	Decreased or no change
Free triiodothyronine (FT$_3$)	No change	Increased or no change	Decreased or no change
T_3 resin uptake (T_3RU)	Decreased	Increased	Decreased
Iodine uptake	Increased	Increased or no change	Decreased or no change

Table 11-8	Indications for Thyroid Function Testing in Pregnancy[a]

Patient on thyroid therapy
Large goiter or thyroid nodularity
History of hyperthyroidism or hypothyroidism
History of neck irradiation
Previous infant born with thyroid dysfunction
Type 1 diabetes mellitus
Family history of autoimmune thyroid disease
Fetal demise in utero

[a]Adapted with permission from Mestman JH. Thyroid diseases in pregnancy other than Graves' disease and postpartum thyroid dysfunction. *Endocrinologist.* 1999;9(4):294-307.

active free T_3 and free T_4 (FT_4). Therefore, serum FT_4 may offer better specificity for thyroid testing during pregnancy. The free T_4 index can be used as an indirect estimation of FT_4, but direct FT_4 measurement is preferred.

- The serum TSH level is more useful for diagnosing primary hypothyroidism than hyperthyroidism in pregnancy. The TSH is not protein bound and does not cross the placenta. Normal TSH with low FT_4 may suggest secondary hypothyroidism from a central hypothalamic pituitary defect.
- The thyroid gland itself is moderately enlarged in normal pregnancy, although nodularity or frank thyromegaly should provoke thorough evaluation.
- There are few strong indications for thyroid testing during pregnancy (Table 11-8). Universal screening is not necessary or recommended.
  - Figure 11-2 outlines a thyroid testing algorithm.
  - Testing for anti-TSH receptor antibodies is indicated in certain circumstances (Table 11-9). Immunoglobulin G antibodies cross the placenta and can affect

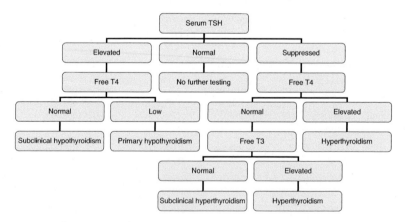

Figure 11-2. Thyroid testing algorithm. TSH, thyroid-stimulating hormone. Adapted from Mestman JH. Thyroid and parathyroid diseases in pregnancy. In: Gabbe SG, Niebyl JR, Simpson JL, eds. *Obstetrics: Normal and Problem Pregnancies.* 5th ed. Philadelphia, PA: Churchill Livingstone; 2007:1011-1037. Copyright © 2007 Elsevier. With permission.

Table 11-9 Indications for TSH Receptor Antibody Testing in Pregnancy[a]

Graves disease (TSI)
  Fetal or neonatal hyperthyroidism in previous pregnancy
  Euthyroid, postablation, in the presence of
    Fetal tachycardia
    IUGR
    Incidental fetal goiter on ultrasound
Incidental fetal goiter on ultrasound (TRAb)
Infant born with congenital hypothyroidism (TRAb)

Abbreviations: IUGR, intrauterine growth restriction; TRAb, TSH receptor–blocking antibodies; TSH, thyroid-stimulating hormone; TSI, TSH receptor–stimulating immunoglobulin.
[a]Adapted from Mestman JH. Hyperthyroidism in pregnancy. *Best Pract Res Clin Endocrinol Metab.* 2004;18(2):267-288. Copyright © 2004 Elsevier. With permission.

the fetal thyroid function. The TSH-stimulating immunoglobulin will stimulate, whereas TSH receptor–blocking antibodies (TRAb) will inhibit fetal thyroid function. The presence of these antibodies in high titers can produce fetal or neonatal goiter and hyperthyroidism or hypothyroidism, respectively.

Hyperthyroid Conditions

- Specific hyperthyroid conditions include Graves disease, hyperemesis gravidarum, gestational trophoblastic disease, struma ovarii, toxic adenoma, toxic multinodular goiter, subacute thyroiditis, TSH-producing pituitary tumor, metastatic follicular cell carcinoma, and painless lymphocytic thyroiditis. Thyrotoxicosis occurs in up to 1 in 500 pregnancies and increases the risk for complications such as preeclampsia, thyroid storm, congestive heart failure, IUGR, preterm delivery, fetal loss, and vasculitis.
  - Clinical signs of thyrotoxicosis include tachycardia, exophthalmos, thyromegaly, onycholysis, heat intolerance, pretibial myxedema, menstrual irregularities, and weight loss. Table 11-7 lists diagnostic test results for normal and hyperthyroid pregnancy.
- Graves disease is the primary cause of thyrotoxicosis in pregnancy, accounting for 95% of cases. It is an autoimmune disease in which thyroid-stimulating antibodies or thyroid-blocking antibodies (TRAb) bind to the thyroid TSH receptors and activate or antagonize thyroid growth and function, respectively. The antibodies can also cross the placenta and affect the fetus. Up to 5% of affected fetuses can develop neonatal Graves disease, which is unrelated to maternal thyroid function. Infants of women who have been previously treated with radioactive iodine or surgery may be at higher risk for neonatal complications because the mothers are not maintained on suppressive medications.
- Hyperemesis gravidarum with high hCG levels in early pregnancy can produce biochemical hyperthyroidism with low TSH and elevated FT_4 (due to the active subunit of hCG mimicking TSH) that typically resolves by the mid-second trimester. Hyperemesis is rarely associated with clinically significant hyperthyroidism, and routine thyroid testing is not recommended in the absence of other findings.

Hyperthyroid Management

- Medical management is with propylthiouracil (PTU) or methimazole. Both cross the placenta and can potentially cause fetal hypothyroidism and goiter. Maintaining high normal range thyroid hormone levels with a minimum drug dosage is the goal.
  - The PTU blocks iodide organification in the thyroid and reduces the peripheral conversion of T_4 to T_3. It is traditionally preferred to methimazole during the first trimester, although placental transfer of the two drugs is nearly equivalent. Both drugs have <0.5% risk of agranulocytosis and <1% risk of thrombocytopenia, hepatitis, and vasculitis. Breastfeeding is allowed for mothers taking PTU because only a small fraction of PTU passes into milk.
    - Initial dose of PTU is 300 to 400 mg daily (divided into an 8-h dosing schedule). The FT_4 should be checked regularly (every 2-4 wk) and the PTU dose adjusted to a maximum of 1200 mg daily to maintain FT_4 levels in the normal range.
  - Methimazole can also be used in pregnancy. The dose is 15 to 100 mg daily (divided into 3 times daily). The association of methimazole with fetal aplasia cutis has largely been refuted. Transition from PTU to methimazole after the first trimester is generally recommended due to the increased risk of hepatic failure associated with use of PTU.
- β-Blockers are used for symptom management in thyrotoxicosis until thyroid hormone levels are normalized with suppressive therapy. Propranolol hydrochloride is the most widely used. Adverse side effects include decreased ventricular function resulting in pulmonary edema. The dose of propranolol is 20 to 80 mg orally every 4 to 6 hours to maintain heart rate below 100 beats per min.
- Iodine 131 thyroid ablation is contraindicated in pregnancy because iodine easily crosses the placenta and can block fetal thyroid uptake, leading to fetal hypothyroidism.
- Surgical management is reserved for severe cases that are unresponsive to medical therapy. Subtotal thyroidectomy may be performed at any time during pregnancy if required.
- **Thyroid storm** is a medical emergency occurring in 1% to 2% of pregnant patients with hyperthyroidism. Heart failure due to the long-term effects of increased T_4 is more frequent and can be exacerbated during pregnancy by preeclampsia, anemia, or infection. Clinical signs include fever higher than 103°F, severe tachycardia, widened pulse pressure, and changes in mentation.
  - Treatment by a standard series of medications is initiated immediately for thyroid storm. Blood work for free T_3, FT_4, and TSH is sent to confirm the diagnosis, but testing should not delay therapy. Oxygen, cooling blankets, antipyretics, and IV hydration are initiated. Fetal monitoring is performed when appropriate.
    - A PTU 1000 mg orally load then 200 mg orally every 6 hours blocks hormone synthesis and conversion.
    - Potassium iodide solution five drops every 8 hours or sodium iodide 500 to 1000 mg IV every 8 hours blocks thyroid hormone release.
    - Dexamethasone 2 mg IV every 6 hours for 24 hours decreases hormone release and peripheral conversion.
    - Propranolol, labetalol, or esmolol is given for tachycardia.
    - Phenobarbital 30 to 60 mg every 6 to 8 hours can relieve extreme restlessness.

Hypothyroid Conditions

- Hypothyroidism in pregnancy is uncommon (2-10 per 1000 pregnancies) because untreated hypothyroidism is associated with infertility. Common causes include Hashimoto thyroiditis, subacute thyroiditis, prior radioablative treatment, and iodine deficiency.

- Type 1 diabetes is associated with 5% incidence of hypothyroidism during pregnancy and has up to a 25% incidence of postpartum thyroid dysfunction.

- Complications of hypothyroidism in pregnancy include preeclampsia, abruptio placentae, anemia, and postpartum hemorrhage. Fetal complications include IUGR, congenital cretinism (growth failure and neuropsychological deficits), and stillbirth. Infants of optimally treated hypothyroid mothers usually have no evidence of thyroid dysfunction.

- The most common etiology of hypothyroidism in the United States is Hashimoto chronic autoimmune thyroiditis, resulting from thyroid antimicrosomal and antithyroglobulin antibodies. Worldwide, the most common cause of hypothyroidism is iodine deficiency.

- Presentation may be asymptomatic or include disproportionate weight gain, lethargy, weakness, constipation, carpal tunnel syndrome, cold sensitivity, hair loss, dry skin, and, eventually, myxedema. Table 11-7 lists test results for hypothyroid pregnancy.

- **Treatment** is initiated if thyroid function testing is consistent with hypothyroidism, regardless of symptoms. Thyroxine replacement is based on the patient's clinical history and laboratory test values and adjusted until TSH remains normal and stable.
  - The starting dose for levothyroxine is 50 to 100 μg daily. It may be several weeks before the full effect is obtained; therefore, TSH should be checked every 4 to 6 weeks after a dose change and then each trimester. The dose may need to be increased in pregnancy due to altered bioavailability/increased metabolism of pregnancy.

Nodular Thyroid

- Nodular thyroid disease should be evaluated when detected during pregnancy. Thyroid cancer occurs in 1 in 1000 pregnancies, and up to 40% of nodules will be malignant. Ultrasonography, fine-needle aspiration, or tissue biopsy can be performed in pregnancy. Surgical excision is the definitive treatment and should not be postponed because of pregnancy, whereas radiation treatment is deferred until after delivery.

PARATHYROID DISORDERS

Parathyroid disorders and calcium dysregulation are uncommon in pregnancy. Calcium requirements do increase during pregnancy, however, so 1000 to 1300 mg calcium and 200 IU vitamin D supplementation are recommended. Fetal calcium uptake, increased plasma volume, renal loss from increased glomerular filtration rate, and hypoalbuminemia lead to lower total maternal serum calcium levels, but ionized calcium remains fairly constant.

- Serum calcium levels are regulated by several hormones:
  - Parathyroid hormone (PTH) increases calcium mobilization from bone, calcium recovery in the kidney, and calcium absorption in the intestine (indirectly via

activation of vitamin D). The PTH increases throughout pregnancy until term, possibly to counteract the inhibitory effects of estrogen on bone.

- Parathyroid hormone–related peptide is produced by the placenta and fetal parathyroid to activate active placental calcium transport and, like PTH, mobilize maternal calcium stores.
- Calcitonin is produced in the parafollicular cells of the thyroid and acts to decrease serum calcium levels.

Hyperparathyroidism

- Hyperparathyroidism produces hypercalcemia. Clinical manifestations include hyperemesis, weakness, constipation, polyuria, polydipsia, nephrolithiasis, mental status changes, arrhythmias, and occasionally pancreatitis. Obstetric and fetal complications include preeclampsia, stillbirth, premature delivery, neonatal tetany, and neonatal death. Poor control of maternal hyperparathyroidism is associated with significant neonatal morbidity and mortality.
- The differential diagnosis of hypercalcemia includes thyrotoxicosis, hypervitaminosis A and D, familial hypocalciuric hypercalcemia, granulomatous disease, and malignancy.
- Laboratory findings include elevated free serum calcium and decreased phosphorus levels. Disproportionately high PTH relative to serum calcium may also be found. Some ECG abnormalities, including arrhythmias, may be present. Ultrasonography is recommended for localization. If radiation exposure is necessary to identify local disease, it should be kept to a minimum.
- Surgical treatment (eg, excision) of a parathyroid adenoma is considered in any patient with symptomatic hyperparathyroidism, following medical stabilization. Hypercalcemic crisis is corrected with IV hydration, furosemide, electrolyte correction, and calcitonin. Oral phosphates can be used as treatment for mild cases or in preparation for surgery.

Hypoparathyroidism

- Hypoparathyroidism is rare and usually occurs iatrogenically after neck surgery. It is the most common cause of hypocalcemia. Patients exhibit cramps, paresthesias, bone pain, hyperacute deep tendon reflexes, tetany, prolonged QT interval, arrhythmias, and laryngospasm. Trousseau sign (carpopedal spasm after blood pressure cuff inflation above systolic pressure for several minutes) or Chvostek sign (upper lip twitching after tapping of the facial nerve) may be present. Fetal skeletal demineralization, subperiosteal resorption, osteitis fibrosa cystica, growth restriction, and neonatal hyperparathyroidism can develop.
- The differential diagnosis of hypocalcemia includes prior parathyroidectomy or thyroid surgery, prior radioactive iodine or radiation treatment, vitamin D deficiency, hypomagnesemia or hypermagnesemia, autoimmune disorders (eg, Addison disease, chronic lymphocytic thyroiditis), eating disorders, renal failure, DiGeorge syndrome, and pseudohypoparathyroidism (ie, PTH resistance).
- Laboratory evaluation shows low serum calcium, low PTH, and elevated serum phosphate levels. The 1,25-dihydroxy vitamin D levels are decreased, and ECG changes include prolongation of the QT interval.
- Treatment is with vitamin D (50 000-150 000 IU/d) and calcium (1000-1500 mg/d) supplementation and low phosphate diet. Doses may need to be increased during

pregnancy and reduced postpartum. Maternal repletion with calcium gluconate during labor and delivery may prevent neonatal tetany. Acute symptomatic hypocalcemia is treated with IV calcium gluconate infusion.

PITUITARY DISORDERS

Pituitary disorders are not common in pregnancy; pituitary dysfunction is commonly associated with anovulatory infertility. See chapters 40 and 43.

- Pituitary hormone release is under hypothalamic control. The anterior pituitary (adenohypophysis) releases adrenocorticotropin (ACTH), TSH, prolactin, growth hormone (GH), follicle-stimulating hormone, luteinizing hormone, and endorphins. The posterior pituitary (neurohypophysis) contains the nerve terminals projecting from the hypothalamus that release oxytocin and antidiuretic hormone (ADH; also called arginine vasopressin).
- During normal pregnancy, the pituitary gland may more than double in size. Lactotroph growth in response to estrogen leads to increased serum prolactin levels, whereas ACTH release increases in response to placental corticotropin-releasing hormone. Luteinizing hormone and follicle-stimulating hormone secretion are decreased in pregnancy. Pituitary GH and TSH decrease as placental GH and hCG rise, respectively. The ADH secretion may be increased in pregnancy, but placental vasopressinase increases degradation, leading to a lowered plasma osmolality set point (ie, 5-8 mOsm/kg decrease).
- The differential diagnosis of pituitary dysfunction includes tumor, infarction, autoimmune/inflammatory disease, infection, infiltrative processes, head trauma, sporadic or familial genetic mutations, prior surgery or radiotherapy, hypothalamic lesions, and empty sella syndrome.

Prolactinoma

- Prolactinoma is the most common pituitary tumor of reproductive age women. Elevated prolactin can cause amenorrhea, anovulation, infertility, and galactorrhea. With increasing size and mass effect, prolactinoma can cause headaches, visual changes, and diabetes insipidus (DI).
- Pituitary adenomas are classified as **microadenomas**, which are ≤10 mm in size, and rarely (<2%) progress to **macroadenomas**, which are >10 mm in diameter, during pregnancy. Up to one third of previously untreated macroadenomas, however, may become symptomatic during pregnancy.
- Initial diagnosis is by history, physical exam, and computed tomography (CT) or magnetic resonance imaging (MRI) of the head. Serum prolactin may not be useful during pregnancy, due to normal pregnancy–induced elevations. Patients with microadenomas can be monitored for symptoms at each prenatal visit, with visual field testing and MRI if visual symptoms develop. Patients with macroadenomas should have baseline visual field testing early in pregnancy, and referral for endocrinology and ophthalmology consults can be considered.
- Treatment of symptomatic prolactinoma is with dopamine agonists, which mimic the prolactin-inhibiting factor activity of hypothalamic dopamine. Bromocriptine or cabergoline can shrink the adenoma and decrease serum prolactin levels. Patients taking these medications should stop them during pregnancy unless they have a symptomatic or large tumor. Transsphenoidal surgical resection of the tumor is

indicated for macroadenomas or high prolactin levels that are not controlled with medication. Radiotherapy can also be used to treat persistent disease. Radiologic evaluation and serum prolactin testing should be followed after treatment.

Acromegaly

- Acromegaly is caused by a GH-secreting pituitary adenoma. Symptoms include coarsened facial features, prominent chin, large feet, spade-like hands, irregular menses, headaches, visual changes, hyperhidrosis, arthralgias, and carpal tunnel syndrome. Usually, these women are infertile, with hyperprolactinemia and anovulation. In the rare patient with acromegaly who becomes pregnant, there are no deleterious or teratogenic effects for the fetus. Carbohydrate intolerance, hypertension, and cardiac abnormalities may complicate pregnancy, however. Laboratory testing shows elevated serum insulin-like growth factor 1 levels and nonsuppressed GH during glucose tolerance testing (100 g glucose load normally suppresses GH release). Diagnosis during pregnancy is complicated by placental GH secretion. Head CT or MRI can localize the tumor. Treatment is with surgical excision, radioablation, or medical treatment with bromocriptine, somatostatin analogues (eg, octreotide or lanreotide), or the newer GH receptor antagonist pegvisomant.

Diabetes Insipidus

- The DI results from abnormal water homeostasis. Central DI results from decreased ADH/vasopressin release due to pituitary tumor, metastases, granuloma, infection, trauma, or global pituitary failure. Nephrogenic DI due to renal resistance to ADH hormone is rare and primarily found in males. Psychogenic DI is due to massive free water consumption. Subclinical DI may be identified during pregnancy when ADH/vasopressin metabolism is increased. Viral hepatitis, preeclampsia, hemolysis, elevated liver enzymes, and low platelets syndrome, and acute fatty liver of pregnancy can also exacerbate or promote DI. Polyuria (>3 L/d) and polydipsia are the clinical hallmarks of DI.
- Diagnosis is by the water deprivation test, showing low urine osmolality and high plasma osmolality with fluid restriction. Desmopressin (DDAVP) injection corrects central DI and can be helpful in confirming the diagnosis. Head CT or MRI may be used to identify pituitary lesions.
- Treatment is with synthetic ADH/vasopressin (ie, DDAVP; L-deamino-I-D-arginine vasopressin) at 10 to 25 μg/d intranasally. Higher doses may be required during pregnancy.

Other Pituitary Disorders

- **Sheehan syndrome** results from pituitary necrosis following massive blood loss. Clinical findings include tachycardia, postural hypotension, hypoglycemia, agalactorrhea, anorexia, nausea, lethargy, weakness, weight loss, decreased pigmentation, periorbital edema, normocytic anemia, and DI. Approximately 4% of patients with obstetric hemorrhage may have mild pituitary dysfunction, but frank Sheehan syndrome can present up to 20 years later. Diagnosis requires laboratory testing for stimulated pituitary hormone secretion (ie, after injecting hypothalamic-releasing hormones). Random blood hormone levels are not useful.

- Lymphocytic hypophysitis is caused by autoimmune lymphocyte and plasma cell infiltration with destruction of the pituitary gland, similar to Sheehan syndrome. Pituitary dysfunction can vary widely, and mass effect may cause headache with visual changes. Head CT or MRI may be helpful in diagnosis. Surgery is reserved for severe symptoms from mass effect.

ADRENAL DISORDERS

Adrenal disorders are not pregnancy induced but do persist during pregnancy, causing significant morbidity without prompt diagnosis. The adrenal gland is profoundly affected by pregnancy and its physiologic changes. Corticotropin-releasing hormone is secreted by the placenta, stimulating ACTH release from the pituitary that increases cortisol production in maternal adrenal glands. Cortisol clearance is also decreased, leading to more than 2-fold increase in total and free serum cortisol levels by the third trimester. Aldosterone production is stimulated by elevated renin/angiotensin II levels in pregnancy; renin activity peaks by the second trimester. Androgen levels are increased 5- to 8-fold, whereas dehydroepiandrosterone sulfate is decreased in pregnancy.

Cushing Syndrome

- Cushing syndrome (see chapter 44) results from long-term exposure to glucocorticoids, either from exogenous steroid use (as in treatment of lupus erythematosus, sarcoidosis, or severe asthma) or from increased endogenous hormone production (from excessive pituitary ACTH production, adrenal hyperplasia, or adrenal neoplasia). Adrenal hyperplasia is the most common cause of Cushing syndrome in pregnancy (up to 50%), with a relative decrease in other etiologies
- Signs and symptoms include moon facies, buffalo hump, truncal obesity, striae, fatigue, weakness, hirsutism, easy bruising, nephrolithiasis, mental status changes, and hypertension.
- Diagnosis is by laboratory testing, showing increased plasma cortisol levels or increased 24-hour urine free cortisol. It can be difficult to identify mild cases due to the normal pregnancy–induced changes in cortisol levels. The dexamethasone suppression test can be used to differentiate a pituitary cause (ie, Cushing disease) from adrenal or exogenous sources of the increased cortisol. Head or abdominal CT or MRI is recommended to localize tumors in the pituitary or adrenal gland.
- Treatment of Cushing syndrome entails medical management of blood pressure and subsequent surgical excision of pituitary or adrenal adenoma. Medical management of the pregnant patient until delivery is usually preferred, although maternal morbidity may be higher with adrenal adenomas, prompting earlier surgical treatment. Metyrapone has been used to block cortisol secretion with adrenal hyperplasia, although it crosses the placenta, may affect fetal adrenal function, and has been associated with preeclampsia. Ketoconazole has been associated with IUGR and may have potential antiandrogen activity; mifepristone is contraindicated in pregnancy.
- Prognosis is improved with early detection and close management, although these patients are at increased risk for maternal complications including hypertension, DM, preeclampsia, cardiac problems, and death. There is increased risk for perinatal complications including IUGR, preterm delivery (up to 50%), stillbirth, and neonatal death.

Hyperaldosteronism

- Hyperaldosteronism can result from adrenal aldosteronoma or carcinoma (about 75%) and bilateral adrenal hyperplasia (about 25%). Symptoms include hypertension, hypokalemia, and weakness. Laboratory testing shows increased serum or urine aldosterone and low plasma renin levels. An MRI can be used to identify and localize an adrenal tumor. Definitive treatment is tumor resection, which can be performed laparoscopically in the second trimester. Medical management is potassium supplementation and treatment of hypertension. Calcium channel blockers or β-blockers are preferred agents for blood pressure control, with spironolactone contraindicated in pregnancy.

Pheochromocytoma

- Pheochromocytoma is a rare catecholamine-secreting tumor of chromaffin cells. Ninety percent arise in the adrenal medulla and 10% in sympathetic ganglia. Ten percent of tumors are bilateral. Ten percent are malignant. It is associated with medullary thyroid cancer and hyperparathyroidism in multiple endocrine neoplasia type 2 syndromes.
- When diagnosed during pregnancy, pheochromocytoma increases maternal mortality to approximately 10%. Fetal mortality increases to nearly 50%, even though the catecholamines do not cross the placenta or directly affect the fetus. The IUGR is common, but there is no increased neonatal mortality after delivery. When the diagnosis is not made before delivery, postpartum maternal mortality increases to about 50%.
- Signs and symptoms of pheochromocytoma include paroxysmal or sustained hypertension, headaches, anxiety, chest pain, visual changes, palpitations, diaphoresis, nausea and vomiting, pallor or flushing, abdominal pain, and seizures. The differential diagnosis should include preeclampsia and other hypertensive diseases.
- Diagnosis is by laboratory testing showing elevated catecholamines, metanephrines, and vanillylmandelic acid in a 24-hour urine specimen. Methyldopa should be discontinued before this test because it will give a false-positive result. Abdominal CT or MRI can be used for localizing the tumor in pregnancy; myocardial perfusion scan can identify extra-adrenal sites.
- Definitive treatment is adrenalectomy, although timing of surgical intervention is controversial: generally, it is recommended either <24 weeks' gestation or following delivery. Medical therapy is primarily with α-adrenergic blockers: phenoxybenzamine (10-30 mg orally 2-4 times daily) or phentolamine (for acute treatment IV). β-Adrenergic blockers are useful to treat tachycardia (eg, propranolol 20-80 mg orally 4 times daily). Cesarean delivery is recommended to avoid the catecholamine surges of labor and delivery, which may increase mortality.

Adrenal Insufficiency

- Adrenal insufficiency may be primary (Addison disease) or secondary to pituitary failure (Sheehan syndrome) or adrenal suppression following exogenous steroids. Destruction of more than 90% of the gland is required to significantly deplete all steroid hormones and cause symptomatic primary failure. When treated, adrenal insufficiency is not associated with adverse fetal or neonatal outcomes.

- Signs and symptoms include hypotension, weakness, fatigue, anorexia, nausea and vomiting, weight loss, and hyperpigmentation of the skin. Pregnancy can exacerbate adrenal insufficiency resulting from Addison disease.
- The differential diagnosis includes idiopathic autoimmune adrenalitis, tuberculosis, histoplasmosis, hemorrhagic necrosis, and infiltrative neoplasms. Other autoimmune disease may also be present, such as Hashimoto thyroiditis, premature ovarian failure, type 1 DM, and Graves disease
- Diagnosis of primary adrenal insufficiency is by laboratory testing showing low plasma cortisol levels and an abnormal ACTH stimulation test (injection of 0.25 mg ACTH without plasma cortisol response at 1 h).
- Treatment includes maintenance replacement of corticosteroids with hydrocortisone (20 mg orally each morning and 10 mg orally each evening) or prednisone (5 mg each morning and 2.5 mg each evening). Fludrocortisone (0.05-0.1 mg orally daily) is given for mineralocorticoid replacement. Patients should continue their usual regimen during pregnancy, with careful follow-up. Stress-dose steroids (eg, hydrocortisone 100 mg IV every 8 h with taper following stress) should be administered during labor and delivery, at the time of major surgical procedures, for severe infection, or other significant stresses.

SUGGESTED READINGS

American College of Obstetricians and Gynecologists Committee on Practice Bulletins—Obstetrics. ACOG Practice Bulletin No. 148: thyroid disease in pregnancy. *Obstet Gynecol.* 2015;125:996-1005. (Reaffirmed 2017)

American College of Obstetricians and Gynecologists Committee on Practice Bulletins—Obstetrics. ACOG Practice Bulletin No. 190: gestational diabetes mellitus. *Obstet Gynecol.* 2018;131:e49-e64.

American College of Obstetricians and Gynecologists Committee on Practice Bulletins—Obstetrics. ACOG Practice Bulletin No. 201: pregestational diabetes mellitus. *Obstet Gynecol.* 2018;132:e228-e248.

Cooper MS. Disorders of calcium metabolism and parathyroid disease. *Best Pract Res Clin Endocrinol Metab.* 2011;25(6):975-983.

De Groot L, Abalovich M, Alexander EK, et al. Management of thyroid dysfunction during pregnancy and postpartum: an Endocrine Society clinical practice guideline. *J Clin Endocrinol Metab.* 2012;97(8):2543-2565.

Karaca Z, Kelestimur F. Pregnancy and other pituitary disorders (including GH deficiency). *Best Pract Res Clin Endocrinol Metab.* 2011;25(6):897-910.

Lekarev O, New MI. Adrenal disease in pregnancy. *Best Pract Res Clin Endocrinol Metab.* 2011;25(6):959-973.

Lowe LP, Metzger BE, Dyer AR, et al. Hyperglycemia and Adverse Pregnancy Outcome (HAPO) Study: associations of maternal A1C and glucose with pregnancy outcomes. *Diabetes Care.* 2012;35(3):574-580.

Nicholson W, Baptiste-Roberts K. Oral hypoglycaemic agents during pregnancy: the evidence for effectiveness and safety. *Best Pract Res Clin Obstet Gynaecol.* 2011;25(1):51-63.

Schnatz PF, Thaxton S. Parathyroidectomy in the third trimester of pregnancy. *Obstet Gynecol Surv.* 2005;60(10):672-682.

Hypertensive Disorders of Pregnancy

Arthur Jason Vaught and Braxton Forde

DEFINITIONS OF HYPERTENSIVE DISORDERS

Hypertensive disorders affect 5% to 10% of all pregnancies.

- **Hypertension** is defined as systolic blood pressure ≥140 mm Hg or diastolic blood pressure ≥90 mm Hg on two separate occasions at least 6 hours but not more than 7 days apart.

- **Chronic hypertension** is high blood pressure diagnosed before pregnancy or before 20 weeks' gestation or first recognized during pregnancy but persisting longer than 12 weeks postpartum. *Note: Chronic hypertension is now defined by the American Heart Association (AHA) as blood pressure ≥130/80 mm Hg; however, in pregnancy, hypertension is still defined by the criteria above.*

- **Gestational hypertension**, formerly known as pregnancy-induced or transient hypertension, is defined as blood pressure ≥140/90 mm Hg on two separate occasions, at least 4 hours apart, after 20 weeks' gestational age. This can also be diagnosed within the first 2 weeks postpartum without a history of chronic hypertension and without the signs and symptoms of preeclampsia. However, if blood pressures remain persistently elevated postpartum, that should warrant a diagnosis of chronic hypertension.

- **Preeclampsia** is diagnosed by elevated blood pressure and proteinuria after 20 weeks' gestation in a patient known to be previously normotensive. Trophoblastic disease or multiple gestation can present with preeclampsia before 20 weeks' gestation.
  - **Mild preeclampsia** is defined by the following criteria:
    - **Blood pressure** ≥140/90 mm Hg confirmed on two measures at least 4 hours apart
    - **Proteinuria** ≥300 mg on a 24-hour urine collection or spot urine protein/creatinine ratio of 0.3 or greater. If neither test is available, a less reliable option is two random urine dipstick results of at least 30 mg/dL ("1+").
    - The 24-hour urine collection remains the gold standard for diagnosing preeclampsia.
  - **Preeclampsia with severe features** is classified by the following criteria:
    - **Blood pressure** of ≥160 mm Hg systolic or ≥110 mm Hg diastolic which is persistent
    - **Signs, symptoms, or lab values** of severe preeclampsia with any elevated
    - Of note, **proteinuria is no longer a diagnostic marker of severe preeclampsia** because level of proteinuria is not associated with maternal or fetal outcomes.
    - **Signs and symptoms** of severe preeclampsia include cerebral or visual disturbances (eg, persistent headache, blurred vision, scotomata), persistent epigastric or right upper quadrant pain, and pulmonary edema.
    - Symptoms that can be seen with severe preeclampsia but are not diagnostic include nausea and vomiting, decreased urine output, hematuria, or rapid weight gain >5 lb in 1 week. An additional sign that does not establish a

diagnosis of preeclampsia but does warrant increased surveillance for pre-eclampsia is the elevation of 15 mm Hg diastolic and 30 mm Hg systolic of the patient's blood pressure from baseline.

- o **Laboratory findings** diagnostic of severe preeclampsia include platelet count below 100 000 platelets per µL, serum creatinine greater than 1.1 mg/dL OR a doubling of the patient's baseline creatinine, liver enzyme (aspartate aminotransferase/alanine aminotransferase) elevation of more than double the upper limit of normal.
- Nondiagnostic, but other lab abnormalities that may be seen are decreased hemoglobin secondary to severe hemolysis in hemolysis, elevated liver enzymes, and low platelets (HELLP) syndrome, microangiopathic hemolytic anemia with abnormal findings on peripheral smear, increased serum bilirubin, elevated serum lactate dehydrogenase, elevated uric acid level, decreased serum haptoglobin, signs of coagulopathy such as prolonged partial thromboplastin time and prothrombin time, and decreased fibrinogen.
- **Fetal findings** associated with preeclampsia may include intrauterine growth restriction (IUGR), oligohydramnios, and other signs of uteroplacental insufficiency. However, none of these findings is diagnostic of preeclampsia or preeclampsia with severe features.
- **Superimposed preeclampsia** is defined as preeclampsia in the setting of maternal chronic hypertension, occurring in 13% to 40% of pregnancies complicated by chronic hypertension. Exacerbation of chronic hypertension versus superimposed preeclampsia can be difficult, especially if there is baseline proteinuria. **Superimposed preeclampsia with severe features** accounts for any of the aforementioned lab abnormalities with elevated blood pressure and new/worsening proteinuria in a patient with chronic hypertension. Persistently elevated blood pressure ($\geq$160 mm Hg systolic or $\geq$110 mm Hg diastolic) without proteinuria in a patient with chronic hypertension is *not* diagnostic of superimposed preeclampsia with severe features.
- **Hemolysis, elevated liver enzymes, and low platelets syndrome** is a variant of preeclampsia defined by the following criteria:
  - o **Hemolysis** identified by burr cells and schistocytes on an abnormal peripheral smear, an elevated serum bilirubin (>1.2 mg/dL), or lactate dehydrogenase level (>600 IU/L), or a low serum haptoglobin
  - o **Thrombocytopenia** with platelets $\leq$100 000/µL is the most consistent finding in HELLP syndrome.
  - o **Elevated liver function tests** (ie, transaminases) more than double the upper limit of normal
  - o Note that hypertension may be absent (12%-18% of cases), mild (15%-50%), or severe (50%). Proteinuria may be absent as well (13%).
- **Eclampsia** is seizure or unexplained coma in a patient with preeclampsia. Eclampsia can rarely present without hypertension (16%) or proteinuria (14%), and if seizure presents without hypertension or proteinuria, other etiologies should be evaluated.

CHRONIC HYPERTENSION

Chronic hypertension carries increased risk for superimposed preeclampsia, preterm delivery, placental abruption, and IUGR. Chronic hypertension is present in up to 5% of pregnancies. The definition for chronic hypertension was adjusted by the

AHA in 2017. This lowered the criteria for chronic hypertension to blood pressure ≥130 mm Hg systolic or ≥80 mm Hg diastolic on two separate occasions, greater than 4 hours apart. This will likely result in a greater number of patients being diagnosed with chronic hypertension. However, the current definition of chronic hypertension affecting pregnancy per American College of Obstetricians and Gynecologists is still blood pressure ≥140 mm Hg systolic or ≥90 mm Hg diastolic on two separate occasions, occurring prior to 20 weeks' gestational age or present prior to conception.

- The **differential diagnosis** of chronic hypertension in pregnancy includes the following:
  - Essential hypertension, which accounts for 90% of hypertension outside of pregnancy
  - Kidney disease, adrenal disorders (eg, primary aldosteronism, congenital adrenal hyperplasia, Cushing syndrome, pheochromocytoma), hyperthyroidism, new-onset collagen vascular disease, systemic lupus erythematosus, aortic coarctation, chronic obstructive sleep apnea, and cocaine use.
- Findings suggestive of secondary hypertension include the following:
  - Hypertension resistant to multiple medications
  - Potassium <3.0 mEq/L
  - Renal dysfunction (creatinine >1.1 mg/dL)
- In pregnancy, worsening chronic hypertension is difficult to distinguish from superimposed preeclampsia, especially in those women who have proteinuria prior to 20 weeks' gestation. Superimposed preeclampsia is more likely in the following scenarios:
  - A sudden exacerbation of hypertension, or a need to escalate the antihypertensive drug dose, especially when previously well controlled
  - A sudden manifestation of other symptoms/signs such as increase in liver enzymes to abnormal levels
  - Platelet levels drop below 100 000/μL
  - Manifestation of symptoms such as right upper quadrant pain and severe headaches
  - Development of pulmonary edema
  - Development of renal insufficiency in women without other renal disease
  - Development of sudden, substantial, and sustained increases in protein excretion
- Ideally, preconception counseling should be performed for chronic hypertensive patients. Patients should be counseled on the risks associated with hypertension and educated on the signs and symptoms of preeclampsia. Patients should be counseled on specific risk factors for superimposed preeclampsia, which include diabetes, obesity, renal disease, history of preeclampsia, or presence of secondary hypertension.
- Patients should also be counseled on medications that could have adverse fetal effects. Specifically, angiotensin-converting enzyme inhibitors, angiotensin receptor blockers, and mineralocorticoid antagonists presently are contraindicated. Statins, used for elevated cholesterol and commonly taken by patients with chronic hypertension, should also be discontinued in pregnancy.
- Obtain **baseline information** early in pregnancy for chronic hypertension, including the following:
  - History of first diagnosis, etiology, duration, and current and prior treatments
  - Complete medical history including cardiovascular risk factors (eg, smoking, increased plasma lipid levels, obesity, and diabetes mellitus) and complicating

medical factors (eg, headaches, history of chest pain, myocardial infarction, stroke, renal disease)
- Complete medication list including vasoactive over-the-counter drugs (eg, sympathomimetic amines, nasal decongestants, diet pills)
- Baseline complete blood count (CBC), complete metabolic panel, urine protein/creatinine ratio (or 24-h urine protein)
- Baseline electrocardiogram (ECG) if not documented within the prior 6 months. Echocardiogram may be indicated if there are abnormalities on ECG or signs of left ventricular hypertrophy.
- **Treatment** is tailored to the severity of illness and presence of comorbidities.
- Lifestyle modification should also be encouraged for patients who meet the AHA criteria for hypertension but not American College of Obstetricians and Gynecologists's criteria for chronic hypertension. This includes reduction of dietary salt (less than 100 mEq/d); diets high in fruits and vegetables; maintenance of ideal body weight; and regular, moderate aerobic exercise. Decreased activity and bed rest should NOT be recommended because they have not been shown to improve pregnancy outcomes. Patients should be encouraged to check blood pressures daily with a home blood pressure cuff monitor.
- If blood pressures remain consistently in the 130s to 140s/80s to 90s, antihypertensives should not be initiated due to concerns for detrimental maternal and fetal effects of hypotension and fetal hypoperfusion. However, for blood pressures that are consistently $\geq$150 mm Hg systolic or $\geq$100 mm Hg diastolic, the following medication can be initiated during pregnancy:
  - **Labetalol**—an α_1 and nonselective β-adrenergic antagonist that can be used as monotherapy or as part of a combination therapy. The typical dose is 200 to 2400 mg/d in two to three divided doses (commonly initiated at 100 mg twice daily). It is contraindicated in patients with greater than first-degree heart block. Labetalol is acceptable but should be used cautiously in patients with severe asthma due to concern for broncho-constrictive side effects. Labetalol is also contraindicated in patients with congestive heart failure. Chronic β-blocker use in pregnancy may have a mild association with IUGR.
  - **Nifedipine**—a calcium channel blocker used commonly in pregnancy that allows convenient daily dosing with the sustained release formulation. A multicenter prospective study of first-trimester drug exposure to calcium antagonists found no increased teratogenicity. The typical dose is 30 to 120 mg/d of an extended-release preparation (commonly initiated at 30-60 mg daily). There is a theoretical risk of neuromuscular blockade and/or pulmonary edema when magnesium and nifedipine are administered together; however, this was not supported in retrospective studies. Some patients will have reflex tachycardia and headaches with nifedipine.
  - **Methyldopa** (Aldomet)—a centrally acting sympathetic outflow inhibitor that decreases systemic vascular resistance and is safe in pregnancy. The typical dose is 500 to 3000 mg/d in two to four divided doses (commonly initiated at 250 mg three times daily). Side effects include hepatic damage; therefore, liver function tests should be performed at least once per trimester. Methyldopa has a high safety profile in pregnancy but frequently fails to control hypertension.
  - **Hydralazine**—a direct peripheral vasodilator that can be combined with methyldopa or a β-blocker. It is not typically considered first line for

hypertension management. The starting oral dose is 10 mg four times a day and may be increased to a maximum of 200 mg/d.

  o **Diuretics** can at times improve blood pressure control if the above medications are failing. Thiazide diuretics have been studied in pregnancy and found to be largely effective; however, consultation with a maternal fetal medicine specialist and serial monitoring of electrolytes should occur if a diuretic is initiated during pregnancy. Loop diuretics can be effective in the acute setting, especially in the setting of the combination of postpartum blood pressure elevations and edema; however, they should not be used first line for blood pressure control.

- Treatment of severe range blood pressures. Elevated sustained blood pressures ≥160 mm Hg systolic or ≥110 mm Hg diastolic can warrant short-term, immediate therapy with intravenous (IV) antihypertensives, including labetalol or hydralazine, for the prevention of acute morbidity from hypertensive urgency. See discussion of "Antihypertensive Therapy" under "Preeclampsia" section.

- **Fetal monitoring:** Antenatal fetal surveillance is recommended, but there is limited data regarding the optimal timing and interval of testing. It is reasonable to perform serial fetal growth ultrasounds every 4 to 6 weeks after the 20-week anatomy scan, particularly for more severe hypertension requiring medication. These patients are often advised to undergo fetal surveillance with nonstress test (NST) or biophysical profile (BPP) and a blood pressure check twice weekly starting at 28 to 32 weeks' gestation (earlier if severe hypertension or suspected IUGR).

- **Delivery:** Timing of delivery should be tailored to the individual patient. In general, those who do not require antihypertensive medications should be delivered at 38 0/7 to 39 6/7 weeks. Those who need antihypertensive medication should be delivered at 37 0/7 to 39 6/7 weeks, and those with difficult to control hypertension at 36 0/7 to 37 6/7 weeks. See below for delivery timing in superimposed preeclampsia.

GESTATIONAL HYPERTENSION

Gestational hypertension is the most common etiology of hypertension in pregnancy, affecting 6% to 7% of nulliparous and 2% to 4% of parous women. The incidence increases with a history of preeclampsia and in multiple gestations. Earlier diagnosis of gestational hypertension increases the risk of preeclampsia; up to 50% of those with hypertension before 30 weeks will progress to preeclampsia.

- **Prognosis and management** depend on timing and severity.
  - If <37 weeks, monitor closely for progression to severe hypertension, preeclampsia, and fetal growth restriction.
  - Delivery is indicated between 37 0/7 weeks and 38 6/7 weeks' gestation for those without severe-range blood pressures and as early as 34 weeks for those with severe-range pressures.
  - If delivery becomes indicated prior to 37 weeks *and* the patient has yet to receive a course of antenatal steroids, then a course of antenatal steroids can be administered. *However*, delivery should NOT be delayed for an antenatal steroid course to be completed, especially in the setting of worsening maternal or fetal status.

- Gestational hypertension may be predictive of chronic hypertension later in life and is important in regard to patient counseling and preventative medical decisions.

PREECLAMPSIA

Preeclampsia occurs in 2% to 7% of healthy nulliparous women and 1% to 5% of parous women. The incidence is higher in twin pregnancies (14%) and for women with a history of preeclampsia (18%). It is the third leading cause of maternal mortality, responsible for over 17% of maternal deaths, and a major cause of neonatal morbidity and mortality.

- **Risk factors** for preeclampsia include the following:
  - Nulliparity
  - Multiple gestation
  - Obesity
  - Chronic hypertension
  - Systemic lupus erythematosus or other autoimmune disorder
  - Thrombophilia
  - Pregestational diabetes
  - Kidney disease
  - History of preeclampsia or eclampsia
  - Low socioeconomic status
  - Family history of preeclampsia, eclampsia, or cardiovascular disease
  - Molar pregnancy
  - Conception via assisted reproductive technologies
  - Advanced maternal age (>40 years)
- The **pathophysiology** of preeclampsia has been studied extensively over the past decade. It is clear that preeclampsia is a systemic disease, and the placenta is the root cause of preeclampsia. The proposed insult to the placenta is an immunologic alteration in trophoblastic function and reduction in trophoblast invasion. This in turn reduces vascular remodeling, reducing perfusion, and increasing velocity of blood in the intervillous space. This leads to both inflammation and endothelial damage and dysfunction. Due to this, angiogenesis and angiogenic factors have been studied extensively. Two particular proteins of interest are soluble fms-like tyrosine kinase 1 (sFlt-1), which is an antiangiogenic agent, and placental growth factor. The sFlt-1 particularly has been shown to be increased 4 to 5 weeks prior to any clinical manifestations of preeclampsia (see "Prediction of Preeclampsia" under "Preeclampsia" section).
- It has also been hypothesized that alteration in the prostacyclin-thromboxane balance plays a role in preeclampsia. Given this, **low-dose aspirin** (81 mg), which blocks thromboxane production, has been studied as a preventative agent for preeclampsia. Small initial studies showed promising results but larger randomized trials showed nonsignificant reduction in preeclampsia. The largest meta-analysis showed a 17% risk reduction in women at high risk for the disease. Patients at high risk for preeclampsia include those with the following:
  - Previous preeclamptic pregnancy
  - Chronic hypertension
  - Renal disease
  - Multifetal pregnancy
  - Pregestational diabetes
  - Systemic lupus erythematosus or other autoimmune disorder (antipospholid syndrome)
- **For pregnancies at high risk for preeclampsia (those that meet the above criteria), we recommend initiating low-dose aspirin between 12 and 28 weeks (ideally before 16 wk) and continue until delivery.** No increased risk of significant bleeding or abruptio placentae has been noted with low-dose aspirin.

- Other factors that increase preeclampsia risk include nulliparity, family history of preeclampsia, low sociodemographic factors (low socioeconomic status, African American ethnicity), maternal age >35 years, obesity, in vitro fertilization, and previously poor pregnancy outcomes. It is unclear if prophylactic aspirin provides any benefit in these conditions. If a patient has two or more of these aforementioned factors, an informed discussion with the patient about the possible benefits of low-dose aspirin should take place.

- Other important measures for preeclampsia prevention are early evaluation and risk reduction through optimizing prepregnancy and maternal health. Women with preeclampsia in the second trimester have a recurrence rate as high as 65%. In patients at high risk for development of preeclampsia, supplementation with fish oil and vitamins C and E has been studied and has been shown to be ineffective. Strict hypertension goals have not been shown to decrease preeclampsia risks either. Calcium supplementation in patients who have a deficiency *has* been shown to decrease the risk of preeclampsia development, although it is very unlikely that a patient would be calcium deficient in the United States and calcium supplementation is, at this time, not recommended. Dietary salt restriction has also been studied in preeclampsia prevention; however, it has not been shown to provide benefit.

- **Prediction** of preeclampsia has been an area of growing research and debate. Uterine artery velocity Doppler and various biomarkers (sFlt-1, soluble endoglin, placental growth factor) have been shown in small studies to be predictive of future preeclampsia development, especially when studied in the second trimester; however, use of these biomarkers has yet to show improvement in either maternal or fetal outcomes during pregnancy and none is approved by the US Food and Drug Administration for clinical use. There are ongoing studies evaluating the combination of biomarkers plus uterine artery Doppler studies to create a prediction algorithm, and ongoing research is warranted.

  - **Uric acid:** A test that is readily available is uric acid, and a recent prospective study showed a uric acid level of 5.2 mg/dL correlated with a positive predictive value of 91.4%. Using uric acid in rare circumstances to evaluate a patient with worsening gestational hypertension for possible progression to preeclampsia is a reasonable option, although regularly checking uric acid levels should not be part of routine care and should not be the principle guiding force in patient management.

- **Diagnosis** of preeclampsia is by symptoms and signs, including elevated blood pressure, proteinuria, and abnormal laboratory findings (described above).

Management of Preeclampsia

- Definitive **management** for gestational hypertension, preeclampsia, and eclampsia is delivery because the placenta is the insulting agent and removal of the placenta will lead to resolution of the disease process.

Management of Preeclampsia Without Severe Features

- In general, **preeclampsia without severe features** (also known as **mild** preeclampsia, see definitions above) at term is treated by delivery, typically at 37 weeks or at time of diagnosis if after 37 weeks.

  - Optimal treatment prior to 37 weeks is usually expectant management. The benefits of antihypertensive medications and early hospitalization are not clearly established. There is no role for bed rest in the management of preeclampsia without severe features.

- Close maternal and fetal observation is essential, but there is no standard protocol for testing or frequency.
- Fetal monitoring can include growth ultrasound and amniotic fluid assessment every 3 to 4 weeks, umbilical artery Doppler velocimetry, and once or twice weekly NST or BPP.
- Maternal monitoring can include weekly or semiweekly blood pressure check and evaluation, and periodic lab testing such as 24-hour urine protein or urine protein/creatinine ratio, serum creatinine, platelet count, and serum transaminases to detect progression to severe preeclampsia.
- A gestational age of >34 weeks with uncontrolled hypertension and abnormal fetal testing should warrant further investigation, and if severe features identified, prompt delivery.

Management of Preeclampsia With Severe Features

- The first priority in treating **preeclampsia with severe features** is to assess and stabilize the mother.
    - **At ≥34 weeks**, delivery is indicated, although immediate cesarean delivery is not usually warranted, rather urgent delivery *after* maternal stabilization is indicated.
        - Patients with a vertex fetus and no contraindication to labor can deliver vaginally.
        - Careful monitoring, at least hourly assessments, and strict intake/output recordings should be maintained. Furthermore, assessment of labs such as CBC and comprehensive metabolic panel should be checked serially (typically every 6-12 h) during an induction of a severely preeclamptic patient to monitor for development of HELLP syndrome.
    - **Between 24 and 34 weeks** expectant management is acceptable if blood pressure is adequately controlled with antihypertensive agents, fetal status is reassuring, and the mother is not developing worsening HELLP syndrome.
        - Magnesium sulfate ($MgSO_4$) and IV antihypertensives may be given initially while betamethasone is administered for fetal lung maturity.
        - Fluid status should be monitored.
        - The CBC, platelets, and liver function tests should be checked daily.
        - Fetal surveillance with NST or BPP should be performed at least weekly, and patients should be instructed regarding maternal assessment of fetal movement.
        - Delivery is indicated by the following: worsening IUGR, nonreassuring fetal tracing, eclampsia, neurologic deficits, pulmonary edema, right upper quadrant/epigastric pain, worsening renal status, disseminated intravascular coagulation, HELLP, placental abruption, or uncontrolled severe blood pressure.
    - **Prior to 24 weeks' gestation**, expectant management is associated with high maternal morbidity and limited perinatal benefit.
- Expectant management of severe preeclampsia with IUGR has been associated with increased risk of fetal death (rate of perinatal death is 5.4%) and should be performed cautiously.
- **Seizure prophylaxis** during labor and for 24-hour postpartum is recommended for patients with preeclampsia. Some patients with severe persistent preeclampsia may need seizure prophylaxis for longer periods *before and after* delivery.
    - **Magnesium sulfate** is the agent of choice for eclamptic seizure prophylaxis. The $MgSO_4$ has been shown to decrease the risk of eclampsia by more than 50%.
        - For prophylaxis, we administer a loading dose of 6 g $MgSO_4$ intravenously over 15 to 20 minutes.

- Maintenance dose is 2 g/hr intravenously (dose should be titrated down if the patient has poor urine output, poor kidney function, or an elevated serum creatinine).
- If there is no IV access, the loading dose is 5 g $MgSO_4$ (50% solution) administered intramuscularly in each buttock (10 g total), with a maintenance dose of 5 g in alternating buttocks every 4 hours.
- The therapeutic serum magnesium level for seizure prophylaxis depends on the laboratory. In general, the therapeutic range is 4.8 to 8.4 mg/dL or 4 to 6 mEq/L. However, it is our practice to follow magnesium levels only for those patients in whom we are unusually concerned for developing supratherapeutic levels. For such patients, check serum magnesium level 4 hours after the loading dose and then every 6 hours as needed or if symptoms suggest magnesium toxicity.
- Patients are monitored hourly for signs and symptoms of magnesium toxicity:
  - Loss of patellar reflexes at 8 to 10 mEq/L
  - Respiratory depression or arrest at 12 mEq/L
  - Mental status changes at >12 mEq/L followed by ECG changes and arrhythmias
  - If magnesium toxicity develops, check the patient's vital signs, stop magnesium and check plasma levels, administer 1-g calcium gluconate IV over 3 minutes, and consider diuretics (eg, furosemide, mannitol).
- **Phenytoin (Dilantin)** is a secondary agent for eclamptic seizure prophylaxis. Magnesium was clearly superior in a large randomized clinical trial and is preferred. It may, however, be contraindicated, as in patients with myasthenia gravis.
  - The loading dose is maternal weight based. For <50 kg, load 1000 mg; for 50 to 70 kg, load 1250 mg; and for >70 kg, load with 1500 mg phenytoin.
  - The first 750 mg of the loading dose should be given at 25 mg/min and the rest at 12.5 mg/min. If the patient maintains normal cardiac rhythm and has no history of heart disease, ECG monitoring is not necessary at this infusion rate.
  - Check the serum phenytoin level at 30 to 60 minutes after infusion.
  - A therapeutic level is >12 μg/mL; recheck level in 12 hours.
  - If the level is <10 μg/mL, reload with 500 mg and check again in 30 to 60 minutes.
  - If the level is 10 to 12 μg/mL, reload with 250 mg and check again in 30 to 60 minutes.
- **Antihypertensive therapy** is indicated for patients with a systolic blood pressure of 160 mm Hg or greater or diastolic blood pressure of 110 mm Hg or greater. Acute treatment aims to reduce blood pressure in a controlled manner without compromising uteroplacental perfusion.
  - It is reasonable to reduce the patient's systolic blood pressure to 140 to 155 mm Hg and the diastolic blood pressure to 90 to 100 mm Hg.
  - While administering magnesium, useful antihypertensive agents for acute management include the following:
    - **Immediate release oral nifedipine:** This is particularly useful in patients without IV access. It has an onset of action of 15 minutes and reaches a peak by 1 hour. Initial dose should be 10 mg orally. Subsequent doses can be given every 20 minutes. Subsequent doses should be 20 mg. A total of three doses every 20 minutes can be attempted to reduce blood pressure. If at any point the patient's blood pressure is reduced below 160/110 mm Hg, she can be observed. While administering short-acting antihypertensives, the blood pressure should be checked at least every 20 minutes. Once blood pressure is below 160/110 mm Hg,

the blood pressure should be checked every 10 minutes for 1 hour, then every 15 minutes for 1 hour, then every 30 minutes for 1 hour, and then every hour for at least the next 4 hours. If three doses of nifedipine do not improve the patient's blood pressures, you should use one of the two following agents.

- **Hydralazine hydrochloride:** Administered intravenously, it has an onset of action within 10 to 20 minutes. The duration of action is 4 to 6 hours.
  - Begin with a 5- to 10-mg IV bolus or push over 2 minutes, and recheck a blood pressure in 20 minutes. If severe blood pressures persist, an additional 10 mg should be administered. No more than 20 mg should be administered over a 20-minute time period. If the blood pressure remains elevated after two doses, an additional antihypertensive should be used. If the blood pressure is reduced below 160/110 mm Hg, the blood pressure monitoring as described above should be initiated.

- **Labetalol hydrochloride:** Administered intravenously, it has an onset of action within 5 to 10 minutes and has a duration of 3 to 6 hours. It is contraindicated in greater than first-degree maternal heart block and should be used cautiously in severe asthmatics.
  - Begin with a 20-mg IV bolus or push over 2 minutes and then check a repeat blood pressure in 20 minutes. If severe range blood pressures persist, 40 mg intravenously should be administered (over 2 or more minutes) and blood pressures checked in 20 minutes. If severe range blood pressures persist, administer 80 mg intravenously. If the blood pressure remains elevated at this time, an additional antihypertensive should be used. If the blood pressure is reduced below 160/110 mm Hg, the blood pressure monitoring as described above should be initiated.
  - When administering IV labetalol, there should be a maximum dosing of 300 mg/24 hr.

- **Fluid management:** Patients with preeclampsia are frequently hypovolemic due to third spacing from low serum oncotic pressure and increased capillary permeability. These same abnormalities also increase risk for pulmonary edema. Diuretics may be used to treat pulmonary edema but should not be used as the primary antihypertensive in preeclamptic patients.
  - Oliguria is defined as urine output of <100 mL in 4 hours. It is treated with 500-mL crystalloid bolus if the lungs are clear. If there is no response, another 500-mL bolus can be administered. If there is no response after 1 L, central hemodynamic monitoring can be considered.
    - Central venous pressure monitoring does not correlate well with pulmonary capillary wedge pressure. Rarely, a Swan-Ganz catheter may be required to help guide fluid management and prevent flash pulmonary edema. More practically, evaluation with lung exam every 2 hours can help identify onset of pulmonary edema.
  - Patients usually begin to effectively diurese about 12 to 24 hours after delivery. In cases of severe renal compromise, it may take 72 hours or more for adequate diuresis to resume.

- **Maternal complications** of severe preeclampsia require a high index of clinical suspicion and include renal failure, acute cardiac failure, pulmonary edema, thrombocytopenia, disseminated intravascular coagulopathy, and cerebrovascular accidents.

- **Perinatal outcome:** There is a high perinatal morbidity and mortality in pregnancies complicated by severe preeclampsia. Fetal mortality rates range from 5% to more than 70% depending on the gestational age.

HELLP SYNDROME

HELLP syndrome often presents with nonspecific complaints such as malaise, abdominal pain, vomiting, shortness of breath, or bleeding.

- The **differential diagnosis** for HELLP syndrome includes the following:
  - Acute fatty liver of pregnancy
  - Thrombotic thrombocytopenic purpura
  - Hemolytic uremic syndrome
  - Immune thrombocytopenic purpura
  - Systemic lupus erythematosus flare
  - Antiphospholipid antibody syndrome
  - Cholecystitis
  - Fulminant hepatitis (of any cause)
  - Acute pancreatitis
  - Disseminated herpes zoster
- **Management** is the same as for severe preeclampsia. Transfusion of red cells, platelets, or factors may be required immediately prior to delivery depending on severity of anemia and thrombocytopenia. Short-term expectant management in order to allow for administration of betamethasone for fetal lung maturity *may* be possible in a very select group of patients with HELLP prior to 34 weeks; however, there are no data suggesting improved perinatal outcomes with this approach.

ECLAMPSIA

Eclampsia should be the presumed diagnosis in obstetric patients with seizures and/or coma without a known history of epilepsy. The incidence of eclampsia is between 1 in 2000 and 1 in 3500 pregnancies in developed countries. Eclampsia occurs in about 1% of patients with preeclampsia. Virtually, all eclampsia is preceded by preeclampsia.

- The **pathophysiology** of eclamptic seizures is unknown but is related to arterial vasospasm and may occur when mean arterial pressure exceeds the capacity of cerebral autoregulation, leading to cerebral edema and increased intracranial pressure.
- Eclampsia can occur antepartum, peripartum, or postpartum and has been reported as late as 3 to 4 weeks postpartum. Patients may have associated hypertension and proteinuria; a small percentage has neither.
- **Management** of eclampsia is an obstetric emergency that requires immediate treatment, including
  - Appropriate management of ABCs (airway, breathing, and circulation) with measures taken to avoid aspiration
  - Seizure control with 6-g $MgSO_4$ IV bolus. If the patient has a seizure during or after the loading dose, an additional 2-g IV bolus of $MgSO_4$ can be given.
  - Treat seizures refractory to $MgSO_4$ with IV phenytoin or a benzodiazepine (eg, lorazepam).
  - Treat *status epilepticus* with lorazepam 0.1 mg/kg IV at a rate ≥2 mg/min. Patients with *status epilepticus* may require intubation to correct hypoxia and acidosis and to maintain a secure airway.
  - Prevent maternal injury with padded bedrails and appropriate positioning.
  - Control of severe hypertension (see medications above)

- **Delivery is indicated after maternal stabilization.**
  - During acute eclamptic episodes, fetal bradycardia is common. It usually resolves in 3 to 5 minutes. Allowing the fetus to recover in utero from the maternal seizure, hypoxia, and hypercarbia before delivery is optimal. However, if fetal bradycardia persists beyond 10 minutes, abruptio placentae should be suspected.
  - Emergency cesarean delivery should always be anticipated in case of rapid maternal or fetal deterioration.
- **Outcomes** depend on the severity of disease. Perinatal mortality in the United States ranges from 5.6% to 11.8%, mainly due to extreme prematurity, placental abruption, and IUGR. The maternal mortality rate is from <1.8% in the developed world to 14% in under-resourced countries. Maternal complications include aspiration pneumonitis, hemorrhage, cardiac failure, intracranial hemorrhage, and transient or permanent retinal blindness.
- Long-term neurologic sequelae of eclampsia are rare. Central nervous system imaging with computed tomography or magnetic resonance imaging should be performed if seizures are of late onset (longer than 48 h after delivery) or if neurologic deficits are clinically evident. The signs and symptoms of preeclampsia usually resolve within 1 to 2 weeks postpartum. Approximately 25% of eclamptic patients develop preeclampsia in subsequent pregnancies, with recurrence of eclampsia up to 2% of cases.

SUGGESTED READINGS

American College of Obstetricians and Gynecologists Committee on Obstetric Practice. ACOG Committee Opinion No. 743: low-dose aspirin use during pregnancy. *Obstet Gynecol.* 2018;132:e44-e52.

American College of Obstetricians and Gynecologists Committee on Obstetric Practice. ACOG Committee Opinion No. 767: emergent therapy for acute-onset, severe hypertension during pregnancy and the postpartum period. *Obstet Gynecol.* 2019;133:e174-e180.

American College of Obstetricians and Gynecologists Committee on Obstetric Practice, Society for Maternal-Fetal Medicine. ACOG Committee Opinion No. 652: magnesium sulfate use in obstetrics. *Obstet Gynecol.* 2016;127:e52-e53. (Reaffirmed 2018)

American College of Obstetricians and Gynecologists Committee on Obstetric Practice, Society for Maternal-Fetal Medicine. ACOG Committee Opinion No. 764: medically indicated late-preterm and early-term deliveries. *Obstet Gynecol.* 2019;133:e151-e155.

American College of Obstetricians and Gynecologists Committee on Practice Bulletins—Obstetrics. ACOG Practice Bulletin No. 202: gestational hypertension and preeclampsia. *Obstet Gynecol.* 2019;133:e1-e25.

American College of Obstetricians and Gynecologists Committee on Practice Bulletins—Obstetrics. ACOG Practice Bulletin No. 203: chronic hypertension in pregnancy. *Obstet Gynecol.* 2019;133:e26-e50.

LaMarca BD, Gilbert J, Granger JP. Recent progress toward the understanding of the pathophysiology of hypertension during preeclampsia. *Hypertension.* 2008;51:982-988.

Ukah UV, De Silva DA, Payne B, et al. Prediction of adverse maternal outcomes from preeclampsia and other hypertensive disorders of pregnancy: a systematic review. *Pregnancy Hypertens.* 2018;11:115-123.

13 Cardiopulmonary Disorders of Pregnancy

Reneé Franklin Moss and Ernest M. Graham

CARDIAC DISORDERS

Cardiac diseases complicate 1% to 4% of pregnancies in women without preexisting cardiac abnormalities. Pregnancy is associated with major alterations in circulatory physiology, and cardiovascular disease contributes to nearly a quarter of pregnancy-related deaths in the United States.

Hemodynamic Changes During Pregnancy

- Profound **hemodynamic alterations** occur during pregnancy, labor, delivery, and the postpartum period. These changes begin during the first 5 to 8 weeks of pregnancy and peak in the late second trimester. Normal pregnancy is associated with fatigue, dyspnea, decreased exercise capacity, peripheral edema, and jugular venous distention. Most pregnant women have audible physiologic systolic murmurs created by augmented blood flow and a physiologic third heart sound (S_3) that reflects the volume-expanded state. The enormous changes in the cardiovascular system during pregnancy carry many implications for management of pregnant patients with cardiac disease.
  - **Blood volume** increases 40% to 50% during normal pregnancy, in part due to estrogen-mediated activation of the renin-aldosterone axis leading to sodium and water retention. The rise in blood volume is greater than the increase in red blood cell mass (20%-30%), contributing to the fall in hemoglobin concentration causing physiologic anemia in pregnancy. Peak dilution occurs at 24 to 26 weeks.
  - **Cardiac output** increases 30% to 50% above baseline by 20 to 26 weeks' gestation, peaks at the end of the second trimester, and then plateaus until delivery. The change in cardiac output is mediated by the following: (1) increased preload due to the rise in blood volume, (2) reduced afterload due to a fall in systemic vascular resistance, and (3) a rise in maternal heart rate of 10 to 15 beats per minute. Stroke volume increases during the first and second trimesters but declines in the third trimester due to caval compression by the gravid uterus. Cardiac output in twin pregnancies is 20% above that of singleton pregnancies. Blood pressure typically falls slightly during the first two trimesters of pregnancy because of reduction in peripheral vascular resistance related to increased progesterone production.
- **Labor and delivery:** During labor and delivery, hemodynamic fluctuations can be profound. Each uterine contraction results in the displacement of 300 to 500 mL of blood into the general circulation. Stroke volume increases, causing a rise in cardiac output of an additional 50% with each contraction. Mean systemic pressure also rises due to catecholamines that are released as a result of the sympathetic nervous system's response to maternal pain and anxiety. Analgesia and anesthesia effectively eliminate this response. Neuraxial blocks can cause maternal hypotension and/or impaired uteroplacental perfusion. If administered to the point of cardiovascular

toxicity, cardiac arrhythmias or a more profound hypotension can occur. Blood loss during delivery can further alter the hemodynamic state.

- **Postpartum:** Immediately postpartum, uterine involution leads to autotransfusion, which increases cardiac output dramatically. In addition, there is a relief of vena caval compression after delivery. Increased venous return augments cardiac output and prompts brisk diuresis. The cardiovascular system returns to the prepregnant baseline within 3 to 4 weeks postpartum.

Cardiac Disease in Pregnancy

- **Signs and symptoms** of cardiac disease overlap common symptoms and findings in pregnancy and include fatigue, shortness of breath, orthopnea, palpitations, edema, systolic flow murmur, and a third heart sound.
- **Evaluation** of cardiac disease includes a thorough history and physical examination. Noninvasive testing includes an electrocardiogram (ECG), a chest radiograph, and an echocardiogram. The ECG may reveal a leftward shift of the electrical axis, especially during the third trimester when the diaphragm is pushed upward by the uterus. Ventricular extrasystoles are a common finding. Routine chest radiographs are used to assess cardiomegaly and pulmonary vascular prominence. Echocardiographic evaluation of ventricular function and structural anomalies is invaluable for diagnosis of cardiac disease in pregnancy. Many changes including mild valvular regurgitation and chamber enlargement are normal findings on echocardiogram during pregnancy.

Management of Patients With Known Cardiac Disease

- **Before conception:** Whenever possible, women with preexisting cardiac lesions should receive preconception counseling regarding maternal and fetal risks during pregnancy and long-term maternal morbidity and mortality. The New York Heart Association (NYHA) functional class (Table 13-1) is used as a predictor of outcome. Women with NYHA class III and IV face a mortality rate of 7% and

Table 13-1	New York Heart Association (NYHA) Functional Classification[a]
NYHA Class	Symptoms
I	No symptoms and no limitation in ordinary physical activity such as shortness of breath when walking or climbing stairs.
II	Mild symptoms (mild shortness of breath and/or angina) and slight limitation during ordinary activity
III	Marked limitation in activity due to symptoms, even during less than ordinary activity such as walking short distances (20-100 m); comfortable only at rest
IV	Severe limitations. Experiences symptoms even while at rest; mostly bedbound

[a]Source: American Heart Association, Inc.

morbidity over 30%. These women should be strongly cautioned against pregnancy. A risk index using four risk factors has been shown to accurately predict a woman's chance of having adverse cardiac or neonatal complications: (1) a prior cardiac event, (2) cyanosis or poor functional class, (3) left heart obstruction, and (4) systemic ventricular dysfunction. With two or more risk factors the chance of cardiac event approaches 75%. The Modified World Health Organization Risk Classification of Cardiovascular Disease and Pregnancy (Table 13-2) is another useful tool for preconceptional counseling as it assesses maternal risk associated with various cardiovascular conditions. Four progressively worsening categories are used to divide maternal risk. Pregnancies are contraindicated for World Health Organization class IV.

- **After conception.** Pregnant patients with significant history require cardiac assessment as early as possible. If the pregnancy poses a serious threat to maternal health, the patient should be counseled about the option of pregnancy termination. Patients need close monitoring and follow-up by both a maternal-fetal medicine subspecialist and a cardiologist, with attention to signs or symptoms of worsening congestive heart failure (CHF) throughout the pregnancy. Each visit should include the following: (1) cardiac examination and cardiac review of systems; (2) documentation of weight, blood pressure, and pulse; and (3) evaluation of peripheral edema.
- **During pregnancy.** The most common cardiac complications of pregnancy include arrhythmia and CHF. If symptoms worsen, hospitalization, bed rest, diuresis, or correction of an underlying arrhythmia may be required. Sometimes, surgical correction during pregnancy becomes necessary. When possible, procedures should be performed during the early second trimester to avoid the period of fetal organogenesis and before more significant hemodynamic changes of pregnancy occur. Pregnancy is also a time of hypercoagulability, and anticoagulation should be started if appropriately indicated.

Antibiotic Prophylaxis for Endocarditis

- American College of Obstetricians and Gynecologists has endorsed the 2007 American Heart Association (AHA) guidelines for prevention of infective endocarditis (IE), which contain marked changes from prior AHA guidelines. Antibiotic prophylaxis is no longer recommended, as IE is more likely to result from frequent random bacteremia with daily activities than from bacteremia caused by specific dental, gastrointestinal, or genitourinary (GU) procedures. Prophylaxis is now based on the risk of adverse outcome with the procedure, and it is not recommended for GU procedures, except in high-risk patients with GU infections, to prevent wound infection and sepsis. Antibiotic prophylaxis for IE is not recommended for vaginal delivery.

Congenital Heart Disease

- During pregnancy, women with **congenital heart disease** are at increased risk for cardiac events including pulmonary edema and symptomatic sustained arrhythmias (supraventricular tachycardia and ventricular tachycardia). Risk factors for cardiac events in these women can be found in Table 13-3. These women also face increased risks of adverse neonatal outcomes including preterm delivery and infants with growth restriction, respiratory distress syndrome, and intraventricular hemorrhage. The risk of intrauterine or neonatal death is approximately 12% and 4%, respectively. Additionally, there is an increased incidence of congenital heart

Table 13-2 Modified World Health Organization Risk Classification of Cardiovascular Disease and Pregnancy[a]

Risk Category	Associated Conditions
WHO I—no detectable increased risk of maternal mortality and no/mild increase in morbidity	Uncomplicated, small, or mild pulmonary stenosis Patent ductus arteriosus Mitral valve prolapse Successfully repaired simple lesions: Atrial or ventricular septal defect Patent ductus arteriosus Anomalous pulmonary venous connection
WHO II—small increase in maternal risk mortality or moderate increase in morbidity	If otherwise well and uncomplicated: Unoperated atrial or ventricular septal defect Unrepaired tetralogy of Fallot
WHO II or III—depends on individual case	Mild left ventricular impairment Native or tissue valvular heart disease not considered WHO I or IV Marfan syndrome without aortic dilation Aorta <45 mm in association with bicuspid aortic valve disease Repaired coarctation
WHO III—significantly increased risk of maternal mortality or severe morbidity. Expert counseling required. If pregnancy is decided on, intensive specialist cardiac and obstetric monitoring needed throughout pregnancy, childbirth, and the puerperium	Mechanical valve Systemic right ventricle Fontan circulation Unrepaired cyanotic heart disease Other complex congenital heart disease Aortic dilation 40-45 mm in Marfan syndrome Aortic dilation 45-50 mm in bicuspid aortic valve disease
WHO IV—extremely high risk of maternal mortality or severe morbidity; pregnancy contraindicated. If pregnancy occurs, termination should be discussed. If pregnancy continues, care as for WHO class III.	Pulmonary arterial hypertension from any cause Severe systemic ventricular dysfunction (LVEF <30%, NYHA functional class III-IV) Severe mitral stenosis; severe symptomatic aortic stenosis Marfan syndrome with aorta dilated >45 mm Aortic dilation >50 mm in aortic disease associated with bicuspid aortic valve Native severe coarctation of the aorta

Abbreviations: LVEF, left ventricular ejection fraction; NYHA, New York Heart Association; WHO, World Health Organization.

[a]Data from Balci A, Sollie-Szarzynska KM, van der Bijl AG, et al., for the ZAHARA-II Investigators. Prospective validation and assessment of cardiovascular and offspring risk models for pregnant women with congenital heart disease. *Heart.* 2014;100(17):1373-1381.

Table 13-3	Risk Factors for Cardiac Events for Patients With Congenital Heart Disease

Prior history of heart failure
NYHA functional class III
Decreased subpulmonary ventricular EF
Severe pulmonary regurgitation
Smoking

Abbreviations: EF, ejection fraction; NYHA, New York Heart Association.

disease in children of women with a congenital abnormality ranging from approximately 3% overall to 50% in women carrying single-gene defects with autosomal dominant inheritance (eg, Marfan syndrome). Because of the heterogeneity of congenital heart lesions, each patient needs individual assessment for ability to tolerate the hemodynamic changes of pregnancy.

- **Minimal-risk lesions** include small ventricular septal defects (VSDs), atrial septal defects (ASDs), and bicuspid aortic valves without stenosis, insufficiency, or aortic enlargement. These patients have near-normal physiology with only minimally increased risk during pregnancy and can receive routine care.
- **Moderate-risk lesions** include repaired tetralogy of Fallot without significant pulmonary insufficiency or stenosis, complex congenital heart disease with anatomic right ventricle serving as systemic ventricle, and mild left side valve stenosis.
- **High-risk lesions** for which patients should be counseled against pregnancy due to the risk of maternal cardiac decompensation and death include Eisenmenger syndrome, severe pulmonary hypertension (HTN), severe aortic stenosis (AS) or left ventricular outflow tract obstruction, Marfan syndrome with aortic dilation >45 mm, or symptomatic ventricular dysfunction with ejection fraction (EF) <40%. Moderate- and high-risk patients should be followed at tertiary care centers with maternal-fetal medicine subspecialists and cardiologists experienced in managing pregnant patients with congenital heart disease.
- **Tetralogy of Fallot**, characterized by right ventricular outflow tract obstruction, VSD, right ventricular hypertrophy, and overriding aorta, is associated with right-to-left shunting and cyanosis. If the defect goes uncorrected, the affected patient rarely lives beyond childhood. In developed countries, almost all patients have had surgical correction with good survival rates (85%-86% at 32-36 years) and good quality of life. Pregnancy is generally well tolerated in patients who have had surgical repair, although these women are at increased risk for right-sided heart failure and arrhythmia.
- **Coarctation of the aorta:** Severe cases of coarctation of the aorta are usually corrected in infancy. Surgical correction during pregnancy is recommended only if dissection occurs. Some studies suggest that patients with a history of coarctation have increased rates of preeclampsia, gestational HTN, and preterm labor. Coarctation of the aorta is associated with other cardiac lesions such as berry aneurysms. Two percent of infants of mothers with coarctation of the aorta may have other cardiac lesions. Coarctation of the aorta is characterized by a fixed cardiac output. Therefore, the patient's heart cannot increase its rate to meet the increased cardiac demands of pregnancy, and extreme care must be taken to prevent hypotension, as with AS.

- **Pulmonary HTN:** Currently, the clinical classification system (Table 13-4) for pulmonary HTN includes five groups of disorders. Group 2 disorders are the most common among pregnant women, whereas groups 3 to 5 are not commonly seen in healthy young women. Pulmonary hypertensive disorders are not all equally dangerous. Among pregnant women, mortality rates as high as 23% with group 1 disorders have been reported, whereas mortality rates around 5% are reported with the remaining groups. Almost 80% of deaths occur during the first month postpartum. Thus, pregnancy is contraindicated with severe disease (mostly from group 1 disorders). Less severe lesions with a better prognosis are now discernible with echocardiography and pulmonary artery catheterization, which can help identify patients who tolerate pregnancy, labor, and delivery well. These women are at greatest risk during labor and delivery when venous return and right ventricular filling are diminished. In order to avoid hypotension, great attention should be given to epidural analgesia induction, blood loss prevention, and treatment at delivery.

- **Septal defects.** Young women with uncomplicated secundum-type ASD or isolated VSD usually tolerate pregnancy well. The ASD is the most common congenital heart lesion in adults. The ASDs are usually very well tolerated unless they are associated with pulmonary HTN. Complications, such as atrial arrhythmias, pulmonary HTN, and heart failure, usually do not arise until the fifth decade of life and are therefore uncommon in pregnancy. The VSDs usually close spontaneously or are closed surgically if the lesion is large. For this reason, significant VSDs are rarely seen in pregnancy. Rarely, uncorrected lesions lead to significant left-to-right shunts with pulmonary HTN, right ventricular failure, arrhythmias, and reversal of the shunt. The incidence of VSD in the offspring of affected parents is 4%; however, small VSDs are often difficult to detect antenatally.

- **Patent ductus arteriosus (PDA):** PDA is not associated with additional maternal risk for cardiac complications if the shunt is small to moderate and if pulmonary artery pressures are normal. Moderate to large PDA may be associated with increased volume, left heart failure, and pulmonary HTN or other pulmonary abnormalities. Therefore, pregnancy is not recommended for patients with large PDA and associated complications.

- **Eisenmenger syndrome** occurs when an initial left-to-right shunt results in pulmonary arterial obliteration and pulmonary HTN, eventually leading to a right-to-left shunt. This serious condition carries a maternal mortality rate of more than 50% if cyanosis is present. In addition, 30% of fetuses exhibit intrauterine growth restriction. Because of increased maternal mortality, pregnancy is generally contraindicated, and termination of the pregnancy should be discussed. If the pregnancy is continued, special precautions must be taken during the peripartum period. Women with Eisenmenger syndrome tolerate hypotension poorly. The patient should be monitored with a Swan-Ganz catheter, and care should be taken to avoid hypovolemia. Postpartum death most often occurs within 1 week after delivery; however, delayed deaths up to 4 to 6 weeks after delivery have been reported.

- **Marfan syndrome** is an autosomal dominant disorder of the fibrillin gene characterized by connective tissue fragility. Cardiovascular manifestations include aortic root dilation and dissection, mitral valve prolapse, and aneurysms. Genetic counseling is recommended. According to the 2010 American College of Cardiology/AHA/American Association of Thoracic Surgeons guidelines, patients with a dilated aortic root >40 mm are considered high risk. If cardiovascular involvement is minor and the aortic root diameter is smaller than 40 mm, the risk in pregnancy is less than 1%. If cardiovascular involvement is more extensive or the aortic root is larger than 40 mm, complications during pregnancy and aortic dissection are increased

Table 13-4	Comprehensive Clinical Classification of Pulmonary Hypertension[a]
Group 1: pulmonary arterial HTN	Idiopathic Heritable Drug and toxin induced Associated with connective tissue disease, HIV infections, portal HTN, congenital heart diseases, schistosomiasis Pulmonary venoocclusive disease and/or pulmonary capillary hemangiomatosis • Idiopathic • Heritable • Drugs, toxins and radiation induced • Associated with connective tissue disease, HIV infection Persistent pulmonary HTN of the newborn
Group 2: pulmonary HTN due to left heart disease	Left ventricular systolic dysfunction Left ventricular diastolic dysfunction Valvular disease Congenital/acquired left heart inflow/outflow tract obstruction and congenital cardiomyopathies Congenital/acquired pulmonary vein stenosis
Group 3: pulmonary HTN due to lung diseases and/or hypoxia	Chronic obstructive pulmonary disease Interstitial lung disease Other pulmonary diseases with mixed restrictive and obstructive pattern Sleep-disoriented breathing Alveolar hypoventilation disorder Chronic exposure to high altitude Developmental lung diseases
Group 4: chronic thromboembolic pulmonary HTN/ other pulmonary artery obstructions	Chronic thromboembolic pulmonary HTN Other pulmonary artery obstructions, that is, tumors, arteritis, pulmonary stenosis, parasites
Group 5: pulmonary HTN with unclear and/ or multifactorial mechanisms	Hematological disorders: chronic hemolysis, myeloproliferative disorders, splenectomy Systemic disorders: sarcoidosis, pulmonary histiocytosis, neurofibromatosis Metabolic disorders: glycogen storage disease, Gaucher disease, thyroid disorders Others: fibrosing mediastinitis, chronic renal failure

Abbreviation: HIV, human immunodeficiency virus; HTN, hypertension.

[a]Adapted from Galiè N, Humbert M, Vachiery JL, et al. 2015 ESC/ERS guidelines for the diagnosis and treatment of pulmonary hypertension: the Joint Task Force for the Diagnosis and Treatment of Pulmonary Hypertension of the European Society of Cardiology (ESC) and the European Respiratory Society (ERS): endorsed by: Association for European Paediatric and Congenital Cardiology (AEPC), International Society for Heart and Lung Transplantation (ISHLT). *Eur Heart J.* 2016;37(1):67-119. Reproduced by permission of European Society of Cardiology & European Respiratory Society.

significantly. Patients should be monitored with serial physical exams as well as echocardiography. The HTN should be avoided. β-Blockade is recommended for patients with Marfan syndrome from the second trimester onward, particularly if the aortic root is dilated. Regional anesthesia during labor is considered safe. Women should labor in the left lateral decubitus position with the second stage shortened by operative vaginal delivery. Cesarean delivery should be reserved for obstetric indications.

- **Idiopathic hypertrophic subaortic stenosis** is an autosomal dominant disorder that manifests as left ventricular outflow tract obstruction secondary to a hypertrophic interventricular septum. Genetic counseling is advised for affected patients. Patients' conditions improve when left ventricular end-diastolic volume is maximized. Pregnant patients fare quite well initially because of an increase in circulating blood volume. There is less progression of disease in those patients who are asymptomatic before pregnancy. Later in pregnancy, however, decreased systemic vascular resistance and decreased venous return may worsen the obstruction. This may cause left ventricular failure as well as supraventricular arrhythmias from left atrial distention. The following labor management points should be kept in mind: (1) inotropic agents may exacerbate obstruction, (2) medications that decrease systemic vascular resistance should be avoided or limited, (3) cardiac rhythm should be monitored and tachycardia treated promptly, and (4) the patient should undergo labor in the left lateral decubitus position with the second stage of labor shortened by operative vaginal delivery.

- **Transposition of the great arteries** is characterized by correct atrioventricular connections and inappropriate ventriculoarterial connections; the aorta arises anteriorly from the right ventricle, and the pulmonary artery arises posteriorly from the left ventricle. The Senning operation (using atrial and septal tissues) and Mustard operation (using extrinsic material such as pericardium) redirect atrial blood via baffles to deliver oxygenated pulmonary venous blood to the systemic right ventricle and deoxygenated systemic venous blood to the pulmonary left ventricle. Long-term follow-up demonstrates an 80% survival at 28 years with the majority of survivors in NYHA class I. Pregnancy in women after Senning or Mustard repair is associated with arrhythmias (ventricular tachycardia, supraventricular tachycardia, atrial flutter), heart failure, and NYHA functional class deterioration as well as a high incidence of serious obstetric complications (65%) and offspring mortality (11.7%).

- **Congenital atrioventricular block:** Although affected patients may need a pacemaker, they usually fare well and do not require special treatment during pregnancy.

Heart Transplant Recipients

- According to the current recommendations from the International Society of Heart and Lung Transplantation, pregnancy is not discouraged in heart transplant recipients who are stable 1-year posttransplant. These patients would require highly specialized care with a multidisciplinary team.

Specific Cardiac Conditions

Cardiomyopathy

- **Cardiomyopathy** can be genetic, idiopathic, or caused by myocarditis or toxins and manifests during pregnancy with signs and symptoms of CHF. These include chest pain, dyspnea, paroxysmal nocturnal dyspnea, and cough. Echocardiography demonstrates chamber enlargement and reduced ventricular function. The heart becomes uniformly dilated, filling pressures increase, and cardiac output decreases. Eventually, heart failure develops and is often refractory to treatment. The 5-year survival rate is approximately 50%; therefore, careful preconception counseling is important, even if the patient is asymptomatic.

- **Hypertrophic cardiomyopathy** with or without left ventricular outflow tract obstruction is an autosomal dominant disorder with a variable phenotype and incidence of 0.1% to 0.5% in pregnancy. Most women with hypertrophic cardiomyopathy do well in pregnancy, and complications are uncommon with prior prepregnancy risk stratification via NYHA functional class and multidisciplinary specialist management. Risk is increased in patients who are symptomatic or if there is significant left ventricular outflow obstruction. The potential exists for poor tolerance of the circulatory overload of pregnancy. Major complications include pulmonary edema secondary to diastolic dysfunction, dysrhythmias secondary to myofibrillar disarray, functional class decline, obstetric complications, and poor fetal outcomes. During pregnancy, β-blockers should be continued and the judicious use of diuretics may be required to treat symptoms of dyspnea.

- **Peripartum cardiomyopathy** is an idiopathic dilated cardiomyopathy that typically develops in the last month of pregnancy or within 5 months of delivery without another identifiable cause of cardiac failure. It is characterized by left ventricular systolic dysfunction with EF <45%. Incidence is 1 in 1300 to 1 in 15 000. Risk factors include advanced maternal age; multiparity; multiple gestations; black race; obesity; malnutrition; gestational HTN; preeclampsia; poor antenatal care; breastfeeding; cesarean delivery; low socioeconomic status; family history; and abuse of tobacco, alcohol, or cocaine. The most common clinical complaints are dyspnea, cough, orthopnea, paroxysmal nocturnal dyspnea, and hemoptysis. Workup and diagnosis are completed with ECG, echocardiography, and lab studies such as brain natriuretic peptide.

  o Of the patients who survive, approximately 50% recover normal left heart function. The mortality rate is 25% to 50%; half of those die within the first month of presentation, and the majority dies within 3 months postpartum. Prognosis is related to left ventricular dysfunction at presentation. Death results from progressive CHF, thromboembolic events, and arrhythmias.

  o Medical management includes fluid and salt restriction, digoxin, diuretics, vasodilators, and anticoagulants; bed rest can predispose to thromboembolism. Cardiac transplantation may be required in advanced unresolving disease. For patients diagnosed antenatally, invasive cardiac monitoring should be considered during labor and until at least 24 hours postpartum. Supplemental oxygen and regional analgesia for pain control should be administered, and a passive second stage of labor facilitated by operative vaginal delivery should take place. Cesarean delivery is reserved for obstetric indications. Intensive care unit monitoring should continue immediately postpartum, including detection and management of possible autotransfusion-induced pulmonary edema.

Valvular Disease

- **Mitral valve prolapse** is the most common congenital heart defect in women. It rarely has implications for maternal or fetal outcomes. It is the most common cause of mitral regurgitation (MR) in women.
- An **MR** is usually well tolerated during pregnancy. The fall in systemic vasoresistance improves cardiac output in pregnancy. Medical management includes diuretics in

the rare event of pulmonary congestion or vasodilators for systemic HTN. Acute, severe worsening of MR can result from ruptured chordae and must be repaired surgically. Women with severe MR before pregnancy should undergo operative repair before conception. Patients with advanced disease may require central monitoring during labor.

- **Aortic regurgitation (AR)** may be encountered in women with rheumatic heart disease, a congenitally bicuspid or deformed aortic valve, IE, or connective tissue disease. An AR is generally well tolerated during pregnancy. Medical management includes diuretics and vasodilators. Ideally, women with severe AR should undergo operative repair before conception; as in MR, surgery during pregnancy should be considered only for control of refractory NYHA functional class III or IV symptoms.

- **Aortic stenosis:** The most common etiology of AS in pregnant women is a congenitally bicuspid valve. Mild AS with normal left ventricular function is usually well tolerated during pregnancy. Asymptomatic severe stenosis can be managed conservatively with bed rest, oxygen, and β-blockade. Moderate to severe AS markedly increases the medical risk of pregnancy; patients are advised to delay conception until correction is performed. Symptoms such as dyspnea, angina pectoris, or syncope usually become apparent late in the second trimester or early in the third trimester. Women with bicuspid aortic valves are also at increased risk for aortic dissection and should be followed carefully. Aortic root enlargement >40 mm or an increase in aortic root size during pregnancy are risk factors for dissection. β-Blockers may be indicated in these patients.

  - Severe symptomatic AS can be managed by percutaneous aortic balloon valvuloplasty prior to labor and delivery but not without significant risk to both mother and fetus. If presenting early in pregnancy, termination should be discussed before surgical correction of severe AS (EF <40%). Spinal and epidural anesthesia are discouraged because of their vasodilatory effects. This disorder is characterized by a fixed afterload; thus, adequate end-diastolic volume, and therefore adequate filling pressure, are necessary to maintain cardiac output. Consequently, great care must be taken to prevent hypotension, tachycardia, and hypoperfusion caused by blood loss, regional anesthesia, or other medications. Patients should be hydrated adequately and placed in the left lateral position to maximize venous return. As with mitral stenosis (MS), hemodynamic monitoring with a pulmonary arterial catheter should be considered during labor and delivery.

- **Pulmonic stenosis** frequently accompanies other congenital cardiac anomalies, but as an isolated lesion, pulmonic stenosis rarely complicates pregnancy. Patients with acyanotic congenital cardiac disease tolerate pregnancy better than those with cyanotic lesions. Echocardiogram-guided percutaneous valvotomy is a potential treatment option.

- **Mitral stenosis** in women of childbearing age is usually due to rheumatic fever. Patients with moderate to severe MS often experience hemodynamic deterioration during the third trimester and/or during labor and delivery. Increased blood volumes and heart rate lead to an elevation of left atrial pressure, resulting in pulmonary edema. Additional displacement of blood volume into the systemic circulation during contractions makes labor particularly hazardous. Mild to moderate MS can be managed with judicious diuresis and β-blockade, although aggressive diuresis should be avoided to preserve uteroplacental perfusion. Cardioselective β-blockers, such as metoprolol and atenolol, are used to treat or prevent tachycardia, optimizing diastolic filling while preventing deleterious effects of epinephrine blockade on myometrial activity. Patients with severe MS who develop NYHA functional class III to IV symptoms during pregnancy should undergo percutaneous balloon valvotomy.

- Atrial fibrillation in pregnant patients with MS may result in rapid decompensation. Digoxin and β-blockers can reduce heart rate, and diuretics may be used to reduce blood volume and left atrial pressure. With atrial fibrillation and hemodynamic deterioration, electrocardioversion can be performed safely and promptly. Atrial fibrillation also increases the risk of stroke and necessitates anticoagulation.
- Most patients with MS can undergo vaginal delivery. However, patients with symptoms of CHF or moderate to severe MS should undergo hemodynamic monitoring with a Swan-Ganz catheter during labor, delivery, and for several hours postpartum. Epidural anesthesia is usually better tolerated hemodynamically than general anesthesia.

Arrhythmias

Premature atrial and/or ventricular complexes are not associated with adverse maternal or fetal outcomes and do not require antiarrhythmic therapy. **Atrial fibrillation** and **atrial flutter** are rare during pregnancy. Rate control can be safely achieved with digoxin or β-blockers. Electrical cardioversion can be performed safely during any stage of pregnancy. Other arrhythmias should be managed with the assistance of a cardiologist. Nonsustained arrhythmias in the absence of organic cardiac disease are best left untreated or managed with lifestyle and dietary modifications (eg, decreasing smoking, caffeine, and stress). Serious, life-threatening arrhythmias associated with an aberrant reentrant pathway should be treated before pregnancy by ablation. If medical therapy is necessary during pregnancy, established drugs such as β-blockers should be used. Artificial pacing, electrical defibrillation, and cardioversion should have no effect on the fetus.

Ischemic Heart Disease

- **Ischemic heart disease** is an uncommon but potentially devastating event in pregnancy. Risk factors include HTN, thrombophilia, diabetes, smoking, transfusion, postpartum infection, obesity, and age >35 years. Anterior wall myocardial infarctions (MIs) are most common. Diagnosis and evaluation of acute cardiac events is similar as in nonpregnant patients. Approximately 67% of MIs during pregnancy occur during the third trimester. If it occurs before 24 weeks' gestation, the option of pregnancy termination should be discussed due to the high incidence of maternal mortality. If delivery takes place within 2 weeks of the acute event, the mortality rate reaches 50%; survival is much improved if delivery takes place more than 2 weeks after the acute event.
- Coronary angioplasty is the preferred reperfusion therapy in cases of ST-elevated MI. Medical therapy for acute MI should be modified in the pregnant patient. Thrombolytic agents increase the risk of maternal hemorrhage to 8% for women who receive thrombolytic therapy shortly after delivery. Low-dose aspirin and nitrates are considered safe. β-Blockers are safe, although some have been linked to a slight decrease in fetal growth. Short-term heparin administration has not been associated with increased maternal or fetal adverse effects. Angiotensin-converting enzyme inhibitors and statins are contraindicated during pregnancy. Hydralazine and nitrates may be used as substitutes for angiotensin-converting enzyme inhibitors.

Cardiovascular Drugs in Pregnancy

- The most commonly used cardiovascular drugs and their potential adverse effects during pregnancy are shown in Table 13-5.
- **Anticoagulation:** Several conditions require the initiation or maintenance of anticoagulation during pregnancy. Anticoagulation choice depends on patient and physician preferences after consideration of the maternal and fetal risks. The three most common agents considered during pregnancy are unfractionated heparin (UFH), low-molecular-weight heparin (LMWH), and warfarin.

Table 13-5	Cardiovascular Drugs in Pregnancy[a]
Drug	**Side Effects**
Amiodarone	Goiter, hypothyroidism and hyperthyroidism, IUGR
ACE inhibitors	Contraindicated; oligohydramnios, IUGR, renal failure, abnormal bone ossification; FDA class X
Aspirin	Baby aspirin not harmful
β-Blockers	Relatively safe; IUGR, neonatal bradycardia and hypoglycemia
Calcium channel blockers	Relatively safe; few data; concern regarding uterine tone at the time of delivery
Digoxin	Safe; no adverse effects
Flecainide	Relatively safe; limited data; used to treat fetal arrhythmias
Hydralazine	Safe; no major adverse effects
Furosemide	Safe; caution regarding maternal hypovolemia and reduced placental blood flow
Lidocaine	Safe; high doses may cause neonatal central nervous system depression
Methyldopa	Safe
Procainamide	Relatively safe; limited data; has been used to treat fetal arrhythmias, no major fetal side effects
Propafenone	Limited data
Quinidine	Relatively safe; rarely associated with neonatal thrombocytopenia; minimal oxytocic effect
Warfarin	Fetal embryopathy, fetal CNS abnormalities, placental and fetal hemorrhage; FDA class X

Abbreviations: ACE, angiotensin-converting enzyme; CNS, central nervous system; FDA, US Food and Drug Administration; IUGR, intrauterine growth restriction.
[a]Adapted from Elkayam U. Pregnancy and cardiovascular disease. In: Braunwald E, ed. *Braunwald's Heart Disease: A Textbook of Cardiovascular Medicine.* 10th ed. Philadelphia, PA: WB Saunders; 2015:1764. Copyright © 2015 Elsevier. With permission.

- The **UFH** does not cross the placenta and is safe for the fetus. Its use, however, has been associated with maternal osteoporosis, hemorrhage at the uteroplacental junction, thrombocytopenia (heparin-induced thrombocytopenia), thrombosis, and a high incidence (12%-24%) of thromboembolic events with older generation mechanical valves. High doses of UFH are often required to achieve the desired activated partial thromboplastin time due to the hypercoagulable state associated with pregnancy. Parenteral infusions should be stopped at least 4 hours before cesarean deliveries. The UFH can be reversed with protamine sulfate.

- The **LMWH**, in comparison to UFH, produces a more predictable anticoagulant response, is less likely to cause heparin-induced thrombocytopenia, is easier to administer and monitor, and has lower risk of osteoporosis and bleeding complications. The LMWH does not cross the placenta and is safe for the fetus. Anti-factor Xa levels can be checked 4 hours after the morning dose and the dose adjusted to attain anti-factor Xa levels of 0.7 to 1.2 U/mL. Although data support the use of LMWH for deep vein thrombosis treatment in pregnant women, there are no data to guide its use in pregnant patients with mechanical valve prostheses, and several small studies have shown increased rates of serious complications.

- **Warfarin**, a vitamin K antagonist, freely crosses the placenta and can harm the fetus. The incidence of warfarin embryopathy (abnormalities of fetal bone and cartilage formation) has been estimated at 4% to 10%; the risk is highest when warfarin is administered during the 6th to 12th week of gestation. Clinically, important embryopathy may be lower if the warfarin dose is <5 mg/d. Fetal central nervous system abnormalities can occur after exposure during any trimester. Some conditions may warrant treatment with warfarin during pregnancy, however. Specifically, in the setting of mechanical prosthetic heart valves, warfarin has been associated with a lower risk of maternal thromboembolic complications compared to heparin (by approximately 2%-4%). Treatment of this high-risk population must balance potentially improved thrombotic prophylaxis against risks of embryopathy. Some groups recommend prophylaxis in patients with mechanical heart valves using heparin agents in the first trimester, with consideration to transitioning to warfarin until the last weeks of pregnancy. The patient must be transitioned back to heparin several weeks before delivery to avoid risk of fetal hemorrhage.

RESPIRATORY DISORDERS

Pulmonary Changes During Pregnancy

- Pregnancy causes mechanical and biochemical changes that affect maternal respiratory function and gas exchange. The most prominent factors are the mechanical effect of the gravid uterus on the diaphragm and the effect of increased circulating progesterone on ventilation. Progesterone is thought to increase the sensitivity of the respiratory center to carbon dioxide.

- Elevation of the diaphragm in the second half of pregnancy decreases functional residual capacity, the resting volume of the lungs at the end of a normal expiration. Despite the alteration in resting diaphragm position, excursion is unaffected and therefore vital capacity is maintained. Airway function is also maintained during pregnancy, as FEV_1 (forced expiratory volume in 1 second) and FEV_1/forced vital capacity are normal. Resting minute ventilation increases by 50% due to increased tidal volume of 40%. Both FEV_1 and peak expiratory flow remain unchanged. As a result of increased minute ventilation, arterial PCO_2 decreases, which is offset by renal bicarbonate excretion, and arterial PO_2 levels are slightly increased. Oxygen consumption increases by 15% to 20% throughout pregnancy, which is compensated by the increased cardiac output. Arterial pH rises slightly from the decrease in PCO_2, resulting in a mild maternal respiratory alkalosis.

Specific Respiratory Disorders

Asthma

- **Asthma** is the most common chronic condition in pregnancy and affects 3% to 12% of gestations. Low birth weight is common in infants born to mothers reporting daily symptoms of moderate asthma. This condition is more likely to worsen in women with prepregnancy severe asthma. For women with severe asthma, a pulmonary examination, peak flow measurement, and review of symptoms should be performed at each visit. Smoking cessation must be encouraged. In addition, patients may monitor their peak flow at home and begin treatment before they become dangerously symptomatic. Pregnant women tend to decrease use of asthma medications, found in Table 13-6, because of fear of fetal malformations. Physicians should provide reassurance that it is safer to take asthma medications in pregnancy than to risk adverse perinatal outcomes from a severe exacerbation. Exacerbations are most frequent between 24 and 36 weeks' gestation and are most commonly precipitated by viral respiratory infections and noncompliance with inhaled corticosteroid regimens. Because asthma exacerbations can be severe, they should be treated aggressively in pregnancy, and the threshold for hospitalization is lower for pregnant patients.
- **Acute asthma exacerbations** that require hospital observation or admission are treated with 40% humidified oxygen and β-agonists initially. Chest radiograph should be obtained. Anticholinergics and inhaled or systemic steroids can be added as needed. Intubation should be considered if the PCO_2 is >40 mm Hg or hypoxia develops.
- **Exacerbations during labor** are rare, perhaps because of the increase in endogenous cortisol. Patients who received steroids throughout their pregnancies may require stress-dose steroids during labor and delivery. General endotracheal anesthesia should be avoided, if possible, because of the increased incidence of bronchospasm and atelectasis.

Influenza

- Every year, 10% of women develop **influenza**. Symptoms, including fever, cough, myalgia, and chills, develop 1 to 4 days after exposure. The most common complication of influenza is pneumonia. Pregnant women are more likely to be hospitalized or admitted to an intensive care unit when affected. See chapter 8 for further discussion, including treatment.

Cystic Fibrosis

- **Cystic fibrosis (CF)** is an autosomal recessive disorder occurring in approximately 1 in 2500 live births and is characterized by abnormal epithelial cell chloride transport and thickened glandular secretions. Diagnosis is confirmed by elevated sweat chloride concentration with pilocarpine iontophoresis or by mutation analysis of

Table 13-6	Asthma Medications in Pregnancy
Inhaled corticosteroids	• Are cornerstone of treatment for persistent asthma of all severities • Remain active locally with little systemic absorption, effectively preventing exacerbations • Reassure patients that side effect profile is not the same as for oral steroids to ensure compliance • Examples: beclomethasone, fluticasone, budesonide, flunisolide, triamcinolone
Oral/IV steroids	• Are indicated for acute exacerbations when patients do not respond to other measures • In acute settings: hydrocortisone 100 mg IV every 8 h or methylprednisolone 125 mg IV every 6 h, followed by oral prednisone taper
β-Sympathomimetics	• Help control asthma via bronchial smooth muscle relaxation • Can be used for symptomatic relief in conjunction with inhaled corticosteroids • Short-acting preparations are safe in pregnancy. • Few data available on long-acting preparations
Anticholinergics	• Are used to treat severe symptoms • Side effects include tachycardia. • Example: aerosolized ipratropium bromide or glycopyrrolate
Cromolyn and leukotriene antagonists	• Useful alternatives for mild persistent asthma • Can be used as additional treatment for more severe exacerbations
Theophylline	• Phosphodiesterase inhibitor • Last treatment option in moderate or severe asthma • Blood levels required during third trimester because clearance increases during this period

Abbreviation: IV, intravenous.

the cystic fibrosis transmembrane conductance regulator (*CFTR*) gene. Due to improved treatment modalities, women with CF are living longer—the median survival age is 37 years—and they are more frequently reaching childbearing age.

• Recent reports are describing better maternal and perinatal outcomes of women with CF. The best predictor of pregnancy and long-term maternal outcome is disease severity, quantified by pulmonary function studies. When matched with nonpregnant women by disease severity, pregnancy does not compromise long-term survival. Poor prognostic factors include FEV_1 <60% of predicted, cor pulmonale, and pulmonary HTN. If prepregnancy FEV_1 is <60% of predicted, the risk for preterm delivery, respiratory complications, and death of the mother within a few years of childbirth is significantly increased.

- Preconception counseling should include offering carrier screening to unaffected partners. If the partner is found to be a carrier, the risk of having an affected child is 50%. A careful discussion should be had between the couple, CF physician, maternal-fetal medicine specialist, and a medical geneticist.
- A multidisciplinary team approach is vital in the care of a pregnant CF patient. Collaboration between the maternal-fetal medicine specialist, CF physician, neonatologist, anesthesiologist, pharmacist, and dietitian should occur throughout the pregnancy.
- The effect of pregnancy on a CF patient is unpredictable; thus, every pregnancy should be regarded as high risk for both mother and fetus. During pregnancy, close monitoring of lung function and sputum microbiology are mandatory. Pulmonary function tests should be performed monthly throughout pregnancy and pulmonary infection should be managed aggressively. Affected patients may also have pancreatic insufficiency manifested as diabetes, malabsorption, or liver cirrhosis. Early diabetes screening in pregnancy is indicated. Due to malabsorption, CF mothers should eat a diet with 120% to 150% of the recommended intake for non-CF patients and should aim for >11 kg of weight gain.
- During labor, fluid and electrolytes should be followed closely. The increased sodium content of sweat in affected patients may make them prone to hypovolemia during labor. Overall, 70% to 80% of pregnant mothers with CF have successful deliveries of healthy infants.
- Breast milk should be evaluated for sodium content before the infant is allowed to breastfeed; in the event of significant sodium elevation, breastfeeding is contraindicated.

Tuberculosis

- **Tuberculosis (TB)** is a worldwide public health issue and highly prevalent in many urban areas.
  - Screening is by subcutaneous injection of purified protein derivative (PPD). Only 80% of results are positive in the setting of reactivation of disease, however, and if a patient previously received the Bacille Calmette-Guérin vaccine, the PPD result may remain positive for life. If the PPD test is positive or TB is suspected, chest radiography with abdominal shielding should be performed, preferably after 20 weeks' gestation. Alternative methods of screening are being developed but have yet to be widely accepted to replace PPD screening.
  - A definitive diagnosis of TB can be made with culture of *Mycobacterium tuberculosis* or acid-fast stain. Sputum samples may be induced using aerosolized saline; the first morning sputum should be collected for 3 consecutive days. If sputum is positive for acid-fast bacilli, antibiotic therapy should be initiated while final culture and sensitivity results are pending.
  - Standard treatment in pregnancy consists of isoniazid (INH) with pyridoxine supplementation, ethambutol, and pyrazinamide. Streptomycin sulfate should be avoided because of the risk of fetal cranial nerve VIII damage. Rifampin should also be avoided during pregnancy unless INH and ethambutol cannot be used. The INH prophylaxis for 6 to 9 months is recommended for asymptomatic patients younger than 35 years with positive PPD results and negative findings on chest radiograph.

- If the patient has converted to positive PPD results within the last 2 years, INH therapy should be initiated during the pregnancy after the first trimester. If the time since conversion is unknown or longer than 2 years, INH is started during the postpartum period. The INH prophylaxis is not recommended for patients older than 35 years due to its hepatotoxicity. If treated, TB should not affect the pregnancy, and pregnancy should not alter the course of the disease.

Acute Respiratory Distress Syndrome

Acute respiratory distress syndrome (ARDS) is an acute lung injury that leads to severe permeability pulmonary edema and respiratory failure. Mortality rates have been reported as high as 25% to 40% in pregnancy.

- Sepsis and diffuse infectious pneumonia are the two most common causes of ARDS in pregnancy. Chorioamnionitis, pyelonephritis, and puerperal pelvic infection are the most common causes of sepsis. Severe preeclampsia and obstetric hemorrhage are also associated with permeability edema.
- Acute respiratory failure is characterized by hypoxemia, dyspnea, and tachypnea. As pulmonary edema increases and lung volume loss results, pulmonary compliance worsens and intrapulmonary blood shunting occurs. Lung abnormalities are heard by auscultation, and a chest radiograph is notable for bilateral lung involvement.
- In the management of ARDS, providing adequate oxygenation is balanced against aggravating further lung injury. Support of systemic perfusion with blood and intravenous crystalloid is vital; however, conservative fluid management rather than liberal is associated with fewer days of mechanical ventilation. Infection should be treated with antimicrobial therapy. Early intubation in pregnancy is preferred if respiratory failure is imminent.

SUGGESTED READINGS

Cunningham FG, Leveno KJ, Bloom SL, et al, eds. Cardiovascular disorders. In: *Williams Obstetrics*. 25th ed. New York, NY: McGraw-Hill; 2018:948-974.

Cunningham FG, Leveno KJ, Bloom SL, et al, eds. Pulmonary disorders. In: *Williams Obstetrics*. 25th ed. New York, NY: McGraw-Hill; 2018:987-1003.

Deen J, Chandrasekaran S, Stout K, Easterling T. Heart disease in pregnancy. In: Gabbe SG, Niebyl JR, Simpson JL, et al, eds. *Obstetrics: Normal and Problem Pregnancies*. 7th ed. Philadelphia, PA: Elsevier; 2017:803-827.

Whitty JE, Dombrowski MP. Respiratory disease in pregnancy. In: Gabbe SG, Niebyl JR, Simpson JL, et al, eds. *Obstetrics: Normal and Problem Pregnancies*. 7th ed. Philadelphia, PA: Elsevier; 2017:828-849.

Wilson W, Taubert KA, Gewitz M, et al. Prevention of infective endocarditis: guidelines from the American Heart Association: a guideline from the American Heart Association Rheumatic Fever, Endocarditis and Kawasaki Disease Committee, Council on Cardiovascular Disease in the Young, and the Council on Clinical Cardiology, Council on Cardiovascular Surgery and Anesthesia, and the Quality of Care and Outcomes Research Interdisciplinary Working Group. *J Am Dent Assoc*. 2007;138:739-745, 747-760.

14 Genitourinary Assessment and Renal Disease in Pregnancy

Lauren M. Kucirka and Cynthia H. Argani

Pregnancy is associated with significant changes in renal and urinary tract structure and function, and renal and urinary tract disorders are common.

KIDNEY AND URINARY TRACT DISORDERS

Renal Physiology in Pregnancy

- The renal system undergoes many physiologic changes during a normal pregnancy. In addition, as the gravid uterus increases in size, it produces a mass effect on the renal system.
- **Structural changes.** During pregnancy, the kidneys increase 1 to 1.5 cm in length and 30% in volume. The collecting system expands more than 80%, with greater dilation on the right side.
  - Mild right-sided physiologic hydronephrosis is seen as early as 6 weeks of gestation. Renal volume returns to normal within the first week postpartum, but hydronephrosis and hydroureter may not normalize until 3 to 4 months after delivery. Elective pyelography should, therefore, be deferred until at least 12 weeks postpartum.
  - These structural changes increase the risk of pyelonephritis in the setting of asymptomatic bacteriuria (ASB) or urinary tract infections (UTIs).
- **Renal filtration.** Blood volume expansion during pregnancy increases renal plasma flow by 50% to 80%, which in turn results in an increased glomerular filtration rate (GFR). Increased GFR can be seen within 1 month after conception, peaking at 40% to 50% above prepregnancy levels by the end of the first trimester.
  - Elevated GFR increases creatinine clearance, so formulas for GFR based on age, height, and weight do not apply; creatinine clearance must be calculated with a 24-hour urine collection in pregnancy.
  - Increased GFR results in lower mean serum blood urea nitrogen (BUN) and serum creatinine during pregnancy (8.5 and 0.46 mg/dL, respectively). A serum creatinine that may be considered normal outside of pregnancy may suggest renal insufficiency in pregnancy.
- **Renal tubular function.** Decreased tubular resorption in pregnancy increases urinary excretion of electrolytes, glucose, amino acids, and protein.
  - Increased calcium clearance is balanced by increased gastrointestinal tract absorption. Ionized calcium remains stable despite decreased total serum calcium because of the lower serum albumin concentration.
  - Physiologic hyponatremia occurs, with plasma sodium concentration falling by 5 mEq/L during pregnancy. Sodium levels return to baseline by 1 to 2 months postpartum.
  - Urinary excretion of glucose increases 10- to 100-fold, and glucosuria is observed routinely in normal pregnancy. Increased urinary glucose increases the risk of bacteriuria and UTIs.

- Renal resorption of bicarbonate decreases to compensate for the respiratory alkalosis of pregnancy, lowering serum bicarbonate by about 5 mEq/L in pregnancy.
- **Routine assessment of renal function.** Although routine antenatal screening for proteinuria is common, there is limited data to support its efficacy. If there is suspicion for preeclampsia, proteinuria can be assessed by either urine protein to creatinine ratio or a 24-hour urine protein test, with ratio $\geq$0.3 mg/dL or proteinuria >300 mg/dL diagnostic in combination with elevated blood pressures.
  - Patients with chronic hypertension, diabetes, preexisting renal disease, or other diseases may have abnormal levels of proteinuria prior to pregnancy and should undergo a baseline 24-hour urine protein collection early in pregnancy.
  - Serum creatinine persistently >0.9 mg/dL should prompt investigation for intrinsic renal disease. The presence of comorbidities should be assessed, and further evaluation should be considered. Renal biopsy during pregnancy should be considered when the results will change management before delivery.

Urinary Tract Disorders in Pregnancy

Urinary Tract Infection

- **Urinary tract infections** are common in pregnancy. Urinary stasis secondary to hydroureter and hydronephrosis, bladder trauma due to compression or edema, vesicoureteral reflux, and increased glucosuria may all contribute to the increased risk of infection. Women with two or more UTIs or a diagnosis of pyelonephritis during pregnancy should be considered for daily suppressive antibiotic therapy until delivery.
  - **Asymptomatic bacteriuria** is the presence of bacteria within the urinary tract, excluding the distal urethra, without signs or symptoms of infection. The prevalence of ASB during pregnancy ranges from 2% to 7%. If left untreated, 20% to 30% of ASB in pregnant women progresses to pyelonephritis; treatment reduces this to 3%. Pyelonephritis is associated with low-birth-weight infants and preterm delivery; as such, its treatment in pregnancy is indicated. Screening for bacteriuria with a urine culture is recommended at the first prenatal visit. Women with sickle cell trait have a 2-fold increased risk of ASB and can be screened every trimester.
    - A clean-catch urine culture with a single bacterial strain >10 000 colonies/mL or catheterized urine culture with >100 colonies/mL warrants treatment.
    - *Escherichia coli* accounts for 75% to 90% of infections. *Klebsiella*, *Proteus*, *Pseudomonas*, *Enterobacter*, and coagulase-negative *Staphylococci* are other common pathogens. Women infected with group B *Streptococcus* bacteriuria should be treated with appropriate antibiotics at the onset of labor or rupture of membranes in order to prevent neonatal infection.
    - Initial therapy is usually empiric and may be altered based on urine culture sensitivities. Short course therapy of 3 to 7 days is as effective as continuous therapy. Repeat urine culture is obtained 1 to 2 weeks after treatment and again each trimester. If bacteriuria persists after two or more treatment courses, suppressive therapy should be considered for the remainder of the pregnancy. Sulfonamides and nitrofurantoin can be used as first line for treatment and suppression during the second and third trimesters. There is mixed evidence regarding associations between these drugs and birth defects when used in the first trimester; however, they may be used when suitable

alternatives are not available. Sulfonamides and nitrofurantoin are contraindicated in women with glucose-6-phosphate deficiency.

- **Acute cystitis** occurs in approximately 1% to 3% of pregnant women. Symptoms include urinary frequency, urgency, dysuria, hematuria, and/or suprapubic discomfort. Empiric treatment regimens are the same as for ASB. If possible, a urine culture should be sent prior to initiating antibiotic therapy.
- **Urethritis** is usually caused by *Chlamydia trachomatis*, and it should be suspected in patients with symptoms of acute cystitis and a negative urine culture. Mucopurulent cervicitis may also be present. The treatment of choice is azithromycin 1 g as a single oral dose for both the patient and her partner. A test of cure should be sent 3 to 4 weeks after treatment.

Pyelonephritis

- **Acute pyelonephritis** occurs in approximately 1% to 2% of all pregnancies and is the leading cause of septic shock in pregnancy. Complications include preterm labor, preterm premature rupture of membranes (PPROM), bacteremia, sepsis, acute respiratory distress syndrome, and hemolytic anemia. Prompt diagnosis and treatment of pyelonephritis in pregnancy are crucial.
  - Symptoms include fever, chills, flank pain, nausea, and vomiting. Frequency, urgency, and dysuria are variably present.
  - Pyelonephritis is a clinical diagnosis. Urine culture, complete blood count, serum creatinine, and electrolytes should be obtained at admission. Blood cultures should be obtained for patients suspected to be in sepsis.
  - Treatment includes administration of intravenous broad-spectrum antibiotics, hydration, and antipyretics. Ceftriaxone is commonly used and is equivalent to ampicillin plus gentamicin. For penicillin-allergic patients, clindamycin plus gentamicin is appropriate. Fluoroquinolones are generally avoided during pregnancy.
  - Pregnant women with pyelonephritis are at increased risk for developing acute respiratory distress syndrome. They should be closely monitored for evidence of respiratory symptomatology with provision of respiratory support as needed.
  - Transition to an oral regimen is appropriate after an afebrile period of greater than 48 hours. Antibiotic regimen should be chosen based on urine culture sensitivities. Oral therapy is continued to complete a 14-day course. Daily suppressive therapy is then initiated for the remainder of pregnancy due to the recurrence risk of approximately 20%.
  - If there is no response to antibiotic treatment within 48 hours, review antibiotic dosing and sensitivities, send repeat urine culture, and obtain renal ultrasonography to evaluate for anatomic anomalies, nephrolithiasis, and intrarenal or perinephric abscess.

Nephrolithiasis

- **Nephrolithiasis** should be considered in a pregnant patient with acute onset of abdominal or flank pain. The incidence is between 0.3 and 4 per 1000 pregnancies. Increased urinary excretion of calcium, urinary stasis, and dehydration are risk factors associated with development of renal stones in pregnancy.
  - Diagnosis is primarily clinical. Classic symptoms include acute onset of colicky flank pain, hematuria, and pyuria. In more than 50% of cases, the stone passes spontaneously after hydration and may be observed directly by filtering

the patient's urine. Renal ultrasonography should be performed to rule out obstruction, but pathologic obstruction from a renal stone must be differentiated from physiologic hydronephrosis of pregnancy. If the diagnosis remains uncertain and there is a negative ultrasound, magnetic resonance urography or noncontrast computed tomography scan can be considered.

- Initial treatment is administration of intravenous hydration and analgesia, with the patient lying on her side with the symptomatic side up. This helps reduce the pressure from the gravid uterus on the affected side. Approximately 75% of stones will pass spontaneously. Associated infections must be treated aggressively. Indications for surgical intervention include impairment of renal function, obstruction, protracted severe pain, or signs of sepsis. Extracorporeal shock wave lithotripsy is contraindicated in pregnancy.

Polycystic Kidney Disease

- Autosomal dominant polycystic kidney disease (ADPKD) afflicts between 1:400 and 1:1000 individuals and is characterized by the presence of large, fluid-filled cysts in the kidneys.
- Complications include hypertension, recurrent UTIs, flank pain, nephrolithiasis, and hematuria. There is an increased risk of developing aortic or berry aneurysms. Pregnant women with ADPKD are at increased risk for hypertensive crisis, preeclampsia, UTIs, and renal dysfunction. It is important to counsel patients that the child has a 50% chance of inheriting ADPKD.

Glomerular Disease

- **Glomerular disease** is caused by a wide spectrum of diseases, and its clinical presentation can vary from no symptoms to renal failure. Clinical syndromes are defined to differentiate these patients, with nephritic and nephrotic syndrome being the most common. Definitive diagnosis ultimately requires a renal biopsy. However, with potential risks, renal biopsy should only be pursued in pregnancy if results will change management.
- **Acute nephritic syndrome**
  - Usually presents with hypertension, hematuria, urinary red cell casts, pyuria, and mild to moderate proteinuria.
  - Causes include poststreptococcal glomerulonephritis, lupus nephritis, immunoglobulin A (IgA) nephropathy, membranoproliferative glomerulonephritis, endocarditis-associated glomerulonephritis, antiglomerular basement membrane disease, Goodpasture syndrome, Wegener syndrome, and Churg-Strauss syndrome.
  - Goodpasture, Wegener, Churg-Straus, Henoch-Schönlein purpura, or cryoglobulinemia can also present as a pulmonary renal syndrome with significant hemoptysis along with glomerulonephritis.
- **Nephrotic syndrome**
  - Usually presents with severe proteinuria (>3.5 g/d), hypertension, edema, hyperlipidemia, and minimal hematuria. Minimal cells or casts, other than fatty casts, are present in urine.
  - Causes include minimal change disease, focal segmental glomerulosclerosis often secondary to human immunodeficiency virus, membranous glomerulonephritis, diabetic nephropathy, hepatitis C, systemic lupus erythematosus, and amyloidosis.

- Complications of glomerular disease in pregnancy include preterm delivery, intrauterine growth restriction (IUGR), stillbirth, maternal hypertension, preeclampsia, and impaired renal function.

Acute Kidney Injury

- **Acute kidney injury** is a sudden loss of renal function. Consensus criteria for diagnosis include an increase in serum creatinine by ≥0.3 mg/dL (27 μmol/L) in 48 hours, an increase to ≥1.5 times baseline within 7 days, or a decrease in urine volume to <3 mL/kg over 6 hours. The utility of these criteria in pregnancy are unknown: Physiologic changes to the renal system result in lower creatinine, and smaller increases in creatinine may represent larger declines in renal function.
  - **Causes:** Causes more common in early pregnancy include hyperemesis gravidarum and septic abortion. Causes more common later in pregnancy and postpartum include severe viral or bacterial infection, severe preeclampsia, hemolytic uremic syndrome (HUS), thrombocytic thrombocytopenic purpura (TTP), acute fatty liver of pregnancy (AFLP), pyelonephritis, ureteral compression or injury, and obstetrical hemorrhage. Nonpregnancy-related causes such as glomerulonephritis or acute tubular necrosis due to drugs or toxins should also be considered.
  - **Management:** General principles of treatment include fluid resuscitation, avoiding nephrotoxins, managing complications such as hyperkalemia, and timely initiation of renal replacement therapy when necessary. Indications for dialysis are the same as in nonpregnant women, with the addition of BUN >50 because BUN is fetotoxic. Identification of the underlying etiology is imperative. Causes of acute kidney injury are typically categorized as (1) prerenal, (2) intrinsic renal, or (3) obstructive.
    - *Prerenal:* Aggressive volume resuscitation and broad-spectrum antimicrobials for infectious causes are paramount. Severe hypotension in the setting of pregnancy is associated with acute cortical necrosis, a pathologic diagnosis that can lead to permanent renal failure.
    - *Intrinsic renal:* Many intrinsic renal causes, such as preeclampsia, hemolysis, elevated liver enzymes, and low platelets (HELLP), AFLP, HUS, and TTP have overlapping features that can make diagnosis difficult. Presence of schistocytes on a peripheral blood smear can help distinguish HUS/TTP from preeclampsia/HELLP, and the mainstay of treatment for HUS is plasmapheresis and eculizumab. Presence of ascites and hypoglycemia suggests AFLP over HELLP; expedient delivery is the mainstay of treatment for both.
    - *Postrenal:* Prompt identification and relief of obstruction or repair of iatrogenic ureteral injury is critical. Management of uterine ureteral compression depends on gestational age; if too early for delivery, amniotomy for polyhydramnios, ureteral stent, nephrostomy tube placement, and dialysis can be considered.

Chronic Kidney Disease

- **Chronic kidney disease** is present in less than 0.2% of all pregnancies. It is defined as impaired renal function or damage for 3 or more months. The most common causes are diabetes, hypertension, glomerulonephritis, and polycystic kidney disease.
- The degree of renal impairment is the major determinant of pregnancy outcome and can be categorized as *mild* (serum creatinine <1.5 mg/dL), moderate (serum

creatinine 1.5-3.0 mg/dL), or severe (serum creatinine >3.0 mg/dL). In general, patients with mild renal dysfunction experience little disease progression during pregnancy, whereas patients with moderate to severe renal insufficiency are at high risk for potentially irreversible loss of renal function. Chronic renal disease in the setting of poorly controlled hypertension markedly increases both maternal and fetal risks. Thus, it is very important to optimize blood pressure in addition to other comorbidities such as diabetes or connective tissue disorders that may worsen renal disease.

- **Pregnancy complications** with chronic renal disease include fetal demise, fetal growth restriction, preeclampsia, eclampsia, and preterm delivery. Maternal and fetal outcomes correlate with severity of baseline renal function and presence of comorbidities.
- **Antepartum management** includes the following:
  - Early pregnancy diagnosis and dating
  - Preconception planning and counseling are encouraged.
  - Baseline laboratory studies including serum creatinine, electrolytes, BUN, 24-hour urine protein and creatinine clearance, urinalysis, and urine culture; serial monitoring of maternal renal function, as clinically indicated
  - Increased frequency of prenatal visits, depending on disease severity
  - Serial ultrasonographic fetal growth examinations
  - Antepartum fetal testing in the third trimester

Renal Dialysis

- Conception occurs in approximately 1% per year of reproductive aged women on dialysis. Between 40% and 75% of these pregnancies result in delivery of a surviving infant. There is a high rate of spontaneous abortion and pregnancy complications. Most infants are born prematurely, usually secondary to severe maternal hypertension or preeclampsia. These patients are also at increased risk for IUGR, polyhydramnios, PPROM, nonreassuring fetal testing, and placental abruption. With significant maternal risks of pregnancies being maintained on dialysis, including severe hypertension, cardiac events, and death, delaying pregnancy until after renal transplantation may be advantageous.
  - Neonatal outcomes are improved with maintenance of the BUN <50 mg/dL on dialysis. This is typically achieved by increasing frequency of dialysis to 5 to 7 days per week.
  - Outcomes are similar with either hemodialysis or peritoneal dialysis. It is therefore reasonable to leave a woman who is well controlled on a particular method on that method.
  - Blood pressure should be controlled, especially during dialysis, to avoid fetal compromise.
  - Electrolytes should be monitored and appropriately corrected. Bicarbonate concentrations, for example, must be managed carefully to avoid dialysis-induced alkalemia. Ultrafiltration goals may be difficult to estimate and should consider fetal and placental growth as well as the plasma volume expansion associated with pregnancy.
  - Continuous fetal monitoring during dialysis after 24 weeks' gestation should be considered to assess fetal tolerance to hemodynamic changes.
  - Anemia is common due to the combined effects of renal failure and pregnancy. Pregnant women may require higher doses of erythropoietin and/or blood transfusions to maintain a hemoglobin of 10 to 11 g/dL.

Renal Transplant

- Approximately 5% to 12% of renal transplant patients who are of reproductive age will become pregnant. The hormonal aberrations associated with end-stage renal disease are usually reversed after kidney transplant, and women often rapidly resume cyclic ovulation and regular menstruation. Pregnancy complications for these patients include increased infections secondary to chronic immunosuppression, hypertension, preeclampsia, preterm labor, PPROM, and IUGR.
  - Transplant patients are generally advised to wait at least 1 year after a living related donor transplant and 2 years after a deceased donor transplant before attempting to become pregnant.
  - Factors associate with favorable outcomes include serum creatinine <1.5 mg/dL, well-controlled blood pressure, proteinuria <500 mg/day, no recent episodes of acute rejection, maintenance level of immunosuppression, and normal appearance of transplanted kidney on ultrasound.
  - Cyclosporine and tacrolimus are commonly used immunosuppressant medications that have favorable safety profiles in pregnancy. Frequent monitoring of drug levels and renal function is imperative to avoid potential toxicity.
  - Mycophenolate mofetil and sirolimus are preferably avoided in pregnancy and have been associated with adverse fetal effects. Patients trying to conceive should be switched from these medications to either tacrolimus or cyclosporine where possible.
  - Mode of delivery is based on obstetric indications. The pelvic allograft does not usually obstruct the birth canal, and vaginal delivery is preferred. When cesarean delivery is indicated, prophylactic antibiotics and careful attention to wound closure are recommended to minimize infectious complications. In addition, knowledge of allograft placement is essential in order to avoid operative injury, although the transplanted kidney is not usually positioned in an area that is vulnerable when using standard approaches to cesarean delivery.

SUGGESTED READINGS

American College of Obstetricians and Gynecologists Committee on Obstetric Practice. ACOG Committee Opinion No. 717: sulfonamides, nitrofurantoin, and risk of birth defects. *Obstet Gynecol*. 2017;130:e150-e152. (Reaffirmed 2019)

American College of Obstetrics and Gynecologists. Hypertension in pregnancy. Report of the American College of Obstetricians and Gynecologists' Task Force on Hypertension in Pregnancy. *Obstet Gynecol*. 2013;122(5):1122-1131.

Henderson JT, Thompson JH, Burda BU, Cantor A. Preeclampsia screening: evidence report and systematic review for the US Preventive Services Task Force. *JAMA*. 2017;317(16):1668-1683

Jim B, Garovic VD. Acute kidney injury in pregnancy. *Semin Nephrol*. 2017;37(4):378-385.

Macejko AM, Schaeffer AJ. Asymptomatic bacteriuria and symptomatic urinary tract infections during pregnancy. *Urol Clin North Am*. 2007;34(1):35-42.

Nevis IF, Reitsma A, Dominic A, et al. Pregnancy outcomes in women with chronic kidney disease: a systematic review. *Clin J Am Soc Nephrol*. 2011;6(11):2587-2598.

Smaill FM, Vazquez JC. Antibiotics for asymptomatic bacteriuria in pregnancy. *Cochrane Database Syst Rev*. 2015;(8):CD000490.

Vidaeff AC, Yeomans ER, Ramin SM. Pregnancy in women with renal disease. Part I: general principles. *Am J Perinatol*. 2008;25(7):385-397.

Vidaeff AC, Yeomans ER, Ramin SM. Pregnancy in women with renal disease. Part II: specific underlying renal conditions. *Am J Perinatol*. 2008;25(7):399-405.

Gastrointestinal Disease in Pregnancy

Steve C. Amaefuna and Abimbola Aina-Mumuney

During pregnancy, anatomic and physiologic changes undergone by the gastrointestinal tract can influence the diagnosis of gastrointestinal disorders. The displacement of the gastrointestinal organs by the gravid uterus changes the location, character, and intensity of gastrointestinal symptoms. This chapter summarizes the normal changes in pregnancy in contrast to pathologic conditions.

NONHEPATIC GASTROINTESTINAL DISORDERS

Nausea and Vomiting of Pregnancy

- Nausea (with or without vomiting) occurs in up to 80% of pregnancies at any time of day, despite the general term *morning sickness*. Mean onset of symptoms is 5 to 6 weeks' gestation. Although symptoms typically abate by 16 to 18 weeks of gestation, they continue into the third trimester in 15% to 20% of pregnant women and until delivery in 5%.
- **Hyperemesis gravidarum** is a severe form of nausea and vomiting in pregnancy, characterized by intractable vomiting, dehydration, alkalosis, hypokalemia, and weight loss usually exceeding 5% of prepregnant body weight. It affects 0.3% to 2% of pregnancies and peaks between the 8th and 12th weeks of pregnancy. The etiology may be multifactorial, involving hormonal, neurologic, metabolic, toxic, and psychosocial factors.
- In true hyperemesis gravidarum, persistent vomiting leads to plasma volume depletion and elevated hematocrit, and metabolic derangements that include increased blood urea nitrogen, hyponatremia, hypokalemia, hypochloremia, and metabolic alkalosis. A complete workup includes a pelvic sonogram to identify multiple gestation or molar pregnancy and thyroid function tests to evaluate for hyperthyroidism. Some patients with hyperemesis gravidarum have transient benign hyperthyroidism most likely due to thyroid stimulation by the human chorionic gonadotropin (hCG) molecule, which is structurally similar to TSH and has been shown in animal studies to be a weak thyrotropin. This usually resolves spontaneously as pregnancy continues.
- **Treatment** depends on the severity of symptoms. Usually, intravenous (IV) hydration and antiemetic therapy are sufficient. Patients may require hospitalization for intractable emesis, electrolyte abnormalities, and severe hypovolemia. Thiamine supplementation (100 mg daily intramuscularly or intravenously) is given prior to administration of glucose to prevent Wernicke encephalopathy. Oral feeding with a bland diet should be introduced slowly as tolerated.
- There are no drugs approved specifically for the treatment of nausea and vomiting in pregnancy; however, the following medications have been shown to be clinically effective (see chapter 5, Figure 5-1):
  - Pyridoxine (vitamin B_6) 10 to 25 mg orally 3 to 4 times daily
  - Doxylamine succinate 20 mg with pyridoxine 20 mg orally at bedtime. A recent formulation consisting of delayed release tablets of 10 mg of doxylamine and

10 mg of pyridoxine has recently become available in the United States, which may be taken as needed, up to four tablets daily: one in the morning, one in the afternoon, and two in the evening.

- Promethazine hydrochloride (Phenergan) 12.5 to 25 mg orally or rectally every 4 to 6 hours
- Prochlorperazine (Compazine) 25 mg rectally twice daily or 5 to 10 mg orally, IV, or intramuscularly 4 times daily
- Metoclopramide hydrochloride (Reglan) 5 to 10 mg orally or intramuscularly 3 times daily
- Ondansetron hydrochloride (Zofran) 4 mg orally or IV 3 times daily
- Methylprednisolone (Medrol) 16 mg orally or IV every 8 hours for 3 days may be used for refractory cases after 10 weeks' gestation. There is a theoretical risk of cleft lip and palate when steroids are administered in the early- to mid-first trimester.
- In severe cases requiring prolonged IV hydration and poor nutritional status, enteral feeds via nasogastric tube is first-line management. Complications from parenteral nutrition, even peripherally inserted central catheters, are common and severe; therefore, parenteral feeding should be used only for the most refractory of patients who cannot tolerate enteral feeding.

Acid Reflux

- **Gastroesophageal reflux disease (GERD)** and the resulting symptom of pyrosis ("heartburn") are common during pregnancy secondary to the altered position of the stomach, decreased lower esophageal sphincter tone (due to elevated progesterone levels), and lower intraesophageal pressures. The incidence is 30% to 50% but may approach 80% in selected populations. Symptoms begin late in the first trimester and become more frequent and severe with increasing gestational age. Risk factors include multiparity and history of GERD before pregnancy.
  - **Treatment** is aimed at neutralizing acid or decreasing reflux.
    - Lifestyle modification is key in treating mild disease. Elevating the head of the bed at night, avoiding meals within 3 hours of bedtime, and consuming smaller but more frequent meals can help. Dietary modification is recommended, including reduced consumption of fatty or acidic foods, chocolate, and caffeine. Cigarette smoking and alcohol consumption can exacerbate GERD.
    - Mild intermittent symptoms can be treated with over-the-counter antacids (eg, calcium carbonate). More persistent and severe symptoms can be treated with H_2 blockers (eg, ranitidine) or proton pump inhibitors (eg, omeprazole).

Peptic Ulcer Disease

- **Peptic ulcer disease (PUD)** is not common in pregnancy, and the hormonal changes of pregnancy usually decrease PUD severity and symptoms.
- **Treatment** during pregnancy is similar to treatment for GERD and consists of diet modification, avoiding nonsteroidal anti-inflammatory drugs, and starting a proton pump inhibitor. Indomethacin for tocolysis in patients with PUD should be avoided. Testing for *Helicobacter pylori* infection is recommended for those with PUD; treatment regimens for *H pylori* should not include tetracycline or levofloxacin during pregnancy.

Effects of Prior Bariatric Surgery on Pregnancy

• Bariatric surgery can be either restrictive (gastric banding or sleeve) or a combination of restrictive and malabsorptive (Roux-en-Y). Rapid weight loss is common following surgery and has been shown to decrease rates of pregestational diabetes, hypertension, gestational diabetes, and preeclampsia. It is recommended that pregnancy after bariatric surgery be delayed for at least 12 to 24 months. Although there is decreased average weight gain during pregnancy, rates of obesity can remain as high as 80% in patients who become pregnant following bariatric surgery. Compared to the general population, obese patients, including those who have had bariatric surgery, are more likely to deliver via cesarean delivery. However, bariatric surgery alone should not be an indication for cesarean delivery. Rates of fetal macrosomia are decreased following Roux-en-Y gastric bypass.

• Nutritional deficiencies following Roux-en-Y gastric bypass may include protein, iron, vitamin B_{12}, folate, vitamin D, and calcium, and individual micronutrient deficiencies should be identified and corrected. Oral multivitamin supplementation should be initiated; however, continued deficiency may require parental supplementation due to malabsorption. An excess of vitamin A can lead to birth defects, and supplementation should not exceed 5000 IU/d during pregnancy. Monitoring the blood count, iron, ferritin, calcium, and vitamin D levels can be considered in each trimester. Nutritional deficiencies can develop in infants who are breastfed by patients who have undergone bariatric surgery.

• Anastomotic leaks, bowel obstruction, internal hernias, ventral hernias, band erosion, and band migration are bariatric-related surgical complications that can occur during pregnancy. Common gastrointestinal complaints during pregnancy like nausea, vomiting, and abdominal pain should be thoroughly evaluated in patients who have had prior bariatric surgery. Abdominal bloating, cramps, nausea, and vomiting can be signs of dumping syndrome, which can occur following the ingestion of refined sugars or high glycemic carbohydrates and result in rapid stomach emptying and small bowel distention. Hyperinsulinemia and consequent hypoglycemia can follow, resulting in tachycardia, palpitations, anxiety, and diaphoresis. Patients who have undergone gastric bypass surgery may not tolerate the 28-week glucose screen used to test gestational diabetes. One week of home glucose monitoring (fasting and 2-hour post prandial) at 24 to 28 weeks of gestation can be considered as an alternative. Extended release preparations of many medications are not recommended in patients who have undergone Roux-en-Y gastric bypass given the decreased intestinal absorptive area. A smaller gastric pouch can lead to gastric ulceration with nonsteroidal anti-inflammatory drug use postpartum in patients who have undergone gastric bypass surgery.

Inflammatory Bowel Disease

• **Inflammatory bowel disease (IBD)**, including **ulcerative colitis** and **Crohn disease**, often presents in reproductive age women. An IBD increases the risk for preterm birth, low birth weight, and fetal growth restriction, particularly if remission is not achieved before or during pregnancy. There is no evidence that pregnancy influences disease activity; however, patients with active disease around the time of conception often fail to achieve remission during the pregnancy.

- **Treatment** is largely pharmacologic. If a patient is well controlled on medications prior to pregnancy, we typically continue treatment, with the few exceptions outlined in the following text. Common medications include 5-ASA formulations and corticosteroids. Because sulfasalazine may interfere with folate absorption, supplemental folate (2 mg orally daily) should be prescribed. Immunosuppressive agents, such as azathioprine, 6-mercaptopurine, cyclosporine, or infliximab, are used for more severe disease. Limited experience shows that all these medications are safe during pregnancy. Methotrexate and mycophenolate are avoided in pregnancy. Antibiotics, particularly metronidazole and cephalosporins, are used for perirectal abscesses/fistulae. There is limited data regarding the safety of antidiarrheal medications such as Kaopectate, Lomotil, and Imodium in pregnancy, but significant teratogenicity is unlikely. Surgical intervention is indicated only for severe complications of IBD.
- The **mode of delivery** may be affected by IBD depending on disease activity and past surgical history. Vaginal delivery can usually be attempted unless there is severe perianal disease or previous colorectal surgery. Operative vaginal delivery or episiotomy should be avoided if possible to prevent excessive perineal trauma. Cesarean delivery may be considered in patients with active perianal disease due to the risk of wound complications and fistulae formation.

Pancreatitis

- **Pancreatitis** is an uncommon cause of abdominal pain in pregnancy, with an incidence of 1 in 1000 to 1 in 10 000 pregnancies.
- The **presentation** is usually midepigastric or left upper quadrant pain with radiation to the back, nausea, vomiting, ileus, and low-grade fever. Cholelithiasis is the most common cause of pancreatitis during pregnancy. Other causes include alcohol abuse, hyperlipidemias, drugs, and autoimmune pancreatitis. Ultrasound is of limited use for acute pancreatitis in pregnancy because of the enlarged uterus and overlying bowel gas. Serum amylase and lipase levels are usually markedly elevated. However, degree of enzyme elevation and disease severity do not reliably correlate.
- **Management** is supportive and consists of IV hydration, analgesics, antibiotics when appropriate, and bowel rest. Most cases of gallstone pancreatitis can be managed medically. In women with gallstone-induced pancreatitis, cholecystectomy should be considered after an acute infection to prevent recurrence.

Appendicitis

- **Appendicitis** can be a challenging diagnosis in the gravid patient due to the changes of pregnancy (see chapter 23).

GALLBLADDER DISORDERS

- **Cholelithiasis** occurs in up to 10% of pregnancies and is often clinically silent. Biliary stasis from progesterone-induced smooth muscle relaxation and the prolithogenic effect of elevated estrogen levels in pregnancy may predispose to gallstone formation. Symptomatic patients typically complain of vague intermittent right upper quadrant discomfort that occurs with meals. Asymptomatic cholelithiasis requires no treatment during pregnancy.
- **Symptomatic cholelithiasis** and **acute cholecystitis**—see chapter 23.

Table 15-1	Liver Function Test Changes During Normal Pregnancy
Alkaline phosphatase	↑
Aminotransferases	↔
Bilirubin	↔
Albumin	↓
Hormone-binding proteins	↑
Lipids	↑
Fibrinogen	↑
PT/aPTT	↔

Abbreviations: aPTT, activated partial thromboplastin time; PT, prothrombin time; ↑, increased or elevated; ↓, decreased; ↔, unchanged.

LIVER DISORDERS

Hepatic Physiology in Pregnancy

- As the gravid uterus expands into the upper abdomen, the liver is displaced posteriorly and to the right, decreasing its estimated size on physical examination. A palpable liver in pregnancy is abnormal, and a workup is indicated. Table 15-1 summarizes the normal changes in liver function tests during pregnancy—some of which are considered abnormal in nonpregnant patients.

Hepatic Disorders Unique to Pregnancy

Cholestasis of Pregnancy

- **Intrahepatic cholestasis of pregnancy (ICP)** is the most common liver disease in pregnancy, with rates ranging from 0.5% to 5.5% in the United States. Globally, it demonstrates significant genetic and geographic variations. Risk factors include a personal or family history of ICP, multiple gestations, in vitro fertilization, advanced maternal age, and chronic hepatitis C infection. Although the cause is poorly understood, it is likely secondary to incomplete bile acid clearance resulting from elevated reproductive hormones in genetically susceptible women. Complications of ICP include preterm labor, meconium ileus, neonatal respiratory distress syndrome, and intrauterine fetal demise. These risks increase progressively with advancing gestational age and are correlated with maternal bile acid levels, regardless of symptoms. Although the cause of fetal demise is unknown, it is thought to be associated with fetal arrhythmias and/or placental vasospasm secondary to high levels of bile acids.
- Initial **diagnosis of ICP** is primarily clinical, with confirmation by laboratory testing to exclude other possible diagnoses. The cardinal symptom is pruritus, especially of the palms and soles that worsens at night. Anorexia, malaise, steatorrhea, and dark urine are also common complaints. Jaundice develops in 15% of patients but resolves quickly after delivery. Fever, abdominal pain, hepatosplenomegaly, and stigmata of chronic liver disease are usually absent. Onset is typically

late in pregnancy (80% after 30 wk), but ICP occasionally occurs in the second trimester.

- **Differential diagnosis** includes preeclampsia, viral hepatitis, and gallbladder disease.
- **Laboratory findings** include elevated total bilirubin, aminotransferases, and fasting serum total bile acids (>10-14 μmol/L). Cholic acid is raised more than chenodeoxycholic acid, which results in an elevation of the cholic/chenodeoxycholic acid ratio compared to pregnant women without ICP. Laboratory abnormalities may arise up to 4.5 weeks after the development of pruritus. Serum alkaline phosphatase and transaminase levels can be moderately elevated. Serum γ-glutamyl transpeptidase, albumin, and prothrombin time remain normal.
- **Treatment** is mainly for symptomatic relief until delivery, which is the definitive therapy. Diphenhydramine and topical emollients can be used to relieve pruritus. Dexamethasone has not been shown to provide symptomatic relief in ICP. Ursodeoxycholic acid (15 mg/kg/d) is the most effective treatment and works by increasing biliary flow, thereby decreasing serum bile acid levels and decreasing pruritus. Cholestyramine (4-16 g, 2-4 times per day) decreases intestinal absorption of bile salts and is effective for mild to moderate symptoms but does not improve laboratory values. It can be considered an adjunct to ursodeoxycholic acid in refractory cases of ICP. Fat-soluble vitamin levels (A, D, E, and K) and prothrombin time should be checked periodically in patients taking cholestyramine for extended treatment.
- ICP at term is associated with <3% risk of fetal demise. Antepartum fetal testing is recommended, although intrauterine demise may occur despite reassuring testing. Delivery should be performed no later than 38 weeks' gestation. Delivery at 36 weeks may be considered in the setting of severe pruritus, jaundice, high total serum bile acids (>100 μm/L), or a history of preterm fetal demise in the context of ICP.
- Recurrence risk in subsequent pregnancies is approximately 70%, and severity varies.

Acute Fatty Liver of Pregnancy

- **Acute fatty liver of pregnancy** is uncommon, occurring in approximately 1 in 10 000 pregnancies. It typically occurs in primigravid women in the third trimester and is associated with multiple gestations, low maternal weight, and with a fetal mitochondrial gene mutation causing long chain 3-hydroxylacyl-CoA-dehydrogenase deficiency. Patients may present with nausea, vomiting, epigastric pain, anorexia, jaundice, or malaise. Intra-abdominal bleeding or altered mental status may indicate disease progression to disseminated intravascular coagulation or hepatic failure. Laboratory tests may reveal hypoglycemia, elevated aminotransferases to 1000 IU/L, leukocytosis, thrombocytopenia, coagulopathy, markedly reduced antithrombin III, metabolic acidosis, hyperuricemia, and renal failure. Treatment includes maternal stabilization with intensive supportive care and prompt delivery, either with induction of labor with close maternal and fetal surveillance or cesarean delivery. Liver function usually normalizes within 1 week postpartum and recurrence in subsequent pregnancy is possible.

Hepatic Disorders Not Directly Related to Pregnancy

Hepatitis

- **Acute and chronic hepatitis**—see chapter 8.

Cirrhosis

- **Hepatic cirrhosis** leads to metabolic and hormonal derangements that usually induce anovulation, amenorrhea, and infertility. Cirrhosis is associated with a spontaneous abortion rate as high as 26%, a preterm delivery rate between 40% and 60%, and a neonatal mortality rate of approximately 15%. Maternal mortality is estimated at 10% but may be up to 50% in patients with portal hypertension who develop gastrointestinal bleeding during pregnancy. Outcomes are generally poor, but hepatic dysfunction before pregnancy and the presence of portal hypertension correlate with worse maternal/fetal prognosis.
- **Esophageal variceal bleeding** is the most common complication of cirrhosis, occurring in 18% to 25% of pregnant women with cirrhosis. To reduce portal pressure and the risk of acute bleeding, β-blockers such as propranolol should be considered. As in nonpregnant patients, endoscopic variceal ligation is the mainstay of therapy for acute episodes of hemorrhage. Portal decompression shunt placement is required when hemorrhage cannot be controlled by endoscopy. If endoscopy is unavailable, balloon tamponade can be employed to control severe bleeding. Other complications include ascites, bacterial peritonitis, splenic artery aneurysm, portal vein thrombosis, portal vein hypertension, hepatic encephalopathy or coma, postpartum uterine hemorrhage, and death.
- Vaginal delivery is preferred over cesarean delivery due to the high rate of intraoperative and postoperative complications. In patients with portal hypertension, however, repetitive Valsalva maneuver in the second stage of labor can increase the risk of significant variceal bleeding. A passive second stage with forceps-assisted delivery may be beneficial. Postpartum hemorrhage is a significant source of morbidity and mortality in this patient population.

Budd-Chiari Syndrome

- **Budd-Chiari syndrome** is a veno-occlusive disease of the hepatic vein that increases hepatic sinusoidal pressure and can result in portal hypertension or hepatic necrosis. The disease presents with abdominal pain and the abrupt onset of ascites and hepatomegaly. Cases are often caused by congenital vascular anomalies, myeloproliferative disorders, or thrombophilic disorders. Diagnosis is made by hepatic Doppler ultrasonography to identify venous occlusion and evaluate the direction and amplitude of blood flow. Acute therapy includes selective thrombolytics and a surgical shunt or transjugular intrahepatic portosystemic shunt for portal hypertension. Chronic Budd-Chiari syndrome is treated with anticoagulation therapy.

SUGGESTED READINGS

Adams TD, Hammoud AO, Davidson LE, et al. Maternal and neonatal outcomes for pregnancies before and after gastric bypass surgery. *Int J Obes (Lond)*. 2015;39(4):686-694.

American College of Obstetricians and Gynecologists Committee on Practice Bulletins—Obstetrics. ACOG Practice Bulletin No. 105: bariatric surgery and pregnancy. *Obstet Gynecol*. 2009;113:1405-1413. (Reaffirmed 2017)

American College of Obstetricians and Gynecologists Committee on Practice Bulletins—Obstetrics. ACOG Practice Bulletin No. 189: nausea and vomiting of pregnancy. *Obstet Gynecol*. 2018;131:e15-e30.

Bacq Y, Sentilhes L, Reyes HB, et al. Efficacy of ursodeoxycholic acid in treating intrahepatic cholestasis of pregnancy: a meta-analysis. *Gastroenterology*. 2012;143(6):1492-1501.

Joshi D, James A, Quaglia A, Westbrook RH, Heneghan MA. Liver disease in pregnancy. *Lancet.* 2010;375(9714):594-605.

Ogura JM, Francois KE, Perlow JH, Elliot JP. Complications associated with peripherally inserted central catheter use during pregnancy. *Am J Obstet Gynecol.* 2003;188(5):1223-1225.

Palatnik A, Rinella ME. Medical and obstetric complications among pregnant women with liver cirrhosis. *Obstet Gynecol.* 2017;129(6):1118-1123.

Poitou Bernert C, Ciangura C, Coupaye M, Czernichow S, Bouillot JL, Basdevant A. Nutritional deficiency after gastric bypass: diagnosis, prevention and treatment. *Diabetes Metab.* 2007;33(1):13-24.

Williamson C, Geenes V. Intrahepatic cholestasis of pregnancy. *Obstet Gynecol.* 2014;124(1):120-133.

16 Autoimmune Disease in Pregnancy

Elizabeth Oler and Donna Maria Neale

Autoimmune disease is characterized by the production of antibodies against self-antigens. Pregnancy creates a unique immune milieu, and with time, there have been major advancements in the understanding of the role of autoimmune components in disease. This chapter aims to review basic immune system adaptation during pregnancy and management of common autoimmune diseases encountered during pregnancy. Many of these illnesses are addressed briefly in this chapter and more fully in their respective system-specific chapters.

PATHOPHYSIOLOGY

During pregnancy, the maternal immune system undergoes a number of changes. Traditional teaching suggests that pregnancy reflects a switch from the normal predominant proinflammatory (type 1 helper T cell) state to an anti-inflammatory (type 2 helper T cell) state. This transition is thought to protect the antigen-distinct fetus from being rejected by its mother. More recent study suggests that the immune changes in pregnancy are not so simplistic but represent a constant interplay between the proinflammatory and anti-inflammatory systems. Because of these changes in the maternal immune profile, autoimmune diseases can present and behave differently during each trimester of pregnancy and also differently from the nonpregnant state. Furthermore, the switch back to the predominant proinflammatory state in the postpartum period can affect disease activity during this time. Clinical applications of these changes help explain exacerbations in type 2 helper T cell–driven diseases such as systemic lupus erythematosus (SLE) and improvement in type 1 helper T cell–driven diseases such as rheumatoid arthritis, multiple sclerosis, and autoimmune thyroiditis during pregnancy, often with increased "flaring" postpartum.

COMMON GENERAL MANAGEMENT CONCERNS

- Care should be taken at the preconception or initial prenatal visit to outline baseline function/disability, recent history, and symptoms of flares. Ideally, patients should have stable disease or remission prior to embarking on pregnancy. If disease is not stable, or pregnancy was unplanned, there should be appropriate vigilance and frequent visits with early referral to Maternal Fetal Medicine and disease-specific specialists. Patients with any autoimmune disease, even if stable at the outset of pregnancy, should be asked about flare symptoms specific to their disorder at every prenatal visit. Care should be taken to ensure that patients with one autoimmune disease have been evaluated for others because they frequently coexist.

- Previously undiagnosed autoimmune disease may be unmasked in pregnancy, frequently in the late first to early second trimester when the hemodynamic changes of pregnancy are most pronounced. Autoimmune disease should be high on the differential for patients with sudden and unexpected deterioration in maternal health.

- Many disease characteristics and complications occur across multiple autoimmune disorders, and prior to addressing these diseases individually, we briefly address these common and important management concerns below.

  - **Anti-Ro and anti-La antibodies**, also known as anti-SSA and anti-SSB antibodies, respectively, are found frequently in patients with SLE and Sjögren disease and occasionally seen in scleroderma and mixed connective tissue disorder. These antibodies have been found to be associated with fetal congenital heart disease (approximately 5%), fetal heart block (approximately 2%), and cutaneous neonatal lupus (15%-20%). If the patient has a history of prior delivery affected by these conditions, the recurrence rate is as high as 25%. The patient should be tested for these antibodies preconceptionally or at the first prenatal visit. If present, fetal echocardiography should be performed at 22 weeks of gestation. PR interval measurements should start at 16 weeks of gestation and repeated weekly until 26 weeks because this is thought to be the most common time for congenital heart block to develop. After 26 weeks of gestation, assessment of the PR interval is carried out biweekly until 34 weeks of gestation to assess for possible fetal heart block. Some evidence suggests decreased risk of recurrent heart block with continuation of hydroxychloroquine, so this should be continued during pregnancy if already on the medication. Maternal dexamethasone administration has previously been recommended to protect the fetal cardiac tissue from further damage; however, follow-up studies have shown that there is probably no benefit. Timing of delivery is dependent on the severity. A referral to a tertiary center with neonatology is strongly recommended. After birth, in the presence of anti-Ro or anti-La, congenital heart block may be present up to a month, and some children will need lifelong pacemaker therapy, particularly if complete heart block is present.

  - **Increased risk of renal dysfunction.** Baseline renal function should be determined in all patients with autoimmune disease because many affect the kidney. The physiologic changes of pregnancy strongly affect renal function, putting women with tenuous renal status at high risk for worsening renal insufficiency and even renal failure. Patients should be carefully evaluated early in pregnancy with 24-hour urine protein and creatinine for baseline function. If abnormal, the patient should be counseled about the high risk of fetal complications as well as maternal morbidity and mortality. Patients with significant renal disease (serum creatinine >2.5 mg/dL) are generally advised against becoming pregnant due to the extremely high risk of maternal and fetal morbidity and mortality.

- **Increased risk of fetal growth restriction (FGR).** Several autoimmune diseases put patients at increased risk for FGR including SLE, scleroderma, mixed connective tissue disease, dermatomyositis/polymyositis, antiphospholipid syndrome, and autoimmune bullous disease. An ultrasound should be performed every 3 to 4 weeks following the anatomy ultrasound. In the presence of FGR, serial fetal umbilical artery Doppler studies should be performed.
- **Increased risk of preeclampsia.** The majority of patients with autoimmune disease have increased risk of preeclampsia, particularly those with baseline renal dysfunction. Patients should have baseline 24-hour urine collection for total protein and creatinine clearance, even in the absence of known renal disease. Serial samples should be collected at least once per trimester in high-risk patients. In women with history of preeclampsia in a prior pregnancy, baby aspirin should be initiated at 12 weeks of gestation.
- **Increased risk of stillbirth.** Antenatal testing is typically initiated at 32 weeks of gestation, unless there is evidence of maternal/fetal compromise prior to this time.
- **Increased risk of premature birth.** Betamethasone should be administered to patients with poor fetal testing results or worsening maternal disease. The timing of administration should be tailored to the individual patient.

AUTOIMMUNE DISORDERS ENCOUNTERED IN PREGNANCY

The sections that follow are organized by disease. For those most commonly encountered, they are further stratified into the three phases: preconception, antenatal, and postpartum periods.

Systemic Lupus Erythematosus

- **Systemic lupus erythematosus** is a multisystem, chronic autoimmune disease which most commonly affects women in their 20s and 30s.
- Organ system involvement is heterogeneous and includes arthritis, photosensitive rash, alopecia, mucocutaneous lesions, lupus nephritis/renal insufficiency, Raynaud phenomenon, pulmonary involvement, gastrointestinal (GI) disease, neurologic symptoms, pericarditis, and hematologic effects. Autoantibodies involved include antinuclear antibody (ANA), anti-Ro antibody, anti-La antibody, anti-Sm antibody, anti-dsDNA antibody, and antiphospholipid antibody (APLA). Complement levels can also be decreased due to consumption in active phases of the disease.
- Lupus is associated with poor obstetric outcomes including FGR, prematurity, stillbirth, and spontaneous abortion. **Active lupus nephritis poses the greatest maternal risk.**

Preconception

- Fertility is *not* intrinsically affected by the disease, but caution must be exercised in women taking teratogenic medications (Table 16-1). Disease should be quiescent, and preferably well-controlled on nonteratogenic agents, for at least 6 months prior to conception.

Table 16-1 Commonly Used Medications in Women of Childbearing Age With Autoimmune Disease

Drug Name	Indications	Pregnancy	Breastfeeding	Notes
Hydroxychloroquine	Lupus Rheumatoid arthritis	✓	✓	• First-line for lupus treatment • Especially important to continue in patients with +SSA/SSB
Tacrolimus	Lupus and lupus flare	✓	✓	• Generally considered second line • Levels should be followed if used.
Prednisone	Many	✓	✓	• Can be used in almost any autoimmune disease flare • Taper is common for outpatient management after initial stabilization.
Methylprednisolone	Many	✓	✓	• IV only medication • Generally used in pulse doses rather than taper
Azathioprine	Lupus Wegener granulomatosis Pemphigus vulgaris Myositis Scleroderma IBD	✓	✓	• First- or second-line treatment for many autoimmune disorders • When breastfeeding, 4-h delay may be safest to mitigate risk of mild asymptomatic neutropenia in exclusively breastfed infants.
Cyclophosphamide	Lupus and lupus flares Polyarteritis nodosa Wegener granulomatosis	✓ (Second and third trimesters only, with caution)	✗	• Considered last line for severe flares only, if other medications have failed • Avoid use during first trimester because it is a known teratogen. • Second and third trimesters have little data for long-term adverse fetal effects, although appears to be less risky.

Drug	Disease			Comments
Methotrexate	Lupus Rheumatoid arthritis Scleroderma	✗	✗	• Known teratogen; discontinue and allow time for wash out prior to conception. • If unplanned pregnancy while taking, discontinue immediately and administer high-dose folic acid. Counsel about high likelihood of birth defects. • Small amounts do get excreted into breast milk, and it may be safe for breastfeeding at low doses.
Mycophenolate mofetil	Lupus Myasthenia gravis Scleroderma	✗	✗	• Known teratogen; discontinue prior to conception.
Sulfasalazine	IBD	✓	✓	• First line with glucocorticoids for IBD flare
Propylthiouracil (PTU)	Graves disease Hyperthyroidism	✓ (First trimester only)	✓	• Risk of maternal hepatotoxicity; liver enzymes should be followed closely.
Methimazole	Graves disease Hyperthyroidism	✓ (Second and third trimesters only)	✓	• Associated with choanal and esophageal atresia and aplasia cutis if used in the first trimester
Pyridostigmine	Myasthenia gravis	✓	✓	• Not required in asymptomatic disease • Myasthenic crisis often requires addition of glucocorticoids, azathioprine, and IVIG or plasmapheresis.

(Continued)

Table 16-1 Commonly Used Medications in Women of Childbearing Age With Autoimmune Disease *(Continued)*

Drug Name	Indications	Pregnancy	Breastfeeding	Notes
Teriflunomide	Multiple sclerosis	✗	✗	• Known teratogen; discontinue and allow time for wash out prior to conception.
Natalizumab	Multiple sclerosis Crohn disease	✓	✗	• Limited data shows a slightly higher rate of birth defects overall when taken 3 mo prior to conception or during pregnancy but nonspecific teratogenesis • Probably safe to take as a second line to interferon β • Occasionally excreted in breast milk; limited data exists. Exercise caution or use alternative agent.
Interferon β	Multiple sclerosis	✓	✓	• Increased risk of low birth weight or preterm birth; no evidence of teratogenic properties • Likely safe in breastfeeding; exercise caution.
Glatiramer acetate	Multiple sclerosis	✓	✓	• Preferred disease-modifying agent during breastfeeding
Mitoxantrone	Multiple sclerosis	✗	✗	• Known teratogen; discontinue and allow time for wash out prior to conception.

Abbreviations: IBD, inflammatory bowel disease; IV, intravenous; IVIG, intravenous immunoglobulin.

- Renal, cardiac, pulmonary, and hematologic systems should be evaluated prior to conception to fully assess disease activity.
- See "Antiphospholipid Syndrome" for management concerns related to this disease subtype.
- Preconception consultation with maternal fetal medicine and rheumatology is strongly recommended when feasible.

Antenatal Period

- Lupus flares occur in one third of patients during pregnancy, and patients should therefore be screened at every visit during pregnancy for disease-specific symptoms. Rheumatology consultation is recommended.
- Pharmacologic agents used in treatment are outlined in Table 16-1.
- When a patient with known lupus presents with hypertension and proteinuria greater than baseline, it may be difficult to distinguish between preeclampsia and a lupus flare. The laboratory and clinical exam findings listed in Table 16-2 may be helpful in differentiating them. Both are characterized by proteinuria, thrombocytopenia, hypertension, or hyperuricemia. Transaminitis supports preeclampsia. Decreased complement levels or urinary red blood cell casts support lupus flare. Maternal fetal medicine, rheumatology, and nephrology consultations are recommended in these cases.
- Serial growth sonograms are recommended in the third trimester because FGR is a common complication of SLE.
- Patients with anti-Ro (SSA) and anti-La (SSB) positive status must be evaluated with serial M-modes to screen for fetal congenital heart block, as described above.

Table 16-2	Distinguishing Between Preeclampsia and Lupus Flare	
Lab or Clinical Test	Lupus Flare	Preeclampsia
Creatinine	Often increased	Often increased
Liver function tests	Rarely increased	Often increased
Serum complement (C3/C4)	Often decreased	Can decrease but usually unchanged
Serum platelets	May be decreased	May be decreased
Serum uric acid	Low to normal	>5.5 highly suggestive
Serum double-stranded DNA	May be increased	Unchanged
Serum antinuclear antibody	May be increased	Unchanged
Peripheral smear	Unchanged	May see schistocytes in HELLP syndrome
Urinalysis	+RBC casts	Acellular urine
Edema/weight gain	Often present	Often present

Abbreviations: HELLP, hemolysis, elevated liver enzymes, and low platelets; RBC, red blood cell.

Postpartum

- Lupus flares can occur postpartum, regardless of disease status in the preconception and antenatal periods. Women are recommended to be screened with routine labs at least once at about 4 to 6 weeks postpartum, and earlier if flare is suspected.
- Breastfeeding is encouraged in women with SLE because most medications are well documented to be safe. Breastfeeding women should be advised to avoid cyclophosphamide (see Table 16-1).
- **Neonatal lupus syndrome** is a rare sequela characterized by skin, hematologic, and other systemic lupus lesions of the neonate. There is a recurrence risk up to 25% in subsequent pregnancies.

Antiphospholipid Syndrome

- **Antiphospholipid syndrome** is present in a subset of SLE. The APLA interfere with coagulation, thrombus formation, and complement pathways.
- Diagnosis requires *positive antibodies on two separate occasions at least 12 weeks apart* plus at least one clinical criterion (Table 16-3). One percent to 5% of healthy individuals may test positive for APLA.

Table 16-3	Diagnostic Criteria for Diagnosis of Antiphospholipid Syndrome[a,b]
	Clinical Criteria
Vascular thrombosis	One or more clinical episodes of arterial, venous, or small vessel thrombosis, in any tissue or organ
Pregnancy morbidity	One or more unexplained, morphologically normal fetal deaths at or beyond 10 wk gestation
	One or more premature births of morphologically normal fetus before 34 wk gestation due to preeclampsia or placental insufficiency
	Three or more unexplained consecutive spontaneous abortions before 10 wk gestation
	Laboratory Criteria
Lupus anticoagulant	Present in plasma on two or more occasions at least 12 wk apart
Anticardiolipin	IgG and/or IgM present in medium or high titer or greater than 99th percentile, at least 12 wk apart
Anti-β_2 glycoprotein I	IgG and/or IgM, present in serum or plasma, greater than 99th percentile, present on two or more occasions at least 12 wk apart

Abbreviations: IgG, immunoglobulin G; IgM, immunoglobulin M.
[a]Antiphospholipid syndrome is present if *at least one clinical and one laboratory criteria* are present.
[b]Adapted from Miyakis S, Lockshin MD, Atsumi T, et al. International consensus statement on an update of the classification criteria for definite antiphospholipid syndrome (APS). *J Thromb Haemost.* 2006;4(2):295-306. Reprinted by permission of John Wiley & Sons, Inc.

- Gravidas are at increased risk for venous or arterial thrombosis, early pregnancy loss, IUGR, second trimester loss, preeclampsia, and pregnancy-induced hypertension.
- Pharmacologic management differs by patient history. During the antepartum period and 6 weeks postpartum, women with
  - **History of thrombosis** should receive prophylactic anticoagulation.
  - **No history of thrombosis** with positive clinical criteria may receive either clinical surveillance or prophylactic anticoagulation.
  - **Recurrent pregnancy loss** should receive prophylactic anticoagulation and low-dose aspirin.
  - Prophylactic anticoagulation with low-molecular-weight heparin, with transition to unfractionated heparin at 36 weeks, is preferred. If patients cannot tolerate heparin analogs, have a history of heparin-induced thrombocytopenia, or have a body weight greater than 150 kg, hematology consultation is recommended.
- **Neonatal thrombosis** attributable to APLA is rare. Fetal factors such as thrombophilia or prematurity often contribute to risk in affected infants.

Sjögren Syndrome

- **Sjögren syndrome** is a chronic inflammatory disorder with diminished lacrimal and salivary gland function and occasional extraglandular symptoms.
- Management and surveillance are similar to that of SLE, depending on which autoantibodies are present. Autoantibodies commonly include Ro; La; ANA; rheumatoid factor; and more rarely, Sm, RNP, anticardiolipin, and lupus anticoagulant.
- Symptomatic management of dry mouth involves diet modifications, regular hydration, and regular dental care. Artificial tears can be given for dry eyes. Extraglandular symptoms may require immunosuppressive therapy similar to the therapies employed in SLE (see Table 16-1).

Addison Disease

- **Addison disease** is an autoimmune disease characterized by adrenal insufficiency.
- Management with glucocorticoid replacement therapy may safely continue throughout pregnancy.
- Prior to the advent of glucocorticoid therapy, maternal mortality was as high as 45%. In general, outcomes are good with adequate glucocorticoid replacement therapy; however, women should be followed closely with frequent electrolyte monitoring.
- As with any patient on chronic corticosteroid therapy, stress dose steroids should be administered in labor or at the time of cesarean delivery.

Autoimmune Thyroid Disease

- **Autoimmune thyroid disease** is characterized by autoantibodies that affect the thyroid gland, leading either to hypo- or hyperthyroidism. Untreated maternal disease can have significant consequences. This spectrum of disorders is more comprehensively discussed in chapter 11.
- **Graves disease** involves thyroid-stimulating immunoglobulins that bind the TSH receptor, causing hyperthyroidism and potential thyrotoxicosis. Thyroidectomy, either medical or surgical, with lifelong thyroid replacement therapy, is the gold standard for treatment.
- **Hashimoto thyroiditis** involves destruction of the thyroid by autoantibodies, resulting in hypothyroidism. Antithyroid peroxidase (anti-TPO) is the most common antibody. Thyroid replacement therapy is the mainstay of treatment.

Type I Diabetes

See chapter 11.

Rheumatoid Arthritis

- **Rheumatoid arthritis** is a chronic polyarthritis of uncertain etiology characterized by morning stiffness and decreased range of motion in affected joints.
- Diagnosis is based on symptoms and lab findings such as rheumatoid factor, anti-CCP, or elevated ESR. Symptoms improve in 50% to 90% of patients during pregnancy; however, up to 90% will experience flares postpartum, particularly in the first 3 months. No obvious adverse fetal effects are known.
- Symptomatic treatment is the cornerstone of management outside of pregnancy and includes nonsteroidal anti-inflammatory drugs, low-dose aspirin, glucocorticoids, and occasionally hydroxychloroquine. Methotrexate is a common treatment for severe cases, and this must be discontinued prior to conception.

Scleroderma

- **Scleroderma** is a chronic inflammatory disorder with nearly universal dermatologic involvement, generally characterized by skin sclerosis (hardening). Patients may also have varying degrees of pulmonary fibrosis, pulmonary hypertension, systemic hypertension, renal insufficiency, GI dysmotility, cardiac manifestations, and musculoskeletal involvement.

Preconception

- The treatment of scleroderma depends on the clinical manifestations in the individual patient (eg, skin, renal, pulmonary involvement). Some medications used to control severe scleroderma, such as methotrexate and mycophenolate mofetil, are teratogenic (see Table 16-1). Patients must be transitioned to nonteratogenic medications prior to conception.
- Renal function should be assessed prior to pregnancy. Whereas there is no clear impact of pregnancy on flaring of scleroderma, renal crises are associated with significant morbidity of both mother and fetus, such as hypertension and FGR.

Antenatal

- Pregnancy often exacerbates GI dysmotility. Proton pump inhibitor may be helpful in these cases.
- When present, perineal/cervical involvement may impacts vaginal delivery and may increase risk of shoulder dystocia. Comprehensive pelvic exam is recommended antenatally. In cases of severe perineal involvement, primary cesarean delivery may be considered.

Postpartum

- There is no increased incidence of flares in the postpartum period.
- Breastfeeding is not contraindicated, dependent on medication usage (see Table 16-1).

Dermatomyositis and Polymyositis

- **Dermatomyositis** and **polymyositis** are heterogeneous, idiopathic inflammatory myopathies characterized by proximal skeletal muscle weakness and muscle inflammation. Dermatomyositis is more associated with skin manifestations.

Some patients have myositis-specific autoantibodies such as anti-Jo 1, anti-Mi-2, or anti-SRP.

- Diagnosis is aided by the presence of these antibodies, elevated muscle enzymes, and abnormal electromyelogram but is confirmed only by biopsy. These disorders are extremely rare, and data is limited even in the nonpregnant population.
- Treatment involves glucocorticoids and/or azathioprine. There is an increased risk of IUGR and perinatal death and active disease is associated with worse outcome, although these conclusions are based on one small case series.

Mixed Connective Tissue Disease

- **Mixed connective tissue disease** is an autoimmune disease associated with anti-U1RNP that is characterized by a combination of symptoms of SLE, scleroderma, rheumatoid arthritis, and myositis. Other autoantibodies sometimes associated with the condition include anti-dsDNA, anti-Sm, and anti-Ro antibodies.
- Presentation is highly variable. Patients with predominately scleroderma or myositis-like features generally having a worse prognosis.
- Treatment is tailored to features of illness. The SLE features are typically glucocorticoid responsive, whereas scleroderma-like features are not.

Crohn Disease and Ulcerative Colitis

- **Crohn disease** and **ulcerative colitis**, collectively termed **inflammatory bowel disease**, are complex disorders characterized by acute and chronic inflammation of the GI tract. Although they are widely understood to be rooted in the immune system, the degree of immune-mediated versus autoimmune components is not well understood and is actively under investigation. Some autoantibodies associated with these diseases include those against intestinal epithelial cells, perinuclear antineutrophil cytoplasmic antibodies in ulcerative colitis, and antibodies against *Saccharomyces cerevisiae* in Crohn disease.
- Medications used to treat these disorders are similar to other autoimmune conditions, including immunomodulators and steroids. Additionally, amino salicylates such as sulfasalazine are utilized in flares and are generally felt to be safe in pregnancy. See chapter 15 for more information on inflammatory bowel disease in pregnancy.

Myasthenia Gravis

- **Myasthenia gravis** is characterized by immunoglobulin G (IgG)-mediated damage to acetylcholine receptors or muscle-specific tyrosine kinase at the neuromuscular junction resulting in contractile muscle weakness of the face, oropharynx, eyes, limbs, and respiratory muscles.
- Women with well-controlled disease can be reassured that flare is unlikely. Women with poorly controlled disease should be counseled of the risk of **myasthenic crisis**, which can be life-threatening, particularly with oropharyngeal or respiratory involvement.
- Pyridostigmine, an anticholinesterase, is used for symptomatic treatment. In severe cases, glucocorticoids and azathioprine can be considered. Plasmapheresis or intravenous immunoglobulin (IVIG) may be needed for crisis. *Magnesium sulfate can precipitate a crisis and is contraindicated.* See chapter 17 for further discussion on myasthenia gravis in pregnancy.

Multiple Sclerosis

- **Multiple sclerosis** is a heterogeneous autoimmune disease of the central nervous system characterized by demyelination, inflammation, and axon degeneration. Various cell types, including T helper 17 and inflammatory T and B cells, have been implicated. The disease exists in relapsing-remitting and progressive forms. Neurologic symptoms such as weakness and visual and sensory loss vary depending on the tissues involved.
- The *Pregnancy In Multiple Sclerosis* study suggests that patients have fewer relapses during pregnancy and tend to flare postpartum. Therefore, many experts recommend discontinuing disease-modifying medications prior to pregnancy (see Table 16-1). See chapter 17 for more information about multiple sclerosis in pregnancy.

Immune Thrombocytopenic Purpura

See chapter 20.

Autoimmune Hemolytic Anemia

- **Autoimmune hemolytic anemia** is characterized by maternal anemia caused by autoantibodies targeting red blood cells. Disease is classified by the type of autoantibody.
- **Cold agglutinin disease** is caused by immunoglobulin M (rarely immunoglobulin A or IgG) antibodies against polysaccharide components of the red blood cell. Symptoms are prominent in cold temperatures. Rapid hemoglobin drops may result in miscarriage or stillbirth. Fetal effects are rare because immunoglobulin M does not cross the placenta. Treatment is supportive, including warm clothing. In severe cases, rituximab is used. Plasmapheresis is rarely necessary. If transfusion is necessary, fluids should be warmed.
- **Warm agglutinin disease** is due to IgG antibodies and may be associated with SLE, viral infection, connective tissue disease, or immune deficiency. When IgG antibodies cross the placenta, fetal effects are usually absent to mild. Maternal treatment options include glucocorticoids and azathioprine. Splenectomy can lead to remission, and IVIG is used for refractory cases. Neonates will transiently be Coombs positive and rarely require transfusion or plasmapheresis.

Autoimmune Neutropenia

- **Autoimmune neutropenia** is characterized by granulocyte specific antibodies and an absolute neutrophil count less than 1500 cells/μL. It is commonly developed in childhood with remission in adulthood. Transplacental passage of antibodies from affected gravidas has been documented. The transient effect on neonates is mild; however, severe infections may occur.

Vasculitic Syndromes

- **Vasculitic syndromes** involve damage to blood vessels, often through immune complexes. Relatively rare in pregnancy, information is limited to small case series and reports.
- **Polyarteritis nodosa** is a necrotizing vasculitis involving small- and medium-sized arteries that is characterized by neuropathy, hypertension, GI disorders, and renal

failure. Treatment consists of glucocorticoids, cyclophosphamide, and angiotensin-converting enzyme (ACE) inhibitors. During pregnancy, this regimen must be reevaluated. Thirty percent of cases are associated with hepatitis B and require antiviral treatment. Although rare, polyarteritis nodosa can be devastating when identified in pregnancy, with morality rates greater than 50%.

- **Wegener granulomatosis** is a necrotizing granulomatous vasculitis with pulmonary, respiratory sinus, and renal involvement. Treatment includes corticosteroids, cyclophosphamide, rituximab, or azathioprine.
- **Takayasu arteritis** is a vasculitis that affects large vessels including the upper aorta and its branches. Surgery prior to pregnancy may improve survival. Most case series report good fetal outcomes; however, the incidence of maternal adverse events varies widely. Baseline function, abdominal aorta involvement, and prenatal care may explain these differences. Hypertension poses significant risk and should be managed aggressively. Invasive monitoring may be necessary.
- **Henoch-Schönlein purpura** is a small-vessel vasculitis characterized by abdominal pain, hematuria, purpura, and arthritis that is more common in childhood. Treatment is supportive, and pregnancy outcomes are generally favorable.
- **Behçet disease** is a systemic vasculitis characterized by uveitis, and oral and genital ulcers. Disease is usually stable during pregnancy; early miscarriage rates are higher.

Autoimmune Bullous Disease

- **Autoimmune bullous disease** is a group of dermatologic conditions caused by antibodies that target maternal skin components.
- **Pemphigus vulgaris** is caused by IgG antibodies against desmogleins, resulting in intraepidermal bullae on the skin and mucous membranes. Its milder variant, pemphigus foliaceus, does not have mucous membrane involvement. Therapy includes systemic glucocorticoids and occasionally azathioprine. Refractory cases are treated with rituximab and IVIG.
- **Bullous pemphigoid** is caused by IgG antibodies against hemidesmosomes in the basement membrane, resulting in subepidermal bullae. When onset occurs during pregnancy, the condition is called *pemphigoid gestationis* or *herpes gestationis*. Exacerbations can occur postpartum and in subsequent pregnancies. Maternal treatment includes topical corticosteroids and antihistamines. Systemic therapy with these agents is used for refractory cases.
- Fetal deaths have been reported in women with high antibody titers in both of these diseases. Titers should be followed closely and, if rising, should prompt aggressive maternal treatment.
- Due to risk of stillbirth, prematurity, and IUGR, antenatal testing may be indicated.
- Neonatal bullous disease occurs in 3% to 40% of infants. Treatment is supportive because lesions resolve as maternal antibodies degrade.

Autoimmune Hepatitis

- **Autoimmune hepatitis** has a heterogeneous presentation ranging from asymptomatic disease to liver failure. Autoantibodies present in type 1 include ANA, antiactin antibody, and anti–smooth muscle antibody. Those in type 2 include anti–liver/kidney microsome type 1 and anti–liver cytosol type 1.
- A healthy pregnancy outcome is possible, although there is an increased risk of prematurity, low birth weight, and stillbirth. Common treatment options include glucocorticoids and azathioprine.

SUGGESTED READINGS

American College of Obstetricians and Gynecologists Committee on Practice Bulletins—Obstetrics. ACOG Practice Bulletin No. 132: antiphospholipid syndrome. *Obstet Gynecol*. 2012;120:1514-1521. (Reaffirmed 2017)

Cunningham F, Leveno KJ, Bloom SL, et al, eds. Connective tissue disorders. In: *Williams Obstetrics*. 25th ed. New York, NY: McGraw-Hill; 2018:chap 59.

Cunningham F, Leveno KJ, Bloom SL, et al, eds. Gastrointestinal disorders. In: *Williams Obstetrics*. 25th ed. New York, NY: McGraw-Hill; 2018:chap 54.

Cunningham F, Leveno KJ, Bloom SL, et al, eds. Preconceptional care. In: *Williams Obstetrics*. 25th ed. New York, NY: McGraw-Hill; 2018:chap 8.

Fischer-Betz R, Specker C. Pregnancy in systemic lupus erythematosus and antiphospholipid syndrome. *Best Pract Res Clin Rheumatol*. 2017;31(3):397-414.

Miyakis S, Lockshin MD, Atsumi T, et al. International consensus statement on an update of the classification criteria for definite antiphospholipid syndrome (APS). *J Thromb Haemost*. 2006;4:295-306.

US National Library of Medicine, National Institutes of Health. Developmental and Reproductive Toxicology Database (DART). US National Library of Medicine Web site. https://www.ncbi.nim.nih.gov.pubmed. Accessed March 3, 2019.

17 Neurologic Diseases in Pregnancy

Ana M. Angarita and Irina Burd

Women with complex preexisting neurologic conditions often achieve pregnancy, necessitating the obstetric provider to be well versed in the treatment of these conditions and their unique implications in the setting of pregnancy. Some conditions are seen more frequently in pregnancy. This section reviews common neurologic complaints and preexisting neurologic conditions and their management during pregnancy.

HEADACHE

- Headache is a common complaint in pregnancy.
- Although most of these headaches are due to benign causes, it is imperative that obstetric providers perform a thorough history and physical examination to identify those headaches that warrant further workup (Table 17-1).
- In the presence of concerning signs or symptoms, neurology consultation and diagnostic workup should be performed.

Imaging/Diagnosis

- Lumbar puncture (LP), magnetic resonance imaging (MRI), and head computed tomography (CT) can be considered for a headache with concerning features.

Table 17-1	History and Physical Exam Findings That Should Prompt Further Headache Workup[a]

History	Physical Exam
• Intense or abrupt onset	• Toxic appearance
• Change in headache characteristics	• Fever
• Atypical aura (>1 h, or with motor weakness)	• Altered mental status
• Visual disturbance/scotoma	• Papilledema
• Prior or coexisting infection	• Any localizing or lateralizing signs
• Onset during exertion	• Neurologic deficit (weakness, sensory loss, dysphagia)
• History of HIV, syphilis, or cancer	
• Environmental exposure	• Meningismus
• No relief from pain medication	

Abbreviation: HIV, human immunodeficiency virus.
[a]Adapted from Contag SA, Bushnell C. Contemporary management of migrainous disorders in pregnancy. *Curr Opin Obstet Gynecol.* 2010;22:437-445.

- MRI poses no radiation exposure risks to the fetus and is the imaging of choice for pregnant patients. However, MRI is expensive and often not readily available.
- Head CT is the imaging of choice for nonpregnant patients because it is less expensive and more readily available in most settings. Although head CT does expose the fetus to some radiation, it is approximately 0.05 rad. This is geometrically below the 5 rad exposure associated with risk of fetal anomalies or pregnancy loss. As such, the diagnostic benefit of a head CT, as with any clinical test, should be weighed against its risks.
- An LP is not contraindicated in pregnancy and should be used if clinically indicated.

Common Obstetric Causes of Headache

- Any headache beyond 20 weeks' gestation and up to 12 weeks' postpartum, especially if not relieved by pain medications, should include evaluation for **preeclampsia**.
- Postdural puncture headache should be considered in postpartum patients particularly if they experience postural headaches (a headache that worsens upon sitting or standing and that improves when the patient lays flat on her back). Although acetaminophen, nonsteroidal anti-inflammatory drugs (NSAIDs), and caffeine are often effective in controlling the pain, anesthesia consultation for blood patching should be considered in patients who are refractory to conservative treatments.

Primary Headaches

Migraine

- Although many chronic migraine sufferers report improved symptoms during pregnancy, it remains a common cause of headache in pregnancy.
- Approximately 2% of women have their first migraine while pregnant.

- **Typical migraine symptoms** include unilateral throbbing headache episodes, which last between 4 and 72 hours and are associated with nausea, vomiting, phonophobia, and photophobia. Some patients also experience a phenomenon known as an aura. It is defined as the development of visual symptoms (ie, a scintillating scotoma, partial loss of visual field) lasting 20 minutes followed by a headache.
- **Imaging:** Noncontrast brain MRI can be used to rule out other causes of headache if alarm symptoms or signs are present.
- **Treatment:** Many of the same pharmacologic and nonpharmacologic treatments that are useful outside of pregnancy are also used during pregnancy. Limit therapy to a maximum of 2 to 3 days per week to avoid a medication-overuse headache.
  - Behavioral and nonpharmacologic therapy: Avoid alcohol and tobacco use. Maintain a regular meal and sleep pattern. Encourage regular exercise and adequate hydration. Other options are relaxation, biofeedback, and acupuncture.
  - Acute symptom management: Treatment of acute migraines can involve a variety of medications (Table 17-2).
    - o Breastfeeding: Women who breastfeed are less likely to have migraine headache recurrence in the postpartum period. Acetaminophen, NSAIDs, metoclopramide, triptans, and opioids can be used. Avoid high-dose aspirin. Ergots are contraindicated.
    - o Prophylaxis therapy: β-Blockers (metoprolol, propranolol, and atenolol), calcium channel blockers (nifedipine), antiepileptics (gabapentin), and antiplatelets (aspirin in doses ≤150 mg/d) can be used in pregnancy. Selective serotonin reuptake inhibitors (citalopram, escitalopram, fluoxetine, sertraline), serotonin-norepinephrine reuptake inhibitors (venlafaxine), and tricyclics (low-dose amitriptyline and nortriptyline) can be used in patients with comorbid depression.

Tension Headaches

- Tension headaches are the most common type of headache.
- Patients describe tightness or tension in their head often with radiation to the neck. There are no associated symptoms or disability.
- The frequency of tension headaches is typically not altered by pregnancy.
- **Treatment:** Behavioral treatment includes avoiding skipping meals, maintaining a regular exercise and sleep pattern, maintaining adequate hydration, and avoiding alcohol and tobacco use. Nonpharmacologic therapies such as heat, massage, relaxation, physical therapy, and acupuncture are often helpful. Pharmacologic treatment with acetaminophen is the first-line therapy. The NSAIDs can be used in the second trimester, but chronic use should be avoided. Muscle relaxants can often be a useful adjunct.

Cluster Headaches

- Cluster headaches are recurrent, unilateral headaches that are accompanied by autonomic symptoms such as nasal stuffiness, tearing, facial swelling, or eyelid edema. They can last up to 2 hours and occur in clusters typically lasting 6 to 8 weeks.
- **Acute treatment:** Oxygen (100% at 10-15 L/min for 10-15 min via nonrebreather face mask) at the onset of attack is first-line therapy. Subcutaneous or intranasal triptans and intranasal lidocaine can also be useful adjunct therapies.
- **Prophylaxis** during pregnancy and breastfeeding includes verapamil and prednisone/prednisolone.

Table 17-2 Treatment Options for Acute Migraine Headache in Pregnancy

Treatment	Comments
First-line therapies	
Acetaminophen	• Extensive evidence of its safety in pregnancy • Inexpensive • May be used in combination with other drugs • Maximum of 4 g daily to avoid liver toxicity
Caffeine	• Up to 200 mg daily considered safe in pregnancy • Can be used in combination with acetaminophen
Metoclopramide	• Often helpful with headache reduction and alleviates associated nausea • Can cause dystonic reaction
Second-line therapies	
NSAIDs/aspirin	• Not used in first trimester due to possible teratogenicity • Safe in second trimester • Use in third trimester should be limited to 48 h or less due to possible premature ductal closure, platelet dysfunction, and oligohydramnios.
Third-line therapies	
Opioids	• Should be used for short duration because dependence can develop in the mother or fetus with high doses over long duration • Can cause constipation and worsen nausea/vomiting associated with migraines • No teratogenic effects associated with opioids
Severe symptoms	
Triptans	• For severe attacks that do not respond to first-line agents • Studies show no association with triptans and birth defects. • Use in third trimester associated with slight increased risk of uterine atony and increased blood loss at delivery
Magnesium sulfate	• 1 or 2 g IV over 15 min
Contraindicated	
Ergotamine	• Associated with hypertonic uterine contractions

Abbreviations: IV, intravenous; NSAIDs, nonsteroidal anti-inflammatory drugs.

Secondary Headaches

Cerebral Venous Thrombosis

- Cerebral venous thrombosis is most common in the postpartum period and in women with thrombophilia.
- It is characterized by progressive, diffuse, unremitting headache. Accompanied by seizures, focal neurologic signs, and funduscopy with signs of elevated intracranial pressure.
- **Imaging:** Noncontrast CT is often unrevealing. Noncontrast brain MRI scan and magnetic resonance venogram show nonarterial territorial infarct.
- **Treatment:** Anticoagulation with intravenous (IV) heparin or low-molecular-weight heparin is recommended during pregnancy. Low-molecular-weight heparin or warfarin should be continued for at least 6 weeks postpartum. Consider thrombophilia workup, especially when there are prior thrombosis episodes or a family history of thrombophilia.

Pseudotumor Cerebri (Idiopathic Intracranial Hypertension)

- Pseudotumor cerebri is characterized by diffuse, nonthrobbing, daily headache aggravated by coughing and straining. It can be associated with papilledema, visual field defect, or sixth nerve palsy.
- **Imaging:** Rule out intracranial mass or cerebral venous thrombosis with a noncontrast head CT and MRI/MR venography, respectively.
- **Diagnosis:** Diagnosis includes LP with increased cerebrospinal fluid pressure with normal cerebrospinal fluid chemistry. Serial LPs are also therapeutic.
- **Treatment:** The mainstay of treatment is to decrease intracranial pressure. Consider acetazolamide and controlled weight gain during pregnancy. Symptomatic management for headaches may be necessary (see Table 17-2).

CARPAL TUNNEL SYNDROME

- Carpal tunnel syndrome is diagnosed clinically. Symptoms include pain and numbness in the median nerve distribution. Pregnant patients are at increased risk due to swelling of carpal tunnel leading to compression of median nerve.
- Symptoms most often present in the third trimester and can remain for up to a year after delivery.
- Treatment with conservative measures such as a wrist brace is usually effective. In rare cases, corticosteroid injections or surgery is indicated.

CHRONIC NEUROLOGIC DISEASES

Multiple Sclerosis

- Multiple sclerosis (MS) predominantly affects women of childbearing age (15-50 y).
- An MS is a demyelinating autoimmune disease characterized by relapsing and remitting neurologic deficits.
- Common symptoms during a flare include optic neuritis, asymmetric numbness, weakness, or ataxia.

Preconception

- Important points to discuss with women include the following:
  - An MS has no meaningful impact on the ability to conceive, or on pregnancy, fetal well-being, or delivery unless the patient has a severe disability.

- Women with MS are not at significantly higher risk for obstetric and neonatal complications.
- The antepartum period is associated with decreased MS flare risk.
- An MS is not an inherited disease and has mainly an environmental component. The risk to a child when a parent has MS is 2% to 2.5%. The risk when a sibling has MS is 2.7%.
- Many of the common treatment options for MS are teratogenic. Women trying to become pregnant are often advised to discontinue disease-modifying drugs due to teratogenic concerns. Interferon β, glatiramer acetate, and dimethyl fumarate are usually stopped approximately 1 month before attempting to conceive. Fingolimod is usually stopped 2 months before and natalizumab 3 months before.

Antepartum

- Relapses decrease in the third trimester of pregnancy.
- **Diagnosis:** MRI can be used during pregnancy. Avoid gadolinium (Figure 17-1).
- **Treatment:** Disease-modifying therapies are usually not used in pregnant women. Consider their use if women have very severe or highly active MS. Acute flares in pregnancy are typically managed with glucocorticoids IV or orally (equivalent of 1 g of methylprednisolone daily for 3-7 d). The glucocorticoids recommended are prednisone, prednisolone, or methylprednisolone. No oral taper is used.
- **Mode of delivery** is not affected by MS and should be based on obstetric indications unless the patient has a severely disabling disease that affects mobility or the ability to push or if the patient has respiratory issues.
- Classically, MS was considered a contraindication for spinal anesthesia. More recently, data has supported individualizing the plan of anesthetic care and spinal anesthesia.

Postpartum

- During the first 3 months postpartum, relapses increase to 70% above prepregnancy level.
- Risk factors for flares in this period include high relapse rate in the year before pregnancy, higher disability prepregnancy, and relapse rate during pregnancy.

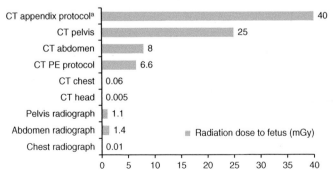

Figure 17-1. Amount of radiation received by the fetus per radiation source. Abbreviations: CT, computed tomography; PE, pulmonary embolus. [a]Range, 20-40. Adapted from Nguyen CP, Goodman LH. Fetal risk in diagnostic radiology. *Semin Ultrasound CT MR.* 2012;33(1):4-10.

- If the patient had a relapse during pregnancy, discuss the need to resume or start disease-modifying therapy after delivery.
- **Breastfeeding:** Disease-modifying therapies should not be used in breastfeeding women.

Epilepsy

Preconception

- Before attempting pregnancy, seizures should be well controlled.
- Many of the drugs used to control epilepsy are teratogenic, and thus, women should be weaned to the lowest effective dose possible before pregnancy or weaned off of the medications entirely.
- Women with epilepsy who are planning a pregnancy or are pregnant should be supplemented with *4 mg folic acid* daily to help prevent neural tube defects.

Antepartum

- Valproate, carbamazepine, phenobarbital, and lamotrigine are commonly used antiepileptics and are all associated with an increased risk of neural tube defects. Monotherapy is associated with less frequent severe congenital defects (Figure 17-2).

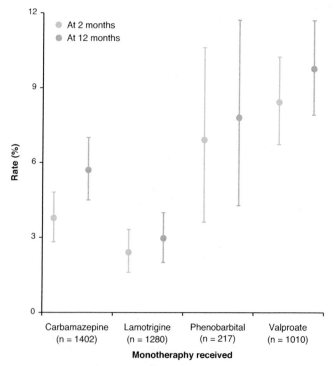

Figure 17-2. The rates of major anomalies associated with in utero exposure to various antiepileptic medications at 2 and 12 months of life. Reprinted with permission from Tomson T, Battino D. Teratogenic effects of antiepileptic drugs. *Lancet Neurol.* 2012;11(9):803-813.

- High hormonal levels and genetic/interindividual variability increase the metabolism of antiepileptic drugs. Hence, some antiepileptic drug levels should be monitored during pregnancy and the dose adjusted as appropriate.
- Nausea and emesis should be well controlled especially in the first trimester to avoid vomiting antiepileptic drugs.
- Pregnancy does not typically affect the frequency of seizures. However, a confounding factor is that pregnant women are often noncompliant with medications for fear of teratogenicity or they cannot take the medications due to nausea and emesis.
- Seizure during pregnancy can cause fetal hypoxia. Fetal monitoring may reflect fetal hypoxia for up to 30 minutes after the seizure. Emergent delivery is not indicated based on this tracing alone.
- Preeclampsia must be considered in the differential in the setting of seizures, particularly in the third trimester.

Postpartum

- A medication plan postpartum should be discussed in advance with the neurologist because dose adjustments of antiepileptic drugs may be required especially in the setting of sleep deprivation and fatigue.
- **Breastfeeding:** Estimates of antiepileptic drug exposure from breast milk are scant, but the available literature suggests that exposure is low for many of these medications. In general, breastfeeding is encouraged.

Myasthenia Gravis

- Myasthenia gravis (MG) is an autoimmune disease characterized by fluctuating skeletal muscle fatigue and weakness due to autoantibodies against acetylcholine receptors.
- Two types:
  - Ocular MG: only eyelids and extraocular muscles affected
  - Generalized MG: ocular, bulbar, limb, and respiratory muscles affected

Preconception

- Women with MG that desire to become pregnant should be counseled that if otherwise healthy, they could have an uneventful pregnancy if they are closely monitored.
- The risk of generalized MG and exacerbations is highest in the first 2 to 3 years after onset. Thus, it is advised to delay pregnancy until at least a couple of years after diagnosis to evaluate the severity of the disease and response to therapy.
- When discontinuing immunosuppressive therapy, birth control should be continued for 6 months before attempting to conceive.
- Initiation of immunosuppressive agents other than prednisone before pregnancy is usually avoided.
- Having MG does not increase the risk of having a neonate with the disease. Up to 10% to 20% of neonates develop transient MG postpartum, lasting for up to 3 months.

Antepartum

- During pregnancy, MG worsens in 40% of women, improves in 30%, and remains stable in 30%. Exacerbations are more likely during the first trimester, in the final 4 weeks of gestation, and immediately postpartum. The clinical status before pregnancy or in prior pregnancies does not predict the course of MG during the actual pregnancy.

- Surgery or infections predispose to disease exacerbation.
- **Treatment:**
  - Acetylcholinesterase inhibitors are first-line therapy for pregnant and nonpregnant patients.
  - Glucocorticoids, azathioprine, and cyclosporine are second-line options and are safe during pregnancy. Methotrexate is contraindicated.
  - Other alternatives if acute exacerbation not responding to first-line medical treatment include plasma exchange and IV immunoglobulin.
  - If thymectomy is considered, it should be performed preconceptionally or postpartum because there is a delayed therapeutic effect.
- Medication interactions: Patients with MG are often challenging to manage because a wide variety of medications can exacerbate symptoms, including the following:
  - Azithromycin and erythromycin
  - Gentamycin
  - Steroids (prednisone)
  - Magnesium salts (magnesium sulfate, milk of magnesia, magnesium-containing antacids). *Magnesium sulfate is contraindicated* in these patients because it may have a paralyzing effect. In the setting of preeclampsia, an alternative antiseizure medication should be used.
  - β-Blockers (propranolol, atenolol, timolol maleate eye drops)
  - Calcium channel blockers
  - Lithium
  - Iodinated contrast agents
- Labor concerns:
  - First stage of labor is not affected by MG because this stage is mediated by smooth muscle. The MG only affects skeletal muscle.
  - Second stage of labor can be affected, and women may develop worsening fatigue with pushing. Consider "laboring down" or operative delivery to minimize fatigue.
  - Mode of delivery: The MG is not an indication for cesarean delivery. Delivery by cesarean should be reserved for standard obstetrics indications.
- Fetal concerns:
  - Immunoglobulin G anti-acetylcholine receptor antibodies can cross the placenta leading to fetal manifestations of MG.
  - Polyhydramnios due to impaired swallowing, decreased fetal movement, and reduced fetal breathing can be observed in fetuses of MG patients.
  - Nonstress test often not reliable because MG can impair fetal movement and therefore accelerations. Contraction stress testing can be useful.

Postpartum

- Women may have disease exacerbation 6 to 8 weeks after delivery.
- Provide contraception counseling for women who begin or continue immunosuppressive therapy after delivery and highlight the importance of effective contraception.
- Birth control should start 4 weeks before starting medical treatment for MG.
- **Breastfeeding:** Acetylcholinesterase inhibitors, prednisone, and prednisolone can be used for the treatment of exacerbations. Immunosuppressants can be used as indicated except for methotrexate, which is contraindicated.

Spinal Cord Injury

Complications of pregnancy in patients with prior spinal cord injuries are often related to the level of the spinal cord lesion.

- Patients with lower lesions (T11 and below) will likely perceive labor pain. Most complications in their pregnancies are related to recurrent urinary tract infections and decubitus ulcers.
- Patients with mid lesions (T5-T10) often have painless deliveries. These patients must be counseled carefully and monitored closely to avoid undetected labor and delivery. Patients can use home uterine monitors or be taught uterine palpation. Weekly cervical examinations should be considered near term.
- Higher lesions (above T6) are associated with **autonomic dysreflexia** leading to potentially life-threatening sympathetic hyperactivity. This is manifested by severe hypertension, loss of consciousness, headache, nasal congestion, facial flushing, sweating, piloerection, bradycardia, tachycardia, or arrhythmia. It can be very challenging to distinguish this condition from preeclampsia. Epidural anesthesia up to T10 is critical in patients with high spinal cord lesions to prevent this complication. In the setting of acute autonomic dysreflexia, labetalol or nifedipine can be used to control blood pressure. Magnesium sulfate has been shown to have some benefit in the setting of autonomic dysreflexia (although it is not first line) and should be considered if preeclampsia cannot be definitively excluded.

Bell Palsy in Pregnancy

- Bell palsy is unilateral facial nerve paralysis. Most of the cases in pregnancy occur during the third trimester and within 7 days after delivery.
- Etiology: It is most likely idiopathic. Infections can also be associated with Bell palsy including herpes simplex or herpes zoster virus activation and Lyme disease.
- Pregnant women are more likely to progress to a complete paralysis than nonpregnant women and men with Bell palsy. However, this difference may be attributed to the fact that fewer women are treated during pregnancy.
- Symptoms include sudden onset, over a day or two. The peak onset of symptoms is within 3 weeks or less from the first day of visible weakness. Patients usually endorse taste changes; dryness of the eye; and difficulty raising the eyebrow, blinking, and closing the eye. No history of trauma, recent surgery, or infection.
- Physical exam: Cranial nerves are intact except for the facial nerve. Findings include an inability to close the eye or generate wrinkles on the forehead, eyebrow sagging, and drooping of the affected corner of the mouth. To rule out infectious etiology, examine the external auditory canal to look for vesicles or scabbing. If associated limb weakness, ophthalmoplegia, or decreased deep tendon reflexes, consider other causes.
- Imaging: indicated if there are atypical physical signs or no improvement in 4 months
- Treatment:
  - Corneal protection with artificial tears and patching of the eye
  - Short course of oral corticosteroid treatment
  - Combined oral corticosteroid and antiviral medications. The latter increases the likelihood of recovery in those cases of concomitant herpetic infection. Treatment should be administered early in the presentation.

Table 17-3	Common Postpartum Nerve Palsies and Mechanisms of Injury	
Nerve Damaged	Common Mechanism of Injury	Deficit
Peroneal nerve	• Prolonged knee flexion during labor • Pressure of fibular head from stirrups • Palmar pressure during pushing	• Inability to dorsiflex the foot, that is, foot drop
Femoral nerve	• Prolonged hip flexion with McRoberts	• Weak quadriceps leading to inability to flex hip • Sensory loss over anterior and medial thigh
Lateral femoral cutaneous	• Prolonged compression	• Purely sensory defect; often paresthesias on outer thigh

POSTPARTUM COMPRESSION NERVE INJURIES

• Risk factors include fetal macrosomia, epidural anesthesia, prolonged second stage, poor positioning in stirrups.
• Prolonged pushing and "over"-aggressive McRoberts during the second stage of labor can be associated with postpartum neuropathies. This is particularly true in patients who have an epidural during the second stage of labor.
• See Table 17-3 for common nerve palsies and the associated mechanism of injury.
• Most patients make a complete recovery. Physical therapy can be helpful.

SUGGESTED READINGS

Coyle PK. Multiple sclerosis in pregnancy. *Continuum (Minneap Minn)*. 2014;20(1):42-59.
Haider B, von Oertzen J. Neurological disorders. *Best Pract Res Clin Obstet Gynaecol*. 2013;27(6):867-875.
Harden CL. Pregnancy and epilepsy. *Continuum (Minneap Minn)*. 2014;20(1):60-79.
Massey JM, De Jesus-Acosta C. Pregnancy and myasthenia gravis. *Continuum (Minneap Minn)*. 2014;20(1):115-127.
Nguyen CP, Goodman LH. Fetal risk in diagnostic radiology. *Semin Ultrasound CT MR*. 2012;33(1):4-10.
O'Neal MA. Headaches complicating pregnancy and the postpartum period. *Pract Neurol*. 2017;17(3):191-202.

Psychiatric Disorders in the Pregnant and Postpartum Patient

Jaden R. Kohn and Lauren M. Osborne

Psychiatric illness and the use of psychotropic medications are not uncommon during pregnancy and lactation. Collaborative care between obstetrician-gynecologists and psychiatrists is essential for comprehensive treatment and can improve patient outcomes.

- Prenatal depression is associated with increased risk of pregnancy and newborn and childhood complications.
- The obstetrician-gynecologist should be able to provide validated screening for psychiatric illness, manage mild to moderate psychiatric illness in the context of perinatal health care, and work collaboratively with psychiatrists and other mental health providers through referral of women with more severe psychiatric illness.
- American College of Obstetricians and Gynecologists now encourages an improved focus on the "fourth trimester"—the postpartum period—during which women are at risk for new or worsening mental health disorders. They recommend that women receive anticipatory guidance regarding signs and symptoms of perinatal depression and anxiety and that women be screened using a validated instrument for depression and anxiety.
- Recommended screening for psychiatric disorders by the obstetrician-gynecologist appears in Table 18-1.
- Useful toolkits and trainings for providers are available from the Massachusetts Child Psychiatry Access Program for Moms (https://www.mcpapformoms.org/).
- Indications for urgent or emergent referral to a psychiatrist are shown in Table 18-2.

MOOD DISORDERS AND PREGNANCY

Major Depressive Disorder

- During the reproductive years, major depressive disorder (MDD) is twice as common in women as men. See Table 18-3 for diagnostic criteria.
- Lifetime risk of a major depressive episode in women is 10% to 25%.
- The 10-item Edinburgh Postnatal Depression Scale is recommended for depression screening during pregnancy and postpartum. Responses are scored 0, 1, 2, or 3. Edinburgh Postnatal Depression Scale score ≥10 indicates substantial depressive symptoms, and ≥13 is likely major depression.
- Screening for personal or family history of mania or hypomania is *essential* prior to initiating antidepressant treatment.
- It is important to assess suicidal thoughts, intent, plans, and ability to attempt suicide. If there is an imminent suicide risk, emergency care in a facility with psychiatric care capabilities is essential.

Postpartum Depressive Disorders

- Postpartum depression (PPD) is the most common complication of childbirth, experienced by nearly 20% of new mothers, with higher rates in those with significant psychosocial stressors.

Table 18-1	Recommended Psychiatric Assessments for OB/GYN Patients
Type of Assessment	**Description/Examples**
Patient history	Previous or current psychiatric symptoms, especially of mania/hypomania if depressive
Family history	Bipolar disorder (strong genetic component) Completed or attempted suicide (increases patient risk)
Mental status exam	Appearance, orientation, speech, mood, suicidal thoughts, hallucinations, delusions, obsessions, compulsions, phobias
Screening for Psychiatric Conditions	
Depression	
Anytime	Patient Health Questionnaire, 2 or 9 items (PHQ-2, PHQ-9)
Perinatal period	Edinburgh Postnatal Depression Scale (EPDS)
Bipolar disorder	Mood Disorder Questionnaire
Anxiety	
Anytime	Generalized Anxiety Disorder 7-item scale (GAD-7) Beck Anxiety Inventory (BAI)
Perinatal specific	Edinburgh Postnatal Depression Score—Anxiety (EPDS-A)[a] Perinatal Anxiety Screening Scale (PASS) Pregnancy-Related Anxiety Questionnaire–Revised (PRAQ-R)
Posttraumatic stress disorder	Posttraumatic Stress Disorder Checklist (PCL-5)
Obsessive-compulsive disorder	Obsessive–Compulsive Inventory-Revised (OCI-R)
IPV	Hurt, Insult, Threaten, Scream (HITS), ACOG IPV Screening Woman Abuse Screening Tool (WAST)

ACOG, American College of Obstetricians and Gynecologists; IPV, intimate partner violence.
[a]Questions 3, 4, and 5 of the general Edinburgh Postnatal Depression Scale comprise a sub-scale to screen for perinatal-specific anxiety.

- Suicide risk markedly increases in the year after delivery, and in many countries, it is the leading cause of death in the first year postpartum.
- Risk factors:
  - Antenatal depression or anxiety
  - Personal or family history of PPD
  - Difficulty breastfeeding

Table 18-2	Indications for Referral to a Psychiatrist

Emergency

- Suicidality (intent, plans, ability, or belief that she may act)
- Homicidality (intent, plans, ability, or belief of action)
- Active psychotic symptoms
- Disorganized behavior or thoughts that impair functioning

Urgent Referral to Psychiatrist

- Failure to respond to multiple antidepressants at maximized dose
- Concern for bipolar disorder
- Suspicion of psychotic symptoms
- Eating disorder
- Suicidality without intent/plans
- Self-injury
- Complicated (personality disorders, trauma, substance use, significant anxiety, major life stressors)

- Fetal or newborn loss
- Lack of personal or community resources
- Financial challenges
- Substance use disorder
- Complications of pregnancy, labor/delivery, or infant's health
- Teen pregnancy
- Unintended pregnancy
- Violent or abusive relationships
- Isolation from family or friends
- Other major life stressors
- Difficult infant temperament
- A woman may be successfully treated with psychotherapy alone if depression is mild; if she is able to care for self/baby; if she has no suicidal ideation; and if she has good social support, access to psychotherapy, an exercise regimen, and protection from sleep deprivation.

Table 18-3	Diagnostic Criteria for Major Depressive Disorder

Depressed mood
Sleep changes (insomnia or hypersomnia)
Interest (loss of interest or loss of pleasure)
Guilt (or feelings of worthlessness)
Energy (lack of energy or fatigue)
Concentration difficulties
Appetite (changes in desire to eat)
Psychomotor retardation or agitation
Suicidal ideation

Note: Patient must have ≥5 of the above symptoms for at least two weeks, plus functional impairment, to meet criteria.

- Pharmacotherapy is indicated if moderate to severe depression (current or historical), suicidal ideation (current or historical), difficulty caring for self or baby, psychotic symptoms, comorbid anxiety, or inability to access nonpharmacologic treatment.
- Indications for hospitalization/immediate care by a psychiatrist: inability to care for self or baby; thoughts of harming baby (nonintrusive, egosyntonic, or nondistressing to the patient); suicidal intent and plan; delusional beliefs; mania; psychosis; distortion of reality.
- Prevention of PPD in nondepressed women with history of PPD: Close monitoring and social support are essential. Antidepressant medication during pregnancy (antenatal depression) or immediately after delivery (euthymic and off medications for pregnancy) may prevent recurrence and prolong time to relapse. The best evidence exists for selective serotonin reuptake inhibitors (SSRIs), but it is important to account for what has worked for the individual woman in the past.

Bipolar Affective Disorders

- Genetic involvement is stronger in bipolar affective disorders (BPAD) than MDD (70% vs 30%-40%), so suspect bipolar disorder if there is a family history of BPAD (although MDD is still the most common mood disorder in those with a family history of BPAD).
- It is important to distinguish BPAD from MDD, anxiety disorders, substance use, and personality disorders. A BPAD may be missed if mania or hypomania not recognized.
- Suspect possible BPAD (rather than MDD) if a patient reports lack of response, or repeated tolerance, to multiple antidepressants.
- Suspect possible BPAD (rather than MDD) if patient presents with a significant history of disrupted relationships or employment or substance use.
- Mania: abnormally and persistently elevated or irritable mood and increased energy (grandiosity, decreased need for sleep, more talkative, flight of ideas, distractible, agitated, goal-directed activity, psychotic symptoms).
- Due to the highly recurrent nature of BPAD (*up to 85% recurrence during pregnancy if mood stabilizers are discontinued*), pharmacotherapy during pregnancy is recommended.
- Patients with confirmed or suspected BPAD should be referred to psychiatry for evaluation.

Postpartum Mania and Psychosis

- Postpartum psychosis is an affective illness that occurs in 1 to 2 women per 1000 births, typically within 2 weeks after delivery.
- Women with preexisting BPAD or a family history of BPAD are at elevated risk.
- A patient with postpartum psychosis as her first psychiatric episode is assumed to have BPAD until proved otherwise. Nevertheless, some women with postpartum psychosis have episodes confined to the postpartum period only.
- Mothers with postpartum psychosis are at greater risk for suicide than those with PPD, and 4% of women with postpartum psychosis have been found to commit infanticide.

- The initial presentation is quite similar to delirium, and it is important to rule out medical causes of delirium. Presentation includes hallucinations; delusions; disorientation to person, place, or time; waxing and waning of consciousness; agitation; insomnia; elevated mood; paranoia; depressive symptoms; mixed symptoms; and inability to care for self and baby.
- Hospitalization, urgent consultation with psychiatry, and treatment with lithium and antipsychotics are essential.

ANXIETY DISORDERS AND PREGNANCY

Pregnancy-Related Anxiety

- Risk factors include elevated general anxiety, nulliparity, and higher education level.
- Associated risks include preterm birth, reduced infant motor and mental development, and alcohol use during pregnancy.
- Screening: Pregnancy-Related Anxiety Questionnaire–Revised
- Supportive psychotherapy can help address this.

Generalized Anxiety Disorder

- Two-thirds of adults with generalized anxiety disorder are women, and median onset occurs in the reproductive years.
- Generalized anxiety disorder is characterized as persistent and excessive worry that is unable to be controlled, associated with physical symptoms (headache, fatigue, muscle tension, gastrointestinal distress, chest pain, palpitations).
- Risk factors include younger age, minimal social support, family history, and stressful life events.
- Treatment: SSRIs, cognitive-behavioral therapy. Benzodiazepines and gabapentin can offer immediate relief but are not appropriate for long-term therapy, whereas SSRIs need titration and time for effect but are the first-line long-term therapy.
- Often associated with substance use as a coping mechanism. It is important to screen for substance use.

Panic Disorder

- Panic attacks are characterized by sudden onset of fear, sweating, palpitations, chest pain, or shortness of breath. They can occur in any psychiatric disorder; those with frequent panic attacks and anxiety about their recurrence have panic disorder. Panic disorder is highly disruptive to functioning and often results in avoidance of potential triggers.
- Patients may have a history of physical or sexual abuse.
- Refer for cognitive-behavioral therapy, treatment with SSRI or serotonin norepinephrine reuptake inhibitor. Benzodiazepines are useful to treat the symptoms of an acute panic attack but do not treat the disorder.

POSTTRAUMATIC STRESS DISORDER AND PREGNANCY

- Posttraumatic stress disorder can occur when a person has a previous experience of actual or threatened death, serious injury, or sexual violence. It is characterized by an emotional response, avoidance of triggers, intense distress with triggers, intrusive event reexperiencing (nightmares, flashbacks), easy startle, and aggressive behavior.

- Acute stress syndrome has the same characteristics but lasts <1 month.
- Anxiety/depression after a stressful or traumatic event does not qualify as posttraumatic stress disorder.
- Women in particular may have experienced rape or intimate partner violence, which can complicate speculum exams, cervical exams, and the process of childbirth.
- Trauma-focused psychotherapy and an SSRI are first line. Women may also experience psychotic symptoms, problematic sleep disturbances, and substance use disorder. Consultation with a psychiatrist in these cases is recommended.

OBSESSIVE-COMPULSIVE DISORDER AND PREGNANCY

- Obsessive-compulsive disorder (OCD) is equally or more common during pregnancy and postpartum compared to the baseline population risk in women. Although data are limited, OCD may be more common in the postpartum period and the presence of PPD may increase risk of both OCD and subthreshold obsessive and compulsive symptoms.
- Obsessions are repetitive, intrusive, unwanted thoughts and can be directed toward the fetus/infant, such as fear of loss or death, fear of contamination, and fear of intentional or accidental harm. The patient recognizes obsessions as irrational and as the product of her own mind but is unable to control them (vs a delusion, which is a false belief the patient firmly believes is true, despite evidence to the contrary).
- Compulsions may include excessive washing or cleaning of self during pregnancy or of the infant postpartum, avoidant behavior, compulsive checking on the infant, or any other ritual behaviors that reduce distress (including ritual mental checking, such as excessive Internet searching about symptoms or excessive need for reassurance from physicians and loved ones).

PRIMARY PSYCHOTIC DISORDERS AND PREGNANCY/POSTPARTUM

- Women with psychosis may be at elevated risk for Cesarean delivery, hemorrhage, abruption, preterm delivery, preterm premature rupture of membranes, poor fetal growth, fetal distress, and fetal demise.
- The physician will need to elicit whether symptoms are primary or substance induced.
- Presentation of schizophrenia includes hallucinations (auditory, visual), delusions, disorganized thought and behavior, apathy, flat affect, limited expression, low energy, and cognitive slowing.
- If the patient has mood symptoms, it may be schizoaffective disorder or BPAD with psychotic features. Those with schizoaffective disorder have distinct episodes of mood symptoms, with psychotic symptoms appearing either with mood symptoms or at times of euthymia. For those with BPAD, psychotic symptoms occur *only* in the setting of a mood episode.
- Women with preexisting psychotic disorders may present with psychosis in the postpartum period; typically, symptoms will be similar to those during prior episodes of psychosis and are less likely to include the hallmarks of postpartum psychosis (elevated mood and delirium-like presentation).

PERIPARTUM TREATMENT OF PSYCHIATRIC ILLNESS

Pharmacotherapy

Common medications used to treat psychiatric illness are reviewed in Table 18-4.

- For all medications, plasma levels will drop 40% to 50% during pregnancy and will rise abruptly in the postpartum, so it is essential to raise doses appropriately during pregnancy and decrease to prepregnancy levels in the postpartum.
- Transport of *all* psychotropic medications through breast milk occurs at less than the 10% cutoff recommended by the American Academy of Pediatrics and thus should generally be considered safe during breastfeeding.
- Pharmacotherapy risks in pregnancy and lactation: From 1979 to 2015, the categories A, B, C, D, and X were used to indicate potential for harm to the fetus/neonate if used during pregnancy and lactation. However, this system was overly simplistic, did not account for the effect of metabolites, and inappropriately grouped drugs with differing levels of risk.
- It is inappropriate to use these old categories to inform decision making about pharmacotherapy in pregnancy and breastfeeding.
- New Pregnancy and Lactation Labeling Rule instituted in 2015 includes "Risk Summary," "Clinical Considerations," and "Data" for both pregnancy and lactation as well as information about "Pregnancy Testing," "Contraception," and "Infertility."

Strategies for Prepregnancy Planning and Unplanned Pregnancy

- Discuss lifestyle modifications that may improve psychiatric disorders (Table 18-5).
- The decision about whether to continue psychiatric medications during pregnancy must be individualized and depends on the severity of illness, adverse effects of specific medications, and illness history during and after previous pregnancies.

Nonpharmacologic Therapies

- Safe and efficacious procedural therapies in pregnancy include electroconvulsive therapy, transcranial magnetic stimulation, and bright light therapy.
- Herbal therapies, supplements, and complementary medicine are not recommended because there is minimal to no evidence regarding their safety or efficacy in pregnancy.

CARE OF THE DIFFICULT PREGNANT PATIENT

- Any of the illnesses described in the preceding sections can present challenges to management due to mood or psychotic symptoms. In addition, some patients without Axis I mental disorders can be challenging to work with, due to personality disorders, interpersonal hostility, or general unpleasantness.
- The following strategies can be effectively used to de-escalate a situation:
  - Respect the patient's physical space (>2 arm lengths when possible) and avoid provocative body language (avoid excessive, direct eye contact; avoid arm folding; keep hands visible and unclenched).
  - Minimize the number of staff members in contact with the patient.
  - Address the patient by her preferred name (first vs last name).
  - Be concise and keep your vocabulary simple, giving her time to process.

Table 18-4 Common Medications Used to Treat Psychiatric Disease With Their Associated Pregnancy and Lactation Risks

| Generic (Brand) | Dosing Considerations in Pregnancy | | | Pharmacokinetics and Monitoring | Pregnancy and Lactation Risks | |
	Starting	Titration	Maximum		Pregnancy Concerns	Lactation Concerns
ANTIDEPRESSANTS						
Selective Serotonin Reuptake Inhibitors						
Citalopram (Celexa)	10-20 mg		20-40 mg		No risk of congenital defects (no conclusive risk of cardiovascular defects, including with paroxetine) Risk of neonatal adaptation syndrome (30%) Low risk of persistent pulmonary hypertension of the newborn Slightly increased risk of spontaneous abortion and preterm birth	Appears to be low risk
Escitalopram (Lexapro)	5-10 mg	10 mg/wk	10-20 mg			
Fluoxetine (Prozac, Sarafem, Selfemra)	10-20 mg		40-120 mg	Onset: 1-4 wk Max effect: 8-12 wk CYP450 family		Not first line in breastfeeding but may be used if previous response in patient
Fluvoxamine (Faverin, Luvox)	25-50 mg	50 mg/wk	100-300 mg			
Paroxetine (Paxil, Pexeva)	10-20 mg	10 mg/wk	40-60 mg			Appears to be low risk
Sertraline (Zoloft)	25-50 mg	25-50 mg/wk	150-250 mg			Lowest transmission in breast milk
Serotonin-Norepinephrine Reuptake Inhibitors						
Desvenlafaxine (Pristiq)	50 mg	After 7 d	100-150 mg	CYP450 family	Limited evidence	Not first line in breastfeeding due to limited evidence

	20-30 mg	20-30 mg/wk	30-120 mg		Limited evidence	Not first line in breastfeeding due to limited evidence
Duloxetine (Cymbalta)	20-30 mg	20-30 mg/wk	30-120 mg	CYP450 family	No evidence of congenital defects Slightly increased risk of spontaneous abortion	Sleepiness and poor weight gain in some case reports only
Venlafaxine (Effexor)	37.5-75 mg	≤75 mg >3 d apart	75-350 mg			

Tricyclic Antidepressants

Clomipramine (Anafranil)			150-250 mg		>300 mg/d increases seizure risk Risk of orthostatic hypotension Possible fetal cardiac risk but poor evidence	Limited evidence
Amitriptyline (Elavil)	25 mg	25 mg q 3-7 d	75-300 mg	Max effect 4-8 wk CYP450 family	Monitor plasma levels Increase dose in third trimester Risk of orthostatic hypotension	Most data regarding amitriptyline; limited evidence for others
Desipramine (Norpramin)			150-300 mg			
Doxepin (Sinequan)			100-300 mg			Not preferred in breastfeeding
Imipramine (Tofranil)			100-300 mg			
Nortriptyline (Pamelor)			75-150 mg		Preferred tricyclic antidepressants due to high quantity of data and fewer side effects (less risk of orthostasis)	No lactation concerns

(Continued)

Table 18-4 Common Medications Used to Treat Psychiatric Disease With Their Associated Pregnancy and Lactation Risks *(Continued)*

| Generic (Brand) | Dosing Considerations in Pregnancy | | | Pharmacokinetics and Monitoring | Pregnancy and Lactation Risks | |
	Starting	Titration	Maximum		Pregnancy Concerns	Lactation Concerns
			ANTIDEPRESSANTS *(continued)*			
			Other Antidepressants			
Bupropion (Wellbutrin)	150 mg XL, 100 mg SR	After 3-7 d	300-450 mg XL, 200-450 mg SR		Decreases seizure threshold Contraindicated in preeclampsia Minimal weight gain or sexual side effects	Theoretical seizure risk in neonate, very limited evidence
Mirtazapine (Remeron)	10-15 mg	After 7 d	15-60 mg	Onset 1-2 wk (bupropion) Onset within 6 wk (trazodone) CYP450 family	Monitor for neutropenia; may be good for hyperemesis gravidarum to increase weight and decrease nausea/ vomiting	Manufacturer recommends using caution.
Trazodone (Desyrel)	25-50 mg	50 mg Every 3-4 d	50-200 mg (sleep), 150-400 mg (MDD, rare)		Limited evidence	Not first line in breastfeeding
Vilazodone (Viibryd)	10 mg	10 mg Every 3-4 d	10-40 mg		No evidence	No evidence
Vortioxetine (Brintellix)	10 mg	Once tolerated	5-20 mg			

ANXIOLYTICS

Benzodiazepines

Alprazolam (Xanax)	0.75-1.5 mg	Every 3-4 d	1-4 mg (anxiety), 5-6 mg IR (panic), 30 mg ER (panic)	half life: 6-27 h CYP450 family	Premature birth, low birth weight, neonatal withdrawal, respiratory distress in case reports No good evidence for increased risk of congenital defects (including no risk of cleft palate)	Use judiciously With chronic use and high dose, increased risk of respiratory depression, sedation, irritability, and poor feeding Low doses of shorter acting benzodiazepine preferred Lorazepam is compatible with breastfeeding
Clonazepam (Klonopin)	0.5-1 mg	Every 3 d	0.5-4 mg, divided	Onset: 20-40 min half life: 17-60 h CYP450 family		
Diazepam (Valium)	2-10 mg, divided	NA	4-40 mg, divided	Onset (IV): 1-3 min half life: >40 h CYP450 family		
Lorazepam (Ativan)	0.5-1 mg, divided	NA	2-6 mg, divided	Onset (IV): 2-3 min half life: 12-14 h CYP450 family		
Temazepam (Restoril)	15 mg (insomnia)	NA	15-30 mg	half life: 4-18 h CYP450 family		

Other

Buspirone (Buspar)	10 mg twice a day	5-10 mg Every 3-7 d	15-60 mg daily	First-pass hepatic metabolism half life: 2-3 h Max effect 2-4 wk CYP450 family	Limited evidence; no controlled human studies

(Continued)

Table 18-4 Common Medications Used to Treat Psychiatric Disease With Their Associated Pregnancy and Lactation Risks *(Continued)*

| Generic (Brand) | Dosing Considerations in Pregnancy | | | | Pregnancy and Lactation Risks | | |
	Starting	Titration	Maximum	Pharmacokinetics and Monitoring	Pregnancy Concerns	Lactation Concerns
			ANTIPSYCHOTICS			
Aripiprazole (Abilify)	2-5 mg (augment) 5-10 mg (mood), 10-15 mg (psychosis)	2 wk	5-10 mg (augment) 10-20 mg (mood) 15-30 mg (psychosis)			Limited evidence for risk of lactation failure Not preferred for breastfeeding
Lurasidone (Latuda)	20-40 mg	1 wk	40-120 mg		Monitor for macrosomia. Neonatal EPS (agitation, abnormal muscle tone or movements, difficulty feeding or breathing, lethargy, tremor)	No human data
Olanzapine (Zyprexa)	2.5-5 mg (augment) 5-10 mg (mood, psychosis)	1 wk	10-15 mg (mood), 20-30 mg (psychosis)	CYP450 family		Preferred in breastfeeding Monitor for sedation.
Quetiapine (Seroquel)	25 mg twice a day	50 mg daily	200-300 mg (BPAD) 100-400 mg (mood) 400-1200 mg (acute mania or psychosis)			Appears to be low risk
Risperidone (Risperdal)	0.5 mg	1 mg daily if tolerated	2-8 mg (acute mania, psychosis)		Risk of orthostatic hypotension Dose-dependent EPS risk	Not preferred for breastfeeding Elevated risk of hyperprolactinemia Risk of neonatal EPS

MOOD STABILIZERS

Drug			Monitoring	Risks	Breastfeeding
Lithium	300 mg	Gradual based on tolerance and response	900-1200 mg (maintenance) 1800 mg (acute)	Monitor serum levels (<1.2 mEq/L, trough goal 0.8-1.2 mEq/L). Titrate dosing throughout pregnancy to maintain level (due to increasing volume of distribution).	Stop 24-48 h prior to delivery; restart when medically stable at prepregnancy dose. 0.7%-1% risk of cardiac malformation (Ebstein anomaly) in first trimester. Risks of polyhydramnios, cardiac arrhythmias, diabetes insipidus, poor thyroid function, premature delivery, floppy infant syndrome	Breastfeeding ok if the parents and pediatrician are very involved. Need to monitor infant for dehydration and lithium toxicity

Antiepileptics

| Carbamazepine (Tegretol) | 200 mg twice a day | 200 mg/wk | 400-1200 mg twice a day | Monitor serum level (4-12 mg/L). | Risk of developmental delay. Neural tube defects (folate 4-5 g daily) Also risks of craniofacial defects, cardiovascular defects, and hypospadias | No concerns |

(Continued)

Table 18-4 Common Medications Used to Treat Psychiatric Disease With Their Associated Pregnancy and Lactation Risks *(Continued)*

Generic (Brand)	Dosing Considerations in Pregnancy			Pharmacokinetics and Monitoring	Pregnancy and Lactation Risks	
	Starting	Titration	Maximum		Pregnancy Concerns	Lactation Concerns
MOOD STABILIZERS *(continued)*						
Antiepileptics *(continued)*						
Gabapentin (Neurontin)	300 mg twice a day	Increase to twice a day over 3 d.	1200-3600 mg 2-3 doses/d	None	Poor fetal growth, developmental delay in animal studies Limited evidence but no findings of risk in human studies	No concerns
Lamotrigine (Lamictal)	25 mg	25 mg daily 2 wk 50 mg daily 2 wk 100 mg daily	100-400 mg	Monitor level in second and third trimester and postpartum. Goal: Titrate dose to maintain prepregnancy level needed for euthymia (need to increase due to estrogen interaction and increasing volume of distribution).	Avoid concomitant use of carbamazepine, phenytoin, primidone, phenobarbital, rifampin, ritonavir, valproic acid. No good evidence suggesting risk of cleft palate	Monitor for risk of Steven-Johnson syndrome rash (rare).

Oxcarbazepine (Trileptal)	300 mg twice a day	600 mg/wk	1200-2400 mg, divided	Monitor level in second and third trimester and postpartum.	Possible craniofacial, cardiac malformations	Limited evidence
Topiramate (Topamax)	25 mg	50 mg/wk	50-300 mg	Monitor level in second and third trimester and postpartum.	Risk if mother develops metabolic acidosis: increased risk of cleft lip/palate, small for gestational age	Limited evidence
Valproic acid (Depakote)	250-500 mg	Can be adjusted as rapidly as possible to treat mania	1200-1500 mg	Monitor level (serum goal 50-125 µg/mL). Need to closely monitor for coagulopathy	Dose-dependent risk of neural tube defects (as much as 10% at doses used for BPAD, need folate 4-5 g daily) Decreased IQ, cognitive defects Only use if other medications have failed to control mood	Risk of neonatal hepatotoxicity Monitor for jaundice.

Abbreviations: BPAD, bipolar affective disorder; CYP450, cytochrome P450; EPS, extrapyramidal symptoms; ER, extended release; IR, immediate release; IV, intravenous; MDD, major depressive disorder; SR, sustained release; XL, extended release.

Table 18-5	Lifestyle Modifications for Treatment of Psychiatric Disorders
Level of Evidence	**Lifestyle Modification**
Substantial evidence	Exercise
	Yoga
	Healthy sleep habits
	Meditation and mindfulness
	Psychotherapy (supportive, interpersonal, cognitive-behavioral, dialectical behavioral, or mindfulness based)
Intermediate evidence	Acupuncture
Limited evidence	Smoking cessation
	Elimination or limitation of caffeine intake and alcohol intake
	Biofeedback
	Relaxation training

- Use active listening and clarifying statements ("What I'm hearing is . . . " or "Tell me if I have this right . . . ").
- Identify the patient's expectations and wants so that you can respond empathically and express a desire to work together with the patient toward her goals. Never deceive a patient by promising something that cannot be provided for her.
- Find something about the patient's position with which you can agree.
- Set clear limits and boundaries about acceptable behavior. Gently but firmly indicate that limits are being set due to your desire to help.

SUGGESTED READINGS

American College of Obstetricians and Gynecologists Committee on Practice Bulletins—Obstetrics. ACOG Practice Bulletin No. 92: use of psychiatric medications during pregnancy and lactation. *Obstet Gynecol*. 2008;111(4):1001-1020. (Reaffirmed 2018)

Byatt N, Straus J, Stopa A, Biebel K, Mittal L, Moore Simas TA. Massachusetts Child Psychiatry Access Program for Moms: utilization and quality assessment. *Obstet Gynecol*. 2018;132(2):345-353.

Eke AC, Saccone G, Berghella V. Selective serotonin reuptake inhibitor (SSRI) use during pregnancy and risk of preterm birth: a systematic review and meta-analysis. *BJOG*. 2016;123(12):1900-1907.

Molyneaux E, Telesia LA, Henshaw C, Boath E, Bradley E, Howard LM. Antidepressants for preventing postnatal depression. *Cochrane Database Syst Rev*. 2018;(4):CD004363.

Osborne LM, Payne JL. Clinical updates in women's health care summary: mood and anxiety disorders: primary and preventive care review. *Obstet Gynecol*. 2017;130(3):674.

Ross LE, Grigoriadis S, Mamisashvili L, et al. Selected pregnancy and delivery outcomes after exposure to antidepressant medication: a systematic review and meta-analysis. *JAMA Psychiatry*. 2013;70(4):436-443.

Russell EJ, Fawcett JM, Mazmanian D. Risk of obsessive-compulsive disorder in pregnant and postpartum women: a meta-analysis. *J Clin Psychiatry*. 2013;74(4):377-385.

19 Substance Use Disorders in Pregnancy

Marielle S. Gross and Lorraine A. Milio

DEFINITIONS AND GENERAL PRINCIPLES

- Substance use disorders (SUDs) have had increased prevalence in many parts of the world in recent years, but especially in the United States, occurring in all racial, ethnic, demographic, and socioeconomic groups. They encompass the use of tobacco and alcohol, misuse of prescription medications, and use of illegal drugs. Together, they contribute substantially to overall morbidity and mortality, including for maternal, fetal, and neonatal populations.

- In the *Diagnostic and Statistical Manual of Mental Disorders* (5th ed.) (*DSM-5*), **substance use disorder** terminology replaces *substance abuse* found in *Diagnostic and Statistical Manual of Mental Disorders* (4th ed.). This change reflects the movement toward considering addiction to be a brain disease with physical and behavioral findings. The *DSM-5* criteria for SUD is listed in Table 19-1.

- The diagnosis of **addiction** follows the criteria for SUD fairly closely and is defined as a primary, chronic disease of brain reward, motivation, memory, and related circuitry as defined by the American Society of Addiction Medicine. **Substance dependence** is present when withdrawal symptoms are precipitated by abrupt discontinuation of the substance use.

- Addiction causes the compulsive use of one or more substances despite significant health and personal sequelae. It disrupts the activity of the brain responsible for reward, motivation, judgment, learning, and memory, and by so doing also disrupts the functioning of families, relationships, and communities. Like diabetes, heart disease, and cancer, addiction is caused by a complex interplay between behavioral, biological, genetic, and environmental factors. An SUD is a **chronic, relapsing disease** and simultaneous use of multiple substances (or "polysubstance abuse") is common. Without treatment, it leads to other physical and mental health disorders, and, over time, may become more severe, disabling, and life-threatening. **Recovery** is the process in which patients abstain from relevant substances and work on improving overall health by leading a self-directed (instead of substance-directed) life.

- An SUD is distinct from chronic pain syndromes, although both involve substance tolerance and physical dependence and the two conditions may co-occur.

EPIDEMIOLOGY, PATHOPHYSIOLOGY, AND MATERNAL/FETAL EFFECTS BY DRUG CATEGORY

Alcohol

- **Epidemiology:** Eleven percent of pregnant women report alcohol use during pregnancy, 4% report binge drinking (>5 drinks/occasion), and 1% report heavy drinking. Ten percent of women ages 15 to 44 years report binge drinking during the first trimester, most before knowing they were pregnant. Alcohol use disorder

Table 19-1	DSM-5 Criteria for Substance Use Disorder

A problematic pattern of use leading to clinically significant impairment or distress is manifested by two or more of the following within a 12-mo period:

- Substance is often taken in larger amounts or over a longer period than was intended.
- A persistent desire or unsuccessful efforts to cut down or control use of the substance
- A great deal of time is spent in activities necessary to obtain, use, or recover from the substance's effects
- Craving or a strong desire or urge to use the substance
- Recurrent use of the substance resulting in a failure to fulfill major role obligations at work, school, or home
- Continued use of the substance despite having persistent or recurrent social or interpersonal problems caused or exacerbated by its effects
- Important social, occupational, or recreational activities are given up or reduced because of use of the substance
- Recurrent use in situations in which it is physically hazardous
- Continued use despite knowledge of having a persistent or recurrent physical or psychological problem that is likely to have been caused or exacerbated by the substance
- Tolerance
- Withdrawal

Mild = 2-3 criteria; moderate = 4-5; severe = 6 or more

Abbreviation: *DSM-5, Diagnostic and Statistical Manual of Mental Disorders* (5th ed.).

is associated with high parity, smoking, history of abuse or incarceration, family history, and other socioeconomic stressors.
- Fetal alcohol syndrome (FAS) affects 1 to 2/1000 US infants versus 3 to 6/1000 with fetal alcohol spectrum disorder. The FAS is the most common cause of mental retardation in the United States.
- **Mechanism of action:** Alcohol produces a wide range of effects dependent on dose, duration, and timing of exposure. It exerts damaging effects on enzymes involved in developmental regulation and factors that dictate neurogenesis. Epigenetic changes in DNA methylation and microRNA expression also occur.
- **Presentation of intoxication**
  - Symptoms: euphoria, impaired memory
  - Signs: cognitive deficits, slurred speech, disinhibited behavior, incoordination, unsteady gait, nystagmus, stupor, and/or coma. Hypotension and tachycardia may occur as a result of both ethanol-induced peripheral vasodilation or dehydration.
- **Presentation of withdrawal**
  - Minor signs/symptoms (6-36 h since last drink): tremulousness, mild anxiety, headache, diaphoresis, palpitations, anorexia, gastrointestinal upset, but mental status is normal

- Seizures (6-48 h after last drink): single or brief flurry of generalized, tonic-clonic seizures with a short post-ictal period; status epilepticus is rare.
- Alcoholic hallucinosis (12-48 h since last drink): visual, auditory, and/or tactile hallucinations with intact orientation and normal vital signs
- Delirium tremens (48-96 h from last drink): delirium, agitation, tachycardia, hypertension, fever, diaphoresis
- **Maternal complications:** hypertension and cardiovascular disease, liver disease, pancreatitis, gastritis, esophagitis, bone marrow suppression, anemia, pneumonia, peripheral neuropathy, cancer (mouth, esophagus, throat, liver, breast); psychiatric complications include depression, anxiety, and irritability; behavioral complications include high-risk sexual practices (increased incidence of human immunodeficiency virus [HIV]/hepatitis B and C), violence, and accidental injuries (eg, motor vehicle accidents, falls). Overall mortality is increased.
- **Fetal and infant effects**
  - **Fetus:** considered to have the most serious neurobehavioral effects of all substances of abuse, with effects dependent on timing and pattern of exposure; alcohol recirculates within the fetal compartment long after maternal intake. There is no threshold alcohol intake during pregnancy that is associated with fetal effects. Risk of fetal death in utero is increased.
  - **Infant/child:** The FAS is diagnosed after birth and includes low birth weight, dysmorphic facial and limb effects, as well as reduced brain size/development. Fetal alcohol spectrum disorder, often underreported, is usually diagnosed in early childhood and manifestations include failure to thrive; impaired intellectual and motor development with deficits in attention, memory, verbal, and executive functioning; reaction time; and motor learning.

Benzodiazepines

- **Epidemiology:** Use in pregnancy has been difficult to quantify. However, benzodiazepine use has increased significantly over the last 20 years. A recent report found benzodiazepine use among approximately 4% of insured pregnant US women. Anxiety disorders affect up to 1 in 3 pregnant women and benzodiazepines are a common treatment, although they are not recommended as first line. Because anxiety is independently associated with adverse perinatal outcome, this may confound interpretation of outcomes associated with benzodiazepine use.
- **Mechanism of action:** Central nervous system effects are mediated by benzodiazepine binding to type A γ-aminobutyric acid (GABA$_A$) receptors, producing a disinhibiting effect by downregulating GABA-mediated inhibition of dopaminergic neurons. This may also induce apoptosis and neuroplasticity resulting in an increased expression of excitatory glutamatergic receptors upon benzodiazepine withdrawal after chronic exposure.
- **Presentation of intoxication**
  - Symptoms: euphoria, disinhibition, relaxation, somnolence
  - Signs: erratic behavior, slurred speech, unsteady gait, incoordination, cognitive impairment (especially anterograde amnesia), nystagmus, stupor or coma, and respiratory depression
- **Presentation of withdrawal:** anxiety/panic attacks, irritability, autonomic hyperactivity, tremor (especially hands), insomnia, diaphoresis, weight loss, headache, muscle pain, poor concentration, palpitations, and nausea, or vomiting. More severe effects include transient hallucinations, generalized tonic-clonic seizures,

psychosis, and delirium. Withdrawal can be *life-threatening* with abrupt discontinuation, especially when higher doses, longer duration of use, or concomitant alcohol or opioid use is present.

- **Maternal complications:** High likelihood of relapse due to underlying neurologic changes from chronic benzodiazepine use; increased all-cause mortality, including overdose death; increased risk of falls and associated injuries. Obstetric risks include increased risk of cesarean delivery.
- **Fetal and infant effects**
  - **Fetus:** spontaneous abortion; preterm delivery; possible increased risk of oral cleft, alimentary tract atresia, and pyloric stenosis
  - **Infant/child:** prematurity; low birth weight with smaller head circumference. Neonatal withdrawal may occur (especially with later pregnancy use) but is less well defined than with opioid exposure. Neonatal withdrawal signs/symptoms are the following: low Apgar score, apnea, hypothermia, hyperreflexia, hypertonia or hypotonia, irritability, lethargy, restlessness, tremor, diarrhea, poor feeding, vomiting.

Club Drugs (Including MDMA [Ecstasy] and LSD [Acid])

- **Epidemiology:** younger, single, white race, binge drinkers, high prevalence of comorbid psychiatric symptoms
- **Mechanism of action:** derivative of amphetamine, induces powerful release of serotonin, norepinephrine, dopamine, and binds adrenaline and serotonin receptors
- **Presentation of intoxication**
  - Symptoms: increased alertness, reduced fatigue, sensation of increased physical and mental powers, euphoria, nausea, blurry vision
  - Signs: hypertension, tachycardia, hyperthermia, agitation, bruxism, ataxia, diaphoresis
- **Presentation of withdrawal:** confusion, depression, sleep difficulty, anxiety, panic attacks
- **Maternal complications:** temperature instability, hyponatremia, risk of seizures, **serotonin syndrome**, rhabdomyolysis, liver, kidney, cardiovascular damage, and potential death. Intensive care unit admission may be necessary and early involvement of intensivist care recommended due to potential for rapid decompensation.
- **Fetal and infant effects**
  - **Fetus:** spontaneous abortion, fetal death due to increased maternal temperature, congenital defects, cardiovascular abnormalities, musculoskeletal anomalies, preterm delivery
  - **Infant/child:** possible impaired intellectual and motor development; outcomes much worse with concurrent alcohol use

Cocaine

- **Epidemiology:** Data varies but may be 0.3% of women of reproductive age or 1.6% of US adults older than age 14; use is highest among those who use other illegal substances, drink heavily, and/or have psychiatric comorbidities. There are significant racial and socioeconomic disparities in use and criminalization of cocaine in powder (insufflated or injected) versus solid "rock" (smoked) form, with the latter, more economical form associated with lower income minorities and higher rates of incarceration.

- **Mechanism of action:** inhibits reuptake of multiple monoamines at the presynaptic junction, increased concentrations of dopamine, serotonin, and norepinephrine in synaptic clefts; causes potent arterial vasoconstrictive effects
- **Presentation of intoxication**
  - Symptoms: increased arousal, improved vigilance and alertness, self-confidence, euphoria, sense of wellbeing, headache
  - Signs: hypertension (**avoid β-blockers**; hydralazine is treatment of choice in pregnancy), tachycardia, psychomotor agitation, hyperthermia, focal neurologic deficits, suicidal behavior
- **Presentation of withdrawal:** prominent psychological features of cravings, potentially severe depression, suicidal ideation, anxiety, fatigue, difficulty concentrating, anhedonia, increased appetite, somnolence, increased rapid eye movement sleep/dreaming, psychomotor retardation. Physical withdrawal is relatively minor, including musculoskeletal pains, tremors, chills, and involuntary motor movements, but also possible coronary vasospasm.
- **Maternal complications:** cardiac ischemia, acute left ventricular heart failure, arrhythmia, seizures, coma, death, ischemic or hemorrhagic stroke, pulmonary complications (with inhalational use) including bronchospasm, pneumothorax, angioedema and pharyngeal burns, rhabdomyolysis
  - With long-term use: atherogenesis, left ventricular hypertrophy, dilated cardiomyopathy, chronic rhinitis, perforation of nasal septum, oropharyngeal ulcers, ischemic colitis, perforated ulcer disease, electrolyte abnormalities, pseudovasculitis skin lesions
  - Obstetric complications include preterm labor, placental abruption, and exacerbation of cardiovascular complications.
- **Fetal and infant effects**
  - **Fetus:** spontaneous abortion, intrauterine growth restriction, preterm birth
  - **Infant/child:** prematurity, small for gestational age, low birth weight, decreased length and head circumference, abnormal behavioral outcomes including lower arousal, poor self-regulation, higher excitability, jitteriness, impaired reflexes, impaired language skills, behavioral issues, poorer executive functioning

Inhalants

- **Epidemiology:** Use is most common among younger adolescents (peak use ages 11-14 years) with increased use in rural areas. Use and associated deaths related to inhalants peaked in the 1990s and has been declining since.
- **Mechanism of action:** Highly lipophilic molecules that rapidly cross into bloodstream, neurons are especially susceptible, taking effect in seconds and lasting 15 to 45 minutes, intoxication maintained via continued inhalation. Central nervous system depression mediated by alteration of neuronal membrane function at glutamate or GABA receptors. Nitrites, which are considered a special class of inhalant that are used for sexual enhancement, produce intense vasodilation, which produces a sensation of heat and warmth. Absorption is rapid across the pulmonary bed and effects are brief, lasting less than 5 minutes.
- **Presentation of intoxication**
  - Symptoms: initial euphoria followed by lethargy, disorientation, headache
  - Signs: impaired judgment and coordination, sweet solvent odor of halogenated hydrocarbons or the "glue" odor may be detectable on the breath; slurred speech, ataxia, hallucinations, agitation, violent behavior, and seizures

- Nitrites: symptoms: enhanced sexual pleasure, increased intracranial pressure causes "rush sensation," headache, nausea, pruritus. Signs: abrupt onset hypotension and reflex tachycardia, possible syncope, possible wheezing.
- **Presentation of withdrawal:** anxiety, irritability, fatigue, headache, craving, aggression, tremors, and poor concentration
- **Maternal complications:** predominant cardiac and neurologic toxicity from hydrocarbons; long-term neurocognitive impairment, cerebellar dysfunction, peripheral neuropathy; decreased brain mass and white matter degeneration, myopathy, parkinsonism, lead poisoning; arrhythmias, myocarditis, or myocardial infarction, pneumonitis, hypoxia, bronchospasm, pulmonary edema, anorexia, weight loss, hepatotoxicity, metabolic acidosis, urinary calculi, glomerulonephritis, aplastic anemia, or hematologic malignancy
  - Nitrites: skin irritation, tracheobronchitis, allergic reactions, polyneuropathy, psychosis, ataxia, megaloblastic anemia, pneumothorax, major depression, suicidality, conduct disorder, acquired methemoglobinemia with potential respiratory depression, altered consciousness, shock, seizures, and death
  - Many vapors are highly flammable and use is associated with burn injury.
- **Fetal and infant effects**
  - **Fetal:** spontaneous abortion, premature delivery, congenital malformations including oral clefts, micrognathia, microcephaly, intrauterine growth restriction
  - **Neonatal/child:** withdrawal in neonates and developmental delay

Marijuana

- **Epidemiology:** Most frequently used illicit substance in the United States, approximately 10% of reproductive-aged women overall, rates in pregnancy range 3% to 34%, with rates highest among pregnant teens; use decreases later in pregnancy; **decriminalization and legalization raises concerns for increased use during pregnancy and breastfeeding**. Criminalization of marijuana use, including during pregnancy, disproportionately affects black women.
- **Mechanism of action:** Δ-9-tetrahydrocannabinol (THC) binds to cannabinoid-1 receptor in central nervous system, induces sedative-like effect by inhibiting release of multiple neurotransmitters presynaptically; concentration of THC in marijuana products has increased greater than 10-fold over the past 30 years.
- **Presentation of intoxication**
  - Symptoms: sedation; euphoria; decreased anxiety/alertness; increased sociability versus social withdrawal; distorted perception of color, sound, space, and time; paranoia; grandiosity; increased appetite
  - Signs: slurred speech, impaired attention, concentration, short-term memory and executive functioning, psychosis
- **Presentation of withdrawal:** irritability, anger, anxiety, depression, and disturbed sleep. Physical symptoms (abdominal pain, headache, muscle tremors, or twitching) are relatively uncommon.
- **Maternal complications:** tachycardia, increased blood pressure and respiratory rate, conjunctival injection, xerostomia, ataxia, nystagmus; may cause acute exacerbations of underlying asthma, pneumomediastinum, and pneumothorax as rare complications of inhalation; increased risk of myocardial infarction
- **Fetal and infant effects**
  - **Fetus:** inconsistent evidence of intrauterine growth restriction; data appears confounded by underlying population risk factors

- **Infant/child:** possible neonatal sleep disturbance, high-pitched cry, altered response to visual stimuli, tremors; differences in infant mental scores (not persisting at >12 mo), attenuated cognitive development (short-term memory, verbal and visual skills), especially **executive function**; increased neuropsychiatric disorders including attention deficit hyperactivity disorder, anxiety, and depression and possible susceptibility to SUD given decreased levels of D2 receptors in reward system demonstrated in animal models

Methamphetamines

- **Epidemiology:** One percent to 2% of US population report using; in high-risk areas, up to 5% of pregnant women report using.
- **Mechanism of action:** increases serotonin, dopamine, norepinephrine, and epinephrine by displacing the stores in presynaptic cytoplasmic vesicles, causing their release and by inhibiting their reuptake from the synapse
- **Presentation of intoxication**
  - Symptoms: increased alertness, chest pain, irritability, agitation, restlessness, dizziness, nausea, insomnia, paranoia, hallucinations, delusions, suicidal or homicidal ideation, formication (skin crawling sensation)
  - Signs: increased blood pressure, increased heart rate, increased temperature, mydriasis, vomiting, diarrhea, profound diaphoresis, abnormal behavior, choreiform movements, breathing problems, nosebleeds; abdominal pain out of proportion to exam may indicate bowel ischemia.
- **Presentation of withdrawal:** initial crash associated with profound cravings and withdrawal syndrome, peaking within 1 to 2 days and lasting up to 3 weeks. Signs and symptoms include dysphoria, depression, suicidal ideation, anhedonia, fatigue, increased sleep, vivid dreams, insomnia or hypersomnia, agitation, anxiety, and increased appetite.
- **Maternal complications:** risk of arrhythmia, heart attack, stroke, pulmonary edema and hypertension, memory loss, seizures brain damage in overdose; stigmata of chronic use include malnourishment, disheveled appearance, agitation, gingival hypertrophy, extensive tooth decay ("meth mouth"), oropharyngeal and mucosal burns, extremities with extensive excoriations and traumatic and thermal injuries
  - Obstetric risks include increased risk of placental insufficiency, vasoconstriction, abruption, premature rupture of membranes, hemorrhage, difficulty breastfeeding due to decreased prolactin
- **Fetal and infant effects**
  - **Fetus:** spontaneous abortion/fetal loss, fetal distress, preterm delivery, intrauterine growth restriction, possible increased risk of cardiovascular, and genitourinary tract abnormalities
  - **Infant/child:** small for gestational age and low birth weight, increased perinatal mortality; if maternal intoxication at delivery, may have irritability, tremors, muscular rigidity, vomiting and diarrhea; dysregulation in infancy, possible learning differences, and neurodevelopmental issues

Opioids

- **Epidemiology:** significantly increased use in the United States over the past 20 years, especially among 18- to 25-year-olds; prevalence of opioid use disorder increased 4-fold among pregnant women from 1999 to 2014, now affecting

6.5 cases per 1000 deliveries; misuse of prescription opioids is most predominant in rural, white populations. Two-thirds of current heroin users began with the misuse of a prescription opioid.

- **Mechanism of action:** Opioid receptors are three types of G protein–coupled receptors (mu, delta, kappa), which initiate intracellular communication; mu activation mediates secondary effects on messenger-generating enzymes (adenylyl cyclase and phospholipase C), leading to decreased cyclic adenosine monophosphate; chronic opioid receptor activation has the opposite effect, leading to upregulation of cyclic adenosine monophosphate. There are opioid receptors in the central (analgesia, miosis, respiratory depression) and peripheral (cough suppression, constipation) nervous system.
- **Presentation of intoxication**
  - Symptoms: euphoria, analgesia, sedation, confusion, lethargy, nausea and anorexia, decreased sex drive, dizziness, headache, agitation, psychosis
  - Signs: miosis (pinpoint pupils) with decrease or absence of pupillary response to light; decreased heart rate and blood pressure, shallow breathing, sweating, emesis, slurred speech
- **Presentation of withdrawal:** flu-like symptoms including nausea, vomiting, diarrhea, sweating, myalgias, chills, rhinorrhea, runny eyes; also insomnia, anxiety, drug cravings, dysphoria, abdominal cramping, uterine irritability
- **Maternal complications:** long-term physical and psychological dependence and tolerance, severe constipation; **IV use increases risk of infections including HIV and hepatitis B/C**, endocarditis, osteomyelitis and soft tissue infections (especially with subcutaneous administration), irregular menses, recurrent mood swings, hyperalgesia, overdose, and trauma-associated death. Methadone can cause arrhythmias, especially prolonged QT, cardiac arrest, hypomagnesemia, pulmonary edema.
  - Obstetric complications include preeclampsia, premature labor, premature rupture of membranes, chorioamnionitis, placental insufficiency, abruption, postpartum hemorrhage, septic thrombophlebitis.
- **Fetal and infant effects**
  - **Fetus:** spontaneous abortion, premature delivery, intrauterine growth restriction, fetal passage of meconium, fetal death in utero, possible increase in congenital heart defects and autonomic dysregulation
  - **Infant/child:** small for gestational age; low birth weight; decreased head circumference; neonatal abstinence syndrome (NAS): sweating, irritability, vomiting, watery stools, high-pitched crying, tremors, seizures, abnormal muscle tone, poor weight gain, and vasomotor and respiratory effects (may be more severe with methadone versus other legal and illegal opiates); increased risk of sudden infant death syndrome; motor and cognitive impairment (memory and special learning); attention deficit hyperactivity disorder; and impaired opiate receptor system

Tobacco

- **Epidemiology:** In the United States, 12.3% of pregnant women smoke throughout pregnancy. Use is highest in the first trimester and decreases as pregnancy progresses, with up to 75% quitting during pregnancy, and most relapsing within 1 year postpartum. Smoking is more common among women who present later for pregnancy care and is more prevalent among white and black women compared to Hispanic women. Five percent to 8% of preterm births, 13% to 19% of term infants with intrauterine growth restriction, 5% to 7% of preterm-related deaths, and 23% to 34% of sudden infant death syndrome deaths were attributed to prenatal smoking. Tobacco use is the leading cause of preventable death in the United States.

- **Mechanism of action:** Nicotine is the primary psychoactive component of tobacco; it is an agonist of the nicotinic acetylcholine receptor and enhances release of neurotransmitters, including epinephrine, norepinephrine, dopamine, acetylcholine, serotonin, vasopressin, glutamate, nitric oxide, calcitonin growth-related peptide, and β-endorphin. Both nicotine and its primary metabolite cotinine readily pass across the placenta, achieving higher concentrations in the fetus than in the mother.
- **Presentation of intoxication**
  - Symptoms: increased alertness and focus, anxiolysis, relaxation, euphoria, improved memory, reduced appetite, decreased pain, nausea, vomiting, diarrhea, chest pain
  - Signs: increased blood pressure, heart rate, respiratory rate
- **Presentation of withdrawal:** Strong physical dependence and tolerance lead to severe withdrawal syndrome, peaking in first 3 days and subsiding over 3 to 4 weeks, although cravings may persist for years. Symptoms of withdrawal include increased appetite, weight gain, dysphoria, depression, anhedonia, insomnia, irritability, frustration, anger, anxiety, difficulty concentrating, and restlessness.
- **Maternal complications:** increased morbidity and mortality from smoking-related conditions including cardiovascular disease, cancers (lung, colorectal and stomach, head and neck, kidney, liver, lower urinary tract, cervical, pancreas), lung disease (chronic obstructive pulmonary disease, acute and chronic lung infections), diabetes, osteoporosis, and postoperative complications
  - Obstetric risks include decreased uterine blood flow, impaired placental function, placenta previa, placental abruption, pregnancy loss, preterm delivery, and preterm premature rupture of membranes.
- **Fetal and infant effects**
  - **Fetus:** intrauterine growth restriction, impaired lung development, accelerated fetal heart rate, decreased fetal breathing, increased risk of chromosomal abnormalities
  - **Infant/child:** disrupted cholinergic system, impaired cardiovascular regulation in neonate

SCREENING AND ROUTINE CARE

- Screening for drug use, including legal and illegal substances, alcohol, and tobacco, should be **universal, nonjudgmental**, and occurs at initial prenatal visit, at least once per trimester, upon admission for delivery, and at postpartum visits. Many cases will be missed if patients are selectively screened or if care is not taken to ensure unbiased assessments. Sensitivity is required because women may be concerned about potential legal risks of disclosure, including child custody concerns. Structured screening should be included in the patient history (may be administered in writing or by interview by the physician or support staff) and may be accompanied by a urine drug screen. The 4P's Plus T is an example of a standardized validated screening tool (Table 19-2). It identifies high-risk patients who screen

Table 19-2	Sample Screening Tool: 4P's Plus T Questionnaire[a]

1. Have you ever used drugs, alcohol, or tobacco during this pregnancy?
2. Have you had a problem with drugs, alcohol, or tobacco in the past?
3. Does your partner have a problem with drugs, alcohol, or tobacco?
4. Do you consider one of your parents to be an addict, an alcoholic, or unable to stop smoking?

[a]The 4P's Plus T tool is a modification of the 4P's tool. Data from Ewing H. *A practical guide to intervention in health and social services with pregnant and postpartum addicts and alcoholics: theoretical framework, brief screening tool, key interview questions, and strategies for referral to recovery resources.* Martinez, CA: The Born Free Project, Contra Costa County Department of Health Services; 1990.

positive for drug, alcohol, or **t**obacco use in the **p**ast, during the current **p**regnancy, in a **p**artner, or in a **p**arent.
- The Screening, Brief Intervention, and Referral to Treatment model has been endorsed by the Institute of Medicine. Screening results should be documented. Any positive responses should prompt further questioning and risk assessment, followed by a brief counseling intervention and referral for further management as needed.
- Patients with certain common neuropsychiatric and biomedical conditions are at especially high risk for concurrent SUDs. These conditions include anxiety, depression, posttraumatic stress disorder, sickle cell disease, and other conditions with a chronic pain component. Poverty, food insecurity, intimate partner violence, and sex work are also all associated with increased risk of SUD. An SUD also increases the risk of sexually transmitted infections including HIV/AIDS, hepatitis B and C, gonorrhea, chlamydia, trichomoniasis, and syphilis. Screening for sexually transmitted infections is recommended during the initial prenatal visit, and rescreening is often indicated.
- Women with SUD during pregnancy should be considered high risk and often benefit from closer maternal and fetal monitoring, including more frequent office visits and additional ultrasound examinations to assess fetal weight if there are concerns such as poor maternal nutritional status or insufficient weight gain. Antenatal fetal testing in the third trimester may be considered, particularly among women whose substance use is associated with placental abnormalities or prior fetal death in utero.
- Postpartum women with SUD are at increased risk for unintended short-interval pregnancy, and patient-centered contraception counseling should be introduced early in prenatal care to give patients the opportunity to develop a well-informed contraception plan.

MANAGEMENT AND REFERRAL

- Counseling should be specific to the individual issues. Intervention should be aimed at helping the patient appreciate the risks of substance use, especially those specific to pregnancy/breastfeeding, and accessing further treatment as indicated.

- **Motivational interviewing** is a useful form of patient-centered counseling in which clinicians collaborate with patients to help explore and resolve their ambivalence about changing unhealthy behaviors, emphasizing the "whether" and "why" rather than the "how." The key processes include engagement, focusing, evoking, and planning. Using a warm, nonjudgmental attitude first elicit how a patient feels about her current substance use and how it fits with her own hopes and values. Then, focus on specific changes she wants to make and what the reasons/rationale are for change (referred to as "change talk"). Finally, when a patient is resolved to make changes, the clinician shifts to supporting the patient in developing and activating a plan for change.

- Patients should be referred for professional substance use treatment when brief intervention is insufficient, the patient has moderate-severe SUD, the patient is using multiple substances, or the patient requires medically supervised withdrawal or maintenance therapy.

  - The first step is to help the patient find a provider who accepts her insurance and set up an initial appointment where a professional counselor will evaluate the appropriate level of care (eg, intensive outpatient vs inpatient treatment). For patients without health insurance, contact the local health department for either direct treatment or referral to a community provider who offers a sliding scale fee schedule.

  - Traditionally, substance use treatment modalities include a combination of counseling, psychotherapy, medications, and mutual help groups. Addiction counseling mainly includes supportive and insight-oriented individual and group therapies aimed at reducing substance use and maintaining recovery. Psychotherapy primarily includes cognitive and behavioral therapies that help the patient identify and correct distorted, maladaptive beliefs and improve functioning by increasing self-observation and decreasing reactivity to stimuli. In pharmacotherapy, medications are applied to reduce substance use. Finally, in mutual help groups, such as 12-step programs like Alcoholics Anonymous, members help one another achieve and maintain abstinence from alcohol and drugs.

  - For patients with opioid use disorder, referral directly to a treatment center for opioid agonist pharmacotherapy, also known as medication-assisted treatment, may be appropriate.

  - For patients suffering from the sequelae of drug or alcohol use, further referral may be indicated (eg, psychiatric referral, dental care, infectious disease consult, gastroenterology consult). **Psychiatric referral** is of particular importance because up to 70% of women with substance misuse have significant concurrent psychiatric illness. Furthermore, roughly half of pregnant women with SUD have posttraumatic stress disorder, often the result of childhood physical and/or sexual abuse. Substance use is often a form of self-medication for those with psychiatric disorders.

  - In addition to referral to medical providers, collaboration with social work and case management is important for optimizing complete care of the pregnant woman with SUD, and these professionals often serve as advocates for patients, helping them navigate the health system, respond to practical obstacles, secure access to other resources she may qualify for, and plan for infant care.

  - Women should also be counseled about the risk of NAS, including what to expect and how to provide supportive care for symptomatic infants. An NAS occurs in 30% to 80% of infants who had chronic in utero opioid exposure (eg, approximately 60% of methadone-exposed neonates are effected, irrespective of maternal maintenance dose). Polydrug use may increase both the severity and duration of NAS. Many nonopioids, such as benzodiazepines, are associated with infant withdrawal symptoms.

- o An NAS is characterized by disturbances in gastrointestinal, autonomic, and central nervous systems, with symptoms including irritability, high-pitched cry, poor sleep, respiratory difficulty, and uncoordinated sucking reflexes with resultant poor feeding and potential failure to thrive. Pharmacologic therapy is indicated for infants with severe NAS symptoms and includes morphine or methadone for opioid-exposed neonates, with possible addition of clonidine or phenobarbital, typically for other substance exposures.

TREATMENT

- See Table 19-3 for descriptions of how to treat acute withdrawal with either a taper (detoxification) or a substitution (maintenance) treatment plan.
- For pregnant women with opioid use disorder, opioid agonist pharmacotherapy (substitution/maintenance) is preferable to medically supervised withdrawal, which often requires management with a taper protocol for gradual detoxification. Those not treated with maintenance pharmacotherapy (eg, methadone, buprenorphine) are at high risk for relapse and worse outcomes.

LABOR AND DELIVERY PAIN MANAGEMENT

- Women on opioid maintenance therapy should continue their maintenance therapy both during labor and the postpartum period. The total daily dose of methadone or buprenorphine may be administered in three to four divided doses every 6 to 8 hours to help alleviate pain during hospitalization. Standard labor pain management such as epidural and spinal anesthesia should be offered; however, partial opioid agonists (eg, butorphanol), which are sometimes included in regional anesthesia preparations, should be avoided to prevent precipitation of withdrawal.
- Postpartum: Continue the same dose of maintenance therapy, consider scheduling nonsteroidal anti-inflammatory drugs (eg, ketorolac) and acetaminophen, and use fast-acting opioids as indicated for each case.
- Studies demonstrate that women on opioid maintenance may require 50% to 70% more opioid medication for adequate pain relief in the immediate postoperative/postpartum setting. The partial antagonism of buprenorphine makes pain control especially difficult in that population. Dose escalations for women on methadone are common in the third trimester, and it is especially important to monitor women receiving both opioid maintenance therapy and opioid pain medication for signs of oversedation.
- For women who have cesarean deliveries or perineal repairs after vaginal delivery, consider using local analgesics to help blunt initial pain response and potentially reduce total pain medication use.
- Discussing the strategy for postoperative pain management with the patient preoperatively creates an opportunity to collaborate on a shared goal of postoperative recovery that is synergistic with the goals of substance treatment.
- As with other patients, care should be taken to avoid sending women home with excess opioid pain medication, and women with underlying SUD are at higher risk of harm from overprescribing. We suggest discharging women with SUD home with no more than 3 to 4 days of opioid pain medication and with a plan for close

Table 19-3 Suggested Pharmacologic Treatment Regimens for Acute Withdrawal and Maintenance Therapy

Substance	Protocol	Notes/Precautions

Alcohol or benzodiazepines	**Taper (Detoxification) Protocols**
	
	• **Thiamine 100 mg orally daily for 3 d**
	First 24 h[a]
	  ○ Diazepam 10 mg IM/orally on admission and repeat in 4 h, followed by
	  ○ Diazepam 10 mg IM/orally every 6 h for three doses; hold for sedation.
	Next 25-48 h[b]
	  ○ Diazepam 5 mg orally every 4 h for six doses; hold for sedation.
	Next 49-72 h[b]
	  ○ Diazepam 5 mg orally every 6 h for four doses; hold for sedation.
	Next 73-96 h[b]
	  ○ Diazepam 5 mg orally every 8 h for three doses as needed
		• Wait until withdrawal symptoms before starting taper unless history of withdrawal seizures or delirium tremens.
		• Hold diphenhydramine and hydroxyzine during taper.
		• Use shorter acting agent (eg, lorazepam) if delivery anticipated within approximately 1 wk.
		• Continue prenatal vitamin and adequate IV/oral hydration.
		• Postpartum detoxification may include other medications: disulfiram, acamprosate, or naltrexone.

Opioids	Buprenorphine (**do not initiate until withdrawal symptoms present**) • Day 1 (induction): 4 mg sublingual; if severe symptoms persist for more than 1 h, can give an additional 4 mg (max total dose 8 mg) • Days 2-4 (stabilization): Dose may be increased in 4-mg increments daily for persisting withdrawal symptoms until 16 mg every day dose. If not well controlled on 16 mg, add adjunctive treatments (eg, clonidine).	• Initiation or titration of *maintenance therapy* is preferred to *detoxification* during pregnancy; however, maintenance therapy is not typically initiated inpatient unless in cooperation with a certified opioid treatment program, which can continue medication-assisted therapy after discharged to home.

(Continued)

Table 19-3 Suggested Pharmacologic Treatment Regimens for Acute Withdrawal and Maintenance Therapy *(Continued)*

Substance	Protocol	Notes/Precautions
	Taper down: after 24 h of well-controlled symptoms, may down-titrate by 2 mg per day **Or** Clonidine 0.1 mg orally • Every 4 h × six doses • Every 6 h × four doses • Every 8 h × three doses • Every 12 h × two doses • One dose on day 5 **Plus** • Dicyclomine (Bentyl) 10 mg orally every 6-8 h as needed for abdominal cramps • Hydroxyzine (Vistaril) 25 mg orally every 6 h as needed for anxiety, restlessness • Loperamide (Imodium) 4 mg orally, followed by 2 mg as needed for loose stools up to 16 mg every day	• Taper should be used only for those not enrolled in medication-assisted therapy, when enrollment is not immediately available or declined by the patient. • Side effects: mild withdrawal symptoms, constipation, sedation, and hypotension with clonidine
Nicotine Nicotine replacement therapy (NRT) Adjunct treatment	• Start nicotine patch 21 mg for >10 cigarettes/d, 14 mg for ≤10 cigarettes/d. • May add one nicotine gum or lozenge every 1-2 h for cravings (up to 24 and 20 daily, respectively) **Or** Bupropion SR orally, particularly if depression is also present	• Smoking cessation counseling is first line. • Caution patients not to smoke while on NRT due to concerns about cardiovascular effects from high doses.

Substitution (Maintenance) Therapy

Methadone
Initiating and titrating
Continuation therapy

Initiating and titrating

- Typically start with 30 mg and may administer 10 mg additional several hours later if severe withdrawal. symptoms persist but do not exceed 40 mg on first day
- Dose may be titrated up by 5-10 mg every 3-5 d until within 60-80 mg range and may then continue to be increased by 5-10 mg every week until patient is stable.

Continuation after missed doses

- Resume usual methadone dose if it can be confirmed (federal regulations require confirmation of *date and amount of last dose* with treatment program before prescribing replacement).
- If usual dose cannot be confirmed, 30 mg can be safely administered to prevent acute withdrawal.
- If patient reports missing interval doses:
  - 1 d missed: Prescribe full dose.
  - 2 d missed: Prescribe half of normal dose.
  - 3 d missed: Do not prescribe until consulting with medical director of her treatment program.

- First line for medication-assisted treatment during pregnancy
- Complete opioid agonist
- Half-life: 24-36 h
- Administered orally (pill or liquid)
- Typical dose: 30-140 mg every day
- Escalation may be required for increasing withdrawal symptoms, especially in third trimester given increased plasma volume, tissue binding, and metabolism as well as reduced protein binding, but dose should not be decreased/tapered during pregnancy unless patient is overly sedated.
- Avoid promethazine (Phenergan) because it "enhances" methadone's effects and benzodiazepines due to respiratory depression.

(Continued)

Table 19-3 Suggested Pharmacologic Treatment Regimens for Acute Withdrawal and Maintenance Therapy *(Continued)*

Substance	Protocol	Notes/Precautions
Buprenorphine (Subutex)/ buprenorphine-naloxone (Suboxone) Initiating and titrating Continuation therapy	**Initiating and titrating: *typically is not initiated during pregnancy*** • Wait until mild to moderate withdrawal symptoms develop before initiating to prevent precipitating acute withdrawal. • Starting dose is 4 mg SL; if withdrawal symptoms persist after 1-2 h, may add 2-4 mg additional dose • Dose may be increased in up to 4-mg increments daily for persisting withdrawal symptoms until 16 mg every day dose. Isolated cases may need higher dosages. **Continuation** after missed doses • Administer usual dose if most recent dose was <3 d ago. • If three doses have been missed, administer 4-mg starting dose and titrate back per protocol above.	• Partial opioid agonist • Half-life: 24-60 h • Sublingual administration • Typical dose: 4-32 mg every day • Severe pain can be difficult to control for women maintained on buprenorphine due to competitive blockade of opioid receptors. • Buprenorphine monotherapy is preferred over the naloxone-containing formulation due to insufficient safety evidence in pregnancy, and women who were on combined therapy when they became pregnant may be transitioned to buprenorphine-only treatment.

Abbreviations: IM, intramuscular; IV, intravenous; SL, sublingual; SR, sustained release.

[a]May add diazepam 10 mg IM/orally every hour as needed for breakthrough alcohol withdrawal for three doses in the first 24 h.

[b]May add diazepam 5 mg orally every 2 h as needed for breakthrough alcohol withdrawal for up to three doses within 25-96 h of protocol initiation.

follow-up in approximately 2 weeks or less depending on comorbidities. Methods to safely dispose of any excess opioids should be reviewed or providers may ask patients to bring any excess medications to their next visit.

BREASTFEEDING AND POSTPARTUM ISSUES

- Most substances discussed in the above section are present in breast milk to some degree; however, the relative concentrations differ and breastfeeding recommendations for women with SUD vary based on the individual circumstances, substance(s) of abuse, and clinician judgment.
- Tobacco use is not a contraindication to breastfeeding. However, breastfeeding women who smoke should be informed about risks of asthma and upper respiratory/ear infections for infants exposed to secondhand smoke. Harm reduction recommendations include smoking away from the baby, ideally outdoors, and wearing protective outerwear to minimize the baby's exposure to chemicals that attach to clothing.
- Women with history of SUD and/or heavy drinking should avoid any alcohol use during breastfeeding; however, small amounts of alcohol consumption are not contraindicated for unaffected women, who should be counseled to wait 3 to 4 hours after a single drink before nursing to ensure negligible infant exposure.
- For women well controlled on methadone or buprenorphine ($\pm$ naloxone) who do not use other substances or illicit opioids, the benefits of breastfeeding generally outweigh the risks. Breastfeeding is associated with decreased rate and severity of NAS.
- For breastfeeding women who require benzodiazepines, it is recommended to use a low dose of drug with a short half-life and no active metabolites (eg, lorazepam, zolpidem). Avoid diazepam and clonazepam due to infant effects.
- Women actively using heroin or other illicit opioids should be advised to avoid breastfeeding due to concerns regarding substance exposure, HIV, and behavioral complications related to polysubstance use (eg, burns, co-sleeping).
- Women actively using cocaine or methamphetamine should not breastfeed because both substances are concentrated in breast milk and may cause life-threatening infant toxicity.
- Breastfeeding women should not use marijuana. Women who use marijuana should be counseled that THC is passed through breast milk and may impair infant neurodevelopment. However, the evidence of harm from perinatal marijuana exposure is limited, and deciding whether the benefits of breastfeeding outweigh the risks of breast milk THC exposure should be individualized to the patient.
- Although most women with SUD significantly decrease or eliminate substance use during pregnancy, many are especially vulnerable to relapse during the postpartum period given hormonal shifts, stress of caring for the newborn, fatigue, and changing family dynamics. Thus, ensuring continuity of substance use treatment and access to supportive services are essential components of postpartum care.
- Women with history of psychiatric disorders and substance use are especially vulnerable to postpartum depression, emphasizing the importance of establishing or reestablishing psychiatric care during pregnancy. Providers should be aware of any state-required reporting of in utero substance exposure for neonates so they may inform/counsel patients appropriately. Postpartum follow-up visits for women with SUD should be scheduled within 1 month and within 2 weeks for women with increased risk of postpartum depression.

SUGGESTED READINGS

American College of Obstetricians and Gynecologists Committee on Obstetric Practice. ACOG Committee Opinion No. 711: opioid use and opioid use disorder in pregnancy. *Obstet Gynecol.* 2017;130:e81-e94. (Reaffirmed 2019)

Landau R. Post-cesarean delivery pain. Management of the opioid-dependent patient before, during and after cesarean delivery. *Int J Obstet Anesth.* 2019;39:105-116.

Reddy UM, Davis JM, Ren Z, Greene MF. Opioid use in pregnancy, neonatal abstinence syndrome, and childhood outcomes: executive summary of a joint workshop by the Eunice Kennedy Shriver National Institute of Child Health and Human Development, American College of Obstetricians and Gynecologists, American Academy of Pediatrics, Society for Maternal-Fetal Medicine, Centers for Disease Control and Prevention, and the March of Dimes Foundation. *Obstet Gynecol.* 2017;130(1):10-28.

Ross EJ, Graham DL, Money KM, Stanwood GD. Developmental consequences of fetal exposure to drugs: what we know and what we still must learn. *Neuropsychopharmacology.* 2015;40(1):61-87.

The Regional Perinatal Advisory Group. Substance use in pregnancy: a clinician's toolkit for screening, counseling, referral and care. Baltimore County Government Web site. https://www.baltimorecountymd.gov/go/perinatal. Accessed September 3, 2019.

20 Hematologic Disorders of Pregnancy

Christopher M. Novak and Rita W. Driggers

MATERNAL HEMATOLOGIC DISORDERS

Anemia

- The Centers for Disease Control and Prevention's definition of **anemia in pregnancy** is hemoglobin (Hb) or hematocrit (Hct) value less than the fifth percentile in a healthy reference population at the same stage of pregnancy. Using this definition, anemia is diagnosed when Hb <11.0 g/dL in the first and third trimesters and <10.5 g/dL in the second trimester.
- Racial differences have been noted, with lower Hb and Hct levels seen in African American women compared with white women. The Institute of Medicine suggests lowering the normal value for Hb by 0.8 g/dL and Hct by 2% in African Americans.
- Anemia is commonly classified according to mean corpuscular volume (MCV) as normocytic (80-100 fL), microcytic (<80 fL), and macrocytic (>100 fL), as the differential diagnosis differs according to MCV (Table 20-1). Anemia can be further classified as hypochromic (low mean corpuscular Hb or hypochromia on peripheral smear) or normochromic.
- Common types of anemia that are encountered during pregnancy include physiologic anemia of pregnancy, iron deficiency anemia, and, less often, megaloblastic anemia (Table 20-2). Iron studies can aid in differentiating various types of anemia (Table 20-3).

Table 20-1	Classification of Anemia by Mean Corpuscular Volume (MCV)[a]	
Microcytic (MCV <80 fL)	**Normocytic (MCV 80-100 fL)**	**Macrocytic (MCV >100 fL)**
Iron deficiency	Early iron deficiency	Vitamin B_{12} deficiency
Thalassemias	Acute blood loss	Folic acid deficiency
Anemia of chronic disease (late)	Sickle cell disease	Drug induced (zidovudine)
Sideroblastic anemia	Anemia of chronic disease	Ethanol abuse
Lead poisoning	Infection (osteomyelitis, HIV, mycoplasma, EBV)	Liver disease
Copper deficiency	Bone marrow disease	Myelodysplastic syndromes
	Chronic renal insufficiency	
	Hypothyroidism	
	Autoimmune hemolytic anemia	

Abbreviations: EBV, Epstein-Barr virus; HIV, human immunodeficiency virus.
[a]Adapted from American College of Obstetricians and Gynecologists Committee on Practice Bulletins—Obstetrics. ACOG Practice Bulletin No. 95: anemia in pregnancy. *Obstet Gynecol.* 2008;112:201-207. (Reaffirmed 2017)

Hemoglobinopathies

- Hemoglobinopathies are genetic abnormalities in the globin portion of the Hb molecule that can either be qualitative, resulting in structural abnormalities like sickle cell anemia, or quantitative, resulting in a decreased number of normal globin chains as in the thalassemias. Normal adult Hb is composed of two α-globin chains and two β-chains (HbA, 96%-97%), two δ-chains (HbA2, 2%-3%), or two γ-chains (HbF, <1%). African, Southeast Asian, and Mediterranean ancestries are associated with a higher risk of being a hemoglobinopathy carrier, and carrier screening should be offered or an Hb electrophoresis obtained at the onset of pregnancy if not previously done.
- **Sickle cell disease (SCD)** describes a group of autosomal recessive hemoglobinopathies resulting from abnormal sickle hemoglobin (HbS) that includes homozygous sickle hemoglobin (HbSS, often called "sickle cell anemia"), sickle cell–hemoglobin C (HbSC), and sickle/β-thalassemia hemoglobin (HbS/β-Thal). The HbS differs from HbA by a substitution of valine for glutamic acid at the sixth position of the β-globin chain. Sickle cell anemia (HbSS) is the most common phenotype, occurring primarily among people from sub-Saharan Africa, South and Central America, Saudi Arabia, India, and Mediterranean countries. Approximately 1 in 12 African Americans has sickle cell trait (HbAS) and 1 in 300 African American newborns have some form of SCD. When deoxygenated, HbS is less soluble and tends to polymerize into rigid aggregates that distort red blood cells (RBCs) into a sickle shape. These sickled cells undergo extravascular hemolysis and affected patients may experience hemolytic anemia, recurrent pain or vasoocclusive crises due to microvascular obstruction by sickled cells, infarction of multiple organ systems, and infection due to being functionally asplenic. Vasoocclusive crises may be triggered by infection, hypoxia, acidosis, dehydration,

Table 20-2 Common Anemias Encounters in Pregnancy

Type of Anemia	Diagnosis	Laboratory Findings	Treatment	Comments
Physiologic anemia	Hemodilution due to greater increase in plasma volume (25%-50%) than RBC mass (10%-25%)	Hct reduced 3%-5%	None	Changes begin by 6 wk gestation and resolve by 6 wk postpartum
Iron deficiency anemia	Microcytic, hypochromic anemia with insidious onset resulting most often in weakness and lethargy; severe cases may cause glossitis, stomatitis, koilonychia, pica, and gastritis.	See Table 20-3. Serum ferritin levels have the greatest sensitivity and specificity; levels <10-15 ng/mL generally indicate iron deficiency anemia.	Start with 60-120 mg of daily oral elemental iron.[a] If unresponsive to or cannot tolerate oral iron or severe anemia, intravenous iron can be given. Transfusion may be indicated in cases of severe anemia (Hb <6 g/dL).	Most common anemia encountered in pregnancy accounting for 50%-75% of cases Caused by increased iron requirement needed to support increased RBC mass and fetal and placental development
Megaloblastic anemia	Macrocytic, hypochromic anemia most often encountered in the third trimester resulting in symptoms of anemia, weight loss, anorexia, roughness of the skin, and glossitis; severe cases can exhibit thrombocytopenia and leukopenia.	Peripheral blood smear shows hypersegmented neutrophils, oval macrocytes, and Howell-Jolly bodies. Low serum folate (<2 ng/mL) or vitamin B_{12} (<200 pg/mL) levels depending on etiology	Folic acid 1 mg/d or Vitamin B_{12} administered orally (1 mg daily) or parentally (1 mg intramuscularly monthly) depending on cause of deficiency	Caused by deficiencies in folate (most common) or vitamin B_{12} resulting in impaired DNA synthesis with ineffective erythropoiesis Deficiencies are often dietary or due to impaired absorption as seen in malabsorptive bariatric surgery procedures.

Abbreviations: Hb, hemoglobin; Hct, hematocrit; RBC, red blood cell.

[a]Ferrous sulfate 325 mg contains 65 mg elemental iron; ferrous gluconate 300 mg contains 34 mg elemental iron.

Table 20-3 Laboratory Studies in Various Anemias[a]

Type of Anemia	Serum Iron	Serum Ferritin	Total Iron Binding Capacity
Iron deficiency anemia	↓	↓	↑
Anemia of chronic disease	↓	↑	↓
Sideroblastic anemia	↑	↑	↓
Thalassemia	↔	↔	↓

Abbreviations: ↓, decreased; ↑, increased; ↔, unchanged.
[a]Adapted with permission from American College of Obstetricians and Gynecologists Committee on Practice Bulletins—Obstetrics. ACOG Practice Bulletin No. 95: anemia in pregnancy. *Obstet Gynecol.* 2008;112(1):201-207. (Reaffirmed 2017). Copyright © 2008 by The American College of Obstetricians and Gynecologists.

or psychological stress and can result in severe pain, fever, organ dysfunction, and tissue necrosis. A serious complication is acute chest syndrome, one of the leading causes of hospitalization and death in patients with SCD. Acute chest syndrome is characterized by a combination of respiratory symptoms with hypoxemia, noninfectious lung infiltrates, and fever.

- **Diagnosis.** Diagnosis is confirmed by Hb electrophoresis, which typically shows 80% to 95% HbS, absent HbA, normal HbA2, and moderately elevated HbF (usually <15%). The anemia is normocytic and normochromic with an Hb concentration of 6 to 10 g/dL and Hct of 18% to 30%. The reticulocyte count is increased to 3% to 15%. Lactate dehydrogenase is elevated, and haptoglobin is decreased. The peripheral blood smear may show sickle cells, target cells, and Howell-Jolly bodies. Jaundice may result from RBC destruction, leading to unconjugated hyperbilirubinemia.
- **Treatment.** Hydroxyurea may be used to reduce intracellular sickling and frequency of painful crises but is not recommended in pregnancy because it is teratogenic in animal studies, although case reports in humans do not suggest a comparable increase in risk. Infections are treated aggressively with antibiotics. Severe anemia is treated with blood transfusion. Pain crises are managed with oxygen, hydration, and analgesia. Controversy surrounds prophylactic exchange transfusion and is reserved for the most severe cases. Additionally, the risks involved with transfusions must be taken into account, such as the risk of maternal alloimmunization, infection, iron overload, and acute and delayed transfusion reactions. Advantages of transfusion are an increase in HbA level, which improves oxygen-carrying capacity and a decrease in HbS-carrying erythrocytes. If a transfusion is given, leukocyte-depleted packed red cells, phenotyped for major and minor antigens, should be used.
- **Pregnancy considerations.** Patients with SCD are at increased risk for sickling during pregnancy because of increased metabolic requirements, vascular stasis, and a relative hypercoagulable state. Complications during pregnancy in women with SCD include an increased risk of spontaneous abortion, intrauterine growth restriction (IUGR), fetal death in utero, low birth weight, preeclampsia, and premature birth. Women with SCD also experience greater risk of urinary

tract infection (UTI), bacteriuria, pulmonary infections and infarction, and, possibly, more painful crises. A multidisciplinary approach involving hematology and anesthesia is recommended to optimize patient care during pregnancy. Due to elevated risk of UTI, a urine culture should be evaluated at minimum in every trimester and treated correspondingly. Women with SCD should receive the pneumococcal vaccine before pregnancy and folate supplementation of 1 to 4 mg/d. Iron supplements should be prescribed only if iron is deficient to avoid iron overload. The intensity of fetal surveillance varies according to the clinical severity of the disease. In severe cases, assessment of fetal well-being should begin at 32 weeks' gestation, and monthly sonography should be performed to evaluate fetal growth. All African American patients should undergo an Hb electrophoresis to assess carrier status. If both the patient and the father of the baby are found to be hemoglobinopathy carriers, genetic counseling is indicated. Amniocentesis or chorionic villus sampling (CVS) may be offered for prenatal diagnosis. Mode of delivery is dictated by usual obstetric indications. After delivery, patients should practice early ambulation and wear thromboembolic deterrent stockings to prevent thromboembolism.

- **Regarding contraception**, the levonorgestrel-containing intrauterine device (IUD) and progestin-only implants are considered excellent contraceptive options for patients with SCD. No well-controlled studies have evaluated oral contraceptives in SCD; however, low-dose combined contraceptives appear to be a good choice in some women with SCD. The benefits of copper-containing IUDs are debated due to a potential for increased blood loss, but copper-containing IUDs are generally considered a safe and effective method of contraception for women with SCD. Progestin-only pills, depot medroxyprogesterone, and barrier devices are also safe for contraception. Medroxyprogesterone acetate (Depo-Provera) injections may decrease the number of pain crises.

- Women with **sickle cell trait** (HbAS) have approximately twice the frequency of UTIs compared to the general population, especially during pregnancy, and should be screened each trimester. No direct fetal compromise exists from maternal sickle cell trait. Partners should be screened because the risk of having a child with SCD becomes one in four if the father is also a carrier.

- The **thalassemias** encompass a group of inherited blood disorders that can cause severe microcytic, hypochromic anemia. α-Thalassemia and β-thalassemia result from absent or decreased production of structurally normal α- and β-globulin chains, respectively, generating an abnormal ratio of α to non-α chains (Table 20-4). The excess chains form aggregates that lead to ineffective erythropoiesis and/or hemolysis. A broad spectrum of syndromes is possible, ranging from no symptoms to transfusion-dependent anemia and death. Both diseases are inherited in an autosomal recessive fashion.

  - **α-Thalassemia** is associated with Southeast Asian, African, Caribbean, or Mediterranean origin and results from a deletion of one to all four α-globin genes, located on chromosome 16. Individuals of Southeast Asian origin are more likely to carry two α-globin gene deletions in cis or on the same chromosome $(- -/\alpha\alpha)$. Their offspring are more likely to be affected by the deletion of three α-globin genes (HbH, $- -/-\alpha$) or four α-globin genes (Hb Barts, $- -/- -$). A fetus would be affected because fetal Hb also requires α chains. Individuals of African origin are more likely to carry two α-globin gene deletions in trans or on each chromosome $(\alpha-/\alpha-)$, and their offspring generally do not develop Hb Barts.

Table 20-4	Findings in Thalassemia[a]		
	Genotype[b]	Lab/Clinical Findings	Specifics
α-Thalassemias			
Silent carrier	−α/αα	Normal or slight microcytosis	Asymptomatic; 25%-30% of African Americans
α-Thalassemia trait	− −/αα (Asian) −α/−α (African)	Mild microcytic, hypochromic Normal Hb electrophoresis	Asymptomatic anemia not treatable with iron Both genotypes identical clinically; position of deleted genes determines severity in offspring (− −/αα at risk for fetus with HbH or hydrops)
HbH disease	− −/−α	Moderate to severe microcytic, hypochromic anemia (Hb 8-10 g/dL) ↑ reticulocytes (5%-10%) HbH = 2%-40%; ↓ HbA2, HbF normal Normal serum iron Heinz bodies on peripheral smear Splenomegaly, bony abnormalities	Anemia worsens during pregnancy, infection, and with oxidant drugs. Treat with long-term transfusion, splenectomy, and iron chelation. May have cholelithiasis
Hydrops fetalis (Hb Bart disease)	− −/− −	Marked anemia (Hb 3-10), ↑ nucleated erythrocytes, 80%-90% Hb Bart; 10%-20% HbH, no HbA Hydrops, heart failure, pulmonary edema, transverse limb reduction defects, hypospadias	Diagnosis often made in pregnancy by sonogram noting hydropic fetus Usually results in death Survival possible with intrauterine transfusion

(Continued)

Table 20-4 Findings in Thalassemia[a] *(Continued)*

	Genotype[b]	Lab/Clinical Findings	Specifics
β-Thalassemias			
β-Thalassemia minor	β^0/β	Asymptomatic or mild microcytic anemia (Hb 8-10 g/dL) ↑ HbA2, ↑ HbF, ↓ HbA	Heterozygous Confers resistance to falciparum malaria Often misdiagnosed as iron deficient
β-Thalassemia trait	$\beta+/\beta$	Mild or no anemia Basophilic stippling ↔ ↑ erythrocytes No splenomegaly, MCV 60 to normal	
β-Thalassemia intermedia	Varies, 2 β mutations (at least 1 mild)	Mild to moderate anemia Prominent splenomegaly, bony deformities, growth retardation, iron overload	Clinical diagnosis May be asymptomatic to severely symptomatic Present with symptoms later in life Chronic transfusions not required
Thalassemia major (Cooley anemia)	β^0/β^0 $\beta+/\beta+$	Hb as low as 2-3 g/dL MCV ,67 fL ↓ reticulocytes ↑↑ HbF, variable HbA2, no HbA ↑ HbF, ↓ HbA, variable HbA2 Splenomegaly; bone changes (increased hematopoiesis), severe iron overload	Homozygous Severity depends on amount of globin produced (β^0/β^0 more severe— no globin) Manifests at age 6-9 months when HbF changes to HbA With transfusions and chelation, may survive into third to fifth decade Die young from infectious or cardiac complications

Abbreviations: ↓, decreased; ↑, increased; ↔, unchanged; Hb, hemoglobin; MCV, mean corpuscular volume.
[a]Adapted with permission from American College of Obstetricians and Gynecologists Committee on Practice Bulletins—Obstetrics. ACOG Practice Bulletin No. 78: hemoglobinopathies in pregnancy. *Obstet Gynecol.* 2007;109(1):229-237. (Reaffirmed 2018). Copyright © 2007 by The American College of Obstetricians and Gynecologists.
[b]Genotype: β and δ—single gene per chromosome. α Gene is duplicated producing two genes per haploid and four per diploid.

- **β-Thalassemia** is associated with Mediterranean, Asian, Middle Eastern, Caribbean, and Hispanic origin. More than 200 alterations (mostly point mutations) in β-globin genes, located on chromosome 11, have been reported. The two consequences of these gene defects are the following: β 0, which is the complete absence of the β chain, and β+, which is decreased synthesis of the β chain. These conditions result in an absence of HbA.

  o **Diagnosis.** Thalassemia is usually microcytic and hypochromic with an MCV of <80 fL, similar to iron deficiency anemia but with important differences in clinical presentation and laboratory testing.

  o **Laboratory findings.** In general, thalassemias, especially the traits, are often misdiagnosed as iron deficiency anemia. However, the anemia is not corrected with iron repletion. A microcytic anemia in the absence of iron deficiency suggests thalassemia and additional testing including electrophoresis and iron studies are warranted. Suspicion for the presence of α-thalassemia is raised by the finding of microcytosis and a normal red cell distribution width with minimal or no anemia in the absence of iron deficiency or β-thalassemia. Pedigree studies are often helpful during workup of patients with α-thalassemia. Molecular genetic testing, such as quantitative polymerase chain reaction, is needed for diagnosis. Quantitative Hb electrophoresis is required for the diagnosis of β-thalassemia and should be suspected in cases of elevated HbA2 (>3.5%) and HbF.

  o **Pregnancy considerations.** Women diagnosed with or at high risk for thalassemia should be offered preconception counseling and information about the availability of prenatal diagnosis. First-trimester, DNA-based prenatal testing (CVS) is available if both members of the couple are carriers. Preimplantation genetic diagnosis may also be an option for affected parents.

    o Women with trait status for either thalassemia require no special care.

    o Pregnancy may exacerbate the anemia, necessitating transfusions, and place women at an increased risk for congestive heart failure and premature delivery.

    o Thalassemia may confer an increased risk of neural tube defects (NTDs) secondary to folic acid deficiency, so up to 4 mg/d periconceptional folic acid supplementation is recommended. Iron supplements should be prescribed only if iron deficiency is present; otherwise, iron overload can result.

    o Women with HbH may have successful pregnancies, with maternal outcome related to the severity of anemia.

    o Pregnancies affected by a fetus with Hb Barts are associated with hydrops fetalis, intrauterine death, and preeclampsia.

    o Information on pregnancy in women with β-thalassemia major or intermedia is more limited, although successful pregnancies have been reported. These women require close medical evaluation and follow-up.

    o If asplenic (HbS/β-Thal), vaccinations for pneumococcus, *Haemophilus influenzae*, and meningococcus need to be up-to-date.

    o Periodic fetal sonography to assess fetal growth in thalassemia patients is recommended. Antepartum fetal testing should be considered in anemic thalassemia patients, especially in cases in which fetal growth is lagging.

    o Ultrasonography is also useful to detect hydrops fetalis but usually at a later gestational age. Intrauterine blood transfusions have shown good success in fetuses with hydrops fetalis.

Thrombocytopenia

- **Thrombocytopenia**, defined as a platelet count <150 000/μL, is caused by increased platelet destruction or decreased platelet production and occurs in about 10% of pregnancies. Clinical signs, such as petechiae, easy bruising, epistaxis, gingival bleeding, and hematuria, are usually not seen until platelets are <50 000/μL. Counts below 50 000/μL may also increase surgical bleeding. The risk of spontaneous bleeding increases only when platelet counts fall below 20 000/μL, and significant bleeding may occur with platelet counts <10 000/μL. Thrombocytopenia, depending on the severity and etiology, may or may not be associated with serious maternal and/or fetal morbidity and mortality. Many conditions can cause thrombocytopenia during pregnancy.

  - **Gestational thrombocytopenia**, also referred to as incidental thrombocytopenia of pregnancy or essential thrombocytopenia, affects up to 8% of pregnancies and accounts for 80% of cases of mild thrombocytopenia during pregnancy. It generally occurs late in gestation and the incidence of fetal or neonatal thrombocytopenia is low. The decreased platelet count is likely due to hemodilution and increased physiologic platelet turnover. Platelet counts usually return to normal within 2 to 12 weeks after delivery. Gestational thrombocytopenia can recur in subsequent pregnancies, although the recurrence rate is unknown.

    - **Diagnosis.** Gestational thrombocytopenia is a diagnosis of exclusion; therefore, the first step is to take a careful history to rule out other causes. Platelet counts obtained before pregnancy and any laboratory data available from prior pregnancies should be reviewed.

      - Four criteria should be present: (1) mild thrombocytopenia (75 000-150 000/μL); (2) no previous history of thrombocytopenia, except during pregnancy; (3) no bleeding symptoms; and (4) platelet counts should return to normal within 2 to 12 weeks postpartum.

      - There are no specific diagnostic tests to distinguish gestational thrombocytopenia from mild idiopathic thrombocytopenic purpura (ITP). In fact, many women with gestational thrombocytopenia have platelet-associated immunoglobulin G (IgG) and serum antiplatelet IgG, making it difficult to distinguish from ITP using platelet antibody testing.

    - **Management.** In gestational thrombocytopenia, no intervention is necessary. Women with gestational thrombocytopenia are not at risk for maternal or fetal hemorrhage or bleeding complications.

      - Monitor platelets closely to detect decreases below 50 000/μL.

      - Document normal neonatal platelet count. Approximately 2% of the offspring of mothers with gestational thrombocytopenia have mild thrombocytopenia (<50 000/μL). However, infants generally do not suffer from severe platelet deficiency.

      - Reevaluate platelet count in the postpartum period to ensure it returns to normal. If thrombocytopenia persists, consider referring patient for evaluation by a hematologist.

- **Hemolysis, elevated liver enzymes, and low platelet (HELLP) syndrome** is the most common pathologic cause of maternal thrombocytopenia. It occurs in approximately 10% to 20% of women who have preeclampsia with severe features, with a platelet count less than 100 000/μL being a hematologic diagnostic criterion for preeclampsia. Platelets usually reach a nadir at 24 to 48 hours after delivery but typically do not drop below 20 000/μL. Clinical hemorrhage rarely occurs unless the patient develops disseminated intravascular coagulopathy, but it is important to note that platelet function may be impaired even if the platelet count is normal. Delivery is recommended following maternal stabilization. Although rare, thrombocytopenia may continue for a prolonged period. Treatment with corticosteroids, however, has not resulted in decreased maternal mortality or morbidity.

- **Idiopathic thrombocytopenic purpura** occurs in approximately 1 in 1000 pregnancies and accounts for 5% of pregnancy-associated thrombocytopenia. The ITP is the most common cause of thrombocytopenia in the first trimester. Antiplatelet antibodies are directed at platelet surface glycoproteins, leading to increased destruction of platelets by the reticuloendothelial system (primarily the spleen) that exceeds the rate of platelet synthesis by the bone marrow. The ITP can be a primary acquired disorder in which no underlying etiology is identified or can be secondary to an underlying disease or drug exposure. The course of ITP is not typically affected by pregnancy.

  o **Diagnosis.** Diagnosis is based on the history, physical exam, complete blood count, and peripheral smear. Women with ITP may report symptoms of easy bruising, petechiae, epistaxis, or gingival bleeding predating pregnancy. The ITP is a diagnosis of exclusion, and there is no diagnostic test. If thrombocytopenia is mild, it is difficult to distinguish ITP from gestational thrombocytopenia; however, a platelet count less than 100 000/μL is more suggestive of ITP. Detection of platelet-associated antibodies is consistent with, but not diagnostic of, ITP because they may also be present in women with gestational thrombocytopenia and preeclampsia. Platelet antibody testing has a fairly low sensitivity (49%-66%). However, the absence of platelet-associated IgG makes the diagnosis of ITP less likely. The ITP is more likely if the platelet count is <50 000/μL or in the presence of an underlying autoimmune disease or history of previous thrombocytopenia. In contrast to gestational thrombocytopenia, ITP-associated thrombocytopenia is typically evident early in pregnancy. Findings include the following:

    o Persistent thrombocytopenia (platelet count <100 000/μL with or without accompanying megathrombocytes on the peripheral smear).

    o Normal or increased megakaryocytes determined from bone marrow.

    o Secondary causes of maternal thrombocytopenia should be excluded (eg, preeclampsia, human immunodeficiency virus [HIV] infection, systemic lupus erythematosus, and drugs).

    o Absence of splenomegaly

  o **Antenatal management.** According to the American Society of Hematology, any adult with a new diagnosis of ITP requires testing for HIV and hepatitis C. Therapy is considered if the platelet counts are below 30 000 to 50 000 μL, or if the patient demonstrates bleeding symptoms, treatment is required. Corticosteroids, intravenous immunoglobulin (IVIG), or both are the first-line treatments for ITP.

    o Glucocorticoids suppress antibody production, inhibit sequestration of antibody-coated platelets and interfere with the interaction between platelets and antibodies. Oral prednisone is started at 0.5 to 2 mg/kg/d and tapered to the lowest dose supporting an acceptable platelet count (usually over 50 000/μL) and tolerable side effect profile. An initial response usually occurs within 4 to 14 days and reaches peak response within 1 to 4 weeks. One-fourth of patients may achieve complete remission. High-dose glucocorticoids, such as methylprednisolone, may be administered at 1 to 1.5 mg/kg IV in divided doses. Very little crosses the placenta. Response is usually seen in 2 to 10 days. Maternal side effects of long-term glucocorticoid treatment include increased risk of hypertension, preeclampsia, weight gain, hyperglycemia, immunosuppression, and gastrointestinal ulceration. Fetal effects include prelabor rupture of membranes and IUGR.

- ○ The IVIG is another therapeutic option, but it is typically reserved for cases refractory to corticosteroids or when a more rapid platelet increase is necessary. The IVIG should be given initially at 1 g/kg as a one-time dose but may be repeated. Initial response usually occurs within 1 to 3 days and peak response is reached within 2 to 7 days. The proposed mechanism of action of IVIG is prolongation of the clearance time of IgG-coated platelets by the maternal reticuloendothelial system.

- ○ Splenectomy is an option in the second trimester in women who fail glucocorticoid and IVIG therapy and are experiencing bleeding associated with platelet counts <10 000/μL. Splenectomy remains the only therapy that provides prolonged remission at 1 year and longer. With splenectomy, remission occurs in 75% of women; however, data in pregnancy are limited. Splenectomy can be performed safely during pregnancy, ideally in the second trimester. Individuals with splenectomies should be immunized against pneumococcus, *H influenzae*, and meningococcus.

- ○ **Intrapartum management.** As pregnancy approaches term, more aggressive measures to increase maternal platelet counts may be indicated to allow for adequate hemostasis during delivery and epidural anesthesia. Platelet counts over 50 000/μL are usually adequate for either vaginal or cesarean delivery. Epidural or spinal anesthesia is considered safe in patients with platelet counts of at least 80 000/μL. Prophylactic platelet transfusion may be appropriate with a maternal platelet count <10 000 to 20 000/μL before vaginal delivery or <50 000/μL before a cesarean delivery or if bleeding is present. For vaginal delivery, the transfusion should begin as close to the timing of delivery as reasonably possible. For cesarean delivery, the transfusion should begin at the time of incision. One "pack" of platelets will increase the platelet count by 5000 to 10 000/μL. Transfused platelets will have a shorter half-life because of circulating antibodies.

- • **Thrombotic microangiopathies** such as thrombotic thrombocytopenic purpura (TTP) and hemolytic uremic syndrome (HUS) can manifest during pregnancy, most often in the third trimester or postpartum, and because of clinical similarities must be differentiated from preeclampsia/HELLP syndrome. Common features of TTP/HUS include hemolytic anemia, marked thrombocytopenia, and severe acute kidney injury. Fever and neurologic impairment can also be seen with TTP. The TTP is marked by an inherited or acquired deficiency in the protease ADAMTS13 that is responsible for cleavage of von Willebrand factor (vWF) multimers to prevent platelet thrombi formation. Atypical HUS resulting from complement dysregulation can be inherited or acquired and is more common in pregnancy than cases of typical HUS that result from the production of Shiga-like toxin in the setting of a diarrheal illness due to *Escherichia coli*. Unlike preeclampsia/HELLP syndrome, TTP/HUS is not definitively treated with delivery and more directed therapy is required. Treatment of these conditions involves appropriate supportive care and therapies directed at the underlying cause. The TTP is treated with plasma exchange (PEX) to remove autoantibodies to ADAMTS13 and restore functional ADAMTS13. Atypical HUS is treated with PEX and anticomplement therapy aimed at blocking the complement cascade.

Thromboembolic Disease

- Thromboembolic disease is linked with both adverse maternal and fetal/ neonatal outcomes. The term *venous thromboembolism* (VTE) encompasses deep vein thrombosis (DVT) and pulmonary embolism (PE). Approximately 80% of VTEs in pregnancy are DVT and 20% are PE. Pregnant women are 4 to 5 times more likely to experience a VTE than age-matched nonpregnant women. Approximately half of all DVT/VTEs occur in the antepartum period and appear to be evenly divided among the three trimesters. Cesarean delivery imparts a 3 to 5 times greater risk than a vaginal delivery. The risk of VTE is greater postpartum.
- Pregnancy is considered a hypercoagulable state. Fibrinogen, coagulation factors, and plasminogen activator inhibitor-1 and plasminogen activator inhibitor-2 levels are increased; free protein S levels are decreased, and fibrinolytic activity is decreased. Additionally, VTE risk is increased by anatomic changes in pregnancy including increased venous stasis and compression of the inferior vena cava and pelvic veins by the enlarging uterus.
- One of the most significant risk factors is a personal history of VTE. Maternal medical conditions including heart disease, SCD, lupus, obesity, diabetes, and hypertension increase risk. Other risk factors include recent surgery, family history of VTE, bed rest or prolonged immobilization, smoking, older than 35 years, multiple gestation, preeclampsia, and postpartum infection.
- **Thrombophilias** may be inherited or acquired. Pregnancy may trigger an event in women with an underlying thrombophilia. Fetal death in utero, severe fetal growth restriction, abruption, and severe early-onset preeclampsia have been correlated with underlying thrombophilias that affect uteroplacental circulation; however, this is controversial, and recent studies fail to reliably establish causal links between thrombophilias and these adverse pregnancy outcomes.
  - **Inherited thrombophilias** (Table 20-5) increase the risk of a maternal thromboembolic event. They are present in up to half of all maternal thrombotic events. Antithrombin deficiency, homozygosity for factor V Leiden mutation, homozygosity for prothrombin G20219A mutation, and compound heterozygosity for both factor V Leiden and prothrombin G20219A are the most potent of the inherited thrombophilias.
  - **Acquired thrombophilias** include persistent antiphospholipid antibody syndromes (lupus anticoagulants, anticardiolipin, or β_2 glycoprotein 1 antibodies). Antiphospholipid antibodies have been associated with arterial and venous thrombosis, autoimmune thrombocytopenia, and obstetric complications that include preeclampsia, IUGR, placental insufficiency, and preterm birth.
- Routine screening for thrombophilias is not recommended in all pregnant women, and screening indications are controversial. American College of Obstetricians and Gynecologists no longer recommends thrombophilia testing in women with recurrent fetal loss, placental abruption, fetal growth restriction,

Table 20-5	Inherited Thrombophilias and Risk of Venous Thromboembolism (VTE) in Pregnancy[a]		
Thrombophilia	VTE Risk per Pregnancy (No History) (%)	VTE Risk per Pregnancy (Previous VTE) (%)	Percentage of All VTE
Factor V Leiden homozygosity	2-14	17	2
Prothrombin G20210A homozygosity	2-4	>17	0.5
Factor V Leiden heterozygous	0.5-3	10	40
Prothrombin G20210A heterozygous	0.4-2.6	>10	17
Protein C deficiency	0.1-1.7	4-17	14
Antithrombin deficiency	0.2-11.6	40	1
Protein S deficiency	0.3-6.6	0-22	3
Factor V Leiden + prothrombin G20210A (compound heterozygosity)	4-8	>20	1-3

[a]Adapted with permission from American College of Obstetricians and Gynecologists Committee on Practice Bulletins—Obstetrics. ACOG Practice Bulletin No. 197: inherited thrombophilias in pregnancy. *Obstet Gynecol.* 2018;132(1):e18-e34. Copyright © 2018 by The American College of Obstetricians and Gynecologists.

or preeclampsia. A thrombophilia workup (Table 20-6) should be considered for the following:

  ○ Personal history of VTE associated with a nonrecurrent risk factor such as prolonged immobilization.
  ○ First-degree relative with a history of high-risk thrombophilia
  ○ Antiphospholipid antibody syndromes screening may be appropriate for women with one or more unexplained fetal deaths at or greater than 10 weeks' gestation of a morphologically normal fetus; one or more premature births of a morphologically normal neonate before 34 weeks due to eclampsia, pre-eclampsia, or placental insufficiency; or three or more unexplained consecutive spontaneous losses before the 10th week.
* Manifestations and diagnosis of VTE in pregnancy
  • DVT
    ○ Over 70% of DVTs in pregnancy develop in the iliofemoral veins, from which they are more likely to embolize, and the majority are on the left side. Diagnosis of DVT is difficult in pregnancy because expected changes in pregnancy may mimic the symptoms of DVT. Additionally, many patients are asymptomatic. If symptoms exist, the most common include calf or lower extremity swelling, pain or tenderness, warmth, and erythema. Homan sign (calf pain with passive dorsiflexion of the foot) is present in <15% of cases, and a palpable cord is present in <10% of cases. Symptoms of an iliac DVT include

Table 20-6	Thrombophilia Testing[a,b]

Primary Tests (Recommended by ACOG)

Factor V Leiden DNA analysis
OR
Activated protein C resistance assay (second generation) followed by DNA analysis for Factor V Leiden if positive
Prothrombin G20210A genotype
Antithrombin activity
Protein C activity
Protein S activity
Lupus anticoagulant
Anticardiolipin antibodies (IgG and IgM)
Anti-β2-glycoprotein (IgG and IgM)

Other Tests (Not Recommended by ACOG)

4G/4G PAI-1 mutation (if not available, plasma PAI-1 activity)
MTHFR mutation screen and/or fasting plasma homocysteine levels

Abbreviations: ACOG, American College of Obstetricians and Gynecologists; IgG, immunoglobulin G; IgM, immunoglobulin M; MTHFR, methylenetetrahydrofolate reductase; PAI-1, plasminogen activator inhibitor-1; PCR, polymerase chain reaction.
[a]Testing should be remote from thrombotic event, not during pregnancy, and while off anticoagulants, except DNA tests.
[b]Adapted with permission from American College of Obstetricians and Gynecologists Committee on Practice Bulletins—Obstetrics. ACOG Practice Bulletin No. 197: inherited thrombophilias in pregnancy. *Obstet Gynecol.* 2018;132(1):e18-e34. Copyright © 2018 by The American College of Obstetricians and Gynecologists.

abdominal pain, back pain, and swelling of the entire leg. In pregnant women with clinical suspicion of DVT, diagnosis is confirmed in <10%.

- o Venous duplex imaging, including compression ultrasound, color, and spectral Doppler sonography, has replaced contrast venography as the gold standard and is the most commonly available noninvasive diagnostic method, with a sensitivity of 97% and specificity of 94% in symptomatic proximal DVT. If the deep venous system is normal, the presence of a clinically significant thrombus is unlikely. Limitations include poor sensitivity for asymptomatic disease and difficulty in detecting iliac vein thromboses.
- o Magnetic resonance imaging is recommended when compression ultrasound results are negative or equivocal and iliac vein thrombosis is suspected. Studies in nonpregnant patients show a sensitivity of 100% and specificity of 98% to 99% for pelvic and proximal DVTs while maintaining a high accuracy in detecting below-the-knee DVTs.
- o D-dimer test is a sensitive but nonspecific test for DVT; however, D-dimer normally increases with gestational age. A normal D-dimer result may be reassuring if clinical suspicion is low, but even a high D-dimer level does not predict VTE in pregnancy.
- The PE remains one of the leading causes of maternal mortality in developed countries, accounting for approximately 20% of deaths. The risk of PE is greatest

immediately postpartum, particularly after cesarean delivery, with a fatality rate of nearly 15%. A PE most commonly originates from DVT in the lower extremities, occurring in nearly 50% of patients with proximal DVT. Symptoms typically associated with PE are all common in pregnancy, such as sudden shortness of breath, chest pain, and cough, or signs of tachypnea and tachycardia. Because of the serious potential consequences of PE and the increased incidence in pregnancy, clinicians must have a low threshold for evaluation.

- o **Diagnosis** starts with a careful history and physical examination, followed by diagnostic tests to rule out other possible etiologies, such as asthma, pneumonia, or pulmonary edema.

- An arterial blood gas, electrocardiogram, and chest x-ray should be performed. Arterial blood gas values are altered in pregnancy and must be interpreted using pregnancy-adjusted normal values. More than half of pregnant women with a documented PE have a normal alveolar-arterial gradient.

- A chest x-ray helps rule out other disease processes and enhances interpretation of the ventilation-perfusion ($\dot{V}/\dot{Q}$) scan. The risks associated with various radiologic tests indicated for PE workup are minimal compared with the consequences of a missed PE.

- Pulmonary angiography is the gold standard for PE diagnosis, but it is expensive and invasive.

- Computed tomographic (pulmonary) angiography (CTA) is becoming the recommended imaging test in pregnant women with suspected PE. The CTA is easier to perform, more readily available, and more cost-effective and provides a lower dose of radiation to the fetus than a $\dot{V}/\dot{Q}$ scan. The CTA is also useful in detecting other abnormalities that may be contributing to the patient's symptoms (eg, pneumonia, aortic dissection). Newer technology, multidetector CTA, allows visualization of finer pulmonary vascular detail and provides greater diagnostic accuracy.

- Historically, the $\dot{V}/\dot{Q}$ scan has been the primary diagnostic test for PE. It is interpreted as low, intermediate, or high probability for PE. High-probability scans (ie, segmental perfusion defect with normal ventilation) confirm PE, with a positive predictive value over 90% when pretest likelihood is high. The $\dot{V}/\dot{Q}$ scans are limited in their usefulness because of the large proportion of indeterminate results. Most fetal radiation exposure occurs when radioactive tracers are excreted in the maternal bladder. Therefore, exposure can be limited by prompt and frequent voiding after the procedure. If patient is postpartum and breastfeeding, breast milk should not be used for 2 days after a $\dot{V}/\dot{Q}$ scan.

- If a pregnant woman has a nondiagnostic lung scan, bilateral venous duplex imaging of the lower extremities is recommended to evaluate for DVT. If DVT is found, PE can be diagnosed. If no DVT is seen, arteriography may be performed for further evaluation before a commitment to long-term anticoagulation is made, or a repeat venous duplex imaging may be repeated in 1 week.

- According to the Centers for Disease Control and Prevention, in all stages of gestation, a dose of <5 rads (0.05 Gy) represents no measurable noncancer health effects. After 16 weeks' gestation, congenital effects are unlikely below 50 rads. The risk for childhood cancer from prenatal radiation exposure is 0.3% to 1% for 0 to 5 rads. Any of the proposed modalities for diagnosis of PE are well below the dose levels that increase congenital abnormalities. Radiation exposure from a two-view chest radiograph is <0.001 rad. A higher dose of fetal radiation is provided with $\dot{V}/\dot{Q}$ scan (0.064-0.08 rad) compared with CTA (0.0003-0.0131 rad). Pulmonary angiography provides approximately 0.2 to 0.4 rad with the femoral approach and <0.05 rad with the brachial approach. Maternal radiation dose is higher with CTA than V̇/Q̇ scan.

- Treatment of VTE in pregnancy
  - When VTE is suspected, anticoagulation with unfractionated heparin (UFH) or low-molecular-weight heparin (LMWH) should be initiated until the diagnosis is excluded. Neither of these heparin anticoagulants crosses the placenta or is secreted into breast milk. Although UFH has been standard treatment for the prevention and treatment of VTE during pregnancy, recent evidence-based clinical practice guidelines now recommend LMWH. Table 20-7 lists dosing regimens. Thromboembolic deterrent compression stockings and leg elevation should be used for DVT.
  - Weight-adjusted LMWH should be used for the treatment of VTE (see Table 20-7). Advantages of LMWH include fewer bleeding complications, lower risk of heparin-induced thrombocytopenia (HIT) and osteoporosis, longer plasma half-life, and more predictable dose-response relationships. Theoretical concerns have been raised regarding once-daily dosing compared to twice-daily dosing (ie, prophylactic or therapeutic) secondary to the increased renal clearance in pregnancy possibly prolonging trough LMWH levels. However, no comparison data of the two regimens are available. Additionally, recent data suggest daily dosing in the treatment of acute VTE is effective. Monitoring of LMWH levels remains controversial. The LMWH cannot be monitored using activated partial thromboplastin time (aPTT) because aPTT will likely be normal. Peak anti-factor Xa activity levels may be measured 4 hours after subcutaneous (SC) injection, with a therapeutic peak goal of 0.6 to 1.0 U/mL (slightly higher if once-daily dosing is used); however, frequent monitoring is not typically recommended, except at extremes of body weight. If trough levels are evaluated with therapeutic dosing (ie, 12 h after dosing), goal level is 0.2 to 0.4 IU/mL. Current guidelines do not provide definitive monitoring recommendations; however, some researchers advocate checking levels periodically (every 1-3 mo).
  - The UFH is administered either IV or SC. The IV UFH may be a better initial therapeutic option in unstable patients (eg, large PE with hypoxia or extensive iliofemoral disease) or patients with significant renal impairment (ie, creatinine clearance <30 mL/min). The goal of the initial bolus dose (typically 80 U/kg) and subsequent maintenance dosing (typically 18 U/kg/h) is to achieve a therapeutic aPTT of 1.5 to 2.5 times normal. Many facilities have standard protocols for heparin titration. The IV treatment should be maintained in the therapeutic range for at least 5 days, after which therapy may be continued with either adjusted-dose SC heparin injections or LMWH. If maintained on UFH, a midinterval (6 h postinjection) aPTT should be monitored every 1 to 2 weeks. Measuring anti-factor Xa heparin levels may assist in evaluating heparin dosing (target level 0.3-0.7 IU/mL). The aPTT response to heparin in pregnant women is often attenuated secondary to elevated heparin-binding proteins and increased factor VIII and fibrinogen. The therapeutic dose may need to be adjusted. Thus, it may be difficult to achieve target aPTT levels late in pregnancy. The major concerns with UFH use during pregnancy are bleeding, osteopenia, and thrombocytopenia. The risk of major bleeding with UFH is approximately 2%. Bone density reductions have been reported in 30% of patients on heparin for over 1 month. The HIT occurs in up to 3% of nonpregnant patients and should be suspected when platelet count decreases to <100 000/μL or <50% of baseline

Table 20-7	Anticoagulation Regimens in Pregnancy[a]	
	Type of Anticoagulation	Dosing Regimen
Prophylactic	LMWH	Enoxaparin 40 mg SC every 24 h Dalteparin 5000 U SC every 24 h Tinzaparin 4500 U SC every 24 h or 75 U/kg SC every 24 h
	UFH	UFH 5000 U SC every 12 h
	Alternative	UFH 5000-7500 U SC every 12 h in first trimester UFH 7500-10 000 U SC every 12 h in second trimester UFH 10 000 U SC every 12 h in third trimester (unless aPTT elevated)
Intermediate dose	LMWH	Enoxaparin 40 mg SC every 12 h Dalteparin 5000 U SC every 12 h
Therapeutic/ treatment (weight-adjusted) dose	LMWH	Enoxaparin 1 mg/kg SC every 12 h Dalteparin 200 U/kg SC every 24 h or 100 U/kg SC every 12 h Tinzaparin 175 U/kg SC every 24 h
	UFH	UFH 10 000 U or more SC every 12 h; doses adjusted to obtain midinterval (6 h postinjection) therapeutic aPTT (often a ratio of 1.5-2.5)
Postpartum anticoagulation (for 4-6 wk)[b]	Warfarin	Adjust dose to target INR of 2.0 – 3.0 with initial UFH or LMWH overlap until INR is > 2.0 for 2 days
	LMWH or UFH	Prophylactic, intermediate, or therapeutic dose

Abbreviations: aPTT, activated partial thromboplastin time; INR, international normalized ratio; LMWH, low-molecular-weight heparin; SC, subcutaneously; UFH, unfractionated heparin.
[a]Adapted from Bates SM, Middeldorp S, Rodger M, James AH, Greer I. Guidance for the treatment and prevention of obstetric-associated venous thromboembolism. *J Thromb Thrombolysis.* 2016;41:92-128 and American College of Obstetricians and Gynecologists Committee on Practice Bulletins—Obstetrics. ACOG Practice Bulletin No. 196: thromboembolism in pregnancy. *Obstet Gynecol.* 2018;132:e1-e17.
[b]Postpartum anticoagulation should be greater or equal to antepartum therapy.

value 5 to 15 days after beginning heparin or sooner with recent heparin exposure. In 25% to 30% of patients who develop HIT, onset occurs rapidly (within 24 h) after starting heparin and is related to recent exposure to heparin. After obtaining a starting platelet level, American College of Obstetricians and Gynecologists recommends checking platelets again on day 5 and then periodically for the first 2 weeks of therapy. Others suggest platelets be monitored at 24 hours and then every 2 to 3 days for the first 2 weeks or weekly for the first 3 weeks. If HIT is acquired and ongoing anticoagulant therapy is required, fondaparinux (Factor Xa inhibitor) or argatroban (direct thrombin inhibitor) can be used. The use of new or direct oral anticoagulants, such as dabigatran, rivaroxaban, apixaban, or edoxaban, is not recommended during pregnancy or during the immediate postpartum period.

- Warfarin sodium crosses the placenta and, therefore, is a potential teratogen and may cause fetal bleeding. Warfarin is likely safe during the first 6 weeks' gestation, but between 6 and 12 weeks' gestation, a risk of skeletal embryopathy exists, consisting of stippled epiphyses and nasal and limb hypoplasia. One-third of fetuses exposed to warfarin late in pregnancy develop central nervous system injuries, hemorrhage, or ophthalmologic abnormalities. Warfarin may be used postpartum and may be given to nursing mothers because it does not enter breast milk. Antepartum use can be considered for women with mechanical heart valves, for which neither LMWH nor heparin provide adequate anticoagulation in the antepartum period.

- Temporary inferior vena cava filters are indicated in women in whom anticoagulants are contraindicated. They may be inserted within a week of elective induction or cesarean delivery and removed at least 6 weeks (for DVT) or up to 4 to 6 months (for PE) postpartum.

- Prophylaxis for VTE in pregnancy
  - **Antepartum.** Limited data exist regarding the use of prophylactic anticoagulation for VTE during pregnancy. Women need to be stratified by risk, and clinical judgment applied when making recommendations for prophylaxis. Although recommendations vary, women at very increased for VTE probably benefit from prophylactic or intermediate dosing of UFH or LMWH throughout pregnancy and postpartum. At a minimum, postpartum prophylaxis is usually recommended in women at elevated risk for VTE.
  - **Intrapartum.** The risk of maternal hemorrhage may be minimized with carefully planned delivery. If possible, induction of labor or scheduled cesarean delivery should be considered in women on therapeutic anticoagulation dosing regimens, so therapy may be discontinued at an appropriate time. When used in therapeutic doses, LMWH should be discontinued 24 hours before elective induction of labor or cesarean delivery. Epidural or spinal anesthesia should not be administered within 24 hours of the last therapeutic dose of LMWH. A common approach is to transition from LMWH to UFH at 36 to 38 weeks' gestation. If the patient goes into spontaneous labor and is receiving SC UFH, she should be able to receive regional analgesia if the aPTT is normal. If significantly prolonged, protamine sulfate may be administered at 1 mg/100 U of UFH. If the patient is at very high risk for VTE, IV UFH can be started and then discontinued 4 to 6 hours before expected delivery. When receiving LMWH once daily for prophylaxis, regional anesthesia can be administered 12 hours after the last dose. Also, LMWH should be withheld for at least 2 to 4 hours after the removal of an epidural catheter.

- **Postpartum.** Postpartum anticoagulation may typically be resumed 6 to 12 hours after cesarean delivery and 4 to 6 hours after vaginal delivery. If at high risk of bleeding postpartum, IV UFH may be chosen initially because its effect dissipates more rapidly and may be reversed with protamine sulfate. Once adequate hemostasis is assured, warfarin can be started by initial overlap with UFH or LMWH until international normalized ratio is 2.0 for 2 consecutive days, with a target international normalized ratio of 2.0 to 3.0. Anticoagulation should be administered for at least 6 weeks postpartum for DVT and 4 to 6 months for PE.
- Birth control options for women with a history of VTE or those with a high-risk thrombophilia
  - Due to the thrombogenic potential of estrogen-containing contraceptives, progestin-only or nonhormonal contraceptive methods are recommended. Natural family planning, condoms, progestin-only pills, levonorgestrel-releasing IUD, copper IUD, and tubal ligation/occlusion are methods that can be discussed with patients at high risk for VTE.

von Willebrand Disease

- von Willebrand disease (vWD) is an inherited congenital bleeding disorder that involves a qualitative or quantitative deficiency of vWF. There are three main types of vWD (Table 20-8). The vWF binds to subendothelium at sites of endothelial injury and is required for proper platelet adhesion. It also serves as a protein carrier for factor VIII increasing its half-life. The vWD is the most common inherited bleeding disorder among American women, with a prevalence of approximately 1%.
  - **Diagnosis.** Clinical suspicion for a diagnosis should exist in any woman with a personal history with or without a family history of easy bruising and heavy or

Table 20-8	von Willebrand Disease Classification[a]		
	Type 1	Type 2	Type 3
Mode of inheritance	AD	AD or AR	AR
Percentage of cases	75	Approximately 25	Rare
Pathophysiology	Partial deficiency of vWF	Qualitatively abnormal vWF	Markedly decreased or absent vWF
Clinical presentation	Asymptomatic to severe bleeding	Moderate to severe bleeding	Severe bleeding

Abbreviations: AD, autosomal dominant. AR, autosomal recessive; vWF, von Willebrand factor.
[a]Adapted from American College of Obstetricians and Gynecologists Committee on Adolescent Health Care. ACOG Committee Opinion No. 580: von Willebrand disease in women. *Obstet Gynecol.* 2013;122:1368-1373. (Reaffirmed 2017)

prolonged bleeding. Clinical findings that warrant further diagnostic evaluation include the following:

o Heavy menstrual bleeding since menarche
o Personal history of postpartum hemorrhage, surgery-related bleeding, or bleeding associated with dental work
o Two or more of the following conditions:
  o Epistaxis, one to two times per month
  o Frequent gum bleeding
  o Family history of bleeding symptoms

- **Laboratory tests.** If diagnostic workup is required following a positive clinical screen, laboratory tests for vWD should be obtained and include vWF antigen, von Willebrand-ristocetin cofactor activity, and factor VIII level. In some cases, genetic testing may be necessary to confirm certain vWD types.
- **Management.** Treatment options for patients with vWD include desmopressin (DDAVP), replacement therapy with vWF-containing concentrates, and antifibrinolytic drugs.

  o The DDAVP is a synthetic analog of antidiuretic hormone that promotes the release of vWF from endothelial storage sites. It can be used in patients with type 1 and some types of type 2 vWD. Administration is IV or by intranasal spray as prophylaxis before invasive procedures or for acute bleeding episodes.

  o The vWF replacement therapy can be used in all types of vWD especially in cases of more serious bleeding situations, when other therapies have failed, or when prolonged treatment is necessary. Therapy is by IV infusion to control bleeding, and dosing is empiric and weight based with the goal to maintain vWF activity above 50%.

  o Antifibrinolytic therapy with aminocaproic acid and tranexamic acid work by inhibiting the conversion of plasminogen to plasmin, thereby preventing fibrinolysis and stabilizing clots to treat bleeding. They are administered IV or orally three to four times a day as needed to control bleeding.

  o **Pregnancy considerations.** Early referral during pregnancy to hematology to confirm diagnosis and establish a management plan is recommended. Anesthesia consultation is also recommended given an increased risk of epidural or spinal hematoma. Genetic counseling should also be offered to discuss the possibility of having an affected child. Periodic assessment of vWF and factor VIII levels can be obtained throughout pregnancy, but it is important to remember that vWF and factor VIII levels increase throughout pregnancy, so many patients with vWD may have normal levels near term. Most invasive procedures (ie, amniocentesis or CVS) are safe with vWF and factor VIII levels maintained above 50%. Invasive fetal procedures, such as fetal scalp electrode placement and operative vaginal delivery, are best avoided, if possible, if the fetal vWD status is unknown. Route of delivery is determined by the usual obstetric indications.

FETAL HEMATOLOGIC DISORDERS

Fetal Anemia and Alloimmunization

- Fetal anemia is an uncommon but life-threatening condition for the developing fetus. Historically, RBC alloimmunization has been the most common cause of fetal anemia. Fetal anemia is defined as a fetal Hb concentration that is greater than 2 standard deviation below the mean for gestational age, as fetal Hb concentration increases with advancing gestation. Alternatively, fetal Hct of less than 30% is also used in clinical care to diagnosis fetal anemia.

- **Alloimmunization** in pregnancy refers to maternal antibody formation against fetal RBC or platelet antigens. These antibodies can cross the placenta, and antibody-coated erythrocytes or platelets are destroyed by the fetal immune system, leading to fetal anemia or thrombocytopenia. Antibodies are formed after uncrossmatched transfusion or fetomaternal hemorrhage (FMH), when foreign or fetal blood components enter the maternal circulation. Untreated alloimmunization can cause significant fetal and newborn morbidity and mortality from hemolytic anemia (hydrops fetalis) or neonatal alloimmune thrombocytopenia (NAIT).

- **Red blood cell alloimmunization** to clinically significant antigens occurs in approximately 25 of 10 000 births. The most common of these antigens is the Rhesus D (or Rh D) antigen. Maternal blood type is usually described as ABO+ or ABO−, signifying the presence (+) or absence (−) of the Rh D antigen. The introduction and routine administration of Rh D immunoglobulin to at risk Rh D− mothers over the last 40 years has greatly decreased the incidence of fetal anemia caused by Rh D alloimmunization. The prevalence of Rh D− blood type varies by ethnicity. Fifteen percent of Caucasians and 8% of African Americans and Hispanic Americans are Rh D−. The Rhesus system also includes the antigens C, c, E, and e. Other important red cell antigens are the ABO blood group antigens and more than 50 other minor antigens. Only some of these are associated with red cell alloimmunization, such as anti-Kell (K, k), anti-Duffy (Fy^a), and anti-Kidd (Jk^a, Jk^b) (Table 20-9).

  - **Pathophysiology.** Exposing a woman who does not carry a red cell antigen to the antigen initiates an immune response that produces immunoglobulin M (IgM) and IgG antibodies against the antigen and results in memory B cells that produce IgG on reexposure to the antigen. This process is termed **red blood cell sensitization**. The FMH with transplacental passage of fetal erythrocytes containing the antigen absent on maternal RBCs into the maternal circulation is the main cause of RBC sensitization. This can occur with delivery, trauma, invasive obstetric procedures, spontaneous or induced abortion, or ectopic pregnancy. The RBC sensitization can also occur with maternal blood transfusion of incompatible blood.

    o During pregnancy, the fetal RBCs are targeted by maternal IgG, which can cross the placenta. Fetal anemia develops as fetal RBCs are sequestered and hemolyzed.

    o The fetal response to anemia includes increased erythropoietin production and hematopoiesis. As hemolysis outpaces production, more immature RBCs appear in the fetal circulation, a condition known as erythroblastosis fetalis. Extramedullary hematopoiesis may occur.

    o If the anemia is left untreated, hydrops fetalis develops.

  - **Prevention.** Prevention is only available for Rh D alloimmunization. Injectable anti-D immunoglobulin (RhoGAM) was developed in the 1960s as a means to prevent Rh D alloimmunization. It is made from pooled sterile human IgG antibodies to the Rh D antigen. With routine screening and use of RhoGAM, only 0.1% to 0.4% of pregnancies in Rh D− mothers are complicated by anti-Rh D antibody production.

    o RhoGAM may prevent alloimmunization by binding to any fetal RBCs that enter the maternal circulation. The fetal cells are then cleared by the mother's immune system.

Table 20-9	Atypical Blood Group Antibodies and Incidence of Hemolytic Disease of the Fetus and Newborn (HDFN)		
Frequency of HDFN	Disease Severity	Blood Group System	Antibody
Common	Mild to severe	Kell	K*
		Rh (non-D)	E*, c*
Uncommon	Mild to severe	Rh (non-D)	C*
		Duffy	Fy^a*
		Kidd	Jk^a
		MNSs	M, S, s, U
		Diego	D1^a, Di^b
	Mild	Duffy	By^3
		Kidd	Jk^b, Jk^3
		Kell	k, Ko, Kp^a, Kp^b, Js^a, Js^b
		MNSs	N
		MSSs	Vw, Mur, Hil, Hut
		Lutheran	Lu^a, Lu^b
	Moderate	MNSs	Mi^a
		MSSs	Mt^a
No occurrence	No occurrence	Lewis	NA
		I	NA
		Duffy	Fy^b

*Associated with hydrops fetalis.

- o In the United States, RhoGAM is routinely administered to Rh D− women at 28 weeks estimated gestational age (EGA), and again postpartum if neonatal Rh D+ status is confirmed. Postpartum administration should ideally occur within 72 hours of delivery for maximal protective effect; however, benefit has been suggested with administration as late as 28 days postpartum.
- The standard RhoGAM dose for routine prophylaxis is 300 μg IM.
- The 300 μg of RhoGAM is sufficient to prevent sensitization from 30 mL of fetal blood entering the maternal system. After an event likely to cause FMH, quantification of FMH with a Kleihauer-Betke test determines whether additional RhoGAM dosing is necessary.
  - o The half-life of RhoGAM is 24 days, but it can be detected on maternal antibody screens for up to 12 weeks.
- **Management of Rh-unsensitized patients**
  - o Pregnant patients are screened for antibodies by indirect Coombs test, in which maternal serum is exposed to Rh D+ RBCs. Lack of agglutination signifies the absence of circulating maternal antibody. If the indirect Coombs test is positive (ie, agglutination occurs), the laboratory must distinguish between sensitization and RhoGAM administration earlier in pregnancy.

- ∘ Rh D− pregnant patients should be screened at the first prenatal visit and again at 28 weeks EGA. If unsensitized, no intervention is required. At 28 weeks, a standard dose of 300 μg of RhoGAM is administered if the screen is negative. RhoGAM should also be administered during pregnancy if an Rh D− mother is exposed to a potential sensitizing event (trauma with significant FMH or invasive obstetrical procedures such as CVS, amniocentesis, or external cephalic version). If maternal sensitization occurs at any point during pregnancy, management is the same as it is for Rh-sensitized patients, as described below.
  - ∘ At the time of delivery, both the patient and infant are screened.
- If the neonate is Rh D−, no RhoGAM is necessary.
- If the neonate is Rh D+ and the mother is antibody negative, the standard dose of RhoGAM is given, and a Kleihauer-Betke test is performed to evaluate the need for additional RhoGAM.
- If the neonate is Rh D+ and the mother is antibody positive, no RhoGAM is given and the mother's next pregnancy is managed as Rh sensitized.
- When in question, RhoGAM is given. The risk of giving RhoGAM to a sensitized person is negligible compared with the consequences of permanent sensitization.
- **Management of Rh-sensitized patients**
  - ∘ If paternity is absolutely certain, paternal blood typing and zygosity testing are performed to determine whether the fetus can inherit the Rh D antigen.
- If the father is heterozygous for Rh D, the fetus has a 50% chance of being Rh D+.
- If the father is homozygous for Rh D, the fetus will be Rh D+ and is at risk.
- If the father is Rh D−, no further testing is indicated.
- Alternatively, cell-free DNA testing for fetal Rh D status can be performed with greater than 99% accuracy reported in the second trimester.
- If fetal Rh D status is unknown and the fetus is at risk for anemia, serial maternal D antibody titers can be followed monthly until 24 weeks and then every 2 to 4 weeks.
- Most Rh-sensitized patients have a chronic low D antibody titer. The fetus is not at risk of anemia until a critical titer is reached. The critical titer varies by laboratory but is usually between 1:8 and 1:16. The tests should be performed in the same laboratory.
- In the first affected pregnancy, titers correlate well with fetal status. In subsequent pregnancies, the titer may be less predictive.
- If the critical titer is reached and the fetus is at risk for anemia based on the paternal genotype, options for management include determination of fetal antigen status by amniocentesis or cell-free DNA testing to assess fetal risk.
- The use of middle cerebral arterial (MCA) Dopplers as a noninvasive test to track fetal anemia has eliminated the need for amniocentesis to assess the amniotic fluid spectrophotometric absorbance at 450 nm (ΔOD450). Most centers follow Dopplers every 1 to 2 weeks to detect evolving anemia. Doppler testing may begin as early as 16 to 18 weeks EGA.
- The MCA peak systolic velocity of blood is increased in severe anemia reflecting a decreased blood viscosity. A peak systolic velocity >1.5 multiples of the median suggests clinically significant anemia with a sensitivity that approaches 100% and a false-positive rate of 12%.
- Reliability of MCA Dopplers decreases after 35 weeks and after fetal blood transfusion.

- Fetal blood sampling via the fetal intrahepatic vein or by cordocentesis (also known as percutaneous umbilical blood sampling) allows direct fetal blood sampling and is the only method to confirm the diagnosis of fetal anemia. It is performed between 18 and 35 weeks' gestation usually in response to elevated MCA Dopplers.

- If the fetus is found to be anemic at the time of sampling, transfusion with $O-$, cytomegalovirus-negative, irradiated, and leukoreduced RBCs may be given with a target fetal Hct posttransfusion of 40% to 50%. Serial intrauterine transfusions are generally necessary once the fetus is found to be anemic, the timing of which are dictated by the expected decline in fetal Hct posttransfusion (approximately 1% per day).

- Fetal testing with serial nonstress tests and/or biophysical profiles may be performed weekly beginning at 28 to 32 weeks EGA in severe red cell alloimmunization.

- Delivery timing is individualized. Most experts recommend delivery at 37 to 38 weeks following a final fetal blood sampling and transfusion no later than 34 to 35 weeks EGA. In severely sensitized pregnancies that require multiple invasive procedures, the risk of continued procedures must be weighed against the risk of prematurity, and timing delivery at 32 to 34 weeks EGA can be considered.

- After birth, the neonate may be anemic or jaundiced secondary to hemolytic disease of the newborn. Mild cases are treated with red cell transfusion for anemia and phototherapy for hyperbilirubinemia. The IVIG or neonatal exchange transfusion may be required for more severe disease.

- Management of women with a previously affected pregnancy differs from management of women with their first affected pregnancy. In general, effects of alloimmunization on the fetus or infant become more severe with each subsequent pregnancy.

- If a patient previously had a significantly affected infant (ie, hydrops fetalis, need for intrauterine transfusion or neonatal exchange transfusion), maternal serum antibody titers are not useful in management because they may not correlate as well with fetal status.

- If necessary, paternal blood type and fetal antigen status are determined as previously described. If the fetus is Rh D+ or at risk to be so, evaluation for fetal anemia with MCA Dopplers begins at 16 to 18 weeks EGA.

- Other antigens in the Rh system include C, c, E, and e. If the mother is sensitized to any of these, management is generally the same as for RhD alloimmunization. The Du antigen, now referred to as weak D, is a clinically important D antigen variant with some weak D–positive patients being capable of producing anti-D antibody, although alloimmunization rarely occurs. Weak D–positive patients are considered Rh D− for the purposes of receiving a blood transfusion and should receive RhoGAM during pregnancy.

- The Kell group is the most common minor RBC antigen. At least seven different Kell antigens have been identified. The most common is K. Kell alloimmunization more often results from prior maternal transfusion. Unlike the other red cell antigens, anti-Kell antibodies cause both hemolysis and suppression of fetal erythropoietin/erythropoiesis; therefore, maternal serum antibody titers are not useful. Serial MCA Dopplers guide clinical management.

- **Other causes of fetal anemia.** Other less common causes of fetal anemia include acute parvovirus infection along with other viral, bacterial, and parasitic infections such as toxoplasmosis, cytomegalovirus, and syphilis; fetal α-thalassemia; fetal blood loss; abnormal myelopoiesis complicating Down syndrome; twin anemia-polycythemia sequence complicating monochorionic twin pregnancies; glucose-6-phosphate de-hydrogenase deficiency and pyruvate kinase deficiency; and genetic disorders such as Fanconi anemia and Diamond Blackfan anemia.

- Acute parvovirus infection is the most common infectious cause of fetal anemia. In cases of fetal parvovirus infection, the anemia is usually transient and the result of viral inhibition of erythropoiesis. Severe cases can require fetal transfusion. The risk for a poor fetal outcome is generally greater with congenital infection prior to 20 weeks of gestation, with a 15% risk of fetal death when infection is acquired between 13 and 20 weeks that decreases to 6% when infection is acquired after 20 weeks.

- Following parvovirus exposure, maternal IgG and IgM antibody status should be determined to assess maternal immune status. If testing indicates acute maternal infection (ie, IgM positive), weekly MCA Dopplers to assess for fetal anemia and ultrasound surveillance to asses for fetal hydrops should be initiated. If maternal serologic tests indicate susceptibility to infection (ie, IgM and IgG negative), repeat testing should occur in approximately 3 to 4 weeks. If either IgM or IgG is subse-quently positive, fetal surveillance should be initiated. The peak risk for hydrops is 4 to 6 weeks after maternal infection, but fetal surveillance generally continues for up to 10 to 12 weeks postexposure.

Fetal Thrombocytopenia

- **Maternal ITP-related thrombocytopenia.** In mothers with ITP, placental trans-fer of the IgG platelet antibodies can result in fetal or **neonatal thrombocytope-nia**. Approximately 8% to 15% of neonates will have severe thrombocytopenia (<50 000/μL). Maternal medical therapies to improve platelet counts in cases of ITP have not been shown to reliably prevent fetal thrombocytopenia or im-prove fetal outcome. The general consensus is that no correlation exists between maternal platelet count, or the presence of maternal platelet antibodies, and fetal platelet count. The most reliable indicator of fetal thrombocytopenia is a history of neonatal thrombocytopenia in a sibling. Fetal platelet count cannot be predicted accurately, and even fetal scalp sampling or percutaneous umbilical blood sampling does not provide reliable estimates. In ITP, the neonatal platelet count declines after delivery, reaching a nadir at 48 to 72 hours of life. Notification of a pediatrician for close monitoring of the neonatal platelet count is very important in preventing the sequelae of neonatal intracranial hemorrhage (ICH), a rare event. Some recom-mend obtaining umbilical cord platelet counts at delivery.
  - **Delivery mode.** Using the fetal platelet count to determine route of delivery is not recommended. This is because ICH appears to be more of a neonatal than an intrapartum event and due to the limitations in obtaining an accurate fetal platelet count. A survey of US perinatologists reported that most prefer not to perform invasive tests to evaluate fetal platelets and support a trial of labor. Unfortunately, no randomized controlled studies have compared delivery mode in these neonates. Previously, the assumption that a fetus with a platelet count lower than 50 000/μL is at significant risk for ICH, coupled with the belief that cesarean delivery is less traumatic than spontaneous vaginal delivery, led to the recommendation of cesarean delivery for severe fetal thrombocytopenia in ITP patients. However, there is no evidence that cesarean delivery decreases the risk of ICH. Cesarean delivery should be performed for obstetric indications only.

Should operative vaginal delivery be necessary, fetal thrombocytopenia is generally an accepted contraindication to vacuum-assisted vaginal delivery given the perceived increased fetal risks and should be approached with caution.

- **Neonatal alloimmune thrombocytopenia**, also called fetal alloimmune thrombocytopenia, is the platelet equivalent of hemolytic Rh disease of the newborn. It affects 1 in 1000 to 3000 live births, although the incidence varies by ethnicity. Over 15 platelet antigens have been identified to date, with varying severity of disease. Antibodies to platelet antigen HPA-1a are implicated in 80% of all NAIT cases and 90% of severe cases. Maternal platelet counts are unaffected.
  - **Pathophysiology.** Similar to RBC alloimmunization, maternal alloimmunization to fetal platelet antigens occurs with transplacental transfer of platelet-specific antibodies resulting in fetal platelet destruction. However, unlike RBC alloimmunization, NAIT can affect a first pregnancy and maternal antibody transfer can occur as early as the first trimester. Antibody-mediated destruction of fetal platelets in the most severe cases can result in fetal ICH or visceral hemorrhage.
    - Ten percent to 20% of fetuses with NAIT and platelet counts less than 50×10^9/L have ICH. Twenty-five percent to 50% of those can be detected in utero by ultrasound. Fetal death in utero occurs in approximately 14% of cases.
    - The same alloantigens are found as endothelial cell surface antigens; it is possible that hemorrhage may be exacerbated by immune-mediated damage to the lining of fetal capillaries.
  - **Diagnosis.** Diagnostic workup is prompted by clinical suspicion. There is currently no routine screening test for NAIT. An evaluation for NAIT may be initiated for any the following: Sonographic detection of in utero fetal hemorrhage, neonatal thrombocytopenia after delivery, or a prior pregnancy affected by NAIT or by fetal hemorrhage. Workup should also be initiated if the mother has a sister whose pregnancy was complicated by NAIT and who is HPA-1a negative.
    - The diagnosis of NAIT begins with determination of paternal HPA type and zygosity. Detection of maternal antiplatelet antibodies specific for paternal platelets and the incompatible antigen confirm the diagnosis. Antiplatelet antibodies are not always present or may be only intermittently present, and therefore, testing should be conducted at a laboratory with special interest and expertise in NAIT. If antigen-specific antiplatelet antibodies are not present in maternal blood, paternal platelet genotype discordance can help to confirm the NAIT diagnosis.
- If the paternal genotype is heterozygous for a platelet-specific antigen that the maternal genotype lacks, there is a 50% probability (for each discordant antigen) that the fetus is at risk for NAIT. Platelet genotyping from fetal blood or amniotic fluid should be performed.
- If the paternal genotype is homozygous for a platelet-specific antigen that the maternal genotype lacks, then all pregnancies are at risk.
- If the maternal and paternal genotypes are the same, the risk of an affected pregnancy is very low.
  - **Management.** Management of pregnancies at risk for NAIT varies among centers and should be individualized. There is no consensus on optimal treatment. The primary goal of management is to prevent ICH. Maternal antibody titers are not useful to guide treatment. Recent expert consensus recommends

stratified management based on prior pregnancy outcomes that include the presence or absence of ICH and gestational age of manifestation. Pregnancies at the highest risk of ICH include those with a previous fetus or neonates affected by ICH. Maternal therapy and guidance is then adjusted accordingly.

o The IVIG with or without corticosteroids (prednisone 0.5-1 mg/kg/d) is currently the recommended noninvasive therapy. In pregnancies at the highest risk for ICH, weekly maternal IVIG dosed at 1 to 2 g/kg/wk may be initiated at 12 weeks' gestation and continued throughout the pregnancy.

o Fetal blood sampling is the only way to determine fetal platelet count in pregnancies at risk for NAIT. Cordocentesis or intrahepatic vein blood sampling may be used. If a patient had a prior pregnancy that was severely affected by NAIT, she can be offered fetal blood sampling at 32 weeks' gestation if planning for a vaginal delivery to verify the fetal platelet response to therapy. Antigen-screened platelets can be transfused for severe fetal thrombocytopenia; however, the short half-life of transfused platelets may require weekly procedures and transfusions that can worsen the alloimmunization. For possible coincident anemia or acute procedure-related hemorrhage, RBC product is also made available during fetal blood sampling.

o Fetal sonographic assessment for growth and for any evidence of fetal hemorrhage is generally performed throughout pregnancy.

o Vaginal delivery is not contraindicated for fetuses with platelet counts greater than 100×10^9/L, but cesarean delivery is recommended for fetuses with platelet counts below this level, although it is not entirely protective against the development of ICH. At the time of delivery, a complete blood count is obtained on the cord blood.

o After delivery, neonatal platelet counts reach a nadir within the first few days after birth, and gradually improve over weeks as maternal antiplatelet antibodies resolve. Cranial ultrasound is performed to rule out ICH if platelets are <50 000/mL at birth.

o The recurrence rate is high in subsequent pregnancies (85%-90%). Fetuses may be affected more severely and at an earlier gestational age in subsequent pregnancies.

SUGGESTED READINGS

American College of Obstetricians and Gynecologists Committee on Adolescent Health Care. ACOG Committee Opinion No. 580: von Willebrand disease in women. *Obstet Gynecol.* 2013;122:1368-1373. (Reaffirmed 2017)

American College of Obstetricians and Gynecologists Committee on Practice Bulletins—Obstetrics. ACOG Practice Bulletin No. 78: hemoglobinopathies in pregnancy. *Obstet Gynecol.* 2007;109:229-237. (Reaffirmed 2018)

American College of Obstetricians and Gynecologists Committee on Practice Bulletins—Obstetrics. ACOG Practice Bulletin No. 95: anemia in pregnancy. *Obstet Gynecol.* 2008;112:201-207. (Reaffirmed 2017)

American College of Obstetricians and Gynecologists Committee on Practice Bulletins—Obstetrics. ACOG Practice Bulletin No. 132: antiphospholipid syndrome. *Obstet Gynecol.* 2012;120(6):1514-1521. (Reaffirmed 2017)

American College of Obstetricians and Gynecologists Committee on Practice Bulletins—Obstetrics. ACOG Practice Bulletin No. 181: prevention of Rh D alloimmunization. *Obstet Gynecol.* 2017;130:e57-e70.

American College of Obstetricians and Gynecologists Committee on Practice Bulletins—Obstetrics. ACOG Practice Bulletin No. 192: management of alloimmunization during pregnancy. *Obstet Gynecol*. 2018;131:e82-e90.

American College of Obstetricians and Gynecologists Committee on Practice Bulletins—Obstetrics. ACOG Practice Bulletin No. 196: thromboembolism in pregnancy. *Obstet Gynecol*. 2018;132:e1-e17.

American College of Obstetricians and Gynecologists Committee on Practice Bulletins—Obstetrics. ACOG Practice Bulletin No. 197: inherited thrombophilias in pregnancy. *Obstet Gynecol*. 2018;132:e18-e34.

American College of Obstetricians and Gynecologists Committee on Practice Bulletins—Obstetrics. ACOG Practice Bulletin No. 207: thrombocytopenia in pregnancy. *Obstet Gynecol*. 2019;133:e181-e193.

Croles FN, Nasserinejad K, Duvekot JJ, Kruip MJ, Meijer K, Leebeek FW. Pregnancy, thrombophilia, and the risk of a first venous thrombosis: systematic review and Bayesian meta-analysis. *BMJ*. 2017;359:j4452. doi:10.1136/bmj.j4452.

Kadir RA, McLintock C. Thrombocytopenia and disorders of platelet function in pregnancy. *Semin Thromb Hemost*. 2011;37(6):640-652.

Kearon C, Akl EA, Ornelas J, et al. Antithrombotic therapy for VTE disease: CHEST guideline and expert panel report. *Chest*. 2016;149(2):315-352.

Mari G, Norton ME, Stone J, et al. Society for Maternal-Fetal Medicine (SMFM) Clinical Guideline #8: the fetus at risk for anemia—diagnosis and management. *Am J Obstet Gynecol*. 2015;212(6):697-710.

Peterson JA, McFarland JG, Curtis BR, Aster RH. Neonatal alloimmune thrombocytopenia: pathogenesis, diagnosis and management. *Br J Haematol*. 2013;161(1):3-14.

Vaught AJ, Gavriilaki E, Hueppchen N, et al. Direct evidence of complement activation in HELLP syndrome: a link to atypical hemolytic uremic syndrome. *Exp Hematol*. 2016;44(5):390-398.

Ware RE, de Montalembert M, Tshilolo L, Abboud MR. Sickle cell disease. *Lancet*. 2017; 390(10091):311-323.

Winkelhorst D, Murphy MF, Greinacher A, et al. Antenatal management in fetal and neonatal alloimmune thrombocytopenia: a systematic review. *Blood*. 2017;129(11):1538-1547.

Neoplastic Diseases in Pregnancy

Meghan McMahon and Jessica L. Bienstock

Cancer in pregnancy is rare, with an incidence of 1 in 1000 (0.1%) pregnant women. The most common malignancies in pregnancy are breast, melanoma, and cervical cancer; however, ovarian and hematologic cancers are also present in this population.

A new diagnosis of cancer in pregnancy can be very challenging for the patient and provider due to the need to balance risks and benefits of treatment for both mother and fetus. In these scenarios, a multidisciplinary approach is critical and should include an obstetrician, maternal fetal medicine specialist, neonatologist, oncologist, pharmacist, social worker, and psychosocial support services. This chapter reviews general management principles as well as focus on specific cancers most common in this population and discusses the long-term outcomes for mother and child. Given the rarity of occurrence, most of the literature is based on expert opinion, case reports, and small studies.

GENERAL TREATMENT CONCEPTS

When there is a suspicion for cancer, the evaluation should not be delayed due to pregnancy. Delay in diagnosis may affect treatment and ultimately prognosis.

Imaging

- In general, imaging should aim to limit radiation exposure.
- Ultrasound is often the first-line imaging modality and the preferred method. Magnetic resonance imaging (MRI) without gadolinium can also safely be used with no increased risk to the fetus. Gadolinium is a class C agent and crosses the placenta into fetal circulation. American College of Obstetricians and Gynecologists recommends the use of gadolinium contrast with MRI if it will significantly enhance diagnostic performance and would improve fetal or maternal outcomes.
- Other imaging modalities such as x-ray, computed tomography (CT), and mammogram require ionizing radiation, which is a teratogen and can potentially harm the fetus. Adverse outcomes include miscarriage, developmental delay, organ malformation, and increased risk of childhood cancer such as leukemia. However, these outcomes are dependent on the dose of radiation and gestational age of exposure.
  - Plain films have a negligible dose of radiation to the fetus if it is not in the field of view and the recommended shield is placed on the abdomen (Table 21-1). Even abdominal and lumbar x-rays have a very low dose of radiation exposure to the fetus (1-3 mGy), especially when compared to the general background radiation exposure (0.5-1 mGy).
  - Table 21-1 also demonstrates the fetal absorbed doses of radiation for CT scans. Even a CT of the abdomen and pelvis is safe in pregnancy because the exposure (25 mGy) remains less than the threshold dose (100-200 mGy) to cause harm. A CT can also be safely performed with intravenous iodinated and oral contrast in pregnancy (class B agent) because little to none crosses the placenta. Studies have shown no adverse effects of intravenous and oral contrast in animal pregnancies.

Surgery

- Surgery may be necessary in the diagnosis or treatment of cancer and can be performed at any gestational age. However, data shows there is an increased risk of miscarriage in the first trimester. In particular, adnexal surgery should be delayed if possible to the second trimester when the placenta has fully taken over progesterone production from the corpus luteum.
- The greatest risk of surgery in pregnancy is preterm labor with subsequent preterm delivery. Fetal assessment should be performed before and after the procedure with Doppler or ultrasound documentation of the presence of a fetal heartbeat (<24 wk) or nonstress test (>24 wk). Patients should be counseled appropriately regarding these risks and the possible need for emergent delivery via cesarean delivery for a nonreassuring fetal heart tracing. If the patient is at a viable gestational age, the treatment team should consider betamethasone administration and a neonatal intensive care unit consult prior to surgery and discuss with the patient her desires regarding potential emergent cesarean delivery.

Table 21-1	Estimated Fetal Radiation Exposure With Common Imaging Modalities

Imaging	Fetal Absorbed Dose (mGy)[a]
Plain radiograph	
Chest (PA, left)	0.001-0.002
Abdominal (AP)	1-3
Extremities	0.001
Cervical spine	<0.001
Thoracic spine	0.003
Lumbar spine (AP, lat)	1
Limited IVP	6
Barium enema	7
Mammogram	0.2
Computed tomography	
Head	0.5
Chest	0.1
Pulmonary angiogram	0.2
Abdomen	4
Abdomen/pelvis	25
KUB	10
Background (control)	0.5-1
Threshold risk	100-200

Abbreviations: AP, anteroposterior; IVP, intravenous pyelogram; KUB, kidneys, ureter, bladder; lat, lateral; PA, posteroanterior.
[a]1 rad = 10 mGy; 1 mGy = 0.001 Gy.
[b]Data from Sadro CT, Dubinsky TJ. CT in pregnancy: risks and benefits. *Appl Radiol.* 2013;42(10):6-16.

- During surgery, special considerations of the physiologic changes of pregnancy and the pharmacologic safety profile of medications can be challenging. The supine position may be detrimental to the fetus primarily in the third trimester secondary to compression of the inferior vena cava with decreased venous return causing reduced uterine perfusion. Pregnant women also experience delayed gastric emptying placing them at higher risk for aspiration. Pregnancy is also a hypercoagulable state, which may warrant thrombo-prophylaxis in high-risk patients and surgeries. Therefore, it is important to work closely with the anesthesia team during surgery to mitigate these risks to mother and fetus.

Radiotherapy

- Compared to imaging studies discussed under "Imaging" within "General Treatment Concepts" section, treatment radiotherapy exposes the fetus to much higher radiation doses. The developing fetus is highly susceptible to the damaging effects of radiation.

It can have severe adverse fetal effects including intrauterine growth restriction (IUGR), developmental delay, malformations, childhood cancer, or even fetal death. These outcomes depend on gestational age, radiation dose, and treatment site.

- During organogenesis, weeks 2 to 8, exposure to radiation has the highest risk of leading to fetal malformation. During weeks 8 to 25 of gestation, the central nervous system is especially sensitive to radiation. Exposure to 100 mGy can cause a decrease in IQ and exposure to doses greater than 500 mGy significantly increase the risk of growth restriction and central nervous system damage. Hiroshima and Nagasaki radiation survivors demonstrated this high risk of brain damage and developmental delay between 8 and 15 weeks of gestation. After 20 weeks' gestation, anomalies in offspring of women exposed to nuclear bomb explosions were not as severe, and the adverse effects of anemia, pigmentation changes, and erythema were seen more often. There are also reports of childhood cancer and sterility in fetuses exposed to radiation.
- Treatment site plays a critical role. Supradiaphragmatic therapy (ie, head, neck, breast, and extremities) with appropriate shielding can have very little fetal exposure. Most cancers that are remote from the pelvis can be treated with radiation in pregnancy when necessary. However, cancers in the pelvis cannot be adequately treated without potential serious or even lethal effects to the fetus. Therefore, radiation therapy directed in the pelvis is often postponed until the postpartum period if possible.

Chemotherapy

- Chemotherapy agents are designed to target cells that are rapidly dividing and are therefore often teratogenic. Systemic treatment in the first trimester carries a high risk of miscarriage and fetal malformations. The risk of congenital malformation in the first trimester is 7% to 17% with a single agent and as high as 25% in combination therapy. Thus, chemotherapy is generally delayed until after the first trimester. However, in aggressive or advanced disease, delaying treatment may have significant adverse consequences and therefore prompt treatment may be recommended even in the first trimester. If treatment is required in the first trimester, the safest agents include anthracycline antibiotics, vinca alkaloids, or single-agent treatment.
- Potential adverse outcomes in the second and third trimester include transient fetal hematologic suppression, growth restriction, prematurity, preterm rupture of membranes, and stillbirth. Fetal surveillance is recommended, including growth scans every 3 weeks and antepartum testing with nonstress tests beginning at 32 weeks or sooner. Unlike radiotherapy, several studies have shown that chemotherapy given in the second and third trimester does not have a significant impact on neurodevelopment and cognitive capabilities, future malignancies, or fertility in offspring.
- In general, alkylating agents (cyclophosphamide) and antimetabolites (methotrexate) have the greatest risk for adverse pregnancy outcomes, whereas platinum adducts (carboplatin), taxanes (paclitaxel), and antibiotic agents (doxorubicin) have the lowest risk. In addition, it is advised to discontinue chemotherapy after 35 weeks to allow the fetus to eliminate the cytotoxic drug in order to avoid fetal myelosuppression at the time of delivery. Delivery should also be avoided 2 to 3 weeks after treatment to avoid the maternal hematologic nadir.

Table 21-2 Common Cancers in Pregnancy[a]

Cancer Type	Incidence	Symptoms	Initial Evaluation
Breast cancer	1:3000-10 000	Palpable, painless mass Bloody nipple discharge Skin changes	Ultrasound Core needle biopsy
Cervical cancer	1-2:2000-10 000	Abnormal cervical cytology Friable exophytic mass	Colposcopy/biopsy Conization
Ovarian cancer	1:10 000	Mass incidentally found on ultrasound Abnormal pain/bloating	Ultrasound Surgery
Melanoma	1-2.6:1000	New or growing skin lesion	Tumor excision/biopsy
Lymphoma	1:1000-6000	Painless lymphadenopathy Systemic symptoms: fevers or chills	Chest radiograph Bone marrow biopsy Abdominal ultrasound
Thyroid cancer	0.2-1.4:10 000	Palpable thyroid nodule	Fine needle aspiration
Colorectal cancer	1:13 000	Bloody stool Abdominal pain Diarrhea	Colonoscopy

[a]Adapted from Salani R, Billingsley CC, Crafton SM. Cancer and pregnancy: an overview for obstetricians and gynecologists. *Am J Obstet Gynecol.* 2014;211:7-14.

SPECIFIC NEOPLASTIC CARCINOMAS

Cervical Carcinoma

- Cervical carcinoma is the most common gynecologic cancer diagnosed in pregnancy (see Table 21-2). Abnormalities on cervical cytology are found in up to 5% to 8% of all pregnancies. However, invasive cervical cancer is only present in about 1 to 10 per 10 000 pregnancies.
- **Diagnosis**
  - Pregnancy routinely involves visualization of the cervix and pelvic examination. For this reason, most patients who are diagnosed in pregnancy are found in early stages. According to Zemlickis (1991), of pregnant women diagnosed with cervical cancer, 69% to 83% were in International Federation of Gynecology and

Obstetrics stage I, 11% to 23% were in stage II, 3% to 8% were in stage III, and 0% to 3% were in stage IV.

- Routine Pap smear screening is recommended during pregnancy. Normal physiologic changes of pregnancy (ie, cervical vascularity, hypertrophy and hyperplasia of endocervical glands) can cause false-positive rates on Pap smears and mimic more severe dysplasia. These changes can also make colposcopy challenging in pregnancy.
- If a Pap smear is abnormal, patients should undergo further management according to American Society for Colposcopy and Cervical Pathology guidelines, except for a few specific recommendations in pregnancy:
  - If Pap smear result is atypical squamous cells of undetermined significance, low-grade squamous intraepithelial lesion, or negative cytology with + human papillomavirus, it is acceptable to defer colposcopy until 6 weeks postpartum.
  - Cervical conization (including loop electrosurgical excision procedure and cold knife cone [CKC]) is generally contraindicated in pregnancy because of the high complication rate (hemorrhage, abortion, premature labor/delivery, infection) and the high incidence of residual lesions. Conization can be used to confirm microinvasive disease when there is a very high suspicion and diagnosis would alter timing or mode of delivery.
  - Endocervical curettage is relatively contraindicated in pregnancy due to concern for disruption of pregnancy.
- Colposcopy and cervical biopsies are safe in pregnancy. Therefore, if Pap smear results are atypical squamous cells, cannot exclude high-grade squamous intraepithelial lesion, and/or atypical glandular cells, colposcopy is recommended. At the time of colposcopy, biopsies should be performed for lesions suspicious for cervical intraepithelial neoplasia (CIN) 2 or 3 or cancer. Otherwise, if lower grade CIN 1 is suspected, repeat cytology and colposcopy can be performed 6 weeks postpartum. If biopsy shows no CIN 2 or 3, then a repeat Pap smear postpartum is recommended. If biopsy shows CIN 2 or 3, colposcopy and Pap test should be repeated every trimester and postpartum. Repeat biopsies should be taken if the lesion worsens or cytology suggests invasive carcinoma.
- Progression of dysplastic lesions to invasive carcinoma in pregnancy is rare (0%-0.4%) and even regression can occur. If more advanced disease is suspected, additional imaging may be required. Chest x-ray (with abdominal shielding) is recommended to evaluate for pulmonary metastasis. Ultrasonography can be used to evaluate the urinary tract, including evaluating for hydronephrosis. An MRI may also be useful to evaluate tumor volume and spread to adjacent organs. However, to evaluate small lymph node involvement, conventional MRI is poor. Laparoscopic lymphadenectomy is the gold standard for lymph node assessment and can be safely performed in pregnancy.

- **Treatment**
  - If invasive carcinoma is diagnosed in pregnancy, a referral to a gynecologic oncologist is imperative. The treatment options in pregnancy depend on the patient's desire for continuation or termination of the pregnancy as well as the clinical stage of the disease. Patients desiring to preserve their pregnancy must be informed it is not the standard of care and must understand those associated risks. For those patients who wish to continue their pregnancy, routine surveillance is crucial to monitor progression of disease. In microinvasive disease, colposcopy

and clinical exams should be performed every trimester. In all other stages, pelvic exams should be performed every 3 to 4 weeks in pregnancy.

- ○ **Microinvasive disease (stage IA1):** The standard of treatment is a CKC or simple hysterectomy.
  - ○ In desired pregnancies, CKC can be performed with counseling regarding the known risks of bleeding and spontaneous abortion. The CKC is generally considered safest in the second trimester. If there are negative margins, the patient can proceed with vaginal delivery at term. If the patient is at more advanced gestational age at diagnosis, delaying treatment until after delivery is appropriate with surveillance (ie, clinical examinations and colposcopy) every trimester.
  - ○ If the pregnancy is undesired, the patient may opt for pregnancy termination followed by CKC or simple hysterectomy, or simple hysterectomy with the fetus in situ.
- ○ **Stage IA2 to IB1 tumor size <2 cm**
  - ○ If previable gestational age, stage IA2 to a subset of IB1 with tumor size <2 cm, a pelvic lymph node dissection is recommended. If node negative, the recommendation is to then perform definitive treatment with conization or simple trachelectomy (radical trachelectomy has been associated with high incidence of fetal loss). If node positive, the recommendation is neoadjuvant chemotherapy.
  - ○ If diagnosed at a later gestational age, surgical lymphadenectomy becomes more challenging with a large uterus and carries an increased risk of complications related to surgery (ie, preterm labor). It is acceptable to delay treatment until after delivery with close surveillance for disease progression. There is evidence to support no change in prognosis or survival with delaying treatment.
  - ○ If the patient desires pregnancy termination, then radical hysterectomy with pelvic lymphadenectomy with the fetus in situ is recommended.
- ○ **Stage IB1 (tumor ≥2 cm) or higher:** For patients diagnosed with stage IB1 with tumor size ≥2 cm, the recommendation is for either lymph node assessment or neoadjuvant chemotherapy. If lymphadenectomy is performed, para-aortic lymph nodes should also be assessed if the tumor size is ≥4 cm. If lymph nodes are negative, then neoadjuvant chemotherapy is acceptable. If lymph nodes are positive, there is a higher risk of disease progression. Recommend further discussion of termination with definitive treatment as an alternative to neoadjuvant chemotherapy. Delaying treatment in patients with stage IB1 with large tumors ≥2 cm is not recommended. If surgery cannot be performed safely, recommend neoadjuvant chemotherapy.
- ○ **Metastatic disease:** The prognosis for metastatic cervical cancer is poor, making this diagnosis in pregnancy extremely challenging for the patient. In general, treatment is medical with the goal to control disease, usually with chemotherapy.
- ○ **Adenocarcinoma:** There is limited evidence or recommendations for adenocarcinoma in pregnancy but in general, stage by stage, can be treated similarly to squamous cell carcinoma with comparable prognosis.
- • The recommended chemotherapy regimen used during pregnancy is the same as for nonpregnant patients and includes cisplatin every 3 weeks for up to six cycles. Chemotherapy is typically given until 34 to 35 weeks of gestation with delivery planned at term (approximately 3 wk after last chemotherapy).

- **Delivery:** There are no randomized trials comparing the mode of delivery (cesarean delivery vs vaginal delivery). Based on case reports and retrospective studies, in patients with microinvasive disease (stages IA1 and IA2) vaginal delivery appears to be safe; however, episiotomy should be avoided because case reports have recounted recurrence at episiotomy sites. Although there is little data, for women with stage IB1 or greater, vaginal delivery is generally avoided because of data to suggest worse outcomes (ie, obstructed labor and hemorrhage). Definitive treatment can also be accomplished at the time of delivery with a radical hysterectomy at the time of cesarean delivery.
- **Prognosis:** The majority of studies, after stratifying by stage, demonstrate there is no difference between the prognosis of pregnant and nonpregnant women. The effect of cervical cancer on the pregnancy is controversial. Some studies suggest no difference in outcomes (ie, preterm delivery, IUGR, and stillbirth), whereas others indicate lower birth rates and preterm delivery. However, most preterm delivery was iatrogenic in these studies.

Ovarian Carcinoma

- Adnexal masses are commonly diagnosed during routine ultrasound evaluation in pregnancy, most of which are benign. Approximately 1% to 3% of adnexal masses will be malignant (see Table 21-2).
- The typical presentation is an incidental finding on ultrasound. However, other clinical presentations, including lower quadrant abdominal pain, bloating, bowel and urinary symptoms, a palpable adnexal mass, and more rarely acute abdominal pain secondary to torsion or rupture. Most adnexal masses in pregnancy can be managed conservatively because there is a low risk of malignancy or complications, and 50% to 90% resolve spontaneously.
- In pregnancy, the most common ovarian malignancies are germ cell (ie, dysgerminomas, endodermal sinus tumors, immature teratomas, and mixed germ cell tumors), sex cord stromal (ie, granulosa and Sertoli-Leydig), borderline (ie, epithelial tumors of low malignant potential), and more rarely invasive epithelial tumors.
- **Diagnosis**
  - Evaluation of adnexal masses is similar to that of nonpregnant patients. Ultrasonography can be used to characterize the adnexal mass. If additional imaging is required, MRI is the imaging of choice. Unfortunately, typical tumor markers such as human chorionic gonadotropin, α-fetoprotein (AFP), cancer antigen 125 (CA 125), and inhibin A can be skewed in pregnancy. The CA 125 levels peak in the first trimester and decrease thereafter, making CA 125 a helpful tumor marker after the first trimester; levels greater than 1000 are unlikely a consequence of pregnancy and more suggestive of cancer. The AFP also normally rises in pregnancy until the third trimester. However, AFP levels are much higher in germ cell tumors than those associated with NTD on the level of above 9 multiples of the mean. Carcinoembryonic antigen, cancer antigen 19-9, and lactate dehydrogenase can be reliably used in pregnancy. Human epididymis protein 4 is being used more often to detect and manage ovarian cancer, but it can have low levels in pregnancy and is less studied.
  - Definitive diagnosis can only be made on pathologic examination. In general, ovarian masses are removed after the first trimester if they have the following

features: (1) >10 cm in diameter or (2) contain features concerning for carcinoma, including papillary or solid components, irregularity, presence of ascites, and high color Doppler flow.

- The optimal timing for surgery is in the second trimester. After the first trimester, almost all functional cysts have resolved, the production of progesterone has been taken over by the placenta, so removing a corpus luteum will not disrupt the pregnancy, and there is a decreased risk of spontaneous miscarriage. In addition, in the second trimester, the uterine size usually does not hinder a laparoscopic approach.

- If there is a high suspicion for cancer, peritoneal washings should be obtained. Ipsilateral salpingo-oophorectomy is recommended and sent to pathology. The contralateral ovary should be examined with biopsy or wedge resection if involvement is present.

- **Treatment:** If cancer is diagnosed on pathology, a gynecology oncology specialist should be consulted. The staging procedure includes free fluid or peritoneal washings for evaluation, systemic evaluation of all intra-abdominal organs and surfaces, peritoneal biopsies, diaphragm biopsy, omentectomy, and evaluation of pelvic and para-aortic lymph nodes. Typically, this is accompanied by total abdominal hysterectomy and bilateral salpingo-oophorectomy. However, in the setting of desired pregnancy, this is not performed. Subsequent treatment is based on histologic type of ovarian malignancy as well as stage and grade.

  - **Epithelial ovarian cancer:** The recommendation for adjuvant treatment and chemotherapy regimen is similar in pregnant and nonpregnant women. Chemotherapy regimens usually include a platinum drug plus taxane (ie, carboplatin and paclitaxel). It is recommended to initiate chemotherapy after the first trimester. In early-stage disease, delay of treatment can be considered until postpartum.

  - **Germ cell ovarian tumors:** Adjuvant chemotherapy is typically recommended except for stage IA dysgerminoma or stage 1 grade 1 immature teratoma. The most commonly used regimen is bleomycin, etoposide, and cisplatin (BEP). However, these are relatively toxic (especially etoposide) and associated with fetal growth restriction and myelosuppression at birth. Acceptable alternative regimens are cisplatin plus paclitaxel, paclitaxel-carboplatin, or cisplatin-vinblastine-bleomycin.

  - **Tumors of low malignant potential (borderline):** Treatment is generally surgical without the need for adjuvant chemotherapy.

  - **Sex cord stromal tumors:** Most of these tumors progress slowly and the benefit of adjuvant chemotherapy is variable. Therefore, the recommendation is surgical management with oophorectomy and decision for additional treatment deferred until the postpartum period.

- **Prognosis:** There is no evidence that pregnancy worsens prognosis when compared to nonpregnant women and tumor stage, grade, and histology are matched. Most ovarian malignancies diagnosed in pregnancy are early-stage cancers and thus have good 5-year survival rates.

Breast Carcinoma

- Breast cancer occurs in about 1 in 3000 pregnant women. Approximately 1% to 2% of women with breast cancer are first diagnosed during pregnancy (see Table 21-2).

- Similar to the general population, breast cancer typically presents with a palpable mass, skin changes, or bloody nipple discharge. Unfortunately, these findings are often attributed to pregnancy-induced breast changes and can result in a delay of treatment by up to 5 months and increased risk of more advanced stage breast cancer at time of diagnosis. One study showed that 42% of patients diagnosed in pregnancy were stage 3.

- **Diagnosis**
  - Often, the first line of evaluation includes breast ultrasonography. Mammography can be safely preformed in pregnancy with a low radiation exposure (0.2 mGy), well below toxic exposure levels. However, the sensitivity may be decreased because of increased glandularity and water content of the breast during pregnancy. If there is high suspicion on imaging, diagnostic measures should be taken with core needle biopsy or excisional biopsy.
  - Evaluation for metastasis should only be conducted if there is a high suspicion based on additional clinical findings and laboratory results, or if it would alter the course of therapy. The most common sites of metastasis are lungs, liver, and bone. The preferred workup for metastasis includes CT scan of the brain, chest radiograph with shielding, hepatic scan with radionucleotides, and radionucleotide bone scan; however, alternatives may be used, such as ultrasound of liver or MRI of spine without contrast.

- **Treatment**
  - In any diagnosis of cancer in pregnancy, if diagnosed early, providers may offer therapeutic abortion. However, for breast cancer, reports do not show an advantage in survival after therapeutic abortion. In general, the treatment of breast cancer should follow the same principles and criteria as those for nonpregnant patients. There are a few special considerations in pregnancy:
    - If the patient is near term, treatment may be delayed until the postpartum period.
    - Chemotherapy is safe but often deferred until the second trimester.
    - Radiation or hormonal therapies are deferred to the postpartum period.
  - A modified radical mastectomy is the treatment of choice for early-stage disease. Breast conservative therapy includes lumpectomy plus radiation therapy and has been shown to be equivalent to mastectomy in nonpregnant women. Radiation therapy is generally not given in pregnancy due to the detrimental effects on the fetus. Therefore, if there is going to be a significant delay in treatment with radiation therapy >6 months, breast conservation therapy may not be recommended because of an increased risk of local recurrence.
  - Axillary lymph node assessment is a routine component of management of breast cancer for prognosis and adjuvant treatment. Sentinel lymph node biopsy (SLNB) accurately predicts lymph node status in clinically node negative patients. However, for positive lymph node involvement, axillary lymph node dissection is necessary. There is little data regarding the safety of SLNB in pregnancy, but there are increasing numbers of case series that show no fetal defects with SLNB and the use of technetium-99.
  - Adjuvant systemic therapy is then based on tumor characteristics such as size, grade, lymph nodes, estrogen or progesterone receptor status, and human epidermal growth factor receptor 2 (HER2) receptors.
    - **Endocrine sensitive:** Typically, hormonal agents (ie, luteinizing hormone-releasing hormone, tamoxifen) are contraindicated in pregnancy. Tamoxifen is associated with miscarriage, congenital malformations, and fetal death.

In addition, the long-term effects on a female fetus are unknown. For node-negative and low-proliferative disease, it is acceptable to observe until delivery and then start hormonal therapy. However, for node-positive signs of aggressive disease, or metastatic cancer, chemotherapy (anthracycline based) is initiated in the second trimester.

- o **HER2 positive:** HER2-targeted agents (ie, trastuzumab) are contraindicated in pregnancy. Exposure to trastuzumab can lead to oligohydramnios/anhydramnios with severe sequela, including pulmonary hypoplasia, skeletal abnormalities, and neonatal death. Treatment generally includes anthracycline, based chemotherapy initiated in the second trimester. Taxanes can also be added. If disease is metastatic and chemotherapy/trastuzumab needs to be initiated in the first trimester, termination should be discussed.
- o **Triple negative:** Recommended treatment includes anthracycline-based chemotherapy. Taxanes can also be added if needed.
- o **Locally advanced breast cancer (subset IIB, IIIA to IIIC):** managed with multimodal therapy with systemic and regional therapy. Patients often undergo neoadjuvant systemic therapy followed by surgery and assessment of regional nodes. Less commonly, patients undergo primary surgery followed by postoperative radiation therapy and adjuvant systemic treatment.
- An anthracycline-based regimen includes doxorubicin plus cyclophosphamide (AC) or fluorouracil, doxorubicin, and cyclophosphamide (FAC). These regimens are overall safe in pregnancy. To date, there are no studies that show an increased risk of fetal cardiotoxicity.
- **Prognosis:** The prognosis has been found to be similar among pregnant and nonpregnant women with breast cancer when matched by age and stage. However, pregnant women have a higher chance of being diagnosed at a later stage and thus may experience a worse prognosis. Also, like most young women, pregnant patients often have estrogen receptor–negative tumors, which are not affected by the circulating hormones of pregnancy but do carry a worse prognosis.

Other Common Carcinoma in Reproductive-Aged Women

Melanoma

- Melanoma is the most common cancer diagnosed in pregnancy, representing 8% of malignancies in pregnancy (see Table 21-2). Melanoma is also increasing in incidence, especially in women aged 15 to 39 years. There is strong evidence to suggest that pregnancy has no adverse effect on the development or prognosis of melanoma.
- Similar to nonpregnant patients, patients should look for asymmetry, border irregularity, nonuniform color, diameter >6 mm, and evolving size of pigmented lesions. However, in pregnancy, hyperpigmentation of lesions is normal and may lead to delay in diagnosis. All concerning lesions require histopathologic evaluation via biopsy.
- The thickness of melanoma is the most important factor in determining the stage of the lesion. The thickness also determines the recommended margin of resection required. Treatment generally includes excision of the tumor. The goal of surgical resection is complete removal with negative margins to reduce the risk of local recurrence. An SLNB is recommended in patients with melanoma in whom there

is a high risk of regional node metastasis. However, SLNB remains controversial in pregnancy secondary to the use of blue dye and technetium-99, but there is growing evidence that these are safe in pregnancy. However, some practitioners still delay SLNB until after delivery.

- In cases where advanced melanoma is present, additional imaging may be considered. The recommended imaging modalities by American College of Obstetricians and Gynecologists include chest radiography with shielding, ultrasonography, and MRI. Common sites of metastasis include lungs, liver, adrenal, brain, kidney, bone, intestine, pancreas, spleen, stomach, and urinary bladder. Malignant melanoma is the most common tumor to metastasize to the placenta, although metastasis still remains a rare occurrence. After delivery, a thorough evaluation of the placenta is recommended to identify metastasis, including microscopic examination, as only 50% of metastases are visible. If metastasis is present, it carries a poor prognosis for both mother and fetus, and the newborn should be monitored closely for malignant disease.

Hematologic

- **Leukemia**
  - The diagnosis of leukemia in pregnancy is rare, occurring in approximately 1 in 75 000 to 100 000 pregnancies. The most common type is acute lymphoblastic leukemia (28%). Leukemia typically presents with lab abnormalities including anemia, granulocytopenia, and thrombocytopenia. Clinically, patients may develop splenomegaly, adenopathy, serious infection, or bleeding diathesis. Acute leukemia requires immediate treatment regardless of gestational age because delay in therapy can negatively affect prognosis.
  - Recommendations for treatment are limited given the rarity of diagnosis in pregnancy. The two largest reviews, one from Mayo Clinic with 17 cases and the other from 13 French centers with 37 cases, included patients treated with vincristine, daunorubicin, idarubicin, cytarabine, cyclophosphamide, asparaginase, mercaptopurine, prednisone, methotrexate, mitoxantrone, and all-trans retinoic acid, which were given in all trimesters. Adverse effects included IUGR, congenital abnormalities, and fetal and neonatal deaths. Generally, daunorubicin is the anthracycline of choice in pregnancy, yet fetal cardiac function should be monitored because of rare cases of fetal cardiotoxocity.
  - Remission rates are high, ranging from 60% to 80%; however, recurrence is common, often with poor outcomes.
- **Lymphoma**
  - Incidence is estimated at approximately 1 in 1000 to 6000 pregnancies (see Table 21-2). Hodgkin lymphoma occurs in younger women, whereas non-Hodgkin lymphoma occurs later in life. Lymphadenopathy is the most common presenting symptom and is often asymptomatic. Other symptoms include fever, night sweats, weight loss, and pruritus.
  - The standard treatment in nonpregnant patients uses radiotherapy combined with chemotherapy with high cure rates. The treatment in pregnant patients depends on trimester and extent of disease. If diagnosed in the third trimester with localized disease, treatment can be postponed until after delivery. However, if diagnosed in the first or second trimester or in patients with poor prognosis, pregnancy termination may be considered to provide nodal irradiation. If pregnancy

continuation is desired, generally, treatment is limited to multiagent chemotherapy. However, radiation may be given, especially in supradiaphragmatic regions.

OUTCOMES AND FOLLOW-UP

Neonatal Outcomes

- There are no prospective clinical studies evaluating the short- and long-term effects of chemotherapy on pregnancy. Therefore, the data is based on case studies and retrospective studies. Neonatal outcomes including miscarriage, congenital abnormalities, preterm delivery, IUGR, and stillbirth are primarily dependent on gestational age and type of chemotherapeutic agent. There are increased rates of spontaneous abortion in the first 4 weeks and birth defects during weeks 5 to 12 when cytotoxic agents are required. Fetuses exposed in the second and third trimester have the same rate of birth defects as the general population, but exposure has been linked to IUGR, prematurity, and stillbirth.
- In the periimplantation and immediate postimplantation period, radiation has an all-or-none effect, resulting in early pregnancy loss or development of normal pregnancy. High-dose radiation exposure is often deferred in pregnancy because it is associated with poor outcomes, including spontaneous abortion, developmental delay, microcephaly, and IUGR. However, radiation has been safely used outside the pelvis with appropriate shielding.
- Antenatal fetal well-being should be closely monitored with the consultation of a maternal fetal medicine specialist. Antenatal testing and serial growth ultrasounds are generally indicated. If delivery is anticipated prematurely, antenatal steroids are also recommended.

Breastfeeding

In general, breastfeeding is contraindicated in women receiving chemotherapy or hormonal therapy because there is no short-term or long-term safety data. An exception to this guidance is azathioprine, which has failed to show accumulation in milk.

Future Pregnancy

- A large proportion of women diagnosed with cancer are less than 40 years of age with future reproductive goals. Subsequent pregnancy rates are 40% lower among cancer survivors compared to the general population, although these rates are dependent on type of cancer, with survivors of breast cancer having the lowest rates of successful pregnancy. Breast cancer survivors who do become pregnant have no difference in neonatal outcomes when compared to the general population. There is no defined timeline for when patients may attempt pregnancy after treatment. However, some specialists recommend a 2-year disease-free period because that is the highest window for recurrence.
- Prior to women starting cancer treatment, the American Society of Clinical Oncology recommends that physicians address future fertility options and outcomes and provide prompt referrals to reproductive specialists. Fertility-sparing techniques include oocyte/embryo banking, ovarian tissue cryopreservation, ovarian suppression with gonadotropin-releasing hormone agonists, fertility preserving surgery, and ovarian transposition.

SUGGESTED READINGS

American College of Obstetricians and Gynecologists Committee on Obstetric Practice. ACOG Committee Opinion No. 723: guidelines for diagnostic imaging during pregnancy and lactation. *Obstet Gynecol.* 2017;130(4):e210-e216. (Reaffirmed 2019)

Cardonick E, Iacobucci A. Use of chemotherapy during human pregnancy. *Lancet Oncol.* 2004;5(5):283-291.

Kal HB, Struikmans H. Radiotherapy during pregnancy: fact and fiction. *Lancet Oncol.* 2005;6:328-333.

Koren G, Carey N, Gagnon R, Maxwell C, Nulman I, Senikas V. Cancer chemotherapy and pregnancy. *J Obstet Gynaecol Can.* 2013;35:263-280.

Peccatori FA, Azim HA Jr, Orecchia R, et al; for ESMO Guidelines Working Group. Cancer, pregnancy and fertility: ESMO clinical practice guidelines for diagnosis, treatment and follow-up. *Ann Oncol.* 2013;24(6):vi60-vi70.

Salani R, Billingsley CC, Crafton SM. Cancer and pregnancy: an overview for obstetricians and gynecologists. *Am J Obstet Gynecol.* 2014;211:7-14.

Yang KY. Abnormal Pap smear and cervical cancer in pregnancy. *Clin Obset Gynecol.* 2012;55(4):838-848.

22 Skin Conditions in Pregnancy

Angela K. Shaddeau and Crystal Aguh

Pregnancy is known to affect all organs and organ systems, and the skin is no exception. The predominant hormonal shifts and physical changes that occur in pregnancy can lead to several common changes in the skin. These changes are so common that they are considered to be normal effects of pregnancy. Additionally, there are several pathologic rashes and diseases that manifest with skin changes that are specific to pregnancy, and patients can have existing conditions that are affected by pregnancy. It is important for the obstetric provider to have a basic knowledge of the normal changes that occur in pregnancy in addition to the pathologic conditions in order to ensure appropriate treatment or referral, when indicated. Additionally, given that some of these conditions are associated with increased fetal or neonatal morbidity or mortality, early recognition can be of utmost importance.

NORMAL AND COMMON CHANGES IN PREGNANCY

Connective Tissue

- Striae (or "stretch marks") and skin tags are conditions that may be exacerbated by, although are not unique to, pregnancy.
  - **Striae** are linear tears in dermal connective tissue that are often initially red or purple in color and occur in approximately 50% to 80% of women. These marks

may be pruritic and can appear in multiple locations including the abdomen (most commonly), breasts, thighs and buttocks, and axilla and groin. Risk factors for development of striae include having a maternal history, young age, race (increased in nonwhite), higher initial body mass index, higher weight gain, increased circumference of abdomen and hips, and fetal macrosomia. Patients with striae have an increased future incidence of pelvic organ prolapse. There is no known effective topical treatment for striae. Many dermatologists recommend frequent use of moisturizer because dry skin is generally more susceptible to wear and tear. Pulsed dye laser is helpful to decrease redness of early striae, but there is currently no evidence whether this treatment has better outcomes than long-term observation.

- **Skin tags** are soft, pedunculated or papular growths consisting of fibrous connective tissue and epithelial tissue that are either similar in color to a person's skin tone or dark brown. They are not unique to pregnancy, but patients may notice an increase in number during the gestational period. Common locations for these to appear are the neck, axilla, or groin, and they tend to persist after delivery. Treatment is relatively simple with electrocautery or sharp removal in the outpatient setting.

Vascular Changes Affecting Skin

- Vascular changes affecting the skin in pregnancy are primarily due to increases in vascular proliferation due to changes in hormone levels. **Telangiectasias** are persistently dilated blood vessels that can be seen through the skin. A **spider angioma** is a central arteriole with radiating vascular "legs" that is most predominant in sun-exposed areas. Most of these regress spontaneously, but persistent lesions can be treated with laser ablation or low-energy electrocoagulation. Many pregnant women also experience **palmar erythema**, which requires no treatment and resolves spontaneously after delivery.
- **Pyogenic granuloma** is a vascular lesion that can present in pregnancy and can cause particular concern because of the symptoms/presentation. These lesions are red, nodular, and often pedunculated. They are often ulcerated and can have a purulent-appearing discharge. They most often appear on the gums, scalp, fingers, toes, and upper trunk but can appear anywhere. The name is a misnomer because a true granuloma is macrophage dominant, and these lesions are composed mostly of proliferating blood vessels and some other inflammatory cells. Treatment is surgical excision or electrocautery but is commonly delayed until after delivery because some lesions will spontaneously regress.

Changes in Skin Pigmentation in Pregnancy

- Pigmentation changes are very common in pregnancy with up to 91% of women experiencing **hyperpigmentation**. The areola and genitals are the most common areas of the skin to be affected. Additionally, many women develop a **linea nigra**, which is hyperpigmentation of the linea alba (the longitudinal line that runs along the midline of the abdomen).
- **Melasma** is a hyperpigmentation of the face that occurs in up to 70% of pregnant women and commonly appears on the forehead, cheeks, and bridge of the nose. Women are advised to use sunscreen (sun protection factor 15 or greater) and avoid sun exposure to prevent melasma and minimize the hyperpigmentation. Discoloration improves for a majority of women shortly after giving birth. In persistent

cases, treatment is available with a variety of topical options but can require a prolonged treatment course.

- Pregnant women can experience changes or enlargement of existing **nevi** or appearance of new nevi during pregnancy. The incidence of changes in or development of new melanoma during pregnancy is no greater in pregnant women than in non-pregnant women. Women should still be encouraged to have any changing or new nevi examined during pregnancy.

SKIN CONDITIONS UNIQUE TO PREGNANCY

In general, rashes or skin conditions specific to pregnancy have some common features. All of them tend to be pruritic in nature, and most resolve within a few weeks of pregnancy. However, some of these conditions can lead to an increased risk of fetal or neonatal mortality, making an accurate and early diagnosis important. Specific diagnoses are discussed below from most to least common.

- **Pruritus gravidarum** is defined as generalized itching during pregnancy without the presence of a rash, although excoriations from persistent itching can occur. This occurs in approximately 14% of pregnant women. This condition typically presents in the third trimester of pregnancy and is characterized as a whole body pruritus. Pruritus gravidarum is associated with twin gestations, infertility treatment, diabetes, and nulliparity. There are no associated adverse perinatal outcomes, and treatment is based on controlling symptoms.
- **Intrahepatic cholestasis of pregnancy.** In some cases, approximately 1.5% to 2% of the time, generalized pruritus experienced in pregnancy is associated with **intrahepatic cholestasis of pregnancy**. These patients may have associated elevations in liver function tests and bile acids, although pruritus commonly precedes elevations in laboratory values. The pruritus associated with cholestasis is classically most prominent in the palms and soles of the feet and described as being worse at night.
  - Unlike pruritus gravidarum, intrahepatic cholestasis of pregnancy is associated with increased risk for intrauterine fetal demise, meconium-stained amniotic fluid, preterm delivery, and neonatal respiratory distress syndrome. The pathophysiology of sudden fetal death is not well understood.
  - Treatment for the symptoms of intrahepatic cholestasis is ursodeoxycholic acid, which is given with the goal of reducing symptoms and helping to reduce the risk of perinatal morbidity and mortality.
- **Pruritic urticarial papules and plaques of pregnancy** (often called "**PUPPP**") is the most common rash seen in pregnancy and is characterized by erythematous plaques, papules, and urticarial lesions that typically arise in the third trimester of pregnancy. In 80% to 90% of women who develop this condition, these lesions start on the abdomen and spare the umbilicus, and the striae are very commonly involved. In 80% of patients, the pruritus is severe. Treatment is typically with topical steroids. PUPPP is associated with twin pregnancies, gestational hypertension, and increased weight gain and does not tend to recur in future pregnancies.
- **Pemphigoid gestationis** is a variant of bullous pemphigoid and is a rare, autoimmune, blistering condition that is seen during pregnancy and the immediate postpartum period. This most commonly presents in the second or third trimesters but can present in the first trimester occasionally as well. The most common location for lesions is the umbilicus, followed by the trunk, buttocks, and extremities. These lesions are most often vesicles and bullae, but patients can also have erythematous,

urticarial plaques appearing similar to those of PUPPPs. Biopsy sent for hematoxylin and eosin staining and immunofluorescence is therefore required to confirm the diagnosis.

- Treatment for this condition varies based on the severity of the symptoms. For mild to moderate cases, potent topical steroids are used. For moderate to severe cases, prednisone 20 to 40 mg per day is used. In the most severe cases, plasmapheresis, intravenous immunoglobulin, and cyclosporine can be used. Treatment with systemic steroids can minimize the risk to the fetus, but a diagnosis of pemphigoid gestationis does increase the risk of preterm birth and small for gestational age infants.
- Postpartum flares of the condition are common and occur in 50% to 75% of women. When a postpartum flare occurs, the treatment is reinstitution of prednisone. It is important to counsel patients that this condition is likely to recur in future pregnancies.
- **Pustular psoriasis of pregnancy** is described as a severe, generalized, pustular dermatosis. This is classically described as hundreds of white, sterile pustules arising on an erythematous base. However, sometimes, this does not initially present in a generalized fashion but rather in scattered clusters of pustules, making it more difficult to diagnose. Typical timing of onset is the second or third trimester, and areas involved can include the axilla, inframammary folds, groin, gluteal cleft, and umbilicus. This condition has a very high mortality and stillbirth rate with reports in literature up to 50%. Patients should be referred to a dermatologist immediately for clinical and histologic confirmation of disease. If confirmed, systemic corticosteroids are required treatment, and systemic antibiotics may be required if secondary bacterial infection develops. Patients should be monitored closely and may require early delivery given the high rate of complications. This condition resolves after pregnancy but is likely to recur in subsequent pregnancies.
- **Autoimmune progesterone dermatitis** is a rare and poorly defined condition. This condition can present with several different types of skin manifestations, including urticaria, papules, or pustules, or it can be eczematous in nature. These reactions are thought to be caused by a hypersensitivity to progesterone and symptoms typically occur cyclically with the luteal phase of the menstrual cycle but a few cases occur with the onset of pregnancy or get significantly worse with pregnancy.

SKIN CONDITIONS OUTSIDE OF PREGNANCY AND THE RESPONSE TO PREGNANCY

- **Acne** can have a variable response to pregnancy. For many women, pregnancy can lead to the development of painful nodules and pustules that can be debilitating. Unfortunately, treatment options are limited during pregnancy because the most effective treatments may have a teratogenic effect. First-line agents in pregnancy are topical agents such as benzoyl peroxide, azelaic acid, topical clindamycin or erythromycin, or colloidal sulfur. For cases requiring oral antibiotics, erythromycin, clindamycin, azithromycin, and cephalexin are common options. It is important to avoid sulfamethoxazole-trimethoprim (Bactrim) near term, tetracyclines, vitamin A derivatives, retinoids, and tazarotene during pregnancy for the treatment of acne.
- **Psoriasis** affects 1% to 3% of the population. The response of this condition to pregnancy can be variable, with some patients seeing improvement in their symptoms. The symptoms are usually mild in pregnancy but can be severe and can

have associated arthritis. Mild cases can be treated with topical corticosteroids and ultraviolet light B therapy, which is safe in pregnancy. Severe cases may require cyclosporine therapy. Additionally, there are several monoclonal antibody therapies available for the treatment of psoriasis.

- **Atopic dermatitis** is often referred to as "the itch that rashes." It is characterized as an intensely pruritic skin eruption with excoriations. The response in pregnancy is variable, but exacerbations in pregnancy have been referred to as "atopic eruption of pregnancy." These patients often have a personal or family history of asthma, eczema, hay fever, etc. Treatment includes topical emollients, topical steroids, oral antihistamines, and systemic corticosteroids in severe patients.

SUGGESTED READINGS

Black MM, McKay M, Braude PR, eds. *Color Atlas and Text of Obstetric and Gynecologic Dermatology*. London, United Kingdom: Mosby-Wolfe; 1995.

Ingber A. *Obstetric Dermatology: A Practical Guide*. Berlin, Germany: Springer-Verlag; 2009.

Kroumpouzos G. *Text Atlas of Obstetric Dermatology*. Philadelphia, PA: Lippincott Williams & Wilkins; 2014.

Rapini RP. The skin and pregnancy. In: Resnik R, Lockwood C, Moore T, et al, eds. *Creasy & Resnik's Maternal Fetal Medicine: Principles and Practice*. 8th ed. Philadelphia, PA: Elsevier; 2019:1258-1268.

23 Surgical Disease and Trauma in Pregnancy
Bernard D. Morris III and Nancy A. Hueppchen

PERIOPERATIVE CONSIDERATIONS FOR NONOBSTETRIC SURGERY

Anatomic and Physiologic Changes in Pregnancy

- The gravid uterus displaces abdominal organs cephalad and brings adnexal structures into the abdomen, which may change traditional presentations of surgical disease.
- Displacement of the diaphragm reduces functional residual capacity and residual lung volume, prompting an increase in tidal volume and a physiologic respiratory alkalosis.
- Uterine compression of the inferior vena cava (IVC) decreases venous return and may cause supine hypotension. This can often be mitigated by placement of the patient in left lateral tilt position to take pressure off the IVC.
- Increased plasma volume, decreased hematocrit, and generally lower blood pressure make acute blood loss assessment more difficult.
- The hypoalbuminemia of pregnancy predisposes the patient to edema and third spacing of fluids.

Timing of Surgery

- Pregnancy should not preclude any indicated surgery, regardless of trimester.
- The decision for surgery must balance the risk to the fetus versus the risk to the mother for delay in intervention and should be considered with a multidisciplinary approach.
- The second trimester is generally considered the preferred period during pregnancy in which to perform nonobstetric surgery. At this time, fetal organogenesis is complete, and the gravid uterus is less likely to require manipulation or obstruct the operative field.
- Historically, there have been concerns regarding nonobstetric surgery performed in the first trimester due to risk of miscarriage, and surgery performed in the third trimester for risk of preterm labor. Recent examination of existing data casts doubt on whether nonobstetric surgery inherently carries risk of these obstetric complications or whether the presence of surgical disease itself, along with delays in otherwise indicated surgical intervention, is the main driver of this risk.

Diagnostic Imaging

- Ultrasonography and magnetic resonance imaging (MRI) are not associated with fetal harm and generally should be considered as first-line imaging modalities in the pregnant patient.
- Gadolinium-based contrast for use with MRI is water-soluble and therefore can cross the placenta and into fetal circulation, raising the potential for teratogenicity. There is no consistent evidence of harm in human studies. However, given theoretical concerns, gadolinium should only be used when its use for a diagnostic study clearly outweighs these potential risks.
- The amount of ionizing radiation that is considered to have clinically significant teratogenic or deleterious effects of the developing fetus is in the range of 5 to 10 rads (50-100 mGy). Radiation exposure via x-ray, computerized tomography (CT) scan, and nuclear medicine studies is, with rare exceptions, under this threshold, and therefore considered safe in pregnancy. See Table 23-1 for estimated fetal radiation exposure from various diagnostic imaging techniques.
- Risks to the fetus from radiation exposure above the aforementioned threshold (50 mGy) include growth restriction, microcephaly, and intellectual disability; the risk is greatest during organogenesis (2-8 wk) and lessens with increasing gestational age.
- Oral iodinated contrast agents are safe in pregnancy. There is theoretical concern regarding use of intravenous iodinated contrast agents that can cross the placenta to fetal circulation, although animal studies have not demonstrated teratogenic or otherwise adverse effects. Therefore, if intravenous contrast is necessary for a particular diagnostic study, the benefits generally outweigh these theoretical risks.
- Breastfeeding may be continued without interruption after use of either iodinated or gadolinium-based contrast.

Anesthesia and Intraoperative Hemodynamics

- Typical anesthetic agents used in standard concentrations for local, regional, and general anesthesia, including sedatives, analgesics, and paralytics, are safe for use in pregnancy.
- Blood pressure support in the normotensive range is critical intraoperatively to maintain perfusion to the fetus.

| Table 23-1 | Fetal Radiation Exposure From Common Radiologic Procedures[a] |

Procedure	Fetal Dose (mGy)
Cervical spine or extremity radiography	<0.001
Head or neck CT	0.001-0.01
Mammography	0.001-0.01
Chest radiography	0.0005-0.01
Abdominal radiography	0.1-3.0
Lumbar spine radiography	1-10
Intravenous pyelography	5-10
Double-contrast barium enema	1-20
Chest CT or CT pulmonary angiography	0.01-0.66
Technetium-99m bone scintigraphy	4-5
Abdominal CT	1.3-35
Pelvic CT	10-50
^{18}F PET-CT whole body	10-50

Abbreviations: CT, computerized tomography; PET, positron emission tomography.
[a]Adapted from the ACOG Committee Opinion, which was adapted from Tremblay E, Thérasse E, Thomassin-Naggara I, Trop I. Quality initiatives: guidelines for use of medical imaging during pregnancy and lactation. *Radiographics*. 2012;32:897-911.

- Oxygen saturation should be maintained greater than 95% in the pregnant patient.
- When possible, a preoperative fluid bolus should be used to guard against a hypotensive episode following an epidural test bolus.

Surgical Technique

- Laparoscopy can be undertaken safely during pregnancy, even at advanced gestational age, and often is the preferred modality for management of a variety of surgical diseases in the pregnant patient.
- Access may be gained with the open (Hasson), closed (Veress needle), or direct optical trocar techniques; however, care must to be taken to note the height of the uterine fundus and adjust entry point and trocar placement accordingly.
- Ultrasound-guided entry has been described as a technique and may be used to reduce the risk of uterine injury.
- Despite historical concerns regarding carbon dioxide and association with fetal toxicity in animal studies, there is no evidence to suggest such harm in humans.
- Insufflation pressures of 10 to 15 mm Hg are recommended for the pregnant patient.

Fetal Monitoring

- The extent of fetal monitoring recommended depends on the gestational age and viability of the fetus, the type of anesthesia being administered, and the nature and acuity of the surgical intervention

- At minimum, fetal status should be documented prior to and after surgery: For a previable fetus less than 23 to 24 weeks, a fetal heart rate is sufficient.
- Continuous intraoperative fetal monitoring may be considered when the following criteria are met: logistically able to use an external monitor without interfering with the surgery or sterile field, staff is available to interpret the results, and a physician is available to intervene if indicated.
- A nonreassuring fetal heart tracing intraoperatively can often be improved by identifying and correcting maternal hypotension and/or maternal hypoxia; it does not necessarily require urgent cesarean delivery.

SURGICAL DISEASES IN PREGNANCY

Acute Appendicitis

- **Acute appendicitis** is the most common disease requiring surgical intervention, occurring in 1/800 to 1/1500 pregnancies. The rate of appendiceal perforation is significantly higher in pregnancy, presumably due to higher rates of atypical presentation and reluctance to perform appropriate imaging with delays in diagnosis and treatment. Timely diagnosis and treatment are critical because ruptured appendicitis is associated with significantly increased rates of fetal loss (36% vs 1.5%) as well as maternal morbidity and mortality compared with nonruptured appendicitis.
- **Clinical presentation** may include any of the following: anorexia, nausea, vomiting, fever, abdominal pain, leukocytosis with or without bandemia, dysuria, and pyuria. It is important to assess for rebound tenderness and other indications of peritonitis during the physical exam, although these findings may only be present in 50% to 80% of pregnant patients. Nonclassical presentations including right upper quadrant or diffuse abdominal pain are more common in the pregnant patient secondary to anatomic changes. Particular care must be taken to expand the typical differential diagnosis for abdominal pain to consider pregnancy-related conditions, including preeclampsia, round ligament pain, ovarian torsion, preterm labor, placental abruption, and chorioamnionitis.
- **Diagnostic evaluation** with graded compression ultrasonography should be the first-choice modality to evaluate for appendicitis in the pregnant patient, with a sensitivity of 67% to 100% and specificity of 83% to 96%. If ultrasound is inconclusive and appendicitis remains suspected, MRI or CT may be considered, although MRI (sensitivity, 94%; specificity, 97%) is generally preferred in an effort to limit fetal radiation exposure.
- **Management**
  - Appendectomy is the standard treatment; medical management with antibiotics alone is not typically recommended due to limited data on this strategy in pregnant patients. Surgery should not be postponed until the presentation of generalized peritonitis.
  - In the case of ruptured appendicitis with active labor, cesarean delivery may be appropriate. A stable, nonseptic patient with a ruptured appendix in the later stages of labor may attempt a vaginal delivery.
  - Perioperative antibiotics with a second-generation cephalosporin, extended spectrum penicillin, or triple antibiotic therapy (ampicillin, gentamicin, clindamycin) are administered in all cases and continued postoperatively until 24 to 48 hours afebrile in cases of peritonitis, perforation, or periappendiceal abscess.

- Laparoscopy may be useful if the diagnosis is uncertain (eg, with history of pelvic inflammatory disease) and especially in the first trimester. An open laparoscopic entry technique is advisable after 12 to 14 weeks' gestation due to the increased risk of uterine perforation on entering the abdomen.
- Laparotomy is indicated if suspicion for ruptured appendicitis is high, regardless of gestational age.

Acute Cholecystitis

- **Acute cholecystitis** is the next most common surgical disease in pregnancy, affecting about 1 in 1000 pregnant women. Delayed gallbladder emptying in response to hormonal changes predisposes to gallstone formation and biliary sludge, which can be seen in 7% of pregnant patients. The large majority of these patients will be asymptomatic. Approximately 10% of symptomatic patients will develop acute cholecystitis, which if left untreated may progress to cause serious complications such as gangrenous cholecystitis, gallbladder perforation, and cholecystoenteric fistulas.
- **Clinical presentation** includes anorexia, nausea, vomiting, fever, and mild leukocytosis, which may also be present at baseline in pregnancy. Symptoms may be localized to the flank, right scapula, or shoulder. Murphy sign is seen less frequently in pregnancy or may be displaced.
- **Diagnostic evaluation** consists of history and physical examination and laboratory tests (leukocyte count, serum amylase and lipase, total bilirubin, and liver function tests). A right upper quadrant ultrasound is highly accurate for the detection of acute cholecystitis and should be considered the first-line imaging modality. If there is high suspicion for a common bile duct stone, endoscopic retrograde cholangiopancreatography may be of both diagnostic and therapeutic benefit.
- **Management**
  - Conservative initial management includes bowel rest, intravenous hydration, analgesia, and fetal monitoring. A short course of indomethacin may be considered to decrease inflammation and relieve pain.
  - Antibiotics are warranted if symptoms persist for 12 to 24 hours or there is suspicion for infection. Recommended empiric antibiotic regimens include ampicillin/sulbactam (Unasyn), piperacillin/tazobactam (Zosyn), or ceftriaxone plus metronidazole (Flagyl).
  - Surgical management is indicated for sepsis, suspected perforation, or failure of conservative therapy. Even in uncomplicated cases, definitive surgery during the initial hospitalization is a reasonable option given the high risk of recurrence when treated conservatively. When feasible, a laparoscopic approach is the preferred technique.
  - Intraoperative cholangiography can be safely performed if necessary with the use of fetal shielding techniques.
  - Percutaneous gallbladder decompression has been reported for management of more severe cases or in poor surgical candidates.

Bowel Obstruction

- **Bowel obstruction** during pregnancy is most commonly caused by adhesions (60%) or volvulus (25%).
- Conservative management includes bowel rest, intravenous hydration, and nasogastric suction. Proceed with surgical management if the patient develops an acute abdomen.

Ovarian Cysts and Torsion

- **Torsion** occurs when an adnexal mass twists on its vascular pedicle. A disproportionate share of these cases occurs in pregnancy (up to one quarter of all torsion cases). Common causes of adnexal torsion include corpus luteum cysts, theca-lutein cysts, paratubal cysts, dermoids, and ovulation induction. Complications of torsion include adnexal infarction, chemical peritonitis, and preterm labor.
- **Clinical presentation** includes acute pain (usually unilateral) with or without diaphoresis, nausea, and vomiting. An adnexal mass may be palpable.
- **Diagnostic evaluation** is by history, physical examination, and ultrasonography with Doppler flow to evaluate the adnexa. It is important to note that normal Doppler flow does not exclude the possibility of torsion.
- **Conservative management** is indicated for ruptured corpus luteum cysts in hemodynamically stable patients. Corpus luteum cysts usually involute by 16 weeks' gestation.
- **Operative management** is indicated for acute abdomen, torsion, or infarction.
  - Cysts that are persistent, larger than 6 cm, or contain solid elements may require surgery. A laparoscopic approach is often used in the management of adnexal masses in pregnancy.
  - If the ovarian corpus luteum is disrupted, progestins can be used up to 10 weeks of pregnancy to prevent miscarriage

Breast Mass During Pregnancy

- About 1 in 3000 pregnant women in the United States are affected by breast cancer. Pregnant patients tend to be diagnosed late. The average delay between symptoms and diagnosis is 5 months.
- **Diagnostic evaluation** is similar to that of nonpregnant patient.
  - Mammography, with abdominal shielding, is safe in pregnancy; however, there is a 50% false-negative rate.
  - Breast ultrasonography may differentiate solid and cystic masses without radiation exposure but may also give false-negative results.
  - A clinically suspicious breast mass, even with negative imaging, should be biopsied, regardless of pregnancy status. Fine needle aspiration and core biopsy are safe in pregnancy.
- **Management:** See chapter 34.

Pregnancy After Bariatric Surgery

- Bariatric surgery is increasingly common among reproductive-age women.
- Conception should be delayed for 12 to 24 months after bariatric surgery, during the period of most rapid weight loss. In patients who undergo bariatric surgery with a malabsorption component, such as a Roux-en-Y, there is a higher rate of oral contraceptive failure.
- Limited data on pregnancy after bariatric surgery suggest that there is no increase in adverse fetal outcomes. Complications such as gestational diabetes, preeclampsia, and fetal macrosomia may be less common in patients following bariatric surgery than in their obese counterparts but may still occur with greater frequency than the general population.
- Patients who have had gastric banding may need band adjustment during pregnancy.

- Bariatric surgery patients should be appropriately counseled about nutritional goals and risks. Vitamin and mineral deficiencies, including vitamin B_1, B_6, B_{12}; folate; vitamin D; iron; and calcium, should be assessed and appropriately treated. In the absence of any deficiencies, blood count, iron, ferritin, calcium, and vitamin D levels can be considered each trimester. Folic acid, vitamin B_{12}, calcium, vitamin D, and iron supplements are recommended.
- Complications of bariatric surgery, such as anastomotic leak, bowel obstruction, and band erosion, may manifest as nausea, vomiting, and abdominal pain.
- Use of nonsteroidal anti-inflammatory drugs should be avoided.

TRAUMA IN PREGNANCY

Trauma complicates approximately 1 in 12 pregnancies and is the leading cause of nonobstetric maternal death during pregnancy. Motor vehicle accidents account for the large majority (70%) of trauma in pregnancy, with other common causes including falls, intimate partner violence, penetrating trauma, and burns.

- During the first trimester, the uterus lies within the bony pelvis and is relatively protected from direct injury.
- Obstetric complications from trauma include early pregnancy loss, preterm labor and birth, prelabor rupture of membranes, placental abruption, uterine rupture, fetal-maternal hemorrhage with risk of alloimmunization, direct fetal injury, and fetal demise.
- Fetal injury can include skull fractures and intracerebral hemorrhage from blunt pelvic trauma or direct injury from a penetrating wound.
- Fetomaternal hemorrhage occurs in 9% to 30% of trauma cases. Signs include fetal tachycardia, fetal anemia, and fetal demise. Due to the risk of fetomaternal hemorrhage, all Rh-negative pregnant women should receive RhoGAM, if appropriate, after trauma.

Specific Traumatic Injuries

Blunt Trauma

- Motor vehicle collision is the most common cause of blunt trauma. Pregnant women should wear seat belts with the lap belt secured as low as possible over the bony pelvis and not across the fundus or middle of the abdomen. The shoulder strap should be placed across the woman's chest.
- Complications include retroperitoneal hemorrhage (more common in pregnancy from the marked engorgement of pelvic vessels), placental abruption, preterm labor, and uterine rupture.
- Placental abruption is identified in 40% of severe blunt abdominal trauma and 3% of minor blunt trauma cases.
- Uterine rupture occurs in <1% of trauma cases, usually from direct high-energy abdominal impact. It often results in fetal death.
- Complications are more likely in the presence of pelvic fractures. Pelvic fracture with retroperitoneal hemorrhage in a pregnant woman causes significantly increased blood loss compared to nonpregnant patients.
- Splenic rupture is the most common cause of intraperitoneal hemorrhage.
- Direct fetal injury complicates <1% of blunt trauma cases in pregnancy.
- Fetal death is most commonly caused by maternal death and correlates with severity of injury, expulsion from the vehicle, and maternal head injury.

Penetrating Trauma

- Gunshot and stab wounds are the most common causes of penetrating trauma.
- The health of the mother is of primary concern and takes precedence over the fetus, unless vital signs cannot be maintained in the mother, in which case perimortem cesarean delivery should be considered.
- Gunshot wounds to the abdomen carry a fetal mortality rate of up to 71%. Evaluation includes thorough examination of all entrance and exit wounds with radiographs or CT to help localize the bullet.
- Stab wounds to the abdomen carry a more favorable prognosis than gunshot wounds to the abdomen and carry a fetal mortality rate of up to 42%. A CT may help assess the extent of injuries.
- Exploratory laparotomy is performed for any penetrating trauma to the abdomen. Laparotomy for maternal indications is not considered a reason to perform a cesarean delivery, unless a fetal indication for cesarean delivery is present or if the gravid uterus prevents appropriate intraabdominal exploration.
- Tetanus prophylaxis should be considered in eligible candidates.

Thermal Injuries/Burns

- Both maternal and fetal outcomes after burn injury are predominantly related to the extent of burn area. As the burn surface area approaches 40%, the maternal and fetal mortality rate approaches 100%. Maternal age and gestational age do not appear to impact maternal or fetal survival in cases of severe burns.

Trauma Assessment in Pregnancy

- **Initial assessment of the pregnant trauma patient** is the same as for the nonpregnant patient. The mother should be stabilized first, a primary survey conducted, oxygen administered as needed, and intravenous access obtained. Intubation should be performed early, if necessary, to maintain fetal oxygenation and reduce the risk of maternal aspiration.
- **Primary assessment**
  - If the estimated gestational age is >20 weeks, place the patient in a 10- to 15-degree left lateral tilt or supine with a wedge under the right hip in order to displace the gravid uterus off the IVC.
  - Two large-bore intravenous catheters should be placed and crystalloid administered in a volume 3 times the estimated blood loss.
  - Initiate blood transfusion for estimated blood loss >1 L. Patients may lose up to 1500 mL of blood before showing signs of hemodynamic instability due to the increased blood volume in pregnancy.
  - Following aggressive fluid resuscitation, vasopressors may be used to maintain adequate perfusion to the uterus, if needed. See chapter 61.
  - If a chest tube is indicated in the case of penetrating injuries, it should be placed one to two intercostal spaces above the typical placement at the fifth intercostal space given cephalad displacement of the diaphragm in pregnancy.
- **Secondary assessment** is performed after initial stabilization.
  - Examine the patient's entire body, particularly the abdomen and uterus.
  - Assess fetal well-being and estimate gestational age with ultrasound.
  - Assess fetal heart rate by doptones or continuous monitoring, depending on gestational age, and place a tocodynamometer for uterine contractions.

- Greater than four contractions per hour during the first 4 hours of monitoring and/or a positive Kleihauer-Betke (KB) test are concerning for abruption. Fewer than four contractions per hour over 4 hours of fetal monitoring and a negative KB are not associated with increased adverse outcomes.
- Perform a pelvic examination to evaluate for bleeding, ruptured membranes, and cervical change.

- **Diagnostic evaluation**
  - A CT scan including clearance of the c-spine should be performed if indicated and the patient is stable. It should not be delayed due to pregnancy.
  - Ultrasonography (focused assessment with sonography for trauma [FAST] scan) may be used to screen for abdominal injury and to evaluate fetal age and viability. Ultrasound in trauma is 61% sensitive and 94% specific in detecting intra-abdominal injury during pregnancy (compared with 71% sensitive and 97% specific in the nonpregnant patient).
  - Diagnostic peritoneal lavage carries increased risk in pregnant patients compared with nonpregnant patients, although the overall complication rate is still <1%. Typically, CT and ultrasound are sufficient, and diagnostic peritoneal lavage is not needed.
  - Laboratory studies include blood type and antibody screen, crossmatch for anticipated needs, complete blood count, KB test, coagulation profile, urinalysis, and toxicology screen including blood alcohol level. Pelvic injuries should be suspected in cases of gross or microscopic hematuria.
  - Cesarean delivery for nonreassuring fetal status, placental abruption, uterine rupture, or unstable pelvic or lumbosacral fracture in labor may be considered if the mother is stable, depending on gestational age, fetal status, and uterine injury.
  - Tocolysis in trauma cases is controversial but not contraindicated. Standard tocolytic agents produce symptoms that can complicate assessments, however, such as tachycardia (betamimetics), hypotension (calcium channel blockers), and altered sensorium (magnesium sulfate).
  - Fetal monitoring protocols after trauma vary among institutions and have not been evaluated rigorously. We typically monitor patients for 2 to 4 hours after any trauma. If contractions persist, continuous monitoring is extended to 24 hours; injuries that are more serious, significant pain, vaginal bleeding, or nonreassuring fetal monitoring warrant extended observations as well.

CARDIOPULMONARY RESUSCITATION IN PREGNANCY

- The most common causes of cardiac arrest in pregnant patients include trauma/hemorrhage, pulmonary embolism, amniotic fluid embolism, stroke, maternal cardiac disease, anesthetic complications, and flash pulmonary edema.
- Standard Advanced Cardiac Life Support protocols should be followed without modification for pregnancy.
- Left lateral tilt to displace the uterus from the IVC should be used during compressions if it will not compromise the quality of chest compressions.
- Administer medications and defibrillation per protocol. Pressors should not be withheld because fetal outcome depends on successful maternal resuscitation.
- Consider early intubation to reduce aspiration risk, which is increased at baseline in pregnancy.

- **Perimortem or emergency cesarean delivery** is rarely required except in patients with a viable fetus who do not respond to resuscitation. In the latter half of gestation, it may improve maternal resuscitation by increasing venous return and cardiac output.
- **The decision to proceed with perimortem cesarean delivery** should be made within 4 minutes of cardiac arrest with delivery as soon as possible for the best outcome.
- **Perimortem cesarean** should be performed immediately at the bedside. A sterile field is unnecessary. Generally, a midline vertical skin incision is made with a scalpel and carried down to the uterus. The hysterotomy is also performed by midline vertical incision. After delivery of the fetus and placenta, the uterus is closed using running locked sutures. It is important to **continue cardiopulmonary resuscitation throughout the procedure**. If maternal survival is possible, start broad-spectrum antibiotics.
- Infant survival has been reported at 67% if delivered within 15 minutes and 40% if delivered between 16 and 25 minutes. Attempt delivery if any signs of fetal life are detected.
- Delivery does not need to be emergent for maternal brain death unless fetal compromise is present.
- Careful documentation of the circumstances and indications for the performance of perimortem cesarean is essential.

SUGGESTED READINGS

American College of Obstetricians and Gynecologists Committee on Obstetric Practice. ACOG Committee Opinion No. 723: guidelines for diagnostic imaging during pregnancy and lactation. *Obstet Gynecol.* 2017;130(4):e210-e216. (Reaffirmed 2019)

American College of Obstetricians and Gynecologists Committee on Obstetric Practice, American Society of Anesthesiologists. ACOG Committee Opinion No. 775: nonobstetric surgery during pregnancy (replaces Committee Opinion No. 696, April 2017). *Obstet Gynecol.* 2019;133:e285-e286.

American College of Obstetricians and Gynecologists Committee on Practice Bulletins—Obstetrics. ACOG Practice Bulletin No. 105: bariatric surgery and pregnancy. *Obstet Gynecol.* 2009;113:1405-1413. (Reaffirmed 2017)

Brown HL. Trauma in pregnancy. *Obstet Gynecol.* 2009;114(1):147-160.

Dietrich CS III, Hill CC, Hueman M. Surgical diseases presenting in pregnancy. *Surg Clin North Am.* 2008;88:403-419.

Mendez-Figueroa H, Dahlke JD, Vrees RA, Rouse DJ. Trauma in pregnancy: an updated systematic review. *Am J Obstet Gynecol.* 2013;209(1):1-10.

Parangi S, Levine D, Henry A, Isakovich N, Pories S. Surgical gastrointestinal disorders during pregnancy. *Am J Surg.* 2007;193(2):223-232.

Tolcher M, Fisher W, Clark S. Nonobstetric surgery during pregnancy. *Obstet Gynecol.* 2018;132:395-403.

Uzoma A, Keriakos R. Pregnancy management following bariatric surgery. *J Obstet Gynaecol.* 2013;33(2):109-141.

Postpartum Care and Breastfeeding

Timothee Fruhauf and Silka Patel

ROUTINE POSTPARTUM CARE

Normal Postpartum Physiology

- **Uterine involution:** Postdelivery, the uterine fundus is typically palpated around the level of the umbilicus and subsequently recedes approximately 1 cm/d, returning to its nonpregnant size by 6 to 8 weeks postpartum. This timeline can vary with overdistention, parity, mode of delivery, and breastfeeding, but uterine size is not predictive of complications.
- **Lochia:** Postpartum vaginal discharge (lochia) changes from lochia rubra, red-brown discharge containing blood and decidua in the first few days postpartum, to watery pinkish brown lochia serosa 2 to 3 weeks postpartum, and subsequently to yellowish white lochia alba. Time to resolution varies but is typically 6 weeks postpartum.
- **Postpartum blues:** Postpartum blues may be difficult to diagnose because many depressive symptoms overlap with normal postpartum changes in sleep, energy, and appetite. However, depressive symptoms should be evaluated in the context of normal postpartum expectations to identify women for whom symptoms of dysphoria, insomnia, fatigue, and impaired concentration affect daily living. In comparison to postpartum depression (see chapter 18), postpartum blues are mild and self-limited, developing within a few days of delivery and resolving within 2 weeks of delivery.
- **Lactational amenorrhea:** Breastfeeding can suppress the secretion of gonadotropin-releasing hormone resulting in anovulation. However, this relationship is modulated by the extent of breastfeeding and the maternal nutritional status and body mass. Only approximately 40% of women remain amenorrheic at 6 months postpartum with exclusive breastfeeding. The mean time to ovulation is 190 days in women who are exclusively breastfeeding as opposed to an average of 45 days in nonbreastfeeding woman.

The Perineum

- Routine perineal care and normal healing: Perineal pain and edema are common during the first 7 to 10 days postpartum. Second-degree perineal lacerations typically take up to 3 weeks to heal, whereas third- or fourth-degree lacerations heal in 4 to 6 weeks. Use of squirt bottles while voiding, frequent sitz baths, topical anesthetics, witch hazel pads, and cold or warm packs can aid with comfort and recovery. Fourth-degree lacerations can be accompanied by fecal incontinence in the immediate postpartum period, but pelvic floor dysfunction is expected to resolve over time.
- Perineal complications and long-term issues
  - **Perineal infection** spans from cellulitis and abscesses to necrotizing fasciitis but typically presents with worsening pain during the first postpartum week and can

be associated with fever, erythema, shiny or tense skin, drainage, and edema. Treatment includes oral antibiotics and may require opening the repair, draining, irrigating, debriding tissue, or packing depending on the depth and size of the infection.

- **Repair separation (dehiscence)** typically occurs 10 to 14 days postpartum in association with infection and is more common for third- and fourth-degree lacerations. It typically presents with increased pain, abnormal discharge, and a "popping" sensation. For deeper lacerations, a delayed secondary repair may be needed.
- **Hematomas** typically occur within 24 hours of delivery with women noting a rapidly expanding and painful bulge in the vagina, vulva, or perineum. These can be managed conservatively with supportive care, with surgical evacuation, or rarely with selective arterial embolization.

Postpartum Immunizations and Injections

- Inactivated and live vaccines (except smallpox and yellow fever) can be safely administered to breastfeeding women without adverse effects.
- **Rh D immunoglobulin:** An unsensitized Rh-negative woman who delivers an Rh-positive infant should receive 300 μg of Rh D immunoglobulin (RhoGAM) within 72 hours of delivery even if Rh immunoglobulin was given antepartum. If there is laboratory evidence of excessive maternal-fetal hemorrhage, additional doses may be required.
- **Rubella vaccine:** Mothers who are rubella nonimmune should receive the measles-mumps-rubella vaccine prior to discharge after delivery. Use of monovalent rubella vaccine (ie, Rubivax) is not preferred because measles-mumps-rubella is more cost-effective and because many women without immunity to rubella also lack immunity to rubeola (measles). This is a live virus and as such is not given during pregnancy.
- **Varicella vaccine:** Mothers who are varicella nonimmune should receive the first dose of the Varivax vaccine prior to discharge after delivery and the second dose 4 to 8 weeks later, often at the time of the postpartum visit. This is a live virus and as such is not given during pregnancy.
- Catch-up immunizations: The **tetanus-diphtheria-and-pertussis** vaccine should be administered postpartum if not given during pregnancy to reduce transmission of maternal pertussis to the newborn, although indirect protection will not be present until 2 weeks postvaccination. The **hepatitis A and B vaccines** can also be offered if indicated.
- **Influenza vaccine:** The influenza vaccine should be administered postpartum during the influenza season if not given during pregnancy (the attenuated influenza vaccine is safe in pregnancy) because influenza infection has been associated with increased morbidity in pregnancy and postpartum.

Discharge From the Hospital

When no complications occur, mothers may be discharged 24 to 48 hours after vaginal delivery and 24 to 96 hours after cesarean delivery. The following criteria should be met:
- Vital signs are stable and within normal limits.
- Uterine fundus is firm and involuting.

- The amount/color of lochia is appropriate—red, less than a heavy period, decreasing.
- Urine output is adequate.
- Perineal pain is adequately controlled.
- Any surgical incision or vaginal repair sites are healing well without signs of infection.
- The mother is able to eat, drink, ambulate, and void without difficulty.
- No medical or psychosocial issues are identified that preclude discharge.
- The mother has demonstrated knowledge of appropriate self-care and care of her infant including feeding method for the infant.
- Postpartum contraception has been addressed.
- Immunizations and Rh D immunoglobulin, if appropriate, have been administered.
- Follow-up care has been arranged for the mother and infant.
- Infant nutritional needs have been addressed.

The Postpartum Care Continuum: The "Fourth Trimester"

- Postpartum guidance and planning *in* the prenatal period.
  - **Anticipatory guidance** should begin during the prenatal period because the development of a postpartum care plan to support women in their transition from pregnancy to parenthood and well-woman care will optimize health outcomes. Expectations regarding infant feeding and other parenting challenges, postpartum emotional and mental health, recovery from delivery, and management of chronic health conditions including identification of a primary care physician should be discussed.
  - Future pregnancy planning: Prenatally, future reproductive intentions should be addressed to discuss risks of short interpregnancy intervals and to guide decisions about postpartum contraception. Information on the full range of contraceptive methods should be provided, so the patient can select the best method to achieve her goals. This should also include the availability of immediate postdelivery long-acting reversible contraceptives placement (intrauterine devices [IUD] and etonogestrel implant).
  - A postpartum care plan should be created during pregnancy and updated after delivery prior to discharge from the hospital. It should include the following:
    - Contact information for all members of the care team, including the obstetrician and any other providers (eg, social worker, psychiatrist).
    - Date, time, and location for postpartum appointments. Ensure that the patient knows the appropriate phone numbers to call for scheduling recommended appointments.
    - Resources pertaining to the intended method of infant feeding, including WIC and lactation consultant. When needed, assist patient in obtaining a breast pump.
    - Reproductive goals and contraceptive information. Review with the patient desired number of children and interval between pregnancies. Review contraceptive options, including risks, benefits, and side effects of offered methods.
    - Manage any pregnancy complications, including cardiovascular disease, diabetes, and hypertension and their associated follow-up plans postpartum and implications for future pregnancies.

- Offer guidance on symptoms and management of depression, anxiety, and/or other psychiatric conditions. Refer to social work and psychiatry as needed.
- Recommendations for management of common postpartum problems including pelvic floor dysfunction and dyspareunia.
- Follow up plans for chronic health conditions. As needed, identify the primary care provider or other health care providers (eg, psychiatry, hematology, endocrinology) who will continue care for the patient's chronic medical conditions after the postpartum period.

- The initial postpartum assessment (within 3 wk): Given that a substantial portion of morbidity occurs in the early postpartum period, it is ideal to conduct an initial in-person or by-phone assessment within the first 3 weeks postpartum to address any acute issues.

  - Follow-up for **hypertensive diseases of pregnancy**: An evaluation of blood pressure (BP) within 7 to 10 days postpartum is recommended for women with hypertensive disorders of pregnancy. Women with severe hypertension should be seen within the first 3 days postpartum and a full stroke assessment should be conducted.

  - Follow-up for high risk women: Other women who are at risk for complications including postpartum depression, wound infection, lactation difficulties, or chronic conditions may also benefit from an in-person postpartum visit before their later comprehensive postpartum visit.

  - Assessments of women without risk factors: Women without any particular risk factors may also benefit from having an initial assessment with a provider in the first 3 weeks postpartum to address any acute postpartum issues. This assessment does not need to be an in-person office visit and could occur via home visit, phone, phone application, or text message.

- The comprehensive postpartum visit (within 12 wk)

  - Physical exam components: BP measurement and breast, abdomen, and pelvic examinations (including vaginal repair assessment) should be performed. By 6 to 8 weeks postpartum, the uterus should return to its nonpregnant size and lochia should be essentially absent.

  - Sexual activity and **contraception**: Sexual activity can be safely resumed once the perineum is healed and bleeding has decreased, typically by 6 weeks postpartum. However, dyspareunia is common in the context of the healing perineum and vaginal dryness caused by the hypoestrogenic state maintained by breastfeeding. Advise the use of water or silicone-based lubricants. Libido may furthermore be lowered as women adjust to caring for a newborn. Any significant or persistent dyspareunia should nevertheless be evaluated. The discussion of contraception should include an explanation of the rationale for birth spacing and avoidance of short interpregnancy intervals. See chapter 28 for contraception options. If the patient selects a long-acting reversible contraceptive, it should be placed during this postpartum visit whenever feasible.

  - **Depression screening** and emotional well-being: The psychosocial well-being of the patient should be assessed, with specific screening for depression and anxiety using a validated instrument such as the **Edinburgh Postnatal Depression Scale**. If there is evidence of depression, antidepressant medication should be considered and the patient should be referred for mental health care (see chapter 18). If you elect to start an antidepressant medication, the patient should also be screened for a personal history or a family history of bipolar disorder. The postpartum visit is also an opportunity to screen for substance use disorder and follow up on preexisting mental health disorders.

- Antenatal complications: Patients with **preeclampsia** should be followed to ensure resolution of symptoms and exclude underlying hypertensive or renal disease. Women with **gestational diabetes** should be screened for diabetes using a fasting plasma glucose test or a 75-g 2-hour oral glucose tolerance test at their postpartum visit due to their increased risk of underlying diabetes outside of pregnancy.

- Chronic medical conditions and health maintenance: Medications for chronic conditions should be reviewed for their safety profile if the patient is breastfeeding and for any postpartum dose adjustment. Referral to a primary care physician or specialist for further management may be indicated. The postpartum visit is also an opportunity to perform any needed health maintenance measures including immunizations, Pap smear, and the well-woman pelvic exam.

- Infant care: The patient's comfort with caring for the newborn should be evaluated including feeding, childcare strategy, and the availability of pediatric care. A reminder about safe infant sleep practices should be reviewed. If the patient is breastfeeding, any related issues should also be addressed.

- Postpartum care for women experiencing miscarriage, stillbirth, neonatal death: Women who experience a pregnancy loss should have a scheduled postpartum visit to discuss emotional support including possible referral to counselors or support groups, bereavement counseling, test or pathology results related to the loss, recurrent risk, and future pregnancy planning. This needs to occur before the typical time for a comprehensive postpartum visit.

COMMON POSTPARTUM COMPLICATIONS

- **Postpartum hemorrhage** is defined as (1) estimated blood loss of greater than 1000 mL for vaginal or cesarean delivery **or** (2) bleeding associated with symptoms of hypovolemia within 24 hours of delivery. Excessive blood loss that occurs within 24 hours of delivery is termed *primary* or *acute* postpartum hemorrhage, whereas bleeding that occurs more than 24 hours after delivery (up to 6 wk) is termed *secondary* or *late* postpartum hemorrhage. The incidence of postpartum hemorrhage is approximately 1% to 5% of all deliveries (see chapter 3).

- **Postpartum febrile morbidity** is defined as a temperature higher than 38.0°C on at least two occasions at least 4 hours apart, after the first 24 hours postpartum. Common causes include breast engorgement, atelectasis, urinary tract infection, endomyometritis, drug reaction (especially with misoprostol use), and wound infection. Less common causes of postpartum fever include retained products of conception, pelvic abscess, infected hematoma, pneumonia (particularly if the patient received general anesthesia), ovarian vein thrombosis, and septic pelvic thrombophlebitis.
  - **Urinary tract infections** are common in pregnancy and after catheterization; culture should be considered based on clinical examination. It should be treated with oral antibiotics.

- **Endomyometritis** complicates 1% to 3% of vaginal deliveries and is 5 to 10 times more common after cesarean delivery. It presents as fever, uterine fundal tenderness, malaise, or foul-smelling lochia and is usually a polymicrobial infection of gram-positive aerobes (groups A and B streptococci, enterococci), gram-negative aerobes (*Escherichia coli*), and anaerobes (*Peptostreptococcus, Peptococcus, Bacteroides*) from the genital tract. Endomyometritis should be treated with intravenous antibiotics until the patient is clinically improved and afebrile for 24 to 48 hours. See chapter 3 for treatment recommendations. Response to antibiotic treatment is usually prompt. Persistent fever after 48 to 72 hours of antibiotic treatment necessitates further evaluation.

- **Septic pelvic thrombophlebitis** is rare and is more frequently associated with cesarean delivery. It is characterized by high-spiking fevers despite appropriate antibiotics. Patients often feel well between fevers and have no complaint of pain. Imaging is frequently obtained to look for an abscess, but the pelvic thromboses with septic pelvic thrombophlebitis are not always seen on computed tomography or magnetic resonance imaging, so the diagnosis is made based on clinical examination and exclusion of other causes. Continuation of intravenous antibiotics and the potential addition of heparin anticoagulation have been suggested for treatment, although this treatment regimen remains controversial (see chapter 3).

- **Hypertension** is defined as BP of 140/90 mm Hg or higher, taken with the patient in a seated position on two or more occasions at least 6 hours apart. Preeclampsia or eclampsia can present postpartum, even in the absence of an antenatal diagnosis. Any pressure reading of 140/90 mm Hg or higher should be evaluated by repeating BP measurement, assessing for other signs and symptoms of preeclampsia, and obtaining preeclampsia labs (platelets, liver function tests, and a measure of urine protein). In those women who had antenatal preeclampsia, spontaneous postpartum diuresis and normalization of BP are generally expected. Hypertension from preeclampsia can persist for up to 6 weeks, however, and may require further evaluation and treatment.

- **Thromboembolic events** are the leading cause of direct maternal mortality and are more common postpartum, especially after cesarean deliveries and in the presence of additional risk factors (previous venous thromboembolism, thrombophilia, obesity, smoking, postpartum hemorrhage, medical comorbidities). The risk is highest immediately postpartum and gradually declines to baseline by 12 weeks postpartum. Prophylaxis should be individualized and is recommended for women at high risk (see chapter 3).

BREASTFEEDING

Recommendations

- The American Academy of Pediatrics advises exclusive breastfeeding for the first 6 months of life and partial breastfeeding (plus complementary foods) for at least 12 months. The World Health Organization recommends continued partial breastfeeding for 2 or more years.
- Feeding preferences should be discussed during the prenatal visits and those desiring to breastfeed postpartum should be counseled throughout the prenatal course.
- Breastfeeding initiation should be encouraged as soon as possible after delivery. Infants and mothers who initiate breastfeeding within the first hour after

delivery have a higher success rate than those who delay. Those who will be separated from their infants in the immediate postdelivery period (neonatal intensive care unit evaluation/admission) should be offered a breast pump to initiate milk production.

- Newborns should be fed every 2 to 4 hours until satiety. Arouse nondemanding newborn infants every 4 hours for feeding. Frequent breastfeeding establishes maternal milk supply, prevents excessive engorgement, and minimizes neonatal jaundice.
- Breastfeeding may be associated with initial discomfort. Painful breasts should be assessed and positioning reevaluated. Nursing on the less sore breast first, rotating stress points on nipples, and breaking suction before removing the infant may help. Nipple tenderness can be treated with cool or warm compresses, application of expressed breast milk to the nipple, or with mild analgesics. Lanolin cream or all-purpose nipple ointment have not been shown to provide benefit but are commonly used.
- Breastfeeding increases maternal caloric requirements by 500 to 1000 kcal/d and increases the risk of deficiencies in magnesium, vitamin B_6, folate, calcium, and zinc. Thus, women should be encouraged to continue taking their prenatal multivitamin supplement. Human milk may not provide adequate iron for premature newborns or for infants older than 6 months. These infants, and babies of mothers with iron deficiency, should receive iron supplements. Infants who are breastfed should also receive vitamin D supplementation because human milk does not provide an adequate supply.
- Table 24-1 lists the benefits of breastfeeding.

Contraindications to Breastfeeding

- Some structural problems make breastfeeding difficult and sometimes impossible. These include tubular breasts, hypoplastic breast tissue, true inverted nipples (rare), and surgical alterations that sever the milk ducts.
- Contraindications to breastfeeding include the following:
  - Mother actively using drugs of abuse, including excessive alcohol
  - Infant with galactosemia
  - Maternal human immunodeficiency virus infection in a developed country. In developing countries, the benefits of breastfeeding may outweigh the small risk of human immunodeficiency virus transmission.
  - Maternal active and untreated tuberculosis or women with human T-cell lymphotropic virus type I or II. Women can give their infant expressed breast milk and can breastfeed once their treatment regimen is well established.
  - Active untreated maternal varicella. Once the infant has been given varicella zoster immunoglobulin, expressed milk is allowed if there are no lesions on the breast. Within 5 days of the appearance of the rash, maternal antibodies are produced, making breast milk beneficial for passive immunity.
  - Active herpes simplex lesions on the breast
  - Mothers receiving diagnostic or therapeutic radioactive isotopes or who have had recent exposure to radioactive materials.
  - Mothers receiving antimetabolites or chemotherapeutic agents
- *Noncontraindications*
  - Healthy term infants with acquired or congenital cytomegalovirus should breastfeed for the benefit of maternal antibodies.

Table 24-1	Benefits of Breastfeeding

Benefits for Newborns

- Excellent nutrition matched to needs (milk content changes with developmental needs [ie, more protein/minerals after delivery and increased water, fat, and lactose later])
- Secretory IgA are at high levels in colostrum providing passive immunity to infant.
- Boosts cellular immunity by promoting phagocytosis by macrophages and leukocytes
- Bifidus factor in milk promotes *Lactobacillus bifidus* proliferation, protecting from diarrheal pathogen proliferation.
- Decreases the rate and/or severity of bacterial meningitis, bacteremia, diarrhea, respiratory tract infection, necrotizing enterocolitis, otitis media, urinary tract infections, and late-onset sepsis in preterm infants
- Infant mortality reduced by 21% in breastfed infants in the United States
- Breast milk proteins are human specific, thus delaying or reducing some environmental allergies.

Benefits for Mothers

- Can support early bonding between mother and infant
- Oxytocin release during milk letdown increases uterine contractions, thereby decreasing postpartum blood loss and facilitating uterine involution.
- Decreased lifetime risk of ovarian and premenopausal breast cancer proportional to duration of breastfeeding
- Decreased incidence of osteoporosis and postmenopausal hip fracture
- Possible lower cost compared with formula feeding
- Facilitates pregnancy spacing due to lactational amenorrhea
- May help with faster postpartum weight loss

Abbreviation: IgA, immunoglobulin A.

- Babies of mothers with hepatitis A or B may breastfeed as soon as the infant receives appropriate immunoglobulin and the first dose of hepatitis vaccine series. Special attention to avoid broken skin on or around the nipples of mothers with hepatitis B is advised.
- Mothers with hepatitis C may breastfeed. There is no evidence for hepatitis C transmission via breast milk. Again, advise no breastfeeding if skin on or around nipples is broken.

Breastfeeding and Maternal Medications

- Most, but not all, drugs are compatible with breastfeeding, and the American Academy of Pediatrics recommends weighing the benefits of breastfeeding for the mother and infant against the risks of an infant's exposure to a drug.
- The most up-to-date information on compatibility of prescription and over-the-counter medications with breastfeeding can be found on the LactMed

database made available by the National Library of Medicine online and via mobile application.

- In general, nearly all antineoplastic, thyrotoxic, and immunosuppressive medications are contraindicated during breastfeeding. Breastfeeding can continue during maternal antibiotic therapy. Although all major anticonvulsants are secreted in breast milk, they need not be discontinued or breastfeeding discouraged unless the infant exhibits excessive sedation.

Breastfeeding and Contraception

- **Lactational amenorrhea method** is 95% to 99% protective against pregnancy in the first 6 months postpartum if amenorrheic and strict criteria are followed. Feedings must be every 4 hours during the day and every 6 hours at night, and supplemental feedings should not exceed 5% to 10%.
- **Progestin-only contraceptive** (eg, mini-pill, progestin injectables, progestin implants, and the levonorgestrel IUD) do not affect the quality of and may increase the volume of breast milk. These contraceptives are among the preferred methods of hormonal contraception in the immediate postpartum period. Progestins are detectable in breast milk, but no evidence suggests adverse effects on the infant. The levonorgestrel IUD or the etonogestrel implant (Nexplanon) are the progestin-only options with the greatest efficacy; either may be inserted immediately postpartum or at the 6-week postpartum visit. Micronor pills must be taken at the same time daily to be effective.
- **Nonhormonal methods** of contraception (eg, condoms, copper IUD, sterilization) will have no impact on milk production.
- The estrogen in **combination estrogen-progestin contraceptives** (pills, patch, ring) can reduce the quantity and duration of breast milk. If combination oral contraceptive pills are the preferred method of contraception, they should be started 6 weeks postpartum and should only be started after lactation is well established and the infant's nutritional status is appropriate. Some providers may initiate oral contraceptive pills as early as 1 month postpartum if lactation is well established, if the patient declines other forms of contraception, if the risk of repeat pregnancy is significant, and if the patient is without other risk factors for venous thromboembolism.

Lactational Mastitis

- **Mastitis** is a breast infection that occurs in 1% to 2% of breastfeeding women, usually between postpartum weeks 1 and 5. It is characterized by a localized sore, reddened, indurated area on the breast and is often accompanied by fever, chills, and malaise. Forty percent of mastitis is due to *Staphylococcus aureus* infection. Other common organisms include B-hemolytic streptococci, *E coli*, and *Haemophilus influenzae*.
- **Differential diagnosis** (Table 24-2)
  - **Nipple pain:** *Nipple sensitivity* typically occurs at initiation of a feed during the first few weeks postpartum often related to injury (abrasion, bruising, cracking, blistering) due to incorrect positioning or latching. *Areolar dermatitis* presents as a red, scaly, itchy rash and can result from exposure to irritants or allergens and may require topical steroids in addition to avoidance of the irritants. *Nipple vasoconstriction* can occur in mothers with Raynaud phenomenon, cold sensitivity, or nipple trauma.

Table 24-2   Postpartum Breast Tenderness[a]

	Engorgement	Mastitis	Plugged Duct
Onset	Gradual	Sudden	Gradual
Location	Bilateral	Unilateral	Unilateral
Swelling	Generalized	Localized	Localized
Pain	Generalized	Intense, localized	Localized
Systemic symptoms	Feels well	Feels ill	Feels well
Fever	No	Yes	No

[a]Reprinted with permission from Beckmann CRB, Ling FW, Barzansky BM, et al. *Obstetrics and Gynecology*. 4th ed. Baltimore, MD: Lippincott Williams & Wilkins; 2002:158.

- **Clogged milk ducts:** a tender lump in the breast not accompanied by systemic symptoms that resolves after application of warm compresses and massage. It is a localized area of milk stasis causing distention of the tissue. Unrelieved, clogged ducts can lead to *galactoceles*, soft cystic masses filled initially with milk that can become a thick cheesy substance that is difficult to drain. Galactoceles rarely require ultrasound treatment or needle aspiration if conservative methods fail.
- **Breast engorgement:** bilateral, generalized tenderness of breasts, often occurring 2 to 4 days postpartum and associated with low-grade fevers. It results from interstitial edema with onset of lactation or accumulation of excess milk. It may be treated with application of warm compresses followed by hand or pump expression of milk and continued breastfeeding.
- **Inflammatory breast cancer:** a rare disease that presents with breast tenderness and breast skin changes and often associated with axillary lymphadenopathy. It should be considered if mastitis does not resolve with appropriate treatment.
- **Breast abscess:** a firm, tender, fluctuant, usually well-circumscribed mass. Breast ultrasound may be required for diagnosis as well as to facilitate guided drainage or surgical incision and drainage (I&D), which may be necessary for treatment.
- **Breast candidiasis:** a frequent clinical diagnosis despite limited evidence on its presentation. It is typically diagnosed on the basis of out-of-proportion breast pain, history of maternal vaginal candida infection or infant infection, shiny or flaky skin around the nipple, and positive areolar or milk candida culture. Treatment can include topical antifungal, gentian violet, or systemic antifungal.
- **Treatment** for mastitis includes continued nursing, nonsteroidal anti-inflammatory pain medication, and antibiotics. Initial antibiotic therapy is often started with **dicloxacillin** 500 mg orally 4 times per day for 10 days. Clindamycin 300 mg orally 4 times per day may be used in patients with an allergy to β-lactams. Women should continue to express milk, starting on the affected side, to encourage complete emptying. If there is no improvement in 48 hours, antibiotic coverage should be changed to cephalexin or ampicillin with clavulanate (Augmentin) and imaging ordered to evaluate for breast abscess.

Decreased Milk Supply

- The normal volume of milk produced at the end of the first postpartum week is 550 mL/d. By 2 to 3 weeks, milk production is increased to approximately 800 mL/d. Production peaks at 1.5 to 2.0 L/d. Frequent breastfeeding and good maternal nutrition help maintain milk stores. Inadequate milk supply can result from poor nutritional status, dehydration, insufficient breast development in pregnancy resulting from congenital abnormality, previous breast surgery or irradiation, insulin resistance, high androgen levels, or endocrine abnormalities. **Sheehan syndrome** (postpartum pituitary necrosis) can result in lack of milk production from low prolactin levels.
- **Treatment:** Interventions to increase the milk supply will vary based on the cause but overall aim to increase the effectiveness and frequency of breastfeeding with the use of breast pumps or manual milk expression. An emphasis on increasing maternal confidence is also often necessary.

Weaning

- Abrupt weaning is likely to lead to engorgement within 3 days and should be avoided as much as possible. Breast binding, ice packs, and avoiding nipple stimulation are recommended for nonbreastfeeding women or women who wean abruptly.
- Routine weaning (usually after 6 mo) typically follows the child's lead and as such occurs gradually thereby avoiding engorgement. Strategies include dropping breastfeeding sessions, shortening sessions, or increasing time between sessions.

SUGGESTED READINGS

American College of Obstetricians and Gynecologists Committee on Obstetric Practice. ACOG Committee Opinion No. 756: optimizing support for breastfeeding as part of obstetric practice. *Obstet Gynecol.* 2018;132:e187-e196.

American College of Obstetricians and Gynecologists Committee on Obstetric Practice, Presidential Task Force on Redefining the Postpartum Visit. ACOG Committee Opinion No. 736: optimizing postpartum care. *Obstet Gynecol.* 2018;131:e140-e150.

American College of Obstetricians and Gynecologists Women's Health Care Physicians, Committee on Health Care for Underserved Women. ACOG Committee Opinion No. 570: breastfeeding in underserved women: increasing initiation and continuation of breastfeeding. *Obstet Gynecol.* 2013;122:423-428. (Reaffirmed 2018)

Curtis KM, Tepper NK, Jatlaoui TC, et al. U.S. medical eligibility criteria for contraceptive use, 2016. *MMWR Recomm Rep.* 2016;65(3):1-103.

Obstetric Anesthesia
Kristen Ann Lee and Jamie Murphy

Options for peripartum pain relief are driven by patient preference and medical indications. Multiple techniques and procedures for pain relief during the birthing process are available. With appropriate counseling of risks and benefits, patients can choose their preferred analgesic treatments.

PAIN PATHWAYS

- In the first stage of labor (cervical dilation), the pain is visceral, produced by the distention of the lower uterus and cervix and ischemia of the uterine and cervical tissues. Visceral pain signals traverse T10-L1 white *rami communicantes* and enter the spinal cord.
- The second stage involves both visceral and somatic pain. The parturient experiences more somatic pain in the late first stage of labor (7-10 cm cervical dilation), entering into the second stage from distention of the vagina, perineum, and pelvic floor. Somatic pain signals traverse the pudendal nerve (S2-S4) and enter into the anterior spinal cord. The parturient also experiences rectal pressure.

OVERVIEW OF OBSTETRIC ANALGESIA/ANESTHESIA

- Delivery type informs the method of analgesia and anesthesia, whether it be local, regional, or systemic. Local and regional methods include local injection, peripheral nerve block, and regional block. Systemic methods can be administered intramuscularly, intravenously, or by inhalation. General anesthesia is often used in cases where total motor and sensory loss is necessary (Table 25-1) or when contraindications to neuraxial anesthesia are present.
- In **vaginal deliveries**, the goal is to block nociceptive pathways while preserving motor function so that the woman is comfortable but can participate actively with second stage expulsive effort. During the first stage of labor, visceral pain is mollified by the preferred use of regional anesthesia, such as an epidural, spinal, or a combination of both. In the second stage of labor, pain derives from the pudendal nerve with descent of fetal parts. Local anesthesia or peripheral nerve block with pudendal injection or spinal/epidural block can be used during the second stage of labor. The third stage of labor, delivery of placenta, is not prolonged by epidural.
- In **cesarean delivery**, anesthetic selection is often determined by the condition of the mother and fetus, the urgency of the procedure, and physician preference. Operative anesthesia requires a denser motor and sensory block than that used for a vaginal delivery. Neuraxial anesthesia is often the preferred method used because it provides adequate pain control while minimizing the maternal risk of aspiration or unanticipated difficult airway. In addition, neuraxial anesthesia decreases systemic catecholamine release and systemic response to surgery, avoids the side effects of postoperative intravenous (IV) narcotics, and allows the mother to interact with

Table 25-1		Use of Anesthesia in Obstetric Situations[a]				
Situation	Local	Peripheral Nerve Blocks	Regional	Systemic	General	Oral Analgesics
Labor—first stage		X (Paracervical)	X	X	N/A	X (morphine PO often used in early 1st stage)
Vaginal delivery	X	X (Pudendal)	X	X	N/A	
Elective Cesarean Delivery	X		X	(X) this is used as an adjuvant to neuraxial anethesia	X	
Urgent/ Emergent Cesarean Delivery	X		X		X	
Postpartum pain			X	X		X
Postoperative pain		(X) (TAP and QL blocks)	X	X		X

X, marks usual options for obstetric anesthesia.
[a]For more information on practice patterns for obstetric anesthesia, see Traynor A, Aragon M, Ghosh D, et al. Obstetric Anesthesia Workforce Survey: a 30-year update. *Anesth Analg.* 2016;122(6): 1939-1946.

the newborn soon after delivery. Effective neuraxial anesthesia can be achieved by epidural, spinal, or combined spinal-epidural (CSE) approaches and also provides the option to rapidly convert to general anesthesia if needed. General anesthesia is appropriate when the patient presents with contraindications to neuraxial anesthesia (see below), medical indications, or in emergency cases where neuraxial anesthesia cannot be administered in a timely manner. Supplemental local anesthesia can be used by the obstetrician on the operative field as well.

TYPES OF OBSTETRIC ANALGESIA/ANESTHESIA

Local Injection (Field Block)

- **Indications.**
  - Used for repairing episiotomies or lacerations after the delivery
    - Common agents include **lidocaine** (1%-2%) or **2-chloroprocaine** (1%-3%), which provide anesthesia for 20 to 40 minutes. The maximum allowed dose of injected lidocaine is 4.5 mg/kg.

- In rare emergency situations where it is not possible to give general anesthesia or neuraxial analgesia is contraindicated, local anesthesia may be safely used in high-risk patients for cesarean delivery.
- **Advantages.** Local anesthesia can provide pain relief without special equipment or personnel. Local block can relieve most of the pain of simple laceration repair. Minimal systemic effect if administered correctly.
- **Limitations.** May not cover entire field well or may not entirely block pain perception
- **Risks/complications.** Inadvertent IV injection can lead to serious systemic complications. Hypotension, arrhythmias, and seizures are rare complications.

Peripheral Nerve Block (Pudendal, Paracervical)

- **Indications. Pudendal block** may be used as supplemental analgesia during the second stage of labor or before operative deliveries if neuraxial anesthesia has not provided adequate relief. **Paracervical blocks** were previously used during the first stage of labor but are no longer commonly used due to increased risk of complications (see below).
- **Technique for pudendal block:** 5 to 10 mL of local anesthetic (eg, 1% lidocaine) is injected transvaginally about 1 cm medial and posterior to the ischial spine along the sacrospinous ligament at a depth of about 1 cm bilaterally. Care must be taken to avoid injecting directly into the pudendal vessels (Figure 25-1).
- **Advantages.** Peripheral nerve block is highly effective. Within 5 minutes of injection, patients may begin to feel its effect.
- **Limitations.** Total anesthetic injection limits apply. In some cases, relief may be inadequate. Pudendal block may be ineffective in up to 50% of patients, is frequently unilateral, and lasts only 30 to 60 minutes.
- **Risks/complications.** Intravascular injection can result in systemic complications including medication toxicity, hematoma formation, and pelvic infection.

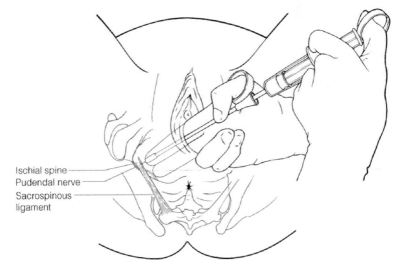

Ischial spine
Pudendal nerve
Sacrospinous
ligament

Figure 25-1. Pudendal block technique. From Callahan T, Caughey AB. *Blueprints: Obstetrics & Gynecology.* 7th ed. Philadelphia, PA: Wolters Kluwer; 2018.

Fetal bradycardia is a known side effect of paracervical block, occurring in approximately 15% of cases. Direct fetal injection is also a risk with paracervical block, resulting in fetal cardiac toxicity. Except in select cases in which other analgesia is not available, paracervical block is usually avoided.

Regional Anesthesia (Epidural, Spinal)

- **Epidural and spinal anesthesia** are the preferred methods for obstetric pain control in the United States. They may be administered separately or as a CSE. Analgesia occurs at or below the T8-T10 dermatomes, with varying degrees of motor blockade.
- **Indications.** Neuraxial anesthesia is the *preferred* method of pain control because of its effectiveness and safety. General anesthesia is associated with increased maternal morbidity associated with increased risk of maternal aspiration and unanticipated difficult intubation. It may be used when there is anticipated difficulty with intubation; a history of malignant hyperthermia, cardiovascular, or respiratory disorders; or a need to prevent autonomic hyperreflexia in women with high spinal cord lesions. Regional anesthesia is preferred in women with preeclampsia because it may increase intravillous blood flow and reduce the need for general anesthesia if cesarean delivery is indicated. *Maternal request* alone is sufficient reason to give regional anesthesia.
- **Technique**
  - Table 25-2 lists agents commonly used for obstetric regional anesthesia.
  - **Epidural** (Figure 25-2): A catheter is introduced into the lumbar epidural space through an epidural needle. The catheter is secured to the patient's back with adhesive tape. Medication is administered via continuous infusion pump (preferred) or intermittent bolus to provide consistent pain relief. Local anesthetic, neuraxial opioid, or a combination of both is used. A test dose (typically 3 mL of 1.5% lidocaine with 1:200 000 epinephrine in bolus) should be given to rule out intrathecal or intravascular catheter placement and avoid complications. Patient-controlled epidural anesthesia allows the patient to self-administer small bolus doses by pressing a dose-demand button. Pain relief may be further improved by a combination of continuous plus patient-controlled dosing.

Table 25-2	Epidural/Spinal Anesthetics	
Class	Action	Examples
Local anesthetics	Block conductance through sodium channels in axons Reversible effect	Amides: lidocaine, bupivacaine, ropivacaine Ester: chloroprocaine
Opioids	Act on opioid receptors in dorsal horn of spinal cord	Morphine, fentanyl, sufentanil, alfentanil
Adrenergic agonists	Bind to α_2 receptors in the spinal cord	Epinephrine, clonidine, dexmedetomidine
Cholinergic agonists	Increase cholinergic effect via muscarinic receptors in the dorsal horn of spinal cord	Neostigmine

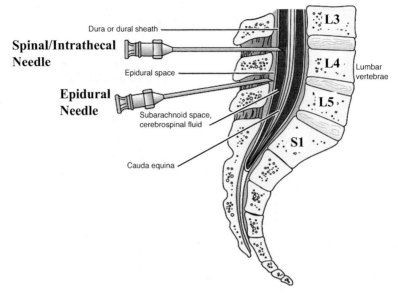

Figure 25-2. Placement of spinal and epidural anesthesia. The spinal cord ends at the conus medullaris near lumbar vertebral bodies L1-L2 in adults, with the cauda equina nerves extending below. Spinal anesthesia is injected directly into the cerebrospinal fluid of the subarachnoid space, whereas epidural anesthesia is deposited in the epidural space (near L3-L4). Combined spinal-epidural analgesia can be administered with a single needle that allows intrathecal injection followed by epidural catheter placement. Adapted with permission from Taylor C, Lillis CA, LeMone P. *Fundamentals of Nursing.* 2nd ed. Philadelphia, PA: JB Lippincott; 1993.

- **Spinal:** A local anesthetic, often in combination with an opioid, is injected into the subarachnoid space. The onset of action is rapid. Continuous spinal anesthesia can be given via an intrathecal catheter, although there is a risk for transient neurologic syndrome especially with infusions of high-dose lidocaine anesthetics.
- **CSE:** This is the needle-through-needle approach in which a smaller bore spinal needle (ie, 25-27 G) is placed inside the epidural needle. A single spinal bolus of opioid, sometimes with local anesthetic, is injected into the subarachnoid space through the spinal needle and then the small needle is withdrawn and an epidural catheter threaded into the epidural space as above. This method combines the rapid onset of spinal anesthesia with the longer lasting relief of an epidural.
- **Advantages.** Regional analgesia provides excellent pain control but allows the patient to participate actively in the labor and delivery process. Increased use of neuraxial anesthesia and the reduction in general anesthesia during deliver has led to significant decreases in anesthesia-associated maternal morbidity and mortality related to aspiration pneumonia and inability to intubate.
- **Limitations.** Regional anesthesia cannot be placed in every case due to time limitations, anatomic considerations, comorbidities, or contraindications. Twenty to 30 minutes are required for full effect of an epidural. Spinal anesthesia lasts only 30 to 250 minutes depending on the drug injected. The CSE is associated with a

higher incidence of fetal bradycardia, with emergency cesarean delivery occurring in 1% to 2% of cases. Failure of the spinal component may occur in 4% of cases in which CSE is used.

- **Contraindications**
  - Patient refusal
  - Coagulopathy
  - Thrombocytopenia is a relative contraindication to neuroaxial blockade, but a safe lower limit for platelet count has not been established. Epidural or spinal anesthesia is considered acceptable, and risk of epidural hematoma is exceptionally low in woman with platelet counts of *70 × 10⁹/L or more*, provided the platelet level is stable, there is no other acquired or congenital coagulopathy, the platelet function is normal, and the patients are not on any antiplatelet or anticoagulant therapy.
  - Infection at injection site
  - Sepsis
  - Hemodynamic instability or refractory hypotension
  - Increased intracranial pressure caused by a mass lesion
- **Risks/complications**
  - **Infection:** meningitis, epidural abscess, reactivation of latent herpes simplex virus (associated with neuraxial morphine use), and maternal fever
  - **Neurologic complications:** epidural hematoma, neural injury, spinal headache, catheter and needle-related complications, back pain, and nerve palsies
    - **Spinal headache.** If the subarachnoid space is entered by the epidural needle, a spinal headache may result in up to 70% of patients. Management includes analgesics, supine positioning, hydration, caffeine, and abdominal binding. More invasive management such as a **blood patch** can be offered if conservative management fails and the patient desires it.
    - **Back pain.** There is no evidence implicating epidural anesthesia as a cause of chronic back pain.
    - **Nerve palsies.** Injuries to the lumbosacral trunk, lateral femoral cutaneous, femoral, and common peroneal nerves have been reported.
  - **Adverse drug reactions.** Local anesthetic toxicity, high spinal block/respiratory distress, allergic reaction, and transient neurologic impairment are possible complications.
    - **Local anesthetic toxicity.** Symptoms include tinnitus, metallic taste, circumoral or tongue numbness, disorientation, and seizures; cardiovascular symptoms include hypotension, dysrhythmias, and cardiac arrest. Management includes the following: Stop injecting local anesthetic, call for rapid response personnel, and secure airway by mask ventilation or, as needed, by more invasive management (eg, intubation or laryngeal mask airway).
    - **High spinal.** Respiratory compromise may result if the block progresses above the C6 dermatome level.
    - **Motor block.** Motor impairment can reduce maternal expulsive efforts and alter the birthing process and parturient experience.
  - Intrathecal opioids can cause **maternal respiratory depression** and hypoxemia.
  - **Hypotension.** Low blood pressure can result from regional anesthesia from sympathetic blockade–induced vasodilation or position-dependent decreased venous return. Hypotension is significant when symptoms develop, such as maternal light-headedness or fetal bradycardia. Episodes can be treated with bolus IV

fluids or low-dose ephedrine (5 mg) or phenylephrine (100 μg). Adequate IV hydration must occur before epidural or spinal access is placed.

- **Fetal complications**
  - **Nonreassuring fetal monitoring.** Bradycardia and transient heart rate decelerations may occur. Hydration is usually adequate treatment, although pressor support (see Hypotension) may be indicated. Repositioning should also be attempted.
  - **Instrumentation.** There is mixed evidence for increased rates of forceps or vacuum delivery with regional anesthesia.

Systemic Analgesia

Opioids (morphine, fentanyl) or mixed opioid agonist-antagonists (butorphanol, nalbuphine) are used for systemic pain relief. They can be administered by intramuscular or IV injection depending on the onset and duration of relief desired. There is no ideal parenteral opioid. Choosing an opioid agent requires careful evaluation of agent characteristics (Table 25-3).

- **Indications:** Maternal request
- **Parenteral agents**
  - **Fentanyl** has a rapid onset, short duration of action, more potent than morphine due to high lipid solubility; repeat exposure can cause fentanyl accumulation, fentanyl has longer half-life.
  - **Morphine** is dose dependent and provides a balance of pain relief with adverse sedation effect.
  - **Nalbuphine (Nubain)** is similar to morphine in analgesic effect but has less risk of severe respiratory depression.
  - **Butorphanol (Stadol)** is more potent than morphine in analgesic relief but has fewer adverse side effects (eg, nausea, vomiting).
  - **Remifentanil** has a rapid onset, short action of duration, and quick elimination of metabolite.
- **Advantages.** Systemic analgesia has a rapid onset and ease of administration and can be administered via IV patient-controlled anesthesia.
- **Limitations.** There are randomized controlled trials that have demonstrated higher pain scores during labor for parenteral compared with regional anesthesia. It is difficult to obtain adequate pain control throughout labor with only narcotic analgesia.
- **Risks/complications**
  - Nausea, vomiting, drowsiness, and pruritus are possible side effects.
  - Maternal respiratory depression requires close monitoring.
  - Sedative effects may increase aspiration risk.
  - All opiates cross the placenta, affecting both fetal and newborn status. Fetal tracings may show decreased variability with maternal narcotic analgesia. Opioid use during labor or delivery may result in newborns with respiratory depression or poor latching.
- **Nitrous oxide** is a systemic analgesia used as supplemental labor analgesia in the United States and worldwide.
  - **Indications.** Useful in situations where patients request pain relief but decline systemic narcotic use or neuraxial anesthesia (or is not available).
  - **Advantages.** There is no limit to patient mobility and no additional monitoring requirement.

Table 25-3 Parenteral Medications for Labor Analgesia[a]

Drug	Usual Dose	Pros	Cons
Morphine	2-5 mg IV or 5-10 mg IM every 4 h	Anxiolytic Sedative	Long onset (10 min IV; 20-40 min IM) Long duration (4-6 h) Neonatal respiratory depression Hypotension (histamine release) Nausea
Fentanyl	1 μg/kg or 50-100 μg IV every 1 h; PCA loading dose 50 μg every 10-25 min	Rapid onset (2-4 min IV) No metabolites Minimal fetal effect Minimal sedation Minimal nausea Can be used as PCA	Short duration (45 min) Potent respiratory depressant Accumulates with repeated doses Minimal sedation
Butorphanol	1-2 mg IV or IM every 4 h	Rapid onset (5-10 min IV; 30-60 min IM) Sedative Minimal fetal effect Minimal nausea "Ceiling" for respiratory depression	Dysphoric reactions "Ceiling" for analgesia Withdrawal in susceptible patients Blocks intrathecal narcotics
Nalbuphine	10-20 mg IM, SC, or IV every 3 h	Rapid onset (5 min IV; 10-15 min IM or SC) Sedative Minimal nausea Can be used as PCA "Ceiling" for respiratory depression Minimal fetal effects	Dysphoric reactions "Ceiling" for analgesia May precipitate withdrawal Blocks intrathecal narcotics
Remifentanil	PCA 0.2 μg/ kg IV every 2 min	Rapid onset (1 min IV) Can be used as PCA	May not provide adequate analgesia in second stage of labor Short duration Potent respiratory depressant Nausea Neonatal respiratory depression

Abbreviations: IM, intramuscular; IV, intravenous; PCA, patient-controlled analgesia; SC, subcutaneous.
[a]Modified from Gibbs RS, Danforth DN (2008). *Danforth's Obstetrics and Gynecology.* 10th ed. Baltimore, MD: Lippincott Williams & Wilkins.

- **Limitations.** It has a lower efficacy as a pain reliever than neuraxial analgesia (causing many to convert to epidural) but does increase maternal satisfaction due to its euphoric effect and change in pain perception.
- **Risks/complications.** Nausea, vomiting dizziness, and drowsiness can occur.

General Anesthesia

- **Indications.** General anesthesia is useful in urgent situations in which epidural/spinal is not available, in cases where regional anesthesia is contraindicated, and in parturients with medical problems that require general anesthesia.
- **Technique**
  - Before intubation, the patient receives a nonparticulate antacid, such as sodium citrate, to neutralize gastric pH and decrease aspiration risk. One hundred percent oxygen is administered for 3 to 5 minutes before induction and intubation, to fortify oxygen reserve.
  - IV agents are used in a rapid sequence induction to minimize aspiration from the abdominal distention/pressure of the gravid uterus.
  - The trachea is intubated quickly with a cuffed endotracheal tube as cricoid pressure is applied to reduce aspiration risk.
- **Maintenance of anesthesia.** Inhaled agents such as isoflurane/desflurane/sevoflurane with an opioid/benzodiazepine adjunct allow a multimodal approach to synergistic analgesia and reduced demand for inhaled agent.
- **Advantages.** Intubation can be performed rapidly in emergent cases. Inhaled fluorinated anesthetics cause rapid uterine relaxation, which may be used to correct uterine inversion or to facilitate internal/external version or release fetal head entrapment. The patient remains still throughout the procedure and does not remember an extensive or prolonged procedure.
- **Limitations.** The parturient is unable to witness the birth of her child. All inhalational agents cross the placenta and can affect the fetus, leading to brief neonatal respiratory depression after delivery.
- **Risks/complications.** There is an **increased maternal morbidity** associated with general anesthesia/intubation. **Aspiration** and hypoxemia can lead to postoperative medical complications. **Neonatal respiratory depression** can occur. Uterine relaxation can increase surgical **blood loss**; therefore, uterotonics should be on hand at the time of obstetric general anesthesia.

Anesthesia Consultation

The following are indications to order a preoperative anesthesia consult:
- **Cardiac disease.** Congenital or acquired disorder, cardiomyopathy, valvular disease, pulmonary hypertension, implanted pacemaker
- **Hematologic abnormalities.** Coagulopathy, on anticoagulation therapy, Jehovah's Witness
  - **Thromboleastography (TEG).** In situations such as obstetric hemorrhage and massive transfusion, a rapid real-time point-of-care test like a TEG can be invaluable in evaluating coagulopathy. A TEG measures the characteristics of a patient's whole blood clot formation and can guide treatment options (eg, fresh frozen plasma, cryoprecipitate, D-amino D-arginine vasopressin, tranexamic acid).
- **Neurologic disease.** Prior spinal cord injury, central nervous system pathology (eg, arteriovenous malformation prior spinal surgeries)
- **Severe hepatic or renal disease.** Hepatitis/cirrhosis, chronic renal insufficiency

- **History of anesthetic complications.** obstructive sleep apnea, malignant hyper-thermia, allergy to local anesthetics, anticipated difficult airway
- **Obstetric complications that may affect anesthesia management.** Placenta accreta, nonobstetric surgery during pregnancy, planned cesarean delivery with concurrent major abdominal procedure
- **Other medical conditions.** Body mass index >50, sickle cell anemia, myasthenia gravis, history of solid organ transplant, neurofibromatosis

SUGGESTED READINGS

American College of Obstetricians and Gynecologists Committee on Practice Bulletins—Obstetrics. ACOG Practice Bulletin No. 209: obstetric analgesia and anesthesia. *Obstet Gynecol*. 2019;133(3):e208-e225.

Bucklin BA, Santos AC. Local anesthetics and opioids. In: Chestnut DH, Wong CA, Tsen LC, et al, eds. *Chestnut's Obstetric Anesthesia: Principles and Practice*. 5th ed. Philadelphia, PA: Mosby Elsevier; 2014.

Nathan N, Wong CA. Spinal, epidural, and caudal anesthesia. In: Chestnut DH, Wong CA, Tsen LC, et al, eds. *Chestnut's Obstetric Anesthesia: Principles and Practice*. 5th ed. Philadelphia, PA: Mosby Elsevier; 2014.

26 Primary and Preventive Care

Sandy R. Truong and Tochi Ibekwe

Obstetrician-gynecologists are in a unique position to interact with women across the reproductive and age spectrum and are seen by many patients as the sole provider of **primary and preventive health care**. The responsibilities of a primary care physician include screening and treatment of selected diseases, counseling, and providing immunizations. Additionally, common nongynecologic conditions that the obstetrician-gynecologist should be familiar with include asthma, allergic rhinitis, respiratory tract infections, urinary tract infections, and skin disorders.

ANNUAL WELL WOMAN VISIT

- History: In addition to a gynecologic history, a thorough history regarding any complaints or symptoms such as breast issues (masses, discharge, pain), menstrual bleeding patterns, sexual function or dysfunction (dyspareunia, discharge), and domestic violence should be obtained. Family history should include risk factors for cardiovascular disease and malignancies.
- Examination: A general head-to-toe examination should be performed with focus on the thyroid (nodules, goiters), breast (masses, discharge, skin changes), and pelvis (lesions, masses).
- Screening: The majority of deaths among women under the age of 65 years is preventable or has modifiable risk factors (Table 26-1). *Primary prevention* is the identification and control of risk factors before disease occurs, and *secondary prevention* is early diagnosis of disease to reduce morbidity/mortality. Screening and counseling on specific issues are discussed below based on patient risk factors.

CANCER

Screening for Breast Cancer

- See chapter 34.
- Excluding skin cancer, breast cancer is the most common cancer in women (a lifetime incidence of 12%) and the second most common cause of cancer-related deaths.

Table 26-1 Leading Causes of Death Among Females of All Races in the United States (2017)[a]

	1-19 y	20-44 y	45-64 y	65-84 y	85+ y	All ages
1	Unintentional injuries	Unintentional injuries	Cancer	Cancer	Heart disease	Heart disease
2	Cancer	Cancer	Heart disease	Heart disease	Alzheimer's disease	Cancer
3	Suicide	Heart disease	Unintentional injuries	Chronic lower respiratory diseases	Cancer	Chronic lower respiratory diseases
4	Homicide	Suicide	Chronic lower respiratory diseases	Stroke	Stroke	Stroke
5	Birth defects	Homicide	Diabetes	Alzheimer's disease	Chronic lower respiratory diseases	Alzheimer's disease

[a]Adapted from Centers for Disease Control and Prevention. Leading causes of death—females—all races and origins—United States, 2017. Centers for Disease Control and Prevention Web site. https://www.cdc.gov/women/lcod/2017/all-races-origins/index.htm. Accessed January 17, 2020.

In 2019, an estimated 268 600 women would be diagnosed with breast cancer, and 41 760 women would die from this disease.

- For average-risk women, screening guidelines for routine mammography and clinical breast examination vary based on organization.
  - The American College of Obstetricians and Gynecologists (ACOG) recommends offering clinical breast examinations every 1 to 3 years for women aged 25 to 39 years and annually for women 40 years and older. Routine mammography should be offered to initiate between 40 and 49 years if patient desires and is recommended every 1 to 2 years at ages 50 to 75 years.
  - The National Comprehensive Cancer Network recommends clinical breast examinations every 1 to 3 years for women aged 25 to 39 years and annually for 40 years and older in conjunction with annual mammography until life expectancy is 10 years or less.
  - The American Cancer Society (ACS) does not recommend clinical breast exams but does recommend
    - *Offering* annual screening mammography for women ages 40 to 44 years
    - Annual screening mammography for women ages 45 to 54 years
    - Annual or biennial screening mammography from 55 years or older until when life expectancy is less than 10 years
  - The US Preventive Services Task Force (USPSTF) does not recommend for or against clinical breast examinations but does recommend biennial mammography from 50 to 74 years.
- The ACOG recommends referral for genetic counseling and testing for patients at increased risk for a hereditary cancer syndrome. See chapter 53 to review who is at increased risk for a hereditary breast cancer syndrome (ie, *BRCA*, Peutz-Jeghers syndrome, Li-Fraumeni syndrome, Cowden syndrome). These patients may need increased surveillance and/or risk-reducing mastectomy.

Screening for Lung Cancer

- In women, lung cancer is the second most commonly diagnosed cancer and is the leading cause of cancer-related deaths. In 2019, an estimated 111 710 women would be diagnosed with lung cancer, and 66 020 women would die from this disease.
- Risk factors include cigarette smoking (associated with 80% of lung cancers in women), radiation therapy, environmental toxins such as asbestos, history of prior lung disease, and family history of lung cancer.
- The majority of studies examining screening modalities for lung cancer (via chest X-ray, sputum cytology, or computerized tomography [CT] scan) have failed to show mortality benefit from early detection of lung cancer. In 2011, the National Lung Screening Trial was the first to show approximately a 20% mortality benefit in asymptomatic heavy smokers (>30 pack-year history) screened with low-dose CT scans. The current recommendation from the ACS is for counseling and informed individual decision making prior to initiation of annual low-dose CT scan screening for high-risk individuals, defined as ages 55 to 74 years with ≥30 pack-year smoking history who smoke or quit smoking within 15 years.
- Smoking cessation, as well as continued abstinence in nonsmokers, is the single most important modifiable risk factor for lung cancer.

Screening for Colorectal Cancer

- In women, colorectal cancer is the third most commonly diagnosed cancer and the third leading cause of cancer-related death. In 2019, an estimated 67 100 women would be diagnosed with colorectal cancer, and 23 380 women would die from this disease. Most colorectal cancers have a long latency period and are curable or readily treatable if detected at an early stage.
- Risk factors include a personal or family history of colorectal cancer or adenomatous colon polyps, smoking, excessive alcohol, obesity, diets high in red meat and low in fruits and vegetables, inflammatory bowel disease, familial adenomatous polyposis, Lynch syndrome, and a history of abdominal radiation. High-risk individuals should be screened with colonoscopy beginning at earlier ages depending on risk.
- For average-risk individuals, the USPSTF recommends screening for colorectal cancer for all persons ages 50 to 75 years, and the decision to screen for colorectal cancer for patients ages 76 to 85 years should be individualized. The decision to stop screening depends on a patient's life expectancy. The USPSTF does not recommend routine colorectal cancer screening for adults 86 years and older. In 2018, the ACS recommended that all adults should begin routine colorectal cancer screening at age 45 years, although this recommendation has not been adopted by other societies to date.
- Many screening protocols exist, divided primarily between stool-based tests and direct visualization tests. Stool-based screening protocols include annual guaiac-based fecal occult blood test, annual fecal immunochemical test, or stool DNA test every 1 to 3 years. Direct visualization tests include colonoscopy every 10 years, CT colonography every 5 years, flexible sigmoidoscopy every 5 years, or flexible sigmoidoscopy every 10 years with fecal immunochemical test every year. The USPSTF recommends shared decision making to identify a regular screening method that best fits a patient's preferences to maximize adherence.
- Women with a diagnosis of Lynch syndrome should initiate screening at ages 20 to 25 years or 10 years before the youngest age of colorectal cancer diagnosis in the family. Colonoscopy is the preferred method of screening.

Screening for Endometrial Cancer

- See chapter 51.
- In women, uterine cancer is the fourth most common cancer diagnosis and the sixth most common cause of cancer-related deaths. Endometrial cancer has a high 5-year survival rate because it often presents at an early stage with abnormal vaginal bleeding.
- No routine screening is recommended for asymptomatic women in the general population.
- Postmenopausal bleeding or significant change in bleeding patterns in premenopausal women with risk factors for endometrial cancer (eg, obesity, unopposed estrogen) should warrant further evaluation such as ultrasound or endometrial sampling.
- Women with Lynch syndrome should undergo endometrial sampling and risk-reducing hysterectomy (see chapter 53).

Screening for Skin Cancer

- Melanoma is the fifth leading cancer in women; risk factors include family history of melanoma, light skin tone, ultraviolet ray exposure, history of radiation treatment for childhood cancer, and immunosuppression. People with between 50 and 100 typical nevi or large congenital nevi are also at increased risk (relative risk of 5-17 and >100, respectively).
- Most groups do not recommend routine skin cancer screening. The ACS suggests routine monthly self-skin examinations for new suspicious lesions especially in higher risk patients. The USPSTF found insufficient evidence for clinician or self-skin examinations but does recommend counseling those with fair skin about minimizing exposure to ultraviolet radiation to reduce risk.
- Guidelines regarding suspicious lesions are as follows:

  - **A**symmetry
  - **B**order irregularities
  - **C**olor variegation
  - **D**iameter >6 mm
  - **E**nlargement/**E**volution of color change, shape, or symptoms

Screening for Ovarian Cancer

- See chapter 52.
- Screening for ovarian cancer is not recommended in women at average risk. It is important to ascertain family and reproductive history to assess a patient's risk for ovarian cancer.
- Women at high risk for ovarian cancer (eg, *BRCA1* or *BRCA2* mutations) can consider screening with transvaginal ultrasound and cancer antigen 125 every 6 months beginning at age 30 years or 5 to 10 years before earliest age of first diagnosis of ovarian cancer in the family (see chapter 53 for further details). Risk-reducing bilateral salpingo-oophorectomy can be performed after completion of childbearing.

Screening for Cervical Cancer

- See chapters 49 and 50.
- The incidence of cervical cancer in the United States has decreased significantly due to routine screening with Papanicolaou (Pap) testing. Routine screening for cervical cancer is recommended starting at age 21 years, regardless of age of first sexual activity. The USPSTF, American Society for Colposcopy and Cervical Pathology, and ACOG recommend that women ages 21 to 29 years should be screened with cytology alone every 3 years, provided the patient does not have a history of cervical intraepithelial neoplasia 2 or worse, is not human immunodeficiency virus (HIV) positive or immunocompromised, and has no history of diethylstilbestrol exposure. Routine human papillomavirus (HPV) testing is not recommended in this age group given the high incidence of transient asymptomatic infection. Women 30 to 65 years can be screened every 5 years with cotesting (cytology and high-risk HPV testing) or high-risk HPV testing alone. Alternatively, Pap screening with cytology alone (without HPV testing) every 3 years may be performed, but this method is the least sensitive.

- Screening for HIV-positive or immunocompromised women should commence within 1 year of onset of sexual activity and no later than 21 years old. Testing should be repeated annually for three consecutive normal tests and then can be spaced to every 3 years.
- After age 65 years, no further screening is recommended if a patient has had adequate negative prior screening results, defined as three consecutive negative cytology results or two consecutive negative cotest results within the last 10 years and the most recent test within last 5 years. Women with prior excisional procedures or cryotherapy should continue age-based screening for at least 20 years from procedure.
- The ACOG and the USPSTF both agree that cervical cancer screening may be discontinued for women who have had a total hysterectomy for benign indications *and* no history of cervical intraepithelial neoplasia 2 or worse.
- Women with abnormal pap smears should be managed per the American Society for Colposcopy and Cervical Pathology guidelines.
- Primary prevention. Gardasil 9 is an HPV vaccine that is approved for the primary prevention HPV-related diseases, including cervical cancer. Gardasil 9 (which covers HPV strains 6, 11, 16, 18, 31, 33, 45, 52, and 58) has been recommended in females ages 9 to 26 years (target ages 11-12 y) and in males ages 9 to 21 years. In late 2018, the vaccine was approved for older patients up to age 45 years. The number of doses of HPV vaccine depends on age at initial HPV vaccination. Women who have received HPV vaccination should be screened for cervical cancer using the same schedule as unvaccinated women. See chapter 49.

HEART AND VASCULAR CONDITIONS

Screening for Coronary Heart Disease

- Coronary heart disease (CHD) is the leading cause of death for women in the United States (cause of 1 in 5 female deaths in 2017). Six percent of women 20 years and older have CHD, and rates of CHD in women increase with age. Risk factors include diabetes, obesity, hypertension, dyslipidemia, smoking, and family history of premature CHD or sudden cardiac death (age <55 y in first-degree male relative or age <65 y in first-degree female relative). A history of preeclampsia and gestational diabetes may also increase risk of cardiovascular disease.
- The USPSTF does not support routine screening of asymptomatic low-risk patients for CHD using resting electrocardiogram (ECG), ambulatory ECG, or exercise ECG. However, a thorough history and physical to assess risk factors for cardiovascular disease is recommended at least every 5 years starting at age 20 years. Counseling for modifiable risk factors (smoking, obesity) and discussion of primary prevention therapies such as aspirin and statins should be initiated if appropriate.
- Primary prevention of cardiovascular disease includes dietary changes; physical activity; management of diabetes, hypertension, and hyperlipidemia; smoking cessation; and low-dose daily aspirin and statin use. Per the 2019 American College of Cardiology (ACC)/American Heart Association (AHA) guidelines, low-dose aspirin might be considered in high-risk patients ages 40 to 70 years who are not at increased bleeding risk.

Screening for Dyslipidemia

- Dyslipidemia is a direct and modifiable risk factor for CHD. Guidelines for screening for dyslipidemia vary. For women with risk factors for CHD, the USPSTF recommends screening for dyslipidemia to start at age 45 years (and perhaps as young as 20). The USPSTF no longer provides recommendations for screening for dyslipidemia in those without risk factors for CHD. The ACOG recommends lipid panel assessment every 5 years, starting at age 45 years.
- Diagnosis of dyslipidemia and calculation of the 10-year atherosclerotic cardiovascular disease (ASCVD) risk requires a lipid panel (see http://tools.acc.org/ASCVD-Risk-Estimator-Plus/#!/calculate/estimate/).
- According to ACC 2018 Guideline on the Management of Blood Cholesterol, primary prevention depends on lifestyle modification and possible statin use, depending on age and risk for ASCVD.
- Lifestyle changes include limiting fat intake (particularly *trans* and saturated fat), increasing dietary fiber and plant sterol intake, losing weight, and increasing physical activity.
- The most commonly used pharmacologic treatments for dyslipidemia include statins, bile acid–binding resins, nicotinic acid, fibric acid derivatives, and cholesterol absorption inhibitors. Decision for treatment initiation and treatment choice depends on the particular lipid profile, risk factors for ASCVD, and calculated 10-year ASCVD risk. Statins are the drug of choice for cardioprotection.

Screening for Hypertension

- Hypertension is a leading risk factor for CHD, congestive heart failure, stroke, ruptured aortic aneurysm, renal disease, and retinopathy. Suboptimal blood pressure has been reported as the number one risk factor for death worldwide. It affects approximately 30% of the adult population.
- Guidelines for the diagnosis of hypertension have recently changed. Previously, hypertension was defined as two or more visits (or home/ambulatory monitoring) with systolic blood pressures ≥ 140 mm Hg and/or diastolic blood pressures ≥ 90 mm Hg. In 2017, the ACC/AHA changed the definition of hypertension to include stage 1 hypertension, defined as systolic 130 to 139 mm Hg and/or diastolic 80 to 89 mm Hg, and stage 2 hypertension, defined systolic ≥ 140 mm Hg and/or diastolic ≥ 90 mm Hg.
- The USPSTF recommends screening for hypertension in adults aged 18 years or older and *annual* screening for adults aged 40 years or older and for those at increased risk for hypertension (individuals with high-normal blood pressure 130 to 139/85 to 89 mm Hg, overweight or obese, or African Americans). Adults between 18 and 39 years with normal blood pressure and no risk factors should be rescreened every 3 to 5 years. The ACOG recommends blood pressure screening annually with well woman visits.
- Essential or primary hypertension may result from excess salt intake, obesity, low fruit/vegetable intake, low potassium, or excessive alcohol use. Secondary causes of hypertension may include chronic renal disease, aortic coarctation, pheochromocytoma, Cushing disease, primary aldosteronism, renovascular disease, sleep apnea, or thyroid disease.
- Lifestyle modifications are encouraged in all patients with suboptimal blood pressure and include weight loss, reduction in dietary sodium intake, moderate alcohol

Table 26-2	American College of Cardiology/American Heart Association Treatment and Follow-up Guidelines for Hypertension (2017)[a]		
Blood Pressure Classification	Drug Therapy	Follow-up
Normal <120/80	Promote optimal lifestyle habits	Reassess in 1 y.
Elevated blood pressure 120-129/<80	Nonpharmacologic therapy	Reassess in 3-6 mo.
Stage I hypertension 130-139/80-89		
No clinical cardiovascular disease or estimated 10-y risk <10%	Nonpharmacologic therapy	Reassess in 3-6 mo.
Clinical cardiovascular disease or estimated 10-y risk ≥10%	Nonpharmacologic therapy AND antihypertensive	Reassess in 1 mo.
Stage 2 hypertension ≥140/80 mm Hg	Nonpharmacologic therapy AND antihypertensive	Reassess in 1 mo.

[a]Data from Whelton PK, Carey RM, Aronow WS, et al. 2017 ACC/AHA/AAPA/ABC/ACPM/AGS/APhA/ASH/ASPC/NMA/PCNA guideline for the prevention, detection, evaluation, and management of high blood pressure in adults: a report of the American College of Cardiology/American Heart Association Task Force on Clinical Practice Guidelines. *Hypertension*. 2018;71(6):e13-e115.

consumption, increased physical activity, and using Dietary Approaches to Stop Hypertension (DASH, a diet high in vegetables, fruits, low-fat dairy products, whole grains, poultry, fish, and nuts).

- The ACC/AHA recommends pharmacologic treatment for patients with blood pressures ≥135 mm Hg systolic or ≥85 mm Hg diastolic and patients with blood pressures ≥130 mm Hg systolic of ≥80 mm Hg with cardiovascular disease, diabetes, chronic kidney disease, age ≥65 years, and an estimated 10-year risk of cardiovascular disease of at least 10% (Table 26-2). Drug choice is determined by comorbid conditions and contraindications and may include single-agent or combination therapy using thiazide diuretics, angiotensin-converting enzyme inhibitors, angiotensin II receptor blockers, β-blockers, or calcium channel blockers.

METABOLIC, ENDOCRINE, AND NUTRITIONAL CONDITIONS

Screening for Diabetes

- The USPSTF recommends screening for type II diabetes in asymptomatic adults aged 40 to 70 years who are overweight or obese. Clinicians can consider screening at a younger age or lower body mass index (BMI) if risk factors are present, such as family history of diabetes, history of gestational diabetes or polycystic ovarian syndrome, or of certain racial or ethnic groups (African American, American Indian or Alaskan Native, Asian American, Hispanic or Latino, or Native Hawaiian or Pacific Islander). The ACOG recommends screening for diabetes every 3 years, starting at age 45 years.

- Screening tests and values, according to the USPSTF
  - Fasting plasma glucose (FPG)
    - Values <5.6 mmol/L or <100 mg/dL are considered normal
    - Values between 5.6 and 6.9 mmol/L or 100 and 125 mg/dL are considered impaired fasting glucose (IFG) or impaired glucose tolerance (IGT)
    - Values ≥7.0 mmol/L or ≥126 mg/dL are considered type 2 diabetes
  - 2-hr 75-g glucose challenge test (GCT)
    - A value of 7.8 mmol/L is considered normal
    - Values between 7.8 and 11.0 mmol/L or 140 and 199 mg/dL are considered IFG or IGT
    - Values ≥11.1 mmol/L or ≥200 mg/dL are considered type 2 diabetes
  - Hemoglobin A_{1C}
    - A value <5.7% is considered normal.
    - Values between 5.7 and 6.4% are considered IFG or IGT
    - A value ≥6.5% is considered type 2 diabetes.
- Patients with impaired glucose tolerance or diagnosis of type 2 diabetes should be referred for counseling on weight loss, diet, and exercise. A trial of lifestyle modifications alone can be considered in those diagnosed with type 2 diabetes with hemoglobin A_{1c} near target (eg, <7.5%). Pharmacologic therapy should otherwise be initiated in type 2 diabetics for improved glycemic control. Upon diagnosis of diabetes, screening should be performed to evaluate for retinopathy, nephropathy, neuropathy, CHD, cerebrovascular disease, peripheral artery disease, and dental disease.

Screening for Thyroid Disorders

- The USPSTF does not recommend screening asymptomatic people for hypothyroidism. The ACOG recommends screening women over age 50 years with thyroid stimulating hormone levels every 5 years. This should also be considered in younger patients with autoimmune disease or strong family history of thyroid disease.

Screening for Osteoporosis

- See chapter 45.
- Approximately one-half of postmenopausal women will have an osteoporotic fracture during their lifetime. Screening for osteoporosis allows for treatment to prevent mortality and morbidity associated with fractures. The USPSTF recommends bone mineral density examinations routinely for women starting at age 65 years. The ACOG recommends testing for all women aged 65 years or older and postmenopausal women <65 years who have one or more risk factors.
- Risk factors for low bone mineral density include low body weight (<70 kg), smoking, family history of osteoporosis, previous fracture, chronic corticosteroid

use, sedentary lifestyle, alcohol or caffeine use, immobilization, use of antiepileptic medications, endocrine disorders (such as hyperparathyroidism, hyperthyroidism, hypogonadism, Cushing syndrome, premature menopause), low calcium or vitamin D intake, malabsorption, inflammatory bowel disease, or chronic liver disease.

- Dual-energy x-ray absorptiometry is the standard of care for measurement of bone density. The most important measurement to consider is the patient's T-score, which reflects the patient's bone density compared to a healthy 30-year-old of the same age and sex.
  - A T-score of −1.0 to −2.5 indicates osteopenia.
  - A T-score of less than −2.5 indicates osteoporosis.
- Repeat screening is recommended every year if the T-score is between −2 and −2.5 or if one has risk factors for ongoing bone loss, every 5 years if T-score is between −1.5 and −2 at any site, and every 15 years if T-score is normal or between −1 and −1.5.
- All postmenopausal women and especially women with osteopenia should be counseled on lifestyle modifications to reduce bone loss. This includes adequate calcium (1200 mg daily) and vitamin D (800 IU daily) intake, reducing alcohol intake, smoking cessation, and exercise at least 30 minutes 3 times a week.
- Pharmacologic therapy is recommended in postmenopausal women with a history of fracture or with osteoporosis based on T-score ≤−2.5. It can also be considered in osteopenic or high-risk women with T-score between −1.0 and −2.5 depending on their Fracture Risk Assessment (FRAX) score (see chapter 45). First-line therapy is bisphosphonate. Other options include parathyroid hormone, selective estrogen receptor modulators, and estrogen/progestin therapy.

Screening for Obesity

- The 2013 to 2014 National Health and Nutrition Examination Survey reported that 40.4% of adult women are obese (BMI ≥30 kg/m^2). It is estimated that 66.5% of American women are either overweight (BMI 25-29.9 kg/m^2) or obese.
- Obesity is associated with an increased risk of morbidity, including type II diabetes, hypertension, infertility, heart disease, gallbladder disease, uterine cancer, colon cancer, and pregnancy-related complications.
- Screening for obesity should include calculation of BMI, measurement of waist circumference, and evaluation of overall risk due to comorbid conditions.
- The BMI is a measure of obesity that correlates with body fat content.
  - Underweight = BMI <18.5 kg/m^2
  - Overweight = BMI 25 to 29.9 kg/m^2
  - Obese = BMI ≥30 kg/m^2
    - Class I obesity = BMI 30 to 34.9 kg/m^2
    - Class II obesity = BMI 35 to 39.9 kg/m^2
    - Class III (morbid) obesity = BMI ≥40 kg/m^2
- The USPSTF recommends that all patients identified as obese be referred for intensive counseling and behavioral interventions to improve diet and physical activity. The ACOG recommends further evaluation and treatment such as bariatric surgery if patient has a BMI ≥40, or 35 with comorbid medical conditions, or has failed prior interventions. In these populations, bariatric surgery may improve outcomes with regard to comorbid conditions such as diabetes.

Counseling on Nutrition

- The 2015 US Department of Agriculture dietary guidelines recommend consumption of a variety of nutrient-dense foods and beverages within an appropriate calorie level. Diet should focus on vegetables from all subgroups (dark green, red and orange, legumes, starchy vegetables); fruits; whole grains; fat-free or low-fat dairy (such as milk, yogurt, cheese, soy beverages); and proteins such as seafood, lean meats and poultry, eggs, legumes, nuts, seeds, and soy products. Additionally, they recommend limiting the intake of saturated and *trans* fats, sodium (2300 mg), cholesterol, added sugars, refined grains, alcohol (up to one drink a day for women).
- Pregnant women and women of childbearing age should consume foods high in iron and folic acid. At least 400 μg of supplemental folic acid per day is recommended in women capable of or considering becoming pregnant. Preferably, iron-rich foods should be taken with vitamin C to enhance absorption. Alcohol consumption should be avoided.
- Older adults, people with darker skin tones, and those with minimal exposure to sunlight should consume at least 600 to 800 IU/day of supplemental vitamin D. Postmenopausal women should consume 1200 mg of calcium daily, either in the form of calcium-rich foods or dietary supplements.
- Estimated caloric requirement for nonpregnant adult women varies between 1800 and 2400 kcal based on level of activity.

INFECTIOUS DISEASES

Women at highest risk for sexually transmitted disease include those with a history of multiple sexual partners, sexually transmitted diseases, inconsistent condom use, commercial sex work, and drug use. Preventive strategies such as abstinence, reduction in number of sexual partners, and barrier contraceptive methods should be discussed with all patients.

Screening for Human Immunodeficiency Virus

- The 2015 Centers for Disease Control and Prevention (CDC) guidelines recommend routine screening in the United States of all adults and adolescents aged 13 to 64 years and all pregnant women, regardless of risk factors, using opt-out screening protocols. Retesting is recommended in women who seek evaluation and treatment for sexually transmitted infections.

Screening for Chlamydia and Gonorrhea

- The 2015 CDC guidelines support chlamydia and gonorrhea screening (with cervical/vaginal swab or urine testing) annually in all sexually active or pregnant women under age 25 years and in women aged 25 years and older with new/multiple sex partners or high-risk behavior. If positive, retesting approximately 3 months after treatment is recommended.
- The USPSTF and CDC recommend against routine screening in asymptomatic individuals for hepatitis B, syphilis, herpes simplex virus, and trichomoniasis in low-risk nonpregnant patients. Women born between 1945 and 1965 with risk factors should be screened at least once for hepatitis C.

SCREENING FOR OTHER MEDICAL CONDITIONS

Screening for Depression

- Depression affects over 30 million American adults yearly. The lifetime risk for women of developing a major depressive disorder is 10% to 25%, 2 to 3 times higher than for men. Rates of depression are higher in women, young and middle-aged adults, and nonwhite persons.
- Factors that may predispose women to depression include perinatal loss, infertility, or miscarriage, physical or sexual abuse, socioeconomic deprivation, lack of support, isolation and feelings of helplessness, personal or family history of mood disorders, loss of a parent during childhood (before age 10 y), history of substance abuse, and menopause.
- The symptoms of depression are summarized by the mnemonic SIG EM CAPS (five out of nine symptoms must be present for over 2 weeks to fulfill the definition of major depression, including either depressed mood or loss of interest).
  - **S**leep—insomnia or hypersomnia
  - **I**nterest—markedly decreased interest or pleasure in activities
  - **G**uilt—feelings of worthlessness or inappropriate guilt nearly every day
  - **E**nergy—fatigue or loss of energy
  - **M**ood—depressed mood most of the day
  - **C**oncentration—diminished ability to think, concentrate, or make decisions
  - **A**ppetite—significant appetite or weight change
  - **P**sychomotor—observable psychomotor retardation or agitation
  - **S**uicide—recurrent thoughts of death or suicide
- The USPSTF recommends screening adults for depression. Many patient questionnaires for self-reporting exist, such as Patient Health Questionnaire (PHQ) and Edinburgh Postnatal Depression Scale (EPDS) in postpartum and pregnant patients. Additionally, in patients who report feelings of depression, direct questioning about suicidal or homicidal ideation is essential.
- Psychosocial treatment may be used alone or in conjunction with antidepressant medication. For patients with mild to moderate depression, psychosocial therapies have been found to be as effective as pharmacologic treatment. Commonly used methods include behavioral therapy, cognitive behavioral therapy, and interpersonal therapy.
- Pharmacologic treatment for depression includes selective serotonin reuptake inhibitors, selective norepinephrine reuptake inhibitors, and tricyclic antidepressants. Patients with severe or chronic depression or failure to respond after 12 weeks of psychotherapy should be started on medication. A large percentage of women experience significant improvement or even complete remission with medical treatment.

Screening for Intimate Partner Violence

- See chapter 37.
- Health maintenance visits should include assessment for intimate partner violence, using direct interview, patient questionnaires, or both (preferably while the patient is alone).

Screening and Counseling for Substance Abuse

Alcohol Abuse

- An estimated 30% of the US population is affected by alcohol misuse, with most of these people engaging in "risky use," which the National Institute on Alcohol Abuse and Alcoholism and the US Department of Agriculture define as consuming more than three drinks on any day or seven drinks per week for women. Alcohol misuse is one of the leading preventable causes of death in the United States.

- All patients aged 18 years or older should be questioned on substance abuse; a number of screening tools exist, for example, the CAGE (Cut down, Annoyed, Guilty, and Eye opener) questions, AUDIT-C, TWEAK, and CRAFFT questionnaires.
- The CAGE questionnaire has been shown to lack sensitivity among women, especially pregnant women, and minorities. Therefore, ACOG recommends modified version, the T-ACE questionnaire, with a positive screen being 2 or more points:
  - Tolerance: How many drinks does it take to feel high? (>2 drinks = 2 points)
  - Annoyed: Have people annoyed you by criticizing your drinking? (Positive response = 1 point)
  - Cut down: Have you ever felt you ought to cut down your drinking? (Positive response = 1 point)
  - Eye opener: Have you ever had a drink first thing in the morning to steady your nerves or get rid of a hangover? (Positive response = 1 point)
- The USPSTF recommends counseling for reducing alcohol consumption; brief 15-minute counseling interventions have been shown to reduce binge drinking. See "Counseling" section for more information.

Tobacco Use

- Tobacco use is the leading cause of preventable deaths in the United States. The USPSTF strongly recommends screening for tobacco use and counseling for cessation because it has been shown that 1 to 3 minutes of counseling significantly increases abstinence rates. The ACOG recommends including e-cigarettes in smoking screening questions as well.
- Behavioral interventions include in-person behavioral support and counseling, telephone counseling, and self-help materials. Medical interventions include nicotine replacement therapy, bupropion, and varenicline.

COUNSELING

- The routine health maintenance visit is an ideal time to counsel patients regarding many health-related behaviors.
- Several techniques for brief physician counseling have been developed, including the five As model, stages of change, and motivational interviewing.
- The Five As model involves
  - *Assess* for problem.
  - *Advise* making a change.
  - *Agree* on action to be taken.
  - *Assist* with self-care support to make the change.
  - *Arrange* follow-up to support the change.
- It is also important to recognize a patient's state of readiness because an estimated 80% of people are unprepared to commit to a lifestyle change at initial encounter. The Stages of Change Model includes the following:
  - Precontemplation: no intention of changing behavior; goal of counseling = introduce ambivalence
  - Contemplation: considering making a change; goal of counseling = explore both sides of the patient's attitude and help resolve behavior
  - Preparation: resolving to make a change; goal of counseling = identify successful strategies for change

- Action: making a change in behavior; goal of counseling = provide solutions to deal with specific relapse triggers
- Maintenance: committed to change; goal of counseling = solidify the patient's commitment to a continued change
- Motivational interviewing is a counseling technique initially used for substance use that can be applied to other goals such as weight loss. The five principles of motivational interviewing are
  - Express empathy through reflective listening
  - Develop discrepancy between clients' goals or values and their current behavior
  - Avoid argument and direct confrontation
  - Adjust to client resistance rather than opposing it directly
  - Support self-efficacy and optimism
- There is evidence that even brief motivational interviewing can trigger significant lifestyle changes.

CARE FOR LESBIANS, BISEXUAL, AND TRANSGENDER WOMEN

- Data from the National Survey of Family Growth suggest that 1.1% to 3.5% of women identify as lesbian or bisexual, respectively. This population faces barriers to health care such as insurance, discriminatory attitudes, and concern for confidentiality and disclosure. Office paperwork should be more inclusive and use terms such as "partners" rather than "husbands" or "spouses."
- All patients should be offered routine screening and counseling as noted above. Routine cervical cancer screening and intimate partner violence screening should not be omitted. In addition, counseling should include contraception and safe sex practices such as condom use on sex toys and avoidance of sharing them. Appropriate referral to fertility specialists should be offered.
- The prevalence of transgender population is not well known, but studies have shown that they are disproportionately more likely to have mental health disorders, substance abuse, and sexually transmitted infections such as HIV. They also experience significant barriers to care with few insurance plans covering the cost of mental health services, hormone therapy, or gender affirmation surgery. Obstetrician-gynecologists may be called on to perform hysterectomies for gender affirmation surgery and should be prepared to refer to appropriate specialists for hormone therapy. Age-appropriate screening for breast, cervical, and prostate cancer should be offered if patient has not undergone mastectomy or hysterectomy.

IMMUNIZATIONS

- Immunizations are an integral component of primary and preventive health care. A patient's vaccination history should be reviewed at regular intervals and updated as appropriate (Figures 26-1 and 26-2).

OTHER PRIMARY CARE PROBLEMS

- **Urinary tract infections (UTIs):** For uncomplicated cystitis, empiric antibiotic treatment without urine culture is appropriate in the nonpregnant patient if the

Recommended vaccination for adults who meet age requirement, lack documentation of vaccination, or lack evidence of past infection

Recommended vaccination for adults with an additional risk factor or another indication

No recommendation

Vaccine	19–21 years	22–26 years	27–49 years	50–64 years	≥65 years
Influenza inactivated (IIV) or Influenza recombinant (RIV) — or	1 dose annually — or				
Influenza live attenuated (LAIV)	1 dose annually				
Tetanus, diphtheria, pertussis (Tdap or Td)	1 dose Tdap, then Td booster every 10 y				
Measles, mumps, rubella (MMR)	1 or 2 doses depending on indication (if born in 1957 or later)				
Varicella (VAR)	2 doses (if born in 1980 or later)				
Zoster recombinant (RZV) (preferred) — or				2 doses — or	
Zoster live (ZVL)				1 dose	
Human papillomavirus (HPV) Female	2 or 3 doses depending on age at initial vaccination				
Human papillomavirus (HPV) Male	2 or 3 doses depending on age at initial vaccination				
Pneumococcal conjugate (PCV13)					1 dose
Pneumococcal polysaccharide (PPSV23)	1 or 2 doses depending on indication				1 dose
Hepatitis A (HepA)	2 or 3 doses depending on vaccine				
Hepatitis B (HepB)	2 or 3 doses depending on vaccine				
Meningococcal A, C, W, Y (MenACWY)	1 or 2 doses depending on indication, then booster every 5 y if risk remains				
Meningococcal B (MenB)	2 or 3 doses depending on vaccine and indication				
Haemophilus influenzae type b (Hib)	1 or 3 doses depending on indication				

Figure 26-1. Recommended adult immunization schedule for ages 19 years or older, United States, 2019. From Centers for Disease Control and Prevention. Recommended adult immunization schedule for ages 19 years or older. Centers for Disease Control and Prevention Web site. https://www.cdc.gov/vaccines/schedules/downloads/adult/adult-combined-schedule.pdf. Accessed January 17, 2020.

□ Recommended vaccination for adults who meet age requirement, lack documentation of vaccination, or lack evidence of past infection

■ Recommended vaccination for adults with an additional risk factor or another indication

■ Precaution—vaccine might be indicated if benefit of protection outweighs risk of adverse reaction

■ Delay vaccination until after pregnancy if vaccine is indicated

■ Contraindicated—vaccine should not be administered because of risk for serious adverse reaction

□ No recommendation

Vaccine	Pregnancy	Immunocompromised (excluding HIV infection)	HIV infection CD4 count <200	HIV infection CD4 count ≥200	Asplenia, complement deficiencies	End-stage renal disease, on hemodialysis	Heart or lung disease, alcoholism[1]	Chronic liver disease	Diabetes	Health care personnel[2]	Men who have sex with men
IIV or RIV / LAIV							1 dose annually			1 dose annually	1 dose annually
Tdap or Td	1 dose Tdap each pregnancy				1 dose Tdap, then Td booster every 10 y						
MMR		CONTRAINDICATED	CONTRAINDICATED		1 or 2 doses depending on indication						
VAR	CONTRAINDICATED	CONTRAINDICATED	CONTRAINDICATED		2 doses						
RZV (preferred) / ZVL	DELAY	CONTRAINDICATED	CONTRAINDICATED					2 doses at age ≥50 y / 1 dose at age ≥60 y			
HPV Female	DELAY	3 doses through age 26 y	3 doses through age 26 y					2 or 3 doses through age 26 y			
HPV Male		3 doses through age 26 y	3 doses through age 26 y					2 or 3 doses through age 21 y			2 or 3 doses through age 26 y
PCV13					1 dose						
PPSV23					1, 2, or 3 doses depending on age and indication						
HepA					2 or 3 doses depending on vaccine						
HepB					2 or 3 doses depending on vaccine						
MenACWY		1 or 2 doses depending on indication, then booster every 5 y if risk remains									
MenB	PRECAUTION	2 or 3 doses depending on vaccine and indication									
Hib		3 doses HSCT[3] recipients only			1 dose						

Figure 26-2. Recommended adult immunization schedule by medical conditions and other indications, United States, 2019. HepA, hepatitis A; HepB, hepatitis B; Hib, *Haemophilus influenzae* type b; HIV, human immunodeficiency virus; HPV, human papillomavirus; HSVCT, hematopoietic stem cell transplant; MenACWY, meningococcal A, C, W, Y; MenB, meningococcal B; MMR, measles, mumps, rubella; PCV13, pneumococcal conjugate; PPSV23, pneumococcal polysaccharide; RZV, zoster recombinant; Td, tetanus and diphtheria; Tdap, tetanus, diphtheria, and pertussis; VAR, varicella; ZVL, zoster recombinant. [1]Precaution for LAIV does not apply to alcoholism. [2]See notes for influenza; hepatitis B; measles, mumps, and rubella; and varicella vaccinations. [3]Hematopoietic stem cell transplant. From Centers for Disease Control and Prevention. Recommended adult immunization schedule for ages 19 years or older. Centers for Disease Control and Prevention Web site. https://www.cdc.gov/vaccines/schedules/downloads/adult/adult-combined-schedule.pdf. Accessed January 17, 2020.

patient displays dysuria and has urine leukocytes and nitrites present on urinalysis. First-line agents include nitrofurantoin 100 mg twice daily for 5 days, trimethoprim-sulfamethoxazole 160/800 mg twice daily for 3 days, or fosfomycin 3 g single dose. If there are any contraindications to first-line treatments, β-lactams and fluoroquinolones are second- and third-line treatments, respectively. The presence of fever or costovertebral angle tenderness is suggestive of an upper tract infection, which requires more aggressive treatment. Recurrent UTIs warrant urine culture for identification of pathogen and targeted antibiotic.

- **Upper respiratory infections:** Typically viral in origin, mild upper respiratory infections should be treated supportively with rest, hydration, humidifier use, and over-the-counter pharmacologic interventions (cough suppressants and decongestants). Antibiotics are not recommended as first line for treatment of uncomplicated upper respiratory illnesses. The presence of secondary bacterial infection is suggested by persistence of rhinosinusitis symptoms for 7 to 10 days and purulent nasal discharge; unilateral tooth, facial, or maxillary sinus pain; or worsening symptoms after initial improvement. Patients with severe pain, fever, and failure of improvement after a period of observation should be treated with narrow-spectrum antibiotics.

- **Asthma:** In addition to monitoring lung function and reducing exposure to triggers, pharmacologic treatment is conducted in a stepwise fashion. Mild intermittent asthma may be treated with quick-acting inhaled β-agonists such as albuterol. For mild persistent asthma, add a low-dose inhaled glucocorticoid or leukotriene blocker. Patients with moderate persistent asthma may be treated with medium-dose inhaled glucocorticoid plus long-acting inhaled β-agonist or a high-dose inhaled glucocorticoid. Severe acute asthma exacerbations may necessitate oral or intravenous corticosteroids or inpatient admission. In addition to vital signs and physical examination, measurement of peak flow can help direct changes in pharmacologic therapy in patients with asthma. Patients with severe asthma should be referred to a pulmonologist or allergist for further management.

- **Acne:** Treatment of acne includes a combination of topical and oral methods and should be referred to dermatologist. Hormonal therapies with oral contraceptives can be effective in the treatment of acne. The US Food and Drug Administration has approved three oral contraceptives for the treatment of acne: ethinyl estradiol 20/30/35 μg/norethindrone 1 mg (Estrostep), ethinyl estradiol 35 μg/norgestimate 180/215/250 μg (Ortho Tri-Cyclen), and ethinyl estradiol 20 μg/drospirenone 3 mg (Yaz). Some treatments for acne are teratogenic so a reliable form of contraception is highly recommended.

SUGGESTED READINGS

American College of Obstetricians and Gynecologists Committee on Gynecologic Practice. ACOG Committee Opinion No. 755: well-woman visit (replaces Committee Opinion No. 534, August 2012). *Obstet Gynecol.* 2018;132:e181-e186.

American College of Obstetricians and Gynecologists Committee on Health Care for Underserved Women. ACOG Committee Opinion No. 512: health care for transgender individuals. *Obstet Gynecol.* 2011;118:1454-1458. (Reaffirmed 2019)

American College of Obstetricians and Gynecologists Committee on Health Care for Underserved Women. ACOG Committee Opinion No. 525: health care for lesbians and bisexual women. *Obstet Gynecol.* 2012;119:1077-1080. (Reaffirmed 2018)

American College of Obstetricians and Gynecologists Committee on Practice Bulletins—Gynecology. ACOG Practice Bulletin No. 168: cervical cancer screening and prevention. *Obstet Gynecol.* 2016;128:e111-e130. (Reaffirmed 2019)

American College of Obstetricians and Gynecologists Committee on Practice Bulletins—Gynecology. ACOG Practice Bulletin No. 179: breast cancer risk assessment and screening in average-risk women. *Obstet Gynecol.* 2017;130(1):e1-e16.

American Diabetes Association. Classification and diagnosis of diabetes mellitus. *Diabetes Care.* 2015;38:S8-S16.

Goff DC Jr, Lloyd-Jones DM, Bennett G, et al. 2013 ACC/AHA guideline on the assessment of cardiovascular risk: a report of the American College of Cardiology/American Heart Association Task Force on Practice Guidelines. *J Am Coll Cardiol.* 2014;63(25, pt B):2935-2959.

Grundy SM, Stone NJ, Bailey AL, et al. 2018 AHA/ACC/AACVPR/AAPA/ABC/ACPM/ADA/AGS/APhA/ASPC/NLA/PCNA guideline on the management of blood cholesterol: a report of the American College of Cardiology/American Heart Association Task Force on Clinical Practice Guidelines. *J Am Coll Cardiol.* 2019;73(24):e285-e350.

Lin JS, Piper MA, Perdue LA, et al. Screening for colorectal cancer: updated evidence report and systematic review for the US Preventive Services Task Force. *JAMA.* 2016;315(23):2576-2594.

US Department of Health and Human Services, US Department of Agriculture. Dietary guidelines for Americans 2015-2020. 8th ed. Washington, DC: Office of Disease Prevention and Health Promotion; 2015. https://health.gov/dietaryguidelines/2015/guidelines/. Accessed March 18, 2018.

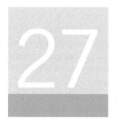

Infections of the Genital Tract

Amanda C. Mahle and Jenell S. Coleman

Sexually transmitted infections (STIs) are common, with approximately 20 million new infections annually in the United States. Most STIs are asymptomatic in women, especially in the initial stages. It is estimated that up to 50% of women with one STI may be coinfected with another infection. Therefore, when infection is confirmed, screening for additional STIs should be considered.

SCREENING

The Centers for Disease Control and Prevention (CDC) recommends prevention of STIs based on five major strategies:

1. Risk assessment and education and counseling on ways to avoid STIs through changes in sexual behaviors and use of recommended prevention services
2. Preexposure vaccination of persons at risk for vaccine-preventable STIs
3. Identification of infected persons with and without symptoms of STIs
4. Effective diagnosis, treatment, counseling, and follow-up of infected persons
5. Evaluation, treatment, and counseling of sexual partners of those infected with an STI

Risk factors for infection include a new partner in the last 60 days, multiple concurrent sexual partners, current or former sex work, prior STI, age less than 25 years old, illicit drug use, incarceration, and lower socioeconomic class. In accordance with the goal of primary prevention, the CDC recommends that health care providers routinely obtain sexual histories from their patients for risk stratification. The importance of effective screening and counseling is underscored by the continued rise in syphilis, gonorrhea, and chlamydia infections over recent years.

INFECTIONS OF THE LOWER FEMALE GENITAL TRACT

Symptoms caused by infections of the lower female genital tract are some of the most common gynecologic complaints. This section reviews infections of the vulva, parasitic infections, vaginitis, ulcerative lesions, and cervicitis.

Vulvar Infections

Human Papillomavirus

- **Human papillomavirus (HPV)** is the most common STI in the United States (see chapter 49). The prevalence of an HPV genital infection is approximately 40% of US adults aged 18 to 59 years old and is highest among teens and young adults. There are over 120 different types of HPV, with approximately 40 types causing a lower genital infection. Most infections will spontaneously resolve within 2 years of initial infection; however, the ability to clear the infection is inversely related to the patient's age.
- There are two main types of HPV infections: oncogenic, high-risk HPV (eg, HPV-16 and HPV-18), and nononcogenic, low-risk HPV (eg, HPV-6 and HPV-11). See chapters 49 and 50 for more information on HPV and cervical dysplasia and cancer. Low-risk HPV types are associated with **condyloma acuminata** (genital warts) and low-grade dysplasia. Ninety percent of cases of genital warts are secondary to HPV-6 and HPV-11 infection.
- **Risk factors** for HPV infection include number of sexual partners, history of other STIs, smoking, immunodeficiency (eg, human immunodeficiency virus [HIV] infection), and use of immunosuppressive medications (eg, chronic steroid use) or solid organ transplant recipient.
- **Signs and symptoms.** Genital warts are soft, sessile, verrucous fleshy raised lesions arising from the vulva, vagina, cervix, urethral meatus, perineum, anus, and oral cavity. Lesions are usually multifocal and asymptomatic but may be associated with itching, burning, bleeding, and/or vaginal discharge and pain.
- **Diagnosis.** The diagnosis is based on gross inspection. A biopsy should be considered if lesions appear hyperpigmented, indurated, fixed, ulcerated, bleeding, or atypical, particularly if the patient is postmenopausal. Furthermore, a biopsy is warranted if the patient does not respond to treatment.
- **Treatment** is indicated for cosmetic and symptomatic relief. Options for treatment are listed in Table 27-1. No single treatment modality has been proven more effective than another. Clinical factors that may influence the choice of treatment modalities include anatomic location, size, morphology, and number of lesions.

Table 27-1 Treatment of Condyloma Acuminata

Therapy	Application	Use in Pregnancy
Patient applied		
Imiquimod 3.75% or 5% cream	Apply 3 times a week at bedtime for up to 16 wk. Wash area with soap and water 6-10 h after application.	Contraindicated
Podofilox 0.5% solution or gel	Apply twice a day for 3 d, no treatment for 4 d, repeat cycle up to 4 times. Do not exceed 0.5 mL volume per day.	Contraindicated
Sinecatechins 15% ointment	Apply 3 times daily for up to 16 wk. Do not use in immunosuppressed or those with genital herpes or open sores.	Contraindicated
Provider administered		
Podophyllin resin at 10%-20% in benzoin	Can be repeated 1 or 2 times weekly as needed	Contraindicated
5-Fluorouracil epinephrine gel	Intralesional injection weekly for up to 6 wk	Contraindicated
Interferons	Inject at edge of and beneath the wart.	Not recommended
Topical trichloroacetic acid (80%-90% solution)	Apply small amount 1 or 2 times weekly. Typical course is six treatments.	Permitted
Excisional procedure	Electrocautery or sharp excision	Only if obstructing vaginal delivery
Cryotherapy with liquid nitrogen	Can be repeated 1 or 2 times weekly until resolved	Permitted
CO_2 laser excision		Not recommended

Abbreviation: CO_2, carbon dioxide.

Additional factors that should be considered are treatment cost, convenience, and treatment side effects.

- Lesions may spontaneously regress and recur, and most lesions will resolve within 3 months of treatment. However, recurrence rates ranges from 30% to 70%, and a combination of treatment modalities may be required. It is important to counsel patients that no modality can ensure complete eradication of the virus and that it remains unclear whether treatment reduces the risk of further transmission.
- See chapter 54 for discussion regarding vulvar intraepithelial neoplasm.

Molluscum Contagiosum

- **Molluscum contagiosum** is a highly contagious DNA poxvirus that infects the skin. The infection is found worldwide; however, it is more prevalent in the developing world. It can be spread by direct skin-to-skin contact (sexual and nonsexual), fomites, and autoinoculation. The incubation period can be from several weeks to months.
- **Signs and symptoms.** Infection is characterized by small, painless dome-shaped papules with a central umbilication. The lesions are often found on the genital region, inner thighs, and buttocks. Multiple lesions may arise; however, often there are fewer than 20. They range in size from 2 to 5 mm in diameter and are typically asymptomatic but can become pruritic, swollen, and inflamed. Often, the infection will spontaneously resolve in 6 months to 1 year; however, but may persist for up to 4 years. Immunocompromised patients may develop very large lesions (>15 mm), which may be resistant to standard therapies.
- **Diagnosis** is often based on gross examination of lesions. If the diagnosis is uncertain, histologic examination can confirm the clinical diagnosis.
- **Treatment.** The infection is usually self-limited, and most studied treatment regimens have not been shown to be effective. Therefore, most experts recommend expectant management. Treatment should be considered, however, in immunocompromised patients and those with sexually transmitted lesions that risk spreading to partners. Additionally, treatment may be prompted by patient preference and lesion visibility. Treatment consists of evacuation of core material with cryofreezing, laser ablation, or curettage. Topical therapies may also be considered, including trichloroacetic acid and benzoyl peroxide.

Parasites

Pediculosis Pubis

- *Pthirus pubis* (**pubic lice**) is an ectoparasite that usually infects the pubic, perineal, and perianal areas but may also involve the eyelids and other body parts. The louse deposits eggs at the base of a hair follicle. The incubation period is 1 week, and the louse can live for as long as 6 weeks. It is transmitted through sexual contact or through shared bedding or clothing.
- **Symptoms** include intense pruritus at the site of infection, which may be accompanied by a maculopapular rash. Systemic symptoms may be present, including fever, malaise, and myalgia.
- **Diagnosis** is made by direct visualization of the lice, larvae, or nits in the pubic hair or microscopic identification of the crab-like louse under oil.

Scabies

- **Scabies** is caused by the mite *Sarcoptes scabiei* var *hominis*. It is high contagious and transmitted via prolonged close contact (sexual or nonsexual) and may infect any part of the body, especially flexural surfaces of the elbows, wrists, finger webs, axilla, breast, genitals, and buttocks. Fomite transmission is possible through clothing, bedding, or towels. The adult female burrows beneath the skin, lays eggs, and travels quickly across the skin.
- **Symptoms.** Scabies often presents with insidious onset of severe intermittent pruritus 3 to 6 weeks after the initial exposure. Subsequent infections can become symptomatic within 24 hours of reinfection. The characteristic lesion is the burrow, a 1- to 10-mm curving track that serves to house the mite. Other lesions include papules and vesicles.

- **Diagnosis.** The appearance of a pruritic eruption with characteristic lesions and distribution is diagnostic. Skin scraping can be obtained, which will reveal the presence of mites, eggs, or feces under oil-immersion microscopic examination.
- **Treatment of pediculosis pubis and scabies.** The first step in management is decontamination of clothing and bed linens with *machine washing and drying on hot* cycle or dry cleaning. Treat pruritus with antihistamines. Other topical treatments are listed in Table 27-2. Treatment should also be provided to sexual and household contacts.

Genital Ulcers

The most common infectious causes of genital ulcers in sexually active women are genital herpes and syphilis. Less common causes include chancroid and donovanosis. Consider the diagnosis of Lipschütz ulcers young women, particularly if they are not yet sexually active.

Genital Herpes

- **Genital herpes** is caused by herpes simplex virus (HSV), a highly contagious DNA virus that infects 1 in 6 people between the ages of 14 and 49 years in the United States. There are an estimated 800 000 new cases annually. There are two types of genital HSV: types 1 and 2. The virus is spread by direct contact with a herpes ulcer, saliva, and genital secretions. The HSV-1 is classically associated with orolabial sores but can spread from the mouth to the genitals through oral sex. The HSV-2 is classically associated with genital infections, but now, HSV-1 is estimated to account for 50% of first-episode genital infections. The HSV-2, more than HSV-1, is associated with intermittent asymptomatic viral shedding and accounts for most HSV transmission.
- **Signs and symptoms.** Genital herpes classically presents as multiple painful, vesicular, or ulcerative lesions. However, some may have mild, subclinical, or asymptomatic presentations. The incubation period is typically 4 days (range of 2-12 d).
  - The primary infection is typically associated with the most severe symptoms, including flu-like symptoms, tender lymphadenopathy, local pain and itching, headaches, and dysuria. Multiple vesicles then appear that may coalesce into painful ulcerations. Outbreaks are self-limiting (can last up to 6 weeks), and lesions heal without scar formation.
  - Recurrent outbreaks are less symptomatic and of shorter duration, typically lasting up to 7 days. They are classically proceeded by prodromal symptoms of localized genital pain, tingling, or shooting pain in the legs, hips, and buttocks, which may occur hours to days before the outbreak of herpetic lesions. The number of recurrent symptomatic outbreaks often decreases over time.
- **Diagnosis.** Clinical suspicion is based on history and the appearance of lesions; however, it is insensitive and nonspecific. Obtain laboratory confirmation with type-specific virology and serologic testing. Determination of HSV-1 or HSV-2 is useful for prognosis and counseling.
  - *Cell culture* and *polymerase chain reaction (PCR) nucleic acid amplitude testing (NAAT)* are the preferred methods for confirmatory diagnosis. The NAAT is more commonly employed due to its increased sensitivity, as compared to viral cell culture. Viral isolates should be typed to determine HSV-1 or HSV-2. Because viral shedding is intermittent, a negative culture or NAAT does not exclude the diagnosis of genital HSV.

Table 27-2 Treatment of Pediculosis Pubis and Scabies

Treatment	Instructions	Special Considerations
Pediculosis pubis		
Permethrin (Nix) 1% cream	Apply to affected areas and wash off after 10 min. Comb the infected areas with a fine-tooth comb.	Safe in pregnancy
Pyrethrins with piperonyl butoxide	Apply to affected area and wash off after 10 min.	Safe in pregnancy
Ivermectin	250 μg/kg orally, repeated in 2 wk	Not recommended in pregnancy
Malathion	0.5% lotion applied for 8-12 h and washed off	Caution in breastfeeding women
Scabies		
Permethrin (Nix) 5% cream	Applied to affected area of the body from the neck down. Wash off after 8-14 h.	Safe in pregnancy
Ivermectin	200 μg/kg orally, repeated in 2 wk	
Lindane (Kwell) lotion	Apply 1 oz of lotion or 30 g of cream in a thin layer to all areas of the body from the neck down and thoroughly wash off after 8 h.	Not safe in pregnancy or if breastfeeding Not recommended for children <10 y Not first line due to side effects including seizures and aplastic anemia
Crusted scabies		
25% topical benzyl benzoate OR 5% permethrin cream PLUS oral ivermectin	Topical treatment: applied to entire body from neck down, applied daily for 7 d and then twice weekly until resolution Ivermectin: 200 μg/kg on days 1, 2, 8, 9, and 15	

- *Serology* can confirm clinical suspicion when culture and NAAT is negative. Antibodies develop within weeks of infection and persist indefinitely. Importantly, immunoglobulin M antibody testing is not type-specific and may be positive during recurrent outbreaks or oral episodes of HSV. Type-specific immunoglobulin G serologic assays that differentiate HSV-1 from HSV-2 are recommended. False negatives may occur, however, in the early stages of infection. Therefore, if there is a high clinical suspicion, the test should be repeated 3 to 4 weeks later.
- Routine serologic screening for HSV is not recommended. The CDC recommends serologic testing in certain scenarios:
  - Recurrent genital symptoms or atypical symptoms with negative HSV NAAT or culture
  - Clinical diagnosis of genital herpes without laboratory confirmation
  - A patient whose partner has genital herpes
  - Patients presenting for evaluation for STIs
  - Persons living with HIV.
- **Treatment.** If untreated, most lesions will spontaneously regress in 2 to 3 weeks. Topical antiviral therapy has not been shown to be efficacious. Systemic antiviral therapy for HSV may reduce symptoms and complications of infection (Table 27-3). The CDC recommends all patients who present with newly acquired HSV receive treatment. Regardless of treatment, the virus cannot be completely eradicated and remains latent in the cell bodies of the sacral nerves S2-S4.
- **Complications** include herpes encephalitis (a rare but potentially life-threatening infection of the brain), aseptic meningitis, pneumonitis, disseminated infection, and urinary tract infections (which can cause severe pain and urinary retention). *Clinicians should differentiate dysuria from urinary retention secondary to loss of sacral sensation due to lumbosacral radiculomyelitis, which is transient but may require use of a Foley catheter.*
- **Counseling.** Patients should be counseled to remain abstinent from the onset of prodromal symptoms until complete reepithelialization of the lesions. Couples should discuss the role of suppressive therapy in decreasing transmission risk. It should be stressed that condoms can reduce but do not eliminate the risk of transmission. There is a 2- to 4-fold increase in acquiring HIV, even without the presence of physical lesions.
- **Special populations**
  - **HIV.** The HSV lesions in persons infected with HIV may be more severe and painful and appear atypical. Additionally, HSV shedding is increased. Therefore, daily suppressive antiviral therapy should be strongly considered in this population (see Table 27-3).
  - **Pregnant** women with an HSV outbreak should be treated. Suppressive therapy, beginning generally at 36 weeks' gestation, is recommended for all women with a history of genital HSV, as cesarean delivery is recommended if a patient reports prodromal symptoms or has an active outbreak at the time of delivery (see chapter 8).

Syphilis

- **Syphilis** is a disease caused by the spirochete *Treponema pallidum*. Transmission is by direct contact with a mucocutaneous lesion, including a chancre, condyloma lata, or mucosal lesion. The incubation period is from 10 days to 3 months. Syphilis has a complex course, characterized by the immunologic response to the spirochete.

Table 27-3   Treatment of Herpes Simplex Virus[a]

Stage	Recommended Treatment Regimens	Duration
Primary outbreak	Acyclovir 400 mg orally 3 times a day Acyclovir 200 mg 5 times per day Famciclovir 250 mg orally 3 times a day Valacyclovir 1 g orally twice a day	7-10 d
Episodic recurrences (begin treatment with onset of prodromal symptoms or within 1 d of lesion outbreak)	Acyclovir 400 mg 3 times a day Acyclovir 800 mg 3 times a day Acyclovir 800 mg twice a day Famciclovir 125 mg twice a day Famciclovir 1 g twice a day Valacyclovir 1 g every day Valacyclovir 500 mg twice a day	5 d 2 d 5 d 5 d 1 d 5 d 3 d
Suppressive therapy	Acyclovir 400 mg twice a day Valacyclovir 500 mg every day Valacyclovir 1 g every day Famciclovir 250 mg twice a day	Per day
Severe disease	5-10 mg/kg IV acyclovir every 8 h Followed by oral antiviral therapy	Continue IV therapy for 2-7 d or until clinical improvement. Oral antivirals continued for total of 10-d course[b]
Persons with HIV, daily suppressive therapy	Acyclovir 400-800 mg twice a day or 3 times a day Valacyclovir 500 mg twice a day Famciclovir 500 mg twice a day	Per day
Persons with HIV, episodic infection	Acyclovir 400 mg 3 times a day Valacyclovir 1 g twice a day Famciclovir 500 mg twice a day	5-10 d
Suppression in pregnancy	Acyclovir 400 mg 3 times a day Valacyclovir 500 mg twice a day	Starting at 36 wk and continuing until delivery

Abbreviations: HIV, human immunodeficiency virus; IV, intravenous.
[a]Adapted from Centers for Disease Control and Prevention. Sexually transmitted diseases treatment guidelines, 2015. *MMWR Recomm Rep.* 2015;64(RR-3):1-137.
[b]Herpes simplex virus encephalitis requires 21 days of total therapy.

- The disease is divided into overlapping stages: primary, secondary, tertiary, and latent syphilis. Patients typically present with primary or secondary syphilis.
  - **Primary syphilis** usually presents as a hard, painless, solitary chancre on the vulva, vagina, or cervix; however, extragenital lesions may occur. Lesions that occur on the cervix or in the vagina often go unrecognized. Nontender inguinal lymphadenopathy is frequently present. The primary chancre usually resolves spontaneously within 2 to 6 weeks.
  - **Secondary syphilis** occurs after hematogenous spread of the spirochete, usually 4 to 8 weeks after primary infection; however, it can occur up to 6 months later. This stage is characterized by generalized nonpruritic papulosquamous rash typically on the palms and soles, irregular rash, mucous patches, patchy alopecia, condyloma lata, and generalized lymphadenopathy. Systemic symptoms such as fever, headache, and malaise also may occur.
  - **Latent syphilis** is defined by seropositivity without evidence of clinical manifestations. Latent syphilis documented as acquired during the previous year is *considered early latent syphilis*. Otherwise, the infection is termed *late latent* or *latent syphilis of unknown duration*. Significantly, late latent is not infectious by sexual transmission.
  - **Tertiary syphilis** develops in up to one-third of the untreated or inadequately treated patients. It is characterized by **gummas**, locally destructive lesions of the bone, skin, or other organs. Cardiovascular involvement in tertiary syphilis includes aortic aneurysm and aortic valve insufficiency.
  - **Neurosyphilis** can occur during any stage of syphilis and is not synonymous with tertiary syphilis. Neurologic symptoms that may present in the first few months to years (up to 10-30 y) following infection include cranial nerve palsy, meningitis, stroke, and auditory and ophthalmic abnormalities. Late neurologic signs may include tabes dorsalis and general paresis. All patients with clinical evidence of CNS involvement, evidence of active tertiary syphilis or serologic treatment failure should have examination of the cerebrospinal fluid (CSF) performed.
- **Screening.** All patients with signs or symptoms of syphilis should have diagnostic testing. Additionally, asymptomatic persons at high risk of acquiring syphilis should be screened for infection. Risk factors include incarceration, commercial sex work, men who have sex with men, HIV infection, and recent diagnosis of another STI. All pregnant women should be screened for syphilis early during their prenatal care. In high-risk patients or in high-prevalence areas, syphilis testing should be repeated during the third trimester and at delivery.
- **Diagnosis.** The *T pallidum* cannot by cultured in vitro. Definitive diagnosis of syphilis is made by identifying the spirochete through dark-field microscopy or by direct fluorescent antibody tests of lesion exudate or tissue. However, most labs make the diagnosis using a combination of nontreponemal serologic tests and treponemal tests. Nontreponemal tests include the Venereal Disease Research Laboratory (VDRL) or rapid plasma reagin. A positive VDRL or rapid plasma reagin test, however, requires confirmation with treponemal testing because false positives are possible. Treponemal tests include fluorescent treponemal antibody absorbed test (FTA-ABS), *T pallidum* passive particle agglutination assay, enzyme immunoassays, and chemiluminescent immunoassays. False-positive nontreponemal tests are associated with HIV infection, older age, pregnancy, autoimmune disorders, chronic active hepatitis, intravenous drug use, febrile illness, and immunization.

Serologic tests become positive 4 to 6 weeks after exposure, usually 1 to 2 weeks after the appearance of the primary chancres.

- Nontreponemal test antibody titers correlate with disease activity and can be used to follow treatment response. A 4-fold change in titer of the same nontreponemal test is considered evidence of treatment response.
- The nontreponemal tests may become nonreactive after treatment; however, for some individuals, these antibodies may persist, a phenomenon referred to as "serofast reaction." The FTA-ABS test will usually remain positive indefinitely, regardless of treatment.
- Most laboratories have begun using a reverse syphilis screening algorithm where the treponemal tests are done first, followed by a nontreponemal test. Treponemal tests will be positive in individuals with previously treated syphilis as well as in those with untreated or incompletely treated syphilis. A positive treponemal test result is then followed by a nontreponemal test with titer. If the nontreponemal test is negative, a different treponemal test should be performed to verify the results of the first test. If the second treponemal test is positive, patients without a history of prior treatment should be offered treatment for late latent syphilis.
- The diagnosis of neurosyphilis cannot be made with a single test but requires a combination of reactive serologic tests, CSF analysis (FTA-ABS testing), and reactive VDRL-CSF with or without clinical symptoms.
- All patients diagnosed with syphilis should be offered HIV and other STI testing.
- **Treatment.** The CDC recommends parenteral benzathine penicillin G as the preferred treatment for all stages of infection. The specific preparation, dose, and duration of treatment are determined by the stage and clinical manifestations (Table 27-4). Penicillin G is the only form of treatment with documented efficacy and recommended in pregnancy. Therefore, pregnant women with a penicillin allergy should be desensitized and treated with penicillin.
- **Jarisch-Herxheimer reaction** (headache, myalgia, fever) is an acute reaction that may occur after initiation of treatment of syphilis (see chapter 8).
- **Follow-up**
  - The CDC recommends serologic and clinical evaluation should be repeated at 6 and 12 months after treatment (or at 3, 6, 9, 12, and 24 mo if HIV positive). Failure of titers to decline 4-fold after therapy for primary or secondary syphilis may be due to treatment failure or reinfection. These patients should have repeat HIV testing and retreated. Additionally, because treatment failure may be from an undiagnosed neurosyphilis, CSF evaluation should be considered.

Acute Genital Ulceration (Lipschütz Ulcers)

Although often considered uncommon, a recent study estimated that up to 30% of all women presenting with acute vulvar ulceration had Lipschütz ulcers. These lesions often occur in nonsexually active adolescent and young women. The most common etiology for these lesions is a systemic viral illness like Epstein-Barr virus infection and less frequently cytomegalovirus. In many cases, however, no specific etiology is identified.

- **Signs and symptoms.** Lipschütz ulcers may present as the sudden onset of one or multiple painful aphthous ulcers of the vulva or lower vagina, with labial edema, fever, and inguinal lymphadenopathy. The lesions are usually greater than 1 cm in diameter and are deep, with a red-violaceous border and a necrotic base, covered with

Table 27-4 Treatment of Syphilis[a]

Stage	Recommended Regimen	Duration
Primary and secondary syphilis		
Primary and secondary syphilis	Benzathine PCN G 2.4 million units IM	Single dose
Retreatment of primary or secondary syphilis	Benzathine PCN G 2.4 million units	Weekly for 3 wk
Nonpregnant primary or secondary infection with PCN allergy	Doxycycline 100 mg twice a day	14 d
	Tetracycline 500 mg 4 times per day	14 d
		10-14 d
	Ceftriaxone 1-2 g daily IM or IV	Single dose (not first line, should not be used for persons with HIV)
	Azithromycin 2 g orally	
Latent syphilis		
Early latent syphilis	Benzathine PCN G 2.4 million units IM	Single dose
Late latent or syphilis of unknown duration	Benzathine PCN G 7.2 million units total	Administered as 3 doses of 2.4 million units IM each at 1-wk intervals
Nonpregnant latent syphilis with PCN allergy	Doxycycline 100 mg twice a day	28 d
	Tetracycline 500 mg 4 times per day	28 d
Tertiary syphilis		
Tertiary syphilis with normal CSF examination	Benzathine PCN G 7.2 million units	Administered as 3 doses of 2.4 million units IM at 1-wk intervals
Neurosyphilis		
Neurosyphilis and ocular syphilis	Aqueous crystalline PCN G 18-24 million units per day	Administered as 3-4 million units IV every 4 h or continuous infusion for 10-14 d
Alternative regimen if compliance can be assured[a]	Procaine PCN G 2.4 million units PLUS probenecid 500 mg orally 4 times a day	Once daily, both for 10-14 d

Abbreviations: CSF, cerebrospinal fluid; HIV, human immunodeficiency virus; IM, intramuscular; IV, intravenous; PCN, penicillin.
[a]Adapted from Centers for Disease Control and Prevention. Sexually transmitted diseases treatment guidelines, 2015. *MMWR Recomm Rep.* 2015;64(RR-3):1-137, with permission.

grayish exudate or an adherent eschar. Other signs and symptoms of an Epstein-Barr virus infection (ie, infectious mononucleosis) may be present, including malaise, headache, pharyngitis, tonsillitis, cervical lymphadenopathy, and transaminitis.

- **Diagnosis.** The diagnosis is made clinically, after excluding other possible etiologies including HSV and syphilis. The proposed criteria include the following:
  - First episode of acute genital ulceration
  - Age less than 20 years old
  - Presence of one or multiple deep, well-demarcated, painful ulcers with a necrotic base on the labia minora or labia majora
  - Bilateral, kissing pattern
  - Absence of any sexual history or absence of sexual contact in the previous 3 months
  - Absence of immunodeficiency
  - Acute course, with abrupt onset and healing within 6 weeks
  - Recent flu-like symptoms
- **Treatment** is aimed at symptom relief, usually with sitz baths and topical anesthetics. The disease is self-limited, typically resolving in 2 to 6 weeks. If a patient presents with multiple, deep, necrotic ulcers, and intense pain, not controlled with topical and oral analgesic medications, a course of steroids may be indicated. Evaluate for evidence of bacterial superinfection and treat as needed.

Other Ulcerative Lesions

- **Chancroid**, rarely occurring in the United States, is caused by *Haemophilus ducreyi*. While still found in Africa and the Caribbean, the incidence is declining worldwide. The presence of a chancroid is a risk factor for HIV transmission. Patients often present with one or more extremely painful genital ulcers, 1 to 2 cm in diameter, with an erythematous base and clearly demarcated borders. The base of the ulcer is usually covered with a gray or yellow purulent exudate, which bleeds when scraped. Some women may present with tender inguinal lymphadenopathy. If present, the lymph nodes may undergo liquefaction and present as fluctuant buboes, which can spontaneously rupture. Definitive diagnosis is with detection of *H ducreyi* on special culture media not widely available. Although probable diagnosis can be made clinically after syphilis and HSV are ruled out. Recommended treatment is azithromycin 1 g oral single dose, ceftriaxone 250 mg intramuscularly single dose, ciprofloxacin 500 mg orally twice a day for 3 days, or erythromycin 500 mg orally 3 times a day for 7 days.
- **Granuloma inguinale (donovanosis)** is another rare cause of genital ulcers in the United States but is endemic in some tropical and developing areas. The disease is a slowly progressive, painless, ulcerative lesion on the perineum or genitals without regional lymphadenopathy. It is caused by *Klebsiella granulomatis*, which is difficult to culture and has no US Food and Drug Administration (FDA)-approved detection assays currently available. The diagnosis is made by dark stain and visualization of Donovan bodies. The first-line treatment regimen is doxycycline 100 mg twice a day up to 3 weeks.
- **Lymphogranuloma venereum (LGV)** is caused by *Chlamydia trachomatis* serovars L1, L2, or L3. The typical manifestation is tender unilateral inguinal and/or femoral lymphadenopathy. A self-limiting ulcer or papule may occur at the initial site of inoculation. Rectal exposure can result in colitis, characterized by mucoid hemorrhagic discharge, anal pain, tenesmus, and systemic symptoms such

as fevers and chills. If left untreated, infection can result in chronic colorectal fistulas and strictures. Diagnosis is based on clinical suspicion, epidemiologic information, and exclusion of other etiologies that may have similar presenting symptoms. Chlamydial testing of genital and lymph node specimens by culture, direct immunofluorescence, or NAAT may be used to confirm the diagnosis. The NAAT-based genotyping to differentiate LGV from non-LGV *C trachomatis* serovars is not widely available; therefore, patients with clinical suspicion for LGV should be treated. The recommended treatment regimen is doxycycline 100 mg twice a day for a total of 21 days.

Vaginitis

- Vaginitis is characterized by pruritus, dyspareunia, and malodorous discharge. The vaginal microbiota is diverse and may include lactobacilli (eg, *Lactobacillus crispatus*, *Lactobacillus gasseri*, and *Lactobacillus jensenii*), diphtheroids, *Candida albicans*, *Gardnerella vaginalis*, *Escherichia coli*, mycoplasmas, and group B streptococci. The physiologic pH is approximately 4, which is primarily influenced by lactic acid produced by *L crispatus*, inhibiting the overgrowth of pathologic bacteria. Physiologic vaginal fluid is typically white, odorless, and seen in dependent areas of the vagina on exam.

- The most common types of vaginitis are bacterial vaginosis (BV), trichomoniasis, and candidiasis (Table 27-5). Diagnosis is based on symptoms, sexual history, and physical exam. A focused history should include information regarding symptoms, duration, relationship to menstrual cycle, use of prior treatment, douching, and sexual history. Physical examination should start with inspection of the vulva and include collection of samples for vaginal pH, amine ("whiff") test, saline wet mount, and potassium hydroxide (KOH) microscopy. The diagnosis is confirmed by microscopic examination of the discharge, including saline wet mount and KOH microscopy, vaginal pH, and commercially available molecular tests.

Table 27-5	Clinical Findings of Vaginitis		
	Bacterial Vaginosis	Trichomoniasis	Vulvovaginal Candidiasis
Vaginal pH	>4.5	5.0-7.0	4.0
Discharge characteristics	Thin, greyish, adherent, fishy odor with KOH application (whiff test)	Thin, frothy, white/gray/yellow-green, copious	Thick, white, curd-like
Wet prep	Clue cells	Trichomonads, WBCs	Hyphae, pseudohyphae, budding yeast (KOH prep)

Abbreviations: KOH, potassium hydroxide; WBCs, white blood cells.

Bacterial Vaginosis

- **Bacterial vaginosis** is the most common cause of vaginitis, although most women meeting diagnostic criteria for BV are asymptomatic. The most common reason for a patient to seek medical care is malodorous discharge. The BV is polymicrobial, not caused by a single specific species of bacteria, but rather a shift in the normal vaginal flora. The shift is characterized by a change in the vaginal microflora from predominance of lactobacilli to anaerobic bacteria, especially *G vaginalis*, *Mycoplasma hominis*, *Bacteroides* species, *Peptostreptococcus* species, and *Fusobacterium* species. Although BV is not considered a sexually transmitted disease, it is associated with multiple male and female partners, a new sex partner, and lack of condom use. Other associations include douching, increased risk of STIs, pelvic inflammatory disease (PID), and postprocedural gynecologic infections.

- **Diagnosis.** The BV is diagnosed by the presence of at least three of four Amsel clinical criteria: (1) homogenous thin discharge coating the vaginal walls, (2) vaginal pH greater than 4.5, (3) greater than 20% clue cells on microscopic examination, and (4) fishy odor before or after the addition of 10% KOH to the sample (whiff test). Detection of three of these criteria has been correlated to Gram stain, which is considered the gold standard for BV diagnosis. Commercially available molecular PCR tests are now available that are microbiome-based assays and may be useful if microscopy is not immediately available. Care should be used when interpreting the results of PCR tests that include only a single organism (eg, *G vaginalis*) because *G vaginalis* may be present in women without BV. Instead, PCR assays that detect multiple organisms are preferred. Some commercially available PCR assays detect BV, vulvovaginal candidiasis (VVC), and trichomoniasis; however, the CDC states that additional validation is necessary before these tests can be used in clinical practice.

- **Treatment.** Treatment of BV is recommended for symptomatic pregnant and nonpregnant patients (Table 27-6). Patients should be counseled to avoid alcohol consumption while taking metronidazole due to the risk of a disulfiram reaction. Partner treatment is controversial because currently there is a lack of evidence that treatment of partners decreases the rate of recurrence.

- **Pregnancy.** The BV in pregnancy has been associated with spontaneous abortion, low birth weight, premature rupture of membranes, and preterm delivery. Women with BV and a susceptible tumor necrosis factor-α genotype have a 6- to 9-fold increase in preterm birth. Although antibiotic therapy has been shown to effectively

Table 27-6	First-Line Therapy for Treatment of Bacterial Vaginosis	
Regimen	Duration
Metronidazole 500 mg orally twice a day	7 d
Metronidazole gel 0.75%, one full applicator (5 g) intravaginally	Once a day for 5 d
Secnidazole 2 g oral granules	Once
Clindamycin cream 2%, one full applicator (5 g) intravaginally	Insert at bedtime for 7 d.

treat BV, treatment trials among asymptomatic women have not shown a reduction in preterm birth risk. Thus, ACOG does not recommend routine screening and treatment of asymptomatic BV in the general obstetrical population. Furthermore, there are insufficient data to recommend screening and treatment among asymptomatic pregnant women with a history of previous preterm delivery. Symptomatic women are treated. Current evidence suggests that treatment of the male partner does not lower recurrence risk.

- **Preoperative patients.** Prior to the use of routine preoperative antimicrobial prophylaxis, older studies showed that BV was a risk factor for surgical site infection and vaginal cuff dehiscence after a hysterectomy. These studies have not been replicated since the routine use of preoperative systemic antibiotic prophylaxis. Given the low risk of BV screening and treatment, however, screening for BV at the preoperative visit and initiation of treatment can be considered in patients undergoing a hysterectomy.

- **Recurrence.** The rate of recurrence of BV is as high as 30% within 3 months and more than 50% within 12 months. If a recurrence does occur, or if symptoms persist despite treatment, retreatment with the same recommended regimen is an acceptable approach. If multiple recurrences occur; however, suppressive long-term therapy should be considered. Suppressive therapy commonly begins with an induction regimen that consists of 0.75% metronidazole gel or an oral nitroimidazole for 7 to 10 days, followed by twice weekly dosing of gel for 4 to 6 months. Alternatively, vaginal boric acid 600-mg suppositories for 30 days can be added to the oral nitroimidazole induction therapy. Monthly oral metronidazole 2 g, given with prophylactic oral fluconazole 150 mg, is also an option.

Trichomoniasis

- **Trichomoniasis** is the most common nonviral STI in the United States, with an estimated 5 million new infections annually. Infection is caused by the unicellular protozoan *Trichomonas vaginalis*, the incubation period for which is 4 to 28 days. Interestingly, unlike other STIs, there are strong racial disparities associated with *T vaginalis* infection, with African American women having a 1.5 to 4 times greater prevalence compared to other racial/ethnic groups. Like other STIs, trichomoniasis is associated with an increased risk of PID and HIV acquisition.

- **Symptoms** include malodorous, yellow-green, copious vaginal discharge that may be associated with vulvar pruritus. Other common complaints include dyspareunia, dysuria, postcoital bleeding, and lower abdominal pain and cramping. However, up to 85% of infected persons will have minimal or no symptoms.

- **Diagnosis.** Exam may reveal frothy, malodorous discolored vaginal discharge. The cervix may appear friable and erythematous, termed a *strawberry* cervix. Saline wet mount may reveal flagellated, motile protozoon; however, the sensitivity is only 55% to 70%. A point-of-care test is available, which may be helpful when microscopy is not readily available. Additionally, NAAT assays are FDA-cleared for detection of *T vaginalis* from vaginal, endocervical, or urine specimens from women. The sensitivity of NAAT is 3 to 5 times greater than a wet mount.

- **Treatment** should be considered for all symptomatic pregnant and nonpregnant women and consists of one oral 2-g dose of either metronidazole or tinidazole. Alternatively, oral metronidazole 500 mg twice daily for 7 days can be used. Although trichomoniasis in pregnancy has been associated with perinatal morbidity (low birth weight, preterm delivery, preterm rupture of membranes), treatment of trichomoniasis in pregnancy has not been shown to decrease the risk of these outcomes.

Metronidazole gel has not been shown to be effective and is not recommended. Patients with an allergy to metronidazole can be referred for desensitization and subsequent treatment with metronidazole. Tinidazole is more expensive than metronidazole; however, it has been shown to reach higher concentrations in the genitourinary tract with fewer gastrointestinal side effects.

- **Treatment of partners.** All patients with recently diagnosed trichomoniasis should be counseled to refrain from intercourse until the patient and her partner have completed treatment. All sexual partners in the past 60 days should be referred for evaluation and presumptive treatment. If evaluation of sexual partners is unlikely, then some states allow for expedited partner therapy (EPT).
- **Follow-up.** The CDC recommends all sexually active women have a test-of-reinfection 3 months after treatment due to the high rate of reinfection. Testing by NAAT can be performed as soon as 2 weeks after treatment. Most organisms respond well to standard treatment, but relative resistance to metronidazole has been documented. If treatment failure occurs and reinfection has been excluded, metronidazole 500 mg orally twice daily for 7 days can be considered. If this treatment regimen fails, either metronidazole or tinidazole 2 g orally for 7 days is recommended.
- **HIV infection.** Up to 50% of women with HIV are also infected with *T vaginalis*. Treatment of symptomatic and asymptomatic, pregnant and nonpregnant, HIV-positive women is recommended because treatment is associated with decreased genital-tract HIV viral load and decreased viral shedding. The recommended treatment for HIV-positive women infected with *T vaginalis* is 500 mg metronidazole twice a day for 7 days.

Vulvovaginal Candidiasis

- The most common species associated with **vulvovaginal candidiasis** is *C albicans*; however, other species of *Candida* or yeast may also cause symptoms. Women often present with vaginal itching, burning, irritation, dyspareunia, external dysuria, and a thick white vaginal discharge. The lifetime incidence of VVC is 75%, with 40% to 45% of women having repeated infections.
- **Diagnosis.** Signs of VVC can include clumpy vaginal discharge, vulvar fissures, excoriations, erythema, and vulvar edema. The vaginal pH is typically normal, between 4 and 4.5. The diagnosis of uncomplicated VVC may be made based on the clinical signs and symptoms, in addition to the presence of hyphae and spores on saline or 10% KOH wet prep, Gram stain of vaginal secretions is positive for yeast, hyphae, or pseudohyphae, or fungal culture is positive. Molecular assays may also be used when microscopy is not readily available. Culture should be performed in women not responding to treatment, in cases where non-albicans species is suspected, or in recurrent VVC to establish species and to test for azole sensitivity.
- Diagnosis should be classified as **uncomplicated** or **complicated VVC** to guide treatment (Table 27-7). Complicated VVC occurs in approximately 5% to 20% of women affected by VVC and are more likely to fail standard therapeutic regimens.
- **Treatment.** Because yeast may be found as part of the endogenous vaginal microbiota, the finding of yeast on wet mount in an asymptomatic woman does not necessarily warrant treatment. All symptomatic patients, including those who are pregnant, should be treated. Empiric treatment of women with clinical signs and symptoms of VVC, but with a negative wet mount, can be considered.
  - Treatment of uncomplicated VVC is listed in Table 27-8. Azole-resistant *C albicans* is extremely rare; however, it should be considered in women with prolonged azole exposure.

Table 27-7	Features of Vulvovaginal Candidiasis[a]
Uncomplicated VVC	Complicated VVC
Sporadic or infrequent episodes	Recurrent VVC (4 or more episodes in year)
AND	OR
Mild to moderate VVC symptoms	Severe VVC symptoms
AND	OR
Likely to be *Candida albicans*	Non-albicans candidiasis (eg, *Candida glabrata*)
AND	OR
Immunocompetent	Diabetes, HIV, immunocompromise, debilitation, immunosuppression, chronic corticosteroid therapy

Abbreviations: HIV, human immunodeficiency virus; VVC, vulvovaginal candidiasis.
[a]From Centers for Disease Control and Prevention. Sexually transmitted diseases treatment guidelines, 2015. *MMWR Recomm Rep.* 2015;64(RR-3):1-137.

- For severe cases of VVC, extended treatment with topical azoles for up to 14 days or fluconazole 150 mg in 2 to 3 doses, 72 hours apart, is recommended. See Table 27-8 for induction and maintenance treatment of complicated VVC. Maintenance therapy is effective in reducing recurrence in up to 50% of women.
- Non-albicans (eg, *Candida glabrata*) VVC optimal treatment remains undefined. The current first-line therapy for non-albicans is a 7- to 14-day course of a non-fluconazole topical azole. If recurrence occurs, there are several options: (1) 600 mg boric acid in gelatin capsule vaginally once daily for 2 weeks, (2) compounded 17% flucytosine cream alone or in combination with 3% amphotericin B vaginally for 2 weeks, or (3) nystatin 100 000 units vaginally for 2 weeks.
- **Treatment of partners** is not indicated unless the partner is symptomatic or in cases of recurrent VVC.

Cervicitis

- **Cervicitis** is characterized by the presence of mucopurulent cervical discharge or cervical bleeding induced with gentle manipulation of the cervix on exam. Patients may be asymptomatic. If symptomatic, patients often complain of abnormal vaginal discharge, intermenstrual bleeding, or postcoital bleeding. Cervicitis may be a manifestation of an upper genital tract infection, including PID. Cervicitis is most commonly caused by *C trachomatis* or *Neisseria gonorrhoeae* infection. Other etiologies include *T vaginalis*, *Mycoplasma genitalium*, and HSV infections; however, in a large majority of patients, no infectious etiology is found.

Table 27-8 Treatment of Vulvovaginal Candidiasis

	Drug	Formulation	Dosage	Duration
Uncomplicated VVC	Clotrimazole (OTC)	1% cream	5 g daily	7 d
		2% cream	5 g daily	3 d
		100-mg vaginal suppository	100 mg daily	7 d
		200-mg vaginal suppository	200 mg daily	3 d
		500-mg vaginal suppository	500 mg daily	1 d
	Miconazole (OTC)	2% cream	5 g daily	7 d
		100-mg vaginal suppository	100 mg daily	7 d
		200-mg vaginal suppository	200 mg daily	3 d
		1200-mg vaginal tablet	1200 mg daily	1 d
	Ticonazole (OTC)	2% cream	5 g intravaginally	3 d
		6.5% ointment	5 g intravaginally	Once
	Butoconazole	2% sustained-release cream	5 g daily	1 d
	Fluconazole	150-mg oral tablet	150 mg once	Once
	Nystatin	100 000 units vaginal tablet	Daily	14 d
	Terconazole	0.4% cream	5 g daily	7 d
		0.8% cream	5 g daily	3 d
Complicated VVC				
Induction	Fluconazole	150 mg orally on day 1, with repeat dose on days 4 and 7		
Maintenance therapy	Fluconazole	150 mg orally weekly for 6 mo		
	Clotrimazole	500 mg intravaginally weekly or 200 mg intravaginally twice a week		

Abbreviations: OTC, over the counter; VVC, vulvovaginal candidiasis.

Chlamydia

- **Chlamydia** is the most commonly reported bacterial STI in the United States. The infection is caused by the intracellular pathogen *C trachomatis*, which preferentially infects the squamocolumnar cells in the transition zone of the cervix. The CDC recommends annual screening of all sexually active women less than 25 years old. Screening is also recommended for older women with risk factors, including a new sex partner, more than one concurrent sexual partner, a sex partner with concurrent partners, or the diagnosis of a recent STI infection in the patient or her partner. Chlamydia infection is associated with PID, and evidence suggests that screening programs have reduced the occurrence of PID.

- **Symptoms.** Chlamydial cervicitis is asymptomatic in approximately 75% of cases; a lack of symptoms leads to its high prevalence. Symptomatic complaints include abnormal vaginal discharge (yellow or mucopurulent), mild dysuria, or postcoital bleeding.

- **Diagnosis.** Chlamydial infections are diagnosed primarily by NAAT. Vaginal swabs are preferred, collected either by patient or clinician. The NAAT can also be performed on a urine sample (ideally first-catch urine). All women who present with symptoms of cervicitis also should be evaluated for gonorrhea and trichomoniasis.

- **Treatment** (Table 27-9) is recommended on diagnosis to prevent adverse sequelae (PID, ectopic pregnancy, chronic pelvic pain, infertility). Presumptive therapy can be initiated based on clinical findings and STI risk assessment.

Table 27-9	Treatment of Chlamydia Infections[a]
Regimen	Duration
Recommended regimen	
Azithromycin 1 g orally	Single dose
Doxycycline 100 mg orally	2 times a day for 7 d
Alternative regimens	
Erythromycin base 500 g orally	4 times a day for 7 d
Erythromycin ethylsuccinate 800 mg orally	4 times a day for 7 d
Levofloxacin 500 mg orally	Once a day for 7 d
Ofloxacin 300 mg orally	2 times a day for 7 d
Pregnancy	
Azithromycin 1 g orally (preferred)	Single dose
Amoxicillin 500 mg	3 times a day for 7 d
Erythromycin base 500 mg orally	4 times a day for 7 d
Erythromycin base 250 mg orally	4 times a day for 14 d
Erythromycin ethylsuccinate 800 mg	4 times a day for 7 d
Erythromycin ethylsuccinate 400 mg	4 times a day for 14 d

[a]Adapted from Centers for Disease Control and Prevention. Sexually transmitted diseases treatment guidelines, 2015. *MMWR Recomm Rep.* 2015;64(RR-3):1-137.

- **Follow-up.** Patients should abstain from intercourse for 7 days after treatment to avoid reinfection. A test-of-cure, 3 to 4 weeks following treatment, is not necessary unless symptoms persist or the patient is pregnant. However, test-of-reinfection is recommended 3 months after treatment. All patients with the diagnosis of chlamydia should also be tested for other STIs, including syphilis, HIV, hepatitis B, trichomoniasis, and gonorrhea.
- **Sexual partners.** All of a patient's sexual partners for the 60 days prior to the onset of symptoms should seek medical advice for evaluation and presumptive treatment. If evaluation of sexual partners is unlikely, then EPT can be considered if allowed by state law.

Gonorrhea

- **Gonorrhea** is the second most commonly reported bacterial STI in the United States. The infection is caused by *N gonorrhoeae*, a gram-negative intracellular diplococcus, which has an incubation period of 3 to 5 days, but it can be as long as 14 days. The most commonly infected site is the endocervix; however, pharyngeal, urethral, and rectal sites can also be infected. Rarely, disseminated infections may occur. Because of the potential for significant complications from an untreated infection, the CDC recommends annual screening for all sexually active women less than 25 years old. Screening is also recommended for older women with risk factors, including those with a new sex partner, more than one concurrent sexual partner, a sex partner with concurrent partners, or the diagnosis of a recent STI infection in the patient or her partner.
- **Signs and symptoms.** Symptoms often go unrecognized, and patients may not present until they develop sequelae of PID. If symptoms do arise, the most common complaints are purulent vaginal discharge, dysuria, intermenstrual bleeding, or cramping.
- **Diagnosis.** The FDA-approved NAATs are available for endocervical, vaginal, and urine samples. The NAAT has greater sensitivity than culture analysis. Vaginal swabs are preferred, collected either by the patient or clinician. Culture should be used when antibiotic sensitivity testing is indicated, especially if treatment failure is suspected.
- **Treatment.** Treatment of gonococcal infections has been complicated by antimicrobial resistance. In 2007, due to the rise in fluoroquinolone-resistance, the CDC recommended against the use of these agents for the treatment of gonorrhea infections. The CDC now recommends treating all persons diagnosed with gonorrhea with a dual therapy regimen using antimicrobials with different mechanisms of action to improve treatment efficacy and minimize the development of resistance (Table 27-10). The current CDC recommendations are ceftriaxone 250 mg intramuscularly plus azithromycin 1 g orally, ideally given on the same day. If a patient reports immunoglobulin E-mediated allergy to cephalosporins (eg, anaphylaxis or Stevens-Johnson syndrome), 240 mg gentamicin intramuscularly plus 2 g azithromycin may be administered.
- **Follow-up.** Patients should be counseled to abstain from intercourse for 7 days following treatment, and until all sexual partners are adequately treated, to reduce the risk of transmission. All patients with the diagnosis of gonorrhea should also be tested for other STIs, including syphilis, HIV, hepatitis B, trichomoniasis, and chlamydia. A test-of-cure, 3 to 4 weeks after treatment, is not necessary unless symptoms persist or if the patient is pregnant. All patients should undergo a test-of-reinfection 3 months after treatment. If treatment failure is suspected,

| Table 27-10 | Treatment of Gonococcal Infections |

Infection	Recommended Regimen
Uncomplicated infections of the cervix, urethra, or rectum	Ceftriaxone 250 mg IM single dose PLUS Azithromycin 1 g oral single dose If ceftriaxone is not available, alternatively: cefixime 400 mg oral single dose PLUS Azithromycin 1 g oral single dose
Disseminated gonococcal infection (arthritis-dermatitis syndrome)	Ceftriaxone 1 g IM or IV every 24 h PLUS Azithromycin 1 g oral single dose Oral follow-up regimen[a]: cefixime 400 mg twice daily to complete 7-d course
Expedited partner therapy	Cefixime 400 mg oral single dose PLUS Azithromycin 1 g oral single dose

Abbreviations: IM, intramuscular; IV, intravenous.
[a]Transition to an oral regimen may be considered 24-48 hours after clinical improvement.

however, then culture and antimicrobial susceptibility testing should be performed.

- **Sexual partners.** All of a patient's sexual partners for the 60 days prior to the onset of symptoms should seek medical advice for evaluation and presumptive treatment. If evaluation of sexual partners is unlikely, then EPT should be considered if allowed by state law.

- **Disseminated gonococcal infection** often presents with a petechial or pustular rash, asymmetric polyarthralgia with or without purulent arthritis, tenosynovitis, or oligoarticular septic arthritis. It may be complicated by perihepatitis and rarely osteomyelitis, vasculitis, endocarditis, or meningitis. Diagnosis may be confirmed with NAAT of genital sites, in addition to specimens obtained from sites of infection, such as joint aspiration, blood, or from a lumbar puncture. Treatment (see Table 27-10) should involve inpatient admission and consultation with an infectious disease specialist.

Mycoplasma genitalium

- ***Mycoplasma genitalium*** is increasingly recognized as a causative agent of cervicitis and PID in women. The *M genitalium* lacks a cell wall and therefore is not amendable to Gram staining. It is also the smallest known self-replicating bacterium and is extremely difficult to culture, requiring up to 2 months to grow. For these reasons, it was only recently recognized as a major causative agent of cervicitis and PID. It is estimated that as many as 1% of reproductive-age adults may be infected with *M genitalium*, making it more prevalent than gonorrhea.

- **Signs and symptoms.** The *M genitalium* infection is associated with mucopurulent cervicitis; however, many may lack any symptoms. Other reported symptoms include vaginal itching, dysuria, and pelvic discomfort. The infection can ascend to the upper genital tract, resulting in signs and symptoms of PID.

- **Diagnosis** is difficult due to a lack of commercially available, FDA-approved diagnostic tests. Some NAAT tests may be locally available. Due to the unique properties of the organism, traditional microbiologic assays, such as culture and staining, are not applicable.
- **Treatment.** The *M genitalium* is susceptible to both azithromycin and doxycycline, which are also used to treat *C trachomatis*. The recommended treatment for documented *M genitalium* infection for those who have not received empiric antibiotic therapy for PID or cervicitis is a single dose of 1 g oral azithromycin. There is increasing concern for azithromycin resistance. If the patient has failed azithromycin, moxifloxacin 400 mg for 7 days should be considered.

INFECTIONS OF THE UPPER GENITAL TRACT

Pelvic Inflammatory Disease

- **Pelvic inflammatory disease** is an infection of the upper genital tract, encompassing endometritis, salpingitis, tubo-ovarian abscess (TOA), and pelvic peritonitis. It arises from an ascending infection from the cervix or vagina. Long-term sequelae of PID include chronic pelvic pain, ectopic pregnancy, infertility, and pelvic adhesive disease.
- Although classically associated with *N gonorrhoeae* and *C trachomatis* infections, recent data suggests that less than 50% of PID cases are associated with positive NAAT for gonorrhea or chlamydia. More often, the etiology is a polymicrobial infection of organisms associated with the vaginal flora including, anaerobes, *G vaginalis*, *Haemophilus influenzae*, enteric gram-negative rods, and *Streptococcus agalactiae*. Additionally, *M genitalium* may have a greater role in PID than previously known. The BV has been associated with the development of PID; however, it is unclear if the incidence of PID would be reduced by universal BV screening and treatment.
- **Risk factors.** The greatest risk factor for PID is a prior diagnosis of PID. Evidence suggests that 10% to 40% of patients with untreated gonococcal or chlamydial infections will develop PID. The risk of PID increases with each subsequent diagnosis of chlamydial infection. Therefore, risk factors associated with STI acquisition are also associated with PID infection. These include new or multiple sexual partners, adolescence and young adulthood, and co-occurring STIs. Prevention and early treatment of STIs can reduce the risk of developing PID. There is no evidence to suggest that intrauterine devices (IUDs) increase the risk of developing PID.
- **Signs and symptoms.** For some women, symptoms of PID may be subtle, if present at all. For others, symptoms may include abdominal or pelvic pain, purulent vaginal discharge, dyspareunia, dysuria, fevers, and chills. With severe infection, the patient may appear acutely ill, with a high fever, tachycardia, nausea, vomiting, and severe abdominal or pelvic pain. If peritoneal involvement is present, the patient may also present with right upper quadrant pain. This symptom is the result of perihepatitis, or **Fitz-Hugh–Curtis syndrome**, which is defined as an ascending infection of the right paracolic gutter leading to localized fibrosis and scarring of the anterior surface of the liver and adjacent peritoneum.
- **Diagnosis.** The PID is a diagnosis of exclusion. No one symptom is diagnostic. The differential includes ectopic pregnancy, acute appendicitis, diverticulitis, and adnexal torsion, which should all be excluded prior to making the definitive

diagnosis of PID. Health care providers should maintain a low threshold for diagnosis of PID to minimize the risk of sequelae.

- **Minimal criteria.** Empiric treatment should be initiated in sexually active young women and in other women at risk for STIs if they are presenting with **pelvic or lower abdominal pain**, if all other diagnoses have been excluded, and if *one or more* of the following clinical signs are present on exam:
    - Cervical motion tenderness
    - Uterine tenderness
    - Adnexal tenderness
- The specificity of the minimal criteria is increased if one or more of the following **additional criteria** are present on exam:
    - Oral temperature of >101°F (38.3°C)
    - Abnormal cervical mucopurulent discharge or cervical friability
    - Presence of abundant numbers of white blood cell on saline microscopy of vaginal fluid
    - Elevated erythrocyte sedimentation rate
    - Elevated C-reactive protein
    - Laboratory documentation of cervical infection with *N gonorrhoeae* or *C trachomatis*
- If on exam, there is normal cervical discharge and a lack of white blood cells on wet prep of vaginal secretions, the diagnosis of PID is unlikely, and alternative diagnoses should be considered.
- The **most specific diagnostic criteria** for PID, however, are listed below:
    - Endometrial biopsy with histopathologic evidence of endometritis
    - Imaging evidence of a hydrosalpinx or a tubo-ovarian complex, or Doppler studies suggesting pelvic infection, such as tubal hyperemia, commonly referred to as "the ring of fire"
    - Laparoscopic findings consistent with PID
- **Treatment.** Goals for PID treatment are to initiate therapy prior to the development of sequelae. Treatment regimens must provide broad-empiric coverage targeting the major etiologic pathogens, including *N gonorrhoeae* and *C trachomatis*, but should also address the polymicrobial nature of the disease. Negative endocervical NAAT for *N gonorrhoeae* and *C trachomatis* does not rule out the possibility of an upper reproductive tract infection.
- Outpatient oral treatment regimens are standard, except for certain high-risk populations. Inpatient treatment should be administered for patients (adolescent and adult) who meet any of the following criteria:
    - Surgical emergencies, such as acute appendicitis, cannot be excluded
    - Evidence of a TOA (minimum of 24 h inpatient observation is recommended)
    - Pregnancy
    - Severe illness, nausea, vomiting, or high fever
    - Unable to adhere to or tolerate an oral regimen
    - Lack of clinical response to an oral regimen
- If a patient is diagnosed with PID and has an IUD in place, there is no evidence to recommend IUD removal. If the patient does not have clinical improvement within 48 to 72 hours after starting treatment, IUD removal may be considered.
- The recommended treatment regimens are listed in Table 27-11. Clinical improvement with parenteral regimens can be expected within 24 to 48 hours of initiation of treatment.

Table 27-11 Treatment of Pelvic Inflammatory Disease, Including Tubo-ovarian Abscess[a]

Route	Regimen	Duration
Parenteral	Cefotetan 2 g IV every 12 h PLUS Doxycycline 100 mg IV or orally[b] every 12 h	After 24-48 h of clinical improvement, patient may be transitioned to doxycycline alone to complete 14-d course.
	Cefoxitin 2 g IV 6 h PLUS Doxycycline 100 mg IV or orally every 12 h	After 24-48 h of clinical improvement, patient may be transitioned to doxycycline alone to complete 14-d course.
	Clindamycin 900 mg IV every 8 h PLUS Gentamicin loading dose IV or IM (2 mg/kg) followed by maintenance dose (1.5 mg/kg) every 8 h (single daily dosing of 3-5 mg/kg may be substituted)	After 24-48 h of clinical improvement, patient may be transitioned to oral clindamycin 450 mg 4 times a day or doxycycline 100 mg twice a day to complete 14-d course. If TOA is present: clindamycin 450 mg 4 times a day, OR Flagyl 500 mg twice a day, in addition to oral doxycycline 100 mg twice a day to complete 14-d course
Alternative parenteral	Ampicillin/sulbactam 3 g IV every 6 h PLUS Doxycycline 100 mg IV or orally every 12 h	14-d course of doxycycline
Intramuscular/ oral regimens	Ceftriaxone 250 mg IM once PLUS Doxycycline 100 mg orally twice a day WITH OR WITHOUT Metronidazole 500 mg orally twice a day	Doxycycline to complete 14-d course Metronidazole to complete 14-d course
	Cefoxitin 2 g IM once PLUS Probenecid 1 g orally administered concurrently	Doxycycline to complete 14-d course Metronidazole to complete 14-d course

(Continued)

Table 27-11	Treatment of Pelvic Inflammatory Disease, Including Tubo-ovarian Abscess[a] (Continued)	
Route	Regimen	Duration
	PLUS Doxycycline 100 mg orally twice a day WITH OR WITHOUT Metronidazole 500 mg orally twice a day	
	Third-generation cephalosporin (ceftizoxime or cefotaxime) PLUS Doxycycline 100 mg twice a day WITH Metronidazole 500 mg orally twice a day	Doxycycline to complete 14-d course Metronidazole to complete 14-d course The recommended third-generation cephalosporins have limited anaerobic coverage and therefore should be used with metronidazole.

Abbreviations: IV, intravenous; TOA, tubo-ovarian abscess.
[a]Adapted from Centers for Disease Control and Prevention. Sexually transmitted diseases treatment guidelines, 2015. *MMWR Recomm Rep.* 2015;64(RR-3):1-137.
[b]Because of pain associated with IV doxycycline infusion, oral formulation is preferred. Oral and IV doxycycline have similar bioavailability.

- **Counseling.** Patients should be advised to refrain from intercourse until completion of the 14-day antibiotic course to limit risk of transmission. Patients should also ensure that their partner is adequately treated for gonococcal and chlamydial infections. Given the high incidence of coinfection with other STIs, all women diagnosed with PID should undergo screening for other STIs including HIV, gonorrhea, chlamydia, hepatitis B, and trichomoniasis.
- **Follow-up.** Clinical improvement is expected within 72 hours of initiation of treatment. All women with a positive gonorrhea or chlamydia NAAT should have a test-of-reinfection 3 months after completion of treatment.
- **Sexual partners.** All sexual partners within 60 days preceding the onset of treatment should be evaluated, tested, and empirically treated for gonorrhea and chlamydia, regardless of etiology of PID. If the patient's last episode of intercourse was greater than 60 days ago, the most recent sexual partner should be treated. As discussed with gonorrhea and chlamydia infections, in states where EPT is permitted, partners can be provided with prescriptions for cefixime 400 mg plus azithromycin 1 g.
- **Sequelae.** Studies suggest that 15% of individuals will develop scarring of the fallopian tubes and intraperitoneal adhesions after a single episode of PID. Infertility due to tubal occlusion affects approximately 10% to 60% of women following an episode of PID, depending on severity. The risk of an ectopic pregnancy following a single episode of PID is increased 7 to 10 times over the general population. The risk increases with each subsequent infection, and approximately 75% of

persons will have adhesive disease after three episodes of PID. Chronic pelvic pain and dyspareunia are associated with adhesive disease.

Tubo-ovarian Abscess

- A **tubo-ovarian abscess** is an inflammatory mass involving the fallopian tube, ovary, and occasionally, other pelvic organs. It is most commonly associated with preceding PID; however, it may also arise in women without a history of PID or STIs. A tubo-ovarian complex is a specific entity in which a collection of pus is associated with agglutination and adhesions between pelvic structures. A TOA and tubo-ovarian complex are both potentially life-threatening, requiring aggressive medical and surgical management. The incidence of true adnexal abscess is approximately 10% in women diagnosed with acute PID.
- The TOAs are usually polymicrobial in etiology, including *E coli*, aerobic bacteria, *Bacteroides fragilis*, *Prevotella*, and other anaerobes. The resultant inflammation can lead to tubal ischemia and necrosis and subsequent pyosalpinx. If treatment of a TOA is delayed, progressive tubal edema and necrosis can lead to increasing agglutination to surrounding tissues, forming a complex mass. Necrosis within the mass facilitates anaerobic bacterial growth and worsening infection, which may result in sepsis.
- **Signs and symptoms.** Patients diagnosed with a TOA classically present with acute lower abdominal pain, fever, chills, and abnormal vaginal discharge. Some report chronic abdominal pain as their only symptom. Approximately 15% of patients presenting with a TOA will by complicated by rupture. These patients often present with acute abdominal pain and signs of sepsis. Immediate surgical exploration is warranted because a ruptured TOA is associated with a 5% to 10% mortality rate if treatment is delayed or inadequate.
- **Diagnosis.** Maintain a low threshold for obtaining pelvic imaging in women diagnosed with PID. A pelvic ultrasound or pelvic computed tomography should be obtained if a woman has any of the following signs or symptoms:
  - Sepsis or acute illness
  - Significant abdominopelvic tenderness precluding pelvic exam
  - Adnexal mass appreciated on pelvic exam, especially if associated with tenderness on exam
  - Lack of improvement, or clinical worsening, despite broad-spectrum antibiotic therapy. If patient previously had negative imaging for TOA, consider reimaging if at least 48 to 72 hours from prior imaging.
- **Treatment.** In a hemodynamically stable patient, inpatient observation and parenteral antibiotic therapy are the mainstay of treatment. First-line therapies are listed in Table 27-11. Add clindamycin or metronidazole for effective anaerobe coverage. Repeat imaging may be considered after 72 hours of antibiotic therapy to ensure reduction in TOA size. Abscess size may be predictive of the antibiotic response. Abscesses greater than 5 to 7 cm in diameter may be more likely to fail conservative management with antibiotics alone. If the TOA is well-localized, then percutaneous drainage of the TOA with subsequent cultures obtained may be considered. In addition to antibiotics, surgical exploration is recommended for the patient with an acute abdomen suggestive of a ruptured TOA or in the patient who is not clinically improving with medical management (including drain placement).
- **Special populations.** A TOA in a postmenopausal woman is concerning for an underlying malignancy. Therefore, the recommended management is surgical exploration with frozen section examination.

Endometritis (Nonpuerperal)

- **Endometritis** is characterized by inflammation of the endometrium. It is thought to arise from an ascending infection from the lower genital tract. In fact, there is a strong correlation between endometritis and chlamydia colonization or infection of the cervix. Endometritis is less associated with gonococcal infections. Organisms that are associated with BV may also cause histologic endometritis, even in asymptomatic women.
- Endometritis can be classified as **acute or chronic**. Acute infection is usually preceded by PID or a recent invasive gynecologic procedure. Chronic infection is more indolent and often associated with *C trachomatis, N gonorrhoeae, Ureaplasma urealyticum, M genitalium,* BV, and tuberculosis.
- **Signs and symptoms.** Chronic endometritis is often asymptomatic. If symptoms are present, patients may complain of intermenstrual bleeding, abnormal uterine bleeding, postcoital bleeding, menorrhagia, or dull, crampy lower abdominal/pelvic pain. Uterine tenderness or cervical motion tenderness may be present on exam. Acute infections often present with more systemic signs and symptoms such as a fever and leukocytosis and are often associated with uterine tenderness and/or cervical motion tenderness on exam.
- **Diagnosis.** The same clinical criteria employed for the diagnosis of PID can also be used to diagnose acute endometritis. An endometrial biopsy is not necessary for the diagnosis of acute infection. A biopsy and culture are necessary, however, for the diagnosis of chronic endometritis. The histologic findings of chronic endometritis are evidence of an inflammatory reaction with monocytes and plasma cells in the endometrial stroma.
- **Treatment.** If acute endometritis is suspected, the treatment is the same as that for PID listed above. Chronic endometritis is treated with doxycycline 100 mg orally twice a day for 10 to 14 days. Broader coverage to include anaerobic organisms may also be considered, especially in the presence of BV.
- See chapter 3 for more information on puerperal endomyometritis.

SUGGESTED READINGS

American College of Obstetricians and Gynecologists Committee on Gynecologic Practice. ACOG Committee Opinion No. 645: dual therapy for gonococcal infections. *Obstet Gynecol.* 2015;126(5):e95-e99. (Reaffirmed 2018)

American College of Obstetricians and Gynecologists Committee on Gynecologic Practice. ACOG Committee Opinion No. 737: expedited partner therapy. *Obstet Gynecol.* 2018;131(6):e190-e193.

Bibbins-Domingo K, Grossman DC, Curry SJ, et al; for US Preventive Services Task Force. Screening for syphilis infection in nonpregnant adults and adolescents: US Preventive Services Task Force recommendation statement. *JAMA.* 2016;315(21):2321-2327.

Centers for Disease Control and Prevention. Sexually transmitted diseases treatment guidelines, 2015. *MMWR Recomm Rep.* 2015;64(RR-3):1-137.

Curry SJ, Krist AH, Owens DK, et al; for US Preventive Services Task Force. Screening for syphilis infection in pregnant women: US Preventive Services Task Force reaffirmation recommendation statement. *JAMA.* 2018;320(9):911-917.

Martens MG. Pelvic inflammatory disease. In: Jones HW, Rock JA, eds. *Te Linde's Operative Gynecology.* 11th ed. Philadelphia: Wolters Kluwer; 2015:631-656.

Wolters V, Hoogslag I, Wout JVT, Boers K. Lipschütz ulcers: a rare diagnosis in women with vulvar ulceration. *Obstet Gynecol.* 2017;130(2):420-422.

28 Contraception and Sterilization
Stacy Sun and Jennifer A. Robinson

Contraception is a key preventive health measure for women. Approximately 60% of all US women and 90% of those at risk for unintended pregnancy report using a contraceptive method. There are numerous noncontraceptive benefits of contraceptives, and an individual woman's priorities regarding contraception use may change over her lifetime.

TIERS OF EFFECTIVENESS

- Table 28-1 lists contraceptive methods available in the United States, along with their perfect-use and typical-use failure rates. Contraceptive methods can also be considered in terms of "tiers of effectiveness" based on pregnancy rates with typical use (Figure 28-1). In this chapter, we discuss methods in approximate descending order of effectiveness.
- Another useful resource is the Centers for Disease Control and Prevention's Medical Eligibility Criteria for Contraceptive Use (CDC MEC), which provides guidance for safe use of contraceptives for women with medical comorbidities. It is available online and as a free downloadable app.

HIGHLY EFFECTIVE CONTRACEPTIVE METHODS

Sterilization (Permanent Contraception)

Female Sterilization

- Female sterilization is a surgical procedure in which the fallopian tubes are occluded, transected, or removed, preventing fertilization by blocking sperm from reaching the oocyte. Sterilization can be performed immediately postpartum (within 48 h after vaginal delivery), at the time of cesarean delivery, or unrelated to pregnancy via laparoscopy or hysteroscopy.
- The Collaborative Review of Sterilization study, a landmark analysis of surgical sterilization in the United States, compared the long-term effectiveness of numerous methods of sterilization and found an overall failure rate of 18.5 pregnancies per 1000 procedures.
- **Advantages:** Female sterilization provides highly effective, permanent contraception to women who do not desire future childbearing. Sterilization decreases the risk of subsequent pelvic inflammatory disease (PID) and may decrease a woman's lifetime risk of ovarian cancer.
- **Disadvantages:** Female sterilization typically requires regional or general anesthesia. There are risks of surgical complications and sterilization failure resulting in intrauterine or ectopic pregnancy. Women sterilized before age 30 years have higher rates of failure and regret compared to older women.
- The reported 10-year cumulative probability of ectopic pregnancy for all female sterilization methods in the Collaborative Review of Sterilization study was 7 in 1000,

Table 28-1 Percentage of Women Experiencing an Unintended Pregnancy During the First Year of Typical Use and the First Year of Perfect Use of Contraception and the Percentage Continuing Use at the End of the First Year, United States[a]

Method	Percentage of Women Experiencing an Unintended Pregnancy Within the First Year of Use		Percentage of Women Continuing Use at 1 Year
	Typical Use	Perfect Use	
No method	85	85	
Spermicides	21	16	42
Female condom	21	5	41
Withdrawal	20	4	46
Diaphragm	17	16	57
Sponge	17	12	36
• Parous women	27	20	
• Nulliparous women	14	9	
Fertility awareness–based methods	15		47
• Ovulation method	23	3	
• Two-day method	14	4	
• Standard days method	12	5	
• Natural cycles	8	1	
• Symptothermal method	2	0.4	
Male condom	13	2	43
Combined and progestin-only pills	7	0.3	67
Evra® patch	7	0.3	67
NuvaRing®	7	0.3	67
Depo-Provera®	4	0.2	56
Intrauterine contraceptives			
• ParaGard®	0.8	0.6	78
(copper T380A)	0.4	0.3	
• Skyla (13.5 mg LNG)	0.2	0.2	
• Kyleena (19.5 mg LNG)	0.1	0.1	
• Liletta (52 mg LNG)	0.1	0.1	80
• Mirena (52 mg LNG)			
Nexplanon®	0.1	0.1	89
Tubal occlusion	0.5	0.5	100
Vasectomy	0.15	0.1	100

Abbreviation: LNG, levonorgestrel.

[a]From Hatcher RA, Nelson AL, Trussell J, et al, eds. *Contraceptive Technology*. 21st ed. New York, NY: Ayer Company Publishers; 2018.

Effectiveness of Family Planning Methods

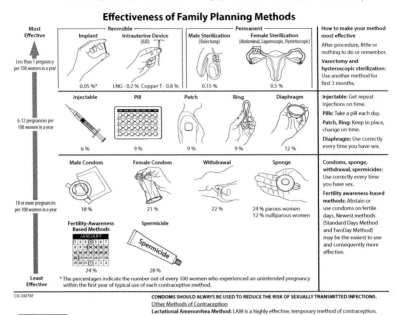

Figure 28-1. Tiers of effectiveness of family planning methods. From Centers for Disease Control and Prevention. Trussell J, Aiken ARA, Micks E, Guthrie KA. Efficacy, safety, and personal considerations. In: Hatcher RA, ed. *Contraceptive Technology*. 21st ed. New York, NY: Ayer Company Publishers, Inc.; 2018.

with greater risk of ectopic pregnancy in younger women. However, whereas the relative risk of ectopic pregnancy (chance that a pregnancy, if it occurs, may be ectopic) may be higher after sterilization, the absolute risk of ectopic pregnancy is lower than in noncontracepting women due to the high efficacy of sterilization.

Bilateral Salpingectomy Versus Bilateral Tubal Occlusion

- Bilateral salpingectomy involves partial or total removal of both fallopian tubes.
- The Parkland and Pomeroy partial salpingectomies are the most common methods used for postpartum sterilization. These involve ligating and excising portions of the fallopian tubes via an infraumbilical incision or during cesarean delivery.
- Laparoscopic sterilization can be performed by banding, clipping, or cauterizing the fallopian tubes or by excising the tubes entirely. Bilateral total salpingectomy requires slightly longer operating time and may have a small increased risk of surgical bleeding compared to bands, clips, or cautery. The advantage of total salpingectomy is potential decreased risks of sterilization failure and ovarian cancer.

Hysteroscopic Tubal Occlusion

- Sterilization via Essure® microinsert is an irreversible method of tubal occlusion in which a stainless steel and nickel-coated coil is inserted into each fallopian tube

under hysteroscopic guidance. A local inflammatory response leads to tissue in-growth around the coil and subsequent tubal occlusion.
- Some women have experienced pelvic pain, abnormal uterine bleeding, or other symptoms following Essure® placement. As of 2019, the Essure® contraceptive system is no longer marketed in the United States.

Male Sterilization

- Vasectomy is the surgical occlusion of the vas deferens, which prevents sperm from being ejaculated. Up to 3 months or 20 postprocedure ejaculations are required before the procedure becomes effective (as determined by two azoospermia results on semen analysis).
- **Advantages:** Vasectomy is highly effective and has no long-term side effects. It is less expensive, has fewer complications than tubal ligation, and can be performed in an office.
- **Disadvantages:** Vasectomy requires an outpatient surgical procedure, is permanent, offers no protection against sexually transmitted infections (STIs), and is not immediately effective.

Long-Acting Reversible Contraception

- **Long-acting reversible contraception (LARC)** refers to reversible methods that are designed to be used for at least 1 year.
- The LARC methods become cost-effective compared to shorter acting methods after 1 year of use and can be considered for women with a wide range of fertility plans, including women who do not desire future childbearing.

Intrauterine Contraception

- Intrauterine contraception, also known as intrauterine devices (IUD) or intrauterine systems, is one of the most effective methods of reversible contraception. The terms *intrauterine contraception*, *IUD*, and *intrauterine system* can be used interchangeably, but the term *IUD* is most common.
- There are two types of IUD available in the United States: hormonal and nonhormonal. All IUDs are flexible plastic devices that are inserted into the uterus and cause a sterile inflammatory reaction that interferes with sperm transport into and within the uterine cavity. Additional contraceptive effects are provided by the active compound in each IUD.

Hormonal Intrauterine Devices

- All hormonal IUDs currently available in the United States include the progestin levonorgestrel (LNG), which causes local uterine effects such as thickening cervical mucus and atrophy of the endometrial lining. These effects contribute to the high efficacy of LNG IUDs.
  - There are four LNG IUDs currently marketed in the United States: 52 mg LNG IUD (Mirena® and Liletta®): initially release 20 µg LNG daily. The Mirena IUD is Food and Drug Administration (FDA)-approved for 5 years and the Liletta is FDA-approved for 6 years but both are likely effective for 7 years. A noncontraceptive benefit is the reduction in menstrual blood loss by up to 90% due to endometrial suppression.
  - 19.5 mg LNG IUD (Kyleena®): initially releases 17.5 µg LNG daily, effective for 5 years
  - 13.5 mg LNG IUD (Skyla®): initially releases 14 µg LNG daily, effective for 3 years
- The 19.5 mg and 13.5 mg LNG IUDs are physically smaller than the 52 mg LNG IUDs, making them potentially more comfortable for nulliparous women.
- The lower dose LNG IUDs are associated with lower rates of amenorrhea than the 52 mg LNG IUDs.

Nonhormonal Intrauterine Devices

The copper T380A (ParaGard®) IUD contains 380 mm^2 of copper, which exerts spermicidal effects. It is effective for at least 10 years and likely up to 12 years. The copper IUD is also the most effective form of postcoital contraception (see "Emergency (Postcoital) Contraception").

Advantages, Disadvantages, Contraindications, Risks

- **Advantages:** The IUDs provide highly effective protection against pregnancy and are easily inserted and removed. The LNG IUDs may correct menstrual bleeding abnormalities and improve anemia. The IUDs may also protect against ascending pelvic infections and endometrial cancer. Return to fertility is rapid after removal. There are no hormonal side effects of the copper IUD.
- **Disadvantages:** In some women, menstrual bleeding may be slightly heavier and/or longer in the initial months after copper IUD insertion. This can generally be managed with nonsteroidal anti-inflammatory drugs. The LNG IUDs may have hormonally related side effects, including irregular bleeding or systemic side effects, which generally correct after a few months of use. Oligomenorrhea or amenorrhea may occur with the 52 mg LNG IUD, which may not be desirable to some women. Insertion and removal of an IUD requires a pelvic exam and a visit with a trained health care provider.
- **Contraindications:** There are few true contraindications to use of IUDs. The IUDs should not be inserted if pregnancy is suspected, if anatomical abnormalities significantly distort the uterine cavity, if there is unexplained vaginal bleeding prior to appropriate medical workup, or if pelvic malignancy is suspected (except in rare cases when a LNG IUD is used to treat early endometrial cancer in patients who are very poor surgical candidates). The IUDs do not need to be removed when cervical dysplasia is discovered and/or treated. Acute pelvic infection is a contraindication to IUD insertion (see below). Women living with human immunodeficiency virus (HIV) can safely use an IUD, although AIDS is a contraindication to IUD use. Women with a known allergy to copper should not use the copper IUD.
- **Risks** of IUD insertion include expulsion (2:100), infection (1:200), uterine perforation (1:1000), and failure resulting in pregnancy (2-8:1000).
- Other considerations:
  - Immediate postpartum or postabortal IUD insertion is safe and may lead to a substantial decrease in unplanned pregnancy. Expulsion risk may be higher compared to interval IUD insertion, but this should be balanced against other concerns (ie, health care access).
  - Pelvic infection: Risk of PID is not increased by IUD use. Progestin IUDs cause thickened cervical mucus, which may decrease the risk of PID by decreasing ascending pelvic infections. The copper IUD does not affect infection risk. Historical associations between IUDs and PID originated with the Dalkon Shield®, an IUD used in the 1970s that had a braided filament string that was associated with increased risk of PID. Modern IUDs have monofilament strings that do not share this risk.
    - Placement of an IUD at the time of active pelvic infection does increase risk of developing PID. Women with evidence of or high suspicion for active STIs should be screened and treated before having an IUD placed. Otherwise, patients with risk factors (as defined by the CDC) can be screened for chlamydia and gonorrhea at the time of placement; IUD insertion does not have to be delayed until test results are available. Asymptomatic, low-risk women do not need additional screening prior to IUD insertion.

- History of PID or prior ectopic pregnancy are not contraindications to IUD use. Diagnosis of uncomplicated chlamydia or gonorrhea infection does not require IUD removal; treatment can be offered with the IUD in place. The PID that is diagnosed with an IUD in place should be treated according to standard guidelines, and the IUD can often be left in place.
- Postinsertion pregnancy: Although the relative risk of ectopic pregnancy is higher among pregnancies occurring with an IUD in place, the overall risk of ectopic pregnancy is reduced because overall pregnancy risk is markedly decreased. If a woman has a desired intrauterine pregnancy with an IUD in place, the IUD should be removed if feasible.

Implantable Contraception

- Nexplanon® is a single radiopaque rod measuring 40×2 mm containing 68 mg etonogestrel that is slowly released over 3 years and suppresses ovulation, thickens cervical mucus, and causes endometrial atrophy.
- The implant is placed under the skin of the inner upper nondominant arm via a preloaded insertion device. The FDA-mandated training is required for providers who wish to insert and remove the implant.
- **Advantages:** The implant provides highly effective protection against pregnancy (see Table 28-1), is relatively easy to insert and remove, and does not require a pelvic exam. Some women may experience decreased menstrual bleeding or amenorrhea. Return to fertility is rapid after removal.
- **Disadvantages/side effects:** Menstrual disturbances are common with Nexplanon®. Bleeding patterns can be unpredictable and may vary over time in the same individual. Dissatisfaction with bleeding is the most common cause for discontinuation. Interventions such as short-term estrogen, oral contraceptive pills, doxycycline, or scheduled nonsteroidal anti-inflammatory drugs have been studied for treatment of bothersome bleeding related to the implant, with mixed results at best. With no intervention, about 50% of women who continue implant use despite unacceptable bleeding will experience improvement over time. There may be other hormonal side effects, such as headache and acne, which may resolve within a few months of insertion because there is an initial burst release of etonogestrel immediately after insertion that then declines to steady-state concentration.
- **Risks:** Implant insertion is generally safe, but rare complications, including infection, nerve injury, migration, allergic reaction, or incorrect placement leading to complicated removal, may occur.
- **Contraindications:** There are few contraindications to the implant; these are discussed below in the review of shorter acting progestin-only methods.

SHORT-ACTING HORMONAL CONTRACEPTIVE METHODS

- Hormonal contraceptives have been used by US women for over 60 years and are extremely safe and effective when used consistently and appropriately.
- In addition to hormonal LARC methods, hormonal contraception includes progestin-only methods (progestin-only pills [POPs] injection) and combined methods containing estrogen and progestin (combined oral contraceptives pills [COCs], transdermal patch, intravaginal ring).

Progestin-only Methods

- Synthetic progestin preparations prevent pregnancy without the use of estrogen.
- All progestin-only methods thicken cervical mucus, making it unfavorable to sperm penetration; only some prevent ovulation.
- Progestin-induced transformation of the endometrium creates an intrauterine environment unfavorable to fertilization and possibly implantation.
- There are few contraindications to these methods, and women who are ineligible to use combined hormonal methods can often use progestin-only methods safely. Progestin-only contraceptives can be initiated immediately postpartum and do not affect breastfeeding.
- **Contraindications:** personal history of breast cancer, complicated diabetes, and severe active liver disease or cirrhosis. Women with most other medical conditions can safely use these methods. For further guidance, refer to the CDC MEC.

Injectable Contraception

- Depot medroxyprogesterone acetate (DMPA) is a progestin-only contraceptive that is injected either intramuscularly (DepoProvera®, 150 mg) or subcutaneously (Depo-SubQ Provera®, 104 mg) every 3 months (12-14 wk). The DMPA provides highly effective contraception, although its potential effectiveness is limited by a discontinuation rate of over 40% in the first year of use.
- **Advantages:** The DMPA is highly effective at preventing pregnancy (see Table 28-1). Some women find the four doses per year more convenient than other shorter acting methods. Noncontraceptive benefits include reduction in menstrual blood loss, improvement in anemia, protection against endometrial cancer, reduced seizure frequency in some women with epilepsy, and reduced frequency of pain crises among some women with sickle cell disease.
- **Disadvantages/side effects:** The DMPA is the only contraceptive associated with weight gain (see below). Other side effects include irregular bleeding, delayed return to fertility, possible hair loss, and change in bone density. Although irregular bleeding is common after the first injection, 50% of women achieve amenorrhea after the first year of use.
- The average timing of return of ovulation is 6 to 10 months after the last injection, but delay of up to 18 months is possible. Patients should be counseled on this potential delay because it can impact future childbearing plans.
- There has long been concern about weight gain with DMPA. In many studies, this weight gain has not proven significant and may reflect overall weight change with age and the US obesity epidemic, especially in adolescents. However, certain subpopulations may be more susceptible than others. Women who gain weight rapidly after initiation of DMPA should be counseled that weight gain is likely to increase with continued use. There does not appear to be a difference in weight gain with intramuscular versus subcutaneous dosing of DMPA.
- In 2004, the FDA added a "black box" warning regarding possible decreased bone mineral density (BMD) with DMPA use, particularly in adolescents. Studies have shown this decrease in BMD is measurable after one injection of DMPA and continues with each subsequent injection. The decrease in BMD is reversible after DMPA discontinuation, is generally <1 standard deviation below the mean, is comparable in magnitude to that which occurs during breastfeeding, and has not been correlated with an increased risk of fracture. The World Health Organization has affirmed that there should be no restrictions on duration of DMPA use based

on bone density concerns. There does not appear to be a role for BMD monitoring in premenopausal DMPA users, and supplementation with estrogen is not advised.

- There has been concern about an increased risk of HIV acquisition associated with DMPA use, although observational studies have yielded mixed results. Research is ongoing to assess whether there is any change in HIV risk associated with DMPA use.

Progestin-Only Pills

- The POPs available in the United States contain 35 μg of norethindrone and are taken daily with no hormone-free interval. They are probably most effective about 6 hours after ingestion, and contraceptive effect diminishes significantly 24 hours after the last dose.
- **Advantages:** The POPs have few medical contraindications. Many women find a daily pill convenient, and the pill can be stopped whenever desired.
- **Disadvantages/side effects:** The most common side effect of POPs is irregular vaginal bleeding. This method is most effective if the pill is taken at the same time each day; variation in the timing of each dose may lead to increased risk of contraceptive failure.

Combined Hormonal Contraceptives

- Combined hormonal contraceptives (CHC) contain both synthetic progestin and estrogen. The CHC prevents pregnancy by suppressing ovulation, thickening cervical mucus, blocking sperm penetration and entry into the upper reproductive tract, and maintaining a thin asynchronous endometrium that inhibits implantation.
- Progestin provides the main contraceptive effects, whereas estrogen maintains the stability of the endometrium and contributes to ovulation inhibition. This allows for predictable monthly withdrawal bleeding and decreases irregular vaginal bleeding.
- Available methods include COCs, the transdermal patch, and the intravaginal ring.
- **Advantages:** Besides providing the contraception, CHC can be used to manage dysmenorrhea, abnormal uterine bleeding, premenstrual symptoms, ovarian cysts, and acne. Use of COCs is associated with 40% to 80% reduced risk of ovarian cancer and 50% to 70% reduced risk of endometrial cancer. Whether these benefits occur with other CHC has not been reported, but it may be possible to extrapolate based on similar components and physiologic effects.
- **Disadvantages/side effects:** Side effects may be associated with either active compound in CHC.
  - Estrogen: bloating, headache, nausea, mastalgia, leukorrhea, hypertension, melasma, telangiectasias
  - Progestin: mood changes, fatigue, mild weight gain, decreased libido
- **Risks:** Systemic use of estrogen increases the risk of venous thromboembolism (VTE). This must be considered in context because the overall risk of VTE in most candidates for hormonal contraception is very low, and the additional risk conferred by CHC is much lower than the risk associated with pregnancy. The risk of VTE in women per year is 4 in 100 000 at baseline, 10 in 100 000 in women using COCs, 20 in 100 000 in women using the contraceptive patch, >100 in 100 000 in pregnant women, and 550 in 100 000 in postpartum women.
- **Contraindications:** Comorbidities that increase the risk of VTE are generally contraindications to CHC use. These include cigarette smoking in women aged 35 years and older, hypertension, personal history of VTE, migraine headaches with aura, presence of multiple risk factors for cardiac disease, and the presence of

antiphospholipid antibodies. Known thrombogenic mutations would also preclude use of CHC, although routine screening for these mutations is not recommended. Personal history of breast and uterine cancer are also contraindications to CHC. For further guidance, providers can refer to the CDC MEC.

Combined Oral Contraceptive Pills

- Current formulations of COCs available in the United States contain 10 to 35 μg of ethinyl estradiol (EE) combined with variable doses of synthetic progestins. Most formulations contain 21 days of active hormones followed by 7 days of placebo. Withdrawal bleeding typically occurs during the week of placebo pills.
- Some formulations provide a longer duration of active pills (eg, 24 or 84 d). Extended-cycle or continuous COCs shorten or eliminate the hormone-free interval. This generally decreases or eliminates withdrawal bleeding. Extended-use preparations also improve menorrhagia, dysmenorrhea, endometriosis, chronic pelvic pain, and menstrual migraines. Spotting or breakthrough bleeding may increase with continuous use. There are no medical advantages to withdrawal bleeding on any schedule, nor are there risks of infrequent or absent bleeding due to use of hormonal contraceptives.
- The COCs may be started at any time during the menstrual cycle. There are no benefits to delaying initiation until menses or a particular day of the week, and the "quick start" method of starting COCs on the day of counseling is associated with improved initiation rates. A week of backup contraception is recommended if pills are started after day 5 of the menstrual cycle.
- **Advantages:** The COCs are the most common reversible contraceptive used in the United States. Many women find daily dosing convenient, and COCs can be stopped without needing to visit a health care provider. They provide predictable bleeding patterns and can improve symptoms of heavy menstrual bleeding, dysmenorrhea, and other menstrual-related symptoms such as acne or headaches.
- **Disadvantages/side effects:** Spotting, irregular menses, and nausea are common after initiation of COCs but generally resolve within the first 3 months. All brands of COCs have equivalent efficacy and side effect profiles. Some women may have idiosyncratic responses to different formulations, in which case it may be appropriate to switch formulations after 3 months of use. Monophasic pills may cause less breakthrough bleeding than bi-, tri-, or quadriphasic preparations.

Transdermal Patch

- The contraceptive transdermal patch releases 150 μg norgestimate (progestin) and 20 μg EE daily. The patch is applied weekly to any body location (other than the breast) for 3 consecutive weeks, followed by a patch-free withdrawal bleeding week.
- **Advantages:** Transdermal delivery avoids hepatic first-pass metabolic effects and maintains steady serum hormone levels without the peaks and troughs seen with pills. Weekly dosing may improve adherence for some women compared to a daily method.
- **Disadvantages:** Local adhesive reactions to the patch are rare (<5%). Clinical trials suggest that the patch is less effective in women who weigh >90 kg (198 lb).
- **Other considerations:** An FDA "black box" warning states that the patch provides approximately 60% more total estrogen than a typical COC containing 35 μg EE. Nonetheless, the daily peak in estrogen is approximately 25% lower with the patch

compared to pills. The clinical significance of this finding, particularly on the risk of VTE, is unclear and studies have not shown an increased risk of fatal blood clots with the patch compared to COCs.

Intravaginal Ring

- The NuvaRing® is a flexible plastic ring measuring 5 cm in diameter and 4 mm in thickness that releases 15 μg of EE and 120 μg of etonogestrel (progestin) daily. It is placed in the vagina for 3 weeks and removed for 1 week, during which withdrawal bleeding occurs. Alternatively, the ring can be kept in the vagina for 4 weeks followed by immediate transition to a new ring for women who desire to use this method continuously.
- Coital problems and expulsion of the ring are rare. If desired, the ring may be removed for up to 3 hours, such as during intercourse, although doing this routinely is not recommended. If the ring is removed for >3 hours, backup contraception should be used until the ring has been back in place for 7 days. The ring achieves a lower steady-state concentration of estrogen compared to the patch and COCs, although it is not known if this difference is clinically significant.
- A new intravaginal ring (Annovera®) containing segesterone acetate and EE was approved by the FDA in August 2018. This ring is designed to be effective for 1 year. The ring is placed vaginally for 3 weeks and then removed for 1 week. This pattern is repeated each month, and the ring is cleaned and stored during each ring-free week.
- **Advantages:** Some women may find monthly ring use more convenient and easier to use consistently than a daily pill. The ring leads to similar menstrual and noncontraceptive effects as COCs. The vaginal ring can be used concurrently with tampons and male condoms but should not be used with female condoms.
- **Disadvantages:** The ring may cause increased vaginal discharge or discomfort during intercourse or may become dislodged. Risks and contraindications are similar to other CHCs.

BARRIER METHODS

Condoms

Male ("Outside") Condom

- Male condoms are made of latex, lambskin, or synthetic material (ie, polyurethane). They should be applied before penetration and should cover the entire length of the erect penis. They should neither be too tight nor too loose, and a reservoir should be left at the tip to retain the ejaculate.
- Adequate lubrication should be used on both the inside and outside of the condom, and the condom should be removed immediately after ejaculation. Condoms with spermicidal lubricant are more effective at preventing pregnancy. The CDC currently suggests that women who are at high risk for HIV infection should not use nonoxynol-9 spermicides because this ingredient may increase the risk of HIV transmission.
- Condoms are highly effective in preventing sexual transmission of HIV and other infections (eg, gonorrhea, chlamydia, trichomonas). However, because condoms do not cover all exposed areas, they may be less effective in preventing infections transmitted by skin-to-skin contact (eg, herpes simplex virus, human papillomavirus, syphilis, chancroid).

- **Advantages:** Male condoms are readily available without a prescription and are relatively inexpensive, making them one of the most accessible contraceptives. In addition to preventing pregnancy, they also provide protection against STIs.
- **Disadvantages:** Condoms must be used correctly and with every act of intercourse to achieve maximum efficacy. They require the cooperation of both partners.

Female ("Inside") Condom

- Female condoms consist of a polyurethane sheath with a flexible ring at either end. The closed end with the upper/inner ring is applied against the cervix and the open end with the lower/outer ring rests against the labia minora outside the introitus. Adequate lubrication is important for function and comfort. Like male condoms, this method decreases STI transmission. It also provides protection on the vulva that may decrease infections transmitted by skin-to-skin contact.
- **Advantages:** Female condoms protect against STIs in addition to preventing pregnancy.
- **Disadvantages:** Female condoms are only available with a prescription and are more expensive than male condoms. Similar to male condoms, they must be used correctly and consistently with every act of intercourse for maximum efficacy and require the cooperation of both partners.

Diaphragm

- A diaphragm is a barrier device that is inserted vaginally and prevents sperm from entering the upper female genital tract. The diaphragm consists of a silicone cup with a flexible ring. The edges of the diaphragm should lie just posterior to the symphysis pubis and deep into the cul-de-sac so that the cervix is completely covered behind the center of the diaphragm. Diaphragms now come in two sizes, nulliparous and parous, and no longer require a pelvic exam for a fitting.
- Although there is no definitive evidence to support the use of a spermicide with the diaphragm, this is a common recommendation in clinical practice. If spermicide is used, it should be applied to the inside of the rubber cup before each act of coitus. The diaphragm should be left in place for a minimum of 6 hours after the last coital act but not >24 consecutive hours. It may be placed hours before intercourse.
- **Advantages:** The diaphragm may be preferable for women who have sex infrequently or who wish to avoid hormonal contraceptives. Diaphragms may offer some protection against STIs.
- **Disadvantages:** Women with uterine prolapse or structural reproductive tract abnormalities may not be able to use a diaphragm. Patients relying on a diaphragm should inspect the diaphragm regularly for holes and should replace the diaphragm at least every 2 years. Their use may increase the risk of urinary tract infection.

FERTILITY AWARENESS–BASED METHODS

- Fertility awareness–based (FAB) methods are those by which a woman voluntarily avoids sexual intercourse during the fertile phase of the menstrual cycle. Effectiveness varies significantly among individuals because these methods rely on regular menses, cooperation of both partners, and periodic abstinence.
- **Advantages:** The FAB methods do not require use of exogenous hormones, and they can be used without involving a health care provider. There are currently many

apps available to help track the menstrual cycle, but these apps may not all be based on rigorous scientific algorithms.

- **Disadvantages:** The FAB methods require regular, predictable menstrual cycles to be most effective and require cooperation of both partners.
- **Calendar method.** Menstrual cycles are charted for 6 months, and this chart is used to calculate the woman's fertile days, based on estimated day of ovulation. Sex is avoided on these fertile days.
- **Cervical mucus.** A woman must monitor the texture and amount of cervical mucus to detect a transition from sticky, yellow-white, scant mucus on nonfertile days to clear, slippery, stretchy mucus at ovulation. Intercourse is avoided from the onset of menses until 3 days after ovulation is predicted.
- **Symptothermal method.** A woman must check her basal body temperature daily and avoid intercourse from the start of menses until 3 days after a rise in temperature occurs. The rise in temperature indicates that ovulation has occurred, and she is no longer at risk for pregnancy during that cycle.
- **Lactational amenorrhea.** During breastfeeding, infant suckling causes hormonal changes at the hypothalamus that interrupt the pulsatile release of gonadotropin-releasing hormone. This, in turn, impairs LH surge and suppresses ovulation. Lactation offers protection against pregnancy only if strict criteria are followed. To be effective contraception, (1) women should be exclusively breastfeeding, (2) breastfeeding (or pumping breast milk) should occur every 3 to 4 hours during the day and every 6 hours at night, (3) the infant should be less than 6 months old, and (4) supplemental feedings should not exceed 5% to 10% of the daily total. Once menses have resumed, it can be assumed that lactation is no longer providing protection against pregnancy.

EMERGENCY (POSTCOITAL) CONTRACEPTION

- Emergency or postcoital contraception (EC) may be used after unprotected intercourse to prevent pregnancy. The EC via insertion of a copper IUD may disrupt implantation. The EC pills (ECP) work mainly through ovulation disruption. There are two types of ECP available in the United States: LNG and ulipristal acetate (UPA).
- There are no contraindications to use of ECP; contraindications to copper IUD use would preclude its use as EC. Use in pregnancy is not advised; however, the use of ECP will not cause termination of existing pregnancy and is not teratogenic. Use of ECP is not an ideal method of routine contraception because it is less effective than other methods. However, repeated use is not dangerous. Irregular bleeding and delay of next menses are common after taking ECP. Patients are encouraged to take a pregnancy test if menses have not resumed within 1 week after expected menstrual timing.

Levonorgestrel Emergency Contraceptive Pills

- The LNG ECP is available over-the-counter without sex or age restrictions. The method includes a total of 1.5 mg LNG that may be taken orally in two doses (0.75 mg 12 h apart) or one dose (1.5 mg). The single-dose regimen has better compliance with fewer side effects and greater efficacy than the two-dose regimen.
- It is effective in preventing pregnancy up to 120 hours after intercourse, but it is most effective when taken within 72 hours after coitus. This regimen is 94% to

98% effective in preventing pregnancy with higher failure rates observed in women who take the dose between 72 and 120 hours after unprotected intercourse. Efficacy is decreased in obese women.

Ulipristal Acetate Emergency Contraceptive Pills

- The UPA (Ella®) is a progesterone receptor antagonist taken as a single 30-mg dose within 120 hours of unprotected intercourse. It works by directly inhibiting follicle rupture and therefore maintains high efficacy even as ovulation nears. The UPA is 92% to 99% effective in preventing pregnancy when taken within 5 days of unprotected intercourse. The UPA has decreased efficacy in obese women but retains better efficacy than LNG ECP in this population.
- Common side effects include gastrointestinal upset, vomiting, breast tenderness, irregular bleeding, dizziness, and headaches. The UPA is only available by prescription.

Copper Intrauterine Device

The copper IUD may be inserted within 5 days of unprotected intercourse to decrease the chance of implantation and is the most effective emergency contraceptive method (99.8%-99.9% effective). It is also the only option that provides ongoing contraception.

SUGGESTED READINGS

American College of Obstetricians and Gynecologists Committee on Practice Bulletins—Gynecology. ACOG Practice Bulletin No. 110: noncontraceptive uses of hormonal contraceptives. *Obstet Gynecol*. 2010;115:206-218. (Reaffirmed 2018)

American College of Obstetricians and Gynecologists Committee on Practice Bulletins—Gynecology. ACOG Practice Bulletin No. 152: emergency contraception. *Obstet Gynecol*. 2015;126:e1-e11. (Reaffirmed 2018)

American College of Obstetricians and Gynecologists Committee on Practice Bulletins—Gynecology. ACOG Practice Bulletin No. 186: long-acting reversible contraception: implants and intrauterine devices. *Obstet Gynecol*. 2017;130:e251-e269.

American College of Obstetricians and Gynecologists Committee on Practice Bulletins—Gynecology. ACOG Practice Bulletin No. 208: benefits and risks of sterilization. *Obstet Gynecol*. 2019;133:e194-e207.

Hatcher RA, Nelson AL, Trussell J, et al, eds. *Contraceptive Technology*. 21st ed. New York, NY: Ayer Company Publishers; 2018.

Peterson HB, Xia Z, Hughes JM, Wilcox LS, Tylor LR, Trussell J. The risk of pregnancy after tubal sterilization: findings from the U.S. Collaborative Review of Sterilization. *Am J Obstet Gynecol*. 1996;174:1161-1170.

29

Abortion

Jessica K. Lee and Chavi Kahn

PREGNANCY TERMINATION

Epidemiology and Safety

- Fifty-six million abortions occur each year worldwide. About half of these are unsafe, resulting in at least 22,800 maternal deaths from abortion and related complications and accounting for 8% of all causes of maternal deaths.
- Safe abortion is very safe in the United States, with a mortality rate of 0.6 per 100 000. Extensive study has shown that safe abortion does not increase future risk of infertility, breast cancer, pregnancy loss, or mental health issues.

Evaluation and Counseling

- Providers caring for patients with unplanned and undesired pregnancy should counsel them on all available options, including parenthood, adoption, and abortion. A nondirective counseling approach should be taken to ensure that they are confident in their decision.
- Obstetrician-gynecologists who do not perform abortions should know how to counsel patients about their options, make appropriate referrals, and manage postabortal complications.
- Induced abortion can be performed medically or surgically, and patients should be counseled about both options.
- A targeted history, physical examination, and limited laboratory testing should be performed prior to abortion.
  - The history should focus on relevant data, such as gynecologic problems (eg, leiomyomata), obstetric history (eg, prior cesarean delivery that can increase risks of abnormal placentation and uterine rupture), and medical problems (eg, asthma, morbid obesity) that might influence the setting and risks of the abortion.
  - Physical examination should include the abdomen and pelvis and also an airway, heart, and lung examination if anesthesia will be used.
  - Although ultrasonography is not necessary on a routine basis, it has become routine in most settings in the United States.
  - Rh status should be determined, and Rh-negative patients should receive Rh immune globulin at the time of induced abortion.
  - A hemoglobin level should be obtained because severe anemia is a contraindication to medication abortion and may require preoperative planning prior to surgical abortion.
- Prior research has shown that antibiotic prophylaxis is important in reducing the risk of infection with surgical abortion. Common antibiotics used are azithromycin, doxycycline, and metronidazole. Oral antibiotics are sufficient.
- Because fertility can return immediately after abortion, contraception counseling should be performed prior to abortion.

SURGICAL ABORTION

Surgical Abortion in the First Trimester

- First-trimester surgical abortion is referred to as *dilation and curettage*. This is the most common method of first-trimester abortion. Principles of care include pain management, cervical dilation, and uterine evacuation via a suction cannula.
- Pain control options include oral analgesia and intravenous (IV) sedation and depend on patient preference and availability of options. General anesthesia is rarely indicated for first-trimester surgical abortion.
- A paracervical block with local anesthesia is also frequently administered to reduce procedural pain.
- Adequate cervical dilation facilitates the procedure and reduces complication rates. In the majority of first-trimester surgical abortions, the cervix can be manually dilated at the time of the procedure.
- For late first-trimester procedures (ie, 12-14 wk), medications such as misoprostol or osmotic dilators can be used for preoperative cervical ripening. The exact gestational age at which this is introduced varies among providers and practice environments and also may depend on the patient's parity. These are discussed further in "Surgical Abortion in the Second Trimester" section.
- Mechanical dilation uses surgical instruments that have progressively increasing diameters (eg, Pratt, Hegar, or Denniston dilators) to open the cervix to a sufficient diameter.
- The suction cannula should be approximately the same diameter in millimeters as the weeks' gestation (ie, a pregnancy measuring 7 weeks' gestational age can be removed with 7-mm cannula).
- Following dilation, electric vacuum aspiration (EVA) or manual vacuum aspiration (MVA) is performed to empty the uterus of products of conception (POCs). Both EVA and MVA use a suction cannula attached to a suction device. The apparatus is advanced through the internal os into the uterine cavity, and uterine contents are aspirated with suction.
- With MVA, a self-locking syringe (50-60 mL) is used as a source of suction, whereas EVA uses tubing attached to an electric suction machine.
- After aspiration, the tissue should be inspected to verify that the POCs are consistent with the gestational age.
- Sharp curettage is generally not necessary. The use of sharp curettage has been associated with increased procedural pain and an increased risk of bleeding and uterine perforation.

Surgical Abortion in the Second Trimester

- The most commonly used surgical procedure for second-trimester abortion is dilation and evacuation (D&E). D&E is considered the preferred method of second-trimester abortion when experienced personnel are available and autopsy of an intact fetus is not required. In experienced hands, D&E is the safest available method of second-trimester abortion.
- Ultrasonographic guidance has become standard in most practice environments in the United States. However, it is not a substitute for competence and does not eliminate risk of complications.

- Preoperative cervical preparation is highly recommended. This can be accomplished via medications that ripen the cervix, such as misoprostol, or by osmotic dilators.
  - Choice of technique depends on provider experience, gestational age, and availability. Osmotic dilators, such as Dilapan-S® (polyacrylonitrile) or laminaria (dried seaweed, *Laminaria japonica*), absorb cervical moisture. As they do so, they gradually enlarge and dilate the cervical canal. They also cause the release of prostaglandins, which ultimately disrupts the cervical stroma, thereby softening the cervix.
  - Osmotic dilators must be placed several hours before the procedure or overnight for maximum effect.
  - For procedures later in the second trimester, dilation is often carried out over 1 to 2 days. Sequential insertion of osmotic dilators may be used.
- An IV sedation is usually recommended for second-trimester surgical abortion depending on availability and patient preference. A paracervical block with local anesthesia in addition to a vasoconstrictive agent (ie, vasopressin, epinephrine) is also frequently administered to reduce procedural pain and postoperative bleeding. General anesthesia is generally not required to perform D&E.
- D&E involves mechanical cervical dilation (with or without preoperative misoprostol and/or osmotic dilators) followed by evacuation of the fetus and placenta via a combination of forceps (ie, Sopher or Bierer forceps) and suction.
- The provider must confirm completion by identifying all major fetal parts (four extremities, spine, and calvarium).

MEDICATION ABORTION

Medication Abortion in the First Trimester

- Evidence-based medication abortion regimens are safe and effective up to 70 days of gestation.
- Medication abortion is most commonly performed using mifepristone (RU-486) followed by misoprostol. Medication abortion can also be performed with methotrexate and misoprostol or misoprostol alone. However, these regimens have fallen out of favor because they are less effective and have more side effects.
  - Mifepristone is a progesterone antagonist and thus blocks the hormone necessary to maintain a pregnancy. Its effects include alterations in the endometrial blood supply and softening the cervix. It also increases uterine contractility and prostaglandin sensitivity.
  - Misoprostol is a prostaglandin that is used to induce uterine contractions, thus promoting expulsion of POCs.
- For pregnancies up to 70 days' gestation, evidence-based recommendations support the use of a 200-mg mifepristone oral dose followed by 800 µg of buccal, sublingual, or vaginal misoprostol 6 to 72 hours later. These regimens are 93% to 99% effective. There are few side effects from mifepristone. Side effects following administration of misoprostol consist primarily of pain, bleeding, fever, and gastrointestinal upset.
- Where access to other options is limited, misoprostol alone can be used in repeat dosing. Effectiveness varies from 47% to 96%.
- With medication abortion, the abortion typically happens at home. Cramping and bleeding usually begin within 1 to 4 hours after taking misoprostol. Blood loss is

typically greater than with surgical abortion. Severe anemia is generally a contraindication to medication abortion.

- Follow-up is necessary to confirm abortion completion. Surgical evacuation is usually advised in cases of medication failure.
- Contraindications to medical abortion include significant anemia, concern for ectopic pregnancy, chronic corticosteroid use, chronic adrenal failure, porphyria, allergy to misoprostol or mifepristone, anticoagulation use, or if an intrauterine device is in place.

Medication Abortion in the Second Trimester (Labor Induction)

- Labor induction is another method of abortion in the second trimester. Advantages of this method are that it does not require IV sedation or a skilled operator. In addition, the fetus remains intact, allowing for a patient to hold the fetus and for fetal examination and autopsy, such as in cases of genetic termination.
- However, labor induction can take 24 hours or longer, major complications and mortality are higher, and fever and severe gastrointestinal side effects are common when higher doses of prostaglandins are used.
- Medications used to induce labor in the second trimester include different preparations of vaginally or buccally administered prostaglandins (prostaglandin E_2 [Prostin E_2] and misoprostol) and high-dose IV oxytocin.
- Mifepristone administered at least 24 hours prior to initiating prostaglandins or oxytocin has been shown to shorten length of induction and increase its success rate.

Follow-up

- Patients can ovulate within 10 days of abortion, and at least half of patients will ovulate within 3 weeks of an abortion procedure. For patients who desire to postpone a future pregnancy, contraception should be initiated immediately.
- Pregnancy symptoms usually resolve within 1 week after abortion. Normal menses may take up to 6 weeks to return. A urine pregnancy test can be positive up to 8 weeks after an abortion.
- Follow-up is traditionally recommended within 2 to 4 weeks to assess for complications, confirm resolution of pregnancy, and readdress contraception.

COMPLICATIONS

- Fortunately, legal abortion is a very safe procedure. However, as with any other procedure, complications can occur.

Complications of Surgical Abortion

- Perforation is a potentially serious but infrequent complication of abortion. The incidence of perforation is about 0.9 per 1000 abortions. Management of perforation is beyond the scope of this chapter.
- Reported rates of hemorrhage vary widely—ranging from 0.05 to 4.9 per 100 abortions—reflecting both diverse definitions and imprecision in estimating volumes of blood loss.
  - Common causes of hemorrhage include cervical injury, uterine perforation, and atony.

- Hemorrhage due to atony can be managed with uterotonics, such as misoprostol, methylergonovine, or carboprost. Bimanual massage and bladder catheterization are also helpful. If hemorrhage continues, tamponade with an intrauterine Foley balloon and/or uterine artery embolization are options. Hysterectomy should be performed if all other options fail.
- Hematometra should be suspected if a patient has intense pain and an enlarged uterus immediately following surgical abortion. Surgical reaspiration is the key to management, and uterotonics can be considered.
- Postabortal endomyometritis may present with fever and abdominal pain postabortion.
  - Oral or IV doxycycline and a cephalosporin, with or without metronidazole, should be administered.
  - The decision to use outpatient versus inpatient management can be made by applying criteria similar to those designated for pelvic inflammatory disease.
  - Oral prophylactic doxycycline administration before surgical abortion can reduce the risk of postabortal endomyometritis by 40%.
- Retained POCs after abortion is a clinical diagnosis. Symptoms include pelvic pain and vaginal bleeding with or without symptoms of infection. Ultrasound can aid in the diagnosis. The treatment is uterine evacuation.

Complications of Medication Abortion

- Complications from medication abortion are rare.
- Patients should be counseled that continuing pregnancy occurs in 1% to 3% of cases.
- Retained products may also occur. This can be managed with surgical evacuation or possibly with an additional dose of misoprostol.
- The risk of hemorrhage requiring blood transfusion is significantly less than 1%.

SUGGESTED READINGS

Borgatta L, Kapp N. Clinical guidelines. Labor induction abortion in the second trimester. *Contraception*. 2011;84(1):4-18.

Chervenak FA, McCullough LB. The ethics of direct and indirect referral for termination of pregnancy. *Am J Obstet Gynecol*. 2008;199(3):232.e1-232.e3.

Fox MC, Krajewski CM. Cervical preparation for second-trimester surgical abortion prior to 20 weeks' gestation: SFP Guideline #2013-4. *Contraception*. 2014;89(2):75-84.

Jabara S, Barnhart K. Is Rh immune globulin needed in early first-trimester abortion? A review. *Am J Obstet Gynecol*. 2003;188:623-627.

The National Academies of Sciences, Engineering, and Medicine. *The Safety and Quality of Abortion Care in the United States*. Washington, DC: The National Academies Press; 2018. doi:10.17226/24950.

30

First and Second Trimester Pregnancy Loss and Ectopic Pregnancy

Jill Edwardson and Carolyn Sufrin

In women presenting with vaginal bleeding and/or abdominal/pelvic pain in pregnancy, providing an accurate diagnosis of pregnancy location and viability is necessary to avoid interruption of a potentially normal, desired pregnancy and to ensure proper management of an abnormal pregnancy. Therefore, this chapter first discusses assessment of pregnancy location and viability in the first trimester, followed by discussion of diagnosis and treatment of pregnancy loss and ectopic pregnancy (EP).

ASSESSMENT OF PREGNANCY LOCATION AND VIABILITY IN THE FIRST TRIMESTER

- Quantitative **β-human chorionic gonadotropin (β-hCG)** serum level
  - Level varies greatly among individuals at the same gestational age and therefore should not be used to estimate gestational age. A single β-hCG value is rarely useful itself and should be interpreted in the context of clinical presentation, pelvic ultrasound, and/or serial β-hCG measurements.
  - The "discriminatory level" is the β-hCG value above, which a normal intrauterine pregnancy (IUP) should be visible on ultrasound. If it is not seen, it raises concern for either abnormal IUP or an extrauterine pregnancy.
  - As a diagnostic aid, the β-hCG level should be conservatively high, to reduce the incidence of a false-positive diagnosis of abnormal pregnancy. Newer recommendations suggest the discriminatory level should be around 3500 mIU/mL for transvaginal ultrasound; however, use of this value should consider the clinical context. In most cases, evidence of an IUP can be seen at lower β-hCG levels.
  - In women with multiple gestations, β-hCG levels are higher than in singletons and may reach levels above the discriminatory level before a pregnancy is visible on ultrasound.
  - Trends in quantitative β-hCG level: Serial β-hCG measurements can differentiate normal from abnormal pregnancies. Although overall, the minimal rate of expected increase in serum β-hCG level is 53% over 48 hours, this rate varies by the initial β-hCG value and gestational age.
  - Normal pregnancy β-hCG levels and trends are listed in Table 30-1.
  - Although 48 hours is a useful timeframe in which to repeat a β-hCG in cases when serial levels are indicated, given variability in trends, it may be more appropriate based on clinical context to recheck levels in less than or greater than 48 hours.
  - Abnormal pregnancy should be suspected when less than the minimal rate of increase is seen over 48 hours. However, an abnormal pregnancy or EP may still be present with apparently normally rising β-hCG levels. Decreasing β-hCG values suggest a failing pregnancy but do not eliminate the possibility of an EP.
  - Once an IUP is visualized on ultrasound, β-hCG levels are not useful in establishing viability, and ultrasound criteria should be used instead.

Table 30-1	Minimal Expected Rate of Increase in β-Human Chorionic Gonadotropin (β-hCG) in 48 Hours by Initial β-hCG Value[a]
Initial β-hCG value	Minimal Expected Rate of Increase in 48 h
<1500 mIU/mL	49%
1500-3000 mIU/mL	40%
>3000 mIU/mL	33%

[a]Adapted with permission from American College of Obstetricians and Gynecologists Committee on Practice Bulletins—Gynecology. ACOG Practice Bulletin No. 193: tubal ectopic pregnancy. *Obstet Gynecol.* 2018;131(3):e91-e103. Copyright © 2018 by The American College of Obstetricians and Gynecologists.

- **Transvaginal ultrasound** milestones and criteria for viability
  - **Intrauterine pregnancy** can only be definitively diagnosed once a **gestational sac** (GS) with either a **yolk sac** (YS) or embryonic pole is seen in the uterus.
  - Typical progression of a *normal IUP*. The GS will appear by the time β-hCG is at the discriminatory level, usually around 5 to 6 weeks; it appears as a small, cystic fluid collection, eccentrically located in the uterus, within the decidua. It will often display a "double decidual sign" or "intradecidual sign": what appear to be two echogenic rings around the GS. After the GS becomes visible, the YS and then embryonic pole will appear.
  - The diagnosis of an *abnormal IUP* should be based on ultrasound milestones, not on weeks gestation. Ultrasound criteria for diagnosis of early pregnancy loss (EPL) were established by the Society of Radiologists in Ultrasound Multispecialty Panel on Early First Trimester Diagnosis of Miscarriage and Exclusion of a Viable Intrauterine Pregnancy to minimize the chances of a false-positive diagnosis of EPL.
    - Diagnostic for EPL:
      - Crown-rump length (CRL) ≥7 mm with no cardiac motion (embryonic demise)
      - Mean sac diameter (MSD) ≥25 mm with no embryo (anembryonic gestation)
      - Absence of embryo with heartbeat ≥14 days after scan showed GS without a YS or ≥11 days after scan that showed GS with YS
    - Suspicious for EPL (generally warrants repeat ultrasound evaluation):
      - CRL <7 mm and no cardiac activity
      - MSD 16 to 24 mm with no embryo
      - Absence of embryo with heartbeat 7 to 13 days after scan that showed GS without YS or 7 to 10 days after scan that showed GS with YS
      - Absence of embryo for ≥6 weeks after LMP
      - YS >7 mm
      - <5 mm difference between MSD and CRL
      - Fetal heart rate <100 beats per minute at 5 to 7 weeks' gestation
- **Ectopic pregnancy:** a pregnancy occurring outside the uterus; definitive diagnosis is possible only if a GS with a YS and/or an embryo is visualized outside the uterus. (See section "Ectopic Pregnancy.")

- **Pregnancy of unknown location** (PUL) describes when there is not a definitive IUP or EP on ultrasound; this **is *not* a diagnosis and should be considered a transient state that requires further evaluation.**
  - Further evaluation of pregnancy of unknown location
  - A stable patient with a desired pregnancy may be **expectantly managed** until a definitive diagnosis is reached. Serum β-hCG is typically repeated in approximately 48 hours and, once the β-hCG level is above the discriminatory level, a TVUS is performed. A β-hCG above the discriminatory level with no IUP on ultrasound or an abnormally rising β-hCG below the discriminatory level is diagnostic of an abnormal pregnancy (intrauterine or ectopic).
  - Diagnostic **dilation and curettage** (D&C), typically with manual uterine aspiration, can be performed for an undesired pregnancy or when the possibility of normal intrauterine gestation is reasonably excluded.
    - Presence of intrauterine chorionic villi visualized on uterine aspirate or pathologic exam are diagnostic for a failed IUP and no further workup is necessary.
    - If villi are *not* identified, repeat β-hCG should be measured 12 to 24 hours after aspiration.
      - A plateau (less than 10%-15% decrease) or increase in β-hCG suggests incomplete evacuation or an EP, and treatment with methotrexate should be considered.
      - A large decrease (≥50%) in β-hCG is consistent with an evacuated IUP and patients can be monitored clinically.
      - A decrease in β-hCG 15% to 50% most likely represents failed IUP, but ectopic is not excluded and close follow-up with serial β-hCG is recommended. Treatment with methotrexate may be considered if subsequent β-hCG levels do not decline.
- Note that it can take up to 35 days (median 19 d) for β-hCG levels to reach zero after a first trimester D&C for EPL and up to 60 days (median 30 d) to reach zero after an induced abortion.
- **Pregnancy of uncertain viability** occurs when TVUS shows an intrauterine GS with no embryonic pole or an embryo without a heartbeat and no findings of definite pregnancy failure.
  - Like PUL, it should be considered a transient state until a final diagnosis is made.
  - The β-hCG values are not helpful in determining the viability of a pregnancy once an IUP has been documented on ultrasound. Viability should be assessed with serial ultrasounds until cardiac activity is visualized or until pregnancy failure is definitively diagnosed (see ultrasound measurement milestones below).

EARLY PREGNANCY LOSS IN THE FIRST TRIMESTER

- EPL encompasses clinical spontaneous abortion and abnormal intrauterine pregnancies on ultrasound. It is defined as a nonviable IUP, with either an empty GS or a GS containing an embryo or fetus without fetal cardiac activity, within the first 12 6/7 weeks' gestation. A patient with EPL may present with symptoms or may be asymptomatic and identified ultrasonographically as an anembryonic gestation or embryonic demise.
- Epidemiology and risk factors
  - EPL is common and occurs in 8% to 20% of clinically recognized pregnancies
  - Risk factors include the following:
    - Maternal age: risk of EPL increases from 9% to 17% at age 20 to 30 years to 20% at age 35 years, 40% at age 40 years, and 80% at age 45 years.

- ○ Risk of EPL increases from 20% in women with one prior EPL to 43% in women with three or more EPL.
- ○ Tobacco, alcohol, or cocaine abuse
- ○ Maternal hypertension, endocrinopathies, uterine anomalies, teratogens, and infection
- ○ Approximately 50% of EPL are due to fetal chromosomal abnormalities. Congenital anomalies also increase the risk of EPL.

- Diagnosis
  - Clinical presentation: Symptoms may include vaginal bleeding and uterine cramping or may be asymptomatic.
  - Spontaneous abortion:
    - ○ **Threatened abortion:** Vaginal bleeding is present, with or without cramping, no fetal tissue has passed, and cervix is closed.
    - ○ **Inevitable abortion:** Fetal tissue has not yet passed, but cervix is open and cramping and bleeding are present.
    - ○ **Incomplete abortion:** Some or all fetal tissue has passed, and bleeding and cramping are present with an open cervix.
    - ○ **Complete abortion:** Fetal tissue has passed, and cervix is closed.
  - Asymptomatic (formerly referred to as a "missed abortion"): Embryonic demise (absence of cardiac activity in a fetus with CRL ≥7 mm) or an anembryonic gestation (MSD ≥25 mm) may be identified on ultrasound in a patient without any symptoms or with vaginal bleeding.
- Vaginal bleeding in early pregnancy
  - Vaginal bleeding is present in 30% of normal pregnancies.
  - Vaginal bleeding and cramping in pregnancy can be associated with EP (up to 20% of cases) or molar pregnancy.
- Assessment
  - Physical exam: Vital signs should be assessed for hemodynamic stability. Pelvic exam should determine if vaginal bleeding is present, if tissue has passed or is passing, the size of uterus, and if the internal cervical os is open or closed.
  - **Septic abortion:** infection of the uterus associated with abortion. Clinical findings can include pelvic or abdominal pain; purulent discharge; open cervix; cervical motion tenderness; uterine tenderness; constitutional symptoms (eg, fever, malaise); tachycardia; and/or tachypnea.
  - Laboratory evaluation should include complete blood count and blood type (for Rh status, see below). Quantitative β-hCG should be obtained and interpreted in the context of ultrasound findings and clinical symptoms.
    - ○ Serial β-hCG can help assess whether a pregnancy is normal or abnormal (as discussed earlier); i.e. if an IUP has previously been documented, drawing β-hCG level is rarely indicated.
  - Ultrasound: EPL diagnosis is certain in a woman with a previously documented IUP who presents with subsequent vaginal bleeding and an empty uterus on ultrasound. Otherwise, TVUS milestones and criteria for viability depend on gestational age, number of fetuses, and β-hCG levels (as discussed earlier).
- Management of EPL
  - General considerations
    - ○ Threatened abortion in a desired pregnancy does not require any treatment because it may progress to be a normal, viable pregnancy.
    - ○ Complete abortion does not require any treatment. If a completed spontaneous abortion is suspected by history and physical exam but no prior IUP was

documented, a repeat β-hCG can be performed, with an expected decrease in β-hCG of 21% to 35% in 48 hours. Based on convenience and other clinical factors, a different interval for repeating β-hCG may be appropriate.

- o **Rh immunoglobulin:** Although the risk of alloimmunization is low, especially early in the first trimester, the consequences can be significant. Therefore, **Rh$_o$(D) immune globulin** (RhoGAM®) administration should be considered for Rh-negative women with EPL, especially if beyond 8 weeks gestation, and is advised to be given within 72 hours of bleeding or uterine evacuation.
- o Treatment options include expectant management, medical management, or surgical evacuation and can generally accommodate patient preferences in the absence of infection or hemorrhage. All treatment options include risks of hemorrhage or infection.

- Expectant management
  - o **Expectant management** may be considered for women presenting in the first trimester without evidence of infection or hemorrhage.
  - o Successful expulsion of pregnancy tissue, defined as expulsion within 4 weeks of diagnosis, occurs in approximately 80% of women. Success rates are highest in women who report tissue passage or have ultrasound evidence of partial expulsion at time of diagnosis. There is no increased risk of infection compared to medical or surgical management.
  - o Advantages: No additional medications or procedures, and a woman can pass the pregnancy in private.
  - o Disadvantages: Patients may experience moderate-to-heavy bleeding and cramping; may take up to 6 weeks to complete
  - o Follow-up generally consists of ultrasound confirmation of an absent GS. Patient report of symptoms, urine pregnancy tests, or serial β-hCG measurements have not been well studied as follow-up methods for women with EPL. If expectant management fails, medical or surgical management is required.

- Medical management
  - o **Medical management** may be considered for women without evidence of infection or hemorrhage. Contraindications include allergy to misoprostol, severe anemia (hemoglobin <10 g/dL is a relative contraindication), or bleeding disorders.
  - o Advantages: decreases the time to expulsion of pregnancy tissue and increases the rate of complete expulsion compared to expectant management; avoids surgical treatment, and a woman can pass the pregnancy in private. Rates of satisfaction are similar to that with surgical management.
  - o Disadvantages: associated with more pain, nausea/vomiting, and bleeding than surgical management. Patients are more likely to experience hemorrhage and a decrease in hemoglobin ≥3 g/dL than women undergoing surgical management, but rates of hemorrhage-related hospitalization are similar (0.5%-1%). Providers should counsel women regarding normal bleeding patterns and to call if soaking 1 to 2 pads per hour for more than 2 hours.
  - o Medical regimens:
    - o **Misoprostol** 800 μg vaginally with a repeat dose 3 hours to 7 days after initial dose if no response
      - Seventy-one percent of women had complete expulsion by day 3 after one dose.
      - Eighty-four percent success rate when a second dose is given as needed.

- The addition of mifepristone 200 mg orally 24 hours prior to misoprostol significantly increases rates of complete expulsion and decreases need for surgical intervention.
  - According to World Health Organization, misoprostol may also be given sublingually (600 μg) for asymptomatic EPL or orally (600 μg) for incomplete abortion. However, oral routes are associated with increased gastrointestinal side effects.
  - Patients may require pain medications (nonsteroidal anti-inflammatory drugs [NSAIDs], consider narcotics) and antiemetics.
  - A follow-up ultrasound is typically performed in 7 to 14 days to confirm the absence of a gestational sac. If expulsion is not completed, the patient may choose expectant management, repeat misoprostol dose, or surgical treatment.
- Surgical management (suction D&C)
  - **Surgical management:** Women presenting with hemorrhage, hemodynamic instability, or signs of infection (septic abortion) should have prompt uterine evacuation. Stable patients may choose surgical management because it provides more immediate completion of the EPL process and does not require follow-up. The success rate approaches 99%.
  - Advantages: completes the process quickly; associated with less bleeding and pain than expectant or medical management
  - Disadvantages: less available than medication if no provider qualified to perform D&C; rare surgical complications, including uterine perforation
  - Procedural considerations (see chapter 29): Suction curettage can be performed in the office, emergency department, or operating room with manual or electric vacuum aspiration. Give antibiotic prophylaxis with doxycycline within 1 hour prior to procedure. Analgesia options include NSAIDs with local anesthesia (generally a paracervical block) with or without oral or intravenous sedation.
  - Follow-up with repeat ultrasound or β-hCG levels is not necessary.
- Counseling should help a woman assess her future pregnancy goals to determine whether she wishes to actively try to conceive or initiate a method of contraception. No data support delaying conception after EPL because there are no differences seen in subsequent EPL or pregnancy complications.
- **Contraception:** After first or second trimester loss management, women who desire to avoid pregnancy may initiate hormonal contraception, including contraceptive implants and, in the absence of uterine infection, hormonal and nonhormonal intrauterine devices (IUDs) immediately after completion of treatment for EPL.

SECOND-TRIMESTER PREGNANCY LOSS

- Second-trimester losses are less common and occur between 13 to 27 weeks of gestation.
- Epidemiology and risk factors
  - Occurs in approximately 1% to 3% of recognized pregnancies
  - Many risk factors are similar to those for first-trimester losses and include maternal medical conditions, chromosomal abnormalities, and teratogenic exposures.
  - Additional risk factors for second-trimester loss include previous second-trimester loss, antiphospholipid syndrome and thrombophilias, cervical insufficiency, preterm premature rupture of membranes, placental abruption, maternal infection, placental insufficiency, and congenital uterine anomalies (see chapter 5).
  - In 50% to 60% of women, the cause of a second-trimester pregnancy loss remains unknown.

- Management of second-trimester pregnancy loss or impending second-trimester loss can be medical or surgical, depending on the patient's clinical stability, clinical exam, risk factors for complications, and patient preferences.
  - Medical management: induction termination
  - Surgical management: D&C or dilation and evacuation
- Counseling on future pregnancy: The risk of recurrence is a function of the underlying etiology of the pregnancy loss.

ECTOPIC PREGNANCY

- An EP is any pregnancy that occurs outside the uterine cavity, most commonly (90%) in the fallopian tube. However, implantation may occur in the abdomen (1%), cervix (<1%), ovary (3%), cesarean scar (<1%), or interstitial area/cornua (2%-3%).
- Epidemiology and risk factors for EP:
  - Approximately 2% of all reported pregnancies are ectopic, and EP accounts for approximately 6% of all pregnancy-related deaths.
  - Heterotopic pregnancy, where EP co-occurs with an IUP, is rare (1 in 4000 to 1 in 30 000) but more common in women undergoing in vitro fertilization (1 in 100).
  - Half of women diagnosed with EP do not have any known risk factors.
  - Women at higher risk for EP include those with a history of EP (approximately 10% risk of recurrence if one prior ectopic and over 25% if two or more), pelvic inflammatory disease, fallopian tube surgery including tubal sterilization, infertility, endometriosis, cigarette smoking, and age over 35 years.
  - Women with an IUD in place have a lower risk of EP than those not using an IUD, but 53% of pregnancies in women with an IUD in place are ectopic.
- Diagnosis
  - Clinical presentation
    - The classical presentation is abdominal pain, vaginal bleeding, and adnexal mass. However, some women with EP may be asymptomatic.
    - Up to 18% of women presenting to the emergency department with first-trimester bleeding vaginal and/or abdominal pain will have an EP. Vaginal bleeding can vary in quantity and pattern. Pain is typically pelvic and may be diffuse or localized.
    - Women with a ruptured EP may present with hemodynamic instability or an acute abdomen. Shoulder pain may be present due to hemoperitoneum irritating the diaphragm.
  - Differential diagnosis
    - In women with a positive pregnancy test and bleeding or pain, the differential diagnosis includes a normal IUP, EPL, EP, or gestational trophoblastic disease.
    - Additional causes of vaginal bleeding and/or abdominal pain (with or without a positive pregnancy test) include cervical, vaginal, or uterine pathology, ovarian torsion, ovarian cyst rupture, or PID.
  - Assessment
    - Physical exam: Patients with EP may have abdominal tenderness with or without rebound, cervical motion tenderness, or a palpable adnexal mass or mass in the cul-de-sac. Ruptured EP may present with peritoneal signs including rebound tenderness, guarding, or rigidity. Symptoms of hypovolemic shock including tachycardia, hypotension, or altered mental status may occur.

- Ultrasound: Definitive diagnosis of EP is possible only if a GS with a YS and/or embryo is visualized outside the uterus.
  - A mass or mass with a hypoechoic area that is separate from the ovary in a woman with a positive pregnancy test and no evidence of an intrauterine GS containing a YS and/or embryo should raise suspicion for an EP.
  - A pseudo-GS, a collection of fluid or blood in the uterine cavity, may be present and should not be confused with a true GS. It tends to be oval in shape with irregular margins and appears centrally in the uterine cavity without an intradecidual sign.
  - Additional radiologic signs of EP include echogenic free fluid in the pelvis (suggesting ruptured EP), a dilated and thick-walled fallopian tube, and increased blood flow to the adnexa containing the EP.
  - **Pregnancy of unknown location:** See above section on PUL for additional diagnostic considerations.
- Laboratory evaluation
  - Serial quantitative β-hCG (see above section)
  - Additional laboratory testing
    - Complete blood count. If the diagnosis of a ruptured EP is uncertain, serial hemoglobin or hematocrit levels may be useful.
    - Creatinine and liver transaminases. Levels should be obtained in preparation for possible methotrexate treatment for EP.
    - Blood type. Rh-negative patients should be treated with $Rh_o(D)$ immune globulin at the time that EP is diagnosed.
- Diagnostic D&C may be performed for PUL, and if chorionic villi are absent in the uterine aspirate, consider medical treatment for EP. If no villi are seen and the postoperative β-hCG plateaus or continues to rise, administer medical treatment for EP.
- Management of EP
  - General considerations
    - Management of the unstable patient requires rapid evaluation, intravenous fluid resuscitation, two large-bore intravenous cannulas, and transfer to the operating room as soon as safely possible.
    - Both intramuscular methotrexate and surgery are safe and effective treatments for EP in appropriately selected patients.
  - Expectant management may be offered in rare circumstances, where β-hCG levels are plateaued or decreasing or an initial β-hCG less than 200 mIU/mL, where the patient is thoroughly counseled and willing to accept the potential risks of tubal rupture and hemorrhage. Expectant management is approximately 57% successful.
  - Medical management of EP with **methotrexate** is successful in 70%-95% of cases.
    - Mechanism of action: Methotrexate is a folate agonist and binds to dihydrofolate reductase to inhibit DNA synthesis and cell repair and replication. It is directly toxic to hepatocytes and is renally excreted.
    - Indications and contraindications (Table 30-2)
      - Relative contraindications indicate women who are more likely to fail medical management with methotrexate; women with relative contraindications who request medical management should be thoroughly counseled on risk of failed treatment and rupture.
      - Complete blood count and metabolic panel including liver and renal function studies must be obtained to see if patient is a candidate for methotrexate administration.

Table 30-2	Absolute and Relative Contraindications to Methotrexate Treatment for Ectopic Pregnancy[a]

Absolute Contraindications	Relative Contraindications
Intrauterine pregnancy	Positive fetal heart motion
Immunodeficiency	Initial β-hCG concentration >5000 mIU/mL
Moderate to severe anemia, leukopenia, or thrombocytopenia	Rapidly increasing β-hCG concentration (>50% in 48 h)
Active pulmonary disease (except asthma)	Ectopic pregnancy measuring >4 cm on transvaginal ultrasonography
Active peptic ulcer disease	Refusal to accept blood transfusion
Significant hepatic dysfunction	
Significant renal dysfunction	
Breastfeeding	
Ruptured ectopic pregnancy	
Hemodynamically unstable patient	
Patient unable/unwilling to follow-up	
Sensitivity to methotrexate	

Abbreviation: β-hCG, β-human chorionic gonadotropin.
[a]Modified from Practice Committee of American Society for Reproductive Medicine. Medical treatment of ectopic pregnancy: a committee opinion. *Fertil Steril.* 2013;100(3):638-644. Copyright © 2013 American Society for Reproductive Medicine. With permission.

- **Dosing** regimens (Table 30-3)—the single-dose regimen has the least side effects but may require an additional dose to be given; it has an approximately 88% success rate. The multiple dose regimen may be slightly more effective (approximately 93%), especially for patients with higher starting β-hCG values (over 5000 mIU/mL), but it has higher rates of side effects; it may be considered for women with a higher risk of treatment failure.
- **Side effects** are seen in systems with rapidly dividing tissues and include nausea, vomiting, stomatitis, dermatitis, diarrhea, gastric distress, dizziness, elevated liver transaminases, pneumonitis, and rarely neutropenia or alopecia. It is common for women treated with methotrexate to experience abdominal or pelvic pain, thought likely to be due to separation of the pregnancy from the underlying tissue. However, patients should be carefully evaluated to rule out rupture of the EP.
- **Follow-up** depends on the dosing regimen chosen (see Table 30-3). Complete resolution of an ectopic generally occurs in 2 to 3 weeks but can take up to 6 to 8 weeks depending on pretreatment β-hCG levels. For any regimen, if β-hCG levels plateau or increase during follow-up, consider uterine aspiration to evaluate for abnormal IUP or consider administering methotrexate for treatment of a persistent EP.
- In addition to counseling regarding side effects and follow-up, counseling should include warning signs for ruptured EP, avoidance of vigorous exercise and sexual intercourse (due to risk of EP rupture), avoidance of

Table 30-3 Methotrexate Dosing Regimens[a]

	Single-Dose Regimen	Two-Dose Regimen	Fixed Multidose Regimen
Initial methotrexate doses	50 mg/m² IM on day 1	50 mg/m² IM on days 1 and 4	1 mg/kg IM on day 1
Scheduled repeat β-hCG level	Days 4[b] and 7	Days 4[b] and 7	Days 3, 5, and 7
Subsequent methotrexate doses	If β-hCG decrease is less than 15% between days 4 and 7, repeat methotrexate 50 mg/m² IM.	If β-hCG decrease is less than 15% between days 4 and 7, readminister methotrexate 50 mg/m² IM and check β-hCG on day 11. If β-hCG decreases less than 15% between day 7 and 11, readminister methotrexate 50 mg/m² IM and check β-hCG on day 14.	Repeat methotrexate 1 mg/kg on days 3, 5, and 7 as needed until β-hCG has decreased by 15% from its previous measurement.
Folinic acid (Leucovorin)	None	None	0.1 mg/kg IM on days 2, 4, 6, and 8
Definition of successful treatment	β-hCG decreases >15% between day 4 and 7.	β-hCG decreases >15% between days 4 and 7, 7 and 11, or 11 and 14.	β-hCG decreases >15% from a previous level.
Definition of treatment failure	β-hCG does not decrease appropriately after 2 doses.	β-hCG does not decrease appropriately after 4 doses.	β-hCG does not decrease appropriately after 4 doses.
Follow-up after successful treatment	Weekly β-hCG until nonpregnant level reached	Weekly β-hCG until nonpregnant level reached	Weekly β-hCG until nonpregnant level reached

Abbreviations: β-hCG, β-human chorionic gonadotropin; IM, intramuscular.
[a]Adapted from Stovall TG, Ling FW. Single-dose methotrexate: an expanded clinical trial. *Am J Obstet Gynecol.* 1993;168(6, pt 1):1759-1762; Barnhart K, Hummel AC, Sammel MD, Menon S, Jain J, Chakhtoura N. Use of "2-dose" regimen of methotrexate to treat ectopic pregnancy. *Fertil Steril.* 2007;87(2):250-256; Rodi IA, Sauer MV, Gorrill MJ, et al. The medical treatment of unruptured ectopic pregnancy with methotrexate and citrovorum rescue: preliminary experience. *Fertil Steril.* 1986;46(5):811-813.
[b]It is common for β-hCG to increase from day 1 to day 4, but this is not clinically important. The change from day 4 to day 7 is clinically important.

folic acid supplements and NSAIDs (which may decrease methotrexate efficacy), and avoidance of new pregnancy until EP resolution is confirmed.

Surgical management

- Surgery is required for any patient with hemodynamic instability, symptoms of an ongoing ruptured EP, or signs of intraperitoneal bleeding or if a patient has absolute contraindications to medical management.
- Surgery should be considered for any patient with a relative contraindication to methotrexate or when methotrexate treatment has failed.
- After an informed discussion with the health care provider, any patient may elect surgery as the primary treatment for EP.
- Procedural considerations
  - Laparoscopy versus laparotomy: Laparoscopy is preferred if possible, whereas laparotomy is typically reserved for an unstable patient, a patient with large volume hemoperitoneum or a patient in whom laparoscopic visualization is compromised.
  - Salpingostomy versus salpingectomy: Salpingectomy is preferred when the fallopian tube is severely damaged or when significant bleeding from the surgical site is present. Salpingostomy should be considered when a patient desires future fertility but has damage to the contralateral fallopian tube making future pregnancy unlikely without assisted reproductive technology. Salpingostomy may be associated not only with higher rates of subsequent IUP but also with higher rates of subsequent EP. Follow-up β-hCG levels are not required unless salpingostomy is chosen.
  - Interstitial/cornual EP may require cornual resection, which can be performed via minimally invasive surgery (laparoscopy) or laparotomy.
- Counseling on future pregnancy: Methotrexate does not affect subsequent fertility or ovarian reserve. Women are recommended to delay pregnancy for at least 3 months after the last dose of methotrexate to reduce risks of fetal death/teratogenicity in the new pregnancy. Counsel on risks of recurrent EP and the need for early medical attention for subsequent pregnancies to assess for recurrent EP.
- Contraception: For women who wish to delay pregnancy, all hormonal methods, including implant and hormonal/nonhormonal IUDs, can be initiated immediately after treatment for an EP.

SUGGESTED READINGS

American College of Obstetricians and Gynecologists Committee on Practice Bulletins—Gynecology. ACOG Practice Bulletin No. 193: tubal ectopic pregnancy. *Obstet Gynecol.* 2018;131:e91-e103.

American College of Obstetricians and Gynecologists Committee on Practice Bulletins—Gynecology. ACOG Practice Bulletin No. 200: early pregnancy loss. *Obstet Gynecol.* 2018;132:e197-e207.

Doubilet PM, Benson CB, Bourne R, et al. Diagnostic criteria for nonviable pregnancy early in the first trimester. *N Engl J Med.* 2013;369:1443-1451.

McNamee KM, Dawood F, Farquharson RG. Mid-trimester pregnancy loss. *Obstet Gynecol Clin North Am.* 2014;41:87-102.

Practice Committee of the American Society for Reproductive Medicine. Evaluation and treatment of recurrent pregnancy loss: a committee opinion. *Fertil Steril.* 2012;98:1103-1111.

Schreiber C, Creinin MD, Atrio J, Sonalkar S, Ratcliffe SJ, Barnhart KT. Mifepristone pretreatment for the medical management of early pregnancy loss. *N Engl J Med.* 2018;378:2161-2170.

31

Abnormal Uterine Bleeding

Katerina Hoyt and Jean R. Anderson

The evaluation of **abnormal uterine bleeding (AUB)** requires consideration of the age and menstrual status of the woman as well as characterization and quantification of the bleeding, specifically the onset, duration, frequency, amount, pattern, and associated symptoms. It is also important to consider bleeding sources outside of the genital tract, including the urinary and gastrointestinal (GI) tracts, that the woman may perceive is coming from the vagina.

MENSTRUAL DIMENSIONS

- The mean menstrual blood loss in women with normal hemoglobin and iron levels is 30 mL, with 95% of women losing <60 mL each menstrual cycle.
- **Normal menstrual bleeding** is as follows:
  - Length of menstrual cycle: 21 to 35 days
  - Duration of menstrual period: 4 to 6 days
  - Blood loss: 5 to 80 mL
- An AUB includes abnormal menstrual parameters (longer or shorter duration or interval, excessive blood loss with menses, intermenstrual bleeding) or other abnormal pattern of bleeding for reproductive-aged women as well as any bleeding in premenarchal or postmenopausal women.

DIFFERENTIAL DIAGNOSIS OF ABNORMAL UTERINE BLEEDING

Causes of uterine bleeding can be organized by age groups (Table 31-1).

Premenarchal Bleeding

- Physiologic premenarchal bleeding may occur in the first few days of life due to the withdrawal of maternal estrogen.
- Other causes include trauma, foreign body, sexual abuse, precocious puberty, infection, and, rarely, neoplasm.
- See chapter 38 for possible causes and evaluation of premenarchal bleeding.

Reproductive-Aged Abnormal Bleeding

- In women of reproductive age with a chief complaint of AUB, pregnancy-related bleeding (eg, ectopic, miscarriage, normal pregnancy) should be ruled out.
- Structural abnormalities, such as leiomyomas and adenomyosis, are common and typically present with heavy menstrual bleeding. Intrauterine polyps classically present with intermenstrual bleeding.
- Ovulatory dysfunction, characterized by either anovulation or oligo-ovulation, typically presents as irregular menstrual bleeding, in which the patient experiences

Table 31-1 Differential Diagnosis of Abnormal Uterine Bleeding by Age Group

Children	Adolescent	Reproductive	Perimenopausal	Menopausal
• Physiologic[a]	• Anovulatory	• Pregnancy (ectopic or intrauterine)	• Anovulatory	• Atrophy
• Vulvovaginitis	• Coagulopathy	• Anovulatory (PCOS)	• Endometrial hyperplasia/neoplasia	• Endometrial hyperplasia/neoplasia
• Foreign body	• Pregnancy (ectopic or intrauterine)	• Vaginitis/cervicitis/PID	• Structural (leiomyomas, polyps)	• Other genital tract neoplasm (benign or malignant)
• Trauma	• Vaginitis/cervicitis/PID	• Structural (leiomyomas, polyps)	• Adenomyosis	• Vaginitis/cervicitis/PID
• Urethral prolapse	• Medications (hormonal contraception, IUD)	• Adenomyosis	• Vaginitis/cervicitis/PID	• Structural (leiomyomas, polyps)
• Endocrinopathies	• Genital tract neoplasm (benign or malignant)	• Endocrinopathies	• Medications (hormonal contraception, IUD, etc)	• Medications (IUD, hormone replacement therapy, etc)
• Precocious puberty	• Müllerian anomalies[b]	• Medications (hormonal contraception, IUD, etc)	• Pregnancy (ectopic or intrauterine)	• Coagulopathy
• Exogenous hormones (eg, ingestion of mother's OCPs)	• Trauma	• Endometrial hyperplasia/neoplasia	• Other genital tract neoplasm (benign or malignant)	• Trauma
• Genital tract neoplasm (benign or malignant)		• Other genital tract neoplasm (benign or malignant)	• Coagulopathy	
• Coagulopathy		• Coagulopathy	• Trauma	
		• Trauma		

Abbreviations: IUD, intrauterine device; OCPs, oral contraceptive pills; PCOS, polycystic ovary syndrome; PID, pelvic inflammatory disease.
[a]Usually occurs during the first 2 weeks of life due to withdrawal from maternal hormones.
[b]Typically present as absence of menstrual bleeding.

phases of no bleeding that may last for 2 or more months as well as phases of heavy and/or prolonged bleeding and/or intermenstrual bleeding. Common causes include polycystic ovary syndrome (PCOS) and hypothyroidism. Anovulatory cycles are common at both extremes of reproductive age.

- Hyperplasia and malignancy (cervical or uterine) are possible causes of abnormal bleeding.
- Adolescents (ages 13-18 years) frequently experience anovulation caused by immaturity or dysregulation of the hypothalamic-pituitary-ovarian axis. For a majority of adolescents, the menstrual cycle will become regular by the third year after menarche. The AUB caused by coagulation disorders is also found more often in this younger population when compared to older women.

Postmenopausal Bleeding

- Postmenopausal bleeding is most commonly caused by endometrial and vaginal atrophy. However, approximately 15% of these women will have some form of hyperplasia and 5% to 10% will have endometrial cancer. Therefore, it is important to rule out malignancy in postmenopausal patients presenting with vaginal bleeding.
- In early menopausal years, polyps and submucosal fibroids are also common etiologies of abnormal bleeding.
- Providers should rule out nongynecologic sources of bleeding, including bleeding from GI tract and urinary tract.

EVALUATION OF ABNORMAL UTERINE BLEEDING

History

A thorough patient history should include the following elements with modifications according to age group:

- Description of bleeding: onset, precipitating factors (trauma, coitus), bleeding pattern (temporal pattern, duration, quantity), and associated symptoms (pain, fever, changes in bowel or bladder function)
- Menstrual history: last menstrual period, age of menarche, menstrual bleeding patterns (frequency, duration, amount of bleeding), associated pain or other symptoms (eg, breast tenderness, irritability, mittelschmerz), age of menopause
- Sexual history: timing of last sexual encounter, male/female partners, number of partners, sexual practices (vaginal, anal, oral), use of barrier protection, and postcoital bleeding
- History of sexually transmitted infections (STIs)
- Contraception
- Gynecologic history: history of fibroids, polyps, pelvic inflammatory disease (PID), or use of a pessary
- Obstetric history
- Review of systems
  - Systemic symptoms: weight loss, fevers, night sweats
  - Gynecologic: dyspareunia, changes in discharge color, consistency, and odor, itching
  - Urinary: frequency, hesitancy, urgency, incontinence, dysuria, hematuria
  - GI: nausea/vomiting, abdominal bloating, early satiety, bowel movement frequency/change, constipation, diarrhea, hematochezia, melena
  - Menopausal symptoms: vasomotor symptoms, sleep disturbances, mood disturbances, and vaginal dryness

- Past medical/surgical history
- Medication regimen, including anticoagulants, hormones, and tamoxifen
- Family history of bleeding disorders as well as breast, colon, ovarian, and endometrial cancer
- Systemic symptoms of bleeding disorder (easy bruising, new onset nose/gum bleeding)
- History of physical/sexual abuse
- In premenarchal children, genitourinary symptoms may be difficult to assess, and parents will be key informants. It is important to consider urinary and GI sources of bleeding. A history should emphasize the following elements: associated vaginal discharge, previous vaginal foreign bodies, history of trauma or suspicion of abuse, recent sore throat or diarrhea, recent streptococcal infection in a household member, abdominal pain or change in appetite, pain with defecation or urination, and medications (and possible ingestion of family member's medications).
- In postmenopausal women, a history should thoroughly assess for signs, symptoms, and risk factors of gynecologic cancers, including use of hormones or tamoxifen; family history of breast, ovarian, colon, or endometrial cancer; and history of abnormal pap smear or endometrial biopsy. It is important to consider urinary and GI sources of bleeding.

Physical Examination

- Notable general physical exam findings include weight/height/body mass index, evidence of hyperandrogenism (eg, hirsutism, acne), thyroid enlargement or nodules, evidence of insulin resistance (eg, acanthosis nigricans), breast discharge, and evidence of bleeding disorders (eg, petechiae, ecchymoses, skin pallor).
- Abdominal exam: tenderness, palpable mass, distention/ascites, hepatosplenomegaly
- Pelvic exam
  - Examine the external genitalia for evidence of trauma (laceration, bruising), masses, and skin lesions (discoloration, ulcers, plaques, verrucous changes, and excoriation).
  - Examine the urethra and anus for evidence of prolapse, hemorrhoids, and anal fissures or masses.
  - Speculum examination with inspection of vaginal vault and cervix may reveal discharge suggestive of infection, evidence of trauma, vaginal or cervical ulcers or masses, polyps, cervical friability, products of conception, or atrophic changes.
  - Bimanual examination should be performed to evaluate presence of cervical motion tenderness, size and contour of uterus and adnexa, presence of any palpable masses, or tenderness. If early pregnancy is documented or suspected, assess whether cervical os is open.
  - Rectovaginal examination should be considered to better palpate the posterior pelvis, rule out rectal masses, and test stool for occult blood, if indicated.
  - Premenarchal children should undergo thorough examination of the external genitalia and perineum. An exam under sedation or anesthesia is often recommended if internal examination is needed; a pediatric cystoscope can be used to visualize the vagina and cervix. See chapter 38.
- Assess for palpable, enlarged lymph nodes, particularly in the groin.
- Evaluate for signs of physical or sexual abuse.
- Premenarchal patients should undergo Tanner staging (see chapter 38) because breast or pubic hair development may suggest normal progressing puberty or precocious puberty (in girls younger than 8 years).
- Neurofibromatosis and McCune-Albright syndrome are rare causes of precocious puberty, so examination of the skin for café au lait spots is recommended.

Laboratory Testing

- Urine (or serum) β-human chorionic gonadotropin to assess for pregnancy, thyroid-stimulating hormone, prolactin, and complete blood count
- In patients with history or physical exam suggesting genital tract infection (or sexual abuse), cervical or vaginal swabs to assess for STIs such as chlamydia, gonorrhea, herpes, or trichomonas should be performed. In premenarchal children, vaginal secretions should be sampled and tested for common pathogens, including group A *Streptococcus* and shigella.
- Cervical cytology should be obtained according to American College of Obstetricians and Gynecologists guidelines. Visible cervical lesions should be biopsied.
- In women with risk factors for endometrial neoplasia, endometrial sampling (ie, endometrial biopsy or dilation and curettage [D&C]) is often indicated. Endometrial sampling may also be helpful in confirming a diagnosis of PID or endometritis. Focal findings on sonographic imaging should prompt consideration of D&C under hysteroscopic guidance.
- Signs or symptoms of androgen excess should prompt androgen testing.
- Urinalysis/urine culture and/or stool hemoccult, if a urinary or GI source of bleeding is suspected
- If a coagulation disorder or hematologic malignancy is suspected, a complete blood count with differential, prothrombin time, and partial thromboplastin time should be obtained. If initial testing is consistent with coagulopathy and/or if the patient history is suggestive of coagulopathy (regardless of the results of initial laboratory testing), referral to a hematologist for follow-up with additional testing for bleeding disorders is recommended.
- In premenarchal children, if the physical examination is suggestive of precocious puberty, initial workup should include serum luteinizing hormone, follicle-stimulating hormone, and estradiol. Referral to a pediatric endocrinologist should be considered for further evaluation.
- If imaging reveals pelvic mass, tumor markers may be indicated. See chapter 52.

IMAGING TECHNIQUES AND TISSUE SAMPLING METHODS

Ultrasonography

- **Transvaginal ultrasonography (TVUS)**
  - A TVUS is useful in evaluating for the presence of fibroids, polyps, intrauterine pregnancy, ectopic pregnancy, and masses within the uterus, adnexa, or cervix.
  - In the workup for possible malignant processes, sonography can be used to measure endometrial thickness to evaluate for endometrial neoplasia in postmenopausal women, in whom an endometrial thickness of >4 mm is considered abnormal. Evaluation of endometrial thickness is less useful in premenopausal women because the endometrial thickness varies throughout the menstrual cycle.
  - Although TVUS is useful as a screening test to assess the endometrial cavity for leiomyomas and polyps, its sensitivity and specificity for evaluating intracavitary pathology are only 56% and 73%, respectively. Sonohysterography and hysteroscopy are superior to TVUS in detection of intracavitary lesions.

- **Saline infusion sonography**, or sonohysterography, involves distention of the uterine cavity with sterile saline to enhance visualization of the endometrial surface during TVUS. Sonohysterography is the most sensitive noninvasive method of diagnosis for endometrial polyps and submucous myomata. However, it does not distinguish between benign and malignant processes.

Computed Tomography

- Computed tomography imaging is often used in the evaluation of metastatic disease of gynecologic malignancies; however, it has no role in routine pelvic assessment for AUB.

Magnetic Resonance Imaging

- Although routine magnetic resonance imaging (MRI) in the evaluation of AUB is not recommended, pelvic MRI can be useful in the diagnosis of adenomyosis and can accurately localize and measure fibroids, thus permitting planning for management (eg, eligibility for embolization, myomectomy, hysterectomy).

Hysteroscopy

- The gold standard for evaluating the endometrial cavity is hysteroscopy. The advantage of this procedure is that it provides direct visualization of the endometrial cavity and can be performed in the office setting or operating room. It can be both diagnostic and operative, allowing for directed biopsies and excision of polyps and submucosal or intracavitary myomas.
- Hysteroscopy with targeted biopsies has a sensitivity and specificity of 98% and 95%, respectively, compared with histologic findings at the time of hysterectomy.

Endometrial Sampling

- Endometrial sampling is typically performed as an office biopsy and is a rapid, safe, and cost-effective procedure to evaluate AUB. Endometrial biopsy has high overall accuracy in diagnosing endometrial cancer when an adequate specimen is obtained and the endometrial process is global. However, a focal lesion occupying less than 50% of the surface area of the endometrial cavity may be missed by blind endometrial biopsy.
- Indications for endometrial sampling in women with AUB vary by age group:
  - Age 45 years or older: In women who are ovulatory, AUB warrants evaluation with endometrial sampling. In postmenopausal women presenting with vaginal bleeding, initial evaluation can include either TVUS or endometrial sampling. Endometrial sampling should also be performed in postmenopausal women with prior TVUS and one or more of the following: endometrial thickness is >4 mm, endometrium demonstrates diffuse or focal increased echogenicity (heterogeneity), endometrium is not adequately visualized, and there is persistent bleeding.
  - Younger than 45 years: Endometrial sampling is recommended in women who have risk factors for unopposed estrogen (eg, obesity, PCOS), have failed medical management, have persistent AUB, or are at high risk of endometrial cancer (eg, tamoxifen therapy, Lynch syndrome).

Dilation and Curettage

- A D&C can be both diagnostic and therapeutic (in the case of certain diagnoses, such as polyps and submucosal myomas) but incurs the cost of an operating room and carries the risks of anesthesia.

- A D&C, generally under hysteroscopic guidance, may be indicated in women with nondiagnostic endometrial biopsies, biopsies with insufficient tissue for analysis, inability to tolerate an office procedure, or cervical stenosis making an office procedure unsuccessful. A D&C with hysteroscopy is also useful in evaluating patients with focal lesions as well as those with prior endometrial biopsy showing hyperplasia. A D&C should also be considered in women with persistent bleeding despite treatment after normal endometrial biopsy.

SPECIFIC CAUSES OF ABNORMAL UTERINE BLEEDING

Pregnancy-Associated Bleeding

- Pregnancy should be ruled out in any woman in her reproductive years.
- Evaluate with urine or serum β-human chorionic gonadotropin testing, followed by physical exam and pelvic ultrasound if indicated. The differential includes normal pregnancy; ectopic pregnancy; and threatened, inevitable, incomplete, or missed abortion. See chapter 30 for evaluation and management of early pregnancy loss and ectopic pregnancy.

Abnormal Uterine Bleeding in Nonpregnant Women

The most common etiologies of AUB in nonpregnant women may be classified according to the International Federation of Gynecology and Obstetrics (PALM-COEIN) classification system shown in Figure 31-1. Causes of AUB are categorized into structural and nonstructural causes.

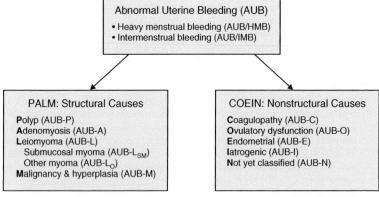

Figure 31-1. International Federation of Gynecology and Obstetrics (PALM-COEIN) classification system for causes of abnormal uterine bleeding in nongravid women of reproductive age. Reprinted with permission from American College of Obstetricians and Gynecologists Committee on Practice Bulletins—Gynecology. ACOG Practice Bulletin No. 128: diagnosis of abnormal uterine bleeding in reproductive-aged women. *Obstet Gynecol.* 2012;120(1):197-206. (Reaffirmed 2016). Copyright © 2012 by The American College of Obstetricians and Gynecologists.

Structural Causes of Abnormal Uterine Bleeding

Polyp (AUB-P)

- Endometrial and endocervical polyps are epithelial proliferations consisting of vascular, glandular, and connective tissue components.
- Although a majority of polyps are benign, a small minority may have malignant features.
- Generally, endometrial polyps tend to be asymptomatic but may be present in 10% to 33% of women with complaints of bleeding, typically in those with heavy menstrual bleeding or intermenstrual bleeding.
- Although ultrasound is generally used as a first-line imaging modality in evaluating a woman with AUB, saline infusion sonogram or hysteroscopy are the most sensitive methods for diagnosing polyps.

Adenomyosis (AUB-A)

- Adenomyosis is a disorder in which endometrial glands and stroma are present within the uterine myometrium. Approximately 60% of women with adenomyosis experience heavy menstrual bleeding.
- A majority of women with adenomyosis will have diffuse uterine enlargement on physical examination.
- Definitive diagnosis is made from histologic examination of uterine tissue after hysterectomy. Preoperatively, adenomyosis can be identified with TVUS or MRI, particularly T2-weighted images. Imaging findings suggestive of adenomyosis include myometrial heterogeneity, asymmetric myometrial thickening, myometrial cysts, subendometrial linear striations, and loss of a clear endomyometrial border.

Leiomyoma (AUB-L)

- Leiomyomas (fibroids) are the most common uterine neoplasm and are the number one indication for hysterectomy in the United States. See chapter 33.
- There is a variety of types of leiomyomas, named primarily for their locations: submucosal, intramural, subserosal, pedunculated, and cervical.
- An AUB is the most common presenting symptom in women who have symptomatic leiomyomas. Submucosal and intramural myomas are commonly associated with heavy or prolonged menstrual bleeding. Subserosal or pedunculated myomas are not considered a major risk for heavy menstrual bleeding. Cervical myomas close to the endocervical canal may cause AUB.
- Leiomyomas can be clinically diagnosed by pelvic examination, typically demonstrating an enlarged, mobile uterus with irregular contour, and pelvic ultrasonography can confirm the diagnosis.

Malignancy and Hyperplasia (AUB-M)

- **Endometrial hyperplasia**, a precursor to endometrial carcinoma, is classified into simple or complex, based on architectural features, and typical or atypical, based on cytologic features. Risk of progression to endometrial cancer is highest with complex atypical hyperplasia/endometrial intraepithelial neoplasia. Endometrial hyperplasia tends to occur during periods of long-term unopposed estrogen exposure, secondary to anovulatory cycles or exogenous use. The AUB is the most common presenting symptom.
  - An endometrial tissue sample, obtained either from an endometrial biopsy or D&C, is required to diagnose endometrial hyperplasia.

- Postmenopausal women diagnosed with endometrial hyperplasia who are on estrogen replacement therapy should discontinue therapy.
- Treatment depends on age, desire for future fertility, surgical risk, and presence of atypia in the pathology specimen. Treatment options include expectant management, progestin therapy, or hysterectomy. Progestin therapy can be an effective treatment for endometrial hyperplasia because progestins promote stromal decidualization and subsequent thinning of the endometrium.
- **Atypical hyperplasia/endometrial intraepithelial neoplasia** is more likely to progress to carcinoma than those cases without atypia; therefore, more aggressive treatment is needed. Atypical hyperplasia concomitantly exists with endometrial carcinoma in up to 25% to 50% of cases. Thus, a significant number of women diagnosed with atypical hyperplasia on curettage will be found to have invasive carcinoma if hysterectomy is performed. Referral to a gynecologic oncologist may be indicated.
  - *Hysterectomy is the treatment of choice* for both premenopausal and postmenopausal women.
  - *Progestin therapy* with Mirena IUD is an option for women who desire to preserve fertility or refuse or cannot tolerate surgery. Mirena IUD may promote regression of atypical hyperplasia in up to 75% to 90% of women. Mirena IUD is preferred over oral progestins. A meta-analysis of women with atypical hyperplasia treated with levonorgestrel IUD demonstrated a regression rate of 90% compared to 69% in those treated with oral progestins.
  - Although Mirena IUD is more effective than oral progestins, megestrol acetate dosed at 80 to 160 mg twice a day may be prescribed for atypical hyperplasia in women who decline/cannot tolerate an IUD or have uterine factors complicating the placement or retention of the IUD (severe distortion of the uterine cavity due to fibroids, a congenital anomaly, or recurrent expulsion). In women treated with progestins, endometrial sampling every 3 to 6 months is recommended to determine the responsiveness of the hyperplasia to therapy. Further treatment will be determined based on the results of repeat endometrial sampling.
  - It must be emphasized that conservative therapy in women with complex atypical hyperplasia involves risk, and close follow-up is necessary.
- **Hyperplasia without atypia/benign endometrial hyperplasia** may be managed conservatively with long-term follow-up and repeat endometrial sampling.
  - Simple hyperplasia without atypia may be managed with progestin-only therapy, oral contraceptives, or expectant management.
    - Expectant management may be used if the inciting factor for the endometrial proliferation has been eliminated (anovulation, now corrected).
    - Progestin therapy includes Mirena, oral progestins, or oral contraceptive pills (OCPs).
    - Follow-up endometrial sampling should be performed to ensure resolution of hyperplasia, and the patient should be reevaluated if bleeding recurs.
  - Complex hyperplasia without atypia may be managed with progestin therapy or hysterectomy.
    - Progestin therapy is standard treatment for women with complex hyperplasia without atypia. Mirena IUD is the preferred treatment, but women unable to tolerate IUD may use megestrol acetate for 3 to 6 months. Repeat endometrial sampling should be performed every 3 to 6 months to determine the

responsiveness of the hyperplasia to therapy. Further treatment will be determined based on the results of repeat endometrial sampling.

- o Hysterectomy is an option for patients who decline or cannot take progestins.
- o If a premenopausal patient desires fertility, pregnancy can be pursued once the biopsy shows resolution of the hyperplasia.
- **Endometrial carcinoma** is rare in patients younger than age 40 years but may be seen in those with chronic anovulation. Postmenopausal bleeding, however, should be assumed to represent endometrial cancer until proven otherwise. Advise pelvic ultrasound and/or endometrial sampling (as indicated; see "Endometrial Sampling" section).
  - Many postmenopausal women who take hormone replacement therapy develop vaginal bleeding initially. Vaginal bleeding can be followed for the first 6 months after beginning continuous combined therapy. However, persistence of bleeding past 6 months warrants evaluation for AUB. Although it may identify focal lesions, TVUS is not as reliable as an endometrial biopsy for excluding endometrial hyperplasia/cancer in women on hormone replacement therapy because endometrial thickness thresholds are not well established in this population. As a result, the preferred diagnostic modality for endometrial hyperplasia and carcinoma is endometrial biopsy or D&C.
- **Cervical carcinoma** is most frequently diagnosed in women between the ages of 35 and 44 years; however, over 15% of cases are found in women over age 65 years. The most common bleeding patterns associated with cervical carcinoma are intermenstrual and postcoital bleeding. See chapters 49 and 50 for screening and treatment.
- Estrogen-producing **ovarian tumors**, such as a granulosa-theca cell tumor, can produce endometrial hyperplasia and AUB. See chapter 52.

Nonstructural Causes of Abnormal Uterine Bleeding

Coagulopathy (AUB-C)

- Approximately 13% of women with heavy menstrual bleeding have a bleeding disorder. Easy bruising and bleeding from multiple sites (eg, nose, gingiva, intravenous sites, GI, and genitourinary tracts) may suggest coagulopathy.
- **Von Willebrand disease (vWD)** is the most common inherited bleeding disorder, affecting 1% to 2% of the population. Low, abnormal, or absent von Willebrand factor leads to a spectrum of disease severity with three main types of vWD (types 1, 2, and 3). In women with vWD, menorrhagia is the most common manifestation, occurring in 60% to 95% beginning at menarche. Women with vWD are also likely to report postpartum or postoperative bleeding or bleeding related to dental work. They may also report easy bruising, epistaxis, or family history of bleeding symptoms.
- Other coagulopathies, including platelet abnormalities, idiopathic thrombocytopenic purpura, and hematologic malignancy (eg, leukemia), may also cause AUB.
- All adolescents with heavy menstrual bleeding and adults with a past medical and family history suggestive of bleeding disorder should undergo laboratory testing for bleeding disorders.
- Initial laboratory testing for bleeding disorders should include complete blood count, prothrombin time, and partial thromboplastin time. If initial testing is consistent with coagulopathy and/or if the patient history is suggestive of coagulopathy (regardless of the results of initial laboratory testing), referral to a hematologist for follow-up with additional testing for vWD or other bleeding disorders is recommended.

- Therapy usually involves treating the underlying cause and may require administration of blood products.
- Little data are available regarding treatment of heavy menstrual bleeding in women with vWD. Oral contraceptives, desmopressin, and antifibrinolytic agents (tranexamic acid) are options. Nasal desmopressin appears to be an effective treatment for vWD.

Ovulatory Dysfunction (AUB-O)

- Women may have either anovulation (the absence of ovulation) or oligo-ovulation (infrequent ovulation).
- Anovulation is multifactorial and related to alterations of the hypothalamic-pituitary-ovarian axis. With long-term anovulation, estrogen production occurs without the progesterone normally produced from a corpus luteum, thus creating an unopposed estrogen state. Therefore, these women are at risk for endometrial hyperplasia and cancer. Anovulation is commonly associated with PCOS and morbid obesity, in which peripheral conversion of androstenedione to estrone occurs in adipose tissue producing elevated estrogen levels.
- Hypothyroidism and hyperprolactinemia are common endocrinopathies that can lead to anovulation.
- The optimal treatment of ovulatory dysfunction depends on the etiology of the anovulation but should relieve symptoms related to AUB, prevent the development of endometrial hyperplasia/cancer, and improve quality of life with minimal side effects. It is directed toward stabilizing the endometrium and treating the underlying hormonal alterations.
- In addition to treatment of associated causes (eg, hypothyroidism, hyperprolactinemia), first-line treatment options for the abnormal bleeding include OCPs, oral progestin therapy, or Mirena IUD.

Endometrial (AUB-E)

- Genital infection, including endometritis or cervicitis, may cause AUB. If present, bleeding associated with endometritis is commonly intermenstrual, whereas bleeding associated with cervicitis is more often postcoital.
- Endometritis should be suspected clinically with uterine tenderness or other signs or symptoms of PID and in women with gonorrhea or chlamydia on vaginal, urine, or cervical testing. Any recent history of instrumentation of the uterus, history of STIs, or recent unprotected sexual contact with a new partner should add to the suspicion of acute endometritis. Chronic endometritis may be more indolent and is diagnosed by endometrial biopsy as evidenced by the presence of plasma cells. Cervicitis is diagnosed by clinical examination and results of STI testing. See chapter 27.
- In the context of a regular menstrual cycle in the absence of other identifiable causes, AUB may be attributed to a primary disorder of the endometrium causing impairment of local endometrial hemostasis. However, there are no available clinical tests to identify such disorders.

Iatrogenic (AUB-I)

- **Psychotropic medications**
  - Certain medications used in the treatment of psychiatric illness can affect the hypothalamic-pituitary axis and interfere with ovulation.

- Antipsychotic medications (ie, dopamine antagonists) commonly cause hyperprolactinemia and subsequent abnormalities in menstruation.
- Phenothiazines and antidepressants, particularly tricyclics, also may interfere with the normal menstrual cycle.
- **Hormonal medications**
  - Progestin-only contraceptives, including depot medroxyprogesterone acetate (Depo-Provera), etonogestrel implant (Nexplanon), and levonorgestrel-releasing IUDs, can be associated with irregular bleeding patterns (increased or decreased duration of menstrual bleeding, intermenstrual bleeding, and amenorrhea), especially in the first few months of use.
  - Combination OCPs: Intermenstrual (breakthrough) bleeding may occur with even one missed contraceptive pill. With long-term use, AUB may result from endometrial atrophy.
  - Other progestational agents: Prolonged use of high doses of progestins, often used in the treatment of AUB and endometrial hyperplasia, may result in endometrial atrophy, which can cause AUB.
- **Copper-containing intrauterine devices**, unlike the levonorgestrel-releasing Mirena intrauterine system, increase average monthly blood loss by approximately 35%. Such bleeding is often treated successfully with antifibrinolytic medications or nonsteroidal anti-inflammatory drugs.
- **Anticoagulants**: The patient can experience AUB at both therapeutic and supratherapeutic dosages.
- **Digitalis**, **phenytoin**, and **corticosteroids** have been implicated as causes of AUB.
- Over-the-counter medications that may contribute to AUB include **motherwort**, **gingko**, and **ginseng**.

Not Yet Classified (AUB-N)

- There may be other contributing factors or causes of AUB, including arteriovenous malformations and myometrial hypertrophy. However, these potential causes have been poorly defined and studied.

MANAGEMENT OF ABNORMAL UTERINE BLEEDING

Medical Therapy

- **Estrogen-progestin contraceptives** are first-line management for many women with AUB, and they may be used in the treatment of both heavy menstrual bleeding (commonly caused by polyps, adenomyosis, and fibroids) and ovulatory dysfunction. Advantages of this method include contraception, menstrual regulation, decreased menstrual flow in patients, and reduced dysmenorrhea. In women with heavy menstrual bleeding, OCPs have been shown to decrease menstrual blood loss by 35% to 65%. Contraindications to OCPs include smoking over the age of 35 years, hypertension, migraines, history of venous thromboembolism, thrombogenic mutations, ischemic heart disease, history of stroke, valvular heart disease, history of breast cancer, liver cirrhosis, and hepatocellular adenoma or malignant hepatoma.
- **Levonorgestrel-releasing intrauterine devices** decrease the risk of hemorrhage, provide protection against endometrial hyperplasia and cancer, and provide contraception. Many women using this method develop scant bleeding or amenorrhea. They may be used in the treatment of heavy menstrual bleeding as well

as ovulatory dysfunction. The 52-mg levonorgestrel-releasing intrauterine device (Mirena) reduces menstrual blood loss by 71% to 95% in women with heavy menstrual bleeding, making it the highest efficacy medical treatment.

- **Depot medroxyprogesterone acetate** (Depo-Provera) is used for women with AUB who have contraindications to estrogen or prefer this as their contraceptive method. It can be used in the treatment of heavy menstrual bleeding and ovulatory dysfunction and reduces menstrual blood loss by 49%. After 12 months of uninterrupted application, 55% of women report amenorrhea.

- **Oral progestins** (megestrol acetate, medroxyprogesterone acetate, and norethindrone acetate) can be used in women with contraindications to estrogen and those who desire pregnancy in a relatively short time frame. They may be used in the treatment of heavy menstrual bleeding, ovulatory dysfunction, and endometrial hyperplasia. They are available in both cyclic and continuous regimens.

- **Antifibrinolytic medications** (eg, tranexamic acid) decrease menstrual blood flow by 50% and need to be taken only during menses. Due to increased thrombotic risk, they are contraindicated in patients with a history of thrombotic events and should not be taken concurrently with OCPs. Although increased risk of thrombosis is a listed potential complication of tranexamic acid, studies have not shown increased incidence of thrombosis in treated women versus the general population. Antifibrinolytics may be especially useful in women who cannot tolerate hormonal treatments.

- **Nonsteroidal anti-inflammatory drugs** may reduce menstrual volume in women with heavy menstrual bleeding by at least 20% to 40% and, like antifibrinolytic medications, need to be taken during menses only.

- Gonadotropin-releasing hormone agonists have limited use for treating AUB long term and can have significant side effects, such as hot flashes, osteopenia, and vaginal dryness due to suppression of estrogen production. Gonadotropin-releasing hormone agonists can be used to induce amenorrhea in patients receiving chemotherapy and can reduce uterine volume by 30% to 50% in women with leiomyomas, which may facilitate less invasive surgery (ie, vaginal or laparoscopic vs abdominal hysterectomy). Add-back therapy, which typically includes a progestin or a progestin plus low-dose estrogen, alleviates menopausal symptoms.

- Danazol has been shown to significantly reduce menstrual blood loss (approximately 50%) and may induce amenorrhea. However, androgenic side effects limit its use.

Surgical Treatment

Surgical treatment may be warranted in patients who fail medical management. The most common indication for surgery is heavy menstrual bleeding due to structural lesions (polyps, leiomyomas, adenomyosis). Etiologies of ovulatory dysfunction are generally treated medically, although surgery is an option for women who desire definitive treatment and wish to avoid the ongoing need for and side effects associated with medication.

- Definitive treatment of polyps consists of surgical removal via operative hysteroscopy. Endocervical polyps can be removed by resection or by grasping them with forceps, twisting them off, and cauterizing the base as needed.

- Myomectomy is an option for women with uterine leiomyomas who have failed medical management and desire to preserve fertility or to retain their uterus. Hysteroscopic myomectomy is a minimally invasive option used for intracavitary myomas.

In women with fibroids in other locations, laparoscopic/robotic and open myomectomy are options.

- Endometrial ablation is a minimally invasive option for treatment of heavy menstrual bleeding and is designed to ablate the full thickness of the endometrium. A variety of modalities are available, including thermal, microwave, laser, cryocautery, and radiofrequency, each with its own advantages and disadvantages.
  - Before performing endometrial ablation, endometrial hyperplasia or carcinoma must be ruled out. It should be only used to treat AUB in women with no intrauterine pathology.
  - Across all methods, the overall success rate is approximately 80% to 90% with 30% to 50% of women reporting amenorrhea 6 months postprocedure. Still, within 5 years, 15% will require a second ablation and 20% will have a hysterectomy. Although endometrial ablation is not recommended in women who desire future fertility, it should not be considered an effective means of contraception and postprocedure contraception should be addressed as part of patient counseling
  - Postablation tubal sterilization syndrome (PATSS) is a complication that may occur following endometrial ablation in women who have undergone prior tubal sterilization. The PATSS consists of cyclic pelvic pain caused by bleeding from active endometrium that is trapped in the uterine cornua. The incidence of PATSS is as high as 10%.
- Uterine artery embolization may be an option for premenopausal women with symptomatic uterine leiomyomas who do not desire future pregnancy. Embolization should not be performed in patients who have PID, uterine malignancy, or subserosal or submucosal fibroids that are pedunculated with a narrow stalk.
- Hysterectomy provides definitive treatment for heavy menstrual bleeding and may be a reasonable option in women with severe bleeding, refractory to medical and less radical surgical therapy, who have completed their childbearing. Minimally invasive approaches are often feasible.

SUGGESTED READINGS

American College of Obstetricians and Gynecologists Committee on Practice Bulletins—Gynecology. ACOG Practice Bulletin No. 128: diagnosis of abnormal uterine bleeding in reproductive-aged women. *Obstet Gynecol.* 2012;120(1):197-206. (Reaffirmed 2016)

American College of Obstetricians and Gynecologists Committee on Practice Bulletins—Gynecology. ACOG Practice Bulletin No. 136: management of abnormal uterine bleeding associated with ovulatory dysfunction. *Obstet Gynecol.* 2013;122(1):176-185. (Reaffirmed 2018)

Bourdel N, Chauvet P, Tognazza E, Pereira B, Botchorishvili R, Canis M. Sampling in atypical endometrial hyperplasia: which method results in the lowest underestimation of endometrial cancer? A systematic review and meta-analysis. *J Minim Invasive Gynecol.* 2016;23(5):692-701.

Matteson KA, Rahn DD, Wheeler TL II, et al. Nonsurgical management of heavy menstrual bleeding: a systematic review. *Obstet Gynecol.* 2013;121(3):632-643.

Munro MG, Critchley HO, Broder MS, Fraser IS. FIGO classification system (PALM-COEIN) for causes of abnormal uterine bleeding in nongravid women of reproductive age. *Int J Gynaecol Obstet.* 2011;113:3-13.

32

Chronic Pelvic Pain

Melissa Pritchard McHale and Khara M. Simpson

Chronic pelvic pain (CPP) is a common problem—an estimated 6% to 27% of women worldwide are affected. These estimates vary tremendously due to lack of consistency regarding the exact definition of CPP. The CPP affects quality of life; increases work absenteeism; decreases overall productivity; and limits normal physical, social, emotional, and sexual function. The differential diagnosis is extensive, and the cause often involves multiple organ systems, with multiple etiologies of pain often present for one patient. The CPP is the diagnosis for 10% to 20% of gynecology office referrals. Up to 90% of patients with CPP will undergo one or more unsuccessful gynecologic procedures. At least 40% of gynecologic laparoscopies are performed for CPP, but only 30% to 60% of those surgeries reveal a cause. Ten percent to 20% of hysterectomies are performed with the primary indication of CPP, but only 50% to 80% of hysterectomies performed for CPP improve symptoms with up to 40% of patients having persistent symptoms.

TYPES OF PELVIC PAIN

There are no standard diagnostic criteria, but a reasonable **definition of CPP** is cyclic or noncyclic pain in the lower abdomen, pelvis, lower back, or buttocks of at least 6 months duration that causes functional disability and motivates the patient to seek medical help. Because of varied definitions, the epidemiology and natural history of CPP are not well described. **Acute pelvic pain** can be defined with the same criteria but lasts <30 days.

- The CPP is most common in younger adult women. Four percent to 15% of reproductive-aged women are affected.
- **Dysmenorrhea** (pain associated with menstrual cycles) occurs in up to 90% of women (see chapter 42). Primary dysmenorrhea is painful menses in the absence of an identified pelvic pathology. Secondary dysmenorrhea is painful menses with an identifiable cause. The most common cause of secondary dysmenorrhea is endometriosis. Risk factors for primary dysmenorrhea include age <30 years, body mass index <20, tobacco use, early menarche, and psychiatric conditions.
- **Dyspareunia** (pain during sexual activity) occurs in 1% to 40% of women. Risk factors include history of pelvic inflammatory disease, anxiety, depression, sexual assault, female circumcision, and postmenopausal status.
- **Noncyclic pelvic pain** (with no relation to menses) occurs in 4% to 40% of women. Risk factors include anxiety, depression, prior cesarean delivery, pelvic adhesions, endometriosis, menorrhagia, and history of miscarriage or physical/sexual abuse.

EVALUATION OF CHRONIC PELVIC PAIN

- **Prior records** (including past history, test results, operative notes, and pathology reports) should be reviewed to avoid redundant tests or procedures and to gauge the effectiveness of prior interventions and progress over time.

- **Pain inventory questionnaires** can be helpful in recording subjective and objective data and may increase the efficiency of initial data gathering. Useful resources are available from the International Pelvic Pain Society at https://www.pelvicpain.org. Pain questionnaires are helpful in allowing the patient to develop a coherent and relevant narrative before appearing at the office and allow rapid review of symptoms, permitting the interview to focus on pain issues. A personal body pain map is extremely helpful in focusing the differential and examination.

- Adequate time should be allotted for a **complete medical and psychosocial history**, without rushing the patient. A detailed review of systems, including genitourinary, gastrointestinal, musculoskeletal, and psychoneurologic questions, is important.
  - Establish a detailed understanding of the intensity, location, character, and duration of the pain and any association with intercourse, menstruation, defecation, recent or distant surgery, radiation treatments, or abdominopelvic infections. Precipitating and relieving factors should be reviewed.
  - Screening for physical or sexual abuse, domestic violence, and other psychosocial stressors (eg, death of loved one, divorce) should be completed. Twenty percent to 60% of patients with CPP report a history of sexual or childhood abuse. A complete mental health history and depression screening are helpful; mood and personality disorders are frequently comorbid with CPP. It is not clear whether these problems are a cause or result of pain. Increased depression scores, however, correlate with increased pain scores, so simultaneous treatment is most effective.
  - Current, usual, and worst pain can be recorded using a pain scale (eg, visual analogue scale). Associated symptoms such as weight loss, hematochezia, and perimenopausal/postmenopausal bleeding should prompt a thorough investigation for malignancy.

- The **physical exam** begins with a general and neurologic assessment. Fully explain the plan and exam techniques to relieve anxiety and promote patient cooperation and comfort. The International Pelvic Pain Society physical exam form or similar tools may be useful for recording the complete assessment. The exam should help narrow the differential, rule out systemic disease or neoplasm, and suggest additional testing.
  - Evaluate the **general appearance**, including dress, nutrition, posture, apparent age, gait, and pain behaviors.
  - Ask the patient to **indicate the precise location** of her pain. If she is able to use a single finger, a discrete source is more likely than if she uses a broad sweeping motion of the entire hand.
  - Note the presence of **scars** or **hernias** on abdominal exam. Gently attempt to elicit pain with palpation of the skin, fascia, or muscle. Especially note any reproducible tenderness. Appropriate **trigger point mapping** should be performed if fibromyalgia is in the differential.
  - Look for **Carnett sign** (ie, increased abdominal tenderness when the patient lifts her head and shoulders in the supine position) suggesting abdominal wall rather than intra-abdominal pathology. Pain with the **Beatty maneuver** (ie, thigh abduction against resistance) may suggest piriformis syndrome. The **obturator sign** (ie, pain with flexion and internal rotation of the hip while lying supine) and the **psoas sign** (ie, pain with hip flexion against resistance) can indicate inflammation or dysfunction within those muscles. The **straight leg raise test** evaluates radiculopathy or intervertebral disk disease. The **FABER test** (ie, pain

with flexion/abduction/external rotation of the hip) assesses hip and sacroiliac joint pathology.

- A thorough **neurologic examination**, including sensation, muscle strength, and reflexes, may be required. Examine the spine for scoliosis while the patient is sitting, standing, walking, and bending at the waist.
- The **gynecologic exam** starts with external observation and then palpation with cotton swabs to define hyperesthetic areas (even if the skin appears normal). Light touch and pinprick sensation testing of the vulva may be required.
  - Start the internal examination with a single-digit vaginal exam if needed. Assess the vestibule, vaginal walls, rectum, urethra, bladder trigone, pubic arch, pelvic floor muscles, cervix, and vaginal fornices. Initial assessment of the uterus and adnexa can be performed with a single digit as well.
  - Visual inspection of the vaginal vault can begin with a single speculum blade. Assess the vaginal cuff or cervix, cervical os, paracervix, and vaginal mucosa.
  - Finally, perform a bimanual exam of the uterus, adnexa, and other pelvic contents followed by rectovaginal exam. The bimanual exam, being the most invasive part of the evaluation, should be performed last. Some patients will be unable to tolerate any additional evaluation following the bimanual exam.

Imaging and Laboratory Testing

Imaging and diagnostic testing are tailored to the differential.

- Pelvic ultrasonography is of little benefit unless uterine or adnexal pathology is suspected. Transvaginal imaging is usually preferred to the transabdominal approach for assessing the pelvic structures.
- Magnetic resonance imaging can be helpful in selected cases, especially if adenomyosis is suspected.
- Plain x-ray of the chest, spine, abdomen, or joints or computed tomography scan is rarely indicated.
- Colonoscopy can assess colorectal cancer, inflammatory bowel disease, diverticulosis, and invasive endometriosis. It is indicated in cases with persistent diarrhea, dyschezia, or hematochezia.
- Cystoscopy can be used for evaluation of bladder symptoms, hematuria or for refractory urinary symptoms in patients with suspected interstitial cystitis (IC)/bladder pain syndrome.
- **Laboratory testing** is guided by the history and physical and may include urine pregnancy test, vaginal pH and wet mount, testing for gonorrhea and chlamydia, complete blood count, erythrocyte sedimentation rate, thyroid-stimulating hormone, rapid plasma reagin, hepatitis B surface antigen, human immunodeficiency virus test, urinalysis/microscopy, and urine culture. There is no standard laboratory panel for CPP. Serum cancer antigen 125 testing is not useful unless a cancer workup is initiated. Endocrine testing for follicle-stimulating hormone, estradiol, and gonadotropin-releasing hormone (GnRH) stimulation test may be indicated for suspected ovarian remnant syndrome.

Laparoscopy and Consults

- Although **pelviscopy** is performed for more than 40% of CPP cases, it should be employed only when noninvasive evaluation is completed and for cases in which a diagnosis can be reasonably anticipated. Laparoscopy is not a substitute for a complete history and physical or for diagnoses that can be made without a procedure. Many causes of CPP are *not* detectable by laparoscopy. It can be performed when a structural cause, such as endometriosis, is known or suspected, and therefore operative management has the potential to provide clinical improvement.

- Selected evaluation by neurology, gastroenterology, anesthesiology, urology, psychiatry, or physical therapy **consultants** can provide important multidisciplinary perspective and assist in forming a complete treatment plan. Often, patients have been through a long, tedious, and piecemeal evaluation by multiple providers followed by redundant diagnostic and treatment failures. Performing a complete and multidisciplinary assessment from the start may reach a successful outcome more efficiently and reassure a demoralized and anxious patient. In addition, some tests are only appropriately obtained via consultation, such as nerve conduction studies or electromyography, if they are necessary.

DIFFERENTIAL DIAGNOSIS OF PELVIC PAIN

The **differential diagnosis** of pelvic pain is extensive, and some patients have multiple diagnoses.

- Selected **causes of chronic pelvic pain** are listed in Table 32-1. Previously undiagnosed medical illness should also be considered, such as neoplasia, sickle cell disease, hyperparathyroidism, urolithiasis, lead/mercury intoxication, lactose intolerance, chronic constipation, chronic appendicitis, and chronic fatigue syndrome.
- Assigning only one unifying diagnosis after a thorough workup for CPP is not always the case; management of multiple disease processes is often required. Therefore, assessment should consider multiple etiologies of pain as well as multidisciplinary approaches to treatment. The following disorders, in addition to being primary etiologies, are frequently comorbid with other causes of CPP and deserve special consideration.
- **Dysmenorrhea** is reported in up to 80% of women with CPP. It is characterized by cramping pelvic or suprapubic pain during menses that radiates to the lower back or thighs, often with mood or behavioral changes (see chapter 42). Nausea/vomiting, diarrhea, irritability, and fatigue may be present. The pathophysiology is inflammatory prostaglandin release upon progesterone withdrawal at the end of the menstrual cycle. Patients with hyperalgesia may experience significantly longer and more intense menstrual pain. Adolescents presenting with dysmenorrhea most commonly have primary dysmenorrhea. Managing menstrual pain that presents without an identifiable pathologic cause can be an important consideration for patients with CPP, and a combination of **nonsteroidal anti-inflammatory drugs** and hormonal suppression of menstrual cycles can be very effective for these patients.
- **Endometriosis** is the most common cause of secondary dysmenorrhea; 6% to 10% of women of reproductive age have endometriosis, and up to 70% of women with CPP have endometriosis. The symptoms of endometriosis are extremely variable, ranging from asymptomatic cases to dysmenorrhea to dysuria to CPP. Significant pain reduction has been observed with hormonal suppressive therapy, although recurrence of pain is generally observed on cessation. Conservative surgical management with excision of endometriosis has been a topic of greater investigation recently, with results demonstrating significant improvements (50%-95%) in short-term pain relief. Care should be individualized (see chapter 42).

Table 32-1 Differential Diagnosis of Chronic Pelvic Pain[a,b]

Category	Etiology	Mechanism	Testing/Diagnosis (in Addition to Physical Exam)	Treatment
Cyclic/ recurrent gynecologic	**Endometriosis**	Ectopic endometrial tissue infiltration and inflammation. Can be cyclic or noncyclic	± imaging, laparoscopy with biopsy	• Ovulation suppression (ie, OCPs, progestins, GnRH agonists), surgical excision of endometriosis lesions, endometriomas, hysterectomy ± BSO
	Adenomyosis	Endometrial stroma and glands deeper than 2 mm within the myometrium results in menorrhagia and dysmenorrhea.	MRI sometimes can be suggested on ultrasound.	• NSAIDs, OCPs, GnRH agonists, progesterone IUD, hysterectomy
	Primary/ secondary dysmenorrhea	Primary = uterine menstrual pain Secondary = menstrual pain due to structural pathology	Rule out other causes.	• NSAIDs, OCPs, GnRH agonists, treatment of secondary causes
	Ovarian remnant syndrome	FSH stimulation of inadequately excised ovarian tissue at time of oophorectomy; similar mechanism if ovaries are purposefully conserved at hysterectomy	Surgical history, serum FSH, and estrogen in premenopausal range	• Adhesiolysis and removal of all ovarian tissue may cure >90%.
	Cervical stenosis	Blocked cervical os results in hematometra, retrograde menstruation.	Ultrasound	• Dilation of cervical os in the office or under sedation in operating room may require hysterectomy if recurrent.

Noncyclic gynecologic	**Abdominopelvic adhesions**	Scar tissue from infection, trauma, endometriosis	Laparoscopy	• Laparoscopy/laparotomy and adhesiolysis may use antiadhesion barriers. • Adhesions may recur despite adhesiolysis.
	Uterine retroversion	Rare cause of deep dyspareunia and dysmenorrhea; very rare cause of uterine pelvic incarceration in early pregnancy	Pelvic exam, ultrasound, pessary test for symptom relief	Hodge pessary or laparoscopic uterine suspension
	Chronic endometritis/ chronic PID	Pelvic tuberculosis, tuboovarian abscess, chronic chlamydial endometritis; more frequent in populations with high rates of STDs	Gonorrhea/chlamydia PCR, endometrial biopsy, ultrasound, laparoscopy	• Antibiotic therapy; azithromycin or doxycycline × 2 wk
	Chronic vulvovaginitis	Recurrent or chronic yeast, trichomonas, or fungal infections	Wet prep, culture, vaginal pH	Antibiotics—treatment followed by a suppressive course, boric acid vaginal suppositories
	Vaginal cuff pain	Posthysterectomy chronic low-grade cuff cellulitis, seroma, neuroma, or nerve entrapment		Antibiotics, cuff resection/ revision, local anesthetic injection, chemical neurolysis
	Contact vulvitis	Contact irritant from lotion, soaps, clothing, etc		Eliminate offending agents; ± apply topical steroids.

(Continued)

Table 32-1 Differential Diagnosis of Chronic Pelvic Pain[a,b] *(Continued)*

Category	Etiology	Mechanism	Testing/Diagnosis (in Addition to Physical Exam)	Treatment
Noncyclic gynecologic	**Vulvodynia**	Vulvar hyperalgesia	Cotton swab test, vaginal pH, wet prep, fungal culture, STI screening, biopsy if clinically indicated	Vulvar care, topical lidocaine, physical therapy, biofeedback, TCAs, SSRIs
	Vulvar vestibulitis	Subset of vulvodynia Nonspecific vestibular inflammation; severe entry dyspareunia	Cotton swab test ± vulvar skin biopsy if clinically indicated	Similar to vulvodynia Vestibulectomy/perineoplasty if conservative management fails
	Pudendal neuralgia	Pudendal nerve injury or entrapment	Diagnostic nerve block	Avoid sitting for prolonged periods of time; pain medications, nerve block, or surgical decompression for severe cases Pudendal nerve block
	Pelvic congestion syndrome	Pelvic vein insufficiency from pelvic varicosities, vascular stasis with tissue edema Pain with increased intraabdominal pressure, prolonged standing Increased risk with collagen vascular disease (eg, Ehlers-Danlos)	Pelvic venography (transuterine contrast injection with real-time radiography), MRA, ultrasound	Ovulation suppression, endovascular embolization, hysterectomy

Gastrointestinal	**Irritable bowel syndrome**	Functional bowel disorder Constipation or diarrhea predominant	Rule out other causes.	Increase dietary fiber, loperamide, stool softeners, dicyclomine. Refer to gastroenterology.
	Inflammatory bowel disease (ulcerative colitis and Crohn disease)	Chronic bowel inflammation	Cramping lower abdominal pain and bloody diarrhea, stool studies, colonoscopy, biopsies	Anti-inflammatory drugs, steroids Refer to gastroenterology.
	Diverticular disease	Colonic outpouchings of mucosa/submucosa due to muscularis weakness at sites of higher pressure; present in >10% of women over age 40 y; can become infected/inflamed	AXR, barium enema, colonoscopy	Antibiotics for infection; increased dietary fiber and hydration
	Intermittent bowel obstruction	Mechanical partial obstruction, usually secondary to adhesions	AXR (upper GI with small bowel follow-through study), CT scan, biopsy of any mass	Bowel decompression and conservative management or surgical adhesiolysis

(Continued)

Table 32-1 Differential Diagnosis of Chronic Pelvic Pain[a,b] *(Continued)*

Category	Etiology	Mechanism	Testing/Diagnosis (in Addition to Physical Exam)	Treatment
Urologic	**Interstitial cystitis/ bladder pain syndrome (IC/BPS)**	Chronic noninfectious cystitis and hyperesthesia	Cystoscopy, hydrodistension	Dietary changes/bladder training Hydrodistension, intravesicle DMSO, oral pentosan polysulfate, low-dose TCAs, antihistamines, hydroxyzine
	Chronic/ recurrent urinary tract infection	Bacterial or fungal infection, often due to anatomic abnormalities, causes irritative voiding symptoms, increases with age and PMP status.	Urinalysis, urine culture, test of cure	Antibiotics ± prophylactic suppression
	Urethral syndrome	Chronic urethral inflammation, infection, or obstruction, similar to IC/BPS	History of dysuria, frequency, urgency, and slow painful urine stream; exam; cystoscopy, urine culture, chlamydia PCR	Hormone replacement therapy in PMP women, biofeedback, DMSO, NSAIDs, muscle relaxants, and alpha antagonists may be useful.

Urethral diverticulum	Herniation of the urethral lining; pocket may become infected/inflamed; a rare cause of chronic pain	History of dysuria, dyspareunia, and postvoid dribbling Anterior vaginal wall mass Urinalysis, urine culture, ± cytology, voiding cystourethrography, double-balloon positive-pressure urethrography, ultrasound, MRI, urethroscopy	Antibiotics for infection, surgical excision
Detrusor-sphincter dyssynergia	Urethral sphincter relaxation does not occur in coordination with detrusor activity causing increased bladder pressure and urine retention; often from CNS injury or multiple sclerosis.	Urodynamics, EMG study	Urethral stent, transurethral sphincterotomy, botulinum toxin injection, and catheterization are possible treatments.

(Continued)

Table 32-1 Differential Diagnosis of Chronic Pelvic Pain[a,b] (Continued)

Category	Etiology	Mechanism	Testing/Diagnosis (in Addition to Physical Exam)	Treatment
Musculoskeletal	**Osteoarthritis**	Referred pelvic pain from chronic degenerative loss of cartilage especially at the hip, knee, sacroiliac, and vertebral joints	Musculoskeletal exam, joint x-rays	Weight loss, lifestyle modification, NSAIDs, physical therapy, joint replacement surgery
	Thoracolumbar syndrome	Hypermobility of thoracolumbar junction in patients with lumbar fusion; referred anterior abdominal and lateral hip pain	Musculoskeletal exam, spinal/hip x-rays	Physical therapy, NSAIDs, orthopedic referral may be appropriate.
	Myofascial pain syndrome/ pelvic floor dysfunction/ levator ani, piriformis syndromes	Irritability, spasm, pain of pelvic floor or abdominal muscles Levator ani syndrome includes chronic or recurrent rectal or vaginal pain or dyspareunia. Piriformis syndrome includes sciatic nerve impingement by piriformis muscle spasm or overuse syndrome; buttock, thigh, leg pain; running and biking can exacerbate.	Pain reproduction or trigger point detection on vaginal or rectal exam Rule out lumbar disk herniation (ie, sciatic root impingement), complete neurologic exam, spinal imaging. EMG testing	Heat packs, muscle relaxants, massage, physical therapy, relaxation techniques, trigger point or botulinum toxin injections

Fibromyalgia	Global myofascial pain syndrome due to abnormal pain processing/ signaling	11 of 18 painful diagnostic trigger points	Exercise, physical therapy, warm packs, massage, NSAIDs, biofeedback, relaxation techniques, low-dose SSRIs, muscle relaxants, trigger point injections
Coccydynia	Trauma to the coccyx can cause S1-S4 nerve pain referred to pelvic floor.	Dynamic spine/ coccygeal x-rays, MRI, diagnostic local anesthetic injection	Local anesthetic or steroid injections, NSAIDs, TCAs, physical therapy, rarely coccygectomy
Hernia	Inguinal, obturator, spigelian, umbilical, etc	CT scan	Manual reduction, binders, avoiding increased intra-abdominal pressure, surgical correction
Lumbar vertebral compression fracture	Osteoporosis, trauma, malignancy; lumbar spine fractures	Spinal x-ray, CT or MRI, DEXA scan	Referral for treatment, physical therapy, rehabilitation, lumbar orthotic brace, occupational therapy, pain medication; surgery for neurologic impairment

(Continued)

Table 32-1 Differential Diagnosis of Chronic Pelvic Pain[a,b] *(Continued)*

Category	Etiology	Mechanism	Testing/Diagnosis (in Addition to Physical Exam)	Treatment
Neurologic	**Nerve entrapment**	Surgical injury of ilioinguinal or iliohypogastric nerve can cause neuroma formation. Obturator internus can press on obturator nerve. Mechanical nerve impingement or stretch can lead to neuropathy.	Anatomic correlation and diagnostic nerve block	Transcutaneous neurolysis, myofascial release procedure, local anesthetic injection, or surgical neurectomy if medical therapy fails
	Peripheral neuropathy/ neuritis/ neuralgia	Numerous local and systemic processes that damage peripheral nerves; persistent numbness, burning, tingling pain	Evaluate for systemic disease and infectious causes (eg, herpes zoster).	TCAs, gabapentin, pregabalin, valproate, transcutaneous electrical nerve stimulation
	Abdominal migraine	Neuronal hyperexcitation; paroxysmal abdominal pain ± nausea/vomiting/flushing; usually in children, rare in adults	H&P, family history; rule out other causes; consider neuroimaging.	Sleep, antiemetics, TCAs; refer to neurology.

Psychiatric[c]			
Posttraumatic disorders	Sexual or physical abuse, especially in childhood	History, psychiatric assessment; rule out organic pathology.	Psychotherapy, treat depression, SSRIs, antidepressants
Somatization disorder	Internal psychological conflict and hypersensitivity to pain stimuli	Four different sites of pain plus two GI, one sexual, and one pseudoneurologic symptom (per diagnostic criteria). Rule out organic pathology.	Psychiatry referral, cognitive-behavioral therapy, antidepressants

Abbreviations: AXR, abdominal x-ray; BSO, bilateral salpingo-oophorectomy; CNS, central nervous system; CT, computed tomography; DEXA, dual-energy x-ray absorptiometry; DMSO, dimethyl sulfoxide; EMG, electromyography; FSH, follicle-stimulating hormone; GI, gastrointestinal; GnRH, gonadotropin-releasing hormone; H&P, history and physical examination; IUD, intrauterine device; MRA, magnetic resonance angiography; MRI, magnetic resonance imaging; NSAIDs, nonsteroidal anti-inflammatory drugs; OCPs, oral contraceptive pills; PCR, polymerase chain reaction; PID, pelvic inflammatory disease; PMP, postmenopausal; SSRIs, selective serotonin reuptake inhibitors; STD, sexually transmitted disease; STI, sexually transmitted infection; TCAs, tricyclic antidepressants.

[a]The evaluation of all pelvic pain should begin with a detailed history and physical exam, including a pelvic exam.

[b]This list is not exhaustive but represents the multiple systems and variety of diagnoses in the workup of chronic pelvic pain. General treatments are listed only to indicate possible therapies used for each condition.

[c]Also include a broader psychiatric differential such as bipolar disorders, personality disorders, depression, and substance abuse.

- **Irritable bowel syndrome (IBS)** is a primary or secondary diagnosis in 40% to 60% of patients with CPP. Associated symptoms of IBS include abdominal distention, bloating, fatigue, and headache. Symptoms are sometimes worse before menses. Although IBS is often comorbid with CPP, it is often a diagnosis of exclusion when considering a primary etiology for CPP.
- **Pelvic adhesions** are eventually diagnosed in about 25% of women with CPP, but a causal relationship is debatable. Pain localization, but not intensity, correlates with the presence of isolated adhesions detected during pelviscopy. Adhesiolysis has not been proven to provide significant relief. Treatment should focus on the causes of adhesions.
- **Bladder pain syndrome (BPS)** (previously described as IC) is a clinical diagnosis that is defined by symptoms of suprapubic pain that are exacerbated by bladder filling and are often accompanied by increased urinary urgency or frequency. The BPS occurs in the absence of urinary infection. It frequently coexists with other causes of CPP, such as vulvodynia and irritable bowel syndrome, as well as other systemic pain conditions such as fibromyalgia. This relationship is often cited as supportive of the theory that pain processing is altered in these patients.
  - Diagnosis of IC has been traditionally made by cystoscopy, with findings of glomerulations or Hunner ulcers. These findings likely represent more severe disease and are not specific or sensitive to IC/BPS. Diagnosis can be made based on symptoms alone with cystoscopy deferred for evaluation of other structural pathology or refractory symptoms from first- or second-line therapy.
  - First-line therapy includes patient education, identification and removal of triggers, and bladder training. Second-line treatment includes oral pentosan sulfate (Elmiron), antihistamines, and low-dose tricyclic antidepressants (eg, amitriptyline). Bladder installation of dimethyl sulfoxide or an anesthetic cocktail of lidocaine, heparin, steroids, and sodium bicarbonate can provide pain relief on an intermittent or continuous basis. Cystoscopy under anesthesia with hydrodistention should be considered in cases refractory to first- and second-line treatment or when the diagnosis is not clear.
- **Myofascial pain** is comorbid with 10% to 20% of cases of CPP. Physical therapy is the mainstay of treatment. Selective serotonin reuptake inhibitors and muscle relaxants may be useful adjuncts.
- **Dyspareunia** can be a primary or secondary symptom in CPP. Additionally, the psychological effect of CPP on relationships and sexual function should be addressed in the evaluation and treatment plan (see chapter 36).
- **Low back pain** is often a separate treatable problem that can exacerbate CPP.
- **Pelvic congestion syndrome** (symptomatic varicose veins of the pelvis) can be objectively diagnosed by transcervical pelvic venogram. This diagnosis can also be suggested by pelvic ultrasound. Randomized trials show correlation between venogram scores and pain, with improvement after treatment. Treatment options include hormonal therapy (progestins, combined oral contraceptives), pelvic vein embolization, and hysterectomy.

MANAGEMENT OF CHRONIC PELVIC PAIN

Management of CPP depends on the etiology and comorbidities (see Table 32-1). The best outcomes may come from a rehabilitation approach with a consistent provider, personalized multidisciplinary treatment, extensive patient education and counseling, and regular office visits. The physician must be open-minded and supportive but offer realistic and explicit goals for therapy. Tailor treatments to the patient and address the underlying etiology, associated pain syndrome, psychological needs, and physical therapy concerns. There is no strong evidence to support medical versus surgical management. At 1 year, about half of surgical patients report improved pain, whereas the rest report no change or worsening symptoms; similar proportions have been reported with medical treatment.

Medical Therapy

- **Medical therapies** are selected to correct or arrest underlying pathology and to relieve pain symptoms. Analgesics should be dosed on noncontingent schedules with additional breakthrough pain treatment as needed. Acetaminophen is a good first-line analgesic.
- **Nonsteroidal anti-inflammatory drugs** (eg, ibuprofen, aspirin, naproxen) are a mainstay of pain treatment, especially if inflammation is present. Contraindications to nonsteroidal anti-inflammatory drug treatment (failure or peptic ulcer disease) must be excluded. Prescribe medications with adequate dosing and frequency. Higher than usual doses may be required.
- **Hormonal treatment** is frequently used for endometriosis and dysmenorrhea.
  - Continuous **oral contraceptive pills (OCPs)** are the first-line treatment for many causes of pelvic pain, particularly for primary dysmenorrhea and endometriosis.
  - **Levonorgestrel intrauterine device.** Suppression of menses can effectively relieve dysmenorrhea, and approximately 20% of patients with a 52-mg levonorgestrel intrauterine device will have amenorrhea following 1 year of use. Even in the absence of amenorrhea, patients can experience relief of symptoms, particularly if some or all of their CPP is due to a uterine cause such as adenomyosis.
  - There is evidence that oral **medroxyprogesterone acetate** and **norethindrone acetate** help control endometriosis symptoms. Depot medroxyprogesterone acetate 150 mg IM every 3 months is another option.
  - **Selective estrogen receptor modulators**, such as letrozole, have demonstrated potential in improving pelvic pain associated with endometriosis. In combination with progestins, OCPs, or GnRH agonists, selective estrogen receptor modulators have demonstrated reduced pain for patients with endometriosis-related pain that is refractory to other medical or surgical treatments when compared to OCPs or GnRH agonists alone.
  - The **GnRH agonists/antagonists** (eg, goserelin, depot Lupron, elagolix) are additional hormonal options. Like OCPs, they prevent ovulation and may help pain associated with menses. The side effect profile of these medications, which often mimics menopausal symptoms, makes them a less appealing option, particularly for younger patients.
- **Tricyclic antidepressants** (eg, amitriptyline, nortriptyline) are effective neuropathic pain medications; they may act by lowering the pain threshold (see Table 32-1). Tricyclics have also been demonstrated to be one of the most effective treatment agents for IBS.
- **Selective serotonin reuptake inhibitor antidepressants** (eg, fluoxetine, sertraline) have not been shown to work well for pain, but they are useful for treatment of comorbid depression or anxiety disorders that can increase pain perception. Serotonin-norepinephrine reuptake inhibitors (**serotonin-norepinephrine reuptake inhibitor**;

eg, duloxetine, venlafaxine, milnacipran) are effective for depression, anxiety, neuropathic pain, and fibromyalgia.

- **Neuromodulatory agents** (eg, gabapentin, pregabalin) are useful for neuropathic pain. Studies have demonstrated superior improvement in pain with gabapentin or pregabalin compared to amitriptyline. Patients experience greatest improvement in control of visceral pain and vulvodynia. There is no data on long-term efficacy of these medications.

- **Muscle relaxants** (eg, cyclobenzaprine, tizanidine baclofen) are sometimes useful for pelvic floor muscle spasm, particularly at the time of initiation of pelvic floor physical therapy, but they should be used as adjuncts or second-line agents with nonsteroidal drugs, until a course of physical therapy can be completed. Diazepam suppositories have been used as a potent muscle relaxant, but the evidence is limited and mixed regarding its efficacy.

- **Thiamine (Vitamin B$_1$)** 100 mg PO daily, **vitamin E** supplementation, and oral **magnesium** supplementation are possible nutritional approaches to dysmenorrhea, although effectiveness data are limited.

- **Opioid analgesia** with oral tramadol, codeine, oxycodone, and hydrocodone may be indicated. Ideally, the use of opioids should be avoided because they can cause hyperalgesia and have addictive potential. If they are needed, it should be in the context of short-course treatment. Intravenous medications are rarely indicated for CPP. In the event that long-term opiate use is initiated, combination long- and short-acting opioids can be beneficial. A chronic pain specialist should be involved when initiating or titrating drug therapy. A thorough review of local prescription drug monitoring programs should be conducted while prescribing opioids, and often a pain contract is helpful to establish the expectation with patients that only one doctor will be responsible for prescribing opioids to them.

Surgical Treatment

- **Surgical therapies** are indicated for specific diagnoses or for patients who do not improve with medical treatments.

- Surgical treatment of severe endometriosis or adhesions can reduce pain in some cases. Patients should understand that there is a strong possibility of recurrence and that additional therapies or medication may be required.

- **Laparoscopic uterosacral nerve ablation** has previously been used for dysmenorrhea in patients with endometriosis who desire to maintain fertility, but several controlled clinical trials show that it is ineffective.

- The superior hypogastric plexus is excised with **presacral neurectomy**. There is some evidence showing modest pain reduction for patients with midline pelvic pain due to dysmenorrhea/endometriosis, although clinical benefit has been demonstrated when the procedure is performed concurrently with excision of endometriosis; therefore, the exact source of clinical improvement is difficult to identify. The procedure can lead to complications such as ureteral injury and uncontrolled bleeding as well as constipation and urinary dysfunction; therefore, the postoperative risks and complications are often thought to outweigh the potential benefits.

- **Pudendal nerve release** from Alcock canal by transgluteal or transperineal approach is performed for some patients with pudendal nerve entrapment, although data is limited regarding its efficacy.

- **Hysterectomy** can be performed for patients with evidence of uterine pain (eg, adenomyosis, some cases of endometriosis) who have completed their childbearing and have not responded well to medical management. Sixty percent to 80% of appropriately selected patients report pain improvement; however, thoughtful consideration of whether the patient's pain is uterine in nature is key.

Other Treatment Options

- Neurologic/pain anesthesia therapies are useful for CPP that can be discretely localized or is due to a specific peripheral nerve injury. Local anesthetic (eg, lidocaine) can be injected for **cutaneous nerve or trigger point block**. Longer acting **peripheral nerve blocks** can benefit some patients. **Botulinum toxin** injection can improve unresponsive spasmodic muscular disorders. Referral to an anesthesia pain specialist may be warranted.

- **Physical therapy** by a provider with expertise in pelvic floor disorders can be helpful in both evaluation and treatment of CPP. Stretching, strengthening, hot/cold applications, pelvic floor training, transcutaneous electrical nerve stimulation, and biofeedback can be used.

- **Psychotherapy** is often beneficial for a patient with chronic pain. Psychological disorders can be diagnosed and managed, and cognitive behavioral therapy, psychotherapy, or counseling can benefit almost all CPP patients. If abuse is reported, the patient should be referred for psychological counseling regardless of the degree to which that history contributes to her pain. In some cases, referral for family or relationship counseling may be indicated as well.

- **Alternative/holistic therapies** such as massage, relaxation techniques, and acupuncture may be appropriate adjunctive interventions for many patients and enhance the effectiveness of traditional medical or surgical therapy. These should be discussed with the patient and integrated in her treatment plan early on.

SUGGESTED READINGS

American College of Obstetricians and Gynecologists Committee on Adolescent Health Care. ACOG Committee Opinion No. 760: dysmenorrhea and endometriosis in the adolescent. *Obstet Gynecol.* 2018;132:e249-e258.

American College of Obstetricians and Gynecologists Committee on Practice Bulletins—Gynecology. ACOG Practice Bulletin No. 114: management of endometriosis. *Obstet Gynecol.* 2010;116:223-236. (Reaffirmed 2018)

Hanno PM, Erickson D, Moldwin R, Faraday MM. Diagnosis and treatment of interstitial cystitis/bladder pain syndrome: AUA guideline amendment. *J Urol.* 2015;193(5):1545-1553.

International Pelvic Pain Society. Professional resources. International Pelvic Pain Society Web site. https://www.pelvicpain.org. Accessed February 1, 2019.

Lamvu G. Role of hysterectomy in the treatment of chronic pelvic pain. *Obstet Gynecol.* 2011;117(5):1175-1178.

Lamvu G, Williams R, Zolnoun D, et al. Long-term outcomes after surgical and nonsurgical management of chronic pelvic pain: one year after evaluation in a pelvic pain specialty clinic. *Am J Obstet Gynecol.* 2006;195:591-600.

Valovska AT, ed. *Pelvic Pain Management.* New York, NY: Oxford University Press; 2016.

33

Uterine Leiomyomas and Benign Adnexal Masses

Esther S. Han and Mostafa A. Borahay

Pelvic masses may present with a wide range of symptoms or may be asymptomatic and discovered incidentally. They may be gynecologic or nongynecologic in etiology (Table 33-1) and may be benign or malignant, posing diagnostic challenges in females of all ages. More than 200 000 women undergo surgery for pelvic masses each year in the United States. A careful patient history and physical exam, along with appropriate laboratory and imaging studies, are essential for proper evaluation.

ADNEXAL MASSES

Adnexal masses—masses of the ovary, fallopian tube, or surrounding tissues—are a common finding, and a thorough evaluation is important to differentiate masses that are gynecologic from those that are nongynecologic in nature and to determine the risk of malignancy. The location of the pelvic mass along with the patient's age and associated symptoms can help narrow the differential.

Evaluation and Diagnosis

- When evaluating a patient who presents with an adnexal mass, it is important to identify acute pathology requiring immediate intervention and evaluate for possible malignancy. It is estimated that there is a 5% to 10% lifetime risk for women undergoing surgery for a suspected ovarian neoplasm. Benign ovarian lesions are found in about 1 in 25 asymptomatic women aged 20 to 39 years. The evaluation of any patient should begin with a thorough history, vital signs, and careful physical examination.

- Past medical history should include detailed menstrual history as well as any history of sexually transmitted infections, previous diagnoses of ovarian cysts, ectopic pregnancies, or endometriosis. History of pelvic pain, dysmenorrhea, abnormal uterine bleeding, as well as obstetric and medication history should be gathered. Nongynecologic causes such as gastrointestinal or renal causes of a pelvic mass must also be considered, and the patient's medical and surgical history can provide important clues and guide decision making regarding the appropriate laboratory and imaging workup. Family history that suggests fibroids, endometriosis, or possible hereditary cancer syndromes should be reviewed.

- A comprehensive physical exam should be performed. Lymph nodes should be palpated for lymphadenopathy, and an abdominal exam should be performed to evaluate for masses or ascites.

- **Transvaginal ultrasound** is the imaging modality of choice for evaluation of pelvic mass. A CT scan and magnetic resonance imaging (MRI) may provide additional information depending on the pathology in question. A CT scan is often employed in working up infection or hemorrhage or to look for metastatic disease in the case of malignancy. The MRI can be helpful in further characterization of fibroid uteri.

Table 33-1 Differential Diagnosis of Pelvic Masses

Benign or Malignant	Location	Type of Mass
Gynecologic		
Benign	Uterus	Leiomyoma
		Adenomyosis
		Adenomyoma
		Müllerian anomalies
	Ovary	Functional cysts: follicular, corpus luteum
		Serous and mucinous cystadenoma
		Theca lutein cyst
		Ovarian torsion
		Mature teratoma (dermoid cyst)
		Endometrioma
	Adnexa	Paratubal/paraovarian cyst
		Hydrosalpinx
		Pyosalpinx
		Ectopic pregnancy
		Tubo-ovarian abscess
		Broad ligament mass or cyst
Malignant	Uterus	Endometrial cancer
		Uterine sarcomas
		Cervical cancer
	Ovary	Borderline tumor
		Epithelial ovarian cancer
		Germ cell tumor
		Sex cord stromal tumors
Nongynecologic		
Benign	Gastrointestinal system	Appendicitis
		Appendiceal abscess or mucocele
		Diverticular abscess
	Urinary system	Ureteral diverticulum
		Pelvic kidney
		Bladder diverticulum
	Other	Nerve sheath tumors
		Peritoneal cysts
Malignant		Gastrointestinal cancers
		Urologic cancers
		Metastatic cancers

Paratubal/Paraovarian Cysts

- Benign paratubal and paraovarian cysts are common and can vary in size. Separate from the ovary, these cysts can be found originating from the fallopian tube itself or arising from the broad ligament. These cysts are often found incidentally on imaging or intraoperatively and are commonly asymptomatic. However, they can sometimes become quite enlarged and cause pain.
- On ultrasound, the cysts are benign appearing with smooth, thin walls and are hypoechoic. Rarely, they can experience torsion or hemorrhage. In these cases, echogenic debris may be seen.
- Malignancy in these cysts is rare, but they are evaluated and monitored similar to ovarian cysts. The presence of solid components within the cyst may indicate neoplasm.

Ovarian Masses

- Ovarian masses are often asymptomatic and found on exam or incidentally found on imaging. Cystic ovarian masses can be histologically divided into functional versus neoplastic cysts. However, without a tissue diagnosis, it is often difficult to differentiate between the two. Very large masses may cause vague pain and pressure. Acute onset of severe pain may indicate torsion or rupture.
- Transvaginal ultrasound is the recommended imaging modality for evaluation of ovarian masses. Benign masses have thin, smooth cyst walls without solid components, septations, or internal blood flow. Such simple cysts are usually benign with malignancy rates of less than 1%.

Functional Ovarian Cysts

- **Functional cysts** are not neoplastic and grow in size due to the accumulation of intrafollicular fluids. Cysts may fill with serous fluid prior to ovulation and form a follicular cyst or fill with blood after ovulation to form a corpus luteum cyst. Benign-appearing functional cysts can be expectantly managed. Simple cysts up to 10 cm may be monitored with serial ultrasounds.

Endometriomas

- **Endometriomas** are commonly found in women with endometriosis (see chapter 42). They are smooth-walled ovarian cysts with ectopic endometrial tissue and filled with chocolate-brown fluid. Endometriomas can grow large in size and cause significant pain, mass effect, or torsion. Endometriomas are also associated with small increased risk of ovarian cancer, particularly endometrioid or clear-cell types. On ultrasound, endometriomas are a rounded cyst within the ovary with homogenous, low-level internal echoes.
- Endometriomas should be surgically excised when the large size puts the patient at risk for ovarian torsion. In women who desire fertility preservation, cystectomy should be considered over oophorectomy. Recurrence of endometriomas is common. Simple drainage has a high recurrence rate. Cystectomy has lower recurrence of pain and endometriomas formation when compared with simple drainage and coagulation of the cyst wall.
- Medical management of endometriomas is limited. However, postoperative medical management is recommended to prevent recurrence. Use of hormonal therapy has been shown to reduce recurrence rates and reduce severity and frequency of dysmenorrhea. However, symptoms may return once medical treatments are discontinued.

Ovarian Teratomas

- **Ovarian teratomas** are germ cell neoplasms that may contain components of all three germ layers—the ectoderm, mesoderm, or endoderm—in a disorganized mass, including various tissues such as fat, hair, bone, and teeth. The vast majority of teratomas are benign. Immature teratomas are malignant and mature teratomas are benign with a 1% to 2% risk of malignant transformation. The most common malignancy associated with dermoid cysts, accounting for 80% of malignant transformation, is squamous cell carcinoma arising from the epithelial lining of the cyst.

- Mature teratomas (dermoid cysts) are the most common benign ovarian neoplasm found in adolescents (10%-25%) and make up 50% of pediatric tumors. They are present bilaterally in 10% of cases.

- On ultrasound, teratomas may display one or more characteristic sonographic signs including fat-fluid or hair-fluid levels, evidence of hair or calcifications suggestive of bone or teeth.

- Teratomas are at increased risk for **ovarian torsion** than other ovarian cysts. Although rare, teratomas may also **rupture**, with greater risk of rupture when torsion occurs. Rupture can lead to chemical peritonitis that can cause a severe inflammatory reaction. As a result, many believe that teratomas >5 cm should be removed.

- When a dermoid cyst in a young patient is benign in appearance, ovarian preservation should be attempted and cystectomy performed. There is some concern regarding whether removal of dermoid cysts should be performed laparoscopically given the increased risk of rupture (and possible chemical peritonitis) during the procedure. However, studies have shown that postoperative peritonitis is rare after laparoscopic cystectomy with copious irrigation and the benefits of minimally invasive surgery outweigh these small risks.

Infectious Etiologies

- Signs and symptoms concerning for an infectious etiology include fevers, chills, nausea, vomiting, pelvic or abdominal pain, vaginal bleeding, purulent discharge, or leukocytosis. A thorough evaluation for pelvic inflammatory disease and tubo-ovarian abscess is warranted in these cases (see chapter 27).

- Adnexal infection may also lead to hydrosalpinx/pyosalpinx secondary to chronic inflammation and edema. Hydrosalpinx may also result from mechanical obstruction secondary to adhesive disease or scarring due to endometriosis. Hydrosalpinx may be asymptomatic and may not require intervention. However, in cases of chronic pelvic pain or infertility, surgical management may be required. The degree of surgical management depends on desire for future fertility and degree of damage to the fallopian tube. In patients seeking assisted reproductive therapies, it may be recommended that damaged fallopian tubes be removed to improve in vitro fertilization success rates.

The Unstable Patient

- In patients presenting with sudden onset of severe pain, acute etiologies including ruptured cysts, ovarian torsion, and ruptured ectopic pregnancy must be considered because these may quickly lead to massive hemorrhage and become surgical emergencies. The unstable patient must be identified quickly for efficient surgical intervention. Pelvic ultrasound remains the imaging modality of choice for initial evaluation of the adnexa. Both benign and malignant cysts can rupture or torse, causing acute pain. Ruptured hemorrhagic cysts may continue to bleed and need surgical intervention.

- Patients with tubo-ovarian abscess should receive parenteral antibiotic therapy until afebrile for at least 24 hours before transitioning to oral antibiotics. Inpatient management may also be required for patients with pelvic inflammatory disease not responding to oral antibiotic therapy or patients with severe nausea and vomiting or otherwise unable to tolerate outpatient therapy as well as pregnant patients (see chapter 27).

The Pediatric and Adolescent Population

- Evaluation of this population should include a thorough menstrual history, and sensitivity and confidentiality should be emphasized when inquiring about sexual activity. When imaging is required, transabdominal ultrasound should be used whenever possible, particularly in very young adolescents or those not yet sexually active (see chapter 38).
- Although malignant masses are uncommon, germ cell tumors are the most common ovarian malignancies seen in children and adolescents. Alpha fetoprotein, β-human chorionic gonadotropin, and lactate dehydrogenase should be collected if there is suspicion for germ cell tumor.
- If required, surgical management is similar to adult populations with emphasis on ovarian preservation. The presence of a gynecologic surgeon rather than a pediatric surgeon alone is associated with higher rates of ovarian preservation.

Pregnancy

- The incidence of adnexal mass in pregnancy varies from 0.05% to 2.4% with an average of 0.19% in the general pregnant population. The rate of torsion of adnexal masses in pregnancy is about 10%, more common in the first trimester and most commonly due to corpus luteum cysts. Evaluation is similar to other premenopausal women with adnexal masses.
- Ultrasound is still the preferred imaging modality. If additional imaging is required, MRI is preferred. In the 1% to 2.3% of adnexal masses requiring surgery during pregnancy, laparoscopic surgery is associated with a significantly lower risk of preterm labor than laparotomy (see chapter 23).

UTERINE MASSES

Leiomyoma

- Uterine leiomyomas, also known as myomas or fibroids, represent the most common pelvic tumors in women. Leiomyomas are benign smooth muscle neoplasms that rarely undergo malignant transformation (<0.5%).
- Fibroids have an incidence of 30% to 70% in reproductive age women, increasing with age. One recent study of women in an urban US health plan showed a cumulative incidence of fibroids by age 50 of nearly 70% in white women and >80% in black women.
- The majority of patients with fibroids are asymptomatic; only about 25% of reproductive age women have symptoms. Symptoms may include pelvic pressure, urinary or fecal complaints, reproductive dysfunction, and abnormal uterine bleeding.
- Leiomyomas represent the single most common indication for hysterectomy. There are many medical and surgical treatment options, including minimally invasive options.

Etiology and Pathophysiology

- Leiomyomas result from monoclonal proliferation of uterine smooth muscle cells or less commonly from smooth muscle cells of uterine blood vessels. They can range in size from millimeters to large tumors filling the abdomen and pelvis and reaching the costal margin. Tumors may be solitary or multiple and are classified by location within the uterus. These cells express estrogen synthetase and aromatase and are capable of converting androgens into estrogen.

- A genetic basis for the presence and growth of uterine leiomyomas appears likely. Family history of leiomyomas increases an individual's risk 1.5- to 3.5-fold. It has been suggested that up to 40% of leiomyomas have associated chromosome abnormalities.

- The growth of uterine leiomyomas is related to circulating estrogen exposure. Progesterone may exert an anti-estrogen effect on the growth of leiomyomas. Fibroids are most prominent and demonstrate maximal growth during the reproductive years and tend to regress after menopause. Whenever leiomyomas grow after menopause, malignancy (eg, leiomyosarcoma) must be considered in the differential diagnosis. Leiomyomas commonly grow during pregnancy, most likely due to the enhanced uterine blood supply that accompanies pregnancy and edematous changes in these tumors.

- As leiomyomas grow, they risk diminution of blood supply, which leads to a continuum of degenerative changes, including calcium deposition. Necrosis, cystic changes, and fatty degeneration are manifestations of compromised blood supply secondary to growth or infarction from torsion of a pedunculated leiomyoma.

- Although malignant degeneration of leiomyomas is possible, most leiomyosarcomas are thought to arise de novo. **Leiomyosarcomas** are diagnosed on the basis of counts of 10 or more mitotic figures per 10 high-power fields (HPFs). Those tumors with 5 to 10 mitotic figures per 10 HPFs are referred to as smooth muscle tumors of uncertain malignant potential. Tumors with <5 mitotic figures per 10 HPFs and little cytologic atypia are classified as cellular leiomyomas.

Classification and Types of Fibroids

- The International Federation of Gynecology and Obstetrics classification system for fibroids categorizes fibroids according to their location in the uterus (Table 33-2).

- **Submucosal fibroids** develop from myometrium just deep to the endometrial lining. These can often protrude into the endometrial cavity or, if pedunculated, can even prolapse through the cervical os. The main symptoms of this subgroup of fibroids include heavy or abnormal bleeding, reduced fertility, miscarriages, and preterm labor.

- **Intramural fibroids**, located within the uterine corpus wall, may distort the uterine cavity.

- **Subserosal fibroids** develop below the serosal layer, can be pedunculated, and occasionally extend between folds of the broad ligament. They do not cause abnormal uterine bleeding but more likely contribute to bulk symptoms.

- **Extrauterine fibroids** are leiomyomas that are found outside of the uterus. They are usually the result of hematogenous spread of neoplastic smooth muscle cells from the uterus. Extrauterine fibroids are histologically identical to intrauterine fibroids. Extrauterine locations most commonly include the genitourinary tract, the gut mesentery, and the cardiopulmonary system. Other rarer locations include the spinal cord and blood vessels.

Table 33-2	International Federation of Gynecology and Obstetrics Classification System for Fibroids[a]
Submucosal Fibroids	
Type 0	Pedunculated, intracavitary
Type 1	<50% intramural
Type 2	≥50% intramural
Nonsubmucosal Fibroids	
Type 3	Contacts the endometrium, 100% intramural
Type 4	Intramural
Type 5	Subserosal, ≥50% intramural
Type 6	Subserosal, <50% intramural
Type 7	Subserosal pedunculated
Type 8	Other (eg, cervical, parasitic)

[a]Adapted from Munro MG, Critchley HO, Fraser IS; and FIGO Menstrual Disorders Working Group. The FIGO classification of causes of abnormal uterine bleeding in the reproductive years. *Fertil Steril.* 2011;95(7):2204-2208.e1-3. Copyright © 2011 American Society for Reproductive Medicine. With permission.

Clinical Manifestations and Diagnosis

- Most patients with leiomyomas are asymptomatic. The most commonly experienced symptoms are abnormal uterine bleeding (eg, heavy, prolonged, frequent, or irregular periods), pelvic pain, pressure, and dyspareunia. Symptoms depend on the size and location of the fibroids and can be affected by compromise of blood supply leading to fibroid degeneration.
- Uterine fibroids have a disproportionate effect on black women. They have been shown to have more fibroids, starting at an earlier age, than their white counterparts. They are 2.4 times more likely to undergo hysterectomy and 6.8 times more likely to undergo myomectomy. At the time of hysterectomy, black women have more fibroids, heavier uteri, and more preoperative anemia and pelvic pain. Unsurprisingly, they also have more severe symptoms including heavy bleeding and anemia, and were more likely to report that fibroids interfered with their daily activities, relationships, and work.
- Various radiologic modalities may be useful for the diagnosis and/or characterization of uterine fibroids (Table 33-3).
- **Abnormal uterine bleeding** including excessive or prolonged menstrual bleeding is the most frequently encountered symptom and may be due to vascular alterations in the endometrium as well as structural alterations affecting normal uterine contractility.
- **Bulk symptoms** include pressure on adjacent organs and increased abdominal girth. Pressure on the bladder may provoke urinary frequency. When the leiomyoma is adjacent to the bladder neck and urethra, incontinence or acute urinary retention with overflow incontinence may occur. Compression from larger leiomyomas may cause ureteral obstruction and hydronephrosis as well as venous compression leading to venous thromboembolism. Posterior fibroids may cause constipation, rectal pressure, or tenesmus. Enlarged fibroids may often present with back pain and pain radiating down one or both legs.

Table 33-3 Diagnostic Imaging for Uterine Leiomyomas

Diagnostic Modality	Advantages	Disadvantages
Pelvic sonogram	Useful for detection and evaluation of fibroid growth	Decreased accuracy in localizing fibroids compared to MRI, especially in patients with a large uterus or multiple fibroids Less sensitive and specific than hysteroscopy and infusion sonohysterography
MRI	Superior to other imaging modalities in evaluating the location of the fibroid and its relationship to the myometrium and uterine serosa; best for surgical planning and before uterine artery embolization Diffusion-weighted MRI along with T2-weighted imaging can lead to 92% accuracy in classifying benign and malignant tumors.	Increased cost
Hysterosalpingogram	Evaluates the contour of the uterine cavity and fallopian tube patency	Does not provide the exact location of fibroids; not appropriate for evaluation of subserosal fibroids Less sensitive and specific than hysteroscopy, infusion sonohysterography, and MRI
Sonohysterography	Characterizes the location and amount of distortion caused by submucosal fibroids	Decreased accuracy in localizing fibroids compared to MRI, especially in patients with a large uterus or multiple fibroids

Abbreviation: MRI, magnetic resonance imaging.

- **Chronic pain** including dysmenorrhea, dyspareunia, and noncyclic pelvic pain often occurs. Acute pain may be a consequence of the torsion of the stalk of a pedunculated leiomyoma or the degeneration of a large leiomyoma.
- Submucosal and intramural fibroids are associated with higher rates of spontaneous miscarriage and **infertility/subfertility** due to impaired implantation, tubal function, or sperm transport. Although it has been shown that removal of submucosal fibroids significantly improves fertility outcomes, there is conflicting evidence regarding the effect of intramural myomectomy on future fertility. Subserosal fibroids are not associated with subfertility.
- **Obstetric complications** that are associated with a fibroid uterus include miscarriage, preterm labor and delivery, malpresentation, cesarean delivery, postpartum hemorrhage, and peripartum hysterectomy. Less common adverse outcomes that may be related to fibroids include intrauterine growth restriction, abnormal placentation, first trimester bleeding, preterm premature rupture of membranes, abruption, and labor dystocia.

Treatment for Leiomyomas

Observation

- No standard size of an asymptomatic myomatous uterus has been determined as an absolute indication for treatment. In a patient with a large asymptomatic myomatous uterus in whom dimensions have not increased and malignancy is unlikely, the patient's age, fertility status, and desire to retain the uterus or avoid surgery must be factored into the treatment plan. Physical and radiologic imaging examinations should be performed initially and may be repeated in 6 months to document the size and growth pattern of the fibroids. If growth is stable, the patient may be followed clinically with annual pelvic examination and imaging as indicated.
- It is difficult to distinguish between benign leiomyomas and **leiomyosarcomas**. Symptoms are nearly identical. Some risk factors for sarcoma differ from risk factors for leiomyomas including postmenopausal status, older age, current or history of previous long-term tamoxifen use, history of retinoblastoma, pelvic irradiation, and hereditary leiomyomatosis and renal cell cancer syndrome. In postmenopausal women with uterine growth or symptomatic fibroids bothersome enough to consider hysterectomy, sarcoma should be considered. Patients with concern for malignancy should not be managed with observation.

Medical Therapy

- Nonhormonal medical therapy is aimed at controlling the symptoms of leiomyomas, specifically excessive menstrual flow or pain. Such therapies include tranexamic acid and nonsteroidal anti-inflammatory drugs.
- Hormonal therapy for fibroids includes contraceptive hormones, progestins including intrauterine devices and gonadotropin-releasing agonists or antagonists. New medical therapies are currently under investigation.
  - Combinations of estrogen and progesterone may control bleeding symptoms while preventing leiomyoma growth. There is conflicting evidence regarding the effect of progestational therapy on changes in fibroid or uterine volume with some small studies showing a decrease in leiomyoma size during treatment. The progestin-releasing intrauterine device has demonstrated good control of heavy menstrual bleeding with little or no change in the size of leiomyomas and

lower treatment failure than oral contraceptive pills. Use of mifepristone, an antiprogestin, has been associated with decrease in the size of leiomyomas with slow rate of regrowth following treatment cessation.

- Gonadotropin-releasing hormone analogues (GnRHa) have been used successfully to achieve hypoestrogenism in various estrogen-dependent conditions. Maximal reduction in tumor volume of approximately 50% has been observed with the use of GnRHa over a 3-month course of treatment. The effects of hormonal treatment are transient, and within 6 months after withdrawal of hormonal therapy, leiomyomas return to their pretreatment state.
  - These agents are useful as a conservative therapy in perimenopausal women or as an adjunct to surgical treatment. Longer than 6 months of GnRHa therapy in young patients is neither practical nor desirable because of the possibility of bone loss. Because they mimic menopause, women can have significant vasomotor side effects.
  - Add-back therapy with concomitant use of low-dose hormone can be used to minimize the adverse effects of GnRHa. Add-back therapy can attenuate the reduction in leiomyoma volume and bleeding, however.
  - Adjunctive presurgical therapy with a 3- to 6-month course of GnRHa can reduce tumor size. Thus, use prior to scheduled hysterectomy may increase the likelihood of success of minimally invasive approach. Additionally, by inducing amenorrhea, GnRHa therapy enables a patient to improve her preoperative hemoglobin levels. However, its preoperative use is associated with obscuring of surgical planes between fibroids and normal myometrium, which may make myomectomy more difficult.
- Aromatase inhibitors have been shown to reduce the volume of fibroids without leading to the side effects caused by systemic hormonal therapy.
- New medical therapies are currently under development. Selective progesterone receptor modulators (SPRM) reduce the progesterone effect on leiomyoma growth and reduce menstrual bleeding with fewer side effects than GnRHas. Ulipristal acetate, a selective progesterone receptor modulator currently being studied in the United States, is approved for repeated intermittent use in Europe, Asia, and Canada.

Surgical Therapy

Myomectomy

- Myomectomy, or surgical excision of the fibroid tissue, is the only surgical option that is available when future childbearing is desired. The location and size of the myoma(s), along with the expertise of the surgeon dictate the approach to myomectomy. Subserosal or intramural fibroids may be resected abdominally or laparoscopically, with or without robotic assistance. Submucosal myomectomy can be performed hysteroscopically. Minimally invasive techniques are preferred whenever appropriate.
- Complications following myomectomy include substantial blood loss, ileus, and pain. Postoperative fever is common on postop day 1. The risk of postoperative adhesive disease following abdominal myomectomy is estimated at 25% to as high as 90%. A laparoscopic approach with the use of an adhesion barrier at the time of surgery may reduce this risk by half. The recurrence risk of leiomyomas is roughly 30% following myomectomy.

- Various interventions have been proven effective in reducing blood loss when compared with placebo during myomectomy. Treatments include misoprostol, vasopressin, bupivacaine plus epinephrine, IV tranexamic acid, gelatin-thrombin matrix, and paracervical tourniquets.
- For patients wishing to conceive, a delay of 3 to 6 months after surgery is advised before attempting pregnancy. The most common obstetric complication following myomectomy includes uterine rupture, abnormal placentation, and preterm delivery. The preferred delivery method after myomectomy with extensive uterine reconstruction is cesarean delivery due to an increased risk of uterine rupture with labor.

Hysterectomy

- Removal of the uterus is the definitive procedure for treatment of symptomatic leiomyomas. Hysterectomy can be performed abdominally, vaginally, and laparoscopically, with or without robotic assistance. However, minimally invasive approaches should be used whenever possible.
- Similar to myomectomy, the method of approach is dictated by the size of the uterus and fibroids, location of fibroids, mobility and ability to safely access vasculature, patient comorbidities, ability to tolerate pneumoperitoneum and Trendelenburg positioning, and surgeon expertise.

Uterine Artery Embolization

- Uterine artery embolization (UAE) decreases the blood supply to the uterus and ultimately causes ischemic necrosis of leiomyomas. The procedure is performed by interventional radiologists and usually involves catheterization of the femoral or radial artery to gain access to the uterine arteries. Under fluoroscopic guidance, the uterine arteries are occluded with one of various available substances.
- The benefits of UAE include short operating and recovery time, use of local anesthesia, and minimal blood loss. Risks of the procedure include infection (4%), complications of angiography (3%), and uterine ischemia or nontarget embolization. Premature ovarian failure secondary to compromise of the ovarian circulation has been reported. Patients typically experience cramping for the first 12 to 18 hours after the procedure. Postembolization syndrome (fever, nausea, vomiting, and severe abdominal pain) has been observed in approximately 30% of patients.
- Outcomes of UAE include a 40% to 60% reduction in uterine size and decreased menstrual bleeding with high rates of patient satisfaction. Patients have significantly less postoperative pain and return to work sooner compared to those undergoing hysterectomy. However, they have increased rates of minor complications. Long-term outcomes may be inferior to myomectomy and hysterectomy, with the rate of reoperation in patients undergoing UAE as high as 30%. Reoperation rate is age dependent, with higher likelihood of success in women older than age 40 years.
- Studies of the impact on postprocedure fertility have suffered from many limitations. Previous studies suggested higher rates of pregnancy complications including miscarriage and postpartum hemorrhage. However, more recent studies have shown comparable pregnancy and preterm delivery rates to the general population with rates of miscarriage that were comparable to patients with untreated fibroids. A 2014 Cochrane review shows low-quality evidence suggesting improved fertility outcomes with myomectomy compared with UAE. The effect of UAE on pregnancy remains understudied and the American College of Obstetricians and Gynecologists advises that it be used with caution in women desiring future pregnancy.

Magnetic Resonance Imaging–Guided Focused Ultrasound Surgery

- With MRI-guided focused ultrasound surgery, fibroid tissue is heated and destroyed using targeted ultrasonic energy passing through the anterior abdominal wall. This procedure is performed with MRI thermal mapping and conducted over several outpatient visits. The MRI-guided focused ultrasound surgery is not appropriate for pedunculated myomas or those adjacent to the bowel or bladder. Although the procedure is currently US Food and Drug Administration approved for premenopausal women who do not desire future fertility, outcome data beyond 24 months is lacking. Potential side effects include skin or nerve burns.

Radiofrequency Ablation

- Radiofrequency ablation technology is currently under investigation for outpatient, minimally invasive fibroid ablation therapy. Transcervical and laparoscopic, ultrasound-guided radiofrequency ablation approaches have shown safety and efficacy in clinical trials.

Congenital Anomalies

- **Hematocolpos/hematometra**: In the adolescent patient, cyclic pain with or without amenorrhea may indicate müllerian anomaly or imperforate hymen and resulting outflow obstruction. When outflow obstruction exists, a mass may form as the result of trapped menstrual blood causing hematocolpos or hematometra of cavitated noncommunicating uterine horn (see chapter 38).

SUGGESTED READINGS

American College of Obstetricians and Gynecologists Committee on Practice Bulletins—Gynecology. ACOG Practice Bulletin No. 96: alternatives to hysterectomy in the management of leiomyomas. *Obstet Gynecol*. 2008;112:387-400. (Reaffirmed 2019)

American College of Obstetricians and Gynecologists Committee on Practice Bulletins—Gynecology. ACOG Practice Bulletin No. 174: evaluation and management of adnexal masses. *Obstet Gynecol*. 2016;128:e210-e226.

Bast RC Jr, Skates S, Lokshin A, Moore RG. Differential diagnosis of a pelvic mass: improved algorithms and novel biomarkers. *Int J Gynecol Cancer*. 2012;22(suppl 1):S5-S8.

Eskander RN, Bristow RE, Saenz NC, Saenz CC. A retrospective review of the effect of surgeon specialty on the management of 190 benign and malignant pediatric and adolescent adnexal masses. *J Pediatr Adolesc Gynecol*. 2011;24:282-285.

Fuldeore MJ, Soliman AM. Patient-reported prevalence and symptomatic burden of uterine fibroids among women in the United States: findings from a cross-sectional survey analysis. *Int J Womens Health*. 2017;9:403-411.

Gupta JK, Sinha A, Lumsden MA, Hickey M. Uterine artery embolization for symptomatic uterine fibroids. *Cochrane Database Syst Rev*. 2014;(12):CD005073.

Kongnyun E, Wiysonge C. Interventions to reduce haemorrhage during myomectomy for fibroids. *Cochrane Database Syst Rev*. 2011;(11):CD005355.

Stewart EA, Nicholson WK, Bradley L, Borah BJ. The burden of uterine fibroids for African American women: results of a national survey. *J Womens Health (Larchmt)*. 2013;22(10):807-816.

Templeman C, Fallat M, Blinchevsky A, Hertweck S. Noninflammatory ovarian masses in girls and young women. *Obstet Gynecol*. 2000;96:229-233.

34 Breast Diseases

Harold Wu and Shriddha Nayak

Breast cancer is a common and devastating health issue for many women. One in 8 women will develop breast cancer in her lifetime. Benign breast disease can be difficult to differentiate from malignant breast disease, and it is important for a gynecologist be able to evaluate and treat breast disease.

ANATOMY

- The **borders of the adult breast** are the second and sixth ribs in the vertical axis and the sternal edge and midaxillary line in the horizontal axis (Figure 34-1). A small portion of breast tissue also projects into the axilla, forming the axillary tail of Spence.
- The breast is composed of **three major tissues**: skin, subcutaneous tissue, and breast tissue. The breast tissue, in turn, consists of parenchyma and stroma. The parenchyma is divided into 15 to 20 segments that converge at the nipple in a radial arrangement. There are between 5 and 10 collecting ducts that open into the nipple. Each duct gives rise to buds that form 15 to 20 lobules, and each lobule consists of 10 to 100 alveoli, which constitute the gland.
- The breast is enveloped by fascial tissue. The superficial pectoral fascia envelops the breast and is continuous with the superficial abdominal fascia of Camper. The undersurface of the breast lies on the deep pectoral fascia, covering the pectoralis major and serratus anterior muscles. Connecting the two fascial layers are fibrous bands (Cooper suspensory ligaments) that are the natural support of the breast.
- The **principal blood supply** to the breast is the **internal mammary artery**, constituting two-thirds of the total blood supply. The additional third, which supplies primarily the upper outer quadrant, is provided by the **lateral thoracic artery**. Nearly all of the lymphatic drainage of the breast is to the axillary nodes. The internal mammary nodes also receive drainage from all quadrants of the breast and are an unusual, but potential, site of metastasis.
- The majority of abnormalities in the breast that result in biopsy are due to benign breast disease. Benign abnormalities can result in pain, a mass, calcifications, and nipple discharge. Similar findings can be present in malignant disease.
- For the purposes of delineating metastatic progression, the **axillary lymph nodes** are categorized into levels. Level I lymph nodes lie lateral to the outer border of the pectoralis minor muscle, level II nodes lie behind the pectoralis minor muscle, and level III nodes are located medial to the medial border of the pectoralis minor muscle.

BREAST EXAM

- Screening guidelines regarding the clinical breast examination vary depending on organization (see chapter 26). The American College of Obstetricians and Gynecologists recommends clinical breast examination be part of the routine gynecologic examination every 1 to 3 years for women aged 25 to 39 years and

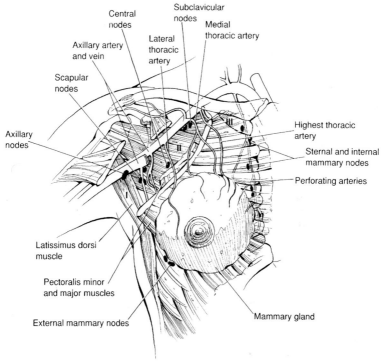

Figure 34-1. Anatomy of the breast. Roman numerals (I, II, III) indicate axillary lymph node levels. Reprinted with permission from Kelley JL, Sukumvanich P. Diseases of the breast. In: Jones HW III, Rock JA, eds. *TeLinde's Operative Gynecology*. 11th ed. Philadelphia, PA: Wolters Kluwer; 2015:1007.

annually for women 40 years and older. It should also be performed if there are any breast-related complaints. The examination consists of the following:

- **Inspection and palpation** of the breasts in the supine and sitting positions, with hands above the head and then on the hips. The supine position flattens the breast tissue against the chest, allowing for a more thorough exam.
- **Observation** of the contour, symmetry, and vascular pattern of the breasts for signs of skin retraction, edema, or erythema in each of the previously mentioned positions
- **Systematic palpation** of each breast, the axilla, and supraclavicular areas in a circular motion using light, medium, and deep pressures. Use the pads of the three middle fingers to palpate for masses. A vertical strip pattern appears more thorough than concentric circles. To ensure that all breast tissue is examined, cover a rectangular area bordered superiorly by the clavicle, laterally by the mid-axillary line, and inferiorly by the bra line.
- Evaluation for nipple discharge, crusting, or ulceration
- For the anatomic location and description of tumors or disease, the surface of the breast is divided into four quadrants and the numbers of the face of a clock are used as reference points. A finding may be described as "a hard mass palpated in

the upper inner quadrant of the right breast at the 2 o'clock position, approximately 2 cm from the nipple."

- The clinical utility of **breast self-examination** is controversial. **Breast self-awareness** is a woman's awareness of the normal appearance and feel of her breasts and may or may not include breast self-examination. She is encouraged to discuss any changes in her breasts with her health care provider.

COMMON BREAST DISORDERS AND COMPLAINTS

Approximately 16% of women ages 40 to 69 years seek a physician's advice for breast-related complaints in any 10-year period, with the most common complaint being a breast lump (40%). Other common complaints include nipple discharge and breast pain. Breast cancer will account for only 10% of these complaints, and the failure to diagnose breast cancer is high on the list of malpractice claims in the United States. The most common reasons for breast-related lawsuits against obstetrician-gynecologists are "physical findings failed to impress" and "failure to refer to the specialist for biopsy." Physicians should be prepared to evaluate, address, and inform patients regarding their concerns.

Mastalgia

- Breast pain may be cyclic or noncyclic. **Cyclic breast pain** is maximal premenstrually and is relieved with the onset of menses. It can be either unilateral or bilateral and may be associated with fibrocystic changes. Fibrocystic pain is primarily localized to the subareolar or upper outer regions of the breast. This pain is likely due to stromal edema, ductal dilation, and some degree of inflammation. Microcysts in fibrocystic disease can progress to form palpable macrocysts.
- **Noncyclic pain** can have various causes, including hormonal fluctuations, firm adenomas, duct ectasia, and macrocysts. It may also arise from musculoskeletal structures, such as soreness in the pectoral muscles from exertion or trauma, stretching of the Cooper ligaments, or costochondritis. Mastitis and hidradenitis suppurativa may present with breast pain. With most noncyclic breast pain, no definite cause is determined. Carcinoma can present with breast pain (<10%), but this is uncommon. The evaluation of breast pain includes a careful history and physical as well as mammography for women over age 35 years. The primary value of mammography is to provide reassurance. Patients with no dominant mass can be reassured.
- In most cases, mastalgia resolves spontaneously, although sometimes only after months or years. Restriction of methylxanthine-containing substances (eg, coffee, tea) has not been shown to be superior to placebo, but some patients may note relief. Pain from a macrocyst may be relieved with aspiration. Symptomatic relief may be achieved with a supportive brassiere, acetaminophen, or a nonsteroidal anti-inflammatory drug. Finally, cyclic pain may be partially relieved with oral contraceptives, thiazide diuretic, danazol, or tamoxifen.

Nipple Discharge

- Nipple discharge is a common complaint and finding on examination of the breast. Nipple discharge is usually benign (95% of cases). The causes of discharge range from physiologic to endocrine related to pathologic. See Figure 34-2 for an algorithm for evaluation of nipple discharge.

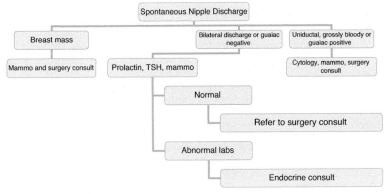

Figure 34-2. Algorithm for evaluation of nipple discharge. TSH, thyroid stimulating hormone.

- **Physiologic secretion** from the nipple during examination or nipple stimulation is a common occurrence. As many as 50% to 80% of women in their reproductive years can express one or more drops of fluid. This benign discharge is usually non-spontaneous, bilateral, and serous in character. If the remainder of the breast exam is normal, reassurance is sufficient, and no further workup is necessary.

- **Galactorrhea** is milk production unrelated to nursing or pregnancy and is typically a bilateral, multiductal discharge. Several endocrine abnormalities give rise to galactor-rhea, such as dopamine inhibitors, hypothalamic/pituitary disease, hypothyroidism, postthoracotomy syndrome, and chronic renal failure. Chronic breast stimulation or exogenous estrogen via oral contraceptive pills may cause galactorrhea. One-third of cases are idiopathic. Evaluation includes a careful history reviewing medications and recent trauma/stimulation of the breast and physical exam. Questioning includes symptoms of amenorrhea, hypothyroid disease, visual field changes, or new-onset headaches, which may suggest the underlying cause of the galactorrhea. Further evaluation includes a prolactin level, thyroid function tests, and brain magnetic reso-nance imaging (MRI) if the prolactin level is elevated. Prolactin levels may be falsely elevated after meals, after breast examination, or based on diurnal variation.

- **Pathologic discharge** is typically unilateral and spontaneous. It may be greenish gray, serous, or bloody. Causes of pathologic discharge are carcinoma, intraductal papilloma (straw colored), duct ectasia, and fibrocystic changes. Only 5% of patho-logic discharge is caused by carcinoma. A physical exam should attempt to identify the area of the breast and the specific duct from which the discharge is expressed. Skin lesions or an associated mass may be identified. If the fluid is not grossly bloody, guaiac testing may be performed to identify subtle bloody fluid. If grossly bloody or guaiac positive, cytology is performed; otherwise, the sensitivity of cytol-ogy is very low for malignancy. In addition, imaging with bilateral mammography is required. If the patient is younger than 35 years, ultrasound may also be used.

Breast Infections

- **Puerperal mastitis** is an acute cellulitis of the breast in a lactating woman. This topic is discussed in detail in chapter 24.

- **Nonpuerperal mastitis** is an uncommon, subareolar infection. In contrast to puerperal mastitis, nonpuerperal mastitis is usually a polymicrobial infection and the woman is generally not systemically ill. Antibiotic coverage typically includes clindamycin or metronidazole in addition to a β-lactam antibiotic. All breast inflammation must raise concern for inflammatory breast cancer, and the threshold for performing a skin biopsy should be low, particularly in the elderly population. Failure to respond to antibiotic treatment should prompt biopsy in any patient. Finally, the patient should be up-to-date with mammography screening.

Breast Mass

- Evaluation of a palpable breast mass requires a careful personal history, family history, physical examination, and radiographic examination. A breast mass reported by the patient should undergo the same evaluation, even if it fails to be appreciated on physical exam.
- In general, breast tissue can be lumpy and irregular. The following are **characteristics concerning for cancerous lesions**: single, hard, immobile, irregular margins, and >2 cm. In the majority of cases, cancerous masses are painless, but 10% of patients with cancer present with some symptoms of breast discomfort. Symptoms that may be associated with breast cancer include nipple discharge, nipple rash or ulceration, diffuse erythema of the breast, adenopathy, or symptoms associated with metastatic disease.
- Diagnostic mammography is recommended in the evaluation of any woman over age 35 years with a palpable breast mass. Findings suspicious for cancer on mammography include increased density, irregular margins, spiculation, or an accompanying cluster of microcalcifications (Figure 34-3).
- In women under age 35 years, ultrasonography may be used to distinguish a simple cyst from a more worrisome complex cyst, solid mass, or tumor.
- Fine-needle aspiration, core-needle biopsy, or excisional biopsy can be used for ultimate tissue diagnosis of the palpable mass. Bloody fluid yielded on aspiration or persistence of a mass after aspiration should prompt excisional biopsy or surgical consultation.
- The combination of physical examination, mammography, and fine-needle aspiration biopsy is referred to as triple diagnosis. Fewer than 1% of breast cancers are missed using this diagnostic approach.
- Benign breast masses include fibroadenomas, breast cysts, or fat necrosis.
  - **Fibroadenoma** is the most common mass lesion found in women younger than 25 years of age. Growth is gradual, and occasional cystic tenderness may be present. If the lesion is palpable, increasing in size, or psychologically disturbing, core or excisional biopsy should be considered. Conservative treatment may be appropriate for small lesions that are not palpable and have been identified as fibroadenomas. Carcinoma within a fibroadenoma is a rare occurrence. A rare malignant tumor that can be confused with fibroadenoma is **cystosarcoma phyllodes**, which is treated by wide resection with negative margins. Local recurrence is uncommon, and distant metastasis is very rare.
  - **Breast cysts** can be found in premenopausal or postmenopausal women. Physical examination cannot distinguish cysts from solid masses. Ultrasonography and cyst aspiration are diagnostic. Simple cysts have a thin wall with no internal echoes and are benign. In these cases, no further therapy is required.

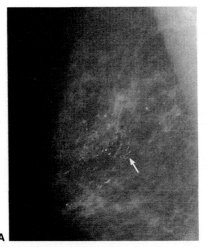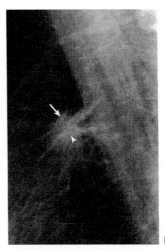

A **B**

Figure 34-3. **A,** A 53-year-old woman with bloody discharge from the nipple. Mediolateral view of the right breast demonstrates casting calcifications involving a large part of the breast extending to the nipple. The calcifications are nonuniform, irregular, and branched (arrow), and they form a dot-dash linear pattern. They are aligned with the ductal system. **B,** A 60-year-old woman with a palpable mass and no other pertinent history. Mediolateral view of the right breast reveals a spiculated mass (arrow) with architectural distortion. Within the center of the mass, irregular (pleomorphic) microcalcifications are present (arrowhead). The diagnosis is carcinoma, largely DCIS, of comedo type (A), and invasive ductal carcinoma, not otherwise specified (B). Reprinted with permission from Pope TL Jr. *Aunt Minnie's Atlas and Imaging Specific Diagnosis.* 2nd ed. Philadelphia, PA: Lippincott Williams & Wilkins; 2003:329.

Complex cysts have a thickened wall or internal septation and are considered suspicious. Complex cysts generally undergo some form of biopsy. If a cyst does not resolve with aspiration, yields a bloody aspirate, recurs within 6 weeks, or is complex on ultrasound evaluation, surgical consultation should be obtained.

• **Fat necrosis** is frequently associated with breast trauma resulting in a breast mass. It can occur after breast biopsy, infection, duct ectasia, reduction mammoplasty, lumpectomy, and radiotherapy for breast carcinoma. Fat necrosis is most common in the subareolar region. This process can be difficult to distinguish from breast cancer on both physical examination and mammography. The lesion needs to be evaluated like any other palpable breast lesion. Only a benign histologic appearance affords reassurance.

BREAST CANCER

Breast cancer is the most common cancer affecting women in the United States and second only to lung cancer in cancer mortality for women. Median age of diagnosis and of death are 61 and 69 years, respectively. Primarily due to improved screening, the prevalence of breast cancer has doubled in the past 50 years. The lifetime risk of breast cancer for a woman is 12.7% (about 1 in 8).

Risk Factors

- The most commonly used model to determine breast cancer risk is the **Gail model**. The number of first-degree relatives with breast cancer, age at menarche, age at first live birth, number of breast biopsies, and presence of atypical hyperplasia on a breast biopsy are its components. Its accuracy is limited because it omits a detailed family history of breast and ovarian cancers and underestimates the risk in African American women and overestimates the risk in Asian American women. *This model should not be used in women who have a personal history of breast cancer or women who are known gene mutation carriers.*

- **Age** is the primary risk factor for breast cancer. Approximately 95% of breast cancers occur in women over 40 years of age.

- **Family history and genetic predisposition.** Family history confers an increased risk for breast cancer, specifically with a history of premenopausal breast cancer in a first-degree relative, male breast cancer, bilateral breast cancer, or a combination of breast and ovarian cancers within a family. Chapter 53 discusses the syndromes below in further detail.
  - *BRCA1* and *BRCA2* are tumor suppressor genes with autosomal dominant inheritance. Inheriting *BRCA1* or *BRCA2* confers a 40% to 70% lifetime risk of breast cancer; yet, these cases account for <10% of all diagnoses. In addition, *BRCA1* confers a 40% risk of ovarian cancer and *BRCA2* a 20% risk for ovarian cancer. Both mutations are more common in the Ashkenazi Jewish population (1 in 40). Women with these mutations have a 35% to 43% chance of developing a second primary breast cancer within the first 10 years of her first breast cancer diagnosis and are at increased risk of pancreatic cancer (see chapter 53).
  - Patients with Li-Fraumeni syndrome, Cowden syndrome (multiple hamartoma syndrome), and Peutz-Jeghers syndrome are also at increased risk of developing breast cancer (see chapter 53).

- **Hormone exposure.** Early menarche (<12 y), late natural menopause (>55 y), older age at first full-term pregnancy, and fewer pregnancies increase a woman's risk of developing breast cancer. Breastfeeding is associated with a lower risk of breast cancer. In addition, moderate alcohol use, which is related to an increase in estrogen, carries a higher risk. Finally, the role of exogenous estrogen use in the development of breast cancer remains controversial. Long-term oral contraceptive use (>10 y) and current hormone therapy use are associated with a nonsignificant increased risk of breast cancer.

- **Diet and lifestyle.** Significant differences in the incidence of breast cancer in different geographic and cultural areas have long raised the suspicion of dietary risk factors. High-fat diets have been implicated, but data are insufficient to support firm dietary advice for reduction in breast cancer risk. Lifestyle activities with protective effects include physical activity and weight control.

- **Personal history.** Women with a history of breast cancer are at a 0.5% to 1% risk per year of developing cancer in the contralateral breast in addition to the risk of recurrence in the treated breast. The majority of recurrences occur within the first 5 years after diagnosis. A personal history of a benign breast biopsy or atypical hyperplasia also yields an increased risk, as does prior radiation therapy (RT) to the chest wall.

Screening and Diagnosis

The main screening modalities include clinical breast exam, breast self-exam, and screening mammography (Table 34-1). The clinical breast exam is best for detecting

Table 34-1 Breast Cancer Screening Techniques and Guidelines

	Application	Sensitivity/Efficacy	Limitations	Guidelines[a]
Mammography	Detects microcalcifications, abnormal shadowing, or soft tissue distortion	Sensitivity: 74%-95% Specificity: 89%-99% Sensitivity is decreased in women under age 50 y and in women with dense breasts. Reduces risk of cancer-related mortality by 16%-35%	Less sensitive for faster growing tumors (young women) Breast density Hormone therapy Breast implants	USPSTF: ≥50-74, every 2 y ACOG: Offer to initiate at age 40 y; recommend no later than age 50 y, every 1-2 y. ACS: Offer at ages 40-45 y; recommend for ages 45-54 y, annually; recommend for age 55 y and older, every 1-2 y.
Clinical breast exam	Inspection and palpation in the supine and sitting positions, including axillary and supraclavicular lymph nodes as well as nipple and areola Recommended 6-10 min	Sensitivity 54% Specificity 94% Detects approximately 5% of cancers missed by mammography Most studies show efficiency in conjunction with mammography—likely that each contributes.	Examiner dependent Less specificity than mammography—higher rate of biopsy for benign disease Limited in obese women	USPSTF: insufficient evidence to recommend for or against ACOG: Offer at ages 25-39 y, every 1-3 y then annually for women age 40 y and older ACS: does not recommend
Breast self-examination	Monthly exams, during approximately 10th day of cycle	Sensitivity 20%-30% Very few randomized trials Failed to show benefit in rate of diagnosis, cancer death, or tumor size	Examiner dependent Higher rate of biopsy for benign disease Studies limited	USPSTF: does not support teaching self-breast exams ACS: not recommended ACOG: not recommended; supports self-breast awareness

Abbreviations: ACOG, American College of Obstetricians and Gynecologists; ACS, American Cancer Society; USPSTF, US Preventive Services Task Force.
[a]Data from American College of Obstetricians and Gynecologists Committee on Practice Bulletins—Gynecology. ACOG Practice Bulletin No. 179: breast cancer risk assessment and screening in average-risk women. *Obstet Gynecol.* 2017;130(1):e1-e16.

tumors greater than 2 cm in size. The National Breast and Cervical Cancer Early Detection Program found that clinical breast exams detect approximately 5% of cancers that are not visible on mammography. Diagnostic modalities include diagnostic mammography and breast biopsy (including fine needle, core, and excisional). Additional imaging diagnostic modalities include ultrasound and MRI.

Mammography

- Mammography remains the primary screening modality for breast cancer. Breast cancers detected by mammography tend to be smaller and have more favorable histologic and biologic features. Limitations to mammography include patient age, rate of tumor growth, density of breast tissue, use of hormone replacement therapy, and breast implants. Approximately 5% to 15% of cancers are not apparent on mammography, and all palpable lesions require biopsy.
- **Screening mammography** is for women with no signs or symptoms of breast disease and consists of bilateral two-view images. Mammography can potentially detect lesions as small as 1 mm. Digital mammography is more effective than film mammography, especially for women younger than 60 years or with dense breasts.
- **Diagnostic mammography** presents various views (eg, spot compression, magnification) and localization techniques and is usually used after the discovery of an abnormal finding on clinical exam, self-exam, or screening mammography. Mammography is an essential part of the evaluation of a patient with clinically evident breast cancer. In this situation, mammography is useful for evaluating other areas of the breast as well as the contralateral breast.

Abnormal Mammogram

- Suspicious radiologic findings require surgical consultation and consideration of breast biopsy, even with an unremarkable physical examination.
- Radiologic findings of concern on mammography
  - Soft tissue density, especially if borders are not well defined
  - Clustered microcalcifications in one area
  - Calcification within or closely associated with a soft tissue density
  - Asymmetric density or parenchymal distortion
  - New abnormality compared with previous mammogram
- When a woman's screening mammography is ambiguous, diagnostic mammography should be performed with possible radiographically directed biopsy. Biopsy techniques for radiographically identified nonpalpable lesions include needle localization, excisional biopsy, and stereotactic core biopsy. If the mammographic studies are inconclusive, a short-term follow-up study at 6 months can be considered (Table 34-2).

Alternate Screening Modalities

- **Ultrasound.** Although ultrasound is not a substitute for mammography, it has become a common tool in the evaluation of breast lesions. Ultrasound is particularly useful in differentiating cystic from solid lesions and is most commonly used in evaluating lesions in young women, especially those younger than age 40 years. It can also be used as an adjunctive screening tool in women with dense or cystic breasts or those with breast implants. Suspicious features include solid masses with ill-defined borders, acoustic shadowing, or complex cystic lesions. Ultrasound guidance also assists in diagnostic procedures, including biopsy or fine-needle aspiration.

Table 34-2 American College of Radiology Breast Imaging Reporting and Data System (BI-RADS) Mammography Assessment Categories[a]

Category	Assessment	Definition	Likelihood of Breast Cancer
1	Negative	Breasts appear normal	Essentially 0%
2	Benign finding(s)	A negative mammogram result, but the interpreter wishes to describe a finding	Essentially 0%
3	Probably benign finding—short interval follow-up suggested	Lesion with a high probability of being benign	>0 but ≤2%
0	Need additional imaging evaluation and/ or previous mammograms for comparison	Lesion noted—additional imaging is needed; used almost always in a screening situation	NA
4	Suspicious abnormality— biopsy should be considered	A lesion is noted for which the radiologist has sufficient concern to recommend biopsy.	>2 but ≤95%
5	Highly suggestive of malignancy— appropriate action should be taken	A lesion is noted that has a high probability of being cancer.	>95%

Abbreviation: NA, not applicable.
[a]Reprinted with permission from Kerlikowske K, Smith-Bindman R, Ljung BM, et al. Evaluation of abnormal mammography results and palpable breast abnormalities. *Ann Intern Med* 2003;139:274-284, with permission; and data from American College of Obstetricians and Gynecologists Committee on Practice Bulletins—Gynecology. ACOG Practice Bulletin No. 164: diagnosis and management of benign breast disorders. *Obstet Gynecol* 2016;127:e141-e56. (Reaffirmed 2018)

- **MRI.** Studies have shown MRI to be more sensitive but less specific and more expensive than mammography in the detection of breast cancers. An MRI screening is recommended for women with a greater than 20% lifetime risk of developing breast cancer. These include women with known *BRCA1* or *BRCA2* mutations, first-degree relatives of those with *BRCA1* or *BRCA2* mutations who have not undergone genetic testing, history of RT to the chest between ages 10 and 30 years and women with certain genetic syndromes (including Li-Fraumeni and Cowden syndrome) or a first-degree relative with one of those syndromes.
  - An MRI screening is not recommended for women at average risk of developing breast cancer.

Premalignant Breast Lesions

- **Atypical hyperplasia** is a proliferative lesion of the breast that possesses some of the features of carcinoma in situ and should be considered premalignant. It carries a 4- to 5-fold increased risk of breast cancer, usually in the ipsilateral breast. Complete excision is recommended. Proliferative lesions, such as sclerosing adenosis, ductal epithelium hyperplasia, and intraductal papillomas, also carry an increased risk of cancer.

- **Lobular carcinoma in situ (LCIS)**, sometimes called *lobular neoplasia*, is a nonpalpable, noninvasive lesion arising from the lobules. The LCIS is more common in premenopausal women and is often an incidental finding on biopsy. It is often multicentric and bilateral, and it is considered an indicator lesion or marker that identifies women at increased risk of subsequent invasive cancer. Absolute risk of developing invasive cancer is approximately 1% per year. Management is controversial and includes observation, tamoxifen administration, or prophylactic mastectomy to reduce the risk of developing subsequent breast cancer.

Malignant Breast Lesions

- Breast cancer most commonly arises in the upper outer quadrant of the breast, taking an average of 5 years to become palpable. It arises in the terminal duct-lobular unit of the breast and can be invasive or noninvasive (in situ). The growth pattern is described as comedo or noncomedo (solid, cribriform, micropapillary, and papillary).

- **Ductal carcinoma in situ (DCIS)**, also called *intraductal cancer*, refers to a proliferation of cancer cells within the ducts without invasion through the basement membrane into the surrounding stroma. Histologically, DCIS can be divided into multiple subtypes: solid, micropapillary, cribriform, and comedo. A DCIS can also be graded as low, intermediate, or high. A DCIS is an early, noninfiltrating form of breast cancer with minimal risk of metastasis and an excellent prognosis with surgical therapy alone with or without RT. The goal of treatment of DCIS is to prevent the development of invasive breast cancer. With the increased use of mammography, DCIS is being diagnosed more often.

- **Invasive cancer.** The two most common types of invasive cancers are lobular and ductal. **Infiltrating lobular** carcinoma is a variant associated with microscopic lobular architecture. These carcinomas account for 10% to 15% of invasive breast cancers, are often multifocal, have a higher incidence of bilaterality, and are less evident on mammography. **Infiltrating ductal** carcinoma accounts for 60% to 75% of all tumors. These cancers account for a group of tumors classified by cell type, architecture, and pattern of spread. These include mucinous, tubular, and medullary carcinomas.

Staging and Prognostic Factors

- **The tumor-node-metastasis (TNM) staging system** for breast cancer from the American Joint Committee on Cancer uses tumor size, axillary node status (incorporating sentinel nodes), and metastasis status.
  - Tumor size (T)
    - TX: Cannot be assessed
    - T0: No evidence of primary tumor
    - Tis: Ductal carcinoma *in situ* or Paget's disease of the nipple without invasive carcinoma

- T1: Greatest dimension of tumor is ≤2 cm
  - T1mi: Greatest dimension is ≤1 mm
  - T1a: Greatest dimension is >1 mm but ≤0.5 cm
  - T1b: Greatest dimension is >0.5 cm but ≤1 cm
  - T1c: Greatest dimension is >1 cm but ≤2 cm
- T2: Greatest dimension is >2 cm but ≤5 cm
- T3: Greatest dimension is >5 cm
- T4: Any size tumor that involves the thoracic wall or skin
  - T4a: Extension to the chest wall
  - T4b: Edema (including *peau d'orange*) or ulceration of the skin of the breast or satellite skin
  - T4c: Both T4a and T4b
  - T4d: Inflammatory carcinoma
- Lymph node metastases (N), pathological classification
  - NX: Cannot be assessed (may have been previously removed)
  - N0: No regional lymph node metastasis
  - N1: Involvement of 1–3 axillary lymph nodes
  - N2: Involvement of 4–9 axillary lymph nodes
  - N3: Involvement of 10 or more axillary lymph nodes, spread to infra/supra-clavicular lymph node(s) or internal mammary lymph node(s)
- Distant metastasis (M)
  - MX: Cannot be assessed
  - M0: No distant metastasis
  - M1: Distant metastasis (including metastasis to ipsilateral supraclavicular lymph)
- Expression of **estrogen and progesterone receptors (ER, PR)** in tumor tissue is associated with a better prognosis and can assist in systemic treatment. Other prognostic factors include tumor grade and expression of the human epidermal growth factor receptor 2 (HER2/neu) oncogene.
- *HER2/neu* is a gene encoding transmembrane receptors for growth factors, thus regulating cellular growth and differentiation. Overexpression of this oncogene leads to a more aggressive subtype of breast cancer, which tends to be poorly differentiated and high grade. They have high rates of lymph node involvement and are more resistant to conventional chemotherapy.
- **In 2018, American Joint Committee on Cancer updated the TNM staging system** to also include tumor grade, ER/PR status, HER2 status, and oncotype DX score (a genomic test that analyzes the activity of a group of genes that can influence tumor growth and response to treatment).
- Prognosis varies based on the stage and the spread of the disease (Table 34-3).

Treatment

Early detection is the key to improved survival rates (see Table 34-3). In general, clinical stages I and II, and certain patients with clinical stage III disease (T3N0), are considered early stages of breast cancer. These patients are generally treated with surgery to the breast and regional lymph nodes with or without RT. Systemic therapy may be offered based on primary tumor characteristics, such as hormone and HER2 receptor status, lymph node involvement, and tumor size and grade. Treatment for locally advanced breast cancers includes multimodal therapy.

| Table 34-3 | 5-Year Breast Cancer Relative Survival Rates Based on the SEER Database[a] |

SEER Stage[b]	Relative Survival[c]
Localized	98.8%
Regional	85.5%
Distant	27.4%
Unknown	54.5%

Abbreviation: SEER, Surveillance, Epidemiology, and End Results.
[a]Adapted from Surveillance, Epidemiology, and End Results Program. Cancer stat facts: female breast cancer. Surveillance, Epidemiology, and End Results Program Web site. https://seer.cancer.gov/statfacts/html/breast.html. Accessed June 6, 2019.
[b]Staging definitions: localized = confined to primary site; regional = spread to regional lymph nodes; distant = cancer has metastasized; unknown = unstaged.
[c]Based on women diagnosed with breast cancer between 2008 and 2014.

Surgical or Local Treatment

- **Mastectomy** involves the complete surgical removal of breast tissue. Mastectomy is recommended if the disease is multicentric, invades skin and chest wall, or has inflammatory features, or if negative margins cannot be achieved with breast preservation. **Radical mastectomy** includes removal of the breast, overlying skin, pectoralis major and minor, and the entire axillary contents. The **modified radical mastectomy** includes removal of the entire breast and underlying fascia of the pectoralis major muscle and levels I and II of the axillary lymph nodes. A **total** or **simple mastectomy** removes the breast with the nipple areolar complex but without lymph nodes. "Skin-sparing" mastectomy provides superior cosmetic results and may be appropriate for patients with DCIS; stages I, II, or III breast cancer; or for prophylactic mastectomy. Nipple-sparing mastectomy is controversial in the treatment of breast cancer. Any type of mastectomy can be performed with or without immediate reconstruction.
- In **breast-conserving therapy** (BCT), a wide local excision or lumpectomy is performed to achieve a 1- to 2-mm negative histologic margin. Adjuvant RT is required. Radiation is delivered to the entire breast with a possible boost dose to the lumpectomy bed. Trials comparing BCT + RT and mastectomy show comparable survival rates.
- Assessing **axillary lymph node status** is important in prognosis, staging, and treatment planning. However, potential complications of axillary dissection include lymphedema (10%-15%), pain, numbness, or weakness of the affected arm.
- Evaluation of the clinically suspicious axillary node can be accomplished with ultrasound plus fine-needle aspiration or core biopsy.
- **Sentinel lymph node biopsy** has evolved into the method of choice for axillary node staging in the clinically negative axilla. The sentinel lymph node is identified using radioactive tracer or dye injected into the periareolar region of the breast. When the isotope and dye are used in combination, the positive predictive value of sentinel node biopsy approaches 100%.
- **Radiation therapy**, although most often administered as part of BCT, can also be used for other indications.

Systemic Therapy

- Systemic therapy given before surgery is termed **neoadjuvant therapy** and is often recommended for patients with locally advanced disease. **Adjuvant therapy**, which is given after surgery, is typically recommended to patients with hormone receptor–positive breast cancer, positive lymph node findings, or other high-risk characteristics.

- **Hormonal therapy** is the most frequently recommended adjuvant systemic therapy and is aimed at targeting ER- and/or PR-positive breast cancer. **Tamoxifen**, a selective ER modulator, has been used most commonly. It blocks the effects of endogenous estrogen at the breast but produces estrogen-like effects in the uterus, bone, liver, and coagulation system. Hormone therapy results in a 26% annual reduction in the risk of recurrence and a 14% annual reduction in the risk of death from breast cancer. Tamoxifen is usually administered for at least 5 years. It is associated with a 2-fold increased risk of endometrial cancer and venous thromboembolic events (approximately 4 cases in 1000 women). Abnormal uterine bleeding in premenopausal women or any postmenopausal bleeding in a woman taking tamoxifen should be assessed with endometrial sampling. However, routine imaging or endometrial sampling is not recommended for tamoxifen users. Risks of venous thromboembolism and endometrial cancer are age related, increasing with advanced age.

  - **Aromatase inhibitors** (eg, letrozole, anastrozole, and exemestane) are potent inhibitors of estrogen synthesis and are therefore typically used in postmenopausal women. They have been shown to be more effective than tamoxifen in treating breast cancer, with virtually no risk of endometrial hyperplasia and a reduced risk of thromboembolic events when compared to tamoxifen. Side effects include osteoporosis, myalgias, elevated cholesterol, and joint pain. These agents are effective as first-line agents or as second-line agents in patients whose cancer has progressed during or after tamoxifen therapy.

- **Biologic therapy.** Trastuzumab (Herceptin) is a genetically engineered monoclonal antibody to the **HER2 protein**. Its use concurrently with chemotherapy in HER2-positive breast cancers results in significant improvement in disease-free and overall survival. There is, however, an increased risk of congestive heart failure and decreased left ventricular ejection fraction in patients receiving trastuzumab, so routine cardiac monitoring is recommended.

- **Chemotherapy** has been shown to improve overall survival and reduce the odds of death by 25% in selected patients. The decision to use cytotoxic chemotherapy depends on tumor histology, tumor size, nodal status, genomic profiling, and benefit-risk calculators.

Metastatic or Advanced Disease

- Although breast cancer is uncommonly found to be metastatic at the time of presentation, approximately one-third of patients subsequently develop distant metastatic disease. Median survival for patients with metastatic disease is 18 to 24 months, but fewer than 5% live beyond 5 years. Breast cancer metastasizes to the bone, liver, and brain. The goal of therapy in metastatic disease is prolongation of survival and palliation of symptoms. Treatments typically include endocrine therapy, chemotherapy, or biologic therapy. Surgery or radiation could be considered for recurrence limited to one organ.

Prevention

- **Chemoprevention** includes treatment with tamoxifen and raloxifene. Appropriate candidates for prophylactic endocrine therapy include women over age 35 years with a history of LCIS, DCIS, or atypical ductal or lobular hyperplasia; women over age 60 years; women between ages 35 and 59 years with Gail model risk of breast cancer $\geq 1.66\%$ over 5 years; or women with known *BRCA1* or *BRCA2* mutations who do not undergo prophylactic mastectomy. **Prophylactic tamoxifen** reduces the risk for ER-positive breast cancer in women without previous breast cancer but does not impact overall survival.
  - **Raloxifene** is a selective ER modulator that has estrogenic effects on lipid and bone but estrogen antagonistic effects on the uterus and breast. It reduces the incidence of hormone-positive breast cancer in postmenopausal women but, like tamoxifen, has no effect on survival. It is slightly less effective than tamoxifen in preventing breast cancer but has lower risks of endometrial cancer/hyperplasia and venous thromboembolism. Its use has not been studied in premenopausal women.
- **Aromatase inhibitors.** Only anastrozole and exemestane have been evaluated in the setting of primary prevention of breast cancer and showed similar results. There was a 50% reduction in number of invasive breast cancers in high-risk women, although with significantly more musculoskeletal side effects, vaginal dryness, vasomotor symptoms, and hypertension when compared with placebo. Although available data indicates that these medications are a reasonable alternative to selective estrogen receptor modulators for postmenopausal women, none are approved for primary prevention of breast cancer in the United States at this time.
- **Surgical prevention** can be considered in two groups of women: (1) patients positive for *BRCA1* or *BRCA2* and (2) patients with a strong family history suggestive of hereditary breast cancer but negative for *BRCA1* or *BRCA2*. Surgical prevention includes contralateral mastectomy, prophylactic bilateral mastectomy, and bilateral salpingo-oophorectomy. Prophylactic bilateral mastectomies have been shown to reduce the risk of breast cancer by 90%. This is increased to 95% if combined with a bilateral salpingo-oophorectomy.

Pregnancy and Breast Cancer

- Pregnancy-associated breast cancer is diagnosed during pregnancy, in the first postpartum year, or any time during lactation. Breast cancer is the most common cancer in pregnancy, with an incidence of 1 in 3000 gestations. The average patient age is 32 to 38 years. Breast cancer can be especially difficult to diagnose during pregnancy and lactation (secondary to increased glandular breast tissue), which may lead to a delay in diagnosis. Thus, cancers are often found at a later stage in pregnant women or immediately postpartum. Mammograms may be performed safely during pregnancy. Pregnant patients do as well as their nonpregnant counterparts at a similar disease stage.
- Treatment during pregnancy is generally the same as that for nonpregnant patients. The tumor can usually be fully excised or mastectomy performed during pregnancy. The agents used to identify the sentinel lymph node are not approved in pregnancy and therefore axillary dissection is commonly performed. Initiation of chemotherapy is generally considered safe after the first trimester.

Radiotherapy should be avoided until after delivery. No evidence has been reported that aborting the fetus or interrupting the pregnancy leads to improved outcome.

SUGGESTED READINGS

American College of Obstetricians and Gynecologists Committee on Practice Bulletins—Gynecology. ACOG Practice Bulletin No. 164: diagnosis and management of benign breast disorders. *Obstet Gynecol*. 2016;127:e141-e156. (Reaffirmed 2018)

American College of Obstetricians and Gynecologists Committee on Practice Bulletins—Gynecology. ACOG Practice Bulletin No. 179: breast cancer risk assessment and screening in average-risk women. *Obstet Gynecol*. 2017;130(1):e1-e16.

American College of Obstetricians and Gynecologists Committee on Practice Bulletins–Gynecology, Committee on Genetics, Society of Gynecologic Oncology. Practice Bulletin No. 182: hereditary breast and ovarian cancer syndrome. *Obstet Gynecol*. 2017;130(3):e110-e126.

Fritz MA, Speroff L, eds. The breast. In: *Clinical Gynecologic Endocrinology and Infertility*. 8th ed. Philadelphia, PA: Lippincott Williams & Wilkins; 2011:621-673.

Leach MO. Breast cancer screening in women at high risk using MRI. *NMR Biomed*. 2009;22:17-27.

Benign Vulvar Disorders

35

Megan E. Lander and Cybill R. Esguerra

ANATOMY OF THE VULVA

- The **vulva** is the external region of the female genitalia, encompassing the area from the labia majora to the hymen.
- The vulva is bounded laterally by the genitocrural folds, anteriorly by the mons pubis, and posteriorly by the perineal body. The space between the labia minora is known as the vulvar vestibule.
  - The transition from the keratinized epithelium of the labia minora to the nonkeratinized vestibular mucosa is demarcated by Hart line.
  - Within the vestibule lie the urethral meatus, vaginal introitus, ostia of Bartholin glands (major vestibular glands), and Skene glands (minor vestibular glands) (see Figure 58-6).
- Branches of the external and internal pudendal arteries provide the vascular supply to the vulva (Figure 35-1).
- Sensory innervation of the anterior vulva is via the genitofemoral nerve and the cutaneous branch of the ilioinguinal nerve. The posterior vulva and the clitoris are innervated by the pudendal nerve.

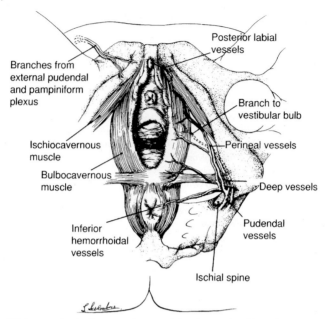

Figure 35-1. Superficial vulvar musculature and vascular supply of the vulva. Reprinted with permission from Rock JA, Jones HW, eds. *Te Linde's Operative Gynecology*. 10th ed. Philadelphia, PA: Wolters Kluwer Health/Lippincott Williams & Wilkins; 2008:505.

INFECTIOUS DISEASES OF THE VULVA

Sexually Transmitted Infections

- **Sexually transmitted infections** are diseases transmitted through sexual contact and can be caused by bacteria, viruses, or parasites. They may be asymptomatic but require prompt treatment, often with antibiotics and education on safer sex practices (see chapter 27).

Bacterial Skin Infections of the Vulva

- **Folliculitis**, **furunculosis**, and **cellulitis** are the most commonly seen bacterial skin infections involving the vulva. These infections are usually caused by *Staphylococcus aureus*; however, *Streptococcus* or enteric species such as *Enterococci* may also be implicated.
- Treatment of initial skin infection is with warm compresses and, in cases of persistent infection or immunosuppression, antibiotic therapy. The antimicrobial agent selected should provide adequate coverage for methicillin-resistant *S aureus*, such as trimethoprim-sulfamethoxazole, doxycycline, or clindamycin.

DERMATOSES AND INFLAMMATORY CONDITIONS

Behçet Syndrome

- **Behçet syndrome** is a rare disease characterized by relapsing aphthous ulcers of the mouth, along with a combination of systemic manifestations, including genital ulcers, ocular inflammation, cutaneous nodules, gastrointestinal ulcers, thrombophlebitis, and arthritis. It is most common in Japanese and Middle Eastern populations.

- Genital ulceration is the most specific finding for Behçet disease, occurring in more than 75% of patients with the disease. Lesions are small, deep, and painful and may be mistaken for herpes. Multiple lesions may result in fenestration of the labia. Ulcers generally heal in 7 to 10 days and recur less frequently than oral ulcers.

- Treatment options include corticosteroids—topical (0.1% betamethasone valerate ointment), intralesional (triamcinolone 5-10 mg/mL injected into the ulcer base), or systemic (prednisone 1 mg/kg)—depending on disease severity. For recurrent lesions, preventive treatment with colchicine (1-2 mg/d) can be offered and should be titrated due to potential for unwanted gastrointestinal effects.

Fox-Fordyce Disease

- **Fox-Fordyce disease** is a rare condition characterized by occlusion of apocrine and apoeccrine sweat glands in the axilla and anogenital region resulting in papular eruption. Patients present with small (2-3 mm), hyperpigmented, clustered papules that are intensely pruritic, often leading to lichenification from chronic scratching. It predominantly affects African Americans. Exacerbations tend to occur before and during menses. Symptoms regress during pregnancy.

- Treatment is with topical corticosteroids, clindamycin, and calcineurin inhibitors (1% pimecrolimus cream). Topical retinoids and intralesional corticosteroids are used as second-line therapy.

Hidradenitis Suppurativa

- **Hidradenitis suppurativa** is a painful apocrine gland disorder resulting from chronic follicular occlusion. This results in deep, pustulent subcutaneous nodules that form sinus tracts and confluent masses. The intertriginous skin areas of the axillae and anogenital region are most frequently involved. Lesions wax and wane and flares commonly occur during menstruation. These lesions vary from inflamed nodules to ulcerating lesions that can result in draining sinuses and extensive scarring. The lesions can be severely malodorous and disfiguring, with the potential for negative psychosocial repercussions in patients inflicted with the disease.

- Disease severity is graded by the Hurley clinical staging system:
  - Stage I: single or multiple abscesses, without sinus tracts or scarring. The majority of patients exhibit stage I disease.
  - Stage II: recurrent abscesses with tract formation and scarring, single or multiple widely separated lesions
  - Stage III: diffuse or near-diffuse involvement, formation of extensive abscesses, sinus tracts, and scarring across an entire region

- Superinfection of hidradenitis suppurativa is polymicrobial, and cultures can help guide treatment. The effectiveness of medical therapy wanes as deeper tissues become involved.

- Treatment options are extensive and are approached in a stepwise fashion, with the goal being to reduce the frequency of new lesions, prevent disease progression, and treat existing lesions and scarring.

- First-line treatment for all patients involves lifestyle modification. Patients are advised to wear loose-fitting clothing, avoid manipulation of lesions, keep the area clean and dry, and use gentle, nonirritating cleansers. Patients should also be counseled on smoking cessation, weight management, and the use of topical antiseptic washes, such as chlorhexidine.

- Hurley stage I disease: Topical clindamycin is the most common first-line treatment for mild disease, with or without adjuvant intralesional corticosteroids. Punch debridement may also be used to eliminate newly inflamed nodules as well as the topical chemical peeling agent resorcinol.
- Hurley stage II and III disease: Therapy with oral tetracyclines (doxycycline 100 mg twice a day) is typically continued for several months. If disease persists, combination therapy with clindamycin (300 mg orally twice a day) and rifampin (600 mg orally daily) can be offered. Other treatment options include dapsone, oral retinoids (acitretin, isotretinoin, alitretinoin), and hormonal therapies. Newer therapies using spironolactone for its antiandrogenic qualities and apremilast, an oral phosphodiesterase 4 inhibitor, are currently being studied with promising results.
- Refractory disease: Patients with any stage of the disease that is nonresponsive to typical medical management as discussed above can sometimes be managed with biologic therapies, including adalimumab and infliximab. Treatment with systemic glucocorticoids (prednisone 40-60 mg/d) can be used in acute inflammatory disease. Surgery can be used to treat individual nodules and sinus tracts, with wide surgical excision reserved for refractory disease.

Atrophic Vulvovaginitis

- Vulvovaginal atrophy, also referred to as genitourinary syndrome of menopause, occurs due to the hypoestrogenic state of menopause. Patients typically present with complaints of vulvovaginal dryness, pain, burning, pruritus, dyspareunia, and dysuria. The vaginal mucosa becomes friable, easily irritated, and more prone to infection. The diagnosis is clinical.
- On physical examination, the labia majora appear lax, whereas the labia minora are significantly atrophied. There may be diminished skin elasticity and narrowing of the introitus. The mucosa is thin, pale, and smooth with loss of the normal vaginal rugae.
- First-line therapy is with nonhormonal vaginal moisturizers and lubricants. Persistent symptoms that do not respond to nonhormonal treatments can be managed with vaginal estrogen therapy in the form of cream, tablet, suppository, or ring (see chapter 45).

Contact Dermatitis

- **Contact dermatitis** is a localized inflammatory skin reaction to an irritant, such as soap, detergent, hygiene product, or clothing material.
- On physical examination, symmetric eczematous lesions are seen in the exposed region.
- Treatment is to identify and remove the offending agent. Oatmeal soaks and sitz baths can be used to help control symptoms. For severe reactions, a mild steroid ointment (eg, betamethasone dipropionate) may be applied.

Psoriasis

- **Psoriasis** typically appears as erythematous plaques with silvery, thick scales involving the labia majora. It is usually accompanied by psoriatic plaques along extensor surfaces of the body but may manifest as isolated vulvar lesions.
- Biopsy may be useful for definitive diagnosis.
- Vulvar psoriasis can be treated with low-potency corticosteroids, such as triamcinolone acetonide.

Lichen Simplex Chronicus

- **Lichen simplex chronicus** is characterized by an intensely pruritic rash often involving the perineum. Chronic scratching leads to bacterial infection and lichenification, producing a thickened, leathery appearance of the vulva.
- Foci of atypical hyperplasia or cancer can develop, with a 3% chance of developing into invasive squamous cell carcinoma. Evaluation should include colposcopy and full-thickness biopsy.
- Initial treatment seeks to break the itch-scratch cycle with topical and intralesional corticosteroids with or without the addition of 6% salicylic acid gel, topical aspirin, and, in some cases, oral gabapentin.

Lichen Planus

- **Lichen planus** is an uncommon, recurrent papulosquamous eruption that can affect the genitalia and oral mucosa. The pathophysiology is thought to involve T-cell autoimmunity to basal keratinocytes.
- Patients present with complaints of increased vaginal discharge, dyspareunia, itching, pain, and burning of the vulva. White papules in a linear or reticular pattern are often seen on the vulva, called Wickham striae.
- A wide range of morphologies are seen. The most common and most difficult to treat is the erosive form in which the tissue becomes denuded and scarred with loss of normal labial and vaginal architecture.
- The use of ultrapotent topical steroids is first-line treatment. Other options include systemic corticosteroids, immunosuppressants, methotrexate, cyclosporine, azathioprine, and hydroxychloroquine. Surgery is not curative and is reserved for treatment of postinflammatory sequelae, such as labial adhesions and introital stenosis.

Lichen Sclerosus

- **Lichen sclerosus** is a progressive dermatologic condition of unknown etiology that is characterized by vulvar epithelial inflammation and atrophy. It is associated with vulvar pruritus (usually most severe at night), pain, and scarring, with gradual loss of the labia minora and prepuce of the clitoris. Patients may also present with complaints of dyspareunia and dysuria.
- Lichen sclerosus is the most common lichen disorder of the vulva. Postmenopausal Caucasian women are most often affected, with a second peak in prepubertal girls.
- On physical exam, lesions appear as thin, white, atrophic papules, likened to cigarette paper. The vaginal mucosa is usually spared. However, narrowing of the introitus and perianal involvement may result in an hourglass or "figure of eight" configuration.
- Women with lichen sclerosis have a 20% risk of having another autoimmune disease, most frequently alopecia areata, vitiligo, or thyroid disease.
- Although lichen sclerosis is not considered a premalignant lesion, patients have a 5% chance of developing vulvar squamous cell carcinoma.
- Vulvar punch biopsies can be performed to confirm the diagnosis but are typically avoided in the prepubertal patient.
- Treatment aims to prevent the progression of the disease and includes chronic use of ultrapotent topical corticosteroid (0.05% clobetasol propionate ointment)

as well as intralesional corticosteroids for hypertrophic lesions. Topical estrogen (0.01% estradiol cream) is indicated for atrophic symptoms. Periodic clinical examinations should be performed. Biopsy should be performed if ulcerations persist or new lesions appear. Surgery is reserved for management of malignancy and postinflammatory sequelae, such as labial adhesions and introital stenosis.

VULVAR PAIN SYNDROMES

Vulvodynia

- See chapter 36.
- **Vulvodynia** is defined as chronic vulvar discomfort, occurring in the absence of focal clinical exam findings or an identifiable neurologic disorder.
- Patients typically complain of burning, stinging, or throbbing pain in the vulvar region. These symptoms may interfere with the ability to have vaginal intercourse, wear tight clothing, exercise, or even sit down. Vulvodynia affects up to 15% of the female population.
- Treatment should be multidisciplinary, with the use of medical and psychological therapies as well as lifestyle modification.

Vulvar Vestibulitis Syndrome

- **Vulvar vestibulitis syndrome** is caused by chronic inflammation of the vestibular glands and is characterized by erythema and severe pain elicited by palpation. The main presenting symptoms are dyspareunia and terminal dysuria.
- Biopsy is of limited utility and usually only demonstrates chronic inflammation.
- Patients with vulvar vestibulitis syndrome benefit from pelvic rest, anti-inflammatory therapy (eg, Burow soaks, sitz baths, Stearin-Lanolin cream application), and pelvic relaxation exercises.
- Vulvar surgery is reserved for patients who fail to respond to conservative therapy or suffer from extensive scarring.

Levator Ani Syndrome

- **Levator ani syndrome** is characterized by painful spasms or pressure sensation high in the rectum, usually worse in the sitting position compared to standing or lying down. It is often the result of trauma to or inflammation of the perineal branch of the pudendal nerve.
- According to the Rome IV criteria, patients must demonstrate all of the following symptoms for the past 3 months with symptom onset at least 6 months prior in order to meet diagnostic criteria:
  - Chronic or recurrent rectal pain or aching
  - Episodes last 30 minutes or longer
  - Tenderness during traction on the puborectalis
  - Exclusion of other causes of rectal pain (eg, inflammatory bowel disease, intramuscular abscess and fissure, thrombosed hemorrhoids, prostatitis, coccygodynia, and major structural alterations of the pelvic floor)
- Patients with mild symptoms may be reassured that episodes are transient. More severe symptoms may require treatment with topical antispasmodics or biofeedback therapy.

Vulvar Neuropathy

- The pudendal, genitofemoral, and ilioinguinal nerves are the main nerves serving the vulvovaginal area. Trauma to or inflammation of these nerves may result in continuous dull, aching, or burning neuropathic pain.
- Anticonvulsants (gabapentin titrated up to 600-900 mg 3 times a day) and tricyclic antidepressants (amitriptyline 0.5-2 mg/kg at bedtime) have been shown to be effective treatments.

BENIGN VULVAR LESIONS

Urethral Caruncle

- A **urethral caruncle** is a benign, fleshy, exophytic papule at the posterior urethral meatus that is most commonly seen in postmenopausal women. Although usually asymptomatic, it can present with vaginal bleeding or dysuria. For symptomatic lesions, treatment is with topical estrogen therapy (0.01% Estrace cream, 2-4 g daily for 1-2 wk). For large or refractory lesions, surgical excision, cryosurgery, or laser vaporization can be performed.

Acrochordon

- **Acrochordons** (ie, skin tags) are common, frequently pedunculated fibroepithelial polyps that have a rubbery, flesh-like consistency. They often arise in areas of chronic irritation or friction, such as the axilla, neck, inframammary, and inguinal regions. Acrochordons do not need treatment unless they are bothersome to the patient, in which case they can be removed via fine-grade scissors, cryosurgery, or electrodessication.

Seborrheic Keratoses

- **Seborrheic keratoses** are flat to slightly raised pigmented lesions that have a characteristic waxy, "stuck-on" appearance. Although benign, providers should have a low threshold to perform excisional biopsy to rule out carcinoma.

Lipoma

- **Lipomas** are benign, painless tumors composed of adipose tissue in the subcutaneous space. They are soft and sometimes pedunculated. They commonly appear on the mons pubis and labia majora. No treatment is necessary unless the lipoma is bothersome, in which case it can be excised with low-risk for recurrence.

BENIGN VULVAR CYSTS

Bartholin Gland Cyst

- **Bartholin gland cysts** occur when the Bartholin glands, which serve to lubricate the vagina and are located deep to the posterior aspect of the labia majora, become occluded. If an obstructed Bartholin gland becomes infected, an abscess may form. Usually polymicrobial, approximately 10% of **Bartholin abscesses** may be caused by *Neisseria gonorrhoeae*.
- Bartholin gland cysts that are asymptomatic do not require treatment. In women age 40 years or older, biopsy is recommended because of the risk of Bartholin

adenocarcinoma. Treatment of Bartholin gland abscesses in patients without signs of systemic infection may include incision and drainage with a Word catheter, marsupialization, or in case of recurrence, resection of the gland. Antibiotic therapy is only administered in the setting of systemic infection, recurrent abscess, or immunosuppression.

Epidermal Inclusion Cysts

- **Epidermal inclusion cysts** are the most common vulvar cysts and occur on the labia majora or minora. They are lined by epithelial cells and contain a white or yellow sebaceous material comprised of keratin and lipid-rich debris. They arise from blockage of pilosebaceous ducts. If traumatized (eg, during vaginal delivery), cysts can become erythematous and tender. Symptomatic cysts can be surgically excised.

Mucus Cysts

- **Mucus cysts** are found within the vestibule and develop from vestigial embryonic structures or from obstruction of the minor vestibular glands. They are lined by mucus-secreting simple columnar epithelium without myoepithelial cells. They are typically asymptomatic.

Gartner Duct Cysts

- **Gartner duct cysts** are benign vaginal cysts that occur in Gartner duct, a remnant of the mesonephric duct. They most often appear as multiple small cysts along the lateral vaginal wall and hymenal ring. These cysts are usually asymptomatic and are discovered incidentally. Treatment is not necessary unless cysts are very large, in which case they can be surgically excised.

Skene Duct Cysts

- **Skene duct cysts** are benign vaginal cysts that occur in the Skene glands (also known as periurethral glands) due to their location adjacent to the distal urethra. Cysts form in these glands when there is obstruction of the duct, which often occurs due to an infection. Most Skene duct cysts are asymptomatic, but some can cause urinary symptoms due to urinary outflow obstruction. Treatment via surgical excision is reserved for symptomatic cysts. If an abscess has formed, broad-spectrum antibiotics (cephalexin for 7-10 d) should be administered.

SUGGESTED READINGS

American College of Obstetricians and Gynecologists Committee on Gynecologic Practice. ACOG Committee Opinion No. 673: persistent vulvar pain. *Obstet Gynecol.* 2015;128(3): e78-e84. (Reaffirmed 2019)

American College of Obstetricians and Gynecologists Committee on Practice Bulletins—Gynecology. ACOG Practice Bulletin No. 93: diagnosis and management of vulvar skin disorders. *Obstet Gynecol.* 2008;111(5):1243-1253. (Reaffirmed 2019)

Baggish MS, Karram M. Atlas of vulvar disorders. In: *Atlas of Pelvic Anatomy and Gynecologic Surgery.* 4th ed. Philadelphia, PA: Elsevier; 2016:841-873.

Haefner HK, Crum CP. Benign conditions of the vagina. In: Crum CP, Nucci MR, Granter SR, et al, eds. *Diagnostic Gynecologic and Obstetric Pathology.* 3rd ed. Philadelphia, PA: Elsevier; 2018:258-274.

36 Female Sexual Function and Dysfunction

Yangshu Linda Pan and Linda C. Rogers

Female sexual dysfunction encompasses a number of conditions characterized by one or more of the following symptoms that result in personal distress: loss of sexual desire, impaired arousal, inability to achieve orgasm, or sexual pain. There is often significant overlap between these conditions, which can make diagnosis and treatment challenging.

EPIDEMIOLOGY

- According to multiple worldwide studies, 40% of women report sexual concerns, with the most common female sexual problem being low desire (26%-43%).
- Difficulty with orgasm was reported next (18%-41%).

PHYSIOLOGY OF SEXUAL FUNCTION

Female sexual function is a complex interplay of the central nervous system, peripheral nervous system, and end organs (Table 36-1).
- The arousal response in women involves increased heart rate, muscle tension, changes in breast sensations, and a subjective state of arousal.
- The vasculature and musculature changes involved in arousal are mediated by dopaminergic stimulation of the peripheral nervous system. Autonomic nerves release nitric oxide and vasointestinal polypeptide that modulate vasodilatation.
- Orgasm is a reflex with involuntary, rhythmic contractions of the pelvic floor muscles (perineal, bulbocavernosus, pubococcygeus), combined with a sudden release of serotonin, prolactin, oxytocin, and endogenous opioids. Contraction of the pelvic floor muscles involves adrenergic and cholinergic mechanisms from the efferent pudendal nerve.
- Estrogen primarily maintains the integrity of the tissues. Androgen levels are associated with libido and arousal, and androgen receptors are found in vulvar and vaginal tissue.

THEORIES OF SEXUAL FUNCTION

- In 2011, Rosemary Basson developed a model of sexual arousal that incorporated psychological and social aspects of women's lives. In her model, desire does not always precede sexual arousal. Instead, women often begin at a state of "sexual neutrality" and respond to or seek sexual stimuli based on many possible psychological motivations. The response to this stimulus is usually arousal, which leads to desire and improved arousal. This model can be explained to patients concerned about lack of desire and can normalize what women commonly experience (a lack of spontaneous desire but the presence of reactive desire).

Table 36-1 Physiologic Female Sexual Response[a]

Phase	Sex Organ Response	General Sexual Response
Excitement	Vaginal lubrication Thickening of vaginal walls and labia Expansion of inner vagina Elevation of cervix and corpus Tumescence of clitoris	Nipple erection Sex-tension flush
Plateau	Orgasmic platform in outer vagina Full expansion of inner vagina Secretion of mucus by Bartholin gland Withdrawal of clitoris	Sex-tension flush Carpopedal spasm Generalized skeletal muscle tension Hyperventilation Tachycardia
Orgasm	Contractions of uterus from fundus toward lower uterine segment Contractions of orgasmic platform at 0.8-s intervals External rectal sphincter contractions at 0.8-s intervals External urethral sphincter contractions at irregular intervals	Specific skeletal muscle contractions Hyperventilation Tachycardia
Resolution	Ready return to orgasm with retarded loss of pelvic vasocongestion Return of normal color and orgasmic platform in primary (rapid) stage Loss of clitoral tumescence and return to position	Diaphoresis Hyperventilation Tachycardia

[a]Reprinted with permission from Beckman CR, Ling F, Barzansky BM, et al. *Obstetrics and Gynecology*. 4th ed. Philadelphia, PA: Lippincott Williams & Wilkins; 2002:610.

DIAGNOSIS OF SEXUAL DISORDERS

Screening

- A few simple questions can initiate the discussion: Are you currently involved in a sexual relationship? Do you have sex with men, women, or both? Do you have any concerns about or pain with sex?
- History should include the nature and frequency of the problem, the degree of distress, whether the problem is lifelong versus newly acquired, situational, or generalized. Additionally, the history can include a discussion of the partner's sexual problems or concerns, partner reaction, and history of prior treatment or intervention.

- Elicit the patient's thoughts concerning the cause of the problems and her expectations from treatment. Also obtain medical history, psychological/psychiatric history, sexual history including abuse or violence, and social history. Inquire about the use of medications that may cause sexual side effects and about the use of personal hygiene products such as soaps or detergents.

Physical Exam

- During visual inspection, note any atrophy, lack of estrogenization, loss of architecture, scarring, hypopigmentation or hyperpigmentation, or possible infection. Examine urethral meatus and anus. Assess for evidence of any vulvovaginal infections, including yeast and bacterial vaginosis. Suspicious skin changes on the vulva warrant biopsy.
- Check the clitoris for phimosis (inability to retract the foreskin over the glans), tenderness, or small masses/foreign bodies. These can sometimes affect sexual function. Clitoral pain is often due to yeast.
- A speculum exam and bimanual exam should be performed to assess for tenderness, adnexal masses, prolapse, and the anal reflex.
- Assessment of the pelvic floor is critical. Note general tone, tender points or bands, and ability to perform a concentric contraction of vaginal muscles.
- Q-tip test: pain mapping with Q-tip best started at nontender site away from introitus, working in toward painful area

SEXUAL DYSFUNCTION DISORDERS

Sexual dysfunction disorders can be divided into four-broad categories: desire, arousal, orgasmic, and pain disorders.

Desire

- **Hypoactive sexual desire disorder (HSDD)** involves >6 months of a decrease in or lack of motivation for sexual activity leading to personal distress.
  - Etiologies: hormonal changes such as adrenal insufficiency, hypopituitarism, inter- and intrapersonal factors, medications (eg, selective serotonin reuptake inhibitors, oral contraceptive pills [OCPs]), medical, and psychiatric conditions (eg, depression, cancer). If situational in etiology (eg, secondary to a situational event), then this is not considered HSDD.
- **Sexual aversion disorder** is a persistent or recurrent aversive response to any genital contact with a sexual partner, emphasizing the role of avoidance.

Arousal

- **Female genital arousal disorder (FGAD)** is defined as the inability to develop or maintain adequate genital response for 6 months or more, including a lack of vulvovaginal lubrication, engorgement of genitalia, and sensitivity of genitalia associated with sexual activity. It can be related to vascular injury or dysfunction and/or neurologic injury or dysfunction. In order to diagnose FGAD, the practitioner must exclude vulvovaginal atrophy, infection, inflammatory disorders of the vulva and vagina, vestibulodynia, and clitorodynia.

- **Female sexual arousal disorder (FSAD)** is an older term, defined in the *Diagnostic and Statistical Manual of Mental Disorders*, 4th edition, as an inability to maintain adequate lubrication-swelling response to sexual excitement through to the completion of the sexual activity. Notably, this definition focuses solely on the genital response. There is ongoing discussion regarding FGAD as a diagnostic revision for FSAD.
- **Female sexual interest/arousal disorder** is a combination of the FSAD and HSDD, according to the *Diagnostic and Statistical Manual of Mental Disorders*, 5th edition (*DSM-5*). It is defined as persistent or recurrent deficient or absent sexual fantasies or desire for sexual activity, and/or inability to attain or to maintain until completion of sexual activity an adequate genital lubrication-swelling response of sexual excitement, and/or delay in or absence of orgasm following a normal sexual excitement phase that causes marked distress or interpersonal difficulty.
- **Persistent genital arousal disorder** involves persistent or recurrent distressing feelings of genital arousal or being on the verge of orgasm not associated with concomitant sexual interest, thoughts, or fantasies for >6 months.
  - Can be concomitant with overactive bladder and/or restless leg syndrome
  - Etiologies: central trigger from perception of increased genital engorgement and subsequent increased sensitivity; Tarlov (perineural) cysts and/or bulging discs compressing genital sensory nerve roots at the site of entry to the sacral spine
  - Examine the clitoris for irritation or foreign bodies because this may lead to stimulation.
  - Treatment goal is to eliminate any excitation from the peripheral genital nerves (S2-S4) or central nervous system pathologies that are misdirected to the hypothalamus and misinterpreted as genital arousal. Consider referral to a center familiar with spinal surgical procedures.
  - Oral medications include zolpidem, tramadol, or varenicline. Other treatment options include pelvic floor physical therapy and transdermal electrical nerve stimulation.
  - Suicidal ideation is possible, and multiple suicides have been reported.

Treatments for Both Desire and Arousal Disorders in Women

Given that there is so much overlap among desire and arousal disorders and that the female sexual response is a complex interaction, treatment must often be multifaceted. Note that treatment of persistent genital arousal disorder differs, as discussed above.

- Flibanserin (Addyi): contraindicated with alcohol, hepatic impairment, and moderate to strong CYP3A4 inhibitors. Side effects include dizziness, fatigue, and nausea. Currently indicated only for premenopausal women. Minimal to modest efficacy; studies showed it increases satisfying sexual encounters by one per month over placebo.
- Bupropion
- Androgens: A 300-mg transdermal testosterone patch has been shown to help certain population of women (status post oophorectomy and hysterectomy) increase sexual fantasies but is not US Food and Drug Administration approved for female sexual dysfunction. There are some concerns over lack of safety data and risks of clitoromegaly, hirsutism, acne, hepatotoxicity, and worsening lipid profile with prolonged use.
- Other treatments: cognitive behavioral therapy, directed masturbation, sex therapy, clitoral suction vacuum device, personal lubricants, self-treatment books

Orgasmic

- **Female orgasm disorder** involves >6 months of distressing compromise of orgasm frequency, intensity, timing, and/or pleasure. It should not be diagnosed if women can achieve clitoral orgasm but not one through vaginal penetration. Also, it should not be diagnosed if there is inadequate stimulation because women show a wide variability in type and intensity of stimulation needed to reach orgasm.
- It can be a consequence of psychosocial issues, medications, medical comorbidities, genital mutilation, pelvic trauma, or hormonal issues.
- **Female orgasmic illness syndrome** is characterized by peripheral and/or central aversive symptoms that occur before, during, or after orgasm.
  - Central aversive symptoms include disorientation, confusion, seizures, insomnia, or headache.
  - Peripheral aversive symptoms include diarrhea, constipation, muscle aches, abdominal pain, fatigue, hot flashes, and chills.
  - If the patient has severe headache with orgasm and no previous history of sexual headaches, consider referral for neurologic exam and imaging because this can be a presenting sign for subarachnoid hemorrhage or other serious pathology.
- **Treatment for orgasmic disorders** includes vibrators to improve blood flow to genitals, "directed masturbation" techniques with the guidance of books (see recommended reading list) or a therapist, and helping patients become more in touch with sexuality and anatomy.

Pain

Genitopelvic Pain/Penetration Disorder

- According to the *DSM-5*, genitopelvic pain/penetration disorder is defined as persistent difficulties leading to significant distress for >6 months with vaginal penetration, pain during penetration attempts, fear and anxiety about penetration, and/or tightening of the pelvic floor muscles during attempted penetration.
- It is essentially a combination of dyspareunia (pain with penetrative intercourse) and vaginismus (high tone pelvic floor dysfunction).
- One very common cause of dyspareunia is vulvodynia. Other causes include sexually transmitted infections, urinary tract infections, and yeast infections.
- The classification and grouping together of dyspareunia and vaginismus as a psychiatric pain disorder in the *DSM-5* is controversial.
- This is a *DSM-5* diagnosis. In a gynecologic clinical setting, the terms *vulvodynia*, *vaginismus*, and *high tone pelvic floor dysfunction* are more commonly used. Vaginismus and high tone pelvic floor dysfunction are essentially synonymous, but the term *vaginismus* is often used for patients who are fearful or phobic about penetration, in addition to having a hypertonic pelvic floor.
- The physician must rule out other causes of pain with intercourse, including vulvovaginal atrophy, pelvic masses, vaginal/vulvar masses or lesions (eg, ulcers, fissures), and dermatologic conditions.

Vaginismus and Vulvodynia

- **Vaginismus** is the persistent or recurrent involuntary spasm of the outer third of the vagina that interferes with sexual intercourse. It often makes any vaginal penetration (tampons, digit, vaginal dilators, gynecologic exam, intercourse) difficult or impossible due to pain and/or fear of pain.

- It is both a psychological disorder manifested by fear and anxiety to penetration and a physical disorder as noted by vaginal spasm. It frequently overlaps with vulvodynia.
- It is one of the more prevalent female sexual dysfunction disorders, with a rate of 5% to 17%.
- Introital hypersensitivity and muscle hypertonicity are commonly identified.
- **Vulvodynia** is vulvar pain most often described as burning pain >3 months in duration that occurs in the absence of relevant visible findings or a specific, clinically identifiable neurologic disorder.

  - Classified into
    - ○ Localized to vestibule (eg, vestibulodynia, vulvar vestibulitis) or clitoris (eg, clitorodynia) or generalized, involving the whole vulva
    - ○ Provoked (by touch), unprovoked (occurs spontaneously), or mixed
  - When a specific disorder can be identified as a cause of the vulvar pain (eg, infectious, inflammatory, neoplastic, trauma, hormonal deficiencies), this is NOT called vulvodynia. Instead, refer to it as *vulvar pain*.
  - The most prevalent subtype is provoked vestibulodynia (PVD), also known as localized provoked vulvodynia or localized PVD.
  - Population-based surveys suggest that between 6% and 8% of women are affected by vulvodynia at any one time, and up to 25% of women are affected in their lifetime. There is a higher incidence in young women, ages 18 to 32 years, with a second peak of vulvar pain around menopause.
  - It often remits spontaneously, but relapse is common.
  - Associated factors: history of candidiasis, comorbid pain conditions, sleep disturbance, mood disorders, posttraumatic stress disorder. Almost half of women with vulvodynia report other chronic pain conditions such as migraine headaches, fibromyalgia, irritable bowel syndrome, and interstitial cystitis.
  - Half of women do not seek medical assistance, and only a small number are diagnosed. The low rate of diagnosis is attributed to practitioner unfamiliarity and patient use of terminology to describe discomfort as "rawness" or "irritation" and not "pain."
  - When perimenopausal or menopausal women present with these symptoms, it is important to first evaluate for and treat vaginal atrophy if indicated. Breastfeeding mothers and OCP users can also present with atrophic vaginitis and pain.

Assessment and Exam for Vaginismus and Vulvodynia

- Understand that there may be extreme anxiety surrounding the examination, to the extent that it might not be possible on a first visit. Ensure patients feel empowered to stop exam at any point and that informed consent is genuine.
- Anxiety during the pelvic exam and cotton-tipped test (Q-tip test) may cause a false-positive for PVD when evaluating for vaginismus.
- Question carefully about hygiene practices. Patients may attribute their symptoms to uncleanliness and overwash with harsh soaps or use over-the-counter products with potential irritants.
- For vaginismus, during a gentle digital exam and speculum exam, attention should be paid to tenderness, adnexal masses or nodularity, pelvic floor muscle tone, prolapse, and the anal reflex.

- For vulvodynia, perform a careful Q-tip test (as described earlier). Use a mirror to help patients understand their own anatomy; localize pain; apply medication more appropriately; and show that painful skin looks normal, illustrating that pain is not due to damage but instead some kind of neural sensitization.

Treatment for Vaginismus and Vulvodynia

- Use a multidisciplinary approach, which includes physical, psychological, and pharmacological therapies.
- Recommend good genital skin care, avoiding irritants; improve moisture; recommend that the patient temporarily stop sexual activity if it causes discomfort; and manage concurrent inflammatory skin conditions.
- Mental health counseling in the form of psychological self-management therapies (relaxation, mindfulness, and meditation) and cognitive behavioral therapy to reduce stress and anxiety have been shown to improve sexual function. Sexual and relationship counseling can help both the patient and her partner.

Vaginismus

- Treatment has a high potential for success.
- Pelvic floor physical therapy performed by a physical therapist with specialized training is effective and recommended. It can include Kegel exercises, pelvic floor rehabilitation, bladder and bowel training, posture, and breathing techniques.
- Vaginal dilator therapy involves daily use of dilators, gradually increasing in size. Dilators can be purchased online and used at home. Patients can also be encouraged to use their own fingers and later their partner's fingers.

Vulvodynia

- Medical treatments are often preferred by patients.
  - Topical medication therapy:
    - Lidocaine 2% to 5% gel or ointment on an as-needed basis (eg, 10-20 min before sex or physical therapy); gels and ointments are better tolerated than creams.
    - Second-line choices include amitriptyline, gabapentin, and baclofen. These are compounded in a neutral base in varying strengths, from 2% to 5% and applied in various regimens (usually at night or twice a day) to the vestibule.
    - Topical steroids are not recommended.
    - Topical therapies promote self-touch, massage, and desensitization, in addition to placebo effect through a therapeutic ritual of application.
  - Oral medication therapy
    - The effectiveness of oral agents is not well understood due to paucity of trials in vulvodynia. If used, it is important to clarify that these medications are being used as pain neuromodulators and not as anticonvulsants or antidepressants.
    - Many of the oral agents, such as tricyclic antidepressants (eg, amitriptyline, desipramine), gabapentin, topiramate, venlafaxine, and duloxetine, are used for other types of neuropathic pain.
  - Surgical treatments
    - Surgery (vestibulectomy) has high rates for success in improving pain and sexual function but is usually pursued only after medical and physical therapies have failed.

- Some international studies show improvement after laser treatment (fractional carbon dioxide) of the vestibule, but more research is needed.
- Other treatments
  - Dilators are widely used even though evidence is limited. They are not used to stretch tissues but to provide proprioceptive feedback and improve sensory tolerance.
  - Electromyography surface or internal biofeedback can help facilitate pelvic floor relaxation, but patients must be able to tolerate an inserted probe to undergo this treatment.
  - Emerging modalities: transcutaneous electrical nerve stimulation, acupuncture, hypnotherapy, deep brain stimulation, and spinal cord stimulators

SEXUAL FUNCTION AND SPECIAL POPULATIONS

- **Postpartum:** Sexual activity postpartum is affected by fatigue, breastfeeding, adjustment to the new baby, hormone changes, pain, and healing. History of an anal sphincter tear may also impact sexual function. In one study of 796 women, 32% resumed intercourse within 6 months and 89% after 6 months.
- **Menopause and premature ovarian failure:** Vulvovaginal atrophy plays a significant role. Atrophy has become an increasingly common cause of sexual pain. Topical estrogen therapy is very effective in appropriate patients (see chapter 45).
- **Nonheterosexual relationships:** Regardless of a patient's sexual orientation, providers should address sexual concerns such as pain, sexually transmitted infections, and intimate partner violence.
- **Transgender patients:** Research suggests there is a complex relationship between gender, bisexuality, and sexual fluidity. Practitioners should have an appreciation for and understanding that sexual attraction can change over short or long periods of time and also toward "more preferred" versus "less preferred" genders.
- **Medical disorders and medications** can affect sexual arousal and function. For example, diabetes and peripheral vascular disease may affect vasocongestion. Depression, substance abuse, and tobacco use can affect sexual function. Medications such as selective serotonin reuptake inhibitors, antipsychotics, antihypertensives, OCPs, and medroxyprogesterone acetate are also known to affect sexual function.
- **Pelvic floor disorders** are associated with decreased arousal, infrequent orgasm, and increased dyspareunia. Patients may have loss of self-esteem, embarrassment, and decreased desire. Urinary or fecal incontinence may additionally cause fear of odor. Surgical management for pelvic floor disorders may increase sexual function, although patients should be counseled about operative risks such as dyspareunia or damage to nerves such as the dorsal nerve of the clitoris.
- **Posthysterectomy:** There are theoretical concerns that total or supracervical hysterectomy can disrupt the complex neurologic and vascular anatomy involved in sexual response. However, sexual function has not been shown to be compromised for most women and may actually be improved once issues such as menorrhagia are resolved.
- **Breast cancer and gynecologic oncology patients:** With the increasing number of cancer survivors, issues of quality of life and survivorship have become more important. Cancer and its treatments can be directly responsible for all types of female sexual disorders. Radiotherapy can cause skin thickening, contractures, vaginal stenosis, and decreased genital sensitivity. Providers should set expectations regarding

sexual health issues after treatment; many women who experience sexual adverse effects state they were not informed in advance. All women who have completed treatment should then be screened for sexual health issues. Symptoms such as vaginal atrophy, dyspareunia, and vaginal stenosis can be specifically addressed. Women can be encouraged to use vaginal moisturizers (applied 2-3 times weekly), lubricants, or coconut oil and engage in regular sexual activity or masturbation to maintain blood flow to the genitals. Use of vaginal estrogen therapy in women with estrogen-sensitive cancers should be decided on a case-by-case basis. Some oncologists are now comfortable with topical estrogen for breast cancer patients unless they are on aromatase inhibitors. For vaginal stenosis, recommendations include dilator therapy to improve elasticity, counseling to modify sexual activity, referral to pelvic physical therapist, or surgery for vaginal adhesions.

- **Infertility:** Many infertile couples think of sexual intercourse as goal oriented and may have trouble finding pleasure in sexual activity.

SUGGESTED READINGS

American College of Obstetricians and Gynecologists Committee on Practice Bulletins—Gynecology. ACOG Practice Bulletin No. 119: female sexual dysfunction. *Obstet Gynecol.* 2011;117:996-1007. (Reaffirmed 2017)

Basson R. Clinical practice. Sexual desire and arousal disorders in women. *N Engl J Med.* 2006;354(14):1497-1506.

Bornstein J, Goldstein AT, Stockdale CK, et al. 2015 ISSVD, ISSWSH, and IPPS consensus terminology and classification of persistent vulvar pain and vulvodynia. *J Sex Med.* 2016;13:607-612.

Carey JC. Pharmacological effects on sexual function. *Obstet Gynecol Clin North Am.* 2006;33:599-620.

Henzell H, Berzins K, Langford JP. Provoked vestibulodynia: current perspectives. *Int J Womens Health.* 2017;9:631-642.

Kammerer-Doak D, Rogers R. Female sexual function and dysfunction. *Obstet Gynecol Clin North Am.* 2008;35:169-183.

Pacik PT, Geletta S. Vaginismus treatment: clinical trials follow up 241 patients. *Sex Med.* 2017;5:e114-e123.

Parish SJ, Goldstein AT, Goldstein SW, et al. Toward a more evidence-based nosology and nomenclature for female sexual dysfunction—part II. *J Sex Med.* 2016;13:1888-1906.

Reed R, Harlow SD, Sen A, Edwards RM, Chen D, Haefner HK. Relationship between vulvodynia and chronic comorbid pain conditions. *Obstet Gynecol.* 2012;120(1):145-151.

Rosen R, Barsky J. Normal sexual response in women. *Obstet Gynecol Clin North Am.* 2006;33:515-526.

Srivastava R, Thakar R, Sultan A. Female sexual dysfunction in obstetrics and gynecology. *Obstet Gynecol Surv.* 2008;63(8):527-537.

Intimate Partner and Sexual Violence

Morgan Mandigo and Orlene Thomas

INTIMATE PARTNER VIOLENCE

Definitions

- **Intimate partner violence (IPV)** may include physical injury, psychological abuse, sexual assault, progressive isolation, stalking, intimidation, and reproductive coercion. Domestic violence is an older term referring to these behaviors within a shared household.
- **Reproductive coercion** is a male behavior to promote pregnancy unwanted by the woman, including "birth control sabotage" or threatening to leave if she does not get pregnant.

Background and Statistics

- The IPV affects all ages, races, sexual orientations, and educational and economic backgrounds.
- It most commonly involves a heterosexual relationship with a female victim, often affected by low socioeconomic status, sexually transmitted infections (STIs), and unintended pregnancy.
- Long-standing abusive relationships develop a cycle in which a violent episode is followed by a period of reconciliation and apology.
- Fear, shame, powerlessness, and social isolation are barriers to escape.
- Eighty-five percent of victims are women.
- In primary care practices, nearly 25% of women endorse current or previous IPV.
- The IPV is the single most common cause of injury to women in the United States and the cause of about 30% of women's emergency room visits.
- One-third of female homicides in the United States are due to IPV.
- Only 54% of IPV is reported to police.
- Reproductive coercion is strongly correlated with (1) ethnic and/or racial minority, (2) low educational achievement, (3) lack of employment, (4) low socioeconomic status, (5) history of STI, (6) history of (or current) unwanted pregnancy, (7) IPV, and (8) increasing age difference between the individual and her partner.

Routine Intimate Partner Violence Screening

- Routine screening for IPV is recommended by the US Department of Health and Human Services, the Institute of Medicine, and the American College of Obstetricians and Gynecologists.
- In a study of trauma victims, a screening protocol increased detection from 5.6% to 30%.
- American College of Obstetricians and Gynecologists recommends screening at (1) new patient visits; (2) annual visits; (3) problem visits for unintended pregnancy or STI; (4) the following obstetric visits: first prenatal visit, once per trimester, and postpartum visit.

Table 37-1	SAFE Questionnaire[a]

- **S**tress/safety: Do you feel that your relationship is safe?
- **A**fraid/abused: Have you ever felt threatened, hurt, or afraid in a relationship?
- **F**riends/family: Do your friends or family know you have been hurt? Could you tell them, and would they be willing to help?
- **E**mergency plan: Do you have a safe place to go and the resources you need in an emergency?

[a]Data from Neufeld B. SAFE questions: overcoming barriers to the detection of domestic violence. *Am Fam Physician*. 1996;53:2575-2582.

- Guidelines for screening
- The environment should be safe, comfortable, and private.
- Realize the aggressor often accompanies the woman to monitor what is said.
- Ensure confidentiality.
- State that your screening is universal.
- Never ask what the patient did wrong or why she remains with her partner and avoid terms such as "abused" and "battered."
- Choose quick screening questions that feel comfortable and make screening routine. Several useful questionnaires have been developed to address abuse:
  - The SAFE questions (Table 37-1).
  - Abuse assessment during pregnancy (Table 37-2).
  - Reproductive coercion script (Table 37-3).
- If you suspect abuse and the patient denies it, readdress the issue during another visit.
- Make sure patients are aware that they can discuss any issues at future visits.

Suspecting Intimate Partner Violence

Maintain a high index of suspicion when there are
- Numerous office or emergency room visits for injury
- Inconsistent explanation for the injuries or a delay in seeking treatment

Table 37-2	Abuse Assessment During Pregnancy[a]

- Has anyone intentionally physically hurt you any time within the last year?
- Has anyone intentionally physically hurt you since you became pregnant?
- Has anyone forced you to engage in sexual activity within the last year?

[a]Data from McFarlane J, Parker B, Soeken K, Bullock L. Assessing for abuse during pregnancy. Severity and frequency of injuries and associated entry into prenatal care. *JAMA*. 1992;267:3176-3178.

Table 37-3	Reproductive Coercion Script[a]

- We've started talking to all patients about safe and healthy relationships because it can have a large impact on your health. Everything here is confidential, so I won't talk to anyone else about what is said unless . . . (modify according to your state laws).
- Has your partner ever forced you to do something sexually that you did not want to do or refused your request to use condoms?
- Does your partner support your decision about when or if you want to become pregnant?
- Has your partner ever tampered with your birth control or tried to get you pregnant when you didn't want to be?

[a]Based on Chamberlain L, Levenson R. *Reproductive Health and Partner Violence Guidelines: an Integrated Response to Intimate Partner Violence and Reproductive Coercion.* San Francisco, CA: Family Violence Prevention Fund; 2010. http://www.futureswithoutviolence.org/userfiles/file /HealthCare/Repro_Guide.pdf. Accessed November 11, 2018.

- Injuries that involve three or more body parts; affect the head, back, breast, and abdomen; or have various stages of healing
- Complaints such as fatigue, headache, gastrointestinal complaints, psychiatric disorders, eating disorders, and substance abuse
- Increased prevalence of sexually transmitted disease or vaginitis, sexual dysfunction, chronic pelvic pain, premenstrual syndrome, unintended pregnancy, medical noncompliance, and late/no prenatal care

Assessment of Risk

If IPV is confirmed, assess your patient's risk. Sample questions include the following:
- How were you hurt?
- Has this happened before?
- When did it first happen?
- How badly have you been hurt in the past?
- Have you ever needed to go to the emergency room for treatment?
- Have you ever been threatened with a weapon, or has a weapon ever been used on you?
- Have you ever tried to get a restraining order against a partner?
- Have your children ever seen or heard you being threatened or hurt?
- Do you know how you can get help for yourself if you are hurt or afraid?
- Is the violence getting worse?
- Are there threats of suicide or homicide?
- Is there a weapon in the home?

Interventions

- Empowerment is the first step because the victim may rely on her abuser for financial support and shelter or may fear repercussions.
- Provide support and do not attempt to make decisions for the patient. Reinforce that she is not to blame.

Table 37-4 Exit Plan for Domestic Violence Intervention[a]

The following exit plan has been proposed for a woman who feels that she or her children are in danger from her partner:

1. Have a change of clothes packed for herself and her children, including toiletries, necessary medications, and an extra set of house and car keys. These can be placed in a suitcase and stored with a friend or neighbor.
2. Cash, a checkbook, and savings account information may also be kept with a friend or neighbor.
3. Have available identification papers, such as birth certificates, social security cards, voter registration card, utility bills, and a driver's license because children will need to be enrolled in school, and financial assistance may be sought. If available, also take financial records, such as mortgage papers, rent receipts, or an automobile title.
4. Take something of special interest to each child, such as a book or toy.
5. Have a plan of exactly where to go, regardless of the time of day or night. This may be a friend or relative's home or a shelter for women and children.
6. Have a separate phone available to make emergency phone calls.

[a]Modified with permission from Helton A. Battering during pregnancy. *Am J Nurs.* 1986;86(8):910-913.

- Treat the patient's injuries and screen for suicidal tendencies, depression, and substance abuse. Document thoroughly, including direct quotations and photographs.
- Use social workers, counselors, and violence prevention programs. Provide resources and offer to let the patient call while in your office. Abusive partners often monitor cell phone usage; therefore, offering a separate cell phone may facilitate leaving an unsafe situation.
- Do not force a woman to leave before she is ready; leaving is associated with increased physical aggression, and resources need to be in place to minimize risk to the woman and her children during this critically vulnerable transition. When applicable, discuss court restraining orders and laws against stalking with the help of legal and social work resources.
- Review an exit plan or exit drill (Table 37-4).

Special Populations

Pregnancy

- Four percent to 8% of pregnant women report abuse during pregnancy.
- One in six abused women reports her partner was first abusive during a pregnancy.
- Abuse often escalates during the course of the pregnancy and postpartum.
- An IPV can result in miscarriage, preterm labor, low birth weight, and fetal injury or death.
- Women with an unintended pregnancy have a 3-fold higher risk of abuse than those with planned pregnancy.
- An IPV-related homicide is the number one cause of death in pregnancy.

Elder Abuse

- Typically perpetrated by adult family members or caregivers
- Affects about 2 million Americans
- Must be reported to the state Elder Abuse Hotline

Child Abuse

- Must be reported to Child Protective Services

Abuse of Disabled Women

- Patients with physical, cognitive, or emotional disabilities are at a higher risk for IPV and sexual abuse and should be screened at each visit.
- Must be reported to the Disabled Persons Protection Commission
- Sample screening questions include the following:
  - Has your partner prevented you from using a wheelchair, cane, respirator, or other assistive device?
  - Has your partner either threatened to deny you or refused to assist you with an important personal need such as taking your medicine, getting to the bathroom, getting out of bed, bathing, getting dressed, or getting food or drink?

Women With Undocumented Immigrant Status

- These patients may be threatened with deportation as a means of coercion, and they should be reassured that this is illegal.
- Give contact information for attorneys familiar with the process for obtaining nonimmigrant visas.

Sex Workers

- Women who trade sex for money and/or drugs are significantly more likely to become victims of coercive behavior and sexual abuse.
- Clinicians should screen for IPV at every encounter.
- Patients should be assured that illegal activity on their part should not prevent them from reporting violence to the authorities.

SEXUAL VIOLENCE

Definitions

- **Sexual violence:** any sexual activity where consent is not given (eg, assault, sexual harassment, threats, sex trafficking, female circumcision)
- **Sexual assault:** any sexual act performed on one person by another without consent
- **Rape:** a legal (not medical) term that should be avoided in medical records

Background

- One in six women will be sexually assaulted in her lifetime.
- Seventy-three percent of sexual assault victims know their offender.
- Approximately one in six sexual assaults is reported to the police.

Evaluation and Management

- A sensitive, yet comprehensive, workup should be done with an awareness of the guidelines for collection of forensic evidence.

- When possible and appropriate, refer to a medical center that can perform a sexual assault forensic exam. The following issues should be addressed:
  - Medical: injuries, STI exposure, pregnancy
  - Emotional: crisis intervention, counseling referrals
  - Forensics: documentation, proper collection and handling of evidence, court appearances

Resources

- Rape crisis centers/hotlines have trained crisis counselors/advocates who provide free 24-hour counseling, referral, and victim support services.
- Sexual assault response teams are multidisciplinary teams composed of law enforcement agents, medical providers, sexual assault advocates, and social workers who optimize both patient care and collection of evidence.
- When possible, physical exams should be performed by sexual assault forensic examiners, or sexual assault nurse examiners, who are trained to care for sexual assault victims, collect forensic evidence, and provide legal resources.
- Sexual assault evidence collection kits describe the steps of obtaining informed consent and performing a history and physical exam with emphasis on appropriate collection of forensic evidence.
- The Violence Against Women Act allows for victims to obtain a forensic exam free of charge even if they choose not to report the assault (ie, "Jane Doe rape kits").

Patient History

- A chaperone of the same gender as the patient should be present.
- Take a targeted gynecologic history, including last menstrual period, contraceptive use, and last consensual intercourse.
- Ask about injuries.
- Elicit specifics regarding oral, vaginal, or rectal penetration as well as condom use.
- Ask what the patient has done since the event (eg, showering, bathing, douching, voiding, defecating, changing clothes).
- Document the patient's exact description of the event without inflammatory language or judgment.

Physical Examination

- Obtain informed consent.
- A chaperone of the same gender as the patient should be present.
- The patient should undress with a sheet beneath her to capture any evidence.
- Collect appropriate clothing from the patient and give it to the proper personnel.
- Perform a full skin examination; evaluate all orifices for evidence of laceration, bruising, bite marks, or use of foreign objects; evaluate for abdominal trauma and broken bones.
- Tools such as a Wood's lamp and colposcope can be used to identify semen and subtle signs of trauma; toluidine blue can be used to stain broken skin.
- Document the patient's emotional state.
- Be thorough and systematic in your documentation; use drawings and photographs.

Diagnostic Testing

- Consider radiographic imaging.
- Obtain gonorrhea and chlamydia tests from all sites of contact.

- Obtain vaginal sample for trichomonas.
- Perform pregnancy test.
- Perform human immunodeficiency virus (HIV) counseling and testing.
- Obtain specimens for hepatitis B and C and syphilis.
- Perform screening for "date rape drugs" flunitrazepam (Rohypnol) and γ-hydroxy butyrate.

Treatment

- Treat traumatic injuries.
- Treat presumptively for STIs.
  - Gonorrhea and chlamydia: ceftriaxone 250 mg intramuscularly *AND* azithromycin 1 g orally *OR* doxycycline 100 mg twice daily for 1 week
  - If pregnancy or allergy: erythromycin 1.5 g orally and then 500 mg 4 times a day for 1 week
  - Trichomoniasis: metronidazole 2 g orally (consider an antiemetic for side effects)
- Provide hepatitis B vaccine if the victim has not received it already.
- In high-risk populations, consider penicillin G 2.4 million units for syphilis.
- Consult National Clinician's Post-Exposure Prophylaxis Hotline and offer antiretroviral therapy against HIV if <72 hours has elapsed since the assault (treatment is most effective if started within 4 h).
- Offer emergency contraception.
  - The chance of pregnancy after assault varies according to the menstrual cycle but is generally 2% to 4% in victims not protected by barrier contraception.
- Schedule follow-up visits: pregnancy testing in 1 to 2 weeks; syphilis and HIV testing in 6, 12, and 24 weeks; hepatitis B vaccination in 1 and 6 months.

Psychosocial Sequelae

- Victims may experience posttraumatic stress syndrome, depression, anxiety, and/or rape-trauma syndrome, which includes feelings of anger, fear, shame, anxiety, hypervigilance, nightmares, and physical symptoms.
- Involve social workers to initiate safety planning and referral to rape crisis programs and 24-hour hotlines.
- Follow up in 1 to 2 weeks.

Special Populations

Children

- Sexual abuse also encompasses nonsexual contact, such as pornography or exhibitionism.
- The majority of childhood sexual abuse occurs between ages 6 and 14 and especially between ages 12 and 14.
- The perpetrator is usually a relative or an acquaintance.
- Sexual abuse should be considered in any child with trauma or lacerations involving the posterior hymen or a vaginal foreign body.
- All suspected victims of child abuse should be referred to Child Protective Services.
- Evaluation and management should be performed by specially trained professionals. It is important to establish rapport with the child and record information in the child's own words. For young children, play-interviews and drawings may

promote communication. Note the child's behavior, mental state, and interactions. Ask about recent changes in sleep (night terrors) and behaviors. The examination should be head to toe, allowing the child to establish trust. Have a low threshold for performing an exam under anesthesia. Until the question of protection can be assured, providing temporary placement for the child is advisable. A trained therapist should be available to assist both victim and family.

Adolescents

- More than 75% of date rape, statutory rape, and incest are committed by an acquaintance.
- A history of nonvoluntary sexual activity has been associated with early initiation of voluntary sexual activity, unintended pregnancy, and poor use of contraceptives.
- Teenagers should be routinely asked: "Have you ever had sex when you didn't want to?"
- Examples of teenage empowerment messages include the following:
  - You have the right to say *no* to sexual activity.
  - You have the right to set sexual limits and insist that your partner honor them.
  - Be assertive. Stay sober. Recognize and avoid situations that may put you at risk.
  - Never leave a party with someone you don't know well.
  - No one should ever be forced or pressured into engaging in any unwanted sexual behavior.

Human Trafficking

- **Definition:** recruiting, harboring, transporting, or obtaining a person for involuntary servitude, peonage, debt bondage, or slavery
- **Background:** at least 15 000 individuals trafficked into the United States annually; 80% are female.
- Suspect human trafficking when you note any of the following:
  - Lack of any official identification
  - Vague answers about their situation
  - Inconsistencies to their stories
  - Avoidance of eye contact
  - No control of their money
- Resources are available at the National Human Trafficking Resource Center hotline: 1-888-373-7888.

Female Genital Mutilation

- Female genital mutilation (FGM), female genital cutting, and female circumcision describe the alteration of female genitalia for nontherapeutic reasons, usually without analgesia or aseptic technique. It represents a form of violence against girls/women and is considered a cultural, not religious, practice. Long-term sequelae of FGM include recurrent vaginal infections, menstrual abnormalities, urinary complications, fistulae, sexual dysfunction, vulvar abscesses, vulvodynia, and depression/anxiety. History of FGM is not an indication for a cesarean delivery.
- An FGM is usually grouped into the following types:
  - Type I: excision of the prepuce, which may also include part of the clitoris
  - Type II: complete excision of the clitoris, which may also include part of the labia minora

- Type III (infibulation): removing part or all of the external genitalia and reapproximating the labia majora to create a smaller introitus
- Type IV: all other procedures on the genitals, including stretching, scraping, pricking, burning, and piercing
- Defibulation may be required early in labor (epidural placement advised) in order to perform cervical assessments. If declined, cervical exams can also be performed rectally; however, the infibulated scar may obstruct the second stage of labor. Women with type III FGM have higher risks of peripartum hemorrhage and infection. The optimal timing for defibulation is during the second trimester.

SUGGESTED READINGS

Abdulcadir J, Catania L, Hindin MJ, Say L, Petignat P, Abdulcadir O. Female genital mutilation: a visual reference and learning tool for health care professionals. *Obstet Gynecol.* 2016;128(5):958-963.

American College of Obstetricians and Gynecologists Committee on Health Care for Underserved Women. ACOG Committee Opinion No. 518: intimate partner violence. *Obstet Gynecol.* 2012;119:412-417. (Reaffirmed 2019)

American College of Obstetricians and Gynecologists Committee on Health Care for Underserved Women. ACOG Committee Opinion No. 787: human trafficking (Replaces Committee Opinion No. 507, September 2011). *Obstet Gynecol.* 2019;134:e90-e95.

Breiding MJ, Armour BS. The association between disability and intimate partner violence in the United States. *Ann Epidemiol.* 2015;25:455-457.

Miller E, Decker MR, McCauley HL, et al. Pregnancy coercion, intimate partner violence, and unintended pregnancy. *Contraception.* 2010;81:316-322.

Roberts TA, Auinger P, Klein JD. Intimate partner abuse and the reproductive health of sexually active female adolescents. *J Adolesc Health.* 2005;36:380-385.

Zeitler MS, Paine AD, Breitbart V, et al. Attitudes about intimate partner violence screening among an ethnically diverse sample of young women. *J Adolesc Health.* 2006;39(1):119.e1-119.e8.

RESOURCES

National Domestic Violence Hotline: 1-800-799-SAFE (7233); https://www.thehotline.org/

Rape, Abuse & Incest National Network Hotline: 1-800-656-HOPE (4673)

National Coalition Against Domestic Violence: www.ncadv.org

Office on Violence Against Women (US Department of Justice): www.usdoj.gov/ovw

National Human Trafficking Resources Center Hotline: 1-888-373-7888

Futures Without Violence: www.futureswithoutviolence.org

National Network to End Domestic Violence: www.nnedv.org

National Resource Center on Domestic Violence: www.nrcdv.org

Pediatric Gynecology

Malorie Snider and Carla Bossano

Pediatric gynecology presents many challenges to the general obstetrician-gynecologist unaccustomed to dealing with these young patients. Most of the obstacles may be overcome by communicating effectively and allowing the patient to feel "in control."

- The interview is the most important aspect in determining the true reason for the visit. Due to different levels of maturity in each age group of children, different approaches to communication may be used. For children, including parental figures in the discussion is key, whereas for adolescents, determining the appropriate extent of parental involvement is more nuanced and requires consideration of patient preferences as well as issues of confidentiality.
- This chapter reviews the most commonly encountered problems in pediatric gynecology. Keep in mind that postpubertal pediatric patients may also present with gynecologic problems similar to women of childbearing age.

GYNECOLOGIC EVALUATION OF A PREPUBERTAL CHILD

- The examination presents a unique set of difficulties that may be overcome by following a few key guidelines:
  - Give the patient a sense of control.
  - Display a caring and gentle attitude at all times; the initial evaluation can set the tone for all future examinations.
  - The physical exam should include an overall assessment of other organ systems. This allows the patient to feel more comfortable in the exam room and the examiner to gain an overall appreciation of height, weight, skin disorders, hygiene, and other indicators of pubertal development.
  - If the child is very young or has suffered physical abuse, she may need to be evaluated under anesthesia.
  - Make it clear to the child that the examination is permitted by her caregiver and that if anyone else tries to touch her genital area, she should tell her caregiver.
  - A chaperone should be present during the physical exam.

General Pediatric Physical Exam

- The abdominal exam can be facilitated by placing the child's hand over the examiner's hand.
- Palpate the inguinal regions to identify potential hernias or gonadal masses.
- Tanner classification of the external genitalia and breast development should be used to quantify pubertal changes (Figure 38-1).

Pediatric Pelvic Exam: Positioning

- **Frog-leg posture:** child supine with feet together and knees bent outward; commonly used in the younger patient

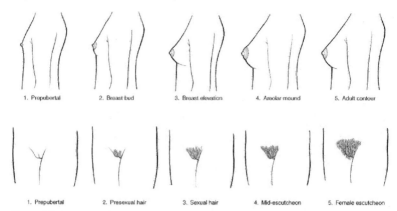

Figure 38-1. Tanner stages of development. Reprinted with permission from Callahan T. *Blueprints of Obstetrics and Gynecology*. 7th ed. Philadelphia, PA: Wolters Kluwer; 2018. Figure 20.3.

- **Knee-chest position:** when combined with a Valsalva maneuver, allows for assessment of the introital area. Using an otoscope for magnification or nasal speculum may help with visualization when the primary complaint is vaginal discharge or foreign bodies.
- **Supine lateral-spread method:** often sufficient enough to allow for visualization of the vestibular structures
- **Mother's lap positioning:** Allow the patient to sit in her mother's lap, knees bent, heels on mom's knees; combine with lateral traction of the labia for adequate exposure.
- When a child is uncooperative or evaluation of the genitalia is not optimal, an **exam under anesthesia** or a return visit may be necessary.

Pediatric Pelvic Exam: Assessment

- Note perineal hygiene, presence of pubic hair, hymenal configuration, size of the clitoris, and the presence of vulvovaginal lesions or vaginal discharge.
- Lateral downward traction of the labia allows visualization of the hymen in prepubertal girls. Sometimes, the cervix can also be visualized using this method as the vagina is very short in prepubertal girls. A colposcope or an ophthalmoscope can also be used to aid examination.
- Specimens, if indicated, may be collected from the vagina. Topical lidocaine jelly can be placed over the introitus by the patient's caregiver. Then, using a moistened small urethral Dacron swab, a vaginal sample can be collected. Alternatively, a butterfly needle/catheter can be altered by cutting off the butterfly/needle section and attaching the remaining tubing to a saline filled syringe. The tubing is then very gently placed past the hymen in the vagina. The vagina can be flushed and aspirated to collect a sample. A pediatric feeding tube attached to a 20-mL syringe also allows for more aggressive vaginal irrigation if needed.
- Internal bimanual exam or traditional speculum exam should not be completed in prepubertal girls without anesthesia. Rectoabdominal exam can be considered in an awake patient if concern for pelvic mass.

- If speculum exam is needed during an exam under anesthesia, a pediatric speculum or even a nasal speculum can be used in rare cases.
- **Common exam findings**
  - Newborn child: It is important to recognize that maternal estrogen influences physical development of the newborn child. Vulvar edema, whitish pink vaginal mucosa, vaginal discharge, and breast enlargement may be normal in the newborn and should regress in the first 8 weeks of life.
  - Toddler-prepubertal child: unestrogenized vaginal mucosa appears thin, hyperemic, and atrophic. Capillary beds may appear like roadmaps and are often mistaken for inflammation, especially around the sulcus of the vestibule and in the periurethral area.

Pediatric Exam: Documentation

- If appropriate, a labeled sketch of the external genitalia should be included in the medical record with a diamond-shaped space used to represent the vestibule of a child in the supine position. Twelve o'clock should represent the clitoris, and 6 o'clock should represent the posterior fourchette.
- The hymen should be described. Of note, there are many variations of a normal hymen and terms such as *intact* or *virginal* should often be avoided. A description of configuration, clefts, tears, tags, etc, should be noted.
- Describe key components include assessing Tanner stage (see Figure 38-1), description of labia majora; labia minora; urethral meatus; hymen; and the presence of any discolorations, hemangiomas, vulvovaginal lesions, or vaginal discharge.

GYNECOLOGIC EVALUATION OF AN ADOLESCENT

Special Considerations in Care of the Adolescent

Although the focus of this chapter is on the evaluation and management of prepubertal pediatric patients, several recommendations should be noted for the evaluation of adolescent patients.

- As many young women first engage in sexual activity during their adolescent years, taking a sexual history is an important part of the adolescent gynecologic assessment.
- Contraceptive counseling and screening for sexually transmitted infections should be routinely offered to adolescents seeking gynecologic care (see chapters 27 and 28).
- It is important to become familiar with federal and state-specific minor consent laws and to educate adolescent patients regarding their confidentiality rights as well as any limitations (eg, parental notification prior to abortion in some states).

Adolescent Gynecologic Exam

- Given changes in pap smear guidelines (see chapter 49), a pelvic exam is not always necessary in the adolescent patient.
- Pelvic exams should be performed in patients under the age of 21 years only if indicated by chief complaint and history.
- An evaluation of external genitalia can still be performed to confirm normal anatomy and development.

- Testing for sexually transmitted infections such as gonorrhea, chlamydia, or trichomoniasis can be performed from urine samples or vaginal swabs.
- If indicated, a Huffman (1/2 × 4 in) or Pederson (7/8 × 4 in) speculum is most appropriate for use in this patient population.
- Although evaluation of Tanner stage may be appropriate at an initial visit, clinical breast exams are not necessary unless indicated by complaint or history until age 25 years.

COMMON PEDIATRIC GYNECOLOGY COMPLAINTS

Vulvovaginitis

- Vaginal discharge is the most common gynecologic complaint in the prepubertal girl and accounts for 40% to 50% of visits to a pediatric gynecology clinic.

History: Key Points

- Note the duration, onset, consistency, quality, and color of the discharge.
- Note other associated symptoms, which commonly include vulvar pruritus/burning/irritation, dysuria, bleeding, foul odor, or perianal itching.
- Inquire regarding visible abnormalities such as rashes, erythema, and lesions.
- Review child's toileting habits including diaper use, potty training status, bowel movement regularity, bedwetting, and cleaning habits (back to front wiping, self-cleaning versus caretaker cleaning).
- Review child's bathing habits, including frequency and types of soaps/lotions/bubble baths used.
- Review general medical history, especially any history of atopy, and recent systemic infections.
- Inquire about frequent swimming/bathing suit use.

Physical Examination

- General physical examination should be completed and should focus on looking for any signs of other skin conditions, such as eczema.
- Pelvic examination should begin with assessment of the vulva and perineum. Assess for presence or absence of visible discharge, skin changes (rashes, erythema, hypo- or hyperpigmentation, excoriations), signs of poor hygiene (stool/debris on vulva or between labia).
- The vagina should then be inspected by downward traction of the labia. Assess for any visible discharge and note appearance of hymen (configuration, signs of trauma), if cervix is visible.
- Collect a sample of any discharge for microscopic examination and culture. Avoid contact with the hymen in prepubertal children.

Etiologies of Vulvovaginitis

Differential diagnosis for vulvovaginitis in a prepubertal child includes nonspecific vulvovaginitis, infections, foreign bodies, dermatoses, systemic illnesses, and anatomic abnormalities.

Nonspecific, Environmental, or Chemical Vaginitis

- Twenty-five percent to 75% of cases are likely caused by poor hygiene, soaps, obesity, association with upper respiratory infections, and irritating clothing in the setting of unestrogenized mucosa.

- Treatment includes discontinuation of the causative agent, perineal hygiene (wiping front to back), sitz baths, loose fitting clothing, cotton underwear, hypoallergenic soaps, wet wipes, and emollients. The child should also be instructed on spreading her legs wide apart and leaning forward during urination to avoid urine pooling in the vagina. Sitting facing the toilet may facilitate this.
- If there is no resolution in 2 to 3 weeks or if initial symptoms are severe, evaluate for a foreign body or infection.
- If symptoms are severe, consider a trial of antibiotics and topical steroid cream.

Infection

- Normal prepubertal vaginal flora includes lactobacilli, α-hemolytic streptococci, *Staphylococcus epidermidis*, diphtheroid, and gram-negative enteric organisms, especially *Escherichia coli*. Candida is present in only 3% to 4% of prepubertal girls.
- Shifts in flora resulting from inoculation by bacteria, viruses, and yeast can result in inflammation and discharge.
- Although many cases of vulvovaginitis may be nonspecific, the most common pathogenic bacteria causing vulvovaginitis include group A *Streptococcus*, *Haemophilus influenzae*, *Staphylococcus aureus*, *Streptococcus pneumoniae*, and *E coli*.
- Sexually transmitted diseases can cause vulvovaginitis in a prepubertal child and if found are typically the result of sexual abuse.
- Children may pass respiratory flora from the nose and oropharynx to the genitalia area, making this a possible etiology of vulvovaginitis.
- Children with chronic, nightly episodes of vulvar or perianal itching should be evaluated for *Enterobius vermicularis* (pinworms).
- Children with malodorous discharge should be evaluated for anaerobic infections.
- Cultures should guide antibiotic therapy (Table 38-1). In addition, treatment should include vulvar hygiene measures as for nonspecific vulvovaginitis.

Foreign Bodies

- The foreign bodies are most common in girls aged 2 to 4 years and can vary from wads of toilet paper, buttons, or coins to peanuts and crayons. Antibiotics should be started before removal.
- Retained foreign bodies in the vagina often present with bloody, brown, or purulent discharge of several weeks' duration. Persistent vaginal discharge in a toddler or young girl warrants an exam under anesthesia.
- If the foreign body remains undetected, peritonitis can develop from ascending infection. The child may present with signs/symptoms of systemic infection such as fever and abdominal pain.
- A careful examination of the vaginal wall for any defects or additional embedded foreign bodies should be performed after the object has been removed.
- Once the foreign body is removed, hygiene measures as for nonspecific vaginitis should be followed and the patient should monitor for resolution of symptoms.

Dermatologic Conditions

- Lichen sclerosis, psoriasis, atopic dermatitis, and contact dermatitis of the vulva may all present with symptoms similar to vulvovaginitis. These conditions may respond to topical corticosteroids.
- Careful history and physical exam can identify nongenital symptoms that could point to the correct diagnosis. Systemic dermatologic conditions such as eczema and psoriasis are generally treated as appropriate.

Table 38-1	Treatment of Specific Vulvovaginal Infections in the Prepubertal Child[a]

Etiology	Treatment
Streptococcus pyogenes	Penicillin V potassium; amoxicillin
Haemophilus influenzae	Amoxicillin; amoxicillin/clavulanate; cefuroxime axetil; cefpodoxime; azithromycin
Staphylococcus aureus	Cephalexin; dicloxacillin; amoxicillin-clavulanate; trimethoprim/sulfamethoxazole; clindamycin
Streptococcus pneumonia	Amoxicillin; amoxicillin/clavulanate; cefdinir; cefpodoxime; cefuroxime
Shigella	Trimethoprim/sulfamethoxazole; ampicillin; ceftriaxone; azithromycin
Chlamydia trachomatis	≤45 kg: erythromycin 50 mg/kg/d (divide in 4 doses/d) × 14 d ≥45 kg: <8 y: azithromycin 1 g once ≥8 y: azithromycin 1 g once OR doxycycline 100 mg twice a day orally × 7 d
Neisseria gonorrhoeae	<45 kg: ceftriaxone 125 mg IM PLUS treat for chlamydia as above >45 kg: treated with adult regimens (see chapter 27)
Candida	Topical nystatin, miconazole, clotrimazole, or terconazole cream; fluconazole orally
Trichomonas	Metronidazole 15 mg/kg/d given 3 times a day (max 250 mg 3 times a day) × 7 d; or 50 mg/kg single dose (max 2 g)
Enterobius vermicularis (pinworms)	Mebendazole (Vermox) chewable 100-mg tablet, repeated in 2 wk

Abbreviation: IM, intramuscularly.
[a]Modified with permission from Emans SJ, Laufer MR, Goldstein DP, eds. *Pediatric and Adolescent Gynecology.* 6th ed. Philadelphia, PA: Wolters Kluwer Health/Lippincott Williams & Wilkins; 2011:49. Table 4-3.

- Lichen sclerosus presents with pruritus/irritation, bleeding, and dysuria. Exam findings include hypopigmentation and erythematous plaques in a figure-eight distribution. Thinning and cigarette paper appearance of the skin may be present. The treatment is high-potency corticosteroids as scarring can cause permanent sexual dysfunction. Diagnosis is made by physical exam and rarely requires biopsy in this population.
- Aphthous ulcers are typically seen girls 10 to 15 years old and are very painful, with a purulent base and raised edges; the patient will frequently have nonspecific systemic symptoms as well. The etiology is idiopathic, but it is thought to be viral (eg, influenza, Epstein-Barr virus, cytomegalovirus). Oral corticosteroids are frequently prescribed. If these ulcers are recurrent, consider Behçet disease.

Systemic Illness

- Varicella, measles, Epstein-Barr virus, Crohn disease, Stevens-Johnson syndrome, diabetes mellitus, Behçet syndrome, and Kawasaki syndrome may all result in vaginal discharge, vesicles, fistulas, ulcers, and inflammation.
- Treatment should be based on etiology.

Anatomic Abnormalities

- An ectopic ureter may result in urinary leakage. It is often detected on prenatal ultrasound. After birth, an ultrasound can be used for diagnosis, followed by magnetic resonance imaging (MRI) if indicated.
- A high hymenal opening may impair vaginal drainage; hymenectomy is curative in these cases.
- Urethral prolapse (see "Urethral Prolapse" below)

Prepubertal Vaginal Bleeding

- Vaginal bleeding prior to menarche can result from a wide array of causes but must be taken seriously because some conditions can be life-threatening. Etiologies may include infection, anatomic abnormalities, genital tumors, hormonal abnormalities, foreign body, trauma, or sexual abuse.

Vulvovaginitis

- Any cause of vulvovaginitis may result in vaginal bleeding. See "Vulvovaginitis" above for evaluation and management.

Urethral Prolapse

- The average age of onset is 5 years, and occurrence is more common in African Americans.
- Medical treatment consists of a short-term course of estrogen cream.
- Urinary retention or a large mass may require resection of the prolapsed tissue and insertion of an indwelling catheter.
- Differential diagnosis includes urethral polyps, caruncles, cysts, and prolapsed ureteroceles.

Genital Tumors

- **Sarcoma botryoides** (rhabdomyosarcoma) is the most common malignant tumor of the genital tract in girls. This fast-growing, aggressive tumor arises from the submucosa of the vagina. Ninety percent of cases are diagnosed before age 5 years, with a peak incidence at ages 2 to 3 years. The physical exam is notable for a polypoid soft mass (resembling a bunch of grapes) protruding through the vagina; this tumor can cause vaginal bleeding and abdominal pain. Prognosis is improved with multimodal treatment including surgery, chemotherapy, and radiation.

Endometrial Shedding

- Causes of endometrial shedding are outlined in Table 38-2 and often relate to a hormonal abnormality. Precocious puberty is often associated with endometrial shedding in this population (see the section "Disorders of Puberty").

Trauma and Sexual Abuse

See chapter 37 and "Traumatic Injuries" section below.

Table 38-2	Causes of Endometrial Shedding in Children

- Physiologic neonatal withdrawal bleed in the first 2 wk of life secondary to maternal estrogen withdrawal
- Isolated premature menarche
- Iatrogenic or factitious precocious puberty caused by medications that contain exogenous estrogens
- Idiopathic precocious puberty
- Functional ovarian cysts
- Ovarian neoplasms
- McCune-Albright syndrome
- Central nervous system lesions
- Hormone-producing neoplasms
- Hypothyroidism

Traumatic Injuries

- The period of highest incidence is between ages 4 and 12 years, with 75% of all genital injuries occurring in young girls. Because of differences in anatomy between a child and an adult, a seemingly innocuous lesion can suggest serious injury. Common injuries include the following:
  - **Straddle injuries**
    - Most present as a swollen area of painful ecchymosis or hematoma over the labia; the mons, clitoris, and urethra can be involved. If hematuria is present, consider a voiding cystourethrogram to rule out bladder or urethra injury. Periurethral injuries can result in swelling and urinary retention. Early placement of a urinary catheter is advised.
    - Treat with observation and cold compresses for the first 6 hours. If the hematoma remains the same size or becomes smaller, warm sitz baths are often all that are required. Analgesics and prophylactic antibiotics can be used when a hematoma at the urethral orifice is causing pain and poor urination.
  - **Accidental penetration**
    - Most frequently seen between ages 2 and 4 years, accidental penetration is often the result of falling on a sharp object (eg, pen or pencil).
    - Presentation often includes hematuria, vaginal discharge, or bleeding. A puncture wound may be intraperitoneal with rectal pain or bleeding as the presenting complaint. In an unstable patient with an injury above the hymen, laparoscopy or laparotomy should be performed.
    - Workup involves examination with abdominal radiography, anoscopy, vaginoscopy, and/or sigmoidoscopy. Microscopic hematuria warrants careful urethral catheterization. Resistance to the passage of a catheter requires a voiding cystourethrogram. Catheterization should not be attempted with gross hematuria.
  - **Lacerations**
    - Often secondary to forceful abduction of the legs, gymnastic exercise, water-skiing, bicycle accidents, or motor vehicle accidents.

- ○ Lacerations of the vaginal orifice frequently extend into the fornix.
- ○ Examination under anesthesia must be performed to determine the extent of the injury and rule out involvement of the rectovaginal septum or peritoneal cavity.

Sexual Abuse

- Suspect with unusual injury patterns or odd behavior as well as the following associated complaints: genital trauma, bleeding, chronic genital pain, sexually transmitted infections, anal inflammation, recurrent urinary tract infections, abdominal pain, enuresis/encopresis, or anorexia.
- Behavioral changes include aggression, self-injury, conduct disorders, sleep disturbances, excessive phobias, depression, substance abuse, problems in school, or inappropriate knowledge of sexual behavior.
- Obtain history separately from the child if possible. Avoid leading questions. A doll may provide the young child with a way to express what has happened. A multidisciplinary approach involving the child's pediatrician and social worker may also be beneficial.
- If abuse is suspected, the patient should be referred to an appropriate emergency department with individuals trained in collecting forensic evidence, preferably within 24 hours of the event. All suspected victims of child abuse, including sexual abuse, should be referred to child protective services (see chapter 37).
- Sexual play involves children of the same age without coercion and is a normal part of development.

Labial Adhesions

- In the low estrogen environment of childhood, the labia may fuse in response to any genital trauma, even diaper rash.
- Adhesive vulvitis caused by chronic irritation is common between ages 2 and 6 years.
- Asymptomatic labial adhesions do not require treatment and will resolve spontaneously with increasing estrogen levels in puberty.
- If urinary retention or urinary tract infections occur, treatment is required and involves application of estrogen cream along the white line of the adhesion, with gentle traction twice daily for 2 to 6 weeks. Recurrence is common after treatment. Acute urinary retention requires surgical excision.

Adnexal Masses/Ovarian Torsion

- See chapter 33 on adnexal masses for full discussion of differential diagnosis of adnexal masses.
- Adnexal masses are frequently identified in postmenarchal adolescent girls and should in general be treated in a similar fashion as women of childbearing age.
- Adnexal masses in prepubertal girls are uncommon and are usually identified by caregivers as an abdominal mass or with increased abdominal girth. Acute abdominal pain can also be seen if torsion occurs. Transabdominal ultrasound is the test of choice for initial evaluation. History and exam should look for signs of a hormonally active tumor resulting in precocious puberty.

- Ovarian torsion is often seen to occur with normal ovaries in prepubertal girls secondary to abdominal location of ovaries and a long utero-ovarian ligament. If torsion is suspected and surgical management is planned, ovarian conservation is most appropriate in almost all cases. Even if prolonged torsion is suspected, reduction of torsion is often all that is indicated. Shortening of the utero-ovarian ligament can be considered as a preventive measure as torsion can be recurrent.

Surgical Considerations for Laparoscopy in Children

- Laparoscopy is preferred whenever possible. In the pediatric population, it should be performed by a surgeon experienced in the surgical care of children.
- Patient positioning is often supine as access to the vagina is most likely not necessary. Uterine manipulators are not necessary in prepubertal children as the uterus is very small and unlikely to interfere with visualization.
- In general, open versus closed techniques for abdominal entry are preferred, given the shorter distance from abdominal wall to major vessels. Trocars or instruments 5 mm or smaller should be used. Because of the high risk of hernia, all fascial incisions should be closed.
- Insufflation pressures vary greatly depending on the size of the patient and the strength of the abdominal wall. In children, pressures of 8 to 10 mm Hg are typical.

DISORDERS OF PUBERTY

Puberty is a result of pulsatile gonadotropin-releasing hormone (GnRH) secretion and activation of the hypothalamic-pituitary-gonadal axis. The onset of puberty is generally between 8 and 13 years old in girls. Tanner stages (see Figure 38-1) are used to describe pubertal development.

Delayed Puberty

- Delay of puberty can be caused by anatomic abnormalities, chromosomal disorders, neoplastic growths, or nutritional deficiencies. It commonly presents as a physical delay in maturation combined with amenorrhea.
- Causes of delayed puberty can be classified based on the level of follicle-stimulating hormone (FSH) present, as outlined in Table 38-3.

Hypergonadotropic Hypogonadism (High Follicle-Stimulating Hormone)

- A sufficient amount of gonadotropins are present, but the ovaries are not responsive and therefore do not produce sex steroids. This lack of negative feedback causes the FSH to be high.
- Gonadal dysgenesis
  - Presents as a phenotypic female with lack of or insufficient pubertal development
  - May have some secondary sex characteristics and spontaneous menstruation; most often associated with primary amenorrhea
  - **Turner syndrome** (45, X) occurs in 1 in 2000 to 2500 girls. Phenotype includes primary amenorrhea and short stature.
  - Patients with **Swyer syndrome** (46, XY) often have a normal-to-tall stature. It is caused by a mutation or structural abnormality of the Y chromosome.

Table 38-3	**An Overview of Causes of Delayed Puberty**

FSH Level	Differential Diagnosis
High (>30 mIU/mL)	• Gonadal dysgenesis syndromes: Turner syndrome, Swyer syndrome • Primary ovarian failure
Low (<10 mIU/mL)	• Constitutional delay • Intracranial neoplasms • Isolated gonadotropin deficiencies • Hormone deficiencies • Kallmann syndrome • Prader-Willi syndrome • Laurence-Moon-Biedl syndrome • Chronic disease and malnutrition
Normal	• *Anatomic deformities* result in normal development with primary amenorrhea. • Imperforate hymen • Transverse vaginal septum • Müllerian agenesis

Abbreviation: FSH, follicle-stimulating hormone.

- Primary ovarian failure
  - Ovaries develop but do not contain oocytes; may be associated with chemotherapy, radiation, galactosemia, gonadotropin resistance, autoimmune ovarian failure, or ovarian failure secondary to previous infection.
  - Treatment involves administration of exogenous estrogen and progesterone to avoid osteoporosis and facilitate development of secondary sexual characteristics.

Hypogonadotropic Hypogonadism (Low Follicle-Stimulating Hormone)

- An insufficient level of gonadotropins is present to permit follicular development, and therefore, sex steroids are not produced.
- **Chronic disease:** Conditions including states of malnutrition (eg, starvation, anorexia nervosa, cystic fibrosis, Crohn disease, diabetes mellitus, and hypothyroidism) may disrupt GnRH production.
- **Constitutional delay:** A delay in the GnRH pulse generator postpones the normal physiologic events of puberty.
- **Intracranial neoplasms:** Craniopharyngiomas and pituitary adenomas may cause delayed puberty. Visual symptoms are often associated with these tumors, as are short stature and diabetes insipidus. Diagnosis is by computed tomography (CT) or MRI of the head.
- **Isolated gonadotropin deficiencies:** often secondary to abnormalities in genes encoding proteins related to GnRH, FSH, or luteinizing hormone (LH).
- **Hormone deficiencies:** Aberrations of growth hormone, thyroid hormone, or prolactin can affect puberty.

- **Kallmann syndrome:** presents with a classic triad of anosmia, hypogonadism, and color blindness. The hypothalamus cannot secrete GnRH due to dysfunction in the arcuate nucleus. Few or no secondary sexual characteristics are present.
- **Prader-Willi syndrome:** An autosomal deletion and imprinting disorder associated with obesity, emotional instability, and delayed puberty due to hypothalamic dysfunction.
- Other uncommon causes include **Laurence-Moon** and **Bardet-Biedl syndromes**.

Eugonadism (Normal Follicle-Stimulating Hormone)

- In cases of eugonadal pubertal delay, the hypothalamic-pituitary-gonadal axis remains intact, but primary amenorrhea occurs secondary to anatomic abnormalities in the genitourinary tract, androgen insensitivity, or inappropriate positive feedback mechanisms.
  - Anatomic abnormalities: See "Congenital Anomalies of the Female Reproductive Tract."
  - Androgen insensitivity: See "Ambiguous Genitalia."
- Other causes of primary amenorrhea with eugonadism include anovulation, androgen-producing adrenal disease, and polycystic ovarian syndrome.

Key Points in Evaluation and Management of Delayed Puberty

- A careful medical, surgical, and family history and exam including Tanner staging are important initial steps of evaluation.
- Initial laboratory workup should include serum FSH, prolactin, thyroid-stimulating hormone, and complete blood count.
- Further workup should be determined by initial findings with management based on etiology.

Precocious Puberty

- **Precocious puberty** occurs in only 1 of 10 000 girls and is defined as the presence of secondary sexual characteristics at an age >2.5 standard deviations below the mean (ie, 6 y old in African Americans and 7 y old in Caucasians).
- Accelerated growth velocity and rapid bone growth can result in short adult stature.
- Causes are divided into gonadotropin-dependent and gonadotropin-independent disorders.

Gonadotropin-Dependent Disorders—Central Precocious Puberty

- Related to premature development of the hypothalamic-pituitary axis.
- Most commonly **idiopathic**; secondary sexual characteristics progress in normal sequence but more rapidly than in normal puberty and may fluctuate between progression and regression.
- Characteristic signs and symptoms include breast development without pubic hair development, an increase in height, acne, oily skin or hair, and emotional changes.
- May be transmitted in an autosomal recessive fashion.
- Often ovarian follicular cysts are present due to elevated levels of LH and FSH.
- Other causes involve **central nervous system disease**, particularly mass effects near the hypothalamus. The most common neoplasm is a hamartoma in the posterior hypothalamus.
  - Disease often involves areas surrounding the hypothalamus; mass effect, radiation, or ectopic GnRH-secreting cells are thought to cause premature activation of pulsatile secretion of GnRH from the hypothalamus.

- Diagnosis by CT or MRI of the head; history may be significant for headache, mental status changes, mental retardation, dysmorphic syndromes, and the premature development of secondary sexual characteristics.
- Treatment should be directed at the underlying cause; the location of many of such tumors makes resection difficult, and, as a result, chemotherapy or radiation may be indicated.
- Treatment with a GnRH agonist can result in a short burst of gonadotropin release, followed by downregulation and a decrease in the level of circulating gonadotropins. Follow estradiol levels to make appropriate dose adjustments.

Gonadotropin-Independent Disorders—Pseudoprecocious Puberty

- Exogenous hormones causing early puberty result from a peripheral source. Development of pubertal characteristics may be more rapid than with central causes due to a faster initial rate of hormone production.
- Differential diagnosis includes estrogen-secreting tumors, benign follicular ovarian cysts, McCune-Albright syndrome, Peutz-Jeghers syndrome, adrenal disorders, and primary hypothyroidism.
- Estrogen-secreting ovarian tumors
  - See chapter 52.
- Benign ovarian cysts
  - Most common form of estrogen-secreting masses in children.
  - May require a diagnostic laparoscopy or possibly exploratory laparotomy to differentiate from a malignant tumor. Removal of the cyst may be therapeutic.
- McCune-Albright syndrome
  - Triad: café au lait spots, polyostotic fibrous dysplasia, and cysts of skull and long bones; precocious puberty is present in 40% of cases.
  - Associated with rapid breast development and early occurrence of menarche
  - Sexual precocity results from recurrent follicular cysts. Removal of cyst is not helpful.
  - Aromatase inhibitors may help control symptoms.
  - Evaluate with serial pelvic sonograms to detect the presence of gonadal tumors.
- Peutz-Jeghers syndrome
  - Commonly characterized by mucocutaneous pigmentation and gastrointestinal polyposis
  - Also associated with rare sex cord tumors, including epithelial tumors of the ovary, dysgerminomas, or Sertoli-Leydig cell tumors, whose estrogen secretion may result in feminization and incomplete sexual precocity
  - Girls with Peutz-Jeghers syndrome should be screened with serial pelvic sonograms.
- Adrenal disorders
  - Some adrenal adenomas secrete estrogen and may result in sexual precocity.
- Primary hypothyroidism
  - Characterized by premature breast development and galactorrhea without an associated growth spurt

Key Points in Evaluation and Management of Precocious Puberty

- Perform a detailed evaluation with Tanner staging.
- Laboratory data should include LH, FSH, prolactin, estradiol, progesterone, 17-hydroxyprogesterone, dehydroepiandrosterone, dehydroepiandrosterone sulfate, thyroid-stimulating hormone, thyroxine, and human chorionic gonadotropin.
- A GnRH stimulation test can definitively diagnose central precocious puberty.

- Obtain an x-ray to determine bone age. Head CT or MRI can rule out an intracranial mass. Abdominal/pelvic ultrasound can be used to evaluate the ovaries.
- Goals for management include maximizing adult height and delaying maturation. Treat the intracranial, ovarian, or adrenal pathology if present and attempt to reduce associated emotional problems.

Premature Thelarche

- **Premature thelarche** is defined as bilateral breast development without other signs of sexual maturation in girls before age 8 years. It commonly occurs by age 2 years and is rare after age 4 years.
- The etiology is unclear, but exogenous estrogen must be excluded.
- Precocious puberty must be ruled out.
- Document the appearance of the vaginal mucosa, breast size, and presence or absence of a pelvic mass.
- Obtain bone age. It is within normal range in premature thelarche.
- Perform pelvic ultrasonography, which should exclude ovarian pathology.
- Obtain plasma estrogen levels. They may be mildly elevated; significant elevations suggest another etiology.
- In idiopathic cases, regression often occurs after a few months but may persist for several years.

AMBIGUOUS GENITALIA

Male Feminization

- Genetic males (XY) undergo feminization related to androgen insensitivity.
- **Complete androgen insensitivity** or **"testicular feminization"**
  - Transmitted in a maternal X-linked recessive fashion
  - Pathophysiology: Androgen presence is incapable of inducing maturation of the Wolffian duct. Antimüllerian hormone is present, and müllerian duct formation remains inhibited. The resulting phenotype is female, with a vagina derived from the urogenital sinus that ends in a blind pouch and testes that often descend through the inguinal canal.
  - Clinical presentation: primary amenorrhea, Tanner stage V breast development, scant axillary and pubic hair
  - Management: Gonadectomy is recommended once sexual maturation is complete secondary to an increased incidence of malignancy; exogenous estrogen therapy is also recommended.
- **Incomplete androgen insensitivity**
  - Less common, with presentation ranging from near complete masculinization to near complete failure of virilization
  - As minimal sensitivity to androgens is present, the Wolffian duct system develops to some extent, although spermatogenesis usually remains absent.
  - Physical exam may include a range of clitoromegaly or ambiguous genitalia.
  - Sex assignment depends on the degree of masculinization.
- **5-α Reductase deficiency**
  - Genotypic males (XY) who are often phenotypically female or have ambiguous genitalia in the prepubertal state and undergo virilization at puberty, becoming more phenotypically male. Testicular function is normal, and there is no breast development.

Female Virilization

- Genetic females (XX) are exposed to increased androgen levels that lead to inappropriate virilization, most often an indicator of organic disease in girls.
- Virilizing **congenital adrenal hyperplasia**: most commonly associated with deficiency of 21-hydroxylase, an autosomal recessive disorder; may present in a newborn with ambiguous genitalia and possible salt wasting due to mineralocorticoid deficiency. Virilization may also be delayed until later childhood in less severe forms.
- **Cushing disease** can manifest as growth failure, with or without virilization, obesity, striae, or moon facies.
- **Ovarian tumors:** Sertoli-Leydig cell tumor (eg, arrhenoblastoma) is the most common virilizing ovarian tumor. Others include lipoid cell tumor and gonadoblastoma.

CONGENITAL ANOMALIES OF THE FEMALE REPRODUCTIVE TRACT

Anatomic disorders may present as primary amenorrhea, chronic pelvic pain, mucocolpos, hematocolpos, or hematometra.

- **Imperforate hymen** may present as a bulging, translucent mass at the introitus in the newborn or as cyclic pain, abdominal mass, hematocolpos, and/or a bluish perineal bulge after menarche. Imperforate hymen may regress over the course of childhood. In cases where there is no regression by menarche, surgical intervention is required to incise the hymen and allow stored debris (hematocolpos) to escape. Additional hymenal abnormalities including microperforate and septate hymen may also require surgical intervention but do not completely obstruct the vaginal introitus, and therefore, symptoms are usually absent or less severe.
- **Transverse vaginal septum** is caused by failure of canalization of müllerian tubules and the sinovaginal bulb, leaving a membrane present. Presentation and examination may be similar to an imperforate hymen; however, 35% to 86% are found in the mid to upper vagina. If the membrane is thin, it can be incised and dilated. If thick, evaluation with ultrasound or MRI can guide surgical decision making.
- **Longitudinal vaginal septum** is often associated with uterine and/or renal anomalies. Complaints include persistent bleeding despite the use of a tampon. Surgical correction is indicated. An obstructed hemivagina is frequently seen with ipsilateral renal agenesis.
- **Müllerian agenesis:** Failure of the müllerian tract to develop results in a blind vaginal pouch without uterus or fallopian tubes present. Ovaries are not of müllerian origin and puberty progresses as usual with primary amenorrhea as a presenting complaint. This must be distinguished from androgen insensitivity, as described previously. One-third of these patients have associated urinary tract anomalies, and 12% have skeletal anomalies. A neovagina can be created by progressive dilation or surgery.
- **Vaginal atresia/agenesis** occurs in 1 in 5 to 10 000. Presentation is similar to that of a transverse septum in adolescent girls. Treatment may involve progressive vaginal dilation or surgical reconstruction. Up to 50% have other congenital anomalies, so a full workup is warranted.

SUGGESTED READINGS

American College of Obstetricians and Gynecologists Committee on Adolescent Health Care. ACOG Committee Opinion No. 598: the initial reproductive health visit. *Obstet Gynecol.* 2014;123:1143-1147. (Reaffirmed 2018)

Bacon JL, Romano ME, Quint EH. Clinical recommendation: labial adhesions. *J Pediatr Adolesc Gynecol.* 2015;28(5):405-409.

Bercaw-Pratt JL, Boardman LA, Simms-Cendan JS. Clinical recommendation: pediatric lichen sclerosus. *J Pediatr Adolesc Gynecol.* 2014;27(2):111-116.

Carel JC, Léger J. Clinical practice. Precocious puberty. *N Engl J Med.* 2008;358:2366-2377.

Chan SH, Lara-Torre E. Surgical considerations and challenges in the pediatric and adolescent gynecologic patient. *Best Pract Res Clin Obstet Gynaecol.* 2018;48:128-136.

Emans SJ, Laufer MR, Goldstein DP, eds. *Pediatric and Adolescent Gynecology.* 6th ed. Philadelphia, PA: Lippincott Williams & Wilkins; 2011.

Jacobs AM, Alderman EM. Gynecologic examination of the prepubertal girl. *Pediatr Rev.* 2014;35:97-104.

Shulman L. Müllerian anomalies. *Clin Obstet Gynecol.* 2008;51(2):214-222.

Zuckerman A, Romano M. Clinical recommendation: vulvovaginitis. *J Pediatr Adolesc Gynecol.* 2016;29(6):673-679.

III Reproductive Endocrinology and Infertility

39 The Menstrual Cycle

Brittany L. Schuh and Chailee Faythe Moss

An understanding of the menstrual cycle is fundamental to most interventions in the field of gynecology and obstetrics. This chapter discusses the physiology of the normal cycle. A thorough understanding of this physiology will illuminate the mechanisms by which pathologic changes in the cycle lead to gynecologic disease. Spontaneous, cyclic menstruation requires an intact and functional hypothalamic-pituitary-ovarian axis, endometrium, and genital outflow tract. Abnormalities in any component of this process lead to pathology including amenorrhea (see chapter 43), abnormal uterine bleeding (see chapter 31), and infertility (see chapter 40).

MENSTRUAL CYCLE OVERVIEW

- The menstrual cycle is the natural and regular change the female reproductive system undergoes that makes a pregnancy possible. The cycle is usually a monthly occurrence that leads to the release of a single mature oocyte prepared for fertilization from thousands of primordial oocytes in the ovaries. This occurs via a tightly coordinated cycle with both stimulatory and inhibitory effects. In the absence of pregnancy, the cycle ends and a new cycle begins with the shedding of the endometrium (menstruation).
- The major hormones of the menstrual cycle include gonadotropins (follicle-stimulating hormone, or **FSH**, and luteinizing hormone, or **LH**), estrogen (**estradiol**) and **progesterone**. These hormones are present in varying levels at different points in the menstrual cycle (Figure 39-1).
- The first day of the menstrual cycle (**day 1**) is the first day of menses. From the perspective of ovarian function, the **follicular phase** is from the onset of menses (day 1) through the time of ovulation and the **luteal phase** is from ovulation until the onset of the next menses, which is the beginning of the next cycle. From the

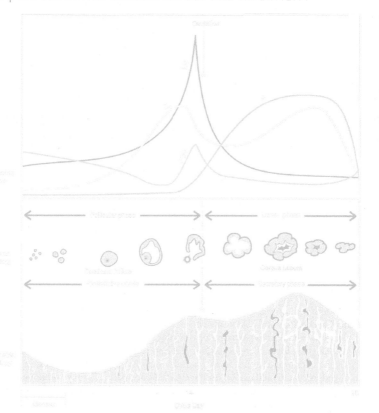

Figure 39-1. The normal menstrual cycle. Changes in serum hormones, ovarian follicle, and endometrial thickness during a 28-day menstrual cycle. Menses occur during the first few days of the cycle. E$_2$, estradiol; FSH, follicle-stimulating hormone; LH, luteinizing hormone; P, progesterone. Reprinted with permission from Berek JS, Berek DL, Hengst TC, et al, eds. *Berek & Novak's Gynecology*. 15th ed. Philadelphia, PA: Wolters Kluwer Health/Lippincott Williams & Wilkins; 2012. Figure 7.9.

perspective of the endometrium, the pre- and postovulatory phases correspond to the proliferative phase and the secretory phase (see Figure 39-1).

- The typical length of a menstrual cycle is **28 ± 7 days**. The follicular phase can vary among women, but a normal phase is considered 10 to 21 days (average is 14 d). Variations in menstrual cycle length are caused by variations in the follicular phase length. The luteal phase is consistently 14 days.

- Although there is typically little menstrual cycle length variability among women aged 20 to 40 years old, more variability is noted for the first 5 to 7 years after menarche and the last 10 years before the cessation of menses. In younger patients, this is usually due to hypothalamic-pituitary axis immaturity; in older patients, this likely reflects diminished ovarian reserve.

PHASES OF THE MENSTRUAL CYCLE

The Early Follicular Phase

- The ovary is least hormonally active during the early follicular phase; thus, this phase is marked by low serum levels of estradiol and progesterone. These low hormone levels lead to a lack of negative feedback on the hypothalamus. Subsequently, the hypothalamus (arcuate nucleus) secretes gonadotropin-releasing hormone with increasing pulsatile frequency and amplitude into the portal circulation, where it travels to the anterior pituitary.
- Gonadotropin-releasing hormone pulses stimulate gonadotrophs in the anterior pituitary to synthesize, store, and secrete the gonadotropic hormones FSH and LH into the systemic circulation.
- The increase in FSH leads to folliculogenesis, which leads to the growth of a cohort of follicles in midfollicular phase.

The Midfollicular Phase

- Each ovarian follicle contains a single oocyte. Granulosa cells surround the oocyte within the follicle. Thecal cells, in turn, enclose the granulosa cell layer.
- According to the **two-cell–two-gonadotropin theory**, LH stimulates thecal cells to synthesize androgens, whereas FSH stimulates granulosa cells to produce estrogens from these androgens. The FSH induces the aromatase enzyme to convert androgens to estrogens (ie, estradiol).
- In response to FSH stimulation, the granulosa cells of the follicles hypertrophy and divide, which further causes an increase in estradiol.
- The FSH stimulates the granulosa cell to produce **inhibin**, another important hormone in the menstrual cycle, which acts to downregulate FSH synthesis and inhibit FSH secretion. It peaks in the early to midfollicular phase (with a second peak at ovulation).
- Estradiol and inhibin exerts negative feedback onto the hypothalamus and pituitary, causing a decrease in FSH and LH.

The Late-Follicular Phase

- During the late-follicular phase, the dominant follicle exerts negative feedback on the other follicles in its ovarian cohort. This mechanism usually permits only one oocyte to mature for release during ovulation.
- In this phase, FSH also induces LH receptors in the ovary, which causes increased ovarian secretion of intrauterine growth factors (ie, insulinlike growth factor 1).
- The elevated levels of estradiol stimulate proliferation and thickening of the endometrium. By the end of the follicular phase, the endometrium typically measures between 8 and 12 mm. A woman may also notice a significant increase in the amount and "stringiness" (Spinnbarkeit test) of cervical mucus.
- Follicular growth continues until the threshold level of systemic estradiol is surpassed, which triggers the **midcycle LH surge**, a phenomenon in which a switch occurs from negative feedback on LH (by estradiol and progesterone) to a sudden positive feedback. This results in a 10-fold increase in serum LH and a smaller rise in FSH.

- The LH surge causes the developing dominant oocyte within the follicle to resume meiosis and ovulate about 36 hours after the midcycle surge.
- Prior to oocyte release during ovulation, the granulosa cells begin to luteinize and produce small amounts of progesterone.

The Luteal Phase

- After ovulation, the remnant of the dominant follicle becomes a **corpus luteum**, rapidly shifting from producing primarily estrogen to primarily progesterone.
- Progesterone causes a slowing of LH pulses and decidualizes the endometrium in preparation for embryo implantation.
- If an oocyte is fertilized, it will implant in the endometrium several days after ovulation and will make human chorionic gonadotropin. This hormone will maintain the corpus luteum (and thus progesterone production) in the absence of LH through the first 4 months of pregnancy until the placenta produces sufficient estrogen and progesterone to maintain the pregnancy.
- In the absence of a fertilized oocyte, the corpus luteum will regress, causing a decline in progesterone and estrogen.
  - Progesterone withdrawal causes the loss of endometrial blood supply, which leads to the sloughing of the endometrium and the onset of menses.
  - The hypothalamic-pituitary axis is released from the negative feedback of estradiol and progesterone, and FSH rises.
  - The onset of menses ends the luteal phase and marks the beginning of the next menstrual cycle.

SUGGESTED READINGS

American College of Obstetricians and Gynecologists Committee on Adolescent Health Care. ACOG Committee Opinion No. 651: menstruation in girls and adolescents: using the menstrual cycle as a vital sign. *Obstet Gynecol*. 2015;126:e143-e146. (Reaffirmed 2019)

Fritz MA, Speroff L. The endocrinology of the menstrual cycle: the interaction of folliculogenesis and neuroendocrine mechanisms. *Fertil Steril*. 1982;38:509-529.

Hoffman BL, Schorge JO, Bradshaw KD, Halvorson LM, Schaffer JI, Corton MM. Reproductive endocrinology. In: Moyer A, Brown RY, eds. *Williams Gynecology*. New York, NY: McGraw-Hill; 2016.

Lenz S. Ultrasonic study of follicular maturation, ovulation and development of corpus luteum during normal menstrual cycles. *Acta Obstet Gynecol Scand*. 1985;64:15-19.

Speroff L, Fritz MA. *Clinical Gynecologic Endocrinology and Infertility*. 8th ed. Philadelphia, PA: Lippincott Williams & Wilkins; 2011.

Treloar AE, Boynton RE, Behn BG, Brown BW. Variation of the human menstrual cycle through reproductive life. *Int J Fertil*. 1967;12:77.

40

Infertility and Assisted Reproductive Technologies

Christina N. Cordeiro Mitchell and Mindy S. Christianson

INFERTILITY

Definitions

- **Infertility:** failure of a couple of reproductive age to conceive after at least 1 year of regular coitus without contraception. Note that for women 35 years and older, a fertility evaluation is recommended if there is no pregnancy after 6 months of trying to conceive.
  - **Primary infertility:** infertility in a woman who has never been pregnant
  - **Secondary infertility:** infertility in a woman who has had one or more previous pregnancies
- **Fecundity:** ability to achieve a live birth within one menstrual cycle
- **Fecundability:** probability of achieving pregnancy within one menstrual cycle. For a normal couple, this is approximately 25%.
- **Primary ovarian insufficiency (POI):** previously referred to as premature ovarian failure. The POI is defined as amenorrhea for 6 months or more plus two follicle-stimulating hormone (FSH) levels over 40 IU/L measured 1 month apart, prior to the age of 40 years.
- **Assisted reproductive technologies (ARTs):** treatments for infertility in which eggs or embryos are handled in the laboratory (eg, in vitro fertilization [IVF])

Incidence

- According to the Centers for Disease Control and Prevention (CDC) (2011-2015 data), 7.3 million US women aged 15 to 44 years have used infertility services (12%).
- Fertility declines with age. Compared to women under 35 years, fertility is 26% to 46% lower in women aged 35 to 39 years and 95% lower in women aged 40 to 45 years.

DIFFERENTIAL DIAGNOSIS

- See Table 40-1 for differential diagnoses for infertility.

Ovarian Factor

- Ovulatory dysfunction causes infrequent or absent ovulation.
- **Types of ovulatory disorders (World Health Organization [WHO] classification)**
  - WHO class I: hypogonadotropic hypogonadal anovulation
    - Hypothalamic amenorrhea attributable to low gonadotropin-releasing hormone (GnRH) levels or pituitary unresponsiveness to hypothalamic GnRH, with resultant low FSH and serum estradiol levels
    - Causes include excessive weight gain or loss, exercise, or emotional stress.

Table 40-1	Infertility Evaluation[a]	
Diagnosis	%	Basic Evaluation
Male factors	30	Semen analysis
Tubal/uterine/peritoneal factors	25	Uterine: TVUS, SIS, HSG, and/or hysteroscopy Tubal/peritoneal: HSG or laparoscopy with chromopertubation
Anovulation/ovarian factors	25	May include midluteal progesterone level, OPKs, AMH, day 3 FSH and estradiol, and/or AFC
Cervical factors	10	Physical examination
Unexplained infertility	10	All of the above

Abbreviations: AFC, antral follicle count; AMH, antimüllerian hormone level; FSH, follicle-stimulating hormone; HSG, hysterosalpingogram; OPKs, ovulation predictor kits; SIS, saline infusion sonohysterography; TVUS, transvaginal ultrasound.
[a]Adapted from Speroff L, Fritz MA. *Clinical Gynecologic Endocrinology and Infertility*. 8th ed. Philadelphia, PA: Lippincott Williams and Wilkins; 2011:1137-1190, with permission.

- WHO class II: normogonadotropic normoestrogenic anovulation
  - Defined by normal levels of estradiol and FSH. Luteinizing hormone (LH) levels, however, may be elevated. This class includes polycystic ovary syndrome (PCOS).
- WHO class III: hypergonadotropic hypoestrogenic anovulation
  - Main causes include POI (premature oocyte depletion) or ovarian resistance.
  - These patients rarely respond to treatment for anovulation.
- **Endocrinopathies**
- Thyroid disorders
  - Hyper- or hypothyroidism can affect normal ovulation by altering concentrations of sex hormone binding globulin and total and free estradiol and testosterone, thereby altering the hypothalamic-pituitary-ovarian axis.
  - Thyroid autoimmunity, even in euthyroid women, may be associated with recurrent miscarriages; its effects on fertility are not clearly defined.
- Hyperprolactinemia
  - May be associated with hypothyroidism; can cause anovulation and amenorrhea by inhibiting normal hypothalamic GnRH pulse rhythm
  - When mild (20-50 ng/mL), patients may have a luteal phase deficiency; when moderate (50-100 ng/mL), they may have irregular menses or amenorrhea; and when severe (>100 ng/mL), patients have amenorrhea.
- **Diminished ovarian reserve**
- Age related: After reaching a peak number of oogonia at 16 to 20 weeks' gestation, female follicular reserve declines over the span of a woman's lifetime. This decline becomes more rapid in the late reproductive years.
  - Women of older reproductive age have decreased oocyte quantity *and* quality, resulting in decreased natural fertility and decreased ovarian

response to controlled ovarian hyperstimulation (COH) during fertility treatment.

o The Society for Assisted Reproductive Technology 2014 National Summary Report reports a singleton livebirth rate per individual patient of 52.6% for women under 35 years, 45.5% for women aged 35 to 37 years, 34% for women aged 38 to 40 years, 19.5% for women aged 41 to 42 years, and 6.7% for women over 42 years.

- Iatrogenic: Prior exposure to chemotherapy and/or radiation can have a detrimental effect on ovarian reserve at a younger age.
- **Primary ovarian insufficiency**
  - Patients who are fragile X permutation carriers or who have Turner syndrome are at risk for POI and may have few or no spontaneous ovulation cycles.
  - Iatrogenic: As above, certain gonadotoxic medications can result in adverse effects that cause patients develop POI and menopausal symptoms after gonadotoxic treatment.

Uterine Factor

- **Müllerian anomalies:** Patients with absent uteri require a gestational carrier with IVF in order to have a genetic child. Patients with other uterine structural abnormalities are able to conceive but may be predisposed to adverse pregnancy outcomes such as preterm delivery.
- **Fibroids** that distort or invade the endometrial cavity can impair implantation or predispose to early pregnancy loss. Depending on the size and location, removal is recommended in patients who wish to conceive.
- **Polyps** can affect implantation in ways similar to fibroids.
- Although the mechanism is unclear, **adenomyosis** has been associated with decreased implantation and clinical pregnancy rates in both spontaneous and IVF cycles as well as an increased risk of miscarriage and preterm delivery.

Tubal Factor

- **Occlusion:** Tubal factor infertility becomes more prevalent with the increased incidence of salpingitis, most often secondary to gonorrhea and chlamydia infection. The frequency of tubal occlusion after one, two, and three episodes of salpingitis is reported to be 11%, 23%, and 54%, respectively. Appendicitis, previous abdominopelvic surgery, endometriosis, and ectopic pregnancy can also lead to adhesion formation and damaged tubes.
- **Hydrosalpinx:** The presence of a hydrosalpinx has been demonstrated to impair IVF outcomes, likely secondary to impaired implantation and a potential toxic effect on the embryo.

Cervical Factor

- **Cervical stenosis** can occur following cervical or uterine surgery such as a loop electrosurgical excision procedure or a cold-knife conization or in patients with a history of amenorrhea and associated hypoestrogenism-induced atrophy of the genitalia.
- **Müllerian anomalies:** Cervical agenesis is a very rare cause of cervical factor infertility.

Male Factor

- **Definitions**
  - **Azoospermia:** absence of sperm in the ejaculate
  - **Oligospermia:** a concentration of fewer than a sperm count of 15 000 000/mL in the ejaculate
  - **Asthenospermia:** reduced sperm motility
  - **Oligoasthenospermia:** reduced sperm concentration and motility
  - **Teratospermia:** abnormal sperm morphology
- **Known causes**
  - **Klinefelter syndrome**
    - Karyotype is 47, XXY.
    - Most common genetic anomaly in azoospermic men
    - Found in 1:500 to 1:1000 live male births
    - Incidence: 3% of infertile men, 3.5% to 14.5% of azoospermic men, 1% of couples referred for intracytoplasmic sperm injection (ICSI).
  - **Congenital absence of the vas deferens**
    - Associated with cystic fibrosis gene mutations in the *cystic fibrosis transmembrane conductance regulator* gene.
    - Partners of men with congenital absence of the vas deferens should be tested for the cystic fibrosis transmembrane conductance regulator mutation prior to pursuing infertility treatment with retrieved sperm.
  - **Y chromosome microdeletions**
    - These occur in up to 7% of men with male factor infertility and in 10% to 15% of men with severe oligo- and azoospermia.
    - Although these men may be able to father children via IVF/ICSI, male offspring would inherit the same microdeletion and be infertile.
  - **Varicocele.** Can cause oligospermia and decreased motility due to in increased intratesticular temperature, decreased testosterone synthesis, altered function and morphology of Sertoli cells, damage to germinal cell membranes, and increased reactive oxygen species

Recurrent Implantation Failure

- Although there is no universally accepted definition, one group has proposed that recurrent implantation failure (RIF) be defined as failure to achieve a clinical pregnancy after transfer of at least four good quality embryos in a minimum of three fresh or frozen cycles in a woman under the age of 40 years.

EVALUATION

Indications for Evaluation

- 1 year of unprotected intercourse without conception if <35 years
- 6 months of unprotected intercourse without conception if 35 years or older
- Patients with known etiologies for infertility such as tubal occlusion
- Patients at risk for infertility, such as those with a history of prior cancer treatment

History and Physical Examination

- History from both partners should include duration of infertility, methods of contraception, previous evaluation and treatment, prior reproductive history, sexual dysfunction, coital frequency and satisfaction, sexually transmitted infections, tobacco and alcohol use, caffeine use, family history of learning disability, and birth defects.

- History from the female partner should also include a complete menstrual history, exercise habits, indices of stress, and presence of dysmenorrhea or menorrhagia, pelvic or abdominal pain, dyspareunia, symptoms of thyroid disease, galactorrhea, or symptoms of hirsutism.
- Physical exam of the female should focus on weight and body mass index, thyroid exam, hirsutism, pelvic or abdominal tenderness, uterine size and mobility, adnexal masses and/or tenderness, and cul-de-sac tenderness or nodularity.
- For men with abnormal semen analyses (see "Evaluation for Male Factor" section and Table 40-2 on page 514), referral to a urologist is indicated.
- **Evaluation components** (see Table 40-1)
  - Female factor evaluation: confirmation of ovulation, ovarian reserve testing, evaluation for endocrine disease as indicated, uterine cavity assessment, evaluation for tubal patency
  - Male factor evaluation: semen analysis

Evaluation for Ovarian Factor

- **Confirmation of ovulation**
  - **Basal body temperature** charting is a simple means of determining whether ovulation has occurred. Daily temperature is taken on waking, before any activity, and recorded on a graph (or in a smartphone app). After ovulation, rising progesterone levels increase the basal temperature by approximately 0.4°F (0.22°C) through a hypothalamic thermogenic effect. Because the rise in progesterone usually occurs 1 to 2 days after ovulation, the temperature elevation does not predict the exact moment of ovulation but offers retrospective confirmation of its occurrence. The temperature elevation is sustained for the remainder of the luteal phase and ends with the onset of the next menses.
  - **Midluteal progesterone:** A progesterone concentration >3.0 ng/mL in a blood sample drawn between cycle day 19 and 23 suggests ovulation has occurred. Normal adequate luteal support usually produces a progesterone concentration >10 ng/mL.
  - **Ovulation predictor kits:** Using a threshold concentration of 40 mIU/mL, positive testing for urinary LH correlates well with the surge of serum LH levels that trigger ovulation. Testing is advised from cycle day 10 through 18; if patients do not obtain a positive result, they are advised to try twice-daily testing next cycle.
  - **Clinical presentation:** Patients with anovulation and/or amenorrhea are by definition classified as having an ovulatory disorder.
- **Assessment of ovarian reserve**
  - **Antimüllerian hormone (AMH)** is a measure of the primordial follicle pool; over a woman's reproductive lifetime, it steadily decreases to undetectable levels by menopause. Typically, an AMH >1.0 ng/mL indicates adequate ovarian reserve.
  - **Day 2 or 3 FSH and estradiol:** Day 2 or 3 FSH values below 10 to 15 mIU/mL suggest adequate ovarian reserve. The exact cutoff depends on the particular laboratory reference standards.
  - **Antral follicle count:** as measured on cycle day 2 or 3 by transvaginal ultrasound (TVUS)

- **Evaluation for other endocrinopathies**
  - For patients with abnormal uterine bleeding or irregular menses, prolactin and thyroid-stimulating hormone levels are indicated. See chapter 44 for more details on further evaluation.

Evaluation for Structural Factor

- Structural factors include uterine, tubal, or cervical factors.
- **Transvaginal ultrasound** has a high specificity and low sensitivity for detecting intrauterine pathology; one study suggests the sensitivity of ultrasound for detecting polyps was 54% with an 80% specificity, and for fibroids sensitivity was 50% with a specificity of 98%.
- **Saline infusion sonohysterography** is an office procedure that involves TVUS after the introduction of sterile water or saline into the uterine cavity (Figure 40-1).
  - Performed in the early follicular phase, within 1 week of cessation of menstrual flow, to minimize chances of interrupting a pregnancy
  - Saline infusion sonohysterography is useful in the assessment of uterine cavity abnormalities such as polyps or submucosal fibroids and can be more accurate than TVUS in the diagnosis of such lesions.

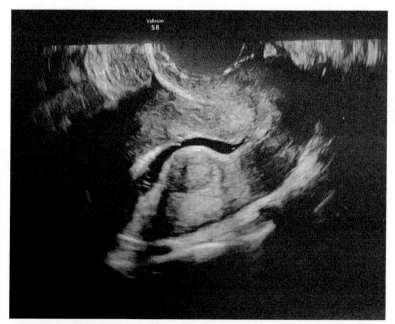

Figure 40-1. Saline infusion sonohysterography demonstrating a posterior submucosal fibroid in the uterine cavity. Original image courtesy of Mindy Christianson, MD, Johns Hopkins Hospital, Department of Gynecology and Obstetrics, Division of Reproductive Endocrinology and Infertility.

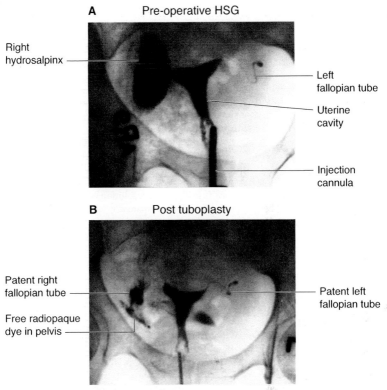

A   Pre-operative HSG

Right hydrosalpinx

Left fallopian tube

Uterine cavity

Injection cannula

B   Post tuboplasty

Patent right fallopian tube

Free radiopaque dye in pelvis

Patent left fallopian tube

Figure 40-2. Hysterosalpingogram (HSG) showing large right hydrosalpinx **(A)** that is re-solved following successful tuboplasty **(B)**. Real-time radiographs are obtained as radiopaque dye is injected through a cannula inserted in the cervical canal. Normal patent tubes demon-strate bilateral spillage from the fallopian tubes into the pelvis. Original images courtesy of Edward Wallach, MD, Johns Hopkins Hospital, Department of Gynecology and Obstetrics, Division of Reproductive Endocrinology and Infertility.

- **Hysterosalpingogram (HSG)** assesses uterine and fallopian tube contour and tubal patency (Figure 40-2).
  - The HSG shows appreciable müllerian anomalies as well as most endometrial polyps, synechiae, and submucosal fibroids. It can also determine tubal patency.
  - Performed in the early follicular phase, within 1 week of cessation of menstrual flow, to minimize chances of interrupting a pregnancy
  - The procedure is performed by injecting a radiopaque contrast through the cervix. As more contrast is injected, it normally passes through the uterine cavity into the fallopian tubes and then spills into the peritoneal cavity. The x-ray films are taken under fluoroscopy to evaluate tubal patency.
  - Nonsteroidal anti-inflammatory drugs may be given preprocedure to prevent cramping.
  - The HSG may have therapeutic effects. Several studies have indicated increased pregnancy rates for several months after the procedure.

- Prophylactic antibiotics (doxycycline) are advisable when the patient has a history of pelvic inflammatory disease or when hydrosalpinges are identified on HSG.
- **Hysteroscopy**
  - Definitive method to evaluate the uterine cavity
  - Can be performed using in-office diagnostic hysteroscopy with little or no anesthesia
- **Diagnostic laparoscopy**
  - Assesses peritoneal and tubal factors, such as endometriosis and pelvic adhesions, and can provide access for simultaneous corrective surgery
  - Laparoscopy should be scheduled in the follicular phase.
  - Today, laparoscopy is most acceptable if patients have another indication for laparoscopy such as pelvic pain. Otherwise, it is often acceptable to move forward with IVF without laparoscopy.
  - Findings on HSG correlate with laparoscopic findings 60% to 70% of the time.
  - **Chromopertubation:** Contrast (usually a dilute solution of indigo carmine) is instilled through the fallopian tubes during laparoscopy to visually document tubal patency.
  - Hysteroscopy may also be included to ensure that no intrauterine abnormalities were missed on the HSG.
- **Physical exam** can assess for abnormal uterine size/contour and müllerian anomalies (including cervical/uterine abnormalities).

Evaluation for Male Factor

- **Semen analysis**
  - Recommended in the initial evaluation of every infertile couple. A comprehensive semen analysis is most useful.
  - Normal semen parameters are typically defined by the WHO guidelines (Table 40-2).
- **Urological evaluation**
  - **Who to refer:** men with any abnormalities on semen analysis, couples with recurrent IVF failure without clear etiology, or in men with a history suspicious for other disease

Table 40-2	World Health Organization Semen Analysis Parameters[a]
Parameter	Standard Lower Limit
Volume	1.5 mL
Total sperm number per ejaculate	39 million/ejaculate
Sperm concentration	15 million/mL
Total motility	40%
Progressive motility	32%
Morphologically normal forms	4%

[a]Adapted from Cooper TG, Noonan E, von Eckardstein S, et al. World Health Organization reference values for human semen characteristics. *Hum Reprod Update*. 2010;16(3):231-245. Reproduced by permission of Oxford University Press.

- Male infertility risk factors: testicular torsion, trauma, tumors, varicocele, cryptorchidism, injuries or surgeries to the pelvis, retrograde ejaculation, prior cancer or prior radiation, use of hot tubs/saunas, smoking, or use of bicycles

TREATMENT FOR INFERTILITY
Treatment of Ovulatory Disorders

- **Clomiphene citrate (CC)**
  - Mechanism of action: a synthetic, nonsteroidal estrogen agonist-antagonist that increases the release of GnRH and subsequent LH and FSH release. Thus, an antiestrogenic effect on hypothalamus results in increased GnRH secretion.
  - Useful in women with oligomenorrhea and amenorrhea, with an intact hypothalamic-pituitary-ovarian axis
  - Patients who are overweight and hyperandrogenic or hypoestrogenic may have decreased responsiveness to CC.
  - See clomiphene-only regimens for dosing on "Controlled Ovarian Hyperstimulation and Protocols for In Vitro Fertilization" section.
  - Adverse effects: vasomotor symptoms such as headache and mood change; rarely, visual symptoms such as transient blurry vision or scotomata have been reported.
  - Complications: cystic ovarian enlargement and multifetal gestations (5%-10% of pregnancies)
- **Letrozole (Femara) or other aromatase inhibitors**
  - Mechanism of action: By inhibiting aromatase activity, the conversion of testosterone to estradiol is decreased. This increases the release of GnRH and subsequent LH and FSH release via negative feedback.
  - Data indicate that letrozole is superior to CC for patients with PCOS for ovulation induction with timed intercourse.
  - Letrozole is quickly metabolized and is generally considered safe for use.
- **Exogenous gonadotropins**
  - Human menopausal gonadotropin (hMG, Menopur) and recombinant FSH (Gonal-F or Follistim) are used primarily in women who fail to respond to CC or who have hypogonadotropic amenorrhea or unexplained infertility.
  - Prescription of these expensive drugs, which are typically used in the more complicated protocols for IVF, should be limited to specialists trained in their use due to risks of ovarian hyperstimulation.
- **Hyperprolactinemia**
  - Bromocriptine is used to induce ovulation in patients with hyperprolactinemia.
    - Bromocriptine is a dopamine agonist that directly inhibits pituitary secretion of prolactin, thereby restoring normal gonadotropin release.
    - The usual starting dose is 2.5 mg at bedtime to prevent dopaminergic side effects, which include nausea, diarrhea, dizziness, and headache.
    - A response is usually seen in 2 to 3 weeks, and 80% of hyperprolactinemic patients ovulate and become pregnant.
  - Cabergoline is an alternative for those who do not tolerate bromocriptine. Benefits include fewer side effects and twice weekly dosing.
- **Thyroid dysfunction:** See chapter 11.
- **Hypothalamic-pituitary-adrenal axis dysfunction**
  - Hypothalamic-pituitary axis problems, including extreme weight gain or loss, excessive exercise, and emotional stress, can all impact the secretion of GnRH from

the hypothalamus and cause ovulatory dysfunction. These must be addressed by appropriate behavioral or psychological intervention.

Treatment of Endometriosis

- Endometriosis is the ectopic growth of hormonally responsive endometrial tissue and accounts for up to 15% of female infertility. Refer to chapter 42 for indications for medical and surgical management.

Treatment of Uterine Factor

- The mainstay treatment for submucous leiomyomas, intrauterine synechiae (Asherman syndrome), and uterine deformities (ie, septae) is operative hysteroscopy with resection of abnormal pathology. In patients with larger fibroids or adenomyomas affecting the uterine lining, a combined abdominal (either laparoscopic or open)/hysteroscopic approach may be indicated.

Treatment of Tubal Factor

- **Tubal occlusion**
  - Proximal tubal obstruction is identified on HSG. Tubal spasm may mimic proximal obstruction, however; thus, tubal obstruction may need to be confirmed by laparoscopy. Treatment consists of tubal cannulation, microsurgical tubocornual reanastomosis, or IVF.
  - Distal tubal disease or distortion can be seen on HSG and laparoscopy. The success of corrective surgery (neosalpingostomy) depends on the extent of disease.
  - For patients with a history of bilateral tubal ligation who desire fertility, options include microsurgical sterilization reversal as well as IVF. Success of tubal reanastomosis depends on age, type, and location of sterilization procedure and requires an adequate remaining length of tubes for successful outcomes.
  - The IVF may be a better option for certain women, particularly those who only want one additional child.
- **Hydrosalpinges:** If IVF is pursued in patients with tubal factor infertility, several studies have shown that success rates of IVF are improved if hydrosalpinges are removed.

Treatment of Recurrent Implantation Failure

- **Endometrial receptivity assay (ERA) testing**
  - **Endometrial receptivity** refers to the finite window of time in which the endometrium is prepared for implantation of an embryo; this is expected to occur 5 days after ovulation.
  - The ERA test was developed to identify endometrial receptivity status based on the gene expression profiles of 238 genes at each stage of the menstrual cycle.
  - The ERA consists of an endometrial biopsy performed during a mock embryo transfer cycle, at the time when embryo transfer would typically occur. Biopsy results can indicate whether the endometrium is receptive, prereceptive, or postreceptive. In the next cycle, the timing of the actual, planned embryo transfer can be adjusted to the time that the endometrium should be receptive, based on the ERA results.
  - Data on patients with RIF of genetically normal embryos demonstrate improved implantation and pregnancy rates with embryo transfer based on ERA testing.

- **Endometrial scratching**
  - Endometrial injury has been theorized to improve implantation by producing an inflammatory response resulting increased release of cytokines involved in the implantation process.
  - Although data is conflicting at present, there is some evidence to date that endometrial injury in the form of hysteroscopy or endometrial scratching with a biopsy pipelle may improve pregnancy rates in subsequent cycles.

Treatment of Male Factors

- Intrauterine insemination (IUI) is recommended for men with a washed total motile sperm count of at least 10 000 000/mL.
- For those men with sperm count <10 000 000/mL, IVF and ICSI can often overcome most other cases of male factor infertility, even in severely oligospermic men.
- Urologic surgery, such as varicocele repair, can improve semen parameters and fertility.

TREATMENTS BEYOND OVULATION INDUCTION WITH TIMED INTERCOURSE

Intrauterine Insemination

- The IUI bypasses the inability of the uterus to tolerate large amounts of unprocessed seminal plasma by washing semen to maximize the number of motile sperm.
  - Components of the ejaculate, including seminal fluid, excess cellular debris, leukocytes, and morphologically abnormal sperm, are removed.
- Timing of the IUI is critical and should optimally occur as follows:
  - The day after detection of the midcycle urinary LH surge in spontaneous or clomiphene/letrozole-induced ovulatory cycles.
  - Thirty-six hours after administration of exogenous human chorionic gonadotropin (hCG)
- Procedure: An IUI cannula is used to bypass the cervix and deliver sperm into the endometrial cavity.

Assisted Reproductive Technologies

- Since the first successful IVF pregnancy delivered in 1978, additional ART advancements have enhanced our ability to overcome infertility.
- **In vitro fertilization**
  - The IVF refers to COH followed by aspiration of oocytes under ultrasound guidance, laboratory fertilization with prepared sperm, embryo culture, and transcervical transfer of the resulting embryos into the uterus. Although most IVF procedures use fresh oocytes from the patient, transfer of embryos derived from frozen/thawed oocytes or fresh/thawed donor eggs are also options.
  - According to the CDC, in 2013, 160 521 oocyte procedures were performed with the intent to perform embryo transfer and 27 564 were performed for fertility preservation.
  - The 2015 Society for ART data indicate an overall live birth rate per egg retrieval cycle of 53.9% for women <35 years of age, 40.2% for women aged 35 to 37 years, 26% for women aged 38 to 40 years, 12.6% for women aged 41 to 42 years, and 3.9% for women aged >42 years.

Table 40-3	In Vitro Fertilization (IVF) Success Rates by Diagnosis[a,b]	
Diagnosis of Patients Undergoing IVF	% of Cycles	% of Cycles That Resulted in Live Birth
Tubal factor	14.3	24.0
Ovulatory dysfunction	13.9	28.8
Diminished ovarian reserve	30.8	13.1
Endometriosis	8.8	27.6
Uterine factor	5.3	17.3
Male factor	34.8	27.1
Other causes	12.8	18.5
Unexplained cause	13.9	29.0
Multiple factors, female only	11.0	17.3
Multiple factors, female + male	17.7	22.0

[a]The total does not equal 100% because more than one diagnosis can be reported per cycle and due to rounding. Success rates are for fresh nondonor eggs or embryos.
[b]Data from Centers for Disease Control and Prevention, American Society for Reproductive Medicine, Society for Assisted Reproductive Technology. *Assisted Reproductive Technology: National Summary Report.* Atlanta, GA: National Center for Chronic Disease Prevention and Health Promotion, Division of Reproductive Health; 2015.
http://www.cdc.gov/art/artdata/index.html. Accessed April 18, 2018.

- See Table 40-3 for IVF success rates by infertility diagnosis.
- **Indications for IVF**
  - Tubal factor: large hydrosalpinges, absent fimbria, severe adhesive disease, recurrent ectopic pregnancies, failed tubal reconstruction, or a history of bilateral tubal ligation that chose IVF over reanastomosis
  - Endometriosis, if other forms of treatment have failed
  - Unexplained infertility, if other forms of treatment have failed (typically at least three failed IUI cycles)
  - Male factor: low sperm count, low sperm motility, and abnormal morphology associated with a reduction in fertilizing ability
  - Uterine malformations precluding conception via intercourse or IUI
  - Human immunodeficiency virus–positive serodiscordant couples: Use of ICSI or sperm washing techniques has enabled human immunodeficiency virus–negative women to safely achieve pregnancy using the sperm of their affected male partners. Processing and handling of these specimens require specialized facilities, protocols, training, and equipment.
  - Men and women seeking fertility preservation: Patients about to undergo chemotherapy or irradiation of their pelvic regions can consider cryopreservation of gametes, embryos, or ovarian tissue for subsequent childbearing via ART.
  - Couples seeking prenatal genetic diagnosis (see "Preimplantation Genetic Testing" section)

- **Intracytoplasmic sperm injection**
  - In ICSI, a single spermatozoon is injected microscopically into each oocyte, and the resulting embryos are transferred transcervically into the uterus. The advent of ICSI has revolutionized fertility treatment for couples confronting male factor infertility refractory to IUI or IVF.

Preimplantation Genetic Testing

- An umbrella term describing all types of genetic testing of the embryo. It is further subdivided into **preimplantation genetic testing (PGT) for aneuploidies (PGT-A)**, **PGT for monogenic disease (PGT-M)**, and **PGT for structural rearrangements (PGT-SR)**.
- The PGT proceeds by biopsy and genetic analysis of one of the following biopsy specimens:
  - Five to 10 cells of trophectoderm tissue from a blastocyst-stage (day 5) embryo. This method is most commonly used today as it has the best outcomes.
  - One to 2 blastomeres of a cleavage-stage (days 2 to 3) embryo derived from IVF. This is currently used less commonly.
  - Polar body biopsy from a metaphase II oocyte obtained after COH. This is useful only for maternally inherited mutations and is unable to detect abnormalities that occur after fusion of the male and female pronuclei; thus, it is rarely used.
- The **PGT-A** is a screening test for de novo aneuploidy (ie, numerical chromosomal abnormalities, including subchromosomal deletions) in embryos from parents who have no known chromosomal abnormality (ie, normal karyotype).
  - Preimplantation genetic screening (PGS) can screen for all 23 chromosomes and can help identify optimal (euploid) embryos for transfer before IVF.
  - Given that 40% to 60% of naturally and artificially conceived embryos are aneuploid, PGS with transfer of only genetically normal embryos can be expected to decrease the rate of miscarriage. However, this process does not improve overall implantation and livebirth rates because PGS cannot increase the number of euploid embryos available prior to transfer.
  - Indications for PGT-A include advanced maternal age, repeated miscarriage, history of an aneuploidy pregnancy, and repeated otherwise unexplained IVF failure.
    - The PGT-A also enables efficient and accurate gender selection by screening selectively for the Y chromosome. This is referred to as elective sex selection or family balancing.
    - Single embryo transfer of PGT-A-normal embryos can be used to decrease the chance of multiple pregnancy.
  - Methods to perform PGT-A include fluorescence in situ hybridization, single-nucleotide polymorphism microarrays, array comparative genomic hybridization, and next generation sequencing.
- The **PGT-M** allows couples with various single-gene disorders and X-linked genetic diseases to avoid transmission of the disorder to their offspring.
  - Method: Single-gene defects are typically detected after amplification by polymerase chain reaction followed by single-nucleotide polymorphism microarray-based technology such as karyomapping or targeted or whole genome sequencing. Only unaffected preimplantation embryos would be transferred to the woman's uterus.

- Indications for PGT-M include the following:
  - ○ Single-gene disorders: Using polymerase chain reaction, DNA extracted from the biopsy specimen is used to screen for a known hereditary disorder (eg, cystic fibrosis, muscular dystrophy, hemophilia, or Huntington disease).
  - ○ Sibling human leukocyte antigen matching: PGT-M was first used in 2000 to screen for Fanconi anemia and simultaneously to select for a preimplantation embryo that was human leukocyte antigen matched to a preexisting sibling afflicted with this disorder.

CONTROLLED OVARIAN HYPERSTIMULATION AND PROTOCOLS FOR IN VITRO FERTILIZATION

- The agents most commonly used to stimulate multiple ovarian follicles are CC, hMG, and recombinant FSH. The particular products and protocols used may be tailored as the treatment progresses to boost the chances of an adequate response and increase the pregnancy rate.
- Follicle maturation during COH is monitored using ultrasound and serial measurement of estradiol levels.
- **Clomiphene-only regimens**
  - These regimens are generally given for 5 days in the early follicular phase of the menstrual cycle
  - The CC is inexpensive and has a low risk of ovarian hyperstimulation syndrome (OHSS) and is most commonly used with timed intercourse at home or IUI. However, it creates a low oocyte yield (only one or two per cycle).
    - ○ Most treatment regimens start with 50 mg/d for 5 days beginning on cycle day 2 or day 5. If a dominant follicle fails to develop, the dose may be increased to 100 mg/d. Maximum dose is 150 mg/d.
  - The hCG, 5000 IU to 10 000 IU, or 250 μg recombinant hCG, may be used to simulate an LH surge. Seventy to 80% of properly selected couples will conceive in the first three cycles after treatment.
  - Potential side effects of CC include vasomotor flushes, blurring of vision, urticaria, pain, bloating, and multiple gestation (5%-7% of cases, usually twins).
- **Gonadotropin regimens**
  - These regimens increase the number of recruited follicles in patients who do not achieve pregnancy with CC and in those patients with endometriosis or unexplained infertility.
  - The hMG, Menopur and Bravelle, which is a combination of LH and FSH, is usually given for 2 to 7 days.
  - Attempts to minimize the potentially deleterious LH component of hMG have led to the manufacture of purified urinary FSH and, more recently, recombinant FSH (recombinant FSH, Follistim, and Gonal-F).
  - To complete oocyte maturation, hCG is administered once at least three follicles have reached 18 mm in diameter.
  - Although gonadotropin injections prove more effective at COH than CC, they are more expensive and can lead to life-threatening OHSS. Other potential disadvantages of gonadotropin use include premature luteinization, spontaneous LH surges resulting in high cancellation rates, and multiple gestations.
- The **GnRH agonist (GnRHa) protocols**
  - The GnRHas increase the number, quality, and synchronization of the oocytes recovered per cycle and thereby improve the fertilization rate, the number of

embryos, and the pregnancy rate. The GnRHas are used via a flare-up protocol or a luteal phase protocol in IVF cycles.

- o The flare-up protocol causes an elevation of FSH in the first 4 days, which increases oocyte recruitment. After 5 days of administration, the GnRHa down-regulates the pituitary to prevent premature luteinization and a spontaneous LH surge.
- o The luteal phase protocol involves starting GnRHa administration on menstrual day 17 to 21 in the cycle before IVF.
- Leuprolide (Lupron) is the most commonly used GnRHa in the United States.
- The **GnRH antagonist (GNRHant) protocols**
  - The GnRHants (Ganirelix and Cetrotide) block LH secretion and the premature LH surges that force cycle cancellation without causing a flare-up effect. Antagonist protocols are very commonly used for COH in IVF cycles.
  - Typically, gonadotropins are given starting on cycle day 2 and GnRHants are started on cycle day 6 or once estradiol levels reach 200 pg/mL or when at least one follicle reaches 13 mm in diameter.
  - Because GnRHants block the periovulatory LH surge, a lower total gonadotropin dose is required to stimulate ovulation and side effects are decreased as compared with GnRHas.

OOCYTE RETRIEVAL, CULTURE, FERTILIZATION, AND TRANSFER

- **Retrieval procedure**
  - This is an ultrasound-guided transvaginal procedure under intravenous sedation, performed 34 to 36 hours after hCG injection. A 17-gauge needle is passed through the vaginal fornix to retrieve oocytes.
  - Potential complications include bowel and bladder injury, infection, and injury to pelvic vessels.
- **Oocyte fertilization**
  - Sperm are diluted, centrifuged, and incubated before 50 000 to 100 000 motile spermatozoa are added to each Petri dish containing an oocyte.
  - Fertilization is documented by the presence of two pronuclei and extrusion of a second polar body at 24 hours.
- **Embryo transfer**
  - Performed 3 to 5 days after oocyte insemination. Day 5 blastocyst transfer is more common today due to higher live-birth rates compared to cleavage-stage (day 3) embryos.
  - Excess embryos not used for transfer can be cryopreserved for an unlimited period, with a survival rate of over 95%.
  - The actual number of embryos transferred depends on the individual's age and other risk factors for multiple pregnancy.
  - Due to compromised corpora lutea function after oocyte retrieval, it is necessary to supplement the luteal phase with progesterone given intramuscularly or by vaginal suppository, beginning the day of oocyte release and continuing into the 12th week of pregnancy
- **Oocyte/embryo freezing**
  - Slow freezing of oocytes and embryos is an older method aimed at avoiding formation of ice crystals, which would typically occur when temperature decreases too quickly.

- Vitrification is a newer method, which allows freezing over a period of seconds, solidifying oocytes or embryos into a glass-like state without ice crystal formation.
- It is becoming widely accepted that vitrification is superior to slow freezing for oocytes and embryos and is becoming the method exclusively used for freezing in IVF centers.

THIRD-PARTY REPRODUCTION

- Includes donor oocytes and sperm, donated embryos, and gestational carriers (surrogates)
- Ethical issues involved include the following maternal, fetal, and long-term effects of ART:
  - Disclosure to children conceived by these technologies regarding their genetic origin
  - Privacy issues for donors
  - Compensation for oocyte donors and gestational carriers

COMPLICATIONS OF ASSISTED REPRODUCTIVE TECHNOLOGIES

Ovarian Hyperstimulation Syndrome

- **Ovarian hyperstimulation syndrome** can be a life-threatening complication of COH characterized by ovarian enlargement and increased capillary permeability. It is potentiated by COH cycles using GnRH analogs for downregulation or hCG to trigger oocyte maturation.
- Presentation: abdominal bloating, ovarian enlargement, ascites, decreased urine output, electrolyte imbalance, hemoconcentration, and hypercoagulability. In severe cases, hydrothorax, acute respiratory distress syndrome, and multiple organ failure can occur.
  - Classified as mild, moderate, or severe according to the presenting symptoms
- Pathophysiology: thought to be mediated by vascular endothelial growth factor, produced by the ovary in response to LH or hCG. Vasodilation and increased capillary permeability result in fluid shifts to extravascular spaces. Severity correlates with hCG levels.
- Risk factors: age <35 years, PCOS, low body mass index, AMH >3.36, antral follicle count >24, >25 follicles at time of retrieval, >24 oocytes retrieved, serum estradiol >3500 pg/mL
- Treatment: Moderate to severe cases of OHSS should be managed as an inpatient.
  - Inpatient treatment includes close monitoring of fluid and renal status, frequent evaluation of electrolytes and coagulation studies, intravascular resuscitation (with crystalloid followed by albumin and furosemide), thrombosis prophylaxis and paracentesis/culdocentesis, and/or thoracentesis, as indicated.
- If impending OHSS is suspected, evidence supports prevention by:
  - The use of GnRHa trigger rather than hCG, elective cryopreservation of all embryos with a delayed embryo transfer, use of metformin at the start of downregulation for PCOS patients, and administration of dopamine agonists (cabergoline) starting at the time of trigger.
  - There is insufficient evidence for prevention by albumin or "coasting" (withholding gonadotropins at the end of stimulation for up to 4 days).

- The OHSS is an entirely iatrogenic entity that can often be avoidable by vigilance and judicious execution and alteration of COH regimen.

Multiple Pregnancy

- **CC/letrozole with timed intercourse or IUI:** The risk of multiple pregnancy is about 7% to 10%. Risk decreases with patient age. Ultrasound monitoring is thought to decrease the risk of multiple pregnancy, by avoiding insemination when follicle counts are high.
- **IVF:** According to CDC data, of the 23 529 pregnancies that resulted from fresh embryo (nondonor egg) transfer procedures in 2016, 21% resulted in a multifetal pregnancies; among all live births from IVF pregnancies, 19% were multiples.
  - In attempting to limit the prevalence of multiple gestation, the American Society for Reproductive Medicine has issued practice recommendations governing the number of embryos transferred. These recommendations are stratified depending on whether cleavage-stage embryos or blastocysts are transferred.
    - o Women aged <35 years: Strong consideration to transfer just one embryo if a favorable prognosis; no more than two embryos (any stage) should be transferred.
    - o Women aged 35 to 37 years: Two cleavage-stage embryos if a favorable prognosis; otherwise, three cleavage-stage embryos may be transferred. No more than two blastocysts may be transferred.
    - o Women aged 38 to 40 years: Three cleavage-stage embryos or two blastocysts if a favorable prognosis; otherwise, four cleavage-stage embryos or three blastocysts may be transferred.
    - o Women >aged 40 years: no more than five cleavage-stage embryos or three blastocysts
  - Should multiple gestation ensue, recourse to selective fetal reduction is available for patients who are comfortable with the ethics and risks of that procedure.

Heterotopic Pregnancy

- Rare complication in which both an intrauterine pregnancy and an extrauterine (ectopic) pregnancy occur simultaneously. This occurs in up to 1% of pregnancies after ART. This incidence is dramatically higher than the corresponding ratio in the general population (1 in 30 000).Women who display signs or symptoms suggesting ectopic pregnancy after ART must be closely followed despite confirmation of an intrauterine pregnancy.

Fetal/Neonatal Effects

- Inconsistent and equivocal evidence links IVF to increased risks of neonatal morbidity, birth defects, developmental disabilities, and certain childhood cancers.
- Conclusive evidence, however, does link IVF to an increased risk of low-birth-weight deliveries even among full-term, singleton neonates. Most recent studies and data suggest that although fetuses resulting from ART are at higher risk of congenital abnormalities when compared to spontaneously conceived fetuses; this associated risk appears to be lower than previously believed and this is in part due to the recognition that some parental factors associated with infertility may play a role in this increased risk (as opposed to simply the practice/inherent science of ART).

Effects of Intracytoplasmic Sperm Injection

- The ICSI has been associated with a statistically significant, but small absolute, increased risk of sex and autosomal chromosome abnormalities and imprinting disorders, such as Beckwith-Wiedemann or Angelman syndromes.
- If a male with a Y chromosome microdeletion undergoes ICSI/IVF, his male offspring will inherit the same microdeletion and, thus, also have male factor infertility.

FERTILITY PRESERVATION

- **Indications** for fertility preservation include the following:
  - Malignancy: Current American Society of Clinical Oncology guidelines recommend discussion of the potential adverse effects of chemotherapy or radiation treatment on future fertility and referral for fertility preservation in any prepubescent or reproductive-aged woman with a new cancer diagnosis.
  - Nonmalignant conditions requiring gonadotoxic or immunosuppressive treatment such as hematologic or rheumatologic diseases
  - Nonmalignant conditions requiring removal of reproductive organs
  - Patients with Turner syndrome or at risk for developing POI
  - Social: patients who elect to delay childbearing

Embryo Cryopreservation

- Requires approximately 2 weeks for COH and oocyte retrieval; requires a male partner/sperm donor
- Frozen embryo livebirth rates are 44.4% for women under 35 years, 40.1% for women 35 to 37 years old, and 35% for women aged 38 to 40 years. Thawing frozen embryos from egg donor embryos have a 39.3% livebirth rate.

Oocyte Cryopreservation

- Requires approximately 2 weeks for COH and oocyte retrieval; requires a male partner/sperm donor
- Typically, a patient should obtain one good quality embryo for every five or six oocytes thawed.
- Oocyte cryopreservation has improved with new vitrification protocols; however, oocyte thaw is not as efficient as embryo thaw. For patients using donor eggs, for example, livebirth rates for fresh eggs are 50.2% versus 38.3% for cryopreserved eggs.
- Oocyte cryopreservation was considered experimental in the United States until 2012 when the experimental label was lifted due to improved outcomes with vitrification.

Ovarian Tissue Cryopreservation

- Ovarian tissue cryopreservation represents the only method for fertility preservation for patients who do not have time to delay for cancer treatment or who are prepubertal.
- Ovarian tissue is harvested via a laparoscopic procedure, typically piggybacked with another cancer-related procedure such as port placement. Ovarian tissue cortex is frozen in strips via a rapid vitrification method. Ovarian tissue can be retransplanted into the ovarian fossa or underneath remaining ovarian cortex, allowing resumption of ovarian function to treat menopausal symptoms.
- To date, at least 130 livebirths have resulted; some spontaneous and some via IVF.

- Future studies may allow for in vitro maturation of immature ovarian follicles, IVF, and retransplant of embryos from patients in whom ovarian tissue transplant may not be oncologically safe (eg, leukemia patients).

Gonadotropin-Releasing Hormone Agonists Treatment Prior to Chemotherapy

- The use of GnRHas, such as leuprolide acetate, is commonly recommended prior to and during chemotherapy in an attempt to protect against ovarian toxicity. However, some studies do not demonstrate that this is truly protective of ovarian reserve and thus should not be considered a reliable method of fertility preservation.
- However, leuprolide acetate therapy can be helpful to prevent significant abnormal uterine bleeding associated with the hematologic effects of chemotherapy (ie, anemia and thrombocytopenia).

Ovarian Transposition

- In patients who require pelvic radiation therapy, the ovary can be transposed to various intra- and retroperitoneal locations such as the paracolic gutters or lateral to the psoas muscles.
- Among women receiving brachytherapy alone, ovarian function was preserved in 90%; in those requiring external beam radiotherapy with or without brachytherapy, ovarian function was preserved in 65%.

SUGGESTED READINGS

Coughlan C, Ledger W, Wang Q, et al. Recurrent implantation failure: definition and management. *Reprod Biomed Online.* 2014;28:14-38.

Donnez J, Dolmans M-M. Fertility preservation in women. *N Engl J Med.* 2017;377:1657-1665.

Hansen M, Kurinczuk JJ, Milne E, de Klerk N, Bower C. Assisted reproductive technology and birth defects: a systematic review and meta-analysis. *Hum Reprod Update.* 2013;19(4):330-353.

Legro RS, Barnhart HX, Schlaff WD, et al; for Cooperative Multicenter Reproductive Medicine Network. Clomiphene, metformin, or both for infertility in the polycystic ovary syndrome. *N Engl J Med.* 2007;356(6):551-566.

Pan MM, Hockenberry MS, Kirby EW, Lipshultz LI. Male infertility diagnosis and treatment in the era of in vitro fertilization and intracytoplasmic sperm injection. *Med Clin North Am.* 2018;337:337-347.

Practice Committee of Society for Assisted Reproductive Technology, Practice Committee of American Society for Reproductive Medicine. Preimplantation genetic diagnosis: a practice committee opinion. *Fertil Steril.* 2008;90:S136-S140.

Practice Committee of the American Society for Reproductive Medicine. Prevention and treatment of moderate and severe ovarian hyperstimulation syndrome: a guideline. *Fertil Steril.* 2016;106:1634-1647.

Practice Committee of the American Society for Reproductive Medicine, Practice Committee of Society for Assisted Reproductive Technology. Criteria for number of embryos to transfer: a committee opinion. *Fertil Steril.* 2013;99:44-46.

Speroff L, Fritz MA. *Clinical Gynecologic Endocrinology and Infertility.* 8th ed. Philadelphia, PA: Lippincott Williams & Wilkins; 2011.

Sunderam S, Kissin DM, Crawford SB, et al. Assisted reproductive technology surveillance–United States, 2013. Centers for Disease Control and Prevention Web site. https://www.cdc.gov/mmwr/preview/mmwrhtml/ss6411a1.htm?s_cid=ss6411a1_w. Accessed April 18, 2018.

Recurrent Pregnancy Loss

Kamaria C. Cayton Vaught and Mindy S. Christianson

41

EPIDEMIOLOGY AND DEFINITION

- Miscarriage, or spontaneous abortion, is classically defined as loss of a fetus weighing <500 g or before the gestational age of 20 weeks. It is the most common complication of early pregnancy, affecting 10% to 25% of pregnancies.
- Recurrent pregnancy loss (RPL) has traditionally been defined as three or more consecutive losses of clinically recognized pregnancies <20 weeks of gestation. The American Society for Reproductive Medicine defines RPL as two or more losses at any gestational age and suggests a thorough evaluation after two or more.
  - Primary RPL: recurrent miscarriages without a previous viable pregnancy
  - Secondary RPL: RPL with previous delivery of a live infant (better prognosis)
- Incidence and risk
  - Five percent of all women will experience two consecutive losses; 1% will have three consecutive losses.
  - Incidence of RPL significantly increases with maternal age, but risks also include genetic factors, uterine pathology, endocrine and metabolic factors, immunologic causes, antiphospholipid antibody syndrome, environmental factors, and infectious agents. At least 50% of all cases remain undiagnosed.
  - Risk of miscarriage increases from 20% in women with a history of one miscarriage to 43% in women with a history of three or more.
  - Studies have shown the overall success rate of achieving a live birth after miscarriage in women with RPL was 66% to 77%.

ETIOLOGIES

Genetic

- **Aging and embryonic aneuploidy.** Age plays a significant role in early pregnancy loss and by default recurrent miscarriages. With increased age, the rate of aneuploidy increases significantly within the oocyte leading to subsequent increases in aneuploid pregnancies.
  - In women <35 years of age, the risk of sporadic miscarriage is 9% to 12% compared to women >35 years of age where the risk of sporadic miscarriage significantly increases to 20%. The highest risk of sporadic miscarriage is seen in women >40 years of age with a rate of approximately 50%.
- **Parental chromosomal abnormalities.** Parental chromosome abnormalities as the cause of RPL is low, at 3% to 5%. However, in couples with RPL, peripheral parental karyotyping should be included in the evaluation.
  - Chromosome structural abnormalities such as translocations and inversions can be assessed by obtaining a parental karyotype. A parental karyotypic abnormality is more likely with young maternal age, ≥3 losses, or a first-degree relative with RPL.
  - Balanced translocations are the most common parental chromosome abnormality diagnosed. As many as 1 in 500 individuals have a balanced translocation.

Parental carriers of balanced translocations can produce either unbalanced (1%-20% of the time) or balanced gametes, with unbalanced gametes resulting in spontaneous abortion 85% of the time.

- Robertsonian translocations, the most common chromosome rearrangement observed in humans, are identified in 2% to 5% of couples with RPL. Parents who are carriers of Robertsonian translocations are at high risk for transmitting an unbalanced chromosome to their offspring. In rare cases, a Robertsonian translocation can involve chromosome 21, resulting in an offspring with trisomy 21.
- A smaller percentage of abnormal parental karyotypes include inversions, microdeletions, and mosaicisms.
- Studies have shown that there is an increased likelihood of a genetic abnormality to be transmitted maternally to the offspring. Given this finding, it is more beneficial to test the mother first followed by the father as needed if unable to test both simultaneously.
- **Genetic counseling** for chromosomal structural abnormalities is warranted in couples with RPL. The subsequent outcomes of future live births depend on which chromosome is involved and the type of rearrangement. Counseling should address whether or not the pregnancy losses were euploid, aneuploid, or affected with a chromosomal rearrangement. If one parent is identified with a structural rearrangement, cell-free DNA, preimplantation genetic testing (PGT), chorionic villus sampling, or amniocentesis should be offered as means of detecting the genetic abnormality in offspring.
- **Cytogenetic analysis of future losses** should be considered in all couples with RPL and may be of psychological value to the couple.
  - Karyotyping is the most common cytogenetic analysis routinely performed. Standard high-resolution karyotyping allows for detection of deletions and duplications greater than approximately 5 to 10 Mb anywhere in the genome.
  - Comparative genome hybridization, array comparative genome hybridization, or microarray allows for genome-wide approaches at a higher resolution (up to 250 kb) compared to conventional karyotyping.
- **Preimplantation genetic diagnosis and aneuploidy screening.** The PGT requires a couple to undergo in vitro fertilization in order to genetically test the embryos for a specific genetic disease or to screen for aneuploidy. To date, there is insufficient data demonstrating that in vitro fertilization with PGT improves the live birth rate in couples with RPL and a structural genetic abnormality. Routine preimplantation embryo testing for aneuploidy is not currently recommended in patients with chromosomal structural abnormalities. However, as technology improves, the ability to accurately identify structural rearrangements will also increase and routine PGT may become recommended in the future.

Uterine Pathology

- Uterine malformations are noted in 10% to 30% of women who experience RPL, compared to approximately 7% in the general population.
- **Congenital anomalies** include developmental defects of the müllerian duct system, such as septate, arcuate, bicornuate, unicornuate, and didelphic uteri. Septate and bicornuate uteri are most commonly associated with RPL and are hypothesized to interfere with uterine distention or abnormal implantation due to decreased vascularity in a septum, increased inflammation, or reduction in sensitivity to hormones. Correction of the uterine tract anomalies may provide benefit in women with RPL.

- **Acquired conditions** that cause abnormalities within the uterus and cervix include uterine synechiae, leiomyoma, polyps, and cervical laxity or shortening.
  - Leiomyomas may be submucosal, intramural, serosal, or pedunculated. Some studies show that submucosal fibroids may be associated with RPL. Vascular supply to the placenta may be affected due to an unfavorable implantation site, whereas large fibroids may distort the uterine cavity. Fibroids may cause alterations in vascular supply of the endometrium or may interfere with gamete or embryo migration. Similarly, observational studies suggest an increased miscarriage rate in patients with large endometrial polyps, whereas the role of small polyps is unclear.
  - Intrauterine synechiae may occur after infections or following instrumentation of the uterus. Aggressive postpartum curettage may lead to significant synechiae formation, or Asherman syndrome, which results in insufficient endometrium to support growth.
  - Cervical insufficiency is associated with pregnancy loss and RPL. Depending on the individual patient, treatment can include progesterone, cervical cerclage, and/or pessary placement (see chapter 5).
- **Workup for uterine pathology**
  - A variety of imaging modalities are used in the evaluation and diagnosis of uterine pathology in relation to reproductive loss. Two-dimensional abdominal or transvaginal pelvic ultrasound and hysterosalpingography are popular screening tools, although they have relatively low rates of accuracy.
  - Hysterosalpingography aids in examination of the intrauterine cavity, but it is unable to reliably detect subtle uterine pathology.
  - Sonohysterography, or saline-infused hysterography, is a more accurate diagnostic tool than plain ultrasound.
  - Office hysteroscopy, with a flexible hysteroscope, is an accurate and well-tolerated method to evaluate the uterine cavity, but it does not differentiate a septate and a bicornuate uterus.
  - Combined hysteroscopy and laparoscopy remain the most definitive diagnostic approach by providing examination of both internal and external abnormalities. This method is also therapeutic because it permits septal resection if needed.
  - Three-dimensional transvaginal ultrasound and magnetic resonance imaging are also promising tools to aid in displaying uterine morphology in women with RPL. Three-dimensional ultrasound seems to be the most accurate imaging modality for the exterior contour of the uterus, which can help differentiate septate and bicornuate uteri.
- **Treatment**
  - The general consensus is that surgical correction of any significant uterine cavity defect should be attempted in women with RPL.
  - Resection of uterine septa (septoplasty), hysteroscopic lysis of adhesions, myomectomy, polypectomy, and cervical cerclage placement are all possible treatments for congenital and acquired uterine abnormalities.

Endocrine/Metabolic Dysfunction

- Endocrine and metabolic factors are implicated in 15% to 60% of RPL cases.
- Abnormal glucose metabolism
  - Poorly controlled diabetes mellitus (hemoglobin $A_{1c} > 8\%$) have been associated with increased risk of miscarriages (see chapter 11).

- Strict glycemic control should be reinforced prior to conception to decrease fetal anomalies. Pregnancy loss is increased in obese women, possibly due to insulin resistance. Weight loss prior to pregnancy improves pregnancy outcome.
- Polycystic ovary syndrome (PCOS)
  - A 20% risk of miscarriage has been noted in this population of women.
  - Proposed mechanisms for explanation of the increased risk of miscarriage with PCOS include hyperandrogenism, elevated luteinizing hormone levels, obesity, hyperinsulinemia, premature or delayed ovulation, metabolic derangements of prostaglandins, growth factors, and elevated cytokines.
  - Metformin has been shown to decrease miscarriage rate in women with PCOS in some studies, but randomized controlled trials offer no definitive evidence. Existing prospective studies show no evidence of teratogenicity or developmental problems in the first 18 months of life in the infants of mothers who used metformin in early pregnancy. Some studies advocate using metformin 500 to 2500 mg by mouth daily through the first trimester in affected women.
- Thyroid dysfunction
  - Clinical and subclinical hypothyroidism are associated with miscarriages and adverse obstetric outcomes. Patients presenting with RPL should be screened for thyroid disease because thyroid supplementation within this population is beneficial.
  - Pathogenesis in patients with RPL include interference with implantation, although exact causation has not been demonstrated.
  - Subclinical hypothyroidism is defined as a thyroid-stimulating hormone (TSH) greater than the upper limits of normal (4.0-5.0 mIU/L) with normal thyroxine (T_4) levels. Currently, there is a lack of consensus on what the normal upper level of TSH is.
  - If TSH levels are within normal limits, there is insufficient evidence to recommend additional T_4 or antithyroid antibody testing.
  - Treating patients with TSH levels between 2.5 and 4.0 mIU/L remains controversial. However, given the minimal risk, it is reasonable to treat, although evidence remains weak.
  - If thyroperoxidase antibodies are present, therapy with T_4 decreases the risk of miscarriage.
  - According to American Society for Reproductive Medicine, if the TSH level is greater than the nonpregnant upper limit of normal (>4.0 mIU/L), patients should be treated with T_4 supplementation to maintain levels <2.5 mIU/L.
  - See chapter 11 for more on thyroid disorders.
- Hyperprolactinemia. Prolactin levels are increased normally in pregnancy. However, routine testing on patients with RPL is not recommended in the absence of cycle abnormalities because there is a lack of evidence that treatment reduces the miscarriage rate. In a study of 64 hyperprolactinemic women treated with bromocriptine, there was a higher rate of pregnancy (86% vs 52%); however, research is limited on whether this intervention leads to higher rates of pregnancies without miscarriage.
- Other hormonal abnormalities
  - Debate on whether other hormonal abnormalities contribute to RPL is controversial.
  - Luteal phase deficiency (LPD), also known as progesterone deficiency. Absence of sufficient progesterone levels can conceptually lead to delayed or late implantation, which in turn, may increase pregnancy loss. Diagnosis of LPD requires histologic endometrial dating that historically is unreliable and not reproducible.

Currently, endometrial biopsy for diagnosing LPD is not recommended. There are some studies that suggest potential benefit with empiric use of progesterone supplementation in women with more than three consecutive pregnancy losses. However, the supporting evidence is of poor methodologic quality.
- Delayed or late implantation

Antiphospholipid Syndrome

- Antiphospholipid syndrome (APS) is associated with RPL. Five percent to 20% of patients with RPL will test positive for antiphospholipid antibodies. Varying pathogenic mechanisms have been attributed to APS-associated pregnancy loss and is trimester specific. In the second trimester, thrombosis within the placental circulation can occur, leading to placental infarction. In the first trimester, studies have suggested that failure of early trophoblastic invasion is more likely because examination of decidua has failed to show correlation with thrombotic events. In APS, antiphospholipid antibodies (eg, lupus anticoagulant, anticardiolipin, or anti-β_2 glycoprotein antibodies) are formed against vascular endothelium and platelets, eventually leading to vascular constriction and thrombosis.
- International consensus classification criteria for APS include one clinical and one laboratory finding to be present.
  - Clinical criteria
    - One or more episodes of arterial, venous, or small vessel thrombosis
    - One or more unexplained pregnancy loss of a morphologically normal fetus of ≥10 weeks of gestation
    - One or more premature births of morphologically normal fetus at ≤34 weeks of gestation due to eclampsia or preeclampsia with severe features or placental insufficiency
    - Three or more consecutive miscarriages before 10 weeks of gestation excluding anatomic, hormonal, parental genetic factors
  - Laboratory criteria
    - Two positive titers of moderate to high dilution at least 12 weeks apart of anticardiolipin or anti-β_2 glycoprotein immunoglobulin G or immunoglobulin M antibodies
    - Lupus anticoagulant (Russell viper venom test) on two occasions at least 12 weeks apart
- Treatment. Studies have shown improved pregnancy outcome in women with APS (particularly those with a prior thrombotic event) who received antithrombotic therapy.
  - Treatment with unfractionated heparin and low-dose acetylsalicylic acid is more effective than acetylsalicylic acid alone in increasing the live birth rate—80% compared to 40%, respectively.
  - Although some studies have suggested that low-molecular-weight heparin (LMWH) also improves APS-associated pregnancy outcomes, comparable efficacy of LMWH to heparin has not been established. The benefit of LMWH is that it carries a decreased risk of heparin-induced thrombocytopenia, heparin-induced osteopenia, and maternal bleeding.

Hereditary Thrombophilias

- Retrospective data suggests a modest association between thrombophilias and RPL. However, prospective studies have failed to give proof to this connection. Therefore, anticoagulation is not recommended for preventing RPL.

- Includes factor V Leiden, prothrombin gene mutations, protein C, protein S, and antithrombin deficiencies
- Screening may be clinically justified in patients with risk factors (personal history of venous thromboembolism, first-degree relative with a known or suspected high-risk thrombophilia).
- Routine screening for thrombophilias in women with RPL without a known risk factor is not recommended.
- Anticoagulation therapy during pregnancy may be considered, although evidence does not support improved pregnancy outcomes.

Immune Dysfunction

- Autoimmune and alloimmune factors may cause RPL similar to graft rejection or defects of the complement system.
- Celiac disease is thought to be associated with RPL and infertility, and treatment appears to prevent these problems; thus, women with RPL should be screened.
- Alloimmunity reflects the theory that pregnancy survival depends on maternal tolerance to foreign fetal antigens instead of maternal sensitization leading to activation of the immune response.
- Historically, attempted therapies have included leukocyte immunization, intra-venous immunoglobulin, third-party donor cell immunization, and trophoblast membrane immunization; however, these are not recommended.
- There are currently no evidence-based methods for clinical use to evaluate or treat possible immune system-related RPL.

Male Factors

- Abnormalities in standard semen analysis parameters (volume, concentration, mo-tility, morphology) are not predictive of RPL.
- Data is conflicting in regard to sperm aneuploidy and DNA fragmentation as an etiology of RPL.
  - Increased rates of sperm sex chromosome disomy has been demonstrated in male partners of couples with RPL. However, sex chromosome aneuploidy was not increased in the products of conception suggesting that cytogenetically abnormal sperm may be selected against during fertilization.
  - Abnormal sperm DNA fragmentation can occur with advanced paternal age or as a result of correctable environmental factors such as varicoceles, toxic exposures, exogenous heat, or increased reactive oxygen species in semen.
  - Routine testing for sperm aneuploidy or DNA fragmentation is not recommended.

Infection and Environmental Exposures

- Infectious agents (listeria, toxoplasma, cytomegalovirus, and primary herpes sim-plex virus) are known causes of miscarriage, but there is no proof of their role in RPL. Therefore, bacterial or viral cultures are not a part of the workup for RPL.
- Chemicals associated with RPL include formaldehyde, pesticides, lead, mercury, benzene, and anesthetic gases, such as nitrous oxide.
- Stress and exercise have not been found to increase the risk of RPL.
- Cigarette smoking has been linked to increased miscarriages by having an adverse effect on trophoblastic function.

- Lifestyle habits such as increased caffeine consumption (>3 cups of coffee, daily) and alcohol consumption (3-5 drinks per week) and cocaine use have also been associated with increased risk of miscarriage.

Psychological Factors

- Pregnancy loss can have a profound effect on emotional well-being. The grief response can include anger, depression, anxiety, guilt, and grief. There is limited data that supports a psychological role in the etiology of pregnancy loss. Studies have shown that emotional support, close surveillance with frequent office visits, phone calls, and even serial ultrasound studies improve pregnancy outcomes. These strategies have been shown in controlled studies to halve the RPL rate (from >50% to 25%) in the absence of any medical or surgical intervention.
- Unexplained RPL. Unfortunately, no identifying causative factor for RPL is present in 50% to 75% of couples with RPL. Counseling of patients should include highlighting their chance of a future successful pregnancy can exceed 50% to 60% depending on maternal age and parity.

EVALUATION

- Table 41-1 describes evaluation for RPL.
- When to evaluate: Women who have experienced two or more clinical losses should have a clinical evaluation for RPL. Pregnancy losses do not have to be consecutive in order to initiate evaluation.
- History and exam
  - A detailed history with pertinent medical history should be obtained.
    - ○ Menstrual history
    - ○ Obstetric history, including paternity and any treatment complications
    - ○ Family history and pedigree analysis
    - ○ Review of systems for detection of underlying medical disorders
    - ○ Identification of inherited thrombophilias
    - ○ Lifestyle assessment including life stressors; weight changes; exercise schedule; caffeine intake; and tobacco, alcohol, or illicit drug use
  - Physical exam should include vital signs, palpation of the thyroid for goiter, breast exam for galactorrhea, and pelvic exam including imaging if necessary to asses uterine size and exclude müllerian anomaly.
- Diagnostic tests
  - Depending on history, TSH; pelvic ultrasound, saline infusion sonography, and/or hysterosalpingogram; parental karyotype; anticardiolipin antibodies; lupus anticoagulant; anti-β_2 glycoprotein I
  - If indicated, factor V Leiden; prothrombin gene mutations: protein C, protein S; antithrombin deficiencies; cytogenetic studies on products of conception; hysteroscopy

TREATMENT PRINCIPLES

- The following principles should be considered when evaluating a patient with a history of RPL:
  - Optimizing lifestyle factors
  - Control of underlying medical conditions

Table 41-1   Evaluation for Recurrent Pregnancy Loss

First-line tests	• Complete medical, surgical, genetic, and family history and a physical examination • Sonohysterography to delineate the internal and external contours of the uterus and distinguishes between septate and bicornuate uteri; other options to evaluate the uterine anatomy include 3-dimensional ultrasound and hysterosalpingography. • Anticardiolipin antibody and anti-β_2 glycoprotein (IgG and IgM) titers and lupus anticoagulant performed twice, 12 wk apart • TSH and thyroid peroxidase antibodies • Prolactin level • Hemoglobin A_{1c} and fasting glucose; consider glucose tolerance testing in obese patients. • Parental karyotype and karyotype of the abortus if the above examinations are normal
Second-line tests	• Hysteroscopy, laparoscopy, or MRI are more invasive than sonohysterography. • Ovarian reserve can be evaluated by measurement of AFC, basal serum FSH, AMH; these tests predict ovarian response in assisted reproductive procedures, but their usefulness in triaging patients for RPL is questionable.
Evidence does not support these tests	• Routine cultures for chlamydia or bacterial vaginosis • ANA titers • Progesterone level; single or multiple serum progesterone levels or endometrial biopsies are not predictive of future pregnancy outcome

Abbreviations: AFC, antral follicle count; AMH, antimüllerian hormone; ANA, antinuclear antibody; FSH, follicle-stimulating hormone; IgG, immunoglobulin G; IgM, immunoglobulin M; MRI, magnetic resonance imaging; TSH, thyroid-stimulating hormone.

- Pregnancy planning with preconceptual counseling
- Genetic counseling if indicated
- Surgical or nonsurgical treatments depending on etiology
- Early pregnancy diagnosis to initiate treatment, if any
- Frequent visits to monitor pregnancy and answer concerns
- If loss recurs, consider cytogenetic studies of products of conception to guide further treatment and prognosis.
- Psychological support and counseling. Stress and anxiety should be considered while caring for couples who experience RPL. Consider psychosocial or spiritual support or counseling.

SUGGESTED READINGS

American College of Obstetricians and Gynecologists. ACOG Practice Bulletin No. 24: management of recurrent pregnancy loss (replaces Technical Bulletin Number 212, September 1995). *Int J Gynaecol Obstet.* 2002;78(2):179-190.

American College of Obstetricians and Gynecologists Committee on Genetics, Society for Maternal-Fetal Medicine. ACOG Committee Opinion No. 682: microarrays and next-generation sequencing technology: the use of advanced genetic diagnostic tools in obstetrics and gynecology. *Obstet Gynecol.* 2016;128:e262-e268. (Reaffirmed 2019)

American College of Obstetricians and Gynecologists Committee on Practice Bulletins—Obstetrics. ACOG Practice Bulletin No. 132: antiphospholipid syndrome. *Obstet Gynecol.* 2012;120:1514-1521. (Reaffirmed 2017)

Atik RB, Christiansen OB, Elson J, et al. ESHRE guideline: recurrent pregnancy loss. *Hum Reprod Open.* 2018;2018(2):hoy004. doi:10.1093/hropen/hoy004.

Jauniaux E, Farquharson RG, Christiansen OB, Exalto N. Evidence-based guidelines for the investigation and medical treatment of recurrent miscarriage. *Hum Reprod.* 2006;21(9): 2216-2222.

Practice Committee of the American Society for Reproductive Medicine. Evaluation and treatment of recurrent pregnancy loss: a committee opinion. *Fertil Steril.* 2012;98(5): 1103-1111.

Robinson L, Gallos ID, Conner SJ, et al. The effect of sperm DNA fragmentation on miscarriage rates: a systematic review and meta-analysis. *Hum Reprod.* 2012;27(10):2908-2917.

Sahoo T, Dzidic N, Strecker MN, et al. Comprehensive genetic analysis of pregnancy loss by chromosomal microarrays: outcomes, benefits, and challenges. *Genet Med.* 2017;19:83-89.

Trott EA, Russell JB, Plouffe L Jr. A review of the genetics of recurrent pregnancy loss. *Del Med J.* 1996;68(10):495-498.

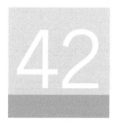

Menstrual Disorders: Endometriosis, Dysmenorrhea, and Premenstrual Dysphoric Disorder

Camilla Yu and Jensara Clay

ENDOMETRIOSIS

* **Endometriosis** is an estrogen-dependent chronic inflammatory disease characterized by the extrauterine presence of functioning endometrial glands and stroma. Most commonly found not only in the ovaries but also in the pouch of Douglas, vesicouterine space, uterosacral ligaments, and surrounding pelvic peritoneum; less commonly seen in laparotomy and episiotomy scars, on bowel, diaphragm, appendix, pleural and pericardial cavities, and the cervix

Theories of the Pathogenesis of Endometriosis

- The etiology of endometriosis is unknown. Several theories involving anatomic, immunologic, hormonal, and genetic factors have been postulated.
- **Sampson's theory of retrograde menstruation:** Retrograde menstruation is the leading theory and suggests that endometriosis is related to the backward flow of endometrial tissue via the fallopian tubes into the peritoneal cavity during menses. Support for this theory is as follows:
  - Blood flowing freely from the fimbriated ends of fallopian tubes has been visualized during laparoscopy (seen in 90% of women with patent fallopian tubes).
  - Endometriosis is most often found in the dependent portions of the pelvis.
  - Incidence of endometriosis is higher in women with obstruction to normal outward menstrual flow (eg, cervical stenosis).
  - Endometriosis is more common in women with shorter menstrual cycles or longer duration of flow, providing more opportunity for endometrial implantation.
- **Coelomic metaplasia:** Totipotential cells of the ovary and peritoneum are transformed into endometriotic lesions by repeated hormonal or infectious stimuli. This may explain the finding of endometriosis in mature teratomas and extraperitoneal sites as well as the incidence of endometriosis in males and premenarchal girls.
- **Lymphatic spread:** One study showed that at time of autopsy, 29% of women with endometriosis had positive pelvic lymph nodes for the disease. Thus, lymphatic spread may be another mechanism to explain endometriotic implants found in remote anatomic areas, such as the lung.
- **Immunologic factors:** Increasing data suggest that specific immunologic factors at the site of endometrial implants play a major role in determining whether and to what extent a patient will develop the disease. These factors are thought to influence the attachment and proliferation of the endometriotic cells. Differences in both humoral and cell-mediated immunity are thought to be involved.
- **Hormonal factors:** Unlike normal endometrial tissue, endometriotic implants can produce aromatase and 17β-hydroxysteroid dehydrogenase type 1, leading to extraovarian estrogen production. Additionally, implants do not adequately express 17β-hydroxysteroid dehydrogenase type 2, the enzyme responsible for inactivating estrogen, leading to a high estrogen environment. Implants demonstrate reduced levels of progesterone receptors and are therefore relatively resistant to the estrogen-antagonizing effects of progesterone seen in normal endometrium.
- **Inflammatory factors:** Elevated levels of interleukin-6 and tumor necrosis factor α have been noted in the peritoneal fluid of endometriosis patients. Interleukin-8 may help in the attachment of endometrial implants in the peritoneum and is also an angiogenic agent. Prostaglandin E_2, a proinflammatory compound, has been shown to be a powerful inducer of aromatase activity in endometriotic implants. Prostaglandin E_2 effects are additionally augmented by estradiol produced by endometriotic aromatase. This positive feedback loop amplifies the proliferative effects of estradiol.
- **Genetic factors:** Women who have a first-degree relative with endometriosis have a 7-fold greater risk of developing endometriosis. The mode of inheritance is most likely multifactorial.

Patient Characteristics

- Mean age at diagnosis is 25 to 30 years. The greatest incidence has been observed in nulliparous women with early age at menarche and shorter menstrual cycles. Increased parity and greater cumulative lactation are protective factors against endometriosis.
- Studies have demonstrated an inverse relationship between incidence of endometriosis and current body mass index (BMI) as well as BMI at 18 years of age. These studies found that women with low BMIs have a statistically significant higher rate of endometriosis compared to women with high BMIs. This relationship appears to be augmented in the subgroup of women who experience infertility.

Clinical Presentation

- Although some women with endometriosis are asymptomatic, the most common symptoms are infertility and pelvic pain.
- **Infertility:** Incidence of endometriosis is believed to up to 50% among infertile couples. Often, asymptomatic patients undergoing laparoscopy for infertility will be diagnosed with mild endometriosis.
- **Pelvic pain:** Up to 70% of women with chronic pelvic pain have endometriosis. Endometrial lesions can lead to chronic inflammation with increases in inflammatory cytokines and subsequent overproduction of prostaglandins, both of which can be a source of pain. Furthermore, endometriotic lesions may express high levels of nerve growth factor and cytokines (eg, tumor necrosis factor α and glycodelin) that stimulate growth and maintenance of functioning nerve roots. Exposure of these nerve roots to the inflammatory milieu within endometriotic implants leads to central sensitization and pain. The severity of pelvic pain does not correlate with the amount of endometriosis present. The pain typically associated with endometriosis is central, deep, and often in the rectal area. Unilateral pain may be compatible with lesions in the ovary or pelvic sidewall. Dysuria or dyschezia can result from urinary or intestinal tract involvement, respectively, and can predict deeply infiltrating endometriosis. Forty-five percent to 50% of patients with deep dyspareunia have been found to have endometriosis. Incidence of endometriosis in patients with **dysmenorrhea** is believed to be 40% to 60%. One study found endometriotic implants in approximately 70% of teenagers who underwent laparoscopy for chronic pelvic pain.
- **Other symptoms:** Depending on site of implantation, patients can experience additional symptoms. Implantation in the anterior abdominal wall or thorax can lead to abdominal pain and chest or shoulder pain, respectively. Implants in the thorax can result in hemoptysis or pneumothorax.

Abnormal Clinical Findings Associated With Endometriosis

- Nodularity of the uterosacral ligaments, which are often tender and enlarged
- Painful swelling of the rectovaginal septum
- Pain with motion of the uterus and adnexa
- Fixed, retroverted uterus and large, immobile adnexa indicative of severe pelvic disease
- Enlarged adnexal mass may be due to ovarian endometrioma.
- Visual evidence of endometriosis may rarely be seen with cervical implants or implants in surgical scars (eg, Pfannenstiel incisions).

Diagnosis of Endometriosis

- **Definitive diagnosis** is made only through **histologic examination** of lesions removed at the time of surgery. Histology reveals endometrial glands and stroma. Hemosiderin-laden macrophages are identified in 77% of endometriosis biopsy specimens.
- **Diagnostic imaging:** Often, an initial diagnostic tool in women with chronic pelvic pain, transvaginal ultrasound is the gold standard to visualize ovarian endometriomas. Although ultrasound can be used to evaluate deep infiltrating endometriosis of the bowel and bladder, this method is highly operator dependent, and magnetic resonance imaging may be needed as confirmatory imaging in equivocal cases. Computed tomography is of limited utility but can help in evaluating thoracic endometriosis and abdominal wall endometriomas. Although the utility of noninvasive imaging in assessing endometriosis is inconsistent, it may be useful in excluding other causes for pelvic pain.
- Experienced clinicians often presumptively diagnose endometriosis based on clinical history and timing of symptoms. When other causes of pelvic pain are excluded, first-line therapy with oral contraceptive pills (OCPs) can be initiated without a surgical diagnosis. If this fails, a thorough survey of the pelvis via laparoscopy or a 3-month course of a gonadotropin-releasing hormone (GnRH) agonist is appropriate.
- **Diagnostic laparoscopy:** Endometriotic lesions classically appear as blue-black powder-burn implants on visual inspection. However, studies report a marked discrepancy in appearance of the lesions and the histology. Nonclassic lesions may appear vesicular, red, white, tan, or nonpigmented. The presence of defects in the peritoneum (usually scarring overlying endometrial implants) is known as Allen-Masters syndrome. Endometriomas, or "chocolate cysts," appear filled with dark brown blood.
  - Surgical staging of endometriosis is done according to the revised American Society for Reproductive Medicine scoring system (1996). Its utility is limited to providing a standardized method to report operative findings. Staging does not correlate with symptomatology or severity of symptoms, nor does it predict future fertility following treatment.

Treatment

- **Expectant management:** Asymptomatic patients or patients with mild symptoms can be managed expectantly.
- **Medical treatment:** Estrogen stimulates the growth of endometriotic implants similar to its effect on normal endometrial tissue. Medical therapy is aimed at suppressing ovarian estrogen stimulation by interrupting the hypothalamic-pituitary-ovarian axis. Inhibition of ovulation by gonadotropin suppression removes the stimulation of endometriosis by cycling sex steroids.
  - **Nonsteroidal anti-inflammatory drugs (NSAIDs)** are a common first-line agent for symptomatic relief of endometriosis-related pain and inflammation. The NSAIDs inhibit prostaglandin production by ectopic endometrium.
  - **Estrogen-progesterone contraceptives:** Combined contraceptives are the treatment of choice for endometriosis-related pain. Combined contraceptives suppress gonadotropin release and subsequently cause decidualization and atrophy of endometrial implants. Symptomatic relief of pelvic pain and dysmenorrhea is

reported in 60% to 95% of patients. However, the estrogenic component may stimulate growth and increase pain during the first few weeks of treatment, and recurrence rates are high after discontinuation of medication. Continuous combined OCPs can provide significant pain relief in patients suffering mainly from dysmenorrhea. Other forms of combined contraception (transdermal patches, vaginal rings) may also be used.

- **Progestins:** Progestins inhibit ovulation by suppressing luteinizing hormone (LH) and, eventually, may induce amenorrhea. They also suppress endometriosis through decidualization and atrophy of endometrial tissue. Progesterone therapy can be continued for suppression of endometriosis symptoms; however, there is a potential for bone demineralization with long-term use. Various forms of progestin can be used, including oral progestin pills, depot medroxyprogesterone acetate, norethindrone acetate, or a levonorgestrel-releasing intrauterine device. Data directly comparing the efficacy of these formulations are limited with most achieving comparable levels of symptomatic relief. However, use and compliance among these methods are limited by side effect profile, and choice of compound should be tailored to individual patient preferences.

- **Gonadotropin-releasing hormone agonists:** When given continuously in a non-pulsatile fashion over the long term, these agents suppress pituitary function by downregulating pituitary GnRH receptors. This interruption of the hypothalamic-pituitary-ovarian axis produces a "medical oophorectomy" or "pseudomenopause." Three available agents are leuprolide acetate (Lupron Depot), nafarelin acetate nasal spray (Synarel), and goserelin acetate (Zoladex). Side effects are related to the hypoestrogenic state. The US Food and Drug Administration has approved up to a 12-month course in combination with add-back therapy to avoid the long-term consequences of the hypoestrogenic state on bone metabolism and lipid profile changes. Recurrence rates following discontinuation of therapy have been quoted as high as 73% after a 5-year follow-up period.

  o **Add-back therapy:** used for minimization of hypoestrogenic side effects and counteracting bone loss. Numerous studies have demonstrated the efficacy of adding back combined estrogen/progesterone or progesterone alone to patients on GnRH agonist therapy. Patients receiving add-back therapy have significantly less vasomotor side effects and bone mineral density loss over a 6-month period while still benefiting from pain relief from endometriosis. Add-back therapies include norethindrone acetate 5 mg daily and conjugated estrogen 0.625 mg together with medroxyprogesterone acetate 5 mg daily.

- The **GnRH antagonists** act similarly to GnRH agonists in suppressing gonadotropin production and thus have similar side effects. The GnRH antagonists, however, provide an immediate effect without the initial agonist effect seen in nonpulsatile dosing of GnRH agonists.

- **Danazol (Danocrine):** A derivative of the synthetic steroid 17α-ethinyltestosterone. It suppresses the midcycle LH surge, inhibits steroidogenesis in the human corpus luteum, and produces a high-androgen and low-estrogen environment that does not support the growth of endometriosis. Approximately 80% of patients experience relief or improvement in symptoms within 2 months of beginning danazol treatment. Androgenic side effects (acne, hirsutism, decrease in breast size, deepening of voice) greatly reduce compliance. Recurrence of symptoms is almost 50% within 4 to 12 months after discontinuation of therapy. Adverse side effects occur in approximately 15% of women taking danazol.

- **Aromatase inhibitors:** Third-generation aromatase inhibitors, letrozole, and anastrozole have been used for treatment of endometriosis refractory to other modalities. They are used alone or combined with GnRH agonists. These medications have been shown to decrease circulating estrogen levels by 50% by inhibiting conversion of androgens to estrogens in ovarian granulosa cells. The most significant side effect is decreased bone density, which is not mitigated with the use of calcium and vitamin D. Additionally, there is evidence to suggest that aromatase inhibitors increase the incidence of ovarian cysts. Additional side effects include vaginal spotting, hot flashes, headaches, and mood swings.

Surgical Treatment

- **Definitive surgery** entails total abdominal hysterectomy with bilateral salpingo-oophorectomy, excision of peritoneal surface lesions or endometriomas, and lysis of adhesions. A "semidefinitive" procedure that preserves an uninvolved ovary is another option because it avoids the long-term risks of surgical menopause. Although there is a 6-fold increased risk of developing recurrent symptoms and an 8-fold reoperation rate to remove the remaining ovary, most women do not require reoperation. Therefore, in women with normal-appearing ovaries, a hysterectomy with ovarian conservation should be considered.
  - Hormone replacement therapy after definitive surgery for the prevention of surgical menopausal symptoms, is considered safe and does not appear to increase the risk for recurrence of endometriosis.
- **Conservative surgery** is usually reserved for patients with endometriosis-related pain but who desire future fertility. Improvement in symptoms is often achieved with laparoscopic excision or destruction of endometrial implants via laser vaporization, electrocoagulation, or thermal coagulation. Although there is significant short-term improvement in pain, a few studies have shown at 3 years postoperation that approximately 30% of patients will require additional surgeries. Postoperative medical suppressive therapy has demonstrated efficacy in treating residual disease and pain as well as increasing pain-free interval following surgery. However, the therapeutic effects do not last beyond discontinuation of the medication.
- **Endometrioma resection:** Surgical resection of endometriomas is pursued to exclude malignancy or treat symptoms refractory to medical therapy. Cystectomy has been shown to be superior to aspiration in studies comparing recurrence rates, pain relief, and rates of subsequent spontaneous pregnancy. Women should be counseled on the risk of reducing ovarian reserve or increasing adhesions, both of which could reduce future fertility.

Endometriosis and Infertility

- The exact incidence of infertility caused by endometriosis is unknown, although endometriosis is found in up to 50% of couples with infertility.
- Theories on the physiologic changes caused by endometriosis that affect fertility potential include abnormal folliculogenesis, elevated oxidative stress, altered immune function, alterations in peritoneal fluid cytokines, and decreased presence of integrins during the implantation phase, thus decreasing endometrial receptivity. Mechanical factors may be attributed to adhesions impairing oocyte transport. Together, these factors decrease oocyte quality and impair fertilization and implantation.

- Fewer oocytes are retrieved when an endometrioma is present, but the pregnancy rate with in vitro fertilization is not greatly altered, and the risk of removing segments of normal ovarian cortex along with the cystectomy must be weighed against the benefits.

Endometriosis and Ovarian Malignancy

- The prevalence of endometriosis in patients with epithelial ovarian carcinoma, especially in endometrioid and clear cell types, is higher than that in the general population. Ovarian carcinoma has been documented in 0.3% to 0.8% of patients with endometriosis.
- The pathology of endometriosis exhibits many of the characteristics of neoplastic lesions: reduced cell cycle inhibitor activity, ability to resist apoptosis, angiogenic potential, and ability to invade surrounding tissue. Although an association exists between endometriosis and certain malignancies, it is considered benign and not a premalignant condition.
- Data shows that there is a 2- to 3-fold increased risk of developing ovarian cancer in women with endometriosis. The overall risk, however, remains low and no additional cancer screening is recommended.
- At present, malignant transformation of endometriotic lesions is a recognized mechanism in the development of ovarian cancer. Definitive surgery to remove all visible evidence of endometriosis is not recommended as a prophylactic means of reducing the development of ovarian malignancy. Rather, long-term use of oral contraceptives is the preferred method of cancer risk reduction because an 80% lower occurrence of ovarian cancer in women with endometriosis has been shown in patients using the drug for >10 years.

DYSMENORRHEA

- **Primary dysmenorrhea** is painful menstruation with no evidence of hormonal or anatomic pathology. **Secondary dysmenorrhea** has an identifiable cause.
- Most commonly reported menstrual disorder, affecting up to 90% of women.
- Risk factors include young age (<20 y), low BMI <20 kg/m^2, menarche <12 years old, longer menstrual cycles and duration of bleeding, heavy menstrual flow, smoking, weight loss attempts, nulliparity, and psychiatric disorders such as depression and anxiety.
- Primary dysmenorrhea presents within 6 months of menarche. If dysmenorrhea does not appear until more than a year after menarche, secondary dysmenorrhea should be suspected (see chapter 32). Primary dysmenorrhea, unlike secondary dysmenorrhea, tends to become less painful as a patient gets older and may also improve after childbirth.

Pertinent Findings in History and Physical Exam

- Defined as spasmodic cramping ("labor-like" pains) beginning 1 to 2 days before or simultaneous with the onset of menses. Cramps are often accompanied by nausea, vomiting, backache, irritability, fatigue, diarrhea, and headache.
- Symptoms with primary dysmenorrhea last only 2 to 3 days; however, pelvic pain and tenderness may persist beyond this interval with secondary dysmenorrhea.

Pain is most intense during first 24 to 36 hours of menstrual flow, consistent with the time of maximal prostaglandin release into the menstrual fluid.

- Clinical presentation with secondary dysmenorrhea varies considerably with its cause. Endometriosis is the most common cause, but other possibilities are pelvic inflammatory disease, adenomyosis, pelvic adhesions, and uterine fibroids.
  - Initial evaluation of dysmenorrhea includes a complete pelvic exam. Microbiologic cultures, ultrasound, and other imaging modalities may be required to identify or rule out secondary dysmenorrhea. Diagnostic laparoscopy may also be indicated in particular situations, for instance, in patients who fail empiric medical therapy for presumed endometriosis-related dysmenorrhea. Primary dysmenorrhea is a clinical diagnosis.

Treatment of Dysmenorrhea

- Three modalities exist: pharmacologic, nonpharmacologic, and surgical. Pharmacologic treatment is preferred for primary dysmenorrhea. Secondary dysmenorrhea is treated by addressing the underlying cause.
  - **Pharmacologic treatments**
    - The NSAIDs are the gold standard of treatment of primary dysmenorrhea. No specific NSAID is most efficacious, but older and generically available NSAIDs are preferred for cost-effectiveness. They relieve primary dysmenorrhea by reducing endometrial prostaglandin production and by exerting a central nervous system analgesic effect. They also have a modest effect in reducing menstrual flow volume.
    - Hormonal treatment: Combined OCPs, contraceptive patch and vaginal ring, single-rod contraceptive progestin implant, depot medroxyprogesterone acetate, and levonorgestrel intrauterine devices can all reduce dysmenorrhea. Levonorgestrel intrauterine device is highly effective in reducing menstrual blood loss with concomitant clinical relief.
    - Glyceryl trinitrate, magnesium, calcium channel antagonists, and vitamin B_6 have been shown to have varying beneficial effects on symptom reduction with primary dysmenorrhea.
  - **Nonpharmacologic treatments**
    - High-frequency transcutaneous electrical nerve stimulation offers significant pain relief by raising pain threshold and increasing the release of endorphins from the spinal cord and peripheral nerves.
    - Although acupressure only has a suggestive role in the reduction of dysmenorrhea, acupuncture has been shown to be equally beneficial to ibuprofen in pain reduction.
    - Continuous suprapubic heat application (heat wrap therapy) has been shown to be more therapeutic than acetaminophen during the initial 8 hours of application.
    - Other nonpharmacologic interventions such as exercise and behavioral and diet modifications have been investigated as possible treatments.
  - **Surgical treatments**
    - Surgical interventions including nerve ablation (uterosacral nerve ablation and presacral neurectomy) and spinal manipulation have shown no long-lasting therapeutic benefit according to Cochrane meta-analyses. Additionally, they carry significant risk of adverse events. Hysterectomy is only considered as a last resort.

PREMENSTRUAL DISORDER: PREMENSTRUAL DYSPHORIA AND PREMENSTRUAL DYSPHORIC DISORDER

- **Premenstrual dysphoria**, or more commonly **premenstrual syndrome (PMS)**, is a cluster of mood, cognitive, and physical disturbances. Symptoms occur cyclically in the second half of the menstrual cycle, most often in the first few days of menses. It is distinct from depression or anxiety disorders and has a prevalence of 3% to 5% among reproductive-aged women.
  - Mood symptoms include irritability, mood swings, depression, and anxiety; cognitive disturbances may be confusion or poor concentration. Physical problems consist of bloating, breast tenderness, appetite changes, hot flashes, insomnia, headache, and fatigue.
- **Premenstrual dysphoric disorder (PMDD)** represents the more severe end of the spectrum. It is composed of the same combination of symptoms but involves an increased severity in perceived symptoms and a marked impairment in daily life. This diagnosis is reserved for patients that meet the *Diagnostic and Statistical Manual of Mental Disorders* (Fifth Edition) criteria set by the American Psychiatric Association.
  - A woman has PMDD when she has five or more of the following symptoms:
    - One (or more) of the following symptoms must be present:
      - Marked depressed mood
      - Marked tension, anxiety or feeling "on edge"
      - Marked mood lability or frequent crying
      - Constant irritability and anger that cause conflict with other people
    - One (or more) of the following symptoms must also be present, to reach a total of five symptoms when combined with the symptoms above:
      - Lack of interest in usual activities
      - Having problems concentrating
      - Marked lack of energy
      - Marked appetite changes, overeating, or cravings
      - Having trouble sleeping or sleeping too much
      - Feeling overwhelmed
      - Physical symptoms such as tender or swollen breasts, headaches, joint or muscle pain, bloating, and weight gain
  - Symptoms must occur in a majority of menstrual cycles, be present in the final week prior to the onset of menses, and resolve in the week postmenses. Symptoms should not be due to the physiological effects of a substance/medication or other medical condition (eg, hyperthyroidism).
- The exact physiologic cause of premenstrual disorders is unknown. Most frequently cited theories include neuroactive progesterone metabolite, γ-aminobutyric acid receptor modulation, and critical reduction in serotonergic function during the luteal phase.

Evaluation and Diagnosis

- Dysmenorrhea, depression and anxiety disorders, menstrual migraine, cyclic mastalgia, irritable bowel syndrome, and hypothyroidism may all present with mood or physical disturbances similar to those that manifest with PMS/PMDD.
- There are no laboratory or physical exam findings required to make the diagnosis. Rather, these tests are used to rule out other causes of similar symptoms. Hormone levels (estrogen, progesterone, LH, FSH) do not vary between women with and without PMS/PMDD; thus, there is little utility in obtaining these values.

- For diagnosis of PMS, symptoms must begin at least 5 days before menses, persist for three menstrual cycles in a row, and end within 4 days after menses starts. It must also interfere with the patient's normal activities.
- Symptom diaries are helpful to determine whether the reported symptoms are limited to the luteal phase or are present throughout the cycle, suggesting a general medical condition. Additionally, they are helpful for patients for instituting self-help strategies and for anticipating symptoms.

Treatment

- Because PMS/PMDD is a chronic problem, adverse effects, cost, and severity of symptoms should all be considered before employing a specific treatment.
- **Lifestyle changes** are most appropriate for mild to moderate PMS/PMDD. Regular aerobic exercise; relaxation therapy; stress reduction; sufficient sleep; dietary limitation of caffeine, alcohol, and salt; and increased consumption of complex carbohydrates during the luteal phase have been shown to reduce the severity of symptoms.
  - **Dietary supplements** (especially St. John's wort but also ginkgo and kava) are somewhat effective for mild to moderate PMS but ineffective for PMDD. However, patients should be aware of their potential adverse effects (especially the effect of St. John's wort on the effectiveness of OCPs).
- In several small randomized trials, **NSAIDs** taken in the luteal phase have been shown to decrease all physical symptoms with the exception of breast tenderness.
- **Selective serotonin reuptake inhibitors** are the most effective pharmacologic treatment for moderate to severe PMS and PMDD. Continuous dosing exerts a greater inhibition of symptoms than intermittent dosing during the luteal phase. Fluoxetine, sertraline, citalopram, and paroxetine all demonstrated a statistically significant improvement in symptoms.
- Combined OCPs can improve PMDD symptoms. **Yaz**, containing drospirenone and 20 mg of ethinyl estradiol, is approved by the US Food and Drug Administration for treatment of PMDD and has been shown effective in treating mood, physical, and behavioral symptoms of PMDD.
- The **GnRH agonists**, such as Lupron, have been used successfully and act by decreasing estrogen and progesterone production by the ovary. Their use should be limited to a short-term course and in women who have not responded to or cannot tolerate selective serotonin reuptake inhibitors or OCPs.
- **Surgical management** of PMDD with bilateral oophorectomy (usually with concomitant hysterectomy) is considered the last resort for rare cases of severely debilitating symptoms refractory to all medical therapy.

SUGGESTED READINGS

American College of Obstetricians and Gynecologists Committee on Practice Bulletins—Gynecology. ACOG Practice Bulletin No. 110: noncontraceptive uses of hormonal contraceptives. *Obstet Gynecol*. 2010;115:206-218. (Reaffirmed 2018)

American College of Obstetricians and Gynecologists Committee on Practice Bulletins—Gynecology. ACOG Practice Bulletin No. 114: management of endometriosis. *Obstet Gynecol*. 2010;116:223-236. (Reaffirmed 2018)

American Psychiatric Association. *Diagnostic and Statistical Manual of Mental Disorders*. 5th ed. Arlington, VA: American Psychiatric Association; 2013.

Brosens I, Puttemans P, Campo R, Gordts S, Brosens J. Non-invasive methods of diagnosis of endometriosis. *Curr Opin Obstet Gynecol*. 2003;15(6):519-522.

Diwadkar GB, Falcone T. Surgical management of pain and infertility secondary to endometiosis. *Semin Reprod Med.* 2011;29(2):124-129.

Gurates B, Bulun SE. Endometriosis: the ultimate hormonal disease. *Semin Reprod Med.* 2003;21(2):125-134.

Latthe P, Mignini L, Gray R, Hills R, Khan K. Factors predisposing women to chronic pelvic pain: systematic review. *BMJ.* 2006;332(7544):749-755.

Shah DK, Correia KF, Vitonis AF, Missmer SA. Body size and endometriosis: results from 20 years of follow-up within the Nurses' Health Study II prospective cohort. *Hum Reprod.* 2013;28(7):1783-1792.

Shakiba K, Bena JF, McGill KM, Minger J, Falcone T. Surgical treatment of endometriosis: a 7-year follow-up on the requirement for further surgery. *Obstet Gynecol.* 2008;111:1285-1292.

Somigliana E, Vigano' P, Parazzini F, Stoppelli S, Giambattista E, Vercellini P. Association between endometriosis and cancer: a comprehensive review and a critical analysis of clinical and epidemiological evidence. *Gynecol Oncol.* 2006;101(2):331-341.

Evaluation of Amenorrhea

Victoire Ndong and Chantel I. Cross

DEFINITION

Amenorrhea is the absence of menses. It is physiologic during pregnancy, lactation, and menopause. The lack of regular, spontaneous menses for any other reason after the expected age of menarche is pathologic.

* **Primary amenorrhea:** no menses by age 14 years in the absence of secondary sexual development or no menstruation by age 16 years with the presence of secondary sexual characteristics
* **Secondary amenorrhea:** the absence of menses in a previously menstruating woman. It is also defined as the lack of menses for 6 months or for three menstrual cycles in women who have experienced menarche. Evaluation, however, need not be deferred solely to conform to these definitions.

EVALUATION OF AMENORRHEA

When to Evaluate for Amenorrhea

* **Evaluation of amenorrhea should begin with a good history as well as physical exam.** Most importantly, **pregnancy should be ruled out** because both primary and secondary amenorrhea require an immediate evaluation for pregnancy.
* Use clinical judgment. The above listed timeline defining amenorrhea does not need to be met prior to initiating an evaluation. Do not overlook gross evidence of a disease process: Turner syndrome (TS), frank virilization, obstructed vagina, or other evidences of a disease process.

- Use a systematic approach, evaluating each critical component of menstruation: hypothalamus, pituitary, ovaries, uterus, and genital outflow tract.

Pertinent History for Amenorrhea

- **Present illness.** Presence of cyclic pelvic or abdominal pain, headache, visual changes, seizure, hot flushes, hot or cold temperature intolerance, vaginal dryness, urinary issues, hirsutism, virilization, galactorrhea, severe physical or emotional stress, changes in weight, diet, athletic training, or trauma.
- **Past medical history.** General health, chronic illnesses (especially autoimmune and thyroid disease); birth defects; all current and recently discontinued medications or supplements; contraception history (especially the use of depot medroxyprogesterone acetate); history of pelvic infection; complications with prior pregnancies or abortions; and any instrumentation of the uterus, abdominal, or pelvic surgeries. Most recent pregnancy, delivery, and lactation history can be significant, as can a personal history of cancer treatment involving radiation therapy and/or chemotherapy.
- **Development.** Age of thelarche, pubarche, and menarche; whether menarche was spontaneous or induced; and cycle regularity
- **Social risk factors.** Severe physical or emotional stress, changes in weight or diet, and athletic training.
- **Family history.** History of late pubertal development, early menopause, mental retardation, or short stature.

Physical Examination for Amenorrhea

- Height, weight, body mass index, waist to hip ratio if obese, blood pressure, and pulse
- General body habitus, looking for disease stigmata of TS, Cushing syndrome, thyroid disease; also gross malnutrition or obesity
- Vision changes or peripheral loss of vision
- Tooth enamel erosion (associated with induced vomiting with bulimia)
- Skin evaluation for hyperpigmentation, acanthosis nigricans, abdominal striae, acne, hirsutism, balding
- Thyroid gland palpation for size, shape, and nodules
- Breast development (Tanner stage), galactorrhea, or other breast discharge
- Abdominal exam for masses, fat distribution, hirsutism, and above listed skin changes (striae, acanthosis nigricans, hyperpigmentation etc).
- External genitalia examined for hair distribution and virilization (clitoromegaly), imperforate hymen, or labial fusion
- Internal genitalia examined for transverse vaginal septum, lateral vaginal obstruction, estrogenized vaginal mucosa, presence of a cervix with visible patent external cervical os
- Rectal exam to evaluate for possible hematocolpos and presence of uterus beyond a vaginal obstruction or absent vaginal orifice. Rectal exam can also assist in evaluating a patient with an intact hymen or infantile vaginal orifice.

Laboratory Evaluation of Amenorrhea

It is important for laboratory evaluation to be guided by the above listed history and physical exam section presenting history and physical examination. Laboratory tests can include the following:
- Human chorionic gonadotropin to evaluate for pregnancy
- Follicle-stimulating hormone (FSH), estradiol (E2), thyroid-stimulating hormone (TSH), and prolactin (PRL)

- 17-Hydroxyprogesterone drawn at 8 AM along with progesterone, testosterone, dehydroepiandrosterone sulfate (DHEA-S) for patients with virilization, hirsutism, or suspected androgen excess
- Testosterone if concern for complete androgen insensitivity
- Karyotype if concern for genitourinary abnormalities, suspicion for gonadal dysgenesis, or complete androgen insensitivity. Also consider if other nonrelated physical malformations are present.

Imaging Evaluation of Amenorrhea

- Pelvic ultrasound for both primary and secondary amenorrhea
- Sonohysterography or hysterosalpingogram (HSG) to evaluate for Asherman syndrome as a cause of secondary amenorrhea; hysteroscopy is definitive.

Further Evaluation and Other Considerations

- Fragile X (FMR1) premutation for patients with primary ovarian insufficiency (POI)
- Antiadrenal antibodies and antithyroid antibodies (antiperoxidase and antithyroglobulin) patients with POI
- Karyotype for patients <30 years with POI
- Cortisol levels (24-h urinary free cortisol, late night salivary cortisol, dexamethasone suppression testing) for patients with suspected Cushing syndrome. Given that Cushing syndrome and polycystic ovarian syndrome (PCOS) share similar symptoms, cortisol testing must be considered in patients suspected to have PCOS who are experiencing symptoms specific to Cushing syndrome (ie, myopathy, weight gain, violaceous striae).
- Antimüllerian hormone (AMH)
- Insulin-like growth factor 1, free T4, morning cortisol level for patients with a pituitary lesion identified by magnetic resonance imaging (MRI)
- Adrenocorticotropin (ACTH) stimulation test for patients with elevated 17-hydroxyprogesterone
- An MRI of the pituitary for hyperprolactinemia or hypogonadotropic hypogonadism, which has no other identifiable etiology (severe physical, emotional stress, malnutrition, medications, hypothyroidism)
- An MRI of pelvis. Obtain when genitourinary abnormalities/anomalies are not well characterized or for surgical planning. An MRI is particularly useful when evaluating for imperforate hymen versus transverse vaginal septum, obstructed hemivagina, and noncommunicating or hypoplastic uterine horn.
- Renal ultrasound and radiographs (computed tomography [CT] or x-ray) of spine for patients with müllerian dysgenesis

Progesterone Withdrawal for Evaluation of Amenorrhea

- Progestin challenge: 5 to 10 mg of medroxyprogesterone (Provera) for 5 to 7 days. Positive response is withdrawal bleed within 2 to 7 days after discontinuation of Provera.
- Approximately 20% of patients with POI, hypothalamic amenorrhea, and hyperprolactinemia experience withdrawal flow depending on the degree of hypoestrogenism.
- Failure to withdraw bleed after sequential estrogen then progestin withdrawal is suggestive of an outflow tract obstruction. Serum E2 level rather than use of progesterone withdrawal may be needed to determine status of estrogen.

- Periodic progesterone-induced withdrawal bleed is indicated as a treatment for amenorrhea to prevent endometrial hyperplasia (particularly when a thickened endometrium is noted on ultrasound).

Differential Diagnosis for Primary Amenorrhea

- History and physical examination to evaluate for genital outflow obstruction
- Keep pregnancy in differential, although less likely.
- Keep the most common causes high on differential (gonadal dysgenesis, müllerian anomalies/dysgenesis, and complete androgen insensitivity).
- To develop a differential diagnosis, categorize the patients into four categories (Table 43-1) based on the presence or absence of a uterus and the presence or absence of breast development (indicative of estrogen).
  - Presence of uterus and absence of breasts likely represent gonadal dysgenesis, hypothalamic failure, or pituitary failure.
  - Absence of uterus and presence of breasts likely represent androgen insensitivity or congenital absence of the uterus.
  - Absence of both uterus and breasts likely represents failure of steroidogenesis to produce sex hormones including 17- or 20-desmolase deficiency, 17α-hydroxylase deficiency, or agonadism. The patient also frequently has 46,XY karyotype combined with gonadal failure.

Table 43-1	Differential Diagnosis of Primary Amenorrhea	
	Breast Development Present	Breast Development Absent
Uterus present	Consider secondary amenorrhea differential. Hypothalamic cause Pituitary cause Ovarian cause Uterine cause	**Gonadal dysgenesis** 45,X 46,X; abnormal X Mosaic X 46,XX or 46,XY: pure gonadal dysgenesis 17-Hydroxylase deficiency with 46,XX Galactosemia **Hypothalamic or pituitary failure** Kallmann syndrome CNS congenital defect Hypothalamic-pituitary tumors CNS infection Physiologic delay
Uterus absent	Müllerian agenesis Androgen insensitivity syndrome	17,20-Desmolase deficiency Agonadism 17-Hydroxylase deficiency with 46,XY

Abbreviation: CNS, central nervous system.

- Presence of both uterus and breast development likely represents pituitary etiology (eg, hyperprolactinemia) or another subcategory that also underlies secondary amenorrhea.

Differential Diagnosis for Secondary Amenorrhea

- Always keep pregnancy high on the differential diagnosis.
- Physiologic explanations include pregnancy, menopause, and postpartum lactation. Also consider medications, including progesterone (depot medroxyprogesterone acetate, intrauterine devices, pills, implants), oral contraceptive pills/rings/patch, and antipsychotic medications.
- See Table 43-2 for pathologic causes of secondary amenorrhea.
- If onset is related to previous pregnancy, abortion, or other surgical procedure, consider cervical stenosis or Asherman syndrome and evaluate further with HSG, hysteroscopy, or sonohysterogram.

Table 43-2   Pathologic Causes of Secondary Amenorrhea

Etiology	Causal Factor
Reproductive tract	
Cervical stenosis	Surgical procedure (ie, LEEP, CKC)
Asherman syndrome	Endometrial scarring
Ovarian	
Primary ovarian insufficiency	Idiopathic, chromosomal abnormality, autoimmune disease, infection
Polycystic ovary syndrome	Inappropriate gonadotropin secretion, insulin resistance
Pituitary	
Hyperprolactinemia	Lactotroph hyperplasia ± prolactinoma, drugs
Pituitary adenomas	Thyrotroph, corticotroph, or other hyperplasia
Sheehan syndrome	Postpartum hemorrhage
CNS	
Hypothalamic amenorrhea	Stress, eating disorders, weight loss, excessive exercise
Brain injury	Interruption of HPOA
Inflammatory or infiltrative process	Interruption of HPOA
Other endocrinopathies	
Hypothyroidism, Cushing syndrome, late-onset adrenal hyperplasia	

Abbreviations: CKC, cold knife cone; CNS, central nervous system; HPOA, hypertrophic osteoarthropathy; LEEP, loop electrosurgical excision procedure.

- A PRL mildly elevated: Repeat in the morning (patient needs to refrain from breast stimulation, intercourse, or exercise prior to test). Also, verify normal TSH to rule out hypothyroidism as etiology of hyperprolactinemia. Obtain brain MRI to evaluate for the presence of a pituitary lesion.
- Normal E2 and FSH levels: likely anovulation; consider further evaluation for PCOS.
- Low E2 and low FSH levels: Consider central nervous system (CNS) lesion or hypothalamic-pituitary failure; consider further evaluation with MRI.
- Low E2 and elevated FSH levels: Consider POI and gonadal dysgenesis.
- Elevated TSH: occult or subclinical hypothyroidism
- Markedly elevated DHEA-S: Rule out adrenal tumor with CT scan.
- Elevated 17-hydroxyprogesterone: Consider late-onset congenital adrenal hyperplasia; confirm with ACTH stimulation test.
- Evidence of androgen excess: with a normal E2, FSH, PRL, TSH, and 17-hydroxyprogesterone; should consider PCOS. Can also see mild elevations of DHEA-S in patients with PCOS. May see polycystic ovaries on pelvic sonogram, however, not required for diagnosis.
- Signs or symptoms of Cushing syndrome: Screen with late-night salivary cortisol (easiest), 24-hour urinary free cortisol, 1 mg overnight dexamethasone suppression, or 2-day, low-dose dexamethasone suppression screening tests.

ETIOLOGIES OF AMENORRHEA— SYSTEMATIC EVALUATION

Genital Outflow Tract and Uterine Abnormalities Resulting in Amenorrhea

- **Imperforate hymen** and **transverse vaginal septum** are outflow tract malformations that typically present with acute cyclic pelvic or abdominal pain in a patient soon after the age of expected menarche. The patient will often have age-appropriate secondary development. Examination of an imperforate hymen reveals no obvious vaginal orifice and often a bulging, thin perineal membrane. In a patient with a transverse septum, physical exam will reveal a normal vaginal orifice but no visible cervix. In some cases, an MRI may be required to distinguish an imperforate hymen from a transverse septum.
- **Müllerian agenesis** and **hypoplasia**, also known as Mayer-Rokitansky-Küster-Hauser (MRKH) syndrome, is a relatively common cause of primary amenorrhea. The incidence ranges from 1:4000 to 1:10 000. Subjects with MRKH commonly present in their late teens with normally developing breasts, pubic hair, and external genitalia because the presence and function of the ovaries are normal. Depending on the location of the müllerian agenesis, the patient can present with no vagina, a portion of a vagina, complete uterine agenesis, or a portion of the uterus. Amenorrhea is generally the only complaint, although 2% to 7% may have rudimentary müllerian structures with functioning endometrium, resulting in cyclic pain. An MRI of the pelvis can assist with classifying the anomalies and surgical planning, if required. Imaging of the urinary tract should be performed in all patients with müllerian abnormalities because approximately 30% have renal anomalies. Skeletal abnormalities are also commonly associated with MRKH. Vaginal dilator therapy or surgical construction of a neovagina can usually create a functional vagina.

- **Complete androgen insensitivity syndrome** (CAIS), previously known as testicular feminization, is an X-linked, recessive disorder that occurs in 46,XY individuals and results in a female phenotype. Testes are present and secrete normal male levels of AMH and testosterone. An AMH results in regression of müllerian structures. Masculinization fails to occur because of an androgen receptor defect. Like MRKH, patients with CAIS typically present in the later teens with normal development of breasts with primary amenorrhea. Physical examination generally demonstrates normal external genitalia, a shortened or absent vagina, and no cervix or uterus. Also, physical exam can often differentiate the two conditions because pubic and axillary hair is sparse in CAIS, and testes may be palpable in the inguinal region. The diagnosis of CAIS is confirmed by documenting serum testosterone in the normal male range and a 46,XY karyotype. Because the incidence of gonadal malignancy is 22% to 33% in CAIS, gonadectomy is often recommended. However, because malignancy rarely occurs before age 20 years, deferring surgery until after pubertal maturation and epiphyseal closure have occurred is preferable. It is no longer common practice to hide the diagnosis of CAIS from the adolescent and most are raised female. Vaginal dilator therapy can usually create a functional vagina.
- **Asherman syndrome** is the most common outflow tract obstruction resulting in amenorrhea and accounts for 7% of patients presenting with secondary amenorrhea. Asherman syndrome (ie, intrauterine synechiae) is most commonly associated with aggressive postpartum curettage or abortion. Other risk factors include uterine or cervical surgeries, such as cesarean delivery, septoplasty, myomectomy, and cone biopsy procedures. Infectious causes include tuberculosis, schistosomiasis, infection associated with intrauterine devices, and other severe pelvic infections. Diagnosis can be confirmed with HSG, sonohysterogram, or hysteroscopy. Treatment requires hysteroscopic lysis of intrauterine adhesions.
- **Cervical stenosis** can be the result of congenital defects or acquired following cervical conization or loop electrosurgical excision and dilation and curettage. If cervical stenosis is the underlying etiology of secondary amenorrhea, hematometra and an enlarged uterus should be detected by physical exam and confirmed with ultrasound. Treatment includes serial dilation of the cervix.

Ovarian Abnormalities Resulting in Amenorrhea (Hypergonadotropic Hypogonadism)

- Primary dysfunction at the level of the ovary. No ovarian response to gonadotropin stimulation results in lack of follicular development and production of E2.
- **Gonadal dysgenesis** is the most common cause of primary amenorrhea, accounting for 43% of such cases. Peripheral blood karyotype aids in diagnosis. Although TS is the most frequent cause of gonadal dysgenesis, any condition resulting in depletion of germ cells can cause gonadal dysgenesis and replacement of the gonads with fibrous streaks.
  - **Turner syndrome** classically results from aneuploidy involving the X chromosome. Approximately 60% of TS patients are 45,X and the other 40% include karyotype abnormalities such as 45,X/46,XX mosaics, 46,XXqi isochromosome, and 46,XXp-short arm deletion. Internal and external genitalia develop as normally females. The cohort of primordial follicles undergoes accelerated atresia so that oocytes are depleted prior to the onset of puberty. A lack of gonadal

E2 production results in a failure of breast development and other secondary sexual characteristics.

- Patients with TS exhibit several cardinal features including webbed neck, shield-shaped chest, short stature, and sexual infantilism. Typically, these patients are identified in the pediatric population due to short stature, prior to noting primary amenorrhea. Some TS patients, especially those with mosaic karyotypes, can undergo spontaneous puberty and conception (16% and 3.6% of cases, respectively).

- **Mosaicism** involving partial deletions or rearrangements of one X chromosome can cause a wide range of gonadal dysfunctions, ranging from gonadal dysgenesis to POI. Determining whether a Y chromosome is present in a mosaic is important because the presence of the SRY portion of the Y chromosome predisposes to tumor formation. Presence of a Y chromosome requires gonadectomy or removal of the gonadal streaks.

- **Pure gonadal dysgenesis** is a term used to describe 46,XX or 46,XY individuals who experience dysgenesis of germinal tissue early in embryonic development. Such dysgenesis likely results from genetic, environmental, or infectious insults, although a specific cause is rarely identified. All subjects are phenotypically female of normal height who fail to undergo puberty. Patients with 46,XY gonadal dysgenesis, also known as **Swyer syndrome**, require removal of their gonadal streaks to prevent malignant transformation.

- **CYP17 deficiency** is a rare disorder that can affect 46,XY or 46,XX individuals. The lack of 17α-hydroxylase and 17,20-lyase activities results in both gonadal and adrenal insufficiencies. Patients with an XY karyotype are phenotypic female (due to lack of androgen production) but also lack a uterus because AMH was secreted in early fetal life. Subjects usually present at the time of puberty with hypertension (due to excess mineralocorticoid production), hypokalemia, and hypergonadotropic hypogonadism. CYP17 deficiency is an autosomal recessive disorder.

- **Luteinizing hormone and FSH receptor mutations** have also been identified preventing the ovaries from responding to gonadotropin stimulation and resulting in POI. They can present with varying levels of secondary sexual development and likely primary amenorrhea. However, these conditions are very rare.

- **Primary ovarian insufficiency** can manifest as primary or secondary amenorrhea. For patients who previously menstruated, POI is defined as amenorrhea associated with a depletion of oocytes and cessation of menses before age 40 years. In those with primary amenorrhea, approximately 50% will have an abnormal karyotype. The various possible etiologies for POI associated with secondary amenorrhea are listed below; however, up to 90% of patients with POI remain unexplained following evaluation.

  - **X chromosome abnormalities**, such as short- or long-arm deletions or mosaicism, not severe enough to cause primary gonadal dysgenesis, may cause POI
  - **Spontaneous POI** is not induced by chemotherapy, radiation, or surgery. The majority of cases are idiopathic; 6% have premutations in the gene responsible for **fragile X syndrome (FMR1)**; 4% have **steroidogenic cell autoimmunity**, placing them at risk for adrenal insufficiency. Because 14% of patients with familial POI and 2% of isolated POI will have the FMR1 premutation, it is important to evaluate for the *FMR1* gene premutation, particularly when there is a family history of POI, fragile X, unexplained mental retardation, tremor/ataxia syndrome, and/or any developmental delay in children. In addition, because up

to 20% of patients with POI develop autoimmune hypothyroidism, they should undergo adrenal and thyroid antibody testing. Those under age 30 years with POI should also have karyotyping performed because 13% will show some chromosomal abnormalities. Inclusion of any Y chromosomal material is an indication for gonadectomy.

- **Iatrogenic POI** can be the result of follicular depletion by radiation, chemotherapy (especially with alkylating agents), or surgical manipulation or removal of ovarian tissue. Prior to undergoing radiation or chemotherapy, measures can be taken to decrease exposure to or mitigate damage. Prior to radiation therapy, oophoropexy can position ovaries outside the radiation field. Prior to and throughout chemotherapy treatment for malignancy or severe autoimmune diseases, gonadotropin-releasing hormone (GnRH) agonists or antagonists can potentially provide protection, although the efficacy of these treatments is still debated. Additionally, some centers offer pretreatment ovarian tissue cryopreservation.

- **Galactosemia** (GALT deficiency) is a rare autosomal recessive metabolic disorder that causes an inability to metabolize galactose sugar. The most common long-term complication for girls and women with GALT deficiency is POI, manifesting as primary or secondary amenorrhea or oligomenorrhea. Incidence is between 80% and 90%. Patients with trace levels of residual GALT activity may demonstrate milder phenotype. AMH, which is produced by granulocyte cells, may provide a meaningful predictor of ovarian function in pubertal girls with classic galactosemia.

- **Treatment of POI** involves estrogen replacement and should be initiated in essentially all patients to prevent the onset of osteopenia and osteoporosis. In addition, these women are at high risk for early-onset cardiovascular disease, genitourinary atrophy, vasomotor symptoms, sleep disturbance, and vaginal dryness. Often, POI patients require twice as much estrogen as compared to postmenopausal women to alleviate symptoms. This can be accomplished with use of oral contraceptive pills or higher doses of traditionally used hormone replacement therapy regimens (eg, micronized E2 1-2 mg daily or conjugated equine estrogens 0.625-1.25 mg daily) or transdermal treatment regimens (0.1 mg/24 h). In patients with short stature or open epiphyseal plates, lower doses of estrogen should be used to avoid closure. If the uterus is intact, adjunct cyclic treatment with progestins is required to prevent endometrial hyperplasia.

- Spontaneous pregnancy following POI is possible, although unlikely (approximately 5%). Treatment of infertility classically requires oocyte donation; however, in rare cases, gonadotropins can augment follicular development.

Hypothalamic Dysfunction Resulting in Amenorrhea (Hypogonadotropic Hypogonadism)

- Underlying etiology is a decrease in GnRH release and stimulation of the pituitary to release gonadotropins resulting in failure of folliculogenesis and production of E2.
- The term **hypothalamic amenorrhea** applies to conditions in which GnRH secretion is diminished in the absence of any organic pathology.
- Physical or **psychological stress**, **anorexia nervosa**, **exercise**, and **weight loss** can contribute to dysfunctional hypothalamic GnRH secretion. Affected women are frequently underweight, >10% below ideal body weight, and/or engage in regular strenuous exercise.

- **Kallmann syndrome** results from a genetic mutation that causes failure of olfactory and GnRH neuronal migration from the olfactory placode. The resultant hypogonadotropic hypogonadism is due to the absence of GnRH pulses to stimulate gonadotropin release from the pituitary. This syndrome is characterized by primary amenorrhea, absent breast development, presence of cervix and uterus, and anosmia.
- **Congenital GnRH deficiency** is a genetic condition resulting in the absence of functional hypothalamic neurons. Unlike Kallmann syndrome, it is not associated with anosmia.
- **GnRH receptor mutations** inhibit signaling of GnRH to release gonadotropins from the anterior pituitary. Patients affected have a broad range of phenotypes, depending on the particular mutation.
- **Other CNS pathologies**, such as hypothalamic neoplasms, trauma, hemorrhage, or cranial irradiation, can interrupt the function of the hypertrophic osteoarthropathy. **Craniopharyngioma** is the most common CNS neoplasm causing delayed puberty. An MRI should be ordered for any patient with hypogonadotropic amenorrhea when no obvious external cause is present.
- **Chronic debilitating disease** can also lead to hypogonadotropic amenorrhea as a result of alterations in GnRH pulsatility. This has been observed in renal disease, liver disease, malignancy, and human immunodeficiency virus. However, virtually any serious chronic illness can undermine the hypothalamic-pituitary-ovarian axis.
- **Treatment** involves correcting the underlying causative behavior if identified. The primary treatment is estrogen/progestin replacement as described in the treatment of POI section.

Pituitary Disorders Resulting in Amenorrhea

- **Pituitary lesions** can present with amenorrhea and low or normal levels of gonadotropins. The most common pituitary lesion is a prolactinoma, but nonfunctioning adenomas, adenomas that secrete other pituitary hormones, or empty sella syndrome may also be present.
- **Hyperprolactinemia** accounts for 14% of secondary amenorrhea and a small portion of primary amenorrhea (see chapter 11). Pregnancy and breastfeeding are physiologic causes of hyperprolactinemia. Medications that can cause hyperprolactinemia include most antipsychotics and antidepressants, H_2 receptor blockers, methyldopa, verapamil, reserpine, and metoclopramide. Other medical causes that must be evaluated include hypothyroidism and renal failure. However, by far, the most common pathologic cause of hyperprolactinemia is a prolactinoma.
  - **Prolactinomas** are classified as either microadenomas (<10 mm) or macroadenomas (≥10 mm). Macroadenomas may be associated with bitemporal hemianopsia; therefore, visual field defects should be evaluated for during physical examination.
  - Excess PRL levels can cause negative feedback on hypothalamic GnRH secretion thereby lowering gonadotropin release. In addition to hypogonadism, most women will experience oligo- or amenorrhea and galactorrhea. Galactorrhea is secretion of a milky fluid, unassociated with childbirth or breastfeeding. Discharge may be white/clear in color but also greenish or even bloody. Bloody discharge requires evaluation for an intraductal papilloma or cancer.
  - Laboratory evaluation of serum PRL: Levels >20 ng/mL are considered elevated. A mildly elevated serum PRL should be repeated in a fasting, nonstressed

environment because PRL concentration can vary with time of the day, level of stress, and other factors. Severe hyperprolactinemia (>100 ng/mL) is associated with amenorrhea, but amenorrhea can also be found with moderate levels (50-100 ng/mL). Occasionally, macroadenomas can produce extremely high serum PRL levels (>1000 ng/mL). Women with pituitary macroadenomas should also have additional evaluation including a serum free T4, insulin-like growth factor 1, and morning cortisol level.

- A confirmed elevation in PRL prompts imaging of the pituitary gland, usually by MRI. At least 30% to 40% of women with hyperprolactinemia have a pituitary adenoma. The incidence of malignancy in prolactinomas is very rare.
- Treatment of hyperprolactinemia is usually successful with dopamine agonist therapy (bromocriptine or cabergoline). Less commonly, surgery is required.
- **Sheehan syndrome** is a condition of pituitary necrosis and hypopituitarism most commonly following severe postpartum hemorrhage and hypotension.
- **Infiltrative disease** is most commonly caused by hemochromatosis, a disorder of excessive deposition of iron in the liver, pancreas, anterior pituitary, and heart. Screen iron studies, fasting transferrin saturation >45% is indicative. Treat with phlebotomy and chelation therapy.
- **Isolated gonadotropin (FSH/luteinizing hormone) deficiency** is a rare condition usually associated with thalassemia major, retinitis pigmentosa, or prepubertal hypothyroidism.

Normogonadotropic Amenorrhea

- Heterogeneous group with normal levels of gonadotropins and E2. Patients have normal secondary sexual development. The underlying etiology of amenorrhea is chronic anovulation. See chapter 42 for further discussion about each of these conditions.
- **Polycystic ovarian syndrome** is the most common cause of amenorrhea associated with hyperandrogenism. Patients generally have normal levels of gonadotropins and E2.
  - The Rotterdam Consensus Criteria is the most commonly used criteria for diagnosis of PCOS.
  - After other causes of amenorrhea and hyperandrogenism have been excluded, evidence of chronic anovulation/oligoovulation, androgen excess, and/or polycystic ovaries on ultrasound generally establishes the diagnosis.
  - Hyperandrogenism should be evaluated with serum testosterone, 17-hydroxyprogesterone, and DHEA-S levels to exclude late-onset congenital adrenal hyperplasia or the presence of an adrenal or other androgen-producing tumor.
  - The PCOS is associated with an increased risk for type 2 diabetes, insulin resistance, hypertension, lipid abnormalities, obesity, metabolic syndrome, and endometrial hyperplasia/cancer.
  - Treatment includes weight reduction and inducing withdrawal bleeding through cyclic progesterone or a combined hormonal contraceptive to decrease risk of unopposed estrogen stimulation of uterine lining. Also, identification and treatment of other underlying medical comorbidities (diabetes, obesity, hyperlipidemia, hirsutism).
- **Late-onset congenital adrenal hyperplasia** generally presents similarly to PCOS with amenorrhea and hyperandrogenism. Initial screening with 17-hydroxyprogesterone followed by ACTH stimulation test establishes the diagnosis. Most patients have an autosomal recessive disorder resulting in 21-hydroxylase deficiency. Treatment of amenorrhea involves glucocorticoid replacement and/or combined contraception.

- **Cushing syndrome** is a clinical state resulting from prolonged, inappropriate hypercortisolism. Etiologies include pituitary tumor (Cushing disease), adrenal hypersecretion of cortisol, or iatrogenic (chronic steroid use). It is characterized by loss of normal hypothalamic-pituitary-adrenal feedback mechanisms and loss of the normal circadian rhythm of cortisol secretion. Screening tests include late night salivary cortisol (evaluated diurnal variation), 24-hour urinary free cortisol (evaluates secretion), and dexamethasone suppression testing (evaluates impaired feedback).
- **Hyperprolactinemia** frequently presents with normal gonadotropin levels and normal to mildly depressed E2 (see above listed in the pituitary disorders leading to amenorrhea section).
- **Thyroid disease** can present with normal levels of gonadotropins and amenorrhea. Classic **hypothyroidism** accounts for 1% to 2% of primary and secondary amenorrhea. Hypothyroidism can lead to hyperprolactinemia. Thyrotropin-releasing hormone stimulates the release of TSH and PRL from the anterior pituitary. Therefore, patients with poorly controlled hypothyroidism may also experience sequelae of hyperprolactinemia. Both PRL and TSH should be routinely evaluated as part of the evaluation for amenorrhea. An elevated TSH and low T4 confirm hypothyroidism. An elevated TSH and normal T4 are diagnostic for subclinical hypothyroidism. Clinical hypothyroidism should be treated. Treatment should be initiated with 25 to 50 μg/d of levothyroxine followed by TSH assessment every 4 to 6 weeks until TSH levels normalize. Treatment of subclinical hypothyroidism is controversial but should be considered in children as well as women with infertility who are trying to conceive.

SUGGESTED READINGS

American College of Obstetricians and Gynecologists Committee on Gynecologic Practice. ACOG Committee Opinion No. 698: hormone therapy in primary ovarian insufficiency. *Obstet Gynecol.* 2017;129:e134-e141.

American College of Obstetricians and Gynecologists Committee on Practice Bulletins—Gynecology. ACOG Practice Bulletin No. 194: polycystic ovary syndrome. *Obstet Gynecol.* 2018;131:e157-e171.

Cox L, Liu JH. Primary ovarian insufficiency: an update. *Int J Womens Health.* 2014;6:235-243. doi:10.2147/IJWH.S37636.

Fritz MA, Speroff L. *Clinical Gynecologic Endocrinology and Infertility.* 8th ed. Philadelphia, PA: Lippincott Williams & Wilkins; 2011.

Gordon CM, Ackerman KE, Berga SL, et al. Functional hypothalamic amenorrhea: an Endocrine Society clinical practice guideline. *J Clin Endocrinol Metab.* 2017;102(5):1413-1439.

Legro RS, Arslanian SA, Ehrmann DA, et al. Diagnosis and treatment of polycystic ovary syndrome: an Endocrine Society clinical practice guideline. *J Clin Endocrinol Metab.* 2013;98(12):4565-4592.

Melmed S, Casanueva FF, Hoffman AR, et al. Diagnosis and treatment of hyperprolactinemia: an Endocrine Society clinical practice guideline. *J Clin Endocrinol Metab.* 2011;96(2):273-288.

Palmert MR, Dunkel L. Clinical practice. Delayed puberty. *N Engl J Med.* 2012;366(5):443-453.

Practice Committee of American Society for Reproductive Medicine. Current evaluation of amenorrhea. *Fertil Steril.* 2008;90:S219-S225.

44

Polycystic Ovary Syndrome and Hyperandrogenism

Jacqueline Y. Maher, Maria Facadio Antero, and Howard A. Zacur

DEFINITION AND ANDROGEN PHYSIOLOGY

- **Hyperandrogenism** is characterized by an abnormally elevated serum concentration of androgens and/or physical findings consistent with androgen excess.
- **Androgens** are necessary for normal ovarian and sexual function. They play an important role in cognition, bone health, muscle mass, body composition, mood, and energy.
- Androgens are precursors for estrogen synthesis. At low levels, androgens are produced by theca cells in the ovary, where cholesterol is converted to progesterone, which is then converted to androgens. Androgens are then converted to estrogens in the granulosa cells through the action of aromatase enzymes. At higher concentrations, androgens are converted to more potent 5α-reduced androgens, which cannot be converted to estrogens. These potent androgens inhibit aromatase activity and follicle-stimulating hormone (FSH) induction of luteinizing hormone (LH) receptors in the granulosa cells preventing oocyte maturation and leading to chronic anovulatory state.
- Androgens also affect skeletal homeostasis. They affect bone metabolism directly via androgen receptors expressed by osteocytes and indirectly via conversion of androgens to estrogen. Multiple studies have shown that women with low androgen concentrations have lower bone density and increased fracture risk.
- When produced in excess, androgens in the female can stimulate abnormal terminal hair growth, voice and muscle changes, hair loss, clitoral enlargement, and reduction in breast size.

SIGNS AND SYMPTOMS OF HYPERANDROGENISM

Normal Hair Growth and Physiology

- During gestation, the hair follicles of the developing fetus produce fine, unpigmented hair known as **lanugo**. The total number of hair follicles is determined late in the second trimester of pregnancy. With time, some of the hair follicles produce thick, darkly pigmented **terminal hair** in response to androgen exposure. The remaining hair follicles produce **vellus hair**, which are finer and not as darkly pigmented.
- **Normal hair growth cycle** follows three stages: **anagen** (growth phase), **catagen** (involution phase), and **telogen** phase (rest phase).

Hirsutism

- **Hirsutism** is excessive male pattern hair growth in women. It refers to the growth of terminal hair on the face, chest, back, lower abdomen, and upper thighs caused by the overactivity or overexpression of circulating androgens. The abnormal hair growth is predominantly midline. Androgens stimulate hair growth, increase the diameter of the hair shaft, and deepen the pigmentation of the hair. In contrast,

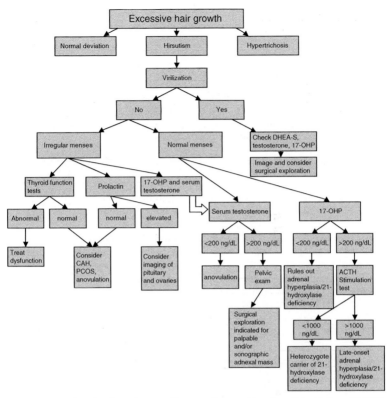

Figure 44-1. Algorithm for evaluation of hirsutism/hyperandrogenism. Abbreviations: 17-OHP, 17-hydroxyprogesterone; ACTH, adrenocorticotropic hormone; CAH, congenital adrenal hyperplasia; DHEA-S, dehydroepiandrosterone sulfate; PCOS, polycystic ovary syndrome.

estrogens slow hair growth and decrease hair diameter and pigmentation. An algorithm for evaluation of hirsutism is seen on Figure 44-1.

- **Idiopathic hirsutism** is the term used when a hirsute individual has normal levels of circulating androgens and has not been diagnosed with polycystic ovary syndrome (PCOS) or another disorder.
- **The Ferriman-Gallwey score** is an objective tool that may be used in the clinical setting to grade hair growth in women. It evaluates nine different androgen-sensitive hair growth sites on a scale from 0 to 4. Ninety-five percent of women will have a score under 8. Scores >8 suggest an excess of androgen-mediated hair growth and should be confirmed with a more extensive hormone evaluation.

Hypertrichosis

- **Hypertrichosis** is the generalized, excessive growth of vellus hair. It may be caused by genetic factors, underlying malignancy, or exposure to drugs such as phenytoin, penicillamine, diazoxide, cyclosporine, and minoxidil. It may also be seen with a number of medical conditions, including anorexia nervosa, hypothyroidism, malnutrition, porphyria, dermatomyositis, and paraneoplastic syndromes. Hypertrichosis should not be mistaken for hirsutism.

Hair Loss

* Recession of hair in the frontal and temporal regions of the scalp and the crown of the head (ie, **male pattern baldness**) in response to androgens is common with aging. This is the most common pattern of hair loss and affects approximately 30% to 40% of men and women alike. However, hair loss is less evident in women because it is typically more diffuse and rarely complete.

Virilization and Clitoromegaly

* This is an appearance of masculine features due to extreme excess androgenic activity. It refers to a constellation of symptoms, including deepening of the voice, male body habitus, male pattern baldness, clitoromegaly, and reduction of breast size.
* **Virilization** is very rare and may be associated with adrenal tumors and hyperplasia or ovarian tumors, such as theca-lutein cysts, luteomas, and Sertoli-Leydig cell tumors.
* **Clitoromegaly** or enlargement of the clitoris may occur. This is a dose-dependent event and is irreversible. It is more commonly seen when the excessive androgen exposure occurs in childhood or around the time of puberty.

Skin Changes

* Androgens stimulate secretions from pilosebaceous glands, resulting in oily skin. **Severe acne** is a manifestation of excessive androgenic hormone activity.
* **Acanthosis nigricans** is a gray-brown, velvety discoloration of the skin that is associated with hyperinsulinemia and obesity. Acanthosis nigricans is typically seen in the groin, neck, axillary, and vulvar regions. Acanthosis nigricans can be seen in patients with PCOS and diabetes mellitus, as well as paraneoplastic syndrome and malignancy, commonly an adenocarcinoma involving the gastrointestinal tract.

Voice Changes

* The vocal cords can undergo irreversible thickening, resulting in a lower tone of the voice.

ANDROGENS IN THE FEMALE

* Circulating androgens found in the blood of premenopausal women include testosterone, androstenedione, dehydroepiandrosterone sulfate (DHEA-S) and its precursor DHEA, and dihydrotestosterone (DHT). Androgens are produced by the adrenal glands and the ovary and arise from peripheral conversion.

Testosterone

* Testosterone is the most potent androgenic hormone.
* In women, nearly 25% of testosterone is secreted from the ovaries and 25% is secreted from the adrenal glands. The remaining one-half is produced from

peripheral conversion of androstenedione to testosterone in the kidneys, liver, and adipose tissue.

- **Normal serum total testosterone concentrations in women range from 20 to 80 ng/dL**, as compared to 300 to 1000 ng/dL in men.
- Total serum testosterone levels in most women with PCOS fall in the range of 30 to 150 ng/dL and levels >150 ng/dL increases the likelihood of a virilizing ovarian or adrenal neoplasm.
- Approximately 65% of testosterone in the circulation is bound to sex hormone–binding globulin (SHBG). Nineteen percent to 33% of testosterone is loosely bound to albumin. The remaining 1% of testosterone circulates in the free and active form. **Free testosterone** is the single most sensitive test to establish the presence of hyperandrogenemia.
- Testosterone levels decrease by 50% from ages 20 to 40 years old. Less testosterone is secreted from the ovary with menopause because the ovarian theca cells are less responsive to LH.

Androstenedione

- Androstenedione is a less potent androgen than testosterone but can produce significant androgenic effects when present in excess amounts.
- It is produced in equal amounts by the adrenal glands (50%) and the ovaries (50%).
- The majority of androstenedione is converted to testosterone.
- Normal serum concentration ranges from 60 to 300 ng/dL, often with a 15% increase at midcycle.

Dehydroepiandrosterone and Dehydroepiandrosterone Sulfate

- Androgen precursors, much less potent than testosterone, are produced predominantly by the adrenal glands, with some component of ovarian production and peripheral conversion.
- The DHEA is metabolized quickly; thus, measurement of its serum concentration does not reflect adrenal gland activity. The DHEA-S has a much longer half-life than DHEA, and measurement of its serum level is used to assess adrenal function.
- Serum hormone concentrations of DHEA-S in women vary widely (normal range of 38-338 μg/dL).

Dihydrotestosterone

- Testosterone is converted DHT by 5α-reductase, an enzyme found in many androgen-sensitive tissues.
- A DHT is a very potent androgen primarily responsible for the androgenic effects on hair follicles.

Sex Hormone–Binding Globulins

- Androgenicity is determined by free hormone concentrations. Thus, SHBG influences the hormonal state. Testosterone and insulin both decrease SHBG levels, whereas estrogen and thyroid hormone increase its levels.
- Patients with low levels of SHBG can develop symptoms of hyperandrogenism due to increase free testosterone levels.

CAUSES OF HYPERANDROGENISM

Five major causes of hyperandrogenism have been identified:
1. **Polycystic ovary syndrome**
2. **Late-onset congenital adrenal hyperplasia (CAH)**
3. **Tumors of the ovary or adrenal glands**
4. **Cushing syndrome or disease**
5. **Idiopathic or drug-induced processes**

DIAGNOSIS OF HYPERANDROGENISM

History and Physical Examination

- Hyperandrogenism may be diagnosed if signs of androgen excess are present (see section on "Signs and Symptoms of Hyperandrogenism").
- A careful medical history should be taken, including a detailed menstrual history asking about age of menarche, regularity of menstrual cycles, pregnancies, oral contraceptive pills (OCP) use, and presence of symptoms of ovulation or menstrual molimina. Patients should also be asked about a history of thyroid disease and hyperinsulinemia.
- A thorough physical examination should be performed.
- Pay particular attention to medications and family history.
- **Transvaginal pelvic ultrasound** should be performed to evaluate for the presence of polycystic ovaries. Polycystic ovaries are defined as having **12 or more follicles in each ovary** measuring 2 to 9 mm and **increased ovarian volume >10 mL**.

Laboratory Evaluation

- Measurement of serum androgen levels may be obtained to diagnose hyperandrogenism (see Figure 44-1). The clinician should check the following:
  - **Testosterone** serum hormone concentrations
  - A **DHEA-S** >700 ng/dL is consistent with abnormal adrenal function.
  - **17α-hydroxyprogesterone (17α-OHP):** normal: 100 to 200 ng/dL
  - **Prolactin:** normal: 1 to 20 ng/mL. Hyperprolactinemia can be associated with hyperandrogenism because it is likely that prolactin receptors are located on the adrenal glands. When prolactin binds to these adrenal receptors, it stimulates the release of DHEA-S.
  - **Thyroid function tests**
- **Diabetes assessment**
  - Normal fasting glucose: <100 mg/dL
  - Impaired fasting glucose or prediabetes: fasting glucose 100 to 125 mg/dL, hemoglobin A_{1c} 5.7% to 6.4%, or 2-hour oral glucose tolerance test (75-g load) 140 to 199 mg/dL.
  - Diabetes mellitus: fasting glucose levels >126 mg/dL, hemoglobin A_{1c} >6.5%, 2-hour oral glucose tolerance test (75-g load) >200 mg/dL, or random plasma glucose >200 mg/dL.

POLYCYSTIC OVARY SYNDROME

- The PCOS is the most common endocrine disorder among reproductive-age women. It affects approximately 4% to 12% of this population.

- It was initially termed *Stein-Leventhal syndrome* based on a cohort of obese amenorrheic women with cystic ovaries. Because of the cystic changes found within the ovaries of affected patients, the terms **hyperandrogenemic chronic anovulation syndrome**, **polycystic ovary syndrome**, and **polycystic ovary disease** are now used to describe these patients. However, polycystic ovaries alone seen on radiologic imaging are a nonspecific finding and may be seen in normal women.
- Individuals with PCOS do not have orderly follicular development. Most cycles fail to lead to the emergence of a dominant follicle or release of an oocyte leading to anovulation. The ovarian cortex becomes populated with numerous small follicles, or "cysts." The hyperandrogenemic state is believed to be both a cause and effect of incomplete follicular development.
- The PCOS is associated with amenorrhea, hyperandrogenism, hyperinsulinemia, and metabolic syndrome. In patients affected by this disorder, it is important to make the appropriate diagnosis early and to closely monitor these individuals because they may be at risk for other comorbidities.

Diagnosis of Polycystic Ovary Syndrome

- There are three recommended diagnostic schemes for PCOS.
  - The **1990 National Institutes of Health criteria** require the presence of hyperandrogenism and irregular menses and allow for a clinical diagnosis without the use of imaging.
  - The most commonly used diagnostic criteria today is the **2003 Rotterdam Consensus Criteria**, which require **any two of the following three manifestations**:
    o Oligomenorrhea and/or anovulation
    o Hyperandrogenism (clinical and/or biochemical signs)
    o Polycystic ovaries on ultrasound
  - In **2009, the Androgen Excess and PCOS Society** defined less inclusive criteria for PCOS, which required **ALL of the following criteria be met**:
    o Hyperandrogenism: hirsutism and/or hyperandrogenemia
    o Ovarian dysfunction: oligo-anovulation and/or polycystic ovaries
    o Exclusion of other androgen excess or related disorders
- Of note, **PCOS is always a diagnosis of exclusion** in all definitions. All other etiologies of hyperandrogenism must be ruled out.
- Patients with PCOS typically present with oligomenorrhea, amenorrhea, hirsutism, obesity, and infertility. All or some of these symptoms may be present. Virilization is not consistent with a diagnosis of PCOS, and other etiologies should be considered.
- Insulin resistance and metabolic syndrome are often associated with PCOS, and these patients should be screened for comorbidities. Providers should check a cholesterol panel, blood pressure, fasting glucose, 2-hour oral glucose tolerance test, and hemoglobin A_{1c}.

Pathophysiology of Polycystic Ovary Syndrome

- The exact cause of PCOS remains unknown. Abnormalities of the hypothalamic-pituitary axis and the ovarian or adrenal steroidogenic pathway, perhaps caused by genetic changes, have been suggested as possible explanations.
- Figure 44-2 outlines the pathophysiology of PCOS.
- **Pituitary and hypothalamus.** At the level of the hypothalamic-pituitary axis, increases in the frequency and amplitude of LH pulses have been recorded. A ratio of serum LH:FSH >2 is observed in PCOS patients.

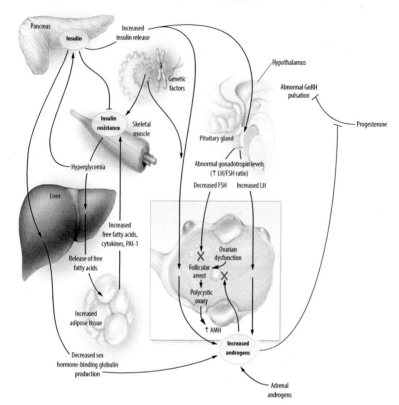

Figure 44-2. Pathophysiology of polycystic ovarian syndrome. Abbreviations: FSH, follicle-stimulating hormone; GnRH, gonadotropin-releasing hormone; LH, luteinizing hormone; PCOM, polycystic ovarian morphology; SHBG, sex hormone–binding globulin. Reprinted and modified from Rosenfield RL. Clinical practice. Hirsutism. *N Engl J Med.* 2005;353:2578-2588.

- **Ovarian androgen production.** Increased secretion of androgens from the ovaries has been observed in patients with PCOS. Elevated LH levels may lead to increased activity of ovarian theca cells, thus producing androgens. Also, elevated insulin may stimulate androgen secretion from both the ovaries and adrenals.
- **Adrenal androgen production.** Some PCOS patients may have mild elevations of DHEA-S levels.

Consequences of PCOS

- **Reproductive complications.** Patients often have **infertility** due to oligo-anovulation, defined as menstrual cycles greater than 35 days. Once they conceive, PCOS patients are not at higher risk for miscarriages but are at increased risk for gestational diabetes, macrosomia, and gestational hypertension.

- **Endometrial hyperplasia and malignancy.** Oligo-anovulation leads to unopposed estrogen and lack of progesterone withdrawal. Over time, this can lead to proliferation of the endometrium that may result in abnormal bleeding and, if untreated, may progress to endometrial hyperplasia and/or endometrial carcinoma.
- **Hyperinsulinemia and insulin resistance.** Insulin resistance is often observed in patients with PCOS, whether or not they are obese. Insulin may cause or contribute to the hyperandrogenic state by activating insulin receptors within the ovary, augmenting androgen secretion, or by acting on insulin-like growth factor receptors. Patients with PCOS are at increased risk for impaired glucose tolerance and 5- to 7-fold more likely to develop type 2 diabetes mellitus.
- **Metabolic syndrome** is characterized by a cluster of conditions such as elevated blood pressure, high serum glucose, increased waist circumference, and abnormal cholesterol or triglyceride levels that, when occurring together, increase the risk of heart disease, stroke, and diabetes. The prevalence of metabolic syndrome in women with PCOS is twice that of controls with similar age and body mass index. Additionally, PCOS patients are at higher risk for nonalcoholic fatty liver disease, which can lead to abnormal liver function tests, steatohepatitis, cirrhosis, and rarely hepatocellular carcinoma.

Treatment for Hyperandrogenism/Polycystic Ovary Syndrome

- Treatment depends on the underlying etiology and the desire for pregnancy.
- **Lifestyle modifications** should be first line in the management of hyperandrogenism. For those individuals who suffer from hirsutism and obesity, weight loss of even 5% can often improve symptoms related to PCOS. Weight loss may result in an elevation of SHBG, a decrease in bioavailable testosterone, and an improvement in insulin sensitivity.
- **Oral contraceptive pills** reduce circulating gonadotropin levels and increase SHBG levels; both work to decrease circulating androgens. The **OCPs are the first line** of treatment of oligomenorrhea, hirsutism, and acne caused by PCOS. Progestins decrease total androgen level by reducing the activity of 5α-reductase. Specific progestins with lower androgenicity include desogestrel, cyproterone acetate, and drospirenone. Overall, OCP usage results in an overall decrease in the formation of new androgen-dependent hair growth and androgen-stimulated acne. All low-dose OCP preparations are believed to have similar results.
- If combination OCPs are contraindicated or not desired, **medroxyprogesterone acetate** may be administered (5-10 mg for 10-12 d) every month or every other month to produce regular withdrawal bleeding. Patients should be cautioned that, unless contraception is used, pregnancy is possible with cyclic progestin therapy.
- **Metformin hydrochloride** is a biguanide antihyperglycemic drug, US Food and Drug Administration (FDA) approved for the management of type 2 diabetes mellitus. Metformin decreases hepatic gluconeogenesis, decreases the intestinal absorption of glucose, and improves insulin sensitivity in the peripheral system, including skeletal muscle, liver, and adipose tissue. In some studies, metformin has been shown to restore menses in approximately 50% of women with PCOS and can improve plasma insulin and insulin sensitivity, reduce serum free testosterone, and increase serum HDL cholesterol.
  - **Dosing:** The optimum dose of metformin for restoration of menses in women with PCOS ranges from **500 mg by mouth 3 times daily to 850 mg by mouth twice daily**. Patients should be titrated up to the appropriate dose of

this medication, starting at the lowest dose once daily, due to the gastrointestinal side effects.

- Metformin has a limited role in the treatment of hirsutism. Other agents may be added to metformin to improve these symptoms.
- Metformin appears to be unique among insulin-sensitizing agents in that it can improve weight loss, hyperandrogenism, and menstrual cycles in individuals with PCOS.

Treatment for hirsutism

- Hirsutism is slow to respond to hormone suppression. Results may not be seen for up to 6 months. Androgen suppression will not alter previous hair growth patterns.
- **OCPs:** as discussed above (see section on Treatment of Hyperandrogenism/Polycystic Ovary Syndrome)
- **Spironolactone** therapy is often initiated if OCP use is not an option for the treatment of hirsutism or if results from OCP therapy are not optimal. Spironolactone, an aldosterone antagonist, is an antihypertensive agent directly inhibits 5α-reductase and decreases androgen synthesis. Because of potential adverse effects on genitalia of male fetuses, spironolactone should be used with contraception in sexually active women. Other side effects include diuresis, orthostatic hypotension, fatigue, dysfunctional uterine bleeding, hyperkalemia, and breast enlargement.
- **Flutamide** is a nonsteroidal antiandrogen (often used for prostate cancer) that blocks the binding of androgen to its receptor, which can cause inhibition of new hair growth. Side effects include dry skin and, rarely, hepatotoxicity. Liver function should be monitored during treatment. Due to adverse fetal effects, effective contraceptive therapy is mandatory.
- **Finasteride:** An inhibitor of mostly type II 5α-reductase, finasteride was developed initially as a treatment for prostate hypertrophy and cancer. By inhibiting 5α-reductase, the drug decreases DHT activity at the level of the hair follicle. Finasteride treatment prevents new hair growth and decreases the terminal hair shaft diameter. No major side effects have been associated with this drug. Again, due to adverse fetal effects, reliable contraception should be used.
- **Minoxidil** is the only drug approved by the FDA for treatment of androgenic alopecia in women. It promotes hair growth by increasing the duration of the anagen phase and enlarging miniaturized and suboptimal follicles. It is available over the counter as a 2% and 5% topical solution.
- **Eflornithine hydrochloride (Vaniqa)** 13.9% cream reduces unwanted facial hair. Eflornithine is a potent antagonist of ornithine decarboxylase, the enzyme necessary for the production of polyamines, organic compounds that stimulate and regulate the growth of hair follicles and other organs. Twice daily topical use has shown improvement after 24 weeks in some clinical trials. The benefit is usually first seen at 8 weeks.
- **Hair removal** by mechanical methods such as shaving, waxing, depilatories, laser, and electrolysis are often used by patients. However, hair regrowth is common. Other adverse effects (including inflammation, blistering, hyperpigmentation, hypopigmentation, and scarring) are more commonly seen in dark-skinned women.

Surgery: Laparoscopic ovarian drilling and wedge resection used to be a standard treatment prior to ovulation-inducing agents. However, because of the high incidence of pelvic adhesions and risk of decreased ovarian reserve, this approach is rarely used today and is now considered second-line therapy.

Fertility Treatment for Polycystic Ovary Syndrome

- **Ovulation induction** medications are frequently required.
- **Clomiphene citrate (Clomid)** is a selective estrogen receptor modulator that functions as an estrogen receptor antagonist in the hypothalamus, thus stimulating gonadotropin-releasing hormone and subsequent FSH secretion. Typical administration is oral doses of 50 to 150 mg/d for 5 days on a monthly basis to induce ovulation in infertile women. It is not used for cycle regulation or as a primary treatment for hirsutism (see chapter 40).
- **Letrozole** is an aromatase inhibitor. It prevents the conversion of androgens to estrogen in the peripheral blood stream. The reduced estrogen levels lead to a subsequent negative feedback to the hypothalamus, which then triggers a compensatory increase in hypothalamic gonadotropin-releasing hormone secretion followed by an increased release of pituitary gonadotropins FSH and LH. Some consider letrozole to be first line for ovulation induction for patients with PCOS when compared to clomiphene. Letrozole resulted in higher pregnancy and live birth rates with no difference in miscarriage or multiple birth rates. However, **caution is advised because letrozole is not FDA approved for ovulation induction and is contraindicated for use during pregnancy**.
- **Gonadotropins** such as recombinant FSH and human menopausal gonadotropins directly stimulate the ovary and may be used to induce ovulation in letrozole- and Clomid-resistant PCOS patients or if undergoing in vitro fertilization (see chapter 40).
- **Metformin** (see "Treatment for Hyperandrogenism/Polycystic Ovary Syndrome" section) is not as effective as monotherapy ovulation-inducing agents letrozole and Clomid but can be used in combination.
- **In vitro fertilization** is the next step if weight loss or ovulation induction with medications are unsuccessful (see chapter 40).

NONCLASSICAL (LATE-ONSET) CONGENITAL ADRENAL HYPERPLASIA

Epidemiology

- The CAH are autosomal recessive disorders that typically present in the neonatal period. A deficiency in the **21-hydroxylase (21-OH)** enzyme due to mutations in the *CYP21A2* gene accounts for approximately 95% of cases.
- Nonclassical congenital CAH (NCCAH) is a less severe form of the disorder and affects 2% to 8% of all hirsute women. In comparison to the classic form of CAH where there is only 0% to 2% enzyme activity, in NCCAH, there is 20% to 50% 21-OH enzyme activity. The NCCAH is more prevalent than classical CAH.
- The enzyme 21-OH converts progesterone to deoxycorticosterone, or 17-hydroxyprogesterone (17-OHP) to 11-deoxycortisol. A decrease in the activity of this enzyme causes diminished cortisol production by the adrenal gland, resulting in increased pituitary secretion of adrenocorticotropic hormone (ACTH). The ACTH stimulates the adrenal gland to produce increased precursor 17-OHP. Higher 17-OHP levels lead to secretion of androstenedione, which is then converted to testosterone (Figure 44-3).

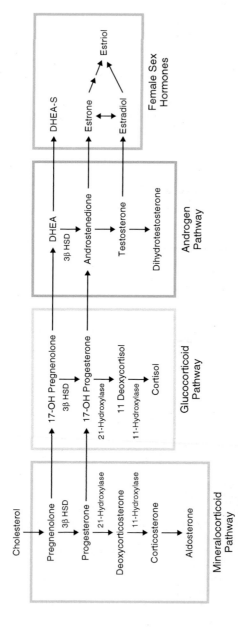

Figure 44-3. Steroid pathway and enzyme mutations associated with Congenital Adrenal Hyperplasia. Abbreviations: DHEA, dehydroepiandrosterone; DHEA-S, dehydroepiandrosterone sulfate; HSD, hydroxysteroid dehydrogenase.

- Enzyme deficiencies of **11β-hydroxylase and 3β-hydroxysteroid dehydrogenase** are other causes but are far less common.
- The prevalence of NCCAH may be as high as 1/1000 to 1/100 in whites, with an even higher prevalence among Ashkenazi Jews and Hispanics.

Signs and Symptoms

- The presentation is often similar to PCOS with oligomenorrhea and signs of hyperandrogenism including hirsutism and acne.
- Unlike typical CAH, symptoms of late-onset CAH are not evident until late childhood or adolescence.
- Salt wasting is absent, and affected females do not have ambiguous genitalia.

Diagnosis

- Measure the basal levels of 17-OHP in the morning during the follicular phase.
  - Normal levels of **17-OHP are <200 ng/dL**.
  - **Levels over 800 ng/dL are virtually diagnostic of CAH.**
  - Levels between 200 and 800 ng/dL require ACTH-stimulation testing (see Figure 44-1). Patients with NCCAH have 17-OHP levels >1500 ng/dL in response to a 250 μg ACTH-stimulation challenge.
- Patients should be tested for 21-OH deficiency, especially when they present with symptoms of hyperandrogenism at a young age or if they have a known family history of CAH. Women of Hispanic or Eastern European Jewish descent should also be tested, where the prevalence of this disorder is higher.

Treatment

- Treatment with **glucocorticoid** agents, such as **hydrocortisone**, **prednisone**, or **dexamethasone**, can restore ovulation and reduce circulating androgen levels; therefore, its use is appropriate for the treatment of infertility and hirsutism in women with NCCAH. In patients with 21-OH deficiency, prednisone 5 mg before bedtime is used to suppress endogenous ACTH.
- The OCPs or antiandrogens may be used to treat hirsutism, alone or in combination with glucocorticosteroids. Ovulation-inducing agents may also be used to treat infertility.

ANDROGEN-PRODUCING OVARIAN OR ADRENAL TUMORS

- Tumors of the ovary or adrenal gland that secrete androgens are rare.
  - In the ovary, causes include **Sertoli-Leydig cell tumors**, **theca-cell (stromal) tumors**, **hilus cell tumors**, and **pregnancy luteomas**. On rare occasions, excess testosterone is produced by malignant cystadenomas, Brenner tumors, and Krukenberg tumors.
  - In the adrenal gland, **adenomas or carcinomas** are the sources of the hyperandrogenism.
- The presence of an **androgen-producing tumor** is suspected on the basis of clinical findings. Palpation of an adnexal mass in a patient with symptoms of

hyperandrogenism or **rapid onset of virilization** even in the presence of normal testosterone levels should prompt a workup for a pelvic tumor. These tumors may often be small and difficult to detect on physical examination alone.

- **Testosterone levels exceeding 150 to 200 ng/dL and DHEA-S levels >700 to 800 μg/dL** are concerning for the presence of an ovarian or adrenal androgen-producing tumor.
- Surgical removal with or without adjuvant therapy is the treatment of choice.

CUSHING SYNDROME

- Cushing syndrome is caused by prolonged exposure to high levels of glucocorticoids.
- **Cushing disease (ACTH dependent)** arises when excessive cortisol secretion is due to excessive release of ACTH from the pituitary. Causes of Cushing disease include an ACTH-secreting adenoma in the pituitary, ectopic ACTH-secreting sources (carcinoid or neuroendocrine tumors), and ACTH-producing pheochromocytoma.
- **Cushing syndrome (ACTH independent)** results from increase cortisol production due to an adenomatous or rarely malignant neoplastic process arising from the adrenals. Other causes of Cushing syndrome include adrenocortical adenomas, pigmented nodular adrenocortical disease, adrenal carcinoma, McCune-Albright syndrome, and exogenous glucocorticoids.

Signs and Symptoms

- Patients have characteristic phenotype on exam, which include rounded face with full cheeks (moon facies); prominent facial skin flushing; short stature; obesity of face and trunk more so than extremities; hirsutism; buffalo hump; purplish striae located in the hips, abdomen, and thighs; ecchymosis; muscle wasting; glucose intolerance; and oligomenorrhea.
- Patients can suffer from hypertension and hyperglycemia, which if severe can progress to diabetes. Osteoporosis is common and may cause pathologic fractures.

Diagnosis

- There are three screening methods that are comparable in accuracy.
  - **24-hour urinary free cortisol excretion measurement:** Levels 3 times the upper limit of normal are deemed abnormal and lower abnormal levels are equivocal. Values **>100 μg/24 h are abnormal and levels >240 μg are almost diagnostic** of Cushing syndrome.
  - **Late night salivary cortisol level:** Levels **>4 nmol/L** are suggestive of Cushing syndrome. Levels maybe falsely elevated in shift workers, older patients, smokers, and people with hypertension or diabetes.
  - **Overnight dexamethasone suppression test:** 1 mg of dexamethasone is given at night and cortisol level are measured at 8:00 to 9:00 AM. **Values <1.8 ng/dL are normal**. If abnormal, a late afternoon ACTH and cortisol should be measured. If low or undetectable ACTH levels, **computed tomography or magnetic resonance imaging** of adrenals should be performed. If ACTH levels are normal or elevated, MRI of the pituitary should be done.

Treatment

- **Surgical excision** of the pituitary or adrenal adenoma is recommended. Radiation can be considered for poor surgical candidates or those who failed surgical treatment.
- **Medical therapy** to diminish hypercortisolism is divided into agents that block steroidogenesis (metyrapone, ketoconazole, etomidate, and mitotane) and inhibit cortisol action by antagonism at the receptor level (mifepristone).

IDIOPATHIC AND DRUG-INDUCED HIRSUTISM

- **Idiopathic hirsutism** is diagnosed in hirsute individuals who have a **negative workup** for other causes of hirsutism. Studies show that 5% to 15% of hirsute patients may have idiopathic hirsutism. An alternative explanation is based on the hypothesis that patients with idiopathic hirsutism demonstrate increased skin sensitivity to androgens. One theory is that patients with idiopathic hirsutism convert testosterone to DHT in greater quantities than normal due to increased activity of 5α-reductase.
- Occasionally, drugs such as **danazol and methyltestosterone** may cause iatrogenic hirsutism.
- The same medications used to treat hirsute PCOS patients may be used to treat idiopathic hirsutism.

SUGGESTED READINGS

American College of Obstetricians and Gynecologists Committee on Practice Bulletins—Gynecology. ACOG Practice Bulletin No. 194: polycystic ovary syndrome. *Obstet Gynecol.* 2018;131(6):e157-e171.

Azziz R. Polycystic ovary syndrome. *Obstet Gynecol.* 2018;132(2):321-336.

Brodell LA, Mercurio MG. Hirsutism: diagnosis and management. *Gend Med.* 2010;7(2): 79-87.

Franik S, Eltrop SM, Kremer JA, Kiesel L, Farquhar C. Aromatase inhibitors (letrozole) for subfertile women with polycystic ovary syndrome. *Cochrane Database Syst Rev.* 2018;(5): CD010287.

Fritz MA, Speroff L, eds. *Clinical Gynecologic Endocrinology and Infertility.* 8th ed. Philadelphia, PA: Lippincott Williams & Wilkins; 2011:498-563.

Nieman LK, Biller BM, Findling JW, et al. Treatment of Cushing's syndrome: an Endocrine Society clinical practice guideline. *J Clin Endocrinol Metab.* 2015;100(8):2807-2831.

Practice Committee of the American Society for Reproductive Medicine. Role of metformin for ovulation induction in infertile patients with polycystic ovary syndrome (PCOS): a guideline. *Fertil Steril.* 2017;108(3):426-441.

Speiser PW, Arlt W, Auchus RJ, et al. Congenital adrenal hyperplasia due to steroid 21-hydroxylase deficiency: an Endocrine Society clinical practice guideline. *J Clin Endocrinol Metab.* 2018;103(11):4043-4088.

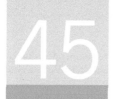

Definitions and Epidemiology of Menopause

Jacqueline Y. Maher and Wen Shen

- **Menopause** is the permanent cessation of menses, dated by the last menstrual period followed by 12 months of amenorrhea.
- The average age of menopause is 51 years, with a normal range of 43 to 57 years. It can also be induced by oophorectomy or iatrogenic ablation of ovarian function.
- **STRAW +10** (Figure 45-1) is considered the gold standard for characterizing reproductive aging in women through menopause. It is an updated guideline from the 2001 Stages of Reproductive Aging Workshop where the concept of a staging system for ovarian aging was developed.
- The transition from reproductive to postreproductive life is divided into several stages, with the final menstrual period (FMP) serving as an anchor. Stages (−5 to −1) precede the FMP and stages (+1 to +2) follow it.
- **Menopausal transition**, traditionally termed *perimenopause* or the *climacteric*, is the transition period from regular menstruation until menopause. It may last for 5 years or more and is highly variable in duration. It is characterized by menstrual cycle changes that include variable cycle length, with skipped periods and increasingly longer intervals of amenorrhea. This transition is associated with the cessation of ovulation, a marked decline in estradiol production, and a modest decline in androgen production.
- Early menopausal transition (−2) is depicted by variable cycle length (>7 d different from the norm) and increased follicle-stimulating hormone (FSH) levels.
- Late menopausal transition (−1) is characterized by two skipped cycles and an interval of amenorrhea >60 days.
- **Diagnosis of menopause is clinical**, without reliance on hormonal measurements.
- When any doubt exists about menopause, other causes of secondary amenorrhea must be ruled out. See chapter 43.

PHYSIOLOGY OF MENOPAUSE

Natural Menopause

- Oocytes undergo atresia throughout a woman's life, with follicular quantity and quality undergoing a critical decline approximately 20 to 25 years after menarche. This follicular decline results in loss of ovarian sensitivity to gonadotropin stimulation.
- During perimenopause, follicular dysfunction can lead to variable menstrual cycle length. The follicular phase is usually shortened due to the decreased number of functional follicles.
- The early menopause transition is typified by increased levels of FSH leading to overall higher estrogen levels.
- As follicular depletion continues, decreased inhibin produced by follicles leads to continued increased FSH. Follicular depletion also leads to recurrent anovulation and subsequent increase in FSH and luteinizing hormone levels.

Stage	-5	-4	-3b	-3a	-2	-1	+1a	+1b	+1c	+2
Terminology	REPRODUCTIVE				MENOPAUSAL TRANSITION		POSTMENOPAUSE			
	Early	Peak	Late		Early	Late	Early			Late
					Perimenopause					
Duration	*variable*				*variable*	1-3 years	2 years (1+1)		3-6 years	*Remaining lifespan*
PRINCIPAL CRITERIA										
Menstrual Cycle	Variable to regular	Regular	Regular	Subtle changes in Flow/Length	*Variable Length* Persistent ≥7-day difference in length of consecutive cycles	Interval of amenorrhea of >=60 days				
SUPPORTIVE CRITERIA										
Endocrine										
FSH			Normal	Variable*	↑ Variable*	↑ >25 IU/L**	↑ Variable*		Stabilizes	
AMH			Low	Low	Low	Low	Low		Very Low	
Inhibin B			Low	Low	Low	Low	Low		Very Low	
Antral Follicle Count 2–10 mm			Low	Low	Low	Low	Very Low		Very Low	
DESCRIPTIVE CHARACTERISTICS										
Symptoms						Vasomotor symptoms *Likely*	Vasomotor symptoms *Most Likely*			*Increasing symptoms of urogenital atrophy*

Menarche → (points to Stage -5)

FMP (0) → (points between Stage -1 and +1a)

*Blood draw on cycle days 2-5

**Approximate expected level based on assays using current pituitary standard

↑ = elevated

Figure 45-1. The Stages of Reproductive Aging Workshop +10 staging system for reproductive aging in women. Abbreviations: AMH, antimüllerian hormone; FMP, final menstrual period; FSH, follicle-stimulating hormone. Reprinted with permission from Harlow SD, Gass M, Hall JE, et al; STRAW 10 Collaborative Group. Executive summary of the Stages of Reproductive Aging Workshop +10: addressing the unfinished agenda of staging reproductive aging. *Menopause.* 2012;19(4):387-395. Copyright ©2012 The North American Menopause Society.

Primary Ovarian Insufficiency

- Primary ovarian insufficiency is cessation of menstrual periods due to failure of the ovaries prior to age 40 years old (also called premature ovarian failure, premature ovarian insufficiency, or premature menopause). It affects 1% of women 40 years or younger. See chapter 43.
- **Diagnosis: <40 years old, amenorrhea >4 months, FSH >40 mIU/mL**

Medical Menopause

- Medical menopause refers to the temporary or permanent amenorrhea result from various medical treatments, such as the following:
  - Ovarian suppression with gonadotropin-releasing hormone agonists
  - Chemotherapy-induced amenorrhea
  - Oncologic radiation therapy

Surgical Menopause

- Surgical menopause occurs after a bilateral oophorectomy in a premenopausal woman and results in an abrupt estrogen withdrawal. It is often associated with more severe symptoms than patients experiencing natural menopause.

SYMPTOMS

Menstrual Cycle Disturbances

- Complaints of irregular bleeding are very common during the menopausal transition. This is due to increasing fluctuations in FSH and estradiol and shortening of the follicular phase from 14 to 10 days. Menstrual irregularities may present as changes in both duration and timing, including skipped cycles and anovulatory cycles.
- If episodes of bleeding occur more often than every 21 days, last longer than 8 days, are very heavy, or occur after a 6-month interval of amenorrhea, evaluation of the endometrium must be undertaken to rule out neoplasm. This may include pelvic ultrasound, endometrial biopsy, and possible dilation and curettage with hysteroscopy.
- **Expectant management** is a reasonable course of action. It is also important to remember that the menopausal transition can vary greatly in length, anywhere from 1 to 3 years.
- **Oral contraceptive pills** can be used during the menopausal transition.

Vasomotor Menopause Symptoms

- Seventy-five percent of menopausal women experience vasomotor symptoms such as hot flashes and night sweats.
- Symptoms begin an average of 2 years before the FMP.
- Eight percent of women who have hot flashes endure them for longer than 1 year, and 50% endure them for longer than 5 years.
- **Pathophysiology:** due to vasomotor instability, thought to be secondary to dysfunction of the thermoregulatory nucleus, which is responsible for maintaining body temperature within a set range known as the thermoregulatory zone
- Characterized by a sudden reddening of the skin over the head, neck, and chest, accompanied by a feeling of intense body heat, palpitations and anxiety, sleep disturbance, and irritability; concludes with profuse perspiration

- **Risk factors:** surgical menopause (up to 90% of women will have vasomotor symptoms), early menopause, low estradiol levels, smoking, and possibly low body mass index
- **Vasomotor menopause symptoms (VMS) treatment** (Table 45-1)
  - **Behavior modification:** use of a fan, dressing in layers, and drinking cool beverages
  - Relaxation techniques, such as slow breathing and yoga
  - Exercise may increase the severity of symptoms by raising core body temperature.
  - **Hormone therapy (HT) is first-line treatment** (see Table 45-1 for dosing). The HT remains the most effective treatment for menopausal signs and symptoms. It should not be used for the prevention of chronic diseases. Health care providers should individualize and treat women with the lowest effective dose for the shortest duration that is needed to relive vasomotor symptoms. Given the variable response to HT, dosage adjustment should be guided by the clinical response.
    - **Women without a uterus** can be given **estrogen therapy alone**, either orally or transdermally for VMS (see Table 45-1 for dosing). Transdermal estrogen delivers estrogen at a relatively constant rate of 50 to 100 mg/dL, comparable to premenopausal endogenous estrogen production. Transdermal administration avoids first-pass liver metabolism effect, which prevents an effect on synthesis of clotting factors (lower risk of venous thromboembolism) and decreases the effect on lipid metabolism.
    - **Women with a uterus** should receive **progestin therapy in addition to their estrogen therapy**. Progestin therapy can be given either daily or for 10 days each month. Unopposed estrogen may increase the incidence of endometrial hyperplasia, which is a precursor to endometrial cancer. Progestins can be given in combination formulations with estrogen or separately. Oral, transdermal, and intrauterine options are available (see Table 45-1 for dosing).
    - **Contraindications for HT:** history of VTE or stroke or those at high risk for developing these conditions, history of breast cancer, or coronary heart disease (CHD)
  - **Alternative medications** include selective serotonin reuptake inhibitors and serotonin-norepinephrine reuptake inhibitors such as **venlafaxine and paroxetine**; **clonidine**, an α-adrenergic agonist; **gabapentin**, an anticonvulsant (see Table 45-1 for dosing).
  - **Alternative therapies** such as soy, black cohosh, red clover, dong quai, and acupuncture have been used to treat hot flashes. However, the limited trials in this area have not shown a benefit compared to placebo. Further investigation is needed to clarify their role in the alleviation of hot flashes and their side effects.

Genitourinary Syndrome of Menopause

- Pathophysiology: The vagina, urethra, and bladder trigone have high estrogen receptor concentrations. Loss of estrogen during menopause thus leads to urogenital atrophy.
- Atrophic vulva loses most of its collagen, adipose tissue, and water-retaining ability and becomes flattened and thin. Sebaceous glands remain intact, but secretions decrease, leading to vaginal dryness. Vaginal shortening and narrowing occur, and the vaginal walls become thin, lose elasticity, and become pale in color.
- Dyspareunia is the most common complaint related to vaginal atrophy.

Table 45-1 Treatment Options for Vasomotor Menopausal Symptoms[a]

Treatment	Dosage/Regimen	Evidence of Benefit*	FDA Approved
Hormonal			
Estrogen-alone or combined with progestin			
• Standard Dose	Conjugated estrogen 0.625 mg/d	Yes	Yes
	Micronized estradiol-17β 1 mg/d	Yes	Yes
	Transdermal estradiol-17β 0.0375–0.05 mg/d	Yes	Yes
• Low Dose	Conjugated estrogen 0.3–0.45 mg/d	Yes	Yes
	Micronized estradiol-17β 0.5 mg/d	Yes	Yes
	Transdermal estradiol-17β 0.025 mg/d	Yes	Yes
• Ultra-Low Dose	Micronized estradiol-17β 0.25 mg/d	Mixed	No
	Transdermal estradiol-17β 0.014 mg/d	Mixed	No
Estrogen combined with estrogen agonist/ antagonist	Conjugated estrogen 0.45 mg/d and bazedoxifene 20 mg/d	Yes	Yes
Progestin	Depot medroxypro-gesterone acetate	Yes	No
Testosterone		No	No
Tibolone	2.5 mg/d	Yes	No
Compound bioidentical hormones		No	No
Nonhormonal			
SSRIs and SSNRIs		No	No
Paroxetine	7.5 mg/d	Yes	Yes
Clonidine	0.1 mg/d	Yes	No

Table 45-1	Treatment Options for Vasomotor Menopausal Symptoms[a] *(Continued)*		
Treatment	Dosage/Regimen	Evidence of Benefit*	FDA Approved
Gabapentin	600–900 mg/d	Yes	No
Phytoestrogens		No	No
Herbal Remedies		No	No
Vitamins		No	No
Exercise		No	No
Acupuncture		No	No
Reflexology		No	No
Stellate-ganglion block		Yes	No

Abbreviations: FDA, US Food and Drug Administration; SSNRIs, selective serotonin-norepinephrine reuptake inhibitors; SSRIs, selective serotonin reuptake inhibitors.
[a]Reprinted with permission from the American College of Obstetrics and Gynecologists Committee on Practice Bulletins—Gynecology. ACOG Practice Bulletin No. 141: management of menopausal symptoms. *Obstet Gynecol*. 2014;123(1):202-216. (Reaffirmed 2018). Copyright © 2014 by The American College of Obstetricians and Gynecologists.

- Estrogen deficiency within the urethra and bladder is associated with urethral syndrome, which is characterized by recurrent episodes of urinary frequency and urgency with dysuria.
- **Genitourinary syndrome of menopause treatments**
  - **Moisturizers and lubricants** include Replens, Astroglide, K-Y jelly, and coconut oil, which can be used to relieve symptoms related to vaginal dryness and dyspareunia.
  - **Local estrogen therapy:** mainstay therapy for urogenital atrophy. Local therapy is advised for the treatment of women with only vaginal symptoms. Local estrogen therapy improves vaginal atrophy and associated symptoms, including dysuria and urinary tract infections. Different forms of local estrogen therapy are available:
    - **Low-dose estrogen creams** (estradiol-17β cream 2 g/d, conjugated equine estrogen cream 0.5-2 g/d) are applied intravaginally from daily to 2 times a week.
    - **Vagifem tablets** (estradiol 25 μg) are given vaginally as one per day for 14 days followed by twice per week.
    - **Estring, estradiol vaginal ring** (estradiol-17β ring 7.5 μg/d), is a silicone ring placed in the vagina for 3 months. It has minimal systemic absorption.

Cognitive Changes

- The incidence of subjective cognitive complaints during the menopausal transition ranges from 31% to 92%.
- Estrogen has a role in supporting memory and prefrontal cortex functioning.
- It has been hypothesized that declines in estrogen during the menopausal transition are associated with reduced cognitive functioning.

- There is an accelerated deterioration of cognitive function once menopause begins. Alzheimer disease is 3 times more common in women than in men.
- In cultured cells and animal models, estrogen has a protective effect on neurons.
- However, studies to date have lacked consistency in testing outcomes and specific aspects of memory function with the use of estrogen replacement.

Depression and Anxiety

- It has been suggested that declines in estrogen occurring around the time of menopause are associated with mood changes.
- **Depression:** Menopause is associated with higher rates of depressive symptoms (2-4 times higher).
  - **Risk factors:** prior depressive episodes, a history of stressful events during childhood, prior premenstrual syndrome, prior postpartum depression, and lengthier menopausal transition
- **Anxiety:** Relatively less is known about the course of anxiety during peri- and postmenopause. The menopausal transition is associated with new-onset anxiety in women without a history of anxiety.
  - **Risk factors:** a history of high premenopausal anxiety
- **Poor sleep maintenance** (nocturnal awakening) occurs in 40% to 60% of menopausal women. Reduced sleep quality in menopause has been linked to depressive symptoms.
- **Treatment**
  - The HT is not currently US Food and Drug Administration approved for treatment of mood dysfunction. The North American Menopause Society's 2017 position statement concludes that there is insufficient evidence to support HT for the treatment of clinical depression, particularly in postmenopausal women.
  - **Selective serotonin reuptake inhibitor/serotonin-norepinephrine reuptake inhibitor** medications that are commonly used for nonhormonal therapy of vasomotor symptoms that may be reasonable to start with include paroxetine (starting dose 7.5 mg/d), citalopram (starting dose 10 mg/d), escitalopram (starting dose 10 mg/d), venlafaxine (starting dose 37.5 mg/d), and desvenlafaxine (starting dose 100 mg/d).

SPECIAL CONCERNS FOR MENOPAUSAL WOMEN

Bone Health

- **Osteoporosis** is the condition of decreased bone mass and bone microarchitectural deterioration with resulting increased risk of skeletal fractures. In the United States, 4 to 6 million women (13%-18% of those over 50 y old) have osteoporosis, resulting in 1.5 million fractures per year. Most common fracture sites include the lumbar vertebrae, wrist (distal radius), and hip (femoral neck). Ninety percent of all hip and spine fractures in Caucasian women aged 65 to 84 years old are secondary to osteoporosis.
- **Pathophysiology:** Estrogen deficiency causes an imbalance of skeletal remodeling, with an increase in resorption that is greater than bone formation. Estrogen binds to receptors on osteoclasts, which break down bone, and inhibits their activity. Decreased serum calcium levels lead to an increase in parathyroid hormone, which stimulates osteoclastic activity.

- **Screening: Bone mineral density (BMD)** testing should routinely start for women at age 65 years old. Postmenopausal women under 65 years old can also benefit from testing if they have risk factors or have an elevated fracture risk assessment (FRAX) risk.
  - **Risk factors** for low BMD: low body weight ($<$127 lb), current smoker, parental family history of osteoporosis, previous fragility fracture (fracture from fall from standing height), chronic corticosteroid use, alcoholism, use of antiepileptic medications, endocrine disorders (such as hyperparathyroidism, hyperthyroidism, hypogonadism, Cushing syndrome, premature menopause), low calcium or vitamin D intake, rheumatoid arthritis, malabsorption, inflammatory bowel disease, or chronic liver disease
  - The **FRAX** tool (https://www.sheffield.ac.uk/FRAX/) is a model used to predict 10-year risk of fracture, taking into account risk factors. Based on the FRAX tool, a 65-year-old woman has a 9.3% 10-year risk for an osteoporotic fracture. Any woman with a greater than 9.3% 10-year risk for fracture should be screened at an earlier age.
- **Diagnosis** is determined by BMD, with **dual-energy x-ray absorptiometry** being the preferred technique. The most important measurement to consider is the patient's *t* **score**, which reflects the patient's bone density compared to a healthy 30-year-old of the same age and sex. *z* Scores correspond to the same measurements using women of the same age as the reference.
  - **Normal** bone *t* scores are above -1.0.
  - **Osteopenia** *t* scores are between -1.0 and -2.5.
  - **Osteoporosis** *t* scores are at/or below -2.5.
- **Prevention and treatment**
  - Universal recommendations: appropriate daily calcium and vitamin D intake/supplementation, weight-bearing exercise, smoking cessation, avoidance of excessive alcohol intake, modifications to reduce fall risks (ie, secure/remove loose rugs)
  - Medical treatment should be initiated in the following groups of women:
    - Any postmenopausal woman with a history of a osteoporotic vertebral or hip fracture
    - Any postmenopausal woman with a BMD score consistent with osteoporosis
    - Any postmenopausal woman with a *t* score of -1.0 to -2.5 and a 10-year FRAX risk of a spine, hip, shoulder fracture of 20%, or a hip fracture risk of at least 3%
- **Treatments.** At the time of this publication, the North American Menopause Society (NAMS) is updating the treatment recommendations and medication dosing for the prevention and treatment of osteoporosis (see http://www.menopause.org/otcharts.pdf). Medications currently in use include the following:
    - Bisphosphonates (alendronate, risedronate, ibandronate, and zoledronic acid) are generally considered first-line treatment. Side effects include heartburn, esophageal irritation, esophagitis, abdominal pain, diarrhea, and osteonecrosis of jaw (rare).
    - Selective estrogen receptor modulators: raloxifene (Evista)
    - Human monoclonal antibody: denosumab (Prolia)
    - Parathyroid hormone: teriparatide (Forteo)
    - Calcitonin
    - Estrogen, oral and transdermal options: Premarin, Climara, Vivelle
    - Combined estrogen-progestins, oral and transdermal options: Prempro, Premphase, Climara Pro

- **Repeat dual-energy x-ray absorptiometry screening**
  - Every 15 years for women with normal bone density or mild osteopenia
  - Every 5 years for women with moderate osteopenia (t score from -1.5 to -1.99)
  - Every year for women with advanced osteopenia (t score from -2.0 to -2.49)
  - Every 1 to 2 years for women undergoing therapy for osteoporosis

Cardiovascular Health

- Cardiovascular disease (CVD) is the single largest killer of American women; approximately 400 000 women die annually from CVD. More women than men die each year from CVD: **1 out of 3 women will die of CVD**.
- The term *atherosclerotic cardiovascular diseases* (ASCVD) broadly encompasses CHD, ischemic stroke, and peripheral arterial disease.
- Coronary artery disease (CAD) is the leading cause of death among postmenopausal women. Women lag 10 years behind men in terms of CAD risk prior to menopause. By age 70, a woman has the same risk of CAD as a male of the same age.
- Women's risk for CVD increases after menopause. The dramatic decline in endogenous estrogens at the menopause transition, which men do not experience, may increase a woman's risk of CVD and explain sex differences in CVD manifestation.
- The Framingham study showed a 2- to 6-fold increased incidence of CAD in postmenopausal women compared to premenopausal women in the same age group.
- Estrogen has a protective effect on reducing CVD risk in premenopausal women. Estrogen aids in vascular smooth muscle relaxation, decreases inflammation, decreases low-density lipoprotein levels, and increases high-density lipoprotein levels.
- An HT as a treatment for CHD is an area of ongoing review and debate. Although HT improved the lipid panel (lowers low-density lipoprotein cholesterol), it did not reduce ASCVD events in older women. As such, **HT should not be used for the sole purpose of ASCVD prevention**, although it was not associated with increased long-term mortality.

HORMONAL REPLACEMENT THERAPY STUDY SUMMARIES

Nurses' Health Study Observational Study

- Nurses' Health Study (NHS) was the largest cohort study of US women, following 121 700 premenopausal women aged 30 to 55 years. This was followed by a 10-year follow-up study that evaluated postmenopausal HT.
- Breast cancer: Current use for >5 years increases risk (higher if age >55). Progestins added to estrogen therapy do not increase risk. Previous use does not significantly increase risk.
- CHD: Current use reduces risk; no substantial increase risk of stroke
- Colon cancer: no increase in risk
- Hip fracture: reduces risk of hip fracture

Women's Health Initiative Prospective Randomized Controlled Trial

- Enrolled postmenopausal women aged 50 to 79 years (mean age, 63; however, approximately 25% of women were >70). In the estrogen plus progestin arm, approximately 33% of women were receiving treatment for hypertension and 13% had high cholesterol. Women with severe menopausal symptoms were discouraged from participating.

- Participants received either estrogen plus progestin, estrogen alone if they had a hysterectomy, or placebo.
- The primary outcome was CHD, with fractures being a secondary outcome.
- Adverse events monitored were breast cancer and venous thromboembolism.
- After 5 years, the estrogen plus progestin arm of the study was stopped early because the number of cases of breast cancer in the treatment group exceeded the predetermined threshold for increased risk.
- In 1 year, of 10 000 postmenopausal women who took estrogen plus progestin, 38 were diagnosed with breast cancer compared to 30 of 10 000 women who took placebo. Women in the estrogen alone group have not shown increased rates of breast cancer.
- Results showed that per 10 000 women annually, the number of heart attacks, strokes, and blood clots were 37, 29, and 34 in the estrogen plus progestin arm compared to 30, 21, and 16 per 10 000 women taking placebo. Women taking estrogen alone also showed increased risk of these events relative to placebo.
- There were fewer bone fractures and diagnoses of colon cancer in both hormone groups.
- A secondary analysis showed that women who initiated HT closer to menopause (within 10 y) had reduced CHD risk compared to women more distant from menopause.
- Lower risk was found for young women and higher risk for older patients.
- **The "Timing Hypothesis":** Given the findings of the NHS and the secondary analyses of the Women's Health Initiative (WHI), it has been theorized that there could be a "window of opportunity" in the early postmenopause stage, when HT can have a protective effect on CVD risk. Further prospective, randomized controlled trials are necessary to evaluate this theory.
- **NHS versus WHI summary:** Data from NHS differs from WHI on breast cancer, CHD, and colon cancer. This may be due to the difference in the age of participants, and their relevance to usual age of starting HT.

Heart and Estrogen/Progestin Replacement Study Prospective Randomized Controlled Trial

- A randomized controlled trial that challenged the generally widely accepted notion that HT reduced the incidence of heart disease in postmenopausal women. The Heart and Estrogen/Progestin Replacement Study trial revealed that HT in women with already established CVD including recent myocardial infarctions, worsened their cardiac outcomes within the first year of treatment.
- Concluded that the use of estrogen plus progestin did not prevent further heart attacks or death from CHD. There were significantly more thromboembolic events in the HT users.

Kronos Early Estrogen Prevention Study

- A double-blinded, placebo-controlled randomized controlled trial of low-dose oral or transdermal estrogen and cyclic monthly progesterone given to healthy women ages 42 to 59 years old within 3 years after menopause over a period of 4 years
- Both HT groups had reduced VMS (night sweat, hot flashes), improved BMD, and decreased genitourinary syndrome of menopause symptoms. Overall, there were similar rates of progression of arterial wall thickness in all treatment groups. There were no statistically significant differences in rates of endometrial cancer,

breast cancer, stroke, transient ischemic attack, venous thromboembolism, or myocardial infarction among treatment groups. Compared to placebo, women in the oral conjugated equine estrogen treatment arm had significant improvement in measures of depression-dejection and anxiety-tension. Neither treatment showed any detectable adverse or beneficial effects on measures of cognition.

- This study concluded that in newly postmenopausal women desiring symptom management and overall better quality of life, hormonal therapy is a safe and viable option for them, understanding that each woman may have different risks factors precluding treatment, making individualization of care important.

Postmenopausal Estrogen/Progestin Interventions Trial Prospective Randomized Controlled Trial

- The Postmenopausal Estrogen/Progestin Interventions trial found that women on HT had greater high-density lipoprotein cholesterol levels than women taking placebo.

Women's Health Initiative Memory Study

- The Women's Health Initiative Memory Study noted a slightly increased risk of cognitive decline and dementia in women 65 years and older taking estrogen alone or with progestin.

SUGGESTED READINGS

American College of Obstetricians and Gynecologists Committee on Gynecologic Practice. ACOG Committee Opinion No. 556: postmenopausal estrogen therapy: route of administration and risk of venous thromboembolism. *Obstet Gynecol.* 2013;121(4):887-890. (Reaffirmed 2019)

American College of Obstetricians and Gynecologists Committee on Gynecologic Practice. ACOG Committee Opinion No. 565: hormone therapy and heart disease. *Obstet Gynecol.* 2013;121(6):1407-1410. (Reaffirmed 2018)

American College of Obstetricians and Gynecologists Committee on Practice Bulletins—Gynecology. ACOG Practice Bulletin No. 129: osteoporosis. *Obstet Gynecol.* 2012;120(3):718-734. (Reaffirmed 2019)

American College of Obstetricians and Gynecologists Committee on Practice Bulletins—Gynecology. ACOG Practice Bulletin No. 141: management of menopausal symptoms. *Obstet Gynecol.* 2014;123(1):202-216. (Reaffirmed 2018)

iMedicalApps. *The Johns Hopkins Menopause Guide.* Baltimore, MD: Johns Hopkins Point of Care Information Technology Center; 2019. https://apps.apple.com/us/app/johns-hopkins -menopause-guide/id1464930929.

Judd HL, Mebane-Sims I, Legault C, et al. Effects of hormone replacement therapy on endometrial histology in postmenopausal women: the Postmenopausal Estrogen/Progestin Interventions (PEPI) Trial. *JAMA.* 1996;275(5):370-375.

Management of osteoporosis in postmenopausal women: 2010 position statement of the North American Menopause Society. *Menopause.* 2010;17(1):25-54.

Manson JE, Aragaki AK, Rossouw JE, et al. Menopausal hormone therapy and long-term all-cause and cause-specific mortality: the Women's Health Initiative randomized trials. *JAMA.* 2017;318(10):927-938.

The NAMS 2017 Hormone Therapy Position Statement Advisory Panel. The 2017 hormone therapy position statement of The North American Menopause Society. *Menopause.* 2017;24(7):728-753.

Female Pelvic Medicine and Reconstructive Surgery

46 Urinary Incontinence and Lower Urinary Tract Symptoms

Prerna Raj Pandya and Chi Chiung Grace Chen

Urinary incontinence is the involuntary leakage of urine. The prevalence of urinary incontinence varies by age and has been estimated as impacting approximately 25% of young women, 44% to 57% of middle-aged and postmenopausal women, and 75% of older women. Urinary incontinence is also a large component of health care expenditure, with the direct cost of care for urinary incontinence in the United States estimated at approximately $19.5 billion. Urinary incontinence can have a significant impact on a woman's health, including physical, psychological, and emotional or social well-being.

IMPACT ON HEALTH

- Urinary incontinence can have a significant impact on a woman's health as a result of its association with depression and anxiety, social isolation and embarrassment, sexual dysfunction, increased risk of falls, perineal infections, loss of independence, increased caregiver burden, nursing home placement, and overall quality of life.

ETIOLOGY AND RISK FACTORS

- Continence is dependent on normal-functioning lower urinary tract anatomic structures, including the bladder and urethra; intact neurologic reflexes, involving the central and peripheral nervous system; and the functional and cognitive ability to voluntarily void. Any disruption in this pathway can lead to urinary incontinence.

- **Risk factors** include age, obesity, parity and childbirth, ethnicity/race, family history, hypoestrogenism, lifestyle factors, previous pelvic surgery of pelvic radiation, impaired functional status, medications, and underlying medical conditions (eg, diabetes, dementia/cognitive impairment, stroke, depression, Parkinson disease, multiple sclerosis).

TYPES OF URINARY INCONTINENCE AND LOWER URINARY TRACT SYMPTOMS

- There are three main types of urinary incontinence in women:
  - **Stress urinary incontinence (SUI)** is the most common type of urinary incontinence among ambulatory community-dwelling women. An SUI is the involuntary loss of urine on effort, physical exertion, sneezing, or coughing. This occurs when abdominal pressure exceeds bladder pressure and should not be confused with physiologic or psychological stress. *Occult or latent stress incontinence* is SUI that is observed only after reduction of coexistent pelvic organ prolapse.
  - **Urgency urinary incontinence (UUI)** is involuntary loss of urine associated with urgency. Many patients complain of inability to reach the toilet in time. Involuntary detrusor contractions are typically the cause.
  - **Mixed urinary incontinence** describes signs and symptoms of both SUI and UUI.
- There are several other subtypes of incontinence and lower urinary tract symptoms (LUTS) that should also be considered during evaluation of a woman with symptoms of urinary incontinence. The following are the relevant definitions as provided by the International Urogynecological Association/International Continence Society Joint Report on the Terminology for Female Pelvic Floor Dysfunction:
  - **Overactive bladder syndrome (OAB)** is urinary urgency usually accompanied by frequency and nocturia, with or without UUI, in the absence of urinary tract infection (UTI) or other obvious pathology. The OAB often results from inappropriate detrusor contraction. When spontaneous or provoked involuntary detrusor contractions are demonstrated on urodynamic testing during bladder filling, this is referred to as **detrusor overactivity**. Detrusor overactivity may be neurogenic (associated with an underlying neurologic process) or idiopathic.
  - **Frequency** is the complaint of voiding too often. In some populations, a cutoff for normal is seven voids during waking hours.
  - **Urgency** is the complaint of a sudden compelling desire to pass urine that is difficult to defer. Urgency can occur with or without incontinence.
  - **Nocturia** is the complaint of waking at night one or more times to void.
  - **Nocturnal enuresis** is the involuntary loss of urine that occurs during sleep.
  - **Postural urinary incontinence** is the involuntary loss of urine associated with change in body position.
  - **Continuous urinary incontinence** is the continuous involuntary loss of urine.
  - **Insensible urinary incontinence** is involuntary loss of urine where the woman has been unaware of how it occurred.
  - **Coital incontinence** is involuntary loss of urine with coitus, which may be further divided into that occurring with penetration and that occurring with orgasm.

- **Functional incontinence** is associated with cognitive, psychological, or physical impairments that make it difficult to reach the toilet and interferes with appropriate toileting.
- **Overflow incontinence** is the involuntary loss of urine when the bladder does not empty completely and is associated with high residual urine volumes or urinary retention.
- **Postmicturition leakage** is the involuntary passage of urine after micturition.
- **Extraurethral urinary incontinence** is urine leakage through channels other than the urethral meatus (ie, genitourinary fistulas or ectopic ureter).
- The LUTS can be grouped into four main categories:
  - **Urinary incontinence symptoms**, as noted above
  - **Bladder storage symptoms**, which are often referred to as "irritative voiding symptoms," include increased daytime urinary frequency, nocturia, urgency, and OAB.
  - **Sensory symptoms** refer to a departure from normal sensation or function experienced by the woman during bladder filling. Increased or decreased sensation causes an earlier or later desire to void in response to a filling bladder.
  - **Voiding and postmicturition symptoms** include changes in normal sensation or function during or following micturition. This consists of symptoms such as hesitancy (delay in initiating micturition), slow stream, intermittency (urine flow that stops and starts during voiding), straining to void, spraying (splitting) of urinary stream, feeling of incomplete bladder emptying, need to immediately revoid, postmicturition leakage, position-dependent micturition, dysuria, and urinary retention.
- **Interstitial cystitis** or **bladder pain syndrome.** The Society for Urodynamics and Female Urology defines interstitial cystitis/bladder pain syndrome as "an unpleasant sensation (pain, pressure, discomfort) perceived to be related to the urinary bladder, associated with LUTS of more than 6 weeks duration, in the absence of infection or other identifiable causes" (see chapter 32).

PATIENT EVALUATION

History

- Any patient evaluation for urinary incontinence should include a thorough medical, surgical, gynecologic, and obstetric history. The clinical evaluation should elicit the patient's symptoms and severity, assess impact on quality of life, evaluate for comorbid medical conditions, identify associated support defects such as a cystocele, and identify potentially reversible causes of urinary incontinence. A useful mnemonic for other causes of urinary incontinence that should be addressed is DIAPPERS: **D**elirium, **I**nfection, **A**trophy, **P**harmacology, **P**sychology, **E**ndocrinopathy, **R**estricted mobility, and **S**tool impaction.
- **Altered sexual functioning and body image.** Patients may complain of dyspareunia, avoidance of intercourse, decreased libido, and decreased self-image.
- Many **validated and reliable questionnaires** can be used to elicit a symptom history from patients, such as the International Consultation on Incontinence Questionnaire, Overactive Bladder Questionnaire, Pelvic Floor Distress Inventory, Urogenital Distress Inventory, Incontinence Severity Index, Incontinence Impact Questionnaire, Pelvic Floor Impact Questionnaire, and the Pelvic Organ Prolapse/Urinary Incontinence Sexual Questionnaire.

- **Bladder diary or frequency volume chart.** The patient records the volume and frequency of fluid intake and voiding as well as symptoms of frequency and urgency and episodes of incontinence for at least 24 hours, ideally for 2 to 3 days.

Physical Exam

A comprehensive **physical examination** should be performed at the first visit, including:
- A **pelvic exam**, including a systematic evaluation of all components of the pelvic floor, pelvic organ support, strength of the levator ani muscles, innervation/ sensation of the perineum, vulvar architecture, and perineal scars.
- Particular attention should be given to urethral anatomy and hypermobility.
  - A **suburethral diverticulum** is an outpouching of the urethra, and patients may complain of dysuria, dyspareunia, postvoid dribbling, and recurrent UTIs.
  - The **Q-tip test** evaluates urethral support. A cotton swab is placed in the urethra to the level of the urethrovesical junction, and the change in axis from rest to strain is measured to assess **urethral hypermobility** (deflection of >30 degrees).
- The **stress test** is performed by looking for urine leakage from the urethral meatus when abdominal pressure is increased, such as with cough or Valsalva. A positive result on a stress test is essential to the diagnosis of SUI. It can be done while standing or in the dorsal lithotomy position, with different bladder volumes, and is a very specific test for SUI. False-negative results can be explained by low bladder volume or lack of patient effort. If pelvic organ prolapse is present, consider performing stress test after prolapse reduction.
- Evaluate for **fistula**. In the United States, gynecologic surgery is the most common cause of **urogenital fistulae** (0.1% of all hysterectomies). Other causes include radiation, trauma, and severe pelvic pathology. In developing countries, obstetric injuries are the most common cause. Patients often report painless and continuous vaginal leakage of urine, usually within the context of recent pelvic surgery (1-2 wk). Instillation of methylene blue dye into the bladder or a Pyridium dye test will stain a vaginal pack if a vesicovaginal fistula is present, which can be confirmed on cystourethroscopy. Intravenous pyelography or computed tomography urography can be performed to evaluate for possible ureterovaginal fistula.

Diagnostic Tests

- **Urinalysis and/or urine culture** can evaluate for microscopic hematuria or UTI.
- **Postvoid residual (PVR)** volume is the volume of urine remaining in the bladder at the completion of micturition and can aid in diagnosing overflow incontinence. Although there are no standard criteria for diagnosing urinary retention, most consider PVR to be abnormal if >150 mL. If an elevated PVR is identified, the test should be repeated.
- **Cystourethroscopy** can be used to assess the anatomy of bladder and urethra.
- **Urodynamic studies** can be used to assess the physiologic function of the bladder during filling, storage, and voiding. Simple cystometric testing can be performed in the office using a straight catheter and syringe to fill the bladder with a known volume of sterile water. At various bladder volumes, the patient is asked to cough and Valsalva in an attempt to demonstrate SUI. Multichannel cystometrics, using one catheter in the bladder and the other either in the vagina or rectum, can be used for

patients with complex symptoms or voiding complaints. Urodynamic evaluation is not required in the assessment of all patients with urinary incontinence symptoms (even those planning for an anti-incontinence procedure) but should be considered as a tool to aid in diagnosis for certain patient populations (prior history of incontinence surgery, history of pelvic radiation, failure to respond to treatments for incontinence, neurogenic voiding dysfunction, mixed incontinence symptoms, or concern for overflow incontinence).

TREATMENT

Conservative Treatment of Lower Urinary Tract Symptoms/ Urinary Incontinence

Conservative treatment options for most types of LUTs, including OAB/UUI, SUI, or mixed incontinence, can be effective as initial strategies. These interventions include the following:

- **Lifestyle modifications** include weight loss, avoidance of dietary triggers including reduction of caffeine intake, smoking cessation, and manipulation of daily fluid intake. Weight loss has been found to be more effective for stress incontinence than OAB/UUI but may be beneficial for both.
- **Bladder retraining** involves scheduled voiding with progressive increases in the interval between voids and urge suppression techniques for women with OAB/UUI.
- **Pelvic floor muscle exercises (PFME)** requiring repeated voluntary pelvic floor muscle training (ie, Kegel exercises) may be used in conjunction with bladder retraining. A PFME performed in a supervised pelvic floor physical therapy program are more effective than exercises performed independently.

Nonsurgical Treatment of Stress Urinary Incontinence

- **Continence pessaries.** Patients can be fit for and taught care for a vaginal support device, known as a continence pessary, for SUI. Pessaries can be used independently or in conjunction with PFME.
- **Pharmacologic** therapy is not recommended for SUI due to lack of efficacy and high rates of adverse side effects.

Surgical Treatment of Stress Urinary Incontinence

- **Suburethral slings** are indicated for SUI with urethral hypermobility, although data also suggest some efficacy in patients with limited urethral mobility. The sling can be placed at the midurethra or bladder neck and provides static stabilization of the urethra at rest and dynamic compression of the urethra with increases in abdominal pressure. Suburethral slings can be created using various biologic and synthetic materials. Typically, autologous fascial slings are placed at the level of the bladder neck, and synthetic slings using polypropylene mesh are placed at the level of the midurethra. *The midurethral sling is now considered the gold standard procedure* and can be placed via retropubic or transobturator approach. Midurethral slings have been found to be as effective as other surgical procedures for SUI (such as fascial slings or colposuspension) with the benefit of shorter operative time and decreased morbidity.

- **Retropubic midurethral sling.** A polypropylene mesh is placed without tension at the midurethra through the retropubic space or space of Retzius. Success rates are similar to that of Burch colposuspension. The UTI is the most common complication (34%), followed by voiding dysfunction, including urinary retention or incomplete bladder emptying (20%-47%), and bladder perforation (5%), with bowel or vascular injuries being the most serious complications (both <1%). Cystoscopy is routinely performed to evaluate for bladder perforation by the placement of sling trocars. Postoperative risks include graft exposure or erosion and urinary retention. Short-term postoperative voiding dysfunction can be seen in up to 47% of cases, but long-term voiding dysfunction requiring sling release is rare (0.6%-2%).
- **Transobturator sling.** A polypropylene mesh is placed without tension at the midurethra through the obturator foramen. This placement avoids the possibility of vascular injury in the space of Retzius or potential bowel injury but could be complicated by the uncommon complication of injury to the obturator vessels, hematoma formation, or hemorrhage (0%-3%). Bladder perforation is less likely than with retropubic approach (<0.1%). Other postoperative risks include groin pain, dyspareunia, mesh exposure, and abscess.
- **Retropubic urethropexy** procedures are indicated for women with SUI and a hypermobile proximal urethra and bladder neck. These are now less commonly performed due to increased morbidity relative to the less invasive midurethral slings.
  - The **Burch retropubic colposuspension** is a well-established surgery for SUI. Via abdominal or laparoscopic approach, permanent sutures are placed in the fibromuscular tissue lateral to the bladder neck/proximal urethra, and the urethrovesical junction is supported by attaching these sutures to the iliopectineal line (ie, Cooper ligament). Reported 5-year success rates have been over 80%.
  - The **Marshall-Marchetti-Krantz** procedure supports the bladder neck and urethra similar to the Burch, except the permanent sutures are placed through the periosteum of the pubic symphysis instead of Cooper ligament. This technique is seldom used now due to the risk of osteitis pubis.
- **Urethral-bulking agent injections** may be appropriate in patients with SUI with or without urethral hypermobility (ie, mobility of less than 30 degrees). Various agents can be used to improve urethral coaptation via cystoscopic injection. These agents include autologous fat, calcium hydroxyapatite particles, ethylene vinyl alcohol copolymer, and polydimethylsiloxane. Symptomatic improvement at 1 year ranges from 60% to 80%, although recurrence of symptoms requiring reinjection within months or years is common. Complications are uncommon but include transient urinary retention.

Conservative Treatment of Overactive Bladder

- Treatment of OAB has included the first-line methods of behavioral and lifestyle modifications, including weight loss, dietary modifications, PFME, and bladder retraining with or without pharmacotherapy.
- If these methods provide unsatisfactory results, advanced therapies can be employed.

Medical Management of Overactive Bladder

- Currently, there are two classes of medications that are typically used for the treatment of OAB, including anticholinergic/antimuscarinic or β_3-agonists. Medications may be combined with behavioral therapies to improve efficacy.

- **Anticholinergic or antimuscarinic** medications inhibit involuntary detrusor contractions. There are six antimuscarinic medications available in various disease and formulations in the United States—darifenacin, fesoterodine, oxybutynin, solifenacin, tolterodine, and trospium.
  - Dry mouth is the most common side effect as well as dry eyes and constipation. These medications are not recommended in patients with closed-angle glaucoma or impaired gastric emptying. Because this class of medications may be associated with a risk of cognitive impairment, dementia, and Alzheimer disease, caution should be taken when prescribing anticholinergic medications in frail or cognitively impaired patients. Providers should prescribe the lowest effective dose or consider alternative medications in high-risk patients.
  - There are minimal differences found in efficacy or side effects between the various anticholinergics available; however, some patients may respond better to one medication in the class and not another.
- Mirabegron is a **β_3-agonist** that relaxes the detrusor muscle during the storage phase and increases bladder capacity by augmenting the sympathetic nervous system stimulation of the bladder. Mirabegron should not be used in patients with uncontrolled hypertension but overall has a favorable side effect profile compared to anticholinergics.
- **Tricyclic antidepressants** such as imipramine improve bladder hypertonicity and compliance. Efficacy is not well established, and adverse effects are common; therefore, imipramine is not commonly used for treatment of OAB.

Surgical Management of Overactive Bladder

- For patients who have failed conservative management or desire to avoid the side effects of medications, surgical management of OAB may be considered.
- Advanced therapies include **sacral nerve root neuromodulation**, **posterior tibial nerve stimulation**, or chemodenervation with intradetrusor **injection of onabotulinumtoxinA**.
- Invasive procedures such as **augmentation cystoplasty** or **urinary diversion** via an ileal conduit are reserved for severe refractory cases.

Treatment of Mixed Urinary Incontinence

- Women with mixed urinary incontinence should be counseled that primary treatment of SUI will not treat UUI symptoms. Patients should be assessed to determine whether symptoms are stress or urge predominant because this will impact treatment. The PFME, behavioral therapy, and lifestyle modifications can impact both types of incontinence, but treatment beyond these should be tailored to the patient's symptoms.

URINARY RETENTION

Urinary retention is the accumulation of urine in the bladder as a result of incomplete bladder emptying, which must be classified as either acute or chronic.

- Acute urinary retention may be seen in a postoperative patient due to the effects of anesthesia or secondary to placement of a suburethral sling. It is important to identify and correct the etiology. This process is generally self-limited. Patients may require a short-term indwelling bladder catheter or clean intermittent catheterization.

- Chronic urinary retention is typically a result of either detrusor underactivity or bladder outlet obstruction and is identified by the measurement of a PVR volume. According to the American Urological Association, chronic urinary retention is defined as an elevated PVR >300 mL recorded on two or more occasions that has persisted for at least 6 months.

Etiology

- **Neurogenic lower urinary tract or pelvic floor dysfunction** is diagnosed after confirming pathology that is neurologic in nature. This could include diabetes mellitus, spinal cord injury, reversible spinal disorders such as disc herniation or compression, progressive neurologic disorders such as multiple sclerosis, or medication side effects. There may be overdistention of the bladder, or neurogenic acontractile detrusor, with resultant involuntary urinary retention. Patients may have absent or delayed sensation to void, increased bladder capacity, and high PVRs. They may complain of overflow incontinence, dribbling, hesitancy, frequency, or nocturia.
- **Detrusor sphincter dyssynergia** is a lack of coordination between bladder contraction and urethral sphincter and pelvic floor relaxation and can result in incomplete bladder emptying and voiding dysfunction commonly associated with neurologic disease.
- **Bladder outlet obstruction** may occur as a result of previous anti-incontinence surgery, anterior vaginal wall prolapse, or other anatomic abnormalities.
- **Fowler syndrome** typically presents as painless urinary retention (often greater than 1 L) in young women (mean age 27 y) without neurologic or anatomic etiology. Urodynamic testing will demonstrate abnormally decreased bladder sensation and failure of urethral sphincter relaxation.

Treatment for Urinary Retention

Management of urinary retention is generally pursued in collaboration with urology colleagues. Treatment may be necessary if there is evidence of elevated bladder pressures and concern for upper urinary tract damage and impaired renal function, recurrent UTIs, or bothersome LUTS (ie, overflow incontinence). Treatment may include the following:

- **Intermittent self-catheterization**
- **Pessaries** to relieve urinary retention caused by obstruction due to prolapse
- **Urethrolysis** if anti-incontinence surgery has resulted in voiding dysfunction and urinary retention secondary to obstruction
- **Sacral nerve root neuromodulation** for idiopathic nonneurogenic refractory detrusor underactivity or less commonly for refractory obstructive chronic urinary retention that is functional in nature
- **Surgical correction** of urethral strictures, diverticula, or caruncles
- **Injection of onabotulinumtoxinA** into the urethral sphincter to relax a neurogenic outlet obstruction

SUGGESTED READINGS

Abrams P, Andersson KE, Birder L, et al. Fourth International Consultation on Incontinence Recommendations of the International Scientific Committee: evaluation and treatment of urinary incontinence, pelvic organ prolapse, and fecal incontinence. *Neurourol Urodyn*. 2010;29(1):213-240.

American College of Obstetricians and Gynecologists Committee on Practice Bulletins—Gynecology, American Urogynecologic Society. ACOG Practice Bulletin No. 155: urinary incontinence in women. *Obstet Gynecol.* 2015;126:e66-e81. (Reaffirmed 2018)

Ford AA, Rogerson L, Cody JD, Ogah J. Mid-urethral sling operations for stress urinary incontinence in women. *Cochrane Database Syst Rev.* 2015;(7):CD006375.

Haylen BT, de Ridder D, Freeman RM, et al. An International Urogynecological Association (IUGA)/International Continence Society (ICS) joint report on the terminology for female pelvic floor dysfunction. *Int Urogynecol J.* 2010;21(1):5-26.

Nager CW, Brubaker L, Litman HJ, et al. A randomized trial of urodynamic testing before stress-incontinence surgery. *N Engl J Med.* 2012;366:1987-1997.

Richter HE, Burgio KL, Brubaker L, et al. Continence pessary compared with behavioral therapy or combined therapy for stress incontinence: a randomized controlled trial. *Obstet Gynecol.* 2010;115(3):609-617.

Schimpf MO, Rahn DD, Wheeler TL, et al. Sling surgery for stress urinary incontinence in women: a systematic review and metaanalysis. *Am J Obstet Gynecol.* 2014;211:71.e1-71.e27.

Visco AG, Brubaker L, Nygaard I, et al. The role of preoperative urodynamic testing in stress-continent women undergoing sacrocolpopexy: the Colpopexy and Urinary Reduction Efforts (CARE) randomized surgical trial. *Int Urogynecol J Pelvic Floor Dysfunct.* 2008;19:607-614.

Visco AG, Brubaker L, Richter HE, et al. Anticholinergic therapy vs. onabotulinumtoxinA for urgency urinary incontinence. *N Engl J Med.* 2012;367:1803-1813.

Pelvic Organ Prolapse

David A. Lovejoy and Chi Chiung Grace Chen

Pelvic organ prolapse (POP) is defined as herniation of the pelvic organs into or out of the vaginal canal. More specifically, POP refers to loss of support of the anterior vaginal wall, the posterior vaginal wall, and/or the vaginal apex, which permits pelvic viscera such as the bladder (cystocele), rectum (rectocele), small bowel (enterocele), sigmoid colon (sigmoidocele), or uterus (apical or uterine prolapse) to protrude into the vagina or through the vaginal introitus. POP does not include rectal prolapse.

EPIDEMIOLOGY

According to the National Health and Nutrition Examination Survey, 3% of women in the United States report symptoms of pelvic pressure or vaginal bulge. There is a noted discrepancy between those patients who report prolapse-related symptoms (3%-6%) and those who demonstrate prolapse on examination (40%-50%), which demonstrates that the majority of women with objective prolapse are asymptomatic. Often, symptoms are not appreciated until prolapse (the leading edge of descent) progresses beyond the introitus. Approximately 300 000 surgeries are performed each year in the United States for POP, and 1 out of 10 women will have surgery for POP in their lifetime.

RISK FACTORS

Risk factors associated with the development of POP include parity, vaginal delivery, age, obesity, connective tissue disorders, menopausal status, and chronic constipation. Most women with pelvic floor disorders and/or POP have multiple risk factors.

- **Race.** Epidemiologic studies have not led to a consensus regarding the relationship between race and POP. However, there is some evidence that Latina and white women have a higher risk of POP when compared to African American women.
- **Age.** The POP increases with age; however, POP is not a normal result of aging.
- **Menopausal status.** Estrogen deficiency can result in urogenital atrophy with resultant thinning of the vaginal submucosa. Estrogen receptors have been identified throughout pelvic floor support structures, including the levator ani and uterosacral ligaments. However, despite the potential impact of estrogen deficiency on the pelvic floor, a recent systematic review only found menopausal status to demonstrate a trend toward a positive association with primary POP, without ever achieving significance.
- **Parity and childbirth.** The incidence of pelvic floor disorders (including POP, urinary incontinence, and anal incontinence) are higher among parous than nulliparous women. Damage to the pelvic tissues during a vaginal delivery is thought to be a key factor in the development of these disorders, which has been demonstrated to be more significant with operative vaginal delivery.
- **Previous pelvic surgery** may increase the risk of pelvic floor disorders.
- Chronically **increased intra-abdominal pressure** (chronic obstructive pulmonary disease, chronic constipation, obesity) may be a risk factor for POP.

PELVIC ORGAN PROLAPSE SIGNS AND SYMPTOMS

- Descent of the following structures:
  - Uterovaginal prolapse (uterine/cervical prolapse)
  - Vaginal vault (cuff scar) prolapse
  - Anterior vaginal wall prolapse (Although the bladder is the most common organ associated with anterior wall POP, avoid using "cystocele" prior to confirming the bladder prolapse is in isolation, as there may be small bowel involvement.)
  - Posterior vaginal wall prolapse (Avoid using "rectocele" prior to confirming rectal involvement in isolation, as small bowel may also be involved.)
  - Other prolapse/findings (urethral mucosal prolapse, urethral caruncle, urethral diverticulum)
- Patients may complain of **pelvic pressure**, heaviness, protruding tissues, or **bulging**.
- **Voiding dysfunction or incontinence** (see chapter 46). Voiding dysfunction may or may not be directly related to objective POP. Patients may complain of day- or nighttime involuntary loss of urine, with or without Valsalva or urgency. Patients who present with more severe anterior wall prolapse are less likely to experience stress urinary incontinence and are more likely to experience symptoms associated with urethral obstruction. They may have urinary hesitancy or incomplete emptying or describe the need for vaginal splinting or Valsalva before successful passage of urine. Furthermore, patients may have associated recurrent or persistent urinary tract infections secondary to urinary retention, and irritative voiding symptoms such as urgency/frequency are not uncommon. Studies show that after anterior colporrhaphy, there is a reduction in urgency incontinence, urinary urgency, and the severity of urinary symptoms; however, de novo voiding dysfunction is also reported. An additional consideration is occult stress incontinence or new-onset stress incontinence

symptoms that are identified only after the prolapse is reduced (eg, after surgery, with manual prolapse reduction on exam, or with pessary placement).

- **Defecatory dysfunction** (see chapter 48). Patients may have symptoms of defecatory dysfunction, especially with apical and posterior compartment prolapse. These include symptoms of incomplete defecation, required splinting or straining, constipation, and pain with defecation. One should be cautioned, however, from assuming reported defecatory dysfunction is directly the result of POP because defecatory dysfunction is both complex and often multifactorial. Studies suggest defecatory complaints resolve approximately 50% of the time following anatomic correction of the posterior wall prolapse.
- **Altered sexual functioning and body image.** Patients may complain of dyspareunia, avoidance of intercourse, decreased libido, and decreased self-image.

RECOMMENDED EVALUATION FOR PATIENT WITH SUSPECTED PROLAPSE

- Obtain detailed **history**, including medical, surgical, obstetric, and gynecologic history. Specific questions targeting bulge-/pressure-related symptoms, dyspareunia, voiding dysfunction (urinary urgency/incontinence, stress incontinence, obstructed voiding), and defecatory dysfunction should be asked as well as the degree of bother and frequency associated with each positive symptom.
- A **physical examination** should be performed. The patient may need to perform a Valsalva maneuver in lithotomy or strain while seated or standing while being examined by the provider. Examination for descent of the anterior and posterior vaginal wall may require the use of a half speculum to depress the opposite wall.
  - A **POP-Q** examination (Pelvic Organ Prolapse Quantification) is recommended; it provides validated, reproducible objective measures that can be used to evaluate and document the degree of prolapse (Figure 47-1 and Table 47-1; for further interactive learning, refer to https://www.augs.org/patient-services/pop-q-tool-interactive).
    - The POP-Q uses the hymen as a fixed point of reference and describes six specific topographic points on the vaginal walls (Aa, Ba, C, D, Bp, and Ap) and three distances (genital hiatus, perineal body, total vaginal length).
    - The prolapse of each segment is measured (centimeter) during Valsalva relative to the hymenal ring with points inside the vagina reported as negative numbers and outside as positive. The numeric values are then translated to a stage as described in Table 47-2.
  - If there is anterior vaginal wall or apical prolapse beyond the hymen/introitus, a postvoid residual should be recorded. If there is urinary urgency with or without additional lower urinary tract symptoms (LUTS), a urinalysis should be obtained at a minimum. Women without bothersome incontinence symptoms but significant apical and or anterior wall prolapse should be evaluated for occult stress incontinence, using either a cough stress test or urodynamics with the prolapse reduced (see chapter 46).

TREATMENT OF PELVIC ORGAN PROLAPSE

The goal of treatment for POP should depend on the patient's goals. The three therapeutic categories are expectant management, nonsurgical, and surgical.

- **Expectant management** is reasonable approach for asymptomatic or mildly symptomatic prolapse as well as in patients without bothersome concomitant LUTS, obstructive voiding, or defecatory dysfunction. Providers can offer reassurance that

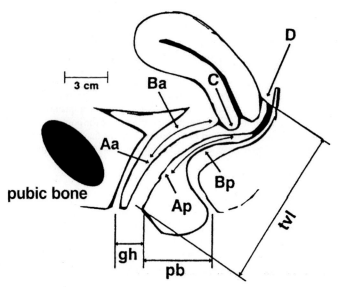

Figure 47-1. The Pelvic Organ Prolapse Quantification (POP-Q) system components and anatomic reference points. For explanation of terms, see Table 47-1. Abbreviations: gh, genital hiatus; pb, perineal body; tvl, total vaginal length. Reprinted with permission from Bent AE, Cundiff GW, Swift SE, et al, eds. *Ostergard's Urogynecology and Pelvic Floor Dysfunction.* 6th ed. Philadelphia, PA: Wolters Kluwer Health/Lippincott Williams & Wilkins; 2007:425.

Table 47-1	Description of the Pelvic Organ Prolapse Quantification System
Point/Distance	Description
Aa	Midline anterior vaginal wall; 3 cm proximal to the urethral meatus
Ba	Anterior vaginal wall; most distal point between Aa and anterior fornix (cuff)
C	Edge of the cervix (or vaginal cuff in posthysterectomy patients)
D	Posterior fornix; not used in patients with hysterectomy
Ap	Midline posterior vaginal wall; 3 cm proximal to the hymenal ring
Bp	Posterior vaginal wall; most distal point between Ap and posterior fornix (cuff)
Genital hiatus	Middle of the urethral meatus to posterior midline hymenal ring
Perineal body	Posterior margin of genital hiatus to the middle anus
Total vaginal length	Greatest depth of vagina with C or D reduced to its normal position

Table 47-2 Description of Pelvic Organ Prolapse Staging System

Staging of the POP-Q System

Stage 0	Perfect support; Aa, Ap at -3; C or D within 2 cm of TVL from introitus
Stage 1	Most distal portion of prolapse is -1 (or more negative) proximal to introitus
Stage 2	Most distal portion within 1 cm of the hymenal ring (between -1 and $+1$)
Stage 3	Most distal portion $>+1$ cm but $<$ (TVL -2) cm distal to introitus
Stage 4	Complete prolapse; most distal portion between TVL and (TVL -2) cm distal to introitus

Abbreviations: POP-Q, Pelvic Organ Prolapse Quantification; TVL, total vaginal length.

treatment is available if and when prolapse becomes bothersome. Risks of expectant management include vaginal epithelial erosion, persistence of LUTS, and defecatory or voiding dysfunction.

- The **nonsurgical approach** may be useful in patients with a mild degree of prolapse who desire future childbearing, have frail health, or are unwilling to undergo surgery.
  - **Pelvic muscle floor training** or **exercises**, also known as Kegel exercises, can alleviate the symptoms of prolapse. These treatments have also been shown in smaller trials to reduce the anatomic severity of mild prolapse.
  - **Pessaries.** The two basic types (Figure 47-2) are supportive (most commonly a ring, with or without support) and space occupying (most commonly a Gellhorn). Pessaries can decrease symptom frequency and severity and delay or avoid surgery. Up to 92% of women can be successfully fitted for a pessary. Risk factors for unsuccessful pessary fitting include a large genital hiatus and a short vaginal length. Treatment with estrogen, either locally or systemically, is associated with decreased vaginal discharge and prolonged pessary use/compliance. Because pessaries can potentially cause vaginal wall erosion, ulceration, and fistula formation if neglected, patients who are unable to remove and replace their pessary independently should be examined routinely (every 3-4 mo). Women who manage their pessary independently (remove, clean with unscented soap, replace) can follow-up annually. Although serious complications are rare, individuals who are unable to independently manage their pessary or whom are unable to follow-up routinely, are at a higher risk. Erosions are reported in 2% to 9% of all patients using pessaries. Complications may be decreased by making sure the pessary does not place excessive pressure on the vaginal epithelium and by emphasizing proper pessary care, as discussed above. A well-fit pessary should not be felt by the patient while in place, and it should remain in place during Valsalva/defecation. If ulceration/erosion or bleeding is documented on examination, the pessary should be removed for a duration of time (2-4 wk) and replaced after resolution of concerning examination findings. Application of local estrogen may promote epithelial healing during the "pessary holiday." More frequent pessary changes should be considered in patients who experience recurrent erosions.

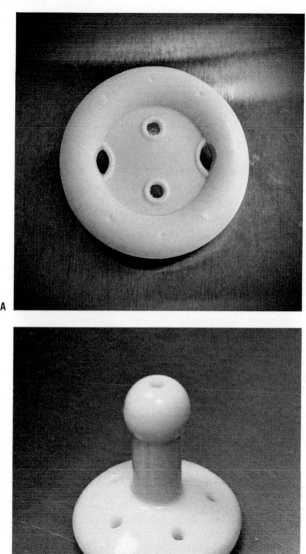

Figure 47-2. **A,** Ring with support pessary. **B,** Gellhorn pessary. Original image courtesy of David A. Lovejoy, MD, Division of Urogynecology, Department of Gynecology and Obstetrics, Johns Hopkins Hospital.

- **Surgery.** The goal of surgery is relief of prolapse symptoms and is recommended for women who have failed or declined expectant or conservative management as described above. *Hysterectomy alone is not an adequate treatment for POP.* Overcorrection should be avoided because it can lead to new symptoms including LUTS or stress urinary incontinence. Although the uterus itself does not contribute to POP, most of the literature on prolapse surgery include hysterectomy concomitantly with POP repair to maximize the opportunity to correct apical support. However, it should be noted that there is a growing body of literature that supports uterine preservation (hysteropexy) versus concomitant hysterectomy at the time of POP repair. Further research is needed before more definitive recommendations can be made.

Surgical Procedures for Pelvic Organ Prolapse

The three categories of POP repair are reconstructive, obliterative, and compensatory.

Reconstructive Surgery

- **Anterior colporrhaphy** involves plicating the layers of the anterior vaginal and pubocervical fibromuscular connective tissue. The 5-year success rate is reported 30% to 40% especially when apical pathology is not concomitantly addressed. No significant difference in risk of recurrence has been demonstrated when comparing native tissue repair with porcine dermis/biologic graft, and although anatomic outcomes are improved with the use of synthetic mesh augmentation of the anterior vagina, their use is complicated by their increased morbidity (increased operative times, blood loss, and 10%-20% risk of mesh exposure). Complications include sexual dysfunction and dyspareunia.
- **Posterior colporrhaphy** is the plication of the rectovaginal fibromuscular connective tissue. De novo dyspareunia may occur and is more common if plication of the puborectalis is performed. No anatomic or subjective benefits compared to native tissue repairs have been demonstrated using synthetic mesh or biologic graft in the repairs.
- **Perineorrhaphy** is the reconstruction of the perineal body and attachment to the rectovaginal septum. The perineum is made up of the confluence of the superficial transverse perineal muscles, bulbocavernosus muscles, and the perineal body. Although genital hiatus size (greater than 3.5-4 cm) is highly predictive of POP recurrence, there is a paucity of data supporting, or arguing against, the routine use of perineorrhaphy at the time of posterior colporrhaphy as a means of preventing recurrence.
- **Sacral colpopexy** replaces normal vaginal support with interposition of a suspensory bridge of synthetic mesh (type 1 polypropylene mesh) or biologic graft between the apical, anterior, and posterior vagina with the anterior sacral promontory. All women with predominantly apical prolapse are considered candidates for this approach, especially those women with a shortened vaginal length, intra-abdominal or ovarian pathology, and/or risk factors for prolapse recurrence (age <60 years, stage III or IV prolapse, or a body mass index >26). Procedure can be performed abdominally or laparoscopically (with or without robotic assistance). Success rates are 78% to 100% for the correction of apical prolapse. Sacral colpopexy results in a lower rate of recurrence and may be more durable than vaginal procedures such as sacrospinous ligament suspension (SSLS) (failure rates: sacral colpopexy 6% vs SSLS 20%). Complications associated with sacral colpopexy include rare intraoperative hemorrhage (1.5%), dyspareunia (7.3%), ileus or small bowel obstruction (2.7%), and mesh/suture complication (4.2%). The Colpopexy and Urinary Reduction Efforts trial reported reoperation rates for mesh erosion as high as 10.5%; however,

many of the participants initially received non–type I mesh. Type I mesh is both monofilamentous and macroporous and is the current surgical standard.

- **Uterosacral ligament suspension** suspends the apex of the vagina to the uterosacral ligaments, restoring the natural axis of the vagina. The Operations and Pelvic Muscle Training in the Management of Apical Support Loss trial found uterosacral ligament suspension and sacrospinous ligament fixation to be comparable anatomically and in terms of adverse outcomes. The most clinically relevant complication is ureteral kinking (3%-5%), in which case, a systematic approach to identifying and releasing the misplaced suture should be implemented.

- **Sacrospinous ligament suspension** anchors the vaginal apex to the sacrospinous ligament, usually on the right side. This approach is faster, less expensive, and associated with earlier return to daily activities than abdominal procedures such as sacral colpopexy, but it has been shown to be not as effective. Success rates are reported between 63% and 97%. There are high rates of postoperative anterior vaginal prolapse (37%), thought to be due to the pronounced posterior deviation of the vaginal axis. Although complications include hemorrhage (2%), nerve injury (1.8%), dyspareunia (3%-10%), and buttock pain (2%-6%), SSLS is unique in that it can be performed without entering the peritoneal cavity, which may be advantageous in patients with a complicated past surgical history.

- **McCall culdoplasty** is a preventative procedure that can be performed concomitantly with any vaginal hysterectomy. The procedure surgically obliterates the cul-de-sac at the time of vaginal hysterectomy and may prevent future enterocele or herniation of the small bowel into the vaginal vault. If identified, an enterocele can be repaired by dissecting the bowel from the vaginal wall and endopelvic connective tissue and obliterating the cul-de-sac.

- **Uterine sparing**
  - **Sacrospinous hysteropexy** is performed by transfixing the cervix or uterosacral ligament to the sacrospinous ligament with permanent or delayed absorbable suture.
  - **Sacral mesh hysteropexy** (attachment of mesh graft to the cervix and uterus and to the anterior longitudinal ligament of the sacrum) and **uterosacral hysteropexy** (plication or shortening of the uterosacral ligaments with uterine preservation) have been described.

Obliterative Procedures

- A **partial colpocleisis (Le Fort)** involves leaving the uterus in place with lateral channels for drainage of potential cervical secretions after the vagina is closed ("obliterated"). In a **total colpectomy**, the vaginal epithelium is removed and the vaginal vault tissue is reduced.
  - Patients should be counseled regarding the risk of regret (5%-10%) because the procedure precludes subsequent vaginal penetrative intercourse. If clinically indicated, preoperative evaluation can include a Pap smear, pelvic sonogram, endometrial biopsy.

- **Colpocleisis** and **colpectomy** involve the closure of the vagina. They may be useful for older patients who do not desire future vaginal intercourse. The benefits include decreased complications, decreased surgical time, and high success rate (86%-100%).

Augmented Surgery

- When native tissue is weak or insufficient, compensatory procedures with graft/mesh placement/augmentation may be then be indicated. Biologic grafts can be **native tissue**, **allografts** (cadaveric tissue), and **xenografts** (porcine, bovine).

- **Anterior and posterior vaginal wall fibromuscular connective tissue replacement.** Various graft materials and synthetic meshes have been used to augment vaginal prolapse repairs. The purpose of the graft is often 2-fold: via replacing the weakened or absent vaginal supports and acting as an absorbable "collagen scaffold" for fibroblast infiltration and scar formation. If the repair is too tight, the loss of flexibility can lead to fecal urgency and dyspareunia.

• **Special consideration**
  • There are many mesh/graft "kits" for anterior and posterior repairs and for apical suspension. Although some of these procedures have resulted in decreased anterior vaginal prolapse recurrence when compared with vaginal restorative procedures without mesh/graft augmentation, the US Food and Drug Administration issued a public health notification in July 2011 regarding adverse events related to transvaginal POP repair with mesh, including mesh erosion (10%-20% within 12 mo), pain, infection, urinary complaints, bleeding, and organ perforation. Therefore, these procedures should only be performed judiciously on selected patients who are thoroughly counseled regarding the data on efficacy and complications and by surgeons specially trained to perform these types of procedures.

Use of Mesh in Vaginal Prolapse Surgery

• Mesh was briefly mentioned during previous discussions of anterior and posterior colporrhaphy. In the past, several mesh/graft kits were available for anterior and posterior vaginal wall repair. However, in April 2019, the FDA ordered all manufacturers of surgical mesh intended for "transvaginal" repair of the anterior and posterior vaginal wall, to stop selling their products immediately. This decision was based upon reported adverse events related to transvaginal POP repair with mesh, including mesh erosion (10% to 20% within 12 mo), pain, infection, urinary complaints, bleeding, and organ perforation. The FDA statement does not include midurethral sling mesh or abdominally place mesh for apical prolapse (Sacrocolpopexy).

SUGGESTED READINGS

Abrams P, Andersson KE, Birder L, et al. Fourth International Consultation on Incontinence Recommendations of the International Scientific Committee: evaluation and treatment of urinary incontinence, pelvic organ prolapse, and fecal incontinence. *Neurourol Urodyn*. 2010;29(1):213-240.

American College of Obstetricians and Gynecologists Committee on Practice Bulletin—Gynecology, American Urogynecologic Society. ACOG Practice Bulletin No. 185: pelvic organ prolapse. *Obstet Gynecol*. 2017;130:e234-e250.

Bradley CS, Zimmerman MB, Qi Y, Nygaard IE. Natural history of pelvic organ prolapse in postmenopausal women. *Obstet Gynecol*. 2007;109:848-854.

Hagen S, Stark D. Conservative prevention and management of pelvic organ prolapse in women. *Cochrane Database Syst Rev*. 2011;(12):CD003882.

Handa VL, Garrett E, Hendrix S, Gold E, Robbins J. Progression and remission of pelvic organ prolapse: a longitudinal study of menopausal women. *Am J Obstet Gynecol*. 2004;190:27-32.

Jelovsek JE, Maher C, Barber MD. Pelvic organ prolapse. *Lancet*. 2007;369:1027-1038.

Madoff RD, Parker SC, Varma MG, Lowry AC. Faecal incontinence in adults. *Lancet*. 2004;364(9434):621-632.

Nygaard I, Barber MD, Burgio KL, et al. Prevalence of symptomatic pelvic floor disorders in US women. *JAMA*. 2008;300:1311-1316.

Swift S, Woodman P, O'Boyle A, et al. Pelvic Organ Support Study (POSST): the distribution, clinical definition, and epidemiologic condition of pelvic organ support defects. *Am J Obstet Gynecol*. 2005;192:795-806.

48 Anal Incontinence

Emily Myer and Tola Fashokun

Anal incontinence (AI) is the complaint of involuntary loss of feces (solid or liquid) or flatus (gas). Fecal incontinence (FI) is the complaint of involuntary loss of feces (solid or liquid). It may be passive, occurring without sensation/warning, or it may be associated with the feeling of difficulty wiping clean or it may be associated with urgency. The AI may also occur with coitus.

- The prevalence of FI varies according to definition, age, and survey method. Systematic reviews of community-dwelling adults show a prevalence of 7.7% to 12.4% with reported ranges from 1.4% to 19.5%.

ETIOLOGY

- Continence of stool depends on a number of integrated factors including the internal and external anal sphincters, puborectalis muscle, intact neurosensory pathway, stool volume and consistency, rectal compliance, and anorectal sensation.
- Anatomically, the main muscles involved in fecal continence include the puborectalis, external anal sphincter, and internal anal sphincter. The puborectalis forms a U-shaped sling around the genital hiatus; when contracted, it pulls the anorectal junction toward the pubic rami, narrowing the genital hiatus. This creates a more acute anorectal angle, which is a critical component for continence of solid stool. The puborectalis muscle fibers blend together with the external anal sphincter. Both muscles rapidly contract when there is a sudden increase in intra-abdominal pressure to prevent FI associated with fecal urgency and stress incontinence. The puborectalis and external anal sphincter muscles optimize function through a combination of cognitive control and involuntary spinal reflexes. The internal anal sphincter is the third muscle of the anal sphincter complex and contributes the majority of resting tone and is essential for passive continence.
- Damage to the anal sphincter complex is a significant risk factor for incontinence with high rates of both flatal incontinence (24%-31%) and FI (9%-19%). Other risk factors for AI include age, diabetes, diarrhea, rectal prolapse, and neurologic disease (eg, stroke, dementia, brain trauma, multiple sclerosis).

PATIENT EVALUATION

- History. In addition to a full medical, surgical, obstetric, and social history, the history should include discussion of onset of incontinence, duration, frequency, association with urgency, and stool consistency. The Bristol stool chart is a useful tool to help determine stool consistency. A bowel diary can help determine associations with urgency, stool consistency, and frequency.
- Questionnaires. Patient intake questionnaires are helpful especially because patients may be reluctant to disclose their FI due to embarrassment. Some recommendations include screening for AI with validated questionnaires including the

Cleveland Clinic Score (Wexner Score) and the St. Marks score. Optional questionnaires to further assess quality of life include the Fecal Incontinence Quality of Life scale and Fecal Incontinence Severity Index.

- Physical exam
  - Assess the skin integrity of the vulva and stool soiling around the anus.
  - In cases of an anal sphincter tear, the "dove tail sign" may be apparent.
  - Ask the patient to squeeze as if holding in gas to evaluate the pelvic floor muscles and then ask the patient to push as if trying to have a bowel movement to evaluate for any ballooning of the perineum, hemorrhoids, and rectal prolapse.
  - Evaluate the S2-S4 nerves by assessing for anal reflex and perianal sensation with a Q-tip gently brushing the perianal and vulvar skin.
  - Perform a vaginal exam to evaluate for pelvic organ prolapse and rectovaginal fistula.
  - Perform a digital rectal examination to assess for resting anal tone and increased tone with voluntary squeeze. During the rectal exam, it is also important to assess for anal hemorrhoids, a gap in the anal sphincter (usually anteriorly), perineal body deficiency, rectal contents, rectal masses, and rectal pain.
- Testing
  - Endoanal or transperineal ultrasound can help identify anal sphincter defects in patients with risk factors for injury to the anal sphincter (eg, forceps-assisted vaginal delivery).
  - Anorectal manometry can provide information regarding resting and squeeze pressures of the anal sphincter and can be used to assess rectal compliance.
  - Pelvic magnetic resonance imaging (static and dynamic) can assess for anatomic reasons for FI such as rectal prolapse or intussusception if these are suspected but not visualized on office evaluation.

TREATMENT

There are multiple treatment options for AI. Conservative treatments should be considered prior to offering more invasive treatment options because these can be successful in 60% to 90% of women. The initial steps are to manage any treatable underlying causes, such as irritable bowel disease, fecal impaction, metabolic disorders, or offending diets. The general gynecologist can provide first-line conservative management and help facilitate some procedural treatments as well. Patients with refractory symptoms should be referred to a specialist (urogynecologist, gastroenterologist, and/or colorectal surgeon).

Conservative Treatments

- Dietary modifications
  - A high-fiber diet (25-40 g daily) can add bulk to the stools and reduce incontinence episodes.
  - Avoid caffeine, artificial sweeteners, and alcohol, which can impact stool transit time.
  - Avoid fructose and lactose, which can contribute to loose stools in some patients.
- Lifestyle modifications
  - Regular toileting especially after meals can help reduce urgency-related leakage.

- Medications
  - Patients with loose stools may benefit from antidiarrheal agents such as loperamide, which decreases transit time in the bowels and increases rectal compliance, which can improve urgency symptoms.
  - If patients have incomplete bowel emptying, they may also benefit from a laxative or enema to improve evacuation and prevent unscheduled bowel leakage.
- Pelvic floor muscle exercises
  - Pelvic floor muscle training may improve AI by improving sensation, coordination, and strength, especially when combined with biofeedback or electrical stimulation.

Procedural Treatments

- Anal plugs are disposable inserts placed in the anus to prevent FI. They can be difficult for patients to tolerate, but if tolerated, they do help prevent fecal leakage. Anal plugs are available by prescription (Deutekom).
- Vaginal bowel control therapy (Eclipse, Pelvalon, Inc, Sunnyvale, California). The Eclipse is a vaginal pessary with an inflatable balloon that provides pressure against the posterior vagina to close off the rectum to help prevent FI. The device is patient controlled, generally well tolerated by patients, and can provide modest improvement of FI symptoms.
- Posterior tibial nerve stimulation. Randomized controlled trials showed mixed results. However, posterior tibial nerve stimulation is not US Food and Drug Administration approved for the indication of FI.
- Rectal irrigation. Scheduled anal irrigation helps to evacuate the rectum and colon to prevent unscheduled bowel leakage. It is also be used to treat constipation. Peristeen by Coloplast is an example of this system.

Surgical Treatments

- Sphincter bulking agents. Injection of bulking material around the anus using needles under direct visualization has been shown to be an effective therapy in the short term with >50% improvement in baseline symptoms noted in 52% of treated patients.
- Sacral neuromodulation. This two-staged minimally invasive procedure has been shown to be an effective therapy for FI in patients with or without anal sphincter defects and is considered a first-line therapy for management of FI by the American Society of Colon and Rectal Surgeons. Large studies have shown significant improvement in incontinent episodes with sacral neuromodulation.
- Anal sphincter repair. For patients with anal sphincter defects on exam or imaging, anal sphincteroplasty can be attempted. Although good success is noted in the short term, in the long term, deterioration and return of FI symptoms occur in 50% of patients.
- Diversion/stoma. Diversion procedures can be used for refractory FI to allow patients the opportunity to resume life activities.

SUGGESTED READINGS

Devroede G, Giese C, Wexner SD, et al. Quality of life is markedly improved in patients with fecal incontinence after sacral nerve stimulation. *Female Pelvic Med Reconstr Surg.* 2012;18(2):103-112.

Hull TL, Zutshi M. Fecal incontinence. In: Walters MD, Karram MM, eds. *Urogynecology and Reconstructive Pelvic Surgery*. 4th ed. Philadelphia, PA: Elsevier; 2015:463-476.

Ng KS, Sivakumaran Y, Nassar N, Gladman M. Fecal incontinence: community prevalence and associated factors—a systematic review. *Dis Colon Rectum*. 2015;58:1194-1209.

Paquette IM, Varma MG, Kaiser AM, Steele SR, Rafferty JF. The American Society of Colon and Rectal Surgeons' clinical practice guideline for the treatment of fecal incontinence. *Dis Colon Rectum*. 2015;58:623-636.

Richter HE, Nager CW, Burgio KL, et al. Incidence and predictors of anal incontinence after obstetric anal sphincter injury in primiparous women. *Female Pelvic Med Reconstr Surg*. 2015;21:182-189.

van der Wilt AA, Giuliani G, Kubis C, et al. Randomized clinical trial of percutaneous tibial nerve stimulation versus sham electrical stimulation in patients with faecal incontinence. *Br J Surg*. 2017;104(9):1167-1176.

Wu JM, Vaughan CP, Goode PS, et al. Prevalence and trends of symptomatic pelvic floor disorders in U.S. women. *Obstet Gynecol*. 2014;123:141-148.

V Gynecologic Oncology

49 Cervical Intraepithelial Neoplasia

Anna L. Beavis and Connie L. Trimble

EPIDEMIOLOGY OF CERVICAL NEOPLASIA

- In the United States, approximately 13 240 women are diagnosed with **cervical cancer** each year, and over 4000 will die from it. It is the second leading cause of cancer death in women aged 20 to 39 years.
- Cervical cancer incidence and mortality disproportionately affect black, Hispanic, American Indian, and Alaska Native women who have rates almost twice as high as white women.
- Approximately 50% of women diagnosed with cervical cancer in the United States have not had adequate screening. Lack of follow-up after screening also likely contributes to the disparity in cervical cancer incidence and mortality.
- Persistent infection with the oncogenic (high risk) **human papillomavirus (HPV)** types 16, 18, 31, 33, 35, 39, 45, 52, 56, 58, 59, and 68 is required but not sufficient to develop cervical cancer and its precursor lesions. The HPV 16 is the most common carcinogenic genotype, followed by HPV 18. Together, they are responsible for 70% of HPV-related cervical cancers. Although approximately 80% of women will be infected through sexual intercourse by an HPV type at some point in their lives, 90% of these infections are transient and will be cleared immunologically within 1 to 2 years.
- Risks for persistent infection include tobacco exposure and immune compromise, including coinfection with human immunodeficiency virus (HIV). An HPV infection in women older than 30 years is more likely to indicate a persistent infection than detectable HPV in younger women. Cervical cancer is thought to occur after a median of 20 to 25 years following the initiation of a persistent HPV infection.
- The conventional cervical cytology smear or the liquid-based cytology (both referred to as **Pap smear**) is used as a screening test to identify the presence of visually abnormal cervical epithelial cells. Either technique is acceptable, but liquid-based cytologic specimens perform better in the presence of blood or mucous and offer the ability to perform reflex or concurrent HPV testing. Oncogenic HPV infection

can be detected on liquid cytology specimens using the digene Hybrid Capture 2 technique, with polymerase chain reaction or in situ hybridization.

- Annually, 4.8 million women have an abnormal Pap smear in the United States. Cytologic abnormalities are categorized using the Bethesda system (see "Diagnostic Categories" in the following text).
- Histologic abnormalities are classified in a two-tiered system of low-grade and high-grade squamous intraepithelial lesions (HSILs). Low-grade squamous intraepithelial lesions (LSILs) include mild dysplasia and cervical intraepithelial neoplasia 1 (CIN 1). The HSILs include moderate and severe dysplasia, carcinoma in situ, and CIN 2/CIN 3.
- A CIN 1 is associated with a high rate of spontaneous regression, whereas untreated CIN 3 has a reported cumulative incidence of invasive cancer of 30.1% at 30 years.

PRIMARY PREVENTION

Vaccination

- The first HPV vaccine directed against HPV types 6, 11, 16, and 18 (Gardasil, Merck, Whitehouse Station, NJ) and was approved for use in 9- to 26-year-old females by the US Food and Drug Administration (FDA) in 2006. This approval was expanded to include males in 2009. In 2014, an expanded nonavalent HPV vaccine was FDA approved, which targets five additional oncogenic HPV types: 31, 33, 45, 52, and 58. This nonavalent vaccine prevents nearly 90% of all cervical cancers and is the only vaccine available in the United States.
- Both the Advisory Committee on Immunization Practices and American College of Obstetricians and Gynecologists (ACOG) recommend administration of the vaccine to females aged 9 to 26 years and males ages 9 to 21 years. High-risk males including men who have sex with men and transgender individuals should be offered the vaccine up to age 26 years. The vaccine is given in three doses at 0, 2, and 6 months part; if the first dose is given before the child's 15th birthday, however, only two doses need to be given, 6 to 12 months apart.
- In late 2018, the vaccine was approved by the FDA for persons ages 26 to 45 years.
- Over a decade of real-world studies have demonstrated that the vaccine is safe and effective, with an over 85% decrease in HSIL lesions in populations where the vaccine was introduced. However, vaccination rates in the United States are low, with only 54% of females and 51% of males as of 2018 in the United States having completed the vaccine series.
- Although the vaccine is not therapeutic, in both HPV-positive and HPV-negative women, it does confer some reduction in risk of high-risk dysplasia.
- Currently, HPV vaccination does not change screening recommendations. However, looking forward, HPV vaccination is likely to influence positive and negative predictive values of the Pap smear by decreasing cervical abnormalities in the population.

Other Primary Prevention

- Smoking cessation. Women who smoke have an increased risk of developing cervical cancer compared to nonsmokers. This is thought to be related to the fact that

smoking triples the likelihood of persistent HPV infection and doubles the risk of progression to CIN 3.
• All women with abnormal Pap smears should be offered testing for HIV and other sexually transmitted infections.

SCREENING GUIDELINES

• Based on the 2018 US Preventive Services Taskforce guidelines endorsed by the American Society for Colposcopy and Cervical Pathology, ACOG, and the Society of Gynecologic Oncology, the current screening recommendations for average-risk women are as follows (Table 49-1):
  • Regular screening should begin at 21 years of age, regardless of the age of first sexual intercourse. Women aged 21 to 29 years should be screened every

Table 49-1	Summary of the USPSTF, ACOG, SGO, and ASCCP Cervical Cancer Screening Recommendations for Average-Risk Women 2018[a]	
Age Group	**Screening Modalities**	**Comments/Considerations**
<21 y	No screening offered	In immunocompromised individuals (eg, those with HIV), screening is recommended to within 1 y of onset of sexual activity.
21-29 y	Cytology alone every 3 y	Reflex HPV testing is recommended for ASC-US Pap smears (acceptable for ages 21-24 y; preferred for women 25 y and older).
30-65 y	Three options: 1. hrHPV testing every 5 y 2. Cytology alone every 3 y 3. Cotesting (hrHPV testing and cytology) every 5 y	Reduction in cervical cancer diagnoses is similar with all three methods, but cotesting results in the most false positives.
>65 y	No screening recommended	Women can stop Pap screenings *only* if they have 10 consecutive y of normal screening and are not high risk.

Abbreviations: ACOG, American College of Obstetricians and Gynecologists; ASCCP, American Society for Colposcopy and Cervical Pathology; ASC-US, atypical squamous cells of undetermined significance; HIV, human immunodeficiency virus; HPV, human papillomavirus; hrHPV, high-risk HPV; SGO, Society for Gynecologic Oncology; USPSTF, US Preventive Services Task Force.
[a]Screening guidelines may continue to change; these are the current guidelines as of the writing of this chapter.

3 years with cytology only. In this age cohort, HPV infections are likely to be transient.

- In women aged 30 to 65 years, screening can be performed every 3 years with cytology alone, or every 5 years with high-risk HPV (hrHPV) testing alone, or every 5 years with cotesting (simultaneous cytology and hrHPV testing). Cotesting results in similar detection rates to the other two screening methods but produces more false-positive results. Cytology alone is the least sensitive method.

- Screening can be stopped at age 65 years if a woman does not have risk factors and has 10 years of negative screening (either three consecutive cytology tests 3 y apart or two cotesting samples 5 y apart). Screening is not recommended to be reinstituted, even in the case of a new sexual partner after the age of 65 years. Annual well-woman exams are still recommended for all adult women.

- In the absence of screening, 8.34 per 1000 women ages 30 to 65 years is diagnosed with cervical cancer; with hrHPV or cotesting every 5 years, the number of women is reduced to 0.29 and 0.30 per 1000, respectively. Cytology every 3 years reduces the rate to 0.76 per 1000.

- Notably, HPV vaccination may change the HPV genotype distribution as well as the positive and negative predictive value of Pap smears. Furthermore, vaccination may influence adherence to screening. However, currently vaccinated women are recommended to undergo routine screening.

Special Populations

- Women who have had a total hysterectomy for benign indications and who do not have a history of high-grade lesion do not require further screening.

- Women with a history of CIN 2/CIN 3 should undergo regular screening for at least 20 years after an initial adequate posttreatment surveillance period, regardless of their age. The same period of vaginal screening is advised for those who underwent a hysterectomy as part of treatment for recurrent CIN 2/CIN 3.

- The ACOG provided screening guidelines for women with **HIV or who are immunocompromised** in their 2016 Practice Bulletin update:
  - Initiate screening within 1 year of onset of sexual activity, 1 year after HIV or immunocompromising diagnosis, or at age 21 years, whichever is earlier.
  - See Figure 49-1 for screening interval recommendations for immunocompromised women under and over the age of 30 years.
  - Cervical cancer screening should continue throughout the woman's lifetime and should not stop at age 65 years.

- The ACOG states that it is reasonable to perform annual cytology on women with in utero exposure to **diethylstilbestrol**.

- In **low-resource settings** where pathology laboratories and personnel are scarce and monetary and/or logistical constraints prohibits follow-up, the World Health Organization and ACOG recommend the use of HPV testing to screen women for cervical cancer. Women with positive HPV testing can either undergo triage to treatment via visual inspection with acetic acid or can undergo direct treatment, either with cryotherapy or the loop electrosurgical excision procedure (LEEP). In areas where HPV testing is not available, visual inspection with acetic acid is the recommended screening modality, followed by treatment for positive findings.

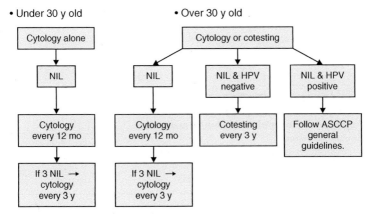

Figure 49-1. Screening recommendations for immunocompromised or HIV-positive women. Abbreviations: ASCCP, American Society for Colposcopy and Cervical Pathology; HPV, human papillomavirus; NIL, negative for intraepithelial lesion or malignancy. Data from American College of Obstetricians and Gynecologists Committee on Practice Bulletins—Gynecology. ACOG Practice Bulletin No. 168: cervical cancer screening and prevention. *Obstet Gynecol.* 2016;128:e111-e130. doi:10.1097/AOG.0000000000001708. (Reaffirmed 2018)

SCREENING METHODS

Pap Smear Cytology

- Pap smears can be collected conventionally either with a fixative on a slide or with liquid-based cytology. They are considered clinically equivalent by the US Preventive Services Taskforce.
- Pap smear reports include specimen type, specimen adequacy, results, and any ancillary testing performed (ie, hrHPV probe).
- Specimen type indicates whether the test is a vaginal or cervical sample.
- Adequacy is reported as satisfactory, unsatisfactory, or endocervical cells not present/lack of transformation zone.
- Unsatisfactory Pap smears should be repeated in 2 to 4 months.
- For average-risk women with cytologically normal Pap smears that lack an endocervical component, screening recommendations and intervals do not change except that HPV testing is recommended (if not already obtained) in women over 30 years of age. Management is then guided by result of the HPV testing.

Human Papillomavirus Testing

- HPV testing can be incorporated as cotesting (done at the time of cytology) or alone, as primary screening.
- The first HPV test approved for cotesting was the digene Hybrid Capture 2 HPV assay (Qiagen Corporation, Gaithersburg, MD). There are now four FDA-approved HPV tests for use with cotesting.
- For cotesting, hrHPV testing can be performed on a liquid cytology sample or with the digene Hybrid Capture 2 DNA collection device.

- The Cobas hrHPV test (Roche Molecular Systems, Pleasanton, CA) is FDA approved for both cotesting *and* primary screening and is able to report HPV genotypes 16 and 18 separately from 12 other high-risk types.

DIAGNOSTIC CATEGORIES: CYTOLOGY

The 2014 update of the 2001 Bethesda System is used to describe normal and abnormal cervical cytology employing the following categories:

- **Negative for intraepithelial lesion or malignancy**
- **Squamous lesions**
  - Atypical squamous cells (**ASC**)
    - of undetermined significance (**ASC-US**)
    - cannot exclude high-grade (**ASC-H**)
  - **LSIL**
  - **HSIL**
    - with features suspicious for invasion
  - Squamous cell carcinoma
- **Glandular lesions**
  - Atypical glandular cells (**AGC**) (endocervical or endometrial)
    - not otherwise specified (**AGC-NOS**)
    - favor neoplasia (**AGC-favor neoplasia**)
  - Adenocarcinoma in situ (**AIS**)
  - Adenocarcinoma

Atypical Squamous Cells

- Approximately 2 million ASC Pap smears a year are recorded in the United States.
- The ASC-US is present in 4.7% of samples and is associated with a 7% to 12% prevalence of CIN 2/CIN 3.
- The ASC-H is present in 0.4% of samples and CIN 2/CIN 3 is present in 26% to 68% of women with this result.
- The risk of invasive cancer associated with an ASC Pap is 0.1% to 0.2%.

Atypical Glandular Cells

- The AGC are found in 0.4% of Pap smears.
- The AGC are associated with significant neoplasia in 9% to 38% (CIN 2/CIN 3, AIS) and in 3% to 17% associated with cancer. One study found that the malignancies of the women with AGC were found in women older than 35 years and were mainly of endometrial origin and therefore suggested endometrial biopsy for every woman with AGC after the age of 35 years.
- An AGC-favor neoplasia has a higher risk of neoplasia (27%-96%) than AGC-NOS (9%-41%).

Low-Grade Squamous Intraepithelial Lesions

- The LSIL is reported in 2.1% of Pap smears and is strongly correlated with HPV infection.
- High-grade dysplasia or neoplasia is found in 12% to 17% of women who undergo colposcopy for LSIL.

High-Grade Squamous Intraepithelial Lesions

- The HSIL is reported in 0.7% of Pap smears.
- A CIN 2/CIN 3 is found in 53% to 97% of women with HSIL cytology. Invasive cancer is identified in 2.0% of women with HSIL cytology.

MANAGEMENT STRATEGIES: CYTOLOGIC ABNORMALITIES

Atypical Squamous Cells of Undetermined Significance

- Reflex testing for hrHPV (preferred): A positive result should be followed by colposcopy. A negative result should be followed by cotesting in 3 years. With this strategy, the sensitivity for detection of CIN 2/CIN 3 is 92%.
- If HPV testing is not available, repeat cytology in 1 year is recommended. If negative, routine screening can resume. If ≥ASC-US, colposcopy is recommended; endocervical curettage (ECC) should be performed if there are no visible lesions or the colposcopy is not satisfactory.

Special Populations

- Adolescents should not be screened for HPV or cervical cancer. They have a higher prevalence of HPV but are likely to clear the infection.
- Delaying first testing until age 21 years in average-risk women is designed to reduce unnecessary diagnostic procedures or interventions and potential iatrogenic morbidity in young women.
- Women ages 21 to 24 years have low rates of high-grade dysplasia; therefore, if ASC-US/HPV is negative, routine screening can be resumed. If ASC-US/HPV is positive, cytology should be repeated at 12 months.
- Pregnant women are tested according to their age group, with the exception that colposcopy can be deferred to 6 weeks postpartum. An ECC is never acceptable in pregnancy.
- Immunosuppressed women or those with HIV who have ASC-US have differential follow-up depending on their age and HPV status (Figure 49-2).

Atypical Squamous Cells Cannot Exclude High-Grade

- These patients require colposcopic examination. Negative colposcopy should be followed by cotesting at 12 and 24 months or can be offered diagnostic excisional procedure.

Atypical Glandular Cells

- All women with AGC should undergo colposcopy with ECC; endometrial sampling is preferred if the woman is ≥35 years old or has risk factors of endometrial neoplasia (eg, unexplained vaginal bleeding, chronic anovulation). An HPV DNA testing is preferred.
- Endometrial and endocervical sampling should be performed routinely for the finding of atypical *endometrial* cells.
- Follow-up for AGC-NOS after negative findings is cotesting at 12 and 24 months.
- Follow-up for AGC-favor neoplasia after a negative evaluation is a diagnostic excisional procedure, preferably cold knife cone (CKC).
- The AIS is managed by a diagnostic excisional procedure, preferably CKC.

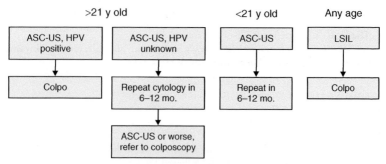

Figure 49-2. Management of atypical squamous cells of undetermined significance (ASC-US) and low-grade squamous intraepithelial lesion (LSIL) in human immunodeficiency virus (HIV)-positive and immunocompromised individuals. Abbreviations: Colpo, colposcopy; HPV, human papillomavirus. Data from American College of Obstetricians and Gynecologists Committee on Practice Bulletins—Gynecology. ACOG Practice Bulletin No. 168: cervical cancer screening and prevention. *Obstet Gynecol.* 2016;128:e111-e130. doi:10.1097/AOG.0000000000001708. (Reaffirmed 2018)

Special Populations

- Pregnant women should be managed in an identical fashion to the general population with the exception that endometrial and endocervical biopsies are unacceptable.
- Benign-appearing endometrial cells on a Pap smear in postmenopausal women should be evaluated with endometrial biopsy.

Low-Grade Squamous Intraepithelial Lesion

- An LSIL carries the same risk of high-grade dysplasia as ASC-US/HPV and is therefore managed identically (colposcopy).
- An ECC is preferred in those with an unsatisfactory or negative colposcopic examination.
- A finding of less than CIN 2/CIN 3 can be followed by cotesting at 12 months.

Special Populations

- Women ages 21 to 24 years with LSIL should be followed by repeat cytology at 12 months and 24 months. A finding of HSIL or greater at 12 months or ASC-US or greater at 24 months merits colposcopy.
- Postmenopausal women can be managed by reflex HPV DNA testing, colposcopy, or repeat cytology at 6 and 12 months.
- Pregnant women with LSIL should have a colposcopic examination. Postpartum follow-up is also acceptable.
- The HIV-positive or immunocompromised women with ASC-US or LSIL should be triaged based on age and HPV status (see Figure 49-2).

High-Grade Squamous Intraepithelial Lesion

- Due to the high risk of significant cervical disease, one approach is to "see and treat" with immediate LEEP in women who are at least 25 years old.

- Colposcopy with ECC is also appropriate. An unsatisfactory colposcopy should be managed by a diagnostic excisional procedure.
- A satisfactory colposcopy that results in a diagnosis of less than CIN 2/CIN 3 can be followed by colposcopy/cytology at 6 and 12 months, excisional diagnostic procedure, or review of the original pathologic material to verify the diagnosis.
- Two consecutive negative Pap smears and no high-grade lesions on colposcopy allow for resumption of a normal screening schedule.
- Persistent HSIL for 24 months should be evaluated with an excisional diagnostic procedure.

Special Populations

- Pregnant women with HSIL should be evaluated by colposcopy. Lesions suspicious for CIN 2/CIN 3 or invasive cancer should be biopsied; it is unacceptable to biopsy other lesions or perform an ECC.
- Evaluation no sooner than 6 weeks postpartum should be performed for women with a diagnosis of less than CIN 2/CIN 3.

MANAGEMENT STRATEGIES: hrHPV POSITIVE ON PRIMARY SCREENING

- Currently, only the Cobas HPV test (Roche Molecular Systems, Pleasanton, CA) is FDA approved for primary HPV cervical cancer screening. This test is able to differentiate types 16 and 18 from 12 other high-risk oncogenic HPV types.
- The recommendations for management of the primary HPV test are as follows:
  - If HPV 16/18 positive, proceed to colposcopy.
  - If positive for 12 other hrHPV types, evaluate cytology (reflex Pap test). If negative for intraepithelial lesion or malignancy, follow-up in 12 months. If ≥ASC-US, proceed with colposcopy.
  - If negative, repeat HPV testing can be performed every 5 years.

DIAGNOSTIC CATEGORIES VIA COLPOSCOPY: HISTOLOGY

- Colposcopy is used for the evaluation of abnormal cervical cytology or for hrHPV testing. The average sensitivity of cytology is only 48%. Therefore, colposcopic examination should include a biopsy of a visible lesion.
- A colposcope is used to examine the cervix after the application of a dilute, 3% acetic acid wash, which dehydrates epithelial cells with a high nuclear-to-cytoplasmic ratio, resulting in acetowhite changes.
- Colposcopy is considered **satisfactory** if the entire squamocolumnar junction is visualized circumferentially and if all lesions are completely visualized.

Cervical Intraepithelial Neoplasia 1

- The CIN 1 is the histologic diagnosis applied to low-grade lesions. However, it is not equivalent to LSIL.
- An estimated 1 million women are diagnosed with CIN 1 annually in the United States, and the annual incidence of CIN 1 is estimated to be 1.2 per 1000 women.
- A CIN 1 progresses in approximately 11% to CIN 2/CIN 3 (Table 49-2).

Table 49-2	Natural History of Untreated Cervical Intraepithelial Neoplasia[a]			
	Regression to Normal (%)	Persistent Dysplasia (%)	Progression to CIN 2/CIN 3 (%)	Progression to CIS (%)
CIN 1	57	30	11	0.3
CIN 2	43	35	—	14-22
CIN 3	32	48-56	—	12

Abbreviations: CIN, cervical intraepithelial neoplasia; CIS, carcinoma in situ.
[a]Data from Mitchell MF, Tortolero-Luna G, Wright T, et al. Cervical human papillomavirus infection and intraepithelial neoplasia: a review. *J Natl Cancer Inst Monogr.* 1996;(21):17-25.

Cervical Intraepithelial Neoplasia 2/3

- The CIN 2/CIN 3 is the histologic diagnosis applied to high-grade lesions. It is not equivalent to HSIL.
- An estimated 500 000 women are diagnosed with CIN 2/CIN 3 annually in the United States, and the annual incidence of CIN 2/CIN 3 is estimated to be 1.5 per 1000 women.

Adenocarcinoma In Situ

- Unlike squamous lesions, AIS lesions are often multifocal. Therefore, negative margins on the excised specimen (LEEP or CKC) do not reliably predict excision of all disease.

MANAGEMENT STRATEGIES: HISTOLOGIC ABNORMALITIES

Treatment Modalities

- Treatment options can be classified as ablative or excisional.
- Ablative procedures do not obtain a sample for pathologic examination.
- Excisional procedures should be performed when invasive cancer cannot be ruled out, microinvasive cancer is suspected on a biopsy, a two-level discrepancy between cytology and histology exists, and whenever concern is raised for endocervical disease.

Ablative Methods

- **Cryotherapy** is performed with a supercooled probe applied directly to the lesion. It is not appropriate for endocervical disease.
- **Carbon dioxide laser** is used to vaporize the tissue to 7-mm depth. Special equipment is necessary, but more irregular areas can be treated.
- Ablative methods are not acceptable for AIS or for unsatisfactory colposcopy.

Excisional Methods

- Excisional procedures may increase a woman's risk of future preterm delivery or premature rupture of the membranes.
- **Loop electrosurgical excision procedure** is an excisional procedure employing a wire with an electrical current. The shape and size of the loop can be altered, and a

second "hat" can be done to obtain further endocervical tissue. Cautery artifact can make interpretation of margins difficult.

- **Cold knife cone** employs a scalpel to excise a cone-shaped wedge of the cervix. The size and shape of the cone can be tailored to the lesion, and this method allows for pathologic determination of margin status. A CKC should be considered over LEEP for cases with AIS, suspected microinvasion, unsatisfactory colposcopy, or a lesion extending into the endocervical canal.

Management of Cervical Intraepithelial Neoplasia 1

- The management of CIN 1 depends on the cytology preceding the diagnosis (see Figure 49-2).
- A CIN preceded by HSIL or AGC (with satisfactory colposcopy, negative ECC)
  - Cotesting at 12 and 24 months with diagnostic excisional procedure if HSIL is encountered again or repeat colposcopy if HPV positive for cytology ≥ASC-US
  - Diagnostic excisional procedure
  - Re-review colposcopic, cytologic, and histologic findings.
- A CIN 1 preceded by ASC-US, ASC-H, or LSIL
  - Cotesting at 12 months
    - o If ≥ASC-US or HPV positive, colposcopy is warranted.
    - o If both negative, age-appropriate screening can resume.
  - Two negative Pap smears or a single negative HPV DNA allows for resumption of standard screening.
- Persistent (>2 y) CIN 1 can be followed as mentioned earlier or treated. Ablative and excisional procedures are acceptable given a satisfactory colposcopy. Ablation is unacceptable after unsatisfactory colposcopy.

Special Populations

- Women ages 21 to 24 years old, management of CIN 1 depends on preceding cytology.
  - A CIN 1 preceded by ASC-US or LSIL, cytology should be performed at 12-month intervals; if ASC-H or HSIL is subsequently encountered, colposcopy is warranted. Routine screening can resume after two negative screens.
  - A CIN preceded by HSIL or ASC-H: colposcopy and cytology every 6 months for 24 months of surveillance
- Pregnant women with CIN 1 should be followed without treatment.

Management of Cervical Intraepithelial Neoplasia 2/3

- A CIN 2/CIN 3 requires excision or ablative treatment after a satisfactory colposcopy. Ablative treatment is only appropriate in nonrecurrent CIN 2/CIN 3 with a satisfactory colposcopy.
- Hysterectomy is not an acceptable initial management for CIN 2/CIN 3.
- After treatment, CIN 2/CIN 3 should be followed by cotesting at 12 and 24 months. Either HPV DNA positivity or ≥ASC-US cytology requires colposcopy with endocervical sampling. If cotesting is normal, cotesting can be performed at 3 years, then normal screening resumed.
- If CIN 2/CIN 3 is identified on the margins of an excision specimen or in the ECC, there are three management options:
  - repeat cytology ECC at 4 to 6 months (preferred)
  - repeat excision (acceptable)
  - hysterectomy if repeat excision not feasible (acceptable)

- After follow-up, routine screening should be continued for at least 20 years.
- Hysterectomy is acceptable for persistent or recurrent CIN 2/CIN 3.

Special Populations

- In younger women, future fertility should be taken into account as well as the fact that CIN 2/CIN 3 can regress spontaneously. For women ages 21 to 24 years, the American Society for Colposcopy and Cervical Pathology recommends colposcopy with cytology at 6-month intervals for 12 months. If CIN 3 is diagnosed on follow-up, or CIN 2/CIN 3 persists for 24 months, treatment is recommended.
- The main goal for pregnant women is to exclude invasive cancer. Biopsy is important if invasion is suspected, and a biopsy during pregnancy is not jeopardizing the pregnancy. An ECC should not be performed. Reassessment with colposcopy should not occur more than every 12 weeks during pregnancy, and deferring reevaluation until 6 weeks postpartum is acceptable.

Management of Adenocarcinoma In Situ

- Cold knife conization is the first-line treatment for AIS, as LEEP is associated with higher rates of positive margins. An ECC should be performed at the time of resection.
- After excision of AIS, if positive margins or ECC are noted, the risk of residual disease is 47% and the risk of cancer is 6%. If margins are negative, the risk of residual disease is still 17% and the risk of occult cancer is 0.6%.
- Hysterectomy is the preferred management for women diagnosed with AIS on diagnostic excisional procedure and who have completed childbearing.

Special Populations

- Women who want to retain fertility should be counseled on the risks associated with that management and should be offered repeat excision and ECC if positive margins are noted on the original excision. Close surveillance including reevaluation at 6 months with cotesting, colposcopy, and ECC is recommended, and close long-term follow-up is recommended per American Society for Colposcopy and Cervical Pathology guidelines.

SUGGESTED READINGS

American College of Obstetricians and Gynecologists Committee on Adolescent Health Care. ACOG Committee Opinion No. 704 summary: human papillomavirus vaccination. *Obstet Gynecol.* 2017;129:1155-1156. doi:10.1097/AOG.0000000000002111.

American College of Obstetricians and Gynecologists Committee on Practice Bulletins—Gynecology. ACOG Practice Bulletin No. 140: management of abnormal cervical cancer screening test results and cervical cancer precursors. *Obstet Gynecol.* 2013;122:1338-1367. (Reaffirmed 2018)

American College of Obstetricians and Gynecologists Committee on Practice Bulletins—Gynecology. ACOG Practice Bulletin No. 168: cervical cancer screening and prevention. *Obstet Gynecol.* 2016;128:e111-e130. doi:10.1097/AOG.0000000000001708. (Reaffirmed 2018)

Arbyn M, Xu L, Simoens C, Martin-Hirsch PP. Prophylactic vaccination against human papillomaviruses to prevent cervical cancer and its precursors. *Cochrane Database Syst Rev.* 2018;(5):CD009069. doi:10.1002/14651858.CD009069.pub3.

Curry SJ, Krist AH, Owens DK, et al. Screening for cervical cancer: US Preventive Services Task Force recommendation statement. *JAMA.* 2018;320:674-686. doi:10.1001/jama.2018.10897.

Garland SM, Kjaer SK, Muñoz N, et al. Impact and effectiveness of the quadrivalent human papillomavirus vaccine: a systematic review of 10 years of real-world experience. *Clin Infect Dis.* 2016;63:519-527. doi:10.1093/cid/ciw354.

Ho GYF, Bierman R, Beardsley L, Chang CJ, Burk RD. Natural history of cervicovaginal papillomavirus infection in young women. *N Engl J Med.* 1998;338:423-428. doi:10.1056/NEJM199802123380703.

Huh WK, Ault KA, Chelmow D, et al. Use of primary high-risk human papillomavirus testing for cervical cancer screening: interim clinical guidance. *J Low Genit Tract Dis.* 2015;19:91-96. doi:10.1097/LGT.0000000000000103.

Markowitz LE, Dunne EF, Saraiya M, et al. Human papillomavirus vaccination: recommendations of the Advisory Committee on Immunization Practices (ACIP). *MMWR Recomm Rep.* 2014;63:1-30.

Massad LS, Einstein MH, Huh WK, et al. 2012 Updated consensus guidelines for the management of abnormal cervical cancer screening tests and cancer precursors. *Obstet Gynecol.* 2013;121:829-846. doi:10.1097/AOG.0b013e3182883a34.

Nayar R, Wilbur DC. The Pap test and Bethesda 2014. "The reports of my demise have been greatly exaggerated" (after a quotation from Mark Twain). *Acta Cytol.* 2015;59:121-132. doi:10.1159/000381842.

Siegel RL, Miller KD, Jemal A. Cancer statistics, 2018. *CA Cancer J Clin.* 2018;68:7-30. doi:10.3322/caac.21442.

Walker TY, Elam-Evans LD, Singleton JA, et al. National, regional, state, and selected local area vaccination coverage among adolescents aged 13-17 years—United States, 2016. *MMWR Morb Mortal Wkly Rep.* 2017;66:874-882. doi:10.15585/mmwr.mm6633a2.

Cervical Cancer

Melissa Pritchard McHale and Kimberly Levinson

Cervical cancer is the fourth most common malignancy among women in the world, and the third most frequent cancer-related cause of death in women. The majority of cervical cancers occur in low- and middle-income nations, accounting for over 90% of cervical cancer deaths. In the United States, cervical cancer is the third most common gynecologic malignancy, and mortality and incidence rates have declined significantly since the introduction of national, standardized screening protocols using routine Papanicolaou smear (Pap test) and, more recently, human papillomavirus (HPV) screening. In recent years, deaths from cervical cancer have decreased at a rate of approximately 2% per year. With primary prevention efforts focused on vaccination with the 9-valent vaccine in addition to secondary prevention efforts with Pap smear and HPV testing, we anticipate further reduction in rates of cervical cancer in the future.

EPIDEMIOLOGY OF CERVICAL CANCER

Approximately 60% of women diagnosed with cervical cancer in developed countries have either never been screened or have not been screened in the preceding 5 years. The mean age for cervical cancer is 48 years old, with most cases diagnosed in women between the ages of 35 and 44 years.

- The primary **risk factor** for cervical cancer is exposure to high-risk human papillomavirus (hrHPV). Other risk factors include smoking, parity, and immunosuppression; race/socioeconomic status; and history of sexually transmitted infections.

  - **hrHPV infection** is present in 99.7% of all cervical cancers. HPV is a nonenveloped, double-stranded DNA virus. The DNA is enclosed in a capsid shell with major L1 and minor L2 structural proteins. The virus is spread through sexual contact. Thus, traditional risk factors for cervical cancer include early age at first coitus, multiple sexual partners, multiparity, lack of barrier contraception, and history of sexually transmitted infection.

    - The hrHPV types 16, 18, 31, 33, 35, 45, 52, and 58 are associated with 95% of squamous cell carcinomas of the cervix. HPV 16 is the most common HPV type associated with squamous cell cervical cancer. Both HPV 16 and HPV 18 are commonly associated with adenocarcinoma of the cervix. Together, HPV types 16 and 18 are responsible for over 70% of cervical cancers.

    - Most HPV infections are transient, resulting in either no change in the cervical epithelium or low-grade intraepithelial lesions that are often spontaneously cleared. Almost all HPV infections are cleared within 6 to 12 months, with only approximately 10% becoming persistent infection. The progression to invasive cancer requires a persistent infection and has a prolonged natural history, most often taking 12 to 15 years, allowing multiple opportunities for detection through screening.

  - **Cigarette smoking** is an independent risk factor in the development of squamous cell carcinoma of the cervix. Although smokers have an increased risk of developing squamous dysplasias and cancer, smoking is not a risk factor for adenocarcinoma of the cervix.

  - **Immunosuppression** increases the risk of developing cervical cancer, with more rapid progression from preinvasive to invasive cancer. Patients with human immunodeficiency virus (HIV) infection are at increased risk for developing cervical cancer and tend to present at a younger age and with more advanced disease than noninfected patients. The Centers for Disease Control and Prevention has described cervical cancer as an AIDS-defining illness. This increased risk also applies to women who are on immunosuppressive medications and women who have undergone organ transplants.

  - **Race and socioeconomic status**

    - The incidence per 100,000 women per year of cervical cancer in the United States was 7.2 from 2011 to 2015. However, this incidence varies by ethnicity and race. Incidence rates per 100,000 women per year for different racial and ethnic groups were as follows: African American, 8.4; white, 7; Native American, 6.2; Hispanic, 9.1; and Asian/Pacific Islander, 5.8. Furthermore, after correction for hysterectomy prevalence, these rates are even more disparate, reaching 53.0 cases per 100,000 women for African American women between the ages of 65 and 69 years, as opposed to white women of the same age, with a rate of 24.7 per 100,000 women.

- These differences are partially accounted for by the increased risk of cervical cancer among women of low socioeconomic status and the barriers to care inherent in this distinction; however, racial disparities remain, independent of socioeconomic status.
- Racial differences are also apparent in survival, which is partially due to the fact that minority women are more commonly diagnosed with cervical cancer at a later stage.

SCREENING, PRESENTATION, AND DIAGNOSIS

Cervical neoplasia is presumed to be a continuum from dysplasia to invasive carcinoma. **Screening** for cervical cancer with the use of the Pap smear, as well as HPV testing and visual inspection with acetic acid (VIA) (particularly in low-income countries), has led to a significant reduction in the incidence, morbidity, and mortality of invasive disease by facilitating the discovery and early treatment of precursor lesions. For further reading on the prevention of cervical cancer and the HPV vaccine, see chapter 49.

Clinical Presentation

- **Early symptoms**
  - Most often, there are no clinical symptoms from early cervical cancer, which is part of the reason why screening for preinvasive or early cancers is so important.
  - Abnormal vaginal bleeding may occur (postcoital, intermenstrual, or postmenopausal bleeding).
  - Serosanguineous or yellowish vaginal discharge, at times foul smelling, may also occur.
  - Dyspareunia can also be a symptom.
- **Late symptoms**
  - Symptomatic anemia
  - Pelvic pain
  - Sciatic and back pain can be related to sidewall extension, hydronephrosis, or metastasis.
  - Bladder or rectal invasion by advanced-stage disease may produce urinary or rectal symptoms (eg, vaginal passage of stool or urine, hematuria, urinary frequency, hematochezia).
  - Lower extremity swelling from occlusion of pelvic lymphatics or thrombosis of the external iliac vein.

Diagnosis of Cervical Cancer

- Some women with cervical cancer will have a visible cervical lesion, whereas others will be detected on routine screening exams and biopsies.
- On **speculum examination**, cervical cancer may appear as an exophytic cervical mass that characteristically bleeds on contact. Endophytic tumors may develop entirely within the endocervical canal, and the external cervix may appear normal. In these cases, bimanual examination may reveal a firm, indurated, and barrel-shaped cervix. The vagina should be inspected for extension of disease. Rectal exam provides information regarding the nodularity of the uterosacral ligaments and helps determine extension of disease into the parametrium.

- On **general physical examination**, advanced cervical cancer may present with enlarged lymph nodes, pleural effusions, ascites, and/or lower extremity edema. Unilateral lower extremity edema may indicate involvement of the pelvic sidewall. Groin and supraclavicular lymph nodes may be indurated or enlarged, indicating spread of disease.
- With obvious exophytic lesions, cervical biopsy is required for histologic confirmation.
- In patients with a grossly normal cervix and abnormal cytology on Pap smear, colposcopic examination with directed biopsies and endocervical curettage (ECC) is necessary (see chapter 49).
- If a definite diagnosis of cervical cancer cannot be made on the basis of office biopsies, further evaluation with a larger cervical conization may be necessary.

DISEASE PROGRESSION, STAGING, AND PROGNOSIS

Routes of Cervical Cancer Spread

- Cervical cancer usually spreads by **direct extension**.
  - **Parametrial extension.** The lateral spread of cervical cancer occurs through the cardinal ligament lymphatics and vessels, and significant involvement of the medial portion of this ligament may result in ureteral obstruction.
  - **Vaginal extension.** The upper vagina may be involved when the primary tumor has extended beyond the confines of the cervix.
  - **Bladder and rectal involvement.** Anterior and posterior spread of cervical cancer to the bladder and rectum is uncommon in the absence of lateral parametrial disease.
- Cervical cancer may also progress via **lymphatic spread** (Figure 50-1).
  - The following are considered first station nodes: obturator, external iliac, hypogastric, parametrial, presacral, and common iliac.
  - Para-aortic nodes are second station, and are rarely involved in the absence of primary nodal disease.
  - Supraclavicular and groin nodes may also be involved with late-stage disease.
  - The percentage of involved lymph nodes increases directly with primary tumor volume and stage of disease.
- **Hematologic metastases** from cervical carcinomas may occur but are less frequent than direct extension or lymphatic spread and are usually seen late in the course of the disease.

Staging of Cervical Cancer

- Cervical cancer is staged according to the **International Federation of Gynecology and Obstetrics (FIGO) system** (Table 50-1 and Table 50-2). As of 2018, **staging of cervical cancer** has changed from primarily a clinically based staging system to a staging system that allows for incorporation of imaging and pathologic findings. Pathologic evaluation, either with biopsy or lymph node dissection is allowable in the current staging system, and when stage is based on pathologic findings, this should be indicated as part of the stage ("p" added to the assigned numeric stage). Lymph-vascular involvement does not alter the classification.

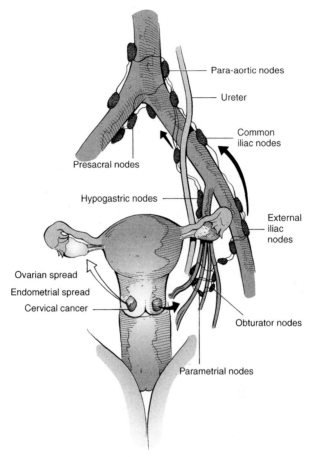

Figure 50-1. Anatomic pathways of spread in invasive cervical cancer. Reprinted with permission from Gibbs RS, Karlan BY, Haney AF, et al, eds. *Danforth's Obstetrics and Gynecology*. 10th ed. Philadelphia, PA: Wolters Kluwer Health/Lippincott Williams & Wilkins; 2008:973. Figure 58.2.

- Routine laboratory studies should include a complete blood count, complete metabolic profile, and urinalysis. No tumor marker has achieved widespread acceptance.
- Inspection and palpation should begin with the cervix, vagina, and pelvis and continue with examination of extrapelvic areas, including the abdomen and groin and supraclavicular lymph nodes.
- Lymphangiograms, arteriograms, computed tomography, magnetic resonance imaging, positron emission tomography, laparoscopy, or laparotomy findings are now used for staging purposes. These imaging studies may help to inform the presence of hydronephrosis as well as nodal metastases in the pelvic or para-aortic regions.
- When doubt exists concerning the stage to which a tumor should be assigned, the earlier stage is chosen. Once a stage has been determined and treatment has begun, subsequent recurrences do not alter the assigned stage.

Table 50-1 International Federation of Gynecology and Obstetrics (FIGO) Staging System for Carcinoma of the Cervix, 2009 Versus 2018[a]

	FIGO Stage 2009	FIGO Stage 2018	5-y Survival by FIGO Stage 2018[b]
Stage I	Cervical carcinoma confined to the uterus (Extension to corpus should be disregarded.)	Cervical carcinoma confined to the uterus (Extension to corpus should be disregarded.)	85.6%
Stage IA	Invasive carcinoma diagnosed by microscopy Stromal invasion ≤5.0 mm/horizontal spread ≤7.0 mm	Invasive carcinoma diagnosed by microscopy Stromal invasion ≤5.0 mm	94.1%
Stage IA1	Stromal invasion ≤3.0 mm/horizontal spread ≤7.0 mm	Stromal invasion ≤3.0 mm	95.8%
Stage IA2	Stromal invasion 3.0-5.0 mm/horizontal spread ≤7.0 mm	Stromal invasion 3.0-5.0 mm	95.0%
Stage IB	Any clinically visible lesion confined to the cervix or microscopic lesion greater than IA1/IA2	Invasive carcinoma Stromal invasion ≥5 mm	75.9%
Stage IB1	Clinically visible lesion ≤4.0 cm	**Stromal invasion 5 mm to <2 cm**	91.6%
Stage IB2	Clinically visible lesion >4.0 cm	**Stromal invasion 2 cm to <4 cm**	83.3%
Stage IB3		**Stromal invasion ≥4 cm**	76.1%
Stage II	Cervical carcinoma invading beyond the uterus but not to the pelvic wall or to lower third of the vagina	Cervical carcinoma invading beyond the uterus but not to the pelvic wall or to lower third of the vagina	56.1%
Stage IIA	Involvement limited to the upper two-thirds of the vagina without parametrial involvement	Involvement limited to the upper two-thirds of the vagina without parametrial involvement	63.4%
Stage IIA1	Clinically visible lesion ≤4.0 cm (+ vaginal involvement)	Clinically visible lesion <4.0 cm (+ vaginal involvement)	70.3%

Stage	FIGO 2009	FIGO 2018[a]	%
Stage IIA2	Clinically visible lesion >4.0 cm (+ vaginal involvement)	Clinically visible lesion ≥4.0 cm (+ vaginal involvement)	65.3%
Stage IIB	Tumor with parametrial invasion but not to the pelvic wall	Tumor with parametrial invasion but not to the pelvic wall	63.9%
Stage III	Tumor extending to the pelvic sidewall and/or involving the lower third of the vagina and/or causing hydronephrosis	Tumor extending to the pelvic sidewall and/or involving the lower third of the vagina and/or causing hydronephrosis	39.3%
Stage IIIA	Tumor involving the lower one-third of the vagina, not extending to the pelvic wall	Tumor involving the lower one-third of the vagina, not extending to the pelvic wall	40.7%
Stage IIIB	Tumor extending to the pelvic wall and/or causing hydronephrosis or nonfunctioning kidney	Tumor extending to the pelvic wall and/or causing hydronephrosis or nonfunctioning kidney	41.4%
Stage IIIC		**Involvement of pelvic and/or para-aortic lymph nodes**	46.3%
Stage IIIC1		**Involvement of pelvic nodes**	60.8%
Stage IIIC2		**Involvement of para-aortic nodes**	37.5%
Stage IV	Carcinoma extends beyond the true pelvis or has involved (biopsy proven) the mucosa of the bladder or rectum.	Carcinoma extends beyond the true pelvis or has involved (biopsy proven) the mucosa of the bladder or rectum.	Not reported
Stage IVA	Tumor invading the mucosa of the bladder or rectum and/or extending beyond the true pelvis (Bullous edema is not sufficient to classify a tumor as T4.)	Tumor invading the mucosa of the bladder or rectum and/or extending beyond the true pelvis (Bullous edema is not sufficient to classify a tumor as T4.)	24.0%
Stage IVB	Distant metastasis (including peritoneal spread or involvement of the supraclavicular, mediastinal, or distant lymph nodes; lung; liver; or bone)	Distant metastasis (including peritoneal spread or involvement of the supraclavicular, mediastinal, or distant lymph nodes; lung; liver; or bone)	14.7%

[a]Bold text indicates changes from 2009.

[b]Reference for FIGO 2009 and 2018 comparison: Wright JD, Matsuo K, Huang Y, et al. Prognostic performance of the 2018 International Federation of Gynecology and Obstetrics cervical cancer staging guidelines. *Obstet Gynecol.* 2019;134(1):49-57.

Table 50-2	Allowable Staging Procedures for Cervical Cancer
Physical examination	Palpation of lymph nodes
	Examination of vagina
	Bimanual rectovaginal examination (under anesthesia recommended)
Radiologic studies	IVP
	Barium enema
	Chest radiograph
	Skeletal radiograph
	Ultrasound
	CT scan
	MRI
	PET scan
Procedures	Biopsy
	Conization
	Hysteroscopy
	Colposcopy
	Endocervical curettage
	Cystoscopy
	Proctoscopy
	Lymph node biopsy
	Lymph node dissection

Abbreviations: CT, computed tomography; IVP, intravenous pyelogram; MRI, magnetic resonance imaging; PET, positron emission tomography.

- Prior to the change in the FIGO staging system, the distribution of stage at presentation was as follows: 38% stage I, 32% stage II, 25% stage III, 4% stage IV, and this did inform 5-year survival, which declined as FIGO stage at diagnosis increased from stage IA (93%) to stage IV (15%). In the prior FIGO staging system, vast discrepancies existed between clinical staging and surgicopathologic findings, such that clinical staging failed to identify extension of disease to the para-aortic nodes in 7% of patients with stage IB disease, 18% with stage IIB, and 28% with stage III. In the new FIGO staging system, these findings are accounted for, it is anticipated that the stage distribution will change, and that prognosis will be more directly associated with stage.
- Only the subclassifications of stage I (IA1, IA2, IB1) require pathologic assessment; however, when pathologic assessment of the nodes is performed (either by biopsy or by lymphadenectomy), this should be indicated as a part of the stage ("p" added to the assigned numeric stage).

Prognostic Factors for Cervical Cancer

- **Prognosis** is directly related to tumor characteristics including histologic subtype, histologic grade, lymph node status, tumor volume, depth of invasion, and lymph-vascular space involvement. Prognosis is also related to FIGO staging (see Table 50-1). Other prognostic variables include age, race, socioeconomic status, and immune status.

Histologic Subtype

- Conflicting data exist on the influence of histologic subtype on tumor behavior, prognosis, and survival. Histologic subtype according to the World Health Organization is as follows:
  - **Squamous cell carcinoma** is the most common histologic type of cervical cancer, comprising about 80% of cases. Squamous cell carcinomas are also subclassified as: **keratinizing, nonkeratinizing, papillary, basaloid, warty, verrucous, squamotransitional**, and **lymphoepithelioma-like** types.
  - **Adenocarcinomas** comprise 17% of invasive cervical carcinomas. Grossly, cervical adenocarcinoma may appear as a polypoid or papillary exophytic mass. However, the lesion may also be located entirely within the endocervical canal and escape visual inspection. Adenocarcinomas may also be subclassified as: **endocervical, mucinous, villoglandular**, and **endometrioid**.
  - **Clear cell carcinomas** are rare and present as nodular, reddish lesions with punctate ulcers and cells with abundant, clear cytoplasm. Diethylstilbestrol exposure is a risk factor.
  - **Adenosquamous carcinoma** has both malignant-appearing glandular and squamous elements. These tumors tend to be aggressive, with studies suggesting lower survival rates than either squamous or adenocarcinomas.
  - Rare subtypes include: **serous carcinoma, glassy cell carcinoma, adenoid cystic carcinoma, adenoid basal carcinoma, undifferentiated carcinoma**, and **small cell carcinoma**.
    - **Small cell neuroendocrine carcinomas** of the cervix are similar to small cell neuroendocrine tumors of the lung and other anatomic locations. These tumors are clinically aggressive, with a marked propensity to metastasize. At diagnosis, disease is often disseminated, with bone, brain, and liver being the most common sites. Because of high metastatic potential, local therapy alone (surgery, radiation, or both) rarely results in long-term survival. Multiagent chemotherapy, in combination with external beam and intracavitary radiation therapy, is the standard therapeutic approach.

Histologic Grade

- Histologic differentiation of cervical carcinomas includes three grades.
  - Grade 1 tumors are **well differentiated** and may form keratinized pearls of epithelial cells. Mitotic activity is low.
  - Grade 2 tumors are **moderately differentiated** carcinomas and have higher mitotic activity and less cellular maturation, accompanied by more nuclear pleomorphism.
  - Grade 3 tumors are composed of **poorly differentiated** cells with less cytoplasm and often bizarre nuclei. Mitotic activity is high. Poorly differentiated tumors have lower 5-year survival rates.

Other Prognostic Factors

- **Node status.** Among surgically treated patients, survival is related to the number and location of involved lymph nodes. With incorporation of node status into the new FIGO staging system (2018), stage should better predict prognosis.

- **Tumor volume.** Lesion size is an important predictor of survival, independent of other factors. Five-year survival rates for lesions <2 cm, 2 to 4 cm, and >4 cm are approximately 90%, 60%, and 40%, respectively. This differentiation has now been incorporated into the FIGO staging system, subclassifying stage IB tumors based on these differences.
- **Lymph-vascular space invasion.** There is mixed data regarding the relationship between lymph-vascular space involvement and survival.

MANAGEMENT OF CERVICAL CANCER

Surgery and chemoradiation therapy are the two modalities most commonly used to treat invasive cervical carcinoma.

Surgical Management

- In general, **primary surgical management** is limited to stages I through IIA.
- Advantages of surgical therapy:
  - It allows for thorough pelvic and abdominal exploration, which can help to identify patients who should be upstaged based on histopathologic findings, and it also allows for individualization of postoperative treatment.
  - Permits conservation of the ovaries with their transposition out of radiation treatment fields.
  - Avoids the use of radiation therapy and the complications associated with it.
  - Despite vaginal shortening, preservation of sexual function is an advantage to surgical management given the effects of radiation therapy on sexual function.
- Disadvantages to surgical therapy:
  - Risks of surgery, including bleeding, infection, damage to organs, vessels, and nerves.
  - Radical hysterectomy results in vaginal shortening; however, with sexual activity, gradual lengthening may occur.
  - Fistula formation (urinary or bowel) and incisional complications related to surgical treatment (when specifically related to surgery, these tend to occur early in the postoperative period and are usually amenable to surgical repair.)
- Other indications for the selection of radical surgery over radiation:
  - concomitant inflammatory bowel disease
  - previous radiation for other disease
  - presence of a simultaneous adnexal neoplasm
- **Surgical approach.** Surgery was often previously performed via a minimally invasive modality including laparoscopic or robotic techniques. Recent randomized data (October 2018) concluded significantly increased risk of recurrence and worse survival in those patients undergoing minimally invasive techniques for radical hysterectomy when compare to those patient undergoing open surgery.
- Once inside the peritoneal cavity, a thorough abdominal exploration should be performed to evaluate for visual or palpable metastases. Particular attention should be paid to the vesicouterine peritoneum for signs of tumor extension or implantation and palpation of the cardinal ligaments and the cervix.
- For those patients undergoing surgical management, lymph node assessment is required for all but stage IA1 tumors with no evidence of lymphvascular space invasion. Sentinel lymph node biopsy for cervical cancer is currently being investigated.

Table 50-3 Classes of Hysterectomy[a]

	Type of Surgery			
	Intrafascial	Extrafascial Class I	Modified Radical Class II	Radical Class III
Cervical fascia	Partially removed	Completely removed	Completely removed	Completely removed
Vaginal cuff	None removed	Small rim removed	Proximal 1-2 cm removed	Upper one-third to one-half removed
Bladder	Partially mobilized	Partially mobilized	Mobilized	Mobilized
Rectum	Not mobilized	Rectovaginal septum partially mobilized	Mobilized	Mobilized
Ureters	Not mobilized	Not mobilized	Unroofed in ureteral tunnel	Completely dissected to bladder entry
Cardinal ligaments	Resected medial to ureters	Resected medial to ureters	Resected at level of ureter	Resected at pelvic side wall
Uterosacral ligaments	Resected at level of cervix	Resected at level of cervix	Partially resected	Resected at postpelvic insertion
Uterus	Removed	Removed	Removed	Removed
Cervix	Partially removed	Completely removed	Completely removed	Completely removed

[a]Adapted with permission from Viswanathan AN. Uterine cervix. In: Halperin EC, Wazer DE, Perez CA, et al, eds. *Perez and Brady's Principles and Practice of Radiation Oncology.* 6th ed. Philadelphia, PA: Wolters Kluwer Health/Lippincott Williams & Wilkins; 2013. Table 69-7.

- Five distinct **classes of hysterectomy** are used in the treatment of cervical cancer (Table 50-3 and Figure 50-2).
  - **Class I** hysterectomy refers to the standard **extrafascial total abdominal hysterectomy**. This procedure ensures complete removal of the cervix with minimal disruption to surrounding structures (eg, bladder, ureters). This procedure may be performed in patients with stage IA1 cervical cancer without lymphvascular space invasion.
  - **Class II** hysterectomy is also referred to as a **modified radical hysterectomy** or **Wertheim hysterectomy** and is well suited for patients with stage IA2 and small lesions (stage IB1 [2018]) that do not distort the anatomy.

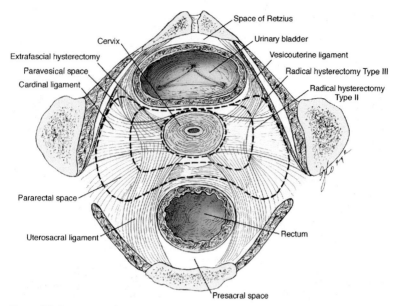

Figure 50-2. Diagram of pelvic anatomy and types of hysterectomy. Reprinted with permission from Berek JS, Hacker NF, eds. *Berek & Hacker's Gynecologic Oncology*. 6th ed. Philadelphia, PA: Wolters Kluwer; 2015:345. Figure 8-10.

- **Class III** hysterectomy, also known as **radical abdominal** or **Meigs hysterectomy**, is recommended for stages IB2, and occasionally for stage IB3 and IIA.
- **Class IV**, or **extended radical hysterectomy**, includes removal of the superior vesical artery, periureteral tissue, and up to three-fourths of the vagina.
- In a **class V**, or **partial exenteration** operation, the distal ureters and a portion of the bladder are resected.
- Classes IV and V procedures may occasionally be used for stage IVA tumors but are rarely performed because these patients are often treated with primary chemoradiation therapy.

Fertility-Preserving Surgical Options

- Fertility-preserving surgeries are used for younger women who have not completed childbearing and require treatment for early stage cervical cancer. These methods include **cervical conization** and **radical trachelectomy** (ie, Dargent operation) and appear to have similar recurrence rates to radical hysterectomy if candidates are selected appropriately.
- Cervical conization is generally reserved for stage IA cervical cancers but is also being investigated with lymphadenectomy for IB1 (FIGO 2018) cancers.
- Radical trachelectomy can be performed for up to stage IB1 (FIGO 2018) tumors with negative nodes. The obstetric outcomes for radical trachelectomy appear to be similar to those for loop electrosurgical excision procedure and conization, which include risk of preterm delivery and low birth weight.
  - Prior to radical trachelectomy, lymph node dissection should be performed to confirm negative lymph node status. To perform the **radical trachelectomy**,

cervical and vaginal branches of the uterine artery are ligated, whereas the main trunk of the uterine artery is preserved. Once the blood supply has been controlled, the cervix is amputated at a point approximately 5 mm caudal to the uterine isthmus. Negative surgical margins should be achieved by frozen section. The uterus is then suspended from the lateral stumps of the transected paracervical ligaments. Once the uterus has been suspended, isthmic cerclage is performed, using a technique similar to that used as prophylaxis against miscarriage. Subsequently, the vaginal and isthmic mucosa are reapproximated.

Primary Chemoradiation Therapy

- **Chemoradiation therapy** can be used for all stages of disease and for most patients, regardless of age, body habitus, or coexistent medical conditions. However, this modality is most commonly used for stage IB3 or greater. Chemoradiation therapy should *not* be used in patients with diverticulosis, tubo-ovarian abscess, or pelvic kidney.
- Radiation therapy should be administered along with concurrent chemotherapy as a radiosensitizer, which results in improved disease-free and overall survival compared with radiation therapy alone.
- Preservation of sexual function is significantly related to the mode of primary therapy. Pelvic radiation produces persistent vaginal fibrosis and atrophy, with loss of both vaginal length and caliber. In addition, ovarian function is lost in virtually all patients who undergo tolerance-dose radiation therapy to the pelvis, unless ovarian transposition has been performed. Fistulous complications associated with radiation therapy tend to occur late and are more difficult to repair because of radiation fibrosis, vasculitis, and poorly vascularized tissues.
- The two main methods for delivering radiation therapy are external photon beam radiation and brachytherapy.
  - **External photon beam radiation** is usually delivered from a linear accelerator. Microscopic or occult tumor deposits from epithelial cancers require 4000 to 5000 cGy for local control. A clinically obvious tumor requires in excess of 6000 cGy. External beam radiation can be delivered via a standard 2- or 4-field technique or is now more commonly delivered via **intensity-modulated radiation therapy**, which is an advanced technology that allows for precise delivery of radiation to the area of the tumor.
  - Once external beam therapy has been completed, **brachytherapy** should be delivered using various intracavitary techniques, including intrauterine tandem and vaginal colpostats, vaginal cylinders, or interstitial needle implants. This is a critical component of curative treatment. Most commonly, a tandem is placed through the cervix into the uterus, and ovoids are placed in the lateral vaginal fornices. Brachytherapy can be delivered as low-dose rates or high-dose rate treatments. Low-dose rate treatments are inpatient over 3 to 4 days and deliver 40 to 70 cGy/h. High-dose rate treatments may be delivered on an outpatient basis over several visits.
  - Classically, two **reference points** were commonly used to describe the dose prescription for cervical cancer:
    - **Point A** is 2 cm lateral and 2 cm superior to the external cervical os and theoretically represents the area where the uterine artery crosses the ureter.
    - **Point B** is 3 cm lateral to point A and corresponds to the pelvic sidewall and to the location of the obturator lymph nodes.
  - The cumulative dose to point A, regardless of method, adequate for central control is usually between 7500 and 8500 cGy. The prescribed dose to point B is

4500 to 6500 cGy, depending on the bulk of parametrial and sidewall disease. The recommendation is to complete radiation therapy within 8 weeks of initiation.

- **Chemoradiation** confers significant survival benefit over radiation alone in the treatment of cervical cancer. When combined with radiation, weekly cisplatin administration reduces the risk of progression for stage IIB through stage IVA cervical cancer. Cisplatin acts as a radiosensitizer, yielding a large reduction in the rate of local recurrence and a more modest reduction in the rate of distant metastases.

Chemotherapy

- **Chemotherapy** is used to treat patients with extrapelvic metastases as well as those with recurrent tumor who have been previously treated with surgery or radiation and are not candidates for exenteration procedures. The best candidates for chemotherapy are those with an excellent performance status and disease that is both outside of the field of radiation and not amenable to surgical resection. Cisplatin has been the most extensively studied agent and has demonstrated the most consistent clinical response rates (20%-25%).
- The most active **combination chemotherapy** regimens for cervical cancer contain cisplatin. The agents most commonly used in combination with cisplatin are paclitaxel and bevacizumab (antiangiogenic therapy). A randomized controlled trial showed a survival benefit with the addition of bevacizumab to cisplatin and paclitaxel alone, and this is the most common regimen used for metastatic cervical cancer. Other agents that have been shown to be active in combination with cisplatin include bleomycin, 5-fluorouracil, mitomycin C, methotrexate, cyclophosphamide, and doxorubicin.

Immunotherapy

- Immunotherapy with Pembrolizumab has also been FDA approved (2018) for advanced cervical cancer for patients with progression after chemotherapy, who are found to have PD-L1 positive tumors.

Combined Modalities

- **Postoperative adjuvant radiation** therapy has been advocated for patients with high-risk features including microscopic parametrial invasion, pelvic lymph node metastases, and positive surgical margins. Postoperative radiation therapy reduces the rate of pelvic recurrence after radical hysterectomy in patients with 2 of 3 intermediate risk factors, including deep stromal invasion, large tumor size, and lymph-vascular space invasion.
- **Neoadjuvant chemotherapy.** Although this strategy may be useful in areas where access to chemoradiation therapy is challenging, a recent randomized clinical trial showed an increased recurrence rate in patients with stage IB2 to IIB disease undergoing neoadjuvant chemotherapy followed by radical hysterectomy when compared to chemoradiation therapy.
- **Adjuvant chemotherapy.** This modality, which consists of additional chemotherapy following definitive chemoradiation therapy is currently being studied in international randomized clinical trials for advanced stage disease.

Management by Stage of Disease

- **Stage IA1** without lymph-vascular invasion is managed with conservative surgery, such as excisional conization or extrafascial hysterectomy. For stage IA1 patients with lymph-vascular invasion, lymphadenectomy and modified radical hysterectomy are recommended. Conization may be used selectively for patients with stage IA1 disease if preservation of fertility is desired, provided that the surgical margins are free of disease.
- **Stage IA2** is associated with positive pelvic lymph nodes in 5% of cases. The preferred treatment of these lesions is modified radical (class II) hysterectomy with pelvic lymphadenectomy. In patients who desire preservation of fertility, cervical conization or radical trachelectomy with lymphadenectomy may be performed.
- Patients treated for microinvasive disease should be followed closely with Pap smear, colposcopy, and ECC every 3 months for the first 2 years and then every 6 months for the following 3 years. For medically inoperable patients, stage IA carcinoma can be effectively treated with chemoradiation.
- **Stages IB1, IB2, IB3, IIA.** Radical hysterectomy (class III hysterectomy) with lymphadenectomy and chemoradiation are equally effective in treating stages IB and IIA carcinoma of the cervix (studies based on 1994 FIGO staging). For stage IB1 disease, radical surgery is preferred because there is a relatively low risk of the need for adjuvant radiation therapy. For women with stage IB1 disease desiring fertility preservation, radical trachelectomy may be performed in women with tumors <2 cm.
  - Management of patients with bulky stage IB disease and stage IIA disease is controversial. The two options are a class III hysterectomy or chemoradiation. Single modality treatment is optimal in this patient population due to the increased risk of morbidity with dual modality treatment; therefore, preoperative determination of intermediate risk features (stromal invasion, tumor size, lymph-vascular space invasion) and high-risk features (parametrial invasion, pelvic lymph node metastases, and positive surgical margins) may be useful to help delineate if surgical therapy alone would be curative.
- **Stages IIB, III, IVA.** Chemoradiation therapy is the treatment of choice for patients with stage IIB and more locally advanced disease. Long-term survival rates with radiation therapy alone are approximately 70% for stage I disease, 60% for stage II disease, 45% for stage III disease, and 18% for stage IV disease. With the routine use of chemoradiation, long-term survival and disease-free progression are increased for all stages of disease.
- **Stage IVB.** Patients with stage IVB disease are usually treated with chemotherapy alone or chemotherapy in combination with local radiation. These patients have a uniformly poor prognosis regardless of treatment modality.

Treatment-Related Complications

- Febrile morbidity can occur after radical hysterectomy due to typical postoperative complications. Major causes of morbidity include lower extremity venous thrombosis, vesicovaginal fistulas (<1%), ureteral fistulas, permanent ureteral stenosis, voiding dysfunction, and pelvic lymphocyst formation.
- The most common acute complications of radiation therapy that occur during or immediately after therapy include uterine perforation, proctosigmoiditis, and acute hemorrhagic cystitis.
- The most common chronic complications that occur months to years after completing therapy include vaginal stenosis, rectovaginal and vesicovaginal fistulas, small bowel obstruction, and radiation-induced second cancers.

Posttreatment Surveillance and Recurrence

- Abdominal exam, leg and groin exam, speculum exam, bimanual rectovaginal examination, and evaluation of lymph nodes should be performed every 3 to 4 months for 2 to 3 years following treatment for cervical cancer. After the first 2 to 3 years, examinations should be done every 6 months until 5 years after treatment completion and then every 1 year thereafter. More frequent examinations are warranted if abnormal signs or symptoms develop. Cervical or vaginal cytology should be completed annually. Performing Pap smears at shorter intervals has not been shown to improve detection of early recurrence, and there is no requirement for routine imaging.

- Treatment of recurrent cervical cancer is dictated by the site of recurrence and by the mode of initial therapy. Only patients with central recurrence and no evidence of disease outside the pelvis are candidates for pelvic exenteration.

Special Management Issues

Cervical Cancer in Pregnancy

- Cervical cancer is the most common malignancy in pregnancy, ranging from 1 in 1200 to 1 in 2200 pregnancies. Cervical cancer coincident with pregnancy requires a multidisciplinary approach; complex diagnostic and therapeutic decisions can be risky for both mother and fetus.

- The symptoms of cervical cancer are the same in pregnant patients and nonpregnant patients. Pregnant women are at risk of delay of diagnosis of cervical cancer. Directed cervical biopsies can be performed safely during pregnancy when high-grade intraepithelial lesions or microinvasion is suspected. The ECC should be avoided due to the risk of rupturing the amniotic membranes. Cervical conization should be performed only if it is strictly indicated and should ideally be performed between 12 and 20 weeks of gestation.

- Pregnant women with cervical cancer should undergo the same evaluation as nonpregnant women. Because the bimanual examination may be difficult in pregnancy, magnetic resonance imaging may be useful to identify extracervical disease.

- In patients with intraepithelial lesions or microinvasive disease stages IA1 and IA2, delaying definitive therapy until after fetal lung maturity has been attained is a reasonable option for desired pregnancies. Patients with less than 3 mm of invasion and no lymph-vascular space involvement may be followed to term and delivered vaginally. The major risk during delivery is hemorrhage due to tearing of the tumor. Recurrences of cervical cancer have been reported at the episiotomy site in women who deliver vaginally.

- Following vaginal delivery, these women should be reevaluated and treated at 6 weeks' postpartum. If delivery is by cesarean section, extrafascial hysterectomy can be performed at the time of delivery or after a delay of 4 to 6 weeks if further childbearing is not desired. Patients with 3 to 5 mm of invasion or lymph-vascular invasion can also be safely followed until fetal lung maturity has been achieved. In these cases, however, surgical treatment should include a modified radical hysterectomy with pelvic lymph node dissection, performed either at the time of cesarean delivery or at 4 to 6 weeks' postpartum. Radiation therapy is associated with survival rates comparable to those after surgical treatment.

- In patients with stages IB and IIA tumors (studies based on 1994 FIGO staging), a delay in therapy *in excess of 6 weeks* may impact survival. If the diagnosis is made after 20 weeks of gestation, consideration may be given to postponing therapy until fetal viability.

- Standard treatment consists of classical cesarean delivery followed by radical hysterectomy with pelvic and para-aortic lymph node dissection; however, this procedure is associated with longer operative time and greater blood loss than in nonpregnant patients. Lower segment transverse cesarean delivery is not recommended because of the increased risk of cervical extension with this procedure that may increase intraoperative bleeding. Radiation therapy results in equivalent survival rates and may be preferable for patients who are poor surgical candidates.
- In patients with more advanced stage disease, delay in treatment may impact survival. Neoadjuvant chemotherapy may be delivered in women for whom definitive treatment delay is planned.

Cervical Cancer in Human Immunodeficiency Virus–Infected Women

- Women with HIV have higher rates of cervical cancer than the general population, and there is an association between low CD4 count and cervical cancer. For this reason, cervical cancer is considered an AIDS-defining illness. For HIV-positive women with normal cytology and a negative HPV test, the risk of cervical cancer is not different from HIV-negative women. However, the risk of progression of an abnormal Pap smear to cervical cancer is much higher in HIV-infected women, including for women with normal cytology and a positive HPV result. Therefore, cervical cancer screening among HIV-infected women is more frequent and the threshold for proceeding to colposcopy is lower (see chapter 49).

Cervical Hemorrhage

- Profuse vaginal bleeding from cervical malignancies is a challenging therapeutic situation. Generally, conservative measures to control cervical hemorrhage are preferable to emergency laparotomy and vascular (ie, hypogastric artery) ligation. Attention must first be directed toward the stabilization of the patient with appropriate intravenous fluid and blood product replacement.
- Immediate control of cervical hemorrhage can usually be accomplished with a vaginal pack soaked in Monsel solution (ferric subsulfate). Topical acetone (dimethyl ketone) applied with a vaginal pack placed firmly against the bleeding tumor bed has also been used successfully to control vaginal hemorrhage from cervical malignancy.
- Definitive control of cervical hemorrhage can be accomplished with external radiation therapy of 180 to 200 cGy/d if the patient has not previously received tolerance doses of pelvic irradiation. Alternatively, arteriography can be used to identify the bleeding vessel(s), and Gelfoam or steel coil embolization can then be performed. Vascular embolization has the disadvantage of producing a hypoxic local tumor environment and potentially compromising the efficacy of subsequent radiation therapy.

Obstructive Uropathy

- The pattern of localized tumor growth seen with cervical cancer often results in complications due to mass effect of the tumor. Most commonly, tumor obstruction of the ureter or ureters can lead to obstructive uropathy.
- Presentation varies depending on whether the obstruction is unilateral or bilateral and how rapidly it develops. In unilateral or partial obstructions, there is typically no change in the volume of urine that is produced. Complete bilateral obstruction

will lead to anuria. Gradual development of obstruction does not lead to pain; however, rapidly developing obstruction of the ureters will lead to flank pain due to acute distension of the renal capsule. Patients may present with symptoms of uremia, such as nausea, vomiting, and altered mental status, due to renal insufficiency.

- In a patient with known cervical cancer, urinary obstruction symptoms should prompt immediate evaluation of the renal system, either with renal ultrasound or noncontrast computed tomography scan for evaluation of hydronephrosis and ureteral dilatation. Management requires expeditious relief of the obstruction, either via percutaneous nephrostomy tubes or ureteral stenting.

Venous Thromboembolism

- Patients with cervical cancer carry many significant risk factors for venous thromboembolism (VTE), most notably a cancer diagnosis. They also routinely undergo surgical procedures or are immobilized for prolonged periods for radiation, which also place them at increased risk for VTE. There is also an increased risk of VTE due to stasis as a result of venous compression. Anticoagulation is recommended in the setting of surgery or prolonged immobility. There are no recommendations for routine anticoagulation outside of those contexts.

CERVICAL CANCER AND GLOBAL HEALTH

- Cervical cancer is a major cause of cancer death in women in developing countries—over 85% of worldwide deaths from cervical cancer are clustered in low-income countries. The World Health Organization estimates that over half a million women will be newly diagnosed with cervical cancer every year, and the majority of these women are between the ages of 15 and 45 years, living in developing nations. Regions at highest risk include East and West Africa with a cumulative risk of 3.9%, South Africa 2.9%, central Asia 2.6%, and Middle Africa. It is estimated that by 2030, an alarming 98% of cervical cancer deaths will occur in developing countries.
- The disparity can be explained by the lack of widespread screening and vaccination for cervical cancer. The Pap screening tool is neither feasible nor practical in most low-resource settings because cytology requires infrastructure, expertise, and resources. Much research has been conducted on the "see and treat" method that makes use of the VIA test as an alternative to the Pap smear in low-resource settings. VIA involves application of acetic acid directly to the cervix followed by visualization and immediate treatment of acetowhite lesions with cryotherapy or cervical conization. Women thus do not need to make several trips for screening and treatment. Across several large studies, VIA has shown varying sensitivities and specificities; with one meta-analysis showing a sensitivity of 82% and a specificity of 60%.
- More recently, HPV screening has emerged as a good alternative or addition to VIA in low-resource settings. Minimal training is required for sample collection, and it may even be performed by the patient.
- An important instrument in the global fight against cervical cancer is the implementation of HPV vaccines in low-income settings. Efforts to decrease the cost of this vaccine would result in increased use in developing nations. Although it will take several decades to see an impact on mortality, this will be an important milestone in overcoming the global cervical cancer burden.

SUGGESTED READINGS

Amant F, Van Calsteren K, Halaska MJ, et al. Gynecologic cancers in pregnancy: guidelines of an international consensus meeting. *Int J Gynecol Cancer*. 2009;19(suppl 1):S1-S12.

Bhatla N, Aoki D, Sharma DN, Sankaranarayanan R. Cancer of the cervix uteri. *Int J Gynaecol Obstet*. 2018;143(suppl 2):22-36.

Bhatla N, Berek JS, Fredes MC, et al. Revised FIGO staging for carcinoma of the cervix uteri. *Int J Gynecol Obstet*. 2019;145(1):129-135.

Green JA, Kirwan JM, Tierney JF, et al. Survival and recurrence after concomitant chemotherapy and radiotherapy for cancer of the uterine cervix: a systematic review and meta-analysis. *Lancet*. 2001;358:781-786.

Hacker NF, Vermorken JB. Cervical cancer. In: Berek JS, Hacker NF, eds. *Berek & Hacker's Gynecologic Oncology*. 6th ed. Philadelphia, PA: Lippincott Williams & Wilkins; 2015:326-389.

Ramirez PT, Frumovitz M, Pareja R, et al. Minimally invasive versus abdominal radical hysterectomy for cervical cancer. *N Engl J Med*. 2018;379:1895-1904.

Schiffman M, Castle PE, Jeronimo J, Rodriguez AC, Wacholder S. Human papillomavirus and cervical cancer. *Lancet*. 2007;370:890-907.

Cancer of the Uterine Corpus

Marla Scott and Amanda Nickles Fader

Uterine cancer is the most common gynecologic malignancy in developed countries and is one of the only solid tumors that is increasing in incidence. In the United States, it is the fourth most common cancer in women and the most common gynecologic malignancy, accounting for 7% of all female cancers.

EPIDEMIOLOGY OF UTERINE CANCER

In the United States and other developed countries, the incidence of uterine cancer is 25 in 100 000 making it the most common gynecologic malignancy in these settings. The American Cancer Society estimated that there were 63 232 new cases and 11 350 deaths from uterine malignancies in 2018.

- The median age at diagnosis is 62 years, and the peak incidence occurs from ages 55 to 70 years. The US women have a 2.8 % lifetime risk of being diagnosed with uterine cancer (2.81% lifetime risk for white women compared to 2.48% for African American women). Despite this similar risk of uterine cancer, African American women are 2 times more likely to die from uterine cancer and have a lower 5-year survival (61% vs 84%) compared to white women.

- Because uterine cancer usually presents with postmenopausal bleeding or irregular bleeding, nearly 70% of uterine cancer is diagnosed at an early stage (confined to primary site), with approximately 20% and 10% of cases presenting with regional or distant metastases, respectively. Most commonly, these are cancers of the endometrium because only 5% of uterine cancers are sarcomas or other subtypes.

- Uterine cancer is stratified by tumor type. These tumors differ in incidence, clinical behavior, and prognosis. **Type I** tumors are endometrioid carcinomas grades 1 and 2 and represent 80% of all uterine cancers. They are typically estrogen responsive, are characterized by mutations in PTEN and KRAS, and have a favorable prognosis. **Type II** tumors include grade 3 endometrioid carcinomas as well as nonendometrioid subtypes of uterine cancers, such as serous, clear cell, carcinosarcoma, and other less common subtypes. These are more aggressive subtypes that are commonly characterized by aberrant p53 expression and have an overall worse prognosis compared to type 1 tumors.

RISK FACTORS FOR UTERINE CANCER

- **Excess exposure to estrogen (endogenous or exogenous)** is the most common risk factor for uterine cancer.
- In the modern era, the most common exposure to **endogenous** estrogen is **obesity**, which increases estrogen by peripheral conversion of androstenedione to estrogen by aromatase in adipose tissues. Nearly 70% of early-stage endometrial cancer patients are obese. The relative risk of death increases with increasing body mass index (BMI), and a BMI >30 kg/m^2 will triple the risk of uterine cancer.
- **Estrogen replacement** without concomitant progesterone is the most common form of **exogenous** estrogen exposure and carries a relative risk of 2.3 to 9.5 for endometrial cancer that may persist for up to 10 years after treatment is stopped (Table 51-1). Additionally, a woman taking **tamoxifen**, a selective estrogen receptor modulator, has

Table 51-1	Risk Factors for Endometrial Cancer[a]
Risk Factor	**Relative Risk**
Older age	2-3
Nulliparity	3
Long-term use of unopposed estrogen therapy	10-20
PCOS	3
Infertility	2-3
Late age at menopause	2-3
Early age menarche	1.5-2
Obesity	2-5
Type 2 diabetes mellitus, hypertension, gallbladder disease, or thyroid disease	1.3-3
Tamoxifen	2-3
Lynch syndrome	6-20

Abbreviation: PCOS, polycystic ovary syndrome.
[a]Modified from Gershenson DM, McGuire WP, Gore M, Quinn MA, Thomas G, eds. *Gynecologic Cancer: Controversies in Management*. Philadelphia, PA: Churchill Livingstone; 2004. Copyright © 2004 Elsevier. With permission.

an annual risk of 2 in 1000 of developing uterine cancer and 40% of women may develop this malignancy more than 12 months after stopping therapy.

- **Age.** A woman's risk of uterine cancer also increases with **age**. Women over 50 years of age account for 90% of endometrial cancer cases, with approximately 5% developing disease before age 40 years.
- **Chronic anovulation** states, such as those seen in **polycystic ovary syndrome**, lead to constant estrogen stimulation of the endometrium and also increase the risk of cancer due to the lack of a corpus luteum to produce progesterone.
- **Nulliparity** (related to infertility) and **diabetes mellitus** are independent risk factors and have a relative risk of two to three for uterine cancer, whereas the association of **hypertension** seems related to obesity.
- Genetic associations (see chapter 53).
  - **Hereditary nonpolyposis colon cancer** or **Lynch syndrome**, is inherited in an autosomal dominant fashion resulting from a germline mutation in one of the mismatch repair genes (*MLH1, MSH2, MSH6*). Patients with Lynch syndrome have a 40% to 60% risk of developing uterine cancer by age 70 years and comprise the majority of inherited cases of uterine cancer. These women are at a significantly higher risk for cancer of the colorectum, renal pelvis, ureter, and ovary.
  - Women with **Cowden syndrome**, an autosomal dominant condition with a mutation in the PTEN tumor suppressor gene, have a 13% to 19% lifetime risk of uterine cancer.
- Some factors can decrease the risk of uterine cancer.
  - Factors that decrease circulating estrogen, such as cigarette smoking and oral contraceptive pill (OCP) use, may be protective; however, use of tobacco products is never encouraged.
  - The **OCPs** decrease endometrial cancer risk by 30% or more, even up to 30 years after discontinuation, and this protection increases with length of use. This is likely related to the progestin effect in OCPs.
  - **Levonorgestrel-releasing intrauterine device (IUD)** use decreases the incidence of endometrial carcinoma (observed to expected ratio 0.5).
  - **Breastfeeding** (at least 3 mo duration) is associated with a 11% risk reduction of uterine cancer.
  - There is a 13% decrease in risk for every 5 years of **increasing age at last birth** when compared to women whose last birth was age of <25 years. This finding was independent of parity.
  - Increased **physical activity**, **weight loss**, and consumption of **coffee** and **tea** have also been shown in some studies to decrease risk of uterine cancer.

SCREENING

- Due to the overall low prevalence of uterine cancer, screening is not recommended in the general population.
- Special populations, however, may benefit from screening.
  - **Lynch syndrome.** The American Cancer Society recommends annual endometrial biopsy (EMB) starting at age 35 years in patients with Lynch syndrome. Due to the high risk of uterine cancer (40%-60%) and increased risk of ovarian cancer (10%-12%) in this population, a risk-reducing hysterectomy with bilateral salpingo-oophorectomy (BSO) is recommended once childbearing is completed (see chapter 53).

- **Cowden syndrome.** There are no guidelines for screening in this population, but it is reasonable to perform EMB with or without transvaginal ultrasound starting at the age of 35 years (see chapter 53).
- **Tamoxifen use.** Routine screening with ultrasound or EMBs is not recommended for tamoxifen users despite the increased risk of developing uterine cancer. A transvaginal ultrasound is not beneficial because tamoxifen use causes subepithelial stromal hypertrophy and therefore increases the thickness of the endometrial stripe, resulting in unnecessary procedures. Women on tamoxifen should be counseled on warning signs and followed with yearly pelvic exams. Any episode of vaginal bleeding should prompt evaluation in this patient population.

PRESENTATION, EVALUATION, AND DIAGNOSIS

Clinical Presentation

- Upward of 90% of uterine cancer cases present with abnormal uterine bleeding (AUB) or postmenopausal bleeding. Although there are many causes of AUB discussed elsewhere in this text, special care should be taken to evaluate women with risk factors and AUB less than age 40 years and anyone with postmenopausal bleeding.
- Approximately 10% of postmenopausal patients who present with bleeding have a diagnosis of cancer on their biopsy. An incidentally discovered thickened endometrial stripe >4 mm without symptoms of postmenopausal bleeding will not necessarily trigger the need for an EMB, but sampling should be considered depending on risk factors. **In women with a thickened endometrial stripe and postmenopausal bleeding, endometrial sampling is advised because the risk of underlying malignancy can be has high as 20%.**
- **Abnormal cervical cytology** may also prompt the workup for uterine cancer. Routine cervical cytology will only detect half of uterine cancer cases and is not a screening test for this disease. A workup should be considered with the following Pap smear results:
  - **Endometrial cells** (remote from menstrual bleeding) in a woman **greater than 40 years old**
  - **Atypical glandular cells of undetermined significance** (The risk of endometrial cancer in women over 35 years with this Pap result is 23%.)
  - **Adenocarcinoma** (Both endometrial and cervical sampling should be performed.)
- Some cases of uterine cancer are discovered **incidentally at the time of hysterectomy**. A recent study revealed that 43% of hysterectomies performed for hyperplasia with atypia will have uterine cancer on final pathology. If a uterine cancer is found at time of surgery, a surgeon skilled with uterine cancer staging procedures (ideally a gynecologic oncologist, if available) should be involved. To avoid this scenario of occult malignancy, it is recommended that all women with AUB have endometrial sampling prior to their hysterectomy.

Evaluation

Women with postmenopausal bleeding should be further evaluated with pelvic ultrasound, EMB, or both.

- **Ultrasound.** On pelvic ultrasound, an endometrial stripe <5 mm portends a low risk for cancer, with a negative predictive value of 99%. However, it provides less information if ≥5 mm; therefore, further diagnostic workup with EMB or dilation and curettage (D&C) is warranted. Those with persistent bleeding should be evaluated with endometrial sampling regardless of stripe measurement.

- **Endometrial sampling**
  - An EMB should be performed in women at high risk for uterine cancer with postmenopausal or AUB. The accuracy of detecting cancer on an EMB is between 91% and 99%. The false-negative rate for EMB is between 5% and 15%.
  - A D&C allows for more complete sampling of the endometrium and has a false-negative rate between 2% and 6%. A D&C is advised when
    - an EMB result is read as "insufficient sample"
    - cervical stenosis prevents office EMB
    - patient is unable to tolerate ambulatory EMB
    - patient has continued bleeding despite prior negative biopsy
    - endometrial polyp or endometrial mass is suspected (D&C with hysteroscopy)

STAGING AND PROGNOSIS

Pretreatment Evaluation

- Complete history, assessing for hereditary cancer syndromes.
- Complete physical exam, including comprehensive pelvic exam assessing the size and mobility of the uterus and assessment for metastasis (ie, supraclavicular lymphadenopathy)
- Consider cancer antigen 125 (CA-125) in patients with uterine serous carcinoma (USC). Elevated CA-125 levels are associated with metastatic disease and can be used to follow the patient if it was elevated at diagnosis.
- Imaging: Chest imaging can be considered. A plain film is reasonable. A computed tomography (CT) or magnetic resonance imaging (MRI) is not necessary in the setting of type I cancers if surgical staging is planned. However, imaging is recommended for women with type II cancers, who have a higher risk of metastatic disease; imaging of the chest, abdomen, and pelvis is warranted preoperatively. If no surgery is planned, an MRI is the best modality to assess myometrial or cervical and lymph node involvement.

Staging of Uterine Cancer

Staging of endometrial cancer is demonstrated in Table 51-2 and is based on surgical findings, as described in the International Federation of Gynecology and Obstetrics 2009 staging criteria. In this new staging system, abdominopelvic cytology is no longer part of the staging criteria.

Surgical Staging Procedures

- Staging for uterine cancer is performed surgically. Because many patients have early-stage disease at the time of diagnosis, this is often the only intervention necessary.
- **Surgical staging** most commonly involves a minimally invasive surgical approach for apparent early-stage disease. The current standard of care is minimally invasive surgery when possible. This is based on eight randomized trials, including the largest trial, the Gynecologic Oncology Group (GOG) LAP-2 phase III study, which demonstrated that a laparoscopic approach to uterine cancer staging is feasible and safe with similar intraoperative complications but fewer postoperative adverse events and a shorter hospital stay. Long-term follow-up data suggest similar recurrence rates

Table 51-2 Staging of and National Comprehensive Cancer Network Management Recommendations for Endometrial Carcinoma by Stage and Grade

Stage[a]	Description	Grade 1	Grade 2	Grade 3
IA	Confined to uterine corpus but <50% myometrial invasion	−RF: Observe +RF: Observe or VBT	−RF: Observe +RF: VBT	−RF: Observe or VBT +RF: Observe or VBT
IB	Confined to uterine corpus but ≥50% myometrial invasion (not to serosa)	−RF: Observe or VBT +RF: Observe or VBT	−RF: Observe or VBT +RF: Observe or VBT	RT: VBT and or EBRT ± systemic therapy
II	Infiltrates cervical stroma but confined to uterus[b]	VBT ± EBRT	VBT ± EBRT	EBRT ± VBT ± systemic therapy
IIIA	Infiltration of uterine serosa or adnexae	EBRT ± VBT ± systemic therapy OR systemic therapy ± VBT		
IIIB	Involvement of vagina and/or parametrium	EBRT ± VBT ± systemic therapy OR systemic therapy ± VBT		
IIIC	Metastasis to pelvic (IIIC1) and/or para-aortic (IIIC2) lymph nodes	EBRT ± VBT ± systemic therapy OR systemic therapy ± VBT		
IVA	Infiltration of bladder and/or bowel mucosa	EBRT ± VBT ± systemic therapy OR systemic therapy ± VBT		
IVB	Distant metastases including in the abdomen and inguinal lymph nodes	Systemic therapy ± EBRT ± VBT		

Abbreviations: EBRT, external beam radiation therapy; RF, risk factors (age >60, depth of invasion and or positive lymphovascular space invasion); RT, radiation therapy; VBT, vaginal brachytherapy.

[a]Staging based on the 2009 International Federation of Gynecology and Obstetrics guidelines and recommendations are based on National Comprehensive Cancer Network Guidelines as presented in the National Comprehensive Cancer Network Guidelines. http://www.nccn.org/professionals/physician_gls/f_guidelines.asp.

[b]Endocervical glandular involvement without stromal involvement is stage I. Endocervical stromal involvement is required for a stage II designation.

and 5-year overall survival in the open and laparoscopic groups with superior short-term quality of life assessments in the laparoscopic cohorts.

- Traditionally, a fully staged procedure includes total extrafascial hysterectomy, BSO, a pelvic and para-aortic lymph node assessment/dissection, and in cases of advanced disease, cytoreduction of all visible disease. Omentectomy should be performed if serous or clear cell histology is suspected.

- **Sentinel lymph node dissection** following lymphatic mapping has become an alternative standard option for the management of lymphatic assessment in low-risk endometrial cancer in lieu of full pelvic and para-aortic lymph node dissection.

  - There is a growing body of both prospective and retrospective data that support the use of sentinel lymph node dissection. This technique is supported in select settings by both the National Comprehensive Cancer Network (NCCN) and Society for Gynecologic Oncology (SGO). Currently, there is ongoing research assessing its utility in higher risk, type II histologies.

  - To complete a sentinel lymph node assessment, either isosulfan blue and technetium-99m or indocyanine green (ICG) alone is injected into the cervix at 3 and 9 o'clock. Approximately 15 to 30 minutes following the injection, the sentinel lymph nodes are identified and removed. This can be done using both laparoscopic and robotic platforms using infrared technology to visualize the ICG dye. There is data to suggest that ICG is superior to isosulfan blue dye; however, both are considered reasonable methods to achieve lymph node mapping.

- If a full **pelvic lymph node dissection** is completed, it involves the removal of nodal tissue from the distal half of each common iliac artery, the anterior and medial proximal half of each external iliac artery and vein, and the distal half of the obturator fat pad anterior to the obturator nerve. **Para-aortic lymph node dissection** involves the removal of nodal tissue over the distal vena cava from the inferior mesenteric artery to the mid common iliac artery and between the aorta and ureter from the inferior mesenteric artery to the left mid common iliac artery.

  - Morbid obesity may render a lymph node dissection more challenging.

  - One pitfall of lymph node dissection is the occurrence of lymphedema (5%-20%). The incidence of this increases with the removal of more nodes and administration of adjuvant radiation.

  - Furthermore, the performance of lymph node dissection is not clearly associated with improved survival. In fact, several prospective randomized trials (A Consolidated Standards of Reporting Trials [CONSORT], A Study in the Treatment of Endometrial Cancer [ASTEC]) have demonstrated no difference in survival when lymph node dissection was performed. However, the retrospective Survival Effect of Para-Aortic Lymphadenectomy (SEPAL) study suggested that women with type II cancers may have a survival benefit from complete pelvic and para-aortic lymphadenectomy.

Cytoreduction

- If visible disease is noted elsewhere in the abdomen, principles of surgical cytoreduction to achieve no gross visible disease should be employed. Complete cytoreduction is associated with a longer median survival.

Histopathologic Factors for Uterine Cancer

- **Type I** endometrial cancers (endometrioid adenocarcinomas grades 1 and 2) are estrogen dependent, arise in a background of hyperplasia with atypia, and account for 80% of uterine cancers. These have a favorable prognosis, are estrogen responsive,

Table 51-3	Classification of Endometrial Hyperplasia[a]
Types of Hyperplasia	**Progressing to Cancer (%)**
Simple (cystic without atypia)	1
Complex (adenomatous without atypia)	3
Atypical	
Simple (cystic with atypia)	8
Complex (adenomatous with atypia)	29

[a]Reprinted with permission from Chi DS, Berchuck A, Dizon DS, et al, eds. *Principles and Practice of Gynecologic Oncology.* 7th ed. Philadelphia, PA: Wolters Kluwer; 2017. Table 21.12.

and may be preceded by an endometrial intraepithelial lesion—atypical and/or complex endometrial hyperplasia. Hyperplasia pathologic type portends a different risk of uterine cancer (Table 51-3).

- **Type II** tumors are not estrogen dependent; arise in a background of endometrial atrophy, are poorly differentiated; and are often of uterine serous, clear-cell and grade 3 endometrioid, undifferentiated, carcinosarcoma, transitional cell, and mesonephric histologies. They account for 10% to 20% of histologies but a disproportionate 40% of the mortality associated with uterine cancers.
- The PTEN tumor suppressor gene, K-ras oncogene, and microsatellite instability resulting from mutations in DNA mismatch repair proteins (eg, MLH1, MSH2, or MSH6) are associated with endometrioid cancer pathogenesis and complex atypical hyperplasia.
- A USC histologically resembles and behaves like ovarian serous cancer. It tends to metastasize early (72% have extrauterine spread at the time of diagnosis) and spreads throughout the peritoneal cavity. Therefore, omentectomy along with upper abdominal and peritoneal biopsies should be performed as part of surgical staging for a known USC. Approximately 30% harbor *HER2* mutations.
- Leiomyosarcoma, endometrial stromal sarcoma (ESS), and other rare histologies makeup the remaining 2% to 5% of uterine cancers.
- **Tumor grade** affects the risk of spread and recurrence and is therefore important in determining the need for adjuvant therapy.
  - **Grade 1** tumors have <5% solid, nonsquamous, or morular component.
  - **Grade 2** tumors are 6% to 50% composed of these features.
  - **Grade 3** tumors have these features in >50% of the tumor.

PROGNOSTIC FACTORS

- The most significant prognostic factors for recurrence and survival are stage, grade, and depth of myometrial invasion. Age, histologic type, lymphovascular space invasion (LVSI), and progesterone receptor activity also have prognostic significance. If LVSI is present it is associated with a 35% rate of recurrence.
- Positive peritoneal cytology is controversial as a prognostic factor. Although multiple large studies show conflicting results, in low-grade disease, it does not

confer worse survival. However, in women with type 2 cancers, an ad hoc study of the LAP-2 trial demonstrated that positive peritoneal cytology was independently associated with worse survival.

- Five-year survival for endometrial cancers are 90% for stage IA cancers, 80% for stage IB and II, 50% to 60% for stage III cancers, and 20% for stage IV.
- Prognosis for the more aggressive histologic types is less favorable. Approximately 70% of patients with USC and 50% with clear cell cancers present with stage III or IV disease. Five-year survival for USC and clear cell carcinoma are 55% and 68%, respectively. Overall, 5-year survival for the aggressive histologic subtypes is 40%.
- Relapses in high-grade histologies tend to occur distally, often in the lungs, liver, or bones, whereas low-risk endometrial cancers tend to recur locally, most commonly in the vagina followed by the pelvis.

MANAGEMENT OF UTERINE CANCER

- Appropriate treatment is determined by stage, grade, histologic type, and the patient's ability to tolerate therapies (see Table 51-2).
- Patients with early-stage, **low-risk endometrial cancer** of endometrioid type require no further therapy beyond surgery, particularly patients with grade 1, stage 1 endometrial cancer and no risk factors.

Management of High-Risk Uterine Cancer

- Treatment for women with higher risk disease is more controversial. Multiple studies have sought to define the appropriate role for adjuvant therapy (see Table 51-2).

Radiation Therapy

- Multiple studies have been performed to assess women who would benefit most from adjuvant radiation. Most patients who receive radiation do so postoperatively; however, women who are not candidates for surgery may receive radiation therapy (RT) upfront.
- Depending on their stage at diagnosis and other risk factors for recurrence, women may receive vaginal brachytherapy, external beam radiation therapy (EBRT), including intensity-modulated RT, or both.
- For uterine-confined disease, patients who most benefit from adjuvant RT are those who are high intermediate risk and high risk. Adjuvant RT should be initiated as soon as the vaginal cuff is healed and no later than 12 weeks after surgery. Adjuvant RT has been shown to reduce vaginal cuff recurrences and improve pelvic control but has not been shown to increase overall survival. There have been four major trials that have evaluated the use of adjuvant radiation in uterine-confined disease. All demonstrated improvement in vaginal or pelvic control with most finding a decrease in locoregional recurrence in those receiving adjuvant RT.

Cytoreductive Surgery

- Stage II uterine cancer significantly increases the risk for vaginal recurrence. If cervical involvement is known preoperatively, a **radical hysterectomy** should be considered, which has been shown to result in a 75% 5-year survival rate. A combination of extrafascial hysterectomy followed by radiation is associated with a 5-year survival rate of 70%. If the diagnosis is made postoperatively, vaginal brachytherapy with or without EBRT may be considered.

- For stage III and IV cancers, **optimal cytoreductive surgery** has been shown to improve survival in retrospective studies. Adjuvant therapy after cytoreduction is advised with systemic therapy, which can be combined with EBRT and or vaginal brachytherapy.

- Complete **salvage cytoreduction** for recurrent disease has been associated with a prolonged progression-free survival (39 mo) versus patients with gross residual disease remaining after surgery (13.5 mo) and may be considered in select patients with a long disease-free interval and who have either oligometastatic or resectable disease.

Chemotherapy and Immunotherapy

- Chemotherapy is often used in the management of women with advanced-stage disease and in select women with type II or high-risk early-stage cancers. Carboplatin and paclitaxel is the regimen of choice for treatment in the upfront setting. Single-agent response rates are low. Multiple trials have been conducted with various regimens.

- Cisplatin and doxorubicin together have a 43% response rate. The addition of paclitaxel to the cisplatin and doxorubicin regimen (TAP) in a randomized trial (GOG 177) resulted in an increase in response rate and survival. There was a significantly higher rate of peripheral neuropathy in the group treated with paclitaxel. Data from the subsequent phase III GOG 209 suggest that carboplatin and paclitaxel may be noninferior and less toxic compared to TAP and has become the standard of care for the treatment of advanced or recurrent/chemo-naive endometrial cancer. In select settings, women with stage III/IVA disease may also benefit from the addition of EBRT with chemotherapy. Recently published GOG 258 demonstrated that chemotherapy with addition of RT did not demonstrate an overall survival benefit but did decrease rate of local recurrence.

- Hormonal therapies (progestins like Megace; selective estrogen receptor modulators like tamoxifen, and aromatase inhibitors) are largely more useful in the palliative setting and are not used with an intention to cure. However, the combination of Megace sequenced with tamoxifen as studied in a phase II GOG trial demonstrated a response rate of >40% in the setting of recurrence.

- Pembrolizumab is an immunotherapy drug that has revolutionized the approach to endometrial cancer care. It was recently approved by the US Food and Drug Administration (FDA) to treat unresectable or metastatic microsatellite instability–high or mismatch repair deficient endometrial cancer that has already been treated with standard therapy. It is a check point inhibitor therapy that targets programmed cell death 1 receptors. The pembrolizumab response rate was an impressive 52%, and overall disease control was 73% in a recent study.

- Targeted therapies that act on the PI3K/AKT/mTor pathway, angiogenesis, and epidermal growth factor receptors are also promising. Bevacizumab and temsirolimus/everolimus are currently under investigation.

- Patients who fail first-line chemotherapy generally have a poor prognosis, with a response rate to second- and third-line agents of <10% and overall survival of <9 months. Recently, there has been data to support everolimus combined with letrozole for recurrent disease with promising results.

Special Considerations

Clear Cell and Uterine Serous Carcinoma

- Type II tumors are notoriously biologically aggressive and are often treated with adjuvant therapy regardless of stage.
- The overall 5-year disease-free survival for clear cell endometrial cancers is only 40%. Relapses are often distant and tend to occur in the abdomen, lungs, and/ or liver.
- As opposed to type I endometrial cancers, the precursor lesion to USC is endometrial intraepithelial carcinoma not endometrial hyperplasia. A USC is associated with LVSI, and 36% of women with no myometrial invasion will have positive lymph nodes. Five-year survival is only 30% to 50% for stage I disease.
- As in ovarian cancer, chemotherapy regimens with carboplatin and paclitaxel have been the most studied and had the most utility. Human epidermal growth factor receptor 2/neu is overexpressed in 30% of USCs. A recent phase II trial found that adding trastuzumab, a monoclonal antibody that targets human epidermal growth factor receptor 2/neu receptors, to the standard regimen of carboplatin/ paclitaxel increased median progression-free survival from 8 months in the control group (carboplatin/paclitaxel without trastuzumab) to 12.8 months in the group that received trastuzumab. This finding was significant in all patients and among patients with stage III or IV disease as well as patients with recurrent disease, making it a promising new treatment option for patients with USC.

Carcinosarcoma

- **Uterine carcinosarcoma** is an aggressive cancer subtype and is associated with previous pelvic radiation. Theses tumors are often large and necrotic. Carcinosarcoma is an independent adverse predictor of survival with a hazard ratio of 3.2 for recurrence compared to the other histologies. Thus, carcinosarcoma should be studied separately from high-risk endometrial cancers given the difference in biologic behavior.
- These tumors are **no longer considered sarcomas but instead are best classified as poorly differentiated endometrial carcinomas**.
- The 5-year survival rate is 50% for stage I tumors and 20% for stage IV.
- Lymph node dissection has not been shown to be therapeutic for these tumors. Stage and mitotic grade are the most predictive of disease course.
- Chemotherapy regimens, including cisplatin, doxorubicin, ifosfamide, and paclitaxel, have been used for carcinosarcoma. Chemotherapy with ifosfamide and paclitaxel resulted in not only an improved response rate, overall survival, and progression-free survival but also more neuropathy compared to ifosfamide alone. Recent data from a phase II trial suggest that **paclitaxel/carboplatin** is also a useful regimen, and the NCCN now considers it the preferred adjuvant therapy for uterine-confined endometrial cancers, including carcinosarcoma.
- Pelvic radiation improves local control but not overall survival in this population.

Fertility Preservation

- Women with very early stage, low-grade uterine cancer (endometrioid histology only) who wish to preserve their fertility may be offered progestin therapy rather than surgery in select cases. However, this is largely based on retrospective and limited phase II data and is not yet considered standard of care.

- Optimal candidates for fertility-sparing treatment include women with the following characteristics:
  - Well-differentiated (grade 1) endometrial adenocarcinoma
  - Tumor with apparent confinement to the endometrium, stage IA (based on MRI)
  - No contraindications to hormone therapy
  - Discussion of risk benefits and understanding that this is not the standard of care
  - Compliance with medical care and willing to undergo interval EMBs
- This should be in conjunction with lifestyle changes and implementing a weight loss plan in patients with a BMI in the overweight or obese category.
- Patients should have their pathology confirmed by D&C specimen and should have an MRI to assess for myometrial or cervical invasion prior to initiating fertility-sparing treatment.
- Acceptable progesterone therapies include megestrol acetate, medroxyprogesterone, or a levonorgestrel-containing IUD. There is limited data to suggest that IUD therapy is as effective as systemic therapy, without the disadvantage of weight gain observed with systemic progestin treatment.
- There have been several meta-analyses on the efficacy of oral progestins for treatment of early endometrial cancer. Regression rates vary between 50% and 84%. Of those with regression of disease, a complete response was noted in 48% to 96%. Median time to response was 6 months (ranges from 8 wk up to 9 mo). The relapse rate varies between 25% and 41%. Fertility rates varied widely between the studies with a range between 28% and 53%.
  - After progestin therapy is initiated, endometrial sampling (EMB or D&C) is performed in 3-month intervals until two negative biopsies are confirmed. Then, the sampling interval can be increased as long as the patient is asymptomatic and there is no evidence of progressive or metastatic disease.
  - After two consecutive negative biopsies, the patient is encouraged to pursue pregnancy.
  - For patients with persistent disease (including endometrial cancer or atypical endometrial hyperplasia), the dose of oral progestin can be increased or if a progestin IUD is being used, then an oral progestin can be added. If there is no response by 9 months, a future response is unlikely and hysterectomy is strongly recommended.

Incomplete Surgical Staging

- Treatment depends on risk factors.
- Grade 1 or 2 tumor with <50% myometrial invasion have a <10% risk of having positive lymph nodes and >90% 5-year survival without any further treatment. However, any grade 3 cancer or grades 1 and 2 cancers with more than 50% invasion pose a >10% risk of positive pelvic lymph nodes, and 5-year survival is decreased to 70% to 85% without further treatment. Therefore, restaging or use of adjuvant radiation is appropriate.
- Laparoscopic node dissection can be used for patients who were incompletely staged at their initial surgery. Additionally, fluorodeoxyglucose positron emission tomography imaging may hold promise for evaluating lymphadenopathy but is not as sensitive as surgical staging.

Medical Contraindications to Surgery

- Women who are medically unable to undergo surgery can be treated with pelvic radiation alone. However, 5-year survival for clinical stage I disease is decreased to 69% with this approach versus 87% for surgery alone.

- It has been shown that for stage I disease with a preoperative CA-125 of <20 U/mL, the risk of extrauterine spread was only 3%. In these cases, vaginal hysterectomy is a therapeutic option for those women unable to undergo a more extensive operation.
- In a small series of patients with a well-differentiated endometrial adenocarcinoma, a progestin-secreting IUD has been shown to be effective therapy.

POSTTREATMENT SURVEILLANCE

- After treatment, surveillance for recurrence should include an examination every 6 months for 2-3 years and then every 6 months or annually per NCCN guidelines.
- The SGO has more specific guidelines that break down surveillance into low risk (stage IA grade 1 or 2), intermediate risk (stage IA grade 2), and high risk (stage III/IV serous or clear cell) (Table 51-4).
- Previously, yearly vaginal cytology was recommended; however NCCN, SGO, and American College of Obstetricians and Gynecologists no longer support this practice because it did not improve survival or outcomes.
- If serum CA-125 is elevated at the time of diagnosis, it can be followed at each visit.
- Most recurrences are diagnosed by symptoms or imaging and occur in the first 2 to 3 years after initial diagnosis. Imaging (CT/MRI/positron emission tomography) should be ordered as needed based on exam or symptoms of recurrence.
- Continue to assess for high-risk features or family diagnoses that might prompt a genetic evaluation.
- An emphasis should be placed on weight loss through dietary modifications and exercise given that a large portion of this population is obese.

Table 51-4	Endometrial Cancer Surveillance Recommendations[a,b]				
	Months			Years	
Variable	0-12	12-24	24-26	3-5	>5
Review of symptoms and physical exam					
Low risk (stage IA grade 1 or 2)	Every 6 mo	Yearly	Yearly	Yearly	Yearly
Intermediate risk (stage IA grade 2)	Every 3 mo	Every 6 mo	Every 6 mo	Every 6 mo	Yearly
High risk (stage III/IV, serous or clear cell)	Every 3 mo	Every 3 mo	Every 6 mo	Every 6 mo	Yearly

[a]Yearly Papanicolaou test or cytologic evaluation is not indicated. There is insufficient evidence of support routinely following cancer antigen 125 or routine chest radiograph, computed tomography, or magnetic resonance imaging. If a recurrence is suspected, computed tomography and/or positron emission tomography is reasonable ± cancer antigen 125.

[b]Adapted from Salani R, Backes FJ, Fung MF, et al. Posttreatment surveillance and diagnosis of recurrence in women with gynecologic malignancies: Society of Gynecologic Oncologists recommendations. *Am J Obstet Gynecol.* 2011;204(6):466-478. Copyright © 2011 Elsevier. With permission.

UTERINE SARCOMA

Sarcoma subtypes include uterine leiomyosarcoma (uLMS), ESS, and undifferentiated uterine sarcoma. The most common subtype is uLMS (63%), followed by ESS and undifferentiated uterine sarcoma. More rare subtypes include adenosarcoma, rhabdomyosarcoma, and perivascular epithelioid cell neoplasm.

- Women with a uterine sarcoma most often present with a rapidly enlarging uterus and are found to have a dominant uterine mass. Some may also present with postmenopausal bleeding.
- No screening is recommended; it is not advised to test for hereditary nonpolyposis colon cancer/Lynch in this population.
- The mainstay of treatment of all soft tissue sarcomas, including uterine, is surgery.
- **Staging of uterine sarcoma.** In 2009, a staging system for uterine sarcomas was developed (Table 51-5). Evaluation should include imaging of the chest, abdomen, and pelvis with CT or MRI/CT.
- If operable, total abdominal hysterectomy with or without BSO is the treatment of choice. The BSO is favored in any postmenopausal woman, in the management of low-grade ESS, and in women with estrogen receptor-positive uLMS. Metastases to the lymph nodes are uncommon and lymphadenectomy is not recommended unless nodes are palpably enlarged.

Leiomyosarcoma

- **Uterine leiomyosarcoma** is an aggressive and rare subtype of uterine sarcoma. The tumors usually arise in the myometrium. Ten percent of patients will have lung metastases at the time of diagnosis. The typical picture is a postmenopausal woman with a rapidly enlarging mass.
- These tumors appear like leiomyomas but have **>10 mitoses per 10 high-power fields**, **diffuse nuclear atypia**, and **coagulative necrosis**. These three factors are collectively known as the Stanford criteria.

Table 51-5	Staging of Endometrial Stromal Sarcoma and Leiomyosarcoma[a]
Stage[b]	Description
IA	Tumor limited to the uterus and ≤5 cm
IB	Tumor limited to the uterus and >5 cm
IIA	Tumor involves the adnexae.
IIB	Tumor involves other pelvic tissues.
IIIA	Tumor infiltrates abdominal tissues at one site.
IIIB	Tumor infiltrates abdominal tissues at more than one site.
IIIC	Metastases in the pelvic and/or para-aortic lymph nodes
IVA	Tumor infiltrates bladder and/or rectum.
IVB	Distant metastases (beyond the adnexa, pelvic, and abdominal tissues)

[a]Carcinosarcomas should be stage as endometrial carcinomas not as a sarcoma.
[b]Staging based on the 2009 International Federation of Gynecology and Obstetrics guidelines as presented in the National Comprehensive Cancer Network Guidelines.

- Hysterectomy with BSO is recommended.
- No survival benefit from adjuvant radiation has been noted in international randomized studies.
- Olaratumab with doxorubicin is FDA approved for treating soft tissue sarcoma not amendable to curative treatment with radiotherapy or surgery. Although this regimen was added to the guidelines as a preferred regimen for treating sarcoma in 2017, a more recent phase III study demonstrated that olaratumab did not lead to a survival advantage when added to doxorubicin, and therefore, this agent was removed recently from the NCCN guidelines as a treatment consideration.
- Trabectedin and pazopanib are two single agents that are approved by the FDA to treatment of recurrent uLMS.
- Either single-agent doxorubicin or fixed-dose rate gemcitabine plus docetaxel demonstrates reasonable response rates as first-line therapy for metastatic uLMS.

Endometrial Stromal Sarcoma

- **Endometrial stromal sarcoma** arise from the endometrium and are considered low grade in most cases. They represent 10% of uterine sarcomas. Even in the setting of low-grade ESS, 36% of patients will relapse and 10% will die from the disease. However, the majority present with early-stage disease and are estrogen and progesterone receptor positive.
- Low-grade ESS often responds to progestins and aromatase inhibitors; gonadotropin-releasing hormone analogs are also an option. Tamoxifen is no longer part of the treatment of ESS because it is contraindicated in women with estrogen receptor-/progesterone receptor-positive tumors.
- Higher grade ESS should be treated with surgery and pelvic radiation. Chemotherapy has not demonstrated much benefit due to the indolent nature of the disease.

Prognosis for Uterine Sarcoma

- A retrospective study including women with all forms of sarcoma showed a 3-year survival rate of 82%, 60%, and 20% for sarcomas with low-, medium-, and high-grade histology, respectively.
- Three-year survival was 56%, 45%, 33%, and 5% for stage I, II, III, and IV sarcomas, respectively. These data may need to be updated in light of the revised staging criteria.

SUGGESTED READINGS

American College of Obstetricians and Gynecologists Committee on Gynecologic Practice. ACOG Committee Opinion No. 601: tamoxifen and uterine cancer. *Obstet Gynecol.* 2014;123:1394-1397. (Reaffirmed 2019)

American College of Obstetricians and Gynecologists Committee on Practice Bulletins—Gynecology. ACOG Practice Bulletin No. 149: endometrial cancer. *Obstet Gynecol.* 2015;125:1006-1026. (Reaffirmed 2017)

Benedetti Panici P, Basile S, Maneschi F, et al. Systematic pelvic lymphadenectomy vs. no lymphadenectomy in earlystage endometrial carcinoma: randomized clinical trial. *J Natl Cancer Inst.* 2008;100(23):1707-1716.

Campos SM, Lee LJ, Del Carmen MG, McMeekin DS. Corpus: epithelial tumors. In: Chi DS, Berchuck A, Dizon DS, Yashar C, eds. *Principles and Practice of Gynecologic Oncology.* 7th ed. Philadelphia, PA: Wolters Kluwer; 2017:511.

Kitchener H, Swart AM, Qian Q, Amos C, Parmar MK; for ASTEC study group. Efficacy of systematic pelvic lymphadenectomy in endometrial cancer (MRC ASTEC trial): a randomised study. *Lancet*. 2009;373(9658):125-136.

Lentao MM Jr, Tornos C, Wolfson AH, O'Cearbhail R. Corpus: mesenchymal tumors. In: Chi DS, Berchuck A, Dizon DS, Yashar C, eds. *Principles and Practice of Gynecologic Oncology*. 7th ed. Philadelphia, PA: Wolters Kluwer; 2017:564.

Mutch DG. The new FIGO staging system for cancers of the vulva, cervix, endometrium and sarcomas. *Gynecol Oncol*. 2009;115:325-328.

Todo Y, Kato H, Kaneuchi M, Watari H, Takeda M, Sakuragi N. Survival effect of para-aortic lymphadenectomy in endometrial cancer (SEPAL study): a retrospective cohort analysis. *Lancet*. 2010;375(9721):1165-1172.

Walker JL, Piedmonte MR, Spirtos NM, et al. Laparoscopy compared with laparotomy for comprehensive surgical staging of uterine cancer: Gynecologic Oncology Group Study LAP2. *J Clin Oncol*. 2009;27:5331-5336.

Ovarian Cancer

Lea A. Moukarzel and Edward J. Tanner III

Ovarian cancer is the tenth most common cancer and the fifth leading cause of cancer-related death in American women. It is the second most common gynecologic cancer following cancer of the uterine corpus and has the highest mortality of all female reproductive system malignancies.

EPIDEMIOLOGY OF OVARIAN CANCER

- For women in the United States, the lifetime risk of developing ovarian cancer is estimated to be 1 in 78 (1.3%). This likelihood increases with age, with a median age at diagnosis of 63 years.
- The risk of malignancy in a solid adnexal mass is 7% in a premenopausal woman and increases to 30% in a postmenopausal woman. Each year, an estimated 22 530 women will be diagnosed with ovarian cancer, and 13 980 will die from their disease.
- Ovarian neoplasms, of which 80% are benign, are divided into three major groups: epithelial, germ cell, and sex cord–stromal tumors (Table 52-1). The ovary can also be a site of metastatic cancer from other sites, particularly from the breast or the gastrointestinal tract (eg, Krukenberg tumors).

EPITHELIAL OVARIAN TUMORS

Tumors derived from the coelomic epithelium are the most common ovarian neoplasms, accounting for 65% of ovarian neoplasms and over 90% of ovarian cancers. Histologic types include serous, mucinous, endometrioid, clear cell, and transitional cell (Brenner tumor). Recent evidence suggests that the precursor lesion for serous carcinomas of the

Table 52-1 Classification of Ovarian Neoplasms

Epithelial Tumors
Serous (histology resembles the lining of the fallopian tube)
Mucinous (histology resembles endocervical epithelium)
Endometrioid (histology resembles endometrial lining)
Clear cell (histology resembles vaginal mucosa)
Transitional cell (Brenner; histology resembles bladder)

Germ Cell Tumors
Dysgerminoma
Endodermal sinus tumor
Embryonal carcinoma
Polyembryoma
Choriocarcinoma
Teratoma
  Immature
  Mature

Sex Cord–Stromal Tumors
Granulosa-stromal cell
  Granulosa cell
  Thecoma-fibromas
Sertoli-Leydig cell
Sex cord tumor
Sex cord tumor with annular tubules
Gynandroblastoma

Unclassified and Metastatic

ovary arise from the fimbriae of the fallopian tube rather than the ovarian epithelium. In support of this theory, patients with high-grade serous ovarian and peritoneal carcinomas are often found to have concurrent serous tubal intraepithelial carcinomas in the mucosa of the fimbria. Furthermore, almost all serous tubal intraepithelial carcinomas demonstrate overexpression of p53 as seen in high-grade serous carcinomas. Nonserous histologies likely still arise from the ovary through other mechanisms.

Risk Factors

- Age over 40 years, white race, nulliparity, infertility, history of endometrial or breast cancer, and family history of ovarian cancer have been consistently found to increase the risk of invasive epithelial cancer. Increased parity, use of oral contraceptive pills (OCPs), history of breastfeeding, tubal ligation, and hysterectomy have been associated with a decreased risk of ovarian cancer.
- Patients with a **family history** of ovarian, breast, endometrial, or colon cancer are at increased risk for developing ovarian carcinoma.
  - Hereditary familial ovarian cancer accounts for approximately 10% of all newly diagnosed cases. Women with one first-degree relative with ovarian cancer have a 5% lifetime risk of developing the disease and those with two first-degree relatives with ovarian cancer have a 7% risk.

- There are three distinct autosomal dominant syndromes that have been termed familial ovarian cancer: site-specific ovarian cancer, hereditary breast and ovarian cancer (*BRCA1* and *BRCA2*), and Lynch syndrome (hereditary nonpolyposis colorectal cancer) (see chapter 53).
- **Lynch syndrome** is an autosomal dominant cancer susceptibility syndrome that describes a familial predisposition to multiple cancers (primarily colon and also endometrial, ovarian, genitourinary tract).
  - Women with Lynch syndrome have a 25% to 60% lifetime risk for endometrial cancer and a 12% to 25% lifetime risk for ovarian cancer.
- **BRCA.** Mutations in the *BRCA1* and *BRCA2* genes, which are involved in DNA repair, have been linked to familial breast cancer, breast-ovary, and site-specific ovarian cancer syndromes.
  - Women with BRCA gene mutations have a lifetime breast cancer risk of 40% to 75%. The lifetime ovarian cancer risks of *BRCA1* and *BRCA2* carriers are 35% to 60% and 10% to 25%, respectively. These women also develop the disease at an earlier age than women without mutations. Additional genes associated with variable ovarian cancer risk have also been identified. These include *CHEK2*, *RAD51*, *BRP1*, and *PALB2*. Genetic screening tests are available.
- **Environmental factors** may play a role in ovarian cancer. A recent meta-analysis does not support a causal relationship between talc exposure and ovarian cancer.
- Reproductive factors play an important role in ovarian cancer risk. Increasing **parity** is associated with a decreased relative risk of developing ovarian cancer, whereas **nulliparity** is associated with an increased risk.
- The use of **OCPs** also has been associated with a decreased relative risk.
- Women with a history of **breastfeeding** have a lower risk of ovarian cancer than nulliparous women and parous women who have not breast-fed.
- Women with **infertility** have an elevated risk of ovarian cancer, independent of nulliparity. Although fertility drugs have been implicated in the development of ovarian cancer, their association has not been clearly separated from the risk that nulliparity and infertility confer.
- **Tubal ligation** and **hysterectomy** with ovarian preservation both appear to lower the risk of ovarian cancer, although the mechanisms remain unclear.

Screening and Prevention

- Early ovarian cancer is often asymptomatic. No available screening test has sufficient positive predictive value for early-stage ovarian cancer.
- **Routine yearly pelvic examination** is still widely used for the general population as a screening tool, but it has poor sensitivity for detecting early-stage disease.
- **Cancer antigen 125 (CA-125)** is a biomarker for ovarian cancer. A level >35 U/mL in postmenopausal women is usually considered abnormal. Approximately 50% of ovarian cancer cases confined to the ovary, and >85% of advanced stage ovarian cancer cases have elevated CA-125 levels. However, this biomarker alone is neither sufficiently sensitive nor specific enough to be diagnostic for ovarian cancer.
  - The CA-125 levels may be elevated in several benign conditions (including pelvic inflammatory disease, endometriosis, fibroids, pregnancy, hemorrhagic ovarian cysts, liver disease, and any other lesion that causes peritoneal irritation) as well as in other malignant conditions (including breast, lung, pancreatic, gastric, and colon cancer). In addition, CA-125 is normal in approximately half of women with stage I ovarian cancer. The most important use is following serial

CA-125 levels to monitor response to treatment and to detect recurrence in women with known ovarian cancer.

- Human epididymis protein 4 (HE4) has similar sensitivity to CA-125 when ovarian cancer patients are compared to healthy controls; however, it has greater sensitivity when compared to those with benign gynecologic disease. Although not yet used for screening, HE4 is currently approved in the United States for monitoring disease progression or recurrence.

- **Other biomarkers.** Cancer antigen 19-9, cancer antigen 15-3, cancer antigen 72-4, carcinoembryonic antigen, lysophosphatidic acid, soluble Fas antigen (sFas), mesothelin, haptoglobin-α, bikunin, HE4, and OVX1 are and have been investigated, with combined biomarker tests commercially available for use in high-risk patients.

- **Transvaginal ultrasonography** has been evaluated as a potential screening tool. Characteristics suggestive of malignancy include complex ovarian cysts with solid components, the presence of septations, papillary projections into the cyst, thick cyst walls, surface excrescences, ascites, and neovascularization. When used to screen the general population, transvaginal ultrasonography has a poor positive predictive value. However, when limited to postmenopausal women with pelvic masses, a sensitivity of 84% and specificity of 78% has been reported.

- **Multimodal screening** using CA-125 measurement with transvaginal ultrasonography yields a higher specificity and positive predictive value than either modality alone. In postmenopausal women, the combination of transvaginal ultrasound and a CA-125 >65 U/mL increased sensitivity to 92% and specificity to 96%. However, this screening approach has not been shown to reduce overall ovarian cancer mortality. At this time, there remains insufficient evidence to support routine screening for ovarian cancer with the use of CA-125 and transvaginal ultrasounds.

- **Current recommendations for screening.** According to the US Preventive Services Task Force, no existing evidence suggests that any screening test, including CA-125, ultrasound, or pelvic examination, reduces mortality from ovarian cancer; therefore, routine screening is not recommended. The American College of Obstetricians and Gynecologists agrees that routine screening tests are not beneficial for low-risk, asymptomatic women. American College of Obstetricians and Gynecologists advises the obstetrician-gynecologist to remain vigilant for the early signs and symptoms of ovarian cancer. The American Cancer Society does not recommend routine screening but states that women at high risk for ovarian cancer should be offered the combination of a pelvic exam, transvaginal ultrasound, and CA-125.

- **Prophylactic bilateral salpingo-oophorectomy.** The decision to perform elective salpingo-oophorectomy largely depends on genetic risk factors. Women at high risk for ovarian cancer (eg, Lynch syndrome, BRCA mutations) should consider prophylactic bilateral salpingo-oophorectomy between ages 35 and 40 years or when childbearing is complete. For other women at population risk (no genetic predisposition for ovarian cancer), age should be incorporated into the decision-making process. There is evidence to suggest that ovarian conservation until the age of 65 years has long-term survival benefits, largely due to reduced risk of cardiovascular disease. After age 65 years, this protection is mitigated and offering concomitant prophylactic bilateral salpingo-oophorectomy is preferred.

- **Opportunistic salpingectomy.** In contrast to the traditional hypothesis that ovarian cancer arises from the ovary's epithelium, more recent data suggest that serous carcinomas of the ovary often arise from the fallopian tube. Given that tubal ligation has been previously demonstrated to protect against epithelial carcinomas of the ovary, salpingectomy at the time of other gynecologic surgery has been suggested as an opportunity to reduce ovarian cancer risk. Opportunistic salpingectomy remains an overall theoretical benefit against the development of ovarian cancer and should only be considered when feasible and does not alter mode of hysterectomy (or other gynecologic surgery).

- The **OCP prophylaxis** is the only documented method of chemoprevention for ovarian cancer, and the effect is substantial. The overall estimate of protection with OCPs is approximately 40%. Increased duration of use appears to be associated with further decreased risk, and the protective effect persists for 10 or more years after discontinuation. The use of OCPs in *BRCA* mutation carriers also confers a decreased risk of ovarian cancer without increasing the risk of breast cancer.

Presentation and Diagnosis

- **Presentation.** Only 15% of ovarian cancer cases are diagnosed while the cancer is localized (stage I), and approximately 68% of patients with epithelial ovarian cancer have advanced disease (stage III or greater) at time of diagnosis. Although some women with early disease experience symptoms, the majority are asymptomatic.
  - When symptoms develop, they are nonspecific and can include abdominal bloating, early satiety, weight loss, constipation, anorexia, urinary frequency, dyspareunia, fatigue, and irregular menstrual bleeding.
  - On physical examination, a pelvic mass is an important sign of disease. In more advanced stages, abdominal distention may develop, and chest examination may reveal evidence of pleural effusion.
- **Workup.** Evaluation of a pelvic mass varies depending on the patient's age, significant medical and family history, and the sonographic characteristics of the mass. Women with pelvic masses that are suspicious for malignancy should be referred to a gynecologic oncologist. In premenopausal women, an adnexal mass less than 8 to 10 cm in diameter with no other concerning features or symptoms is typically monitored with serial sonograms. If the decision is made to proceed with surgical evaluation, the preoperative evaluation should include a full history and physical examination, including a pelvic examination and a Pap smear.
  - Criteria for gynecologic oncology referral include the following:
    - In premenopausal women, CA-125 >200 U/mL, ascites, and evidence of abdominal or distant metastasis
    - In postmenopausal women, CA-125 >35 U/mL, ascites, evidence of abdominal or distant metastasis, and a nodular or fixed pelvic mass
  - Additional tests should be performed on the basis of a patient's risk factors and underlying medical status. Consideration should be given to performing a computed tomography (CT) scan of the chest, abdomen, and pelvis to evaluate for metastatic disease. If surgery is necessary, a surgeon capable of performing an adequate staging procedure should be available, preferably a gynecologic oncologist, to optimize outcomes in cases of malignancy.

Staging and Prognosis

- Epithelial ovarian tumors are classified by cell type and behavior as benign, atypically proliferating, or malignant. Atypically proliferating tumors are also referred to as tumors of low malignant potentials (LMPs) or "borderline" tumors.
- Ovarian cancer is **surgically staged** (Table 52-2). The importance of complete surgical staging in treatment planning and prognosis cannot be overemphasized.

Table 52-2 International Federation of Gynecology and Obstetrics (FIGO) Staging System for Carcinoma of the Ovary, Fallopian Tube, and Primary Peritoneal Cancer[a]

TNM Categories	FIGO Stages	Definition
TX		Primary tumor cannot be assessed
T0		No evidence of primary tumor
T1	I	Tumor limited to the ovaries (one or both) or fallopian tube(s)
T1a	IA	Tumor limited to one ovary; capsule intact, no tumor on ovarian surface of fallopian tube surface; no malignant cells in ascites or peritoneal washings
T1b	IB	Tumor limited to both ovaries or fallopian tubes; capsule intact, no tumor on ovarian or fallopian tube surface; no malignant cells in ascites or peritoneal washings
T1c	IC	Tumor limited to one or both ovaries or fallopian tubes with any of the following:
T1c1		Surgical spill
T1c2		Capsule ruptured before surgery or tumor on ovarian or fallopian tube surface
T1c3		Malignant cells in ascites or peritoneal washings
T2	II	Tumor involves one or both ovaries or fallopian tubes with pelvic extension (below the pelvic brim) or primary peritoneal cancer
T2a	IIA	Extension and/or implants on uterus and/or fallopian tube(s) and/or ovary(ies)
T2b	IIB	Extension to other pelvic tissues, including bowel within the pelvis
T3 and/or N1	III[b]	Tumor involves one or both ovaries or fallopian tubes or primary peritoneal carcinoma with cytologically or histologically confirmed spread to the peritoneum outside the pelvis and/or metastasis to the retroperitoneal lymph nodes
N1		Retroperitoneal lymph node metastasis only
N1a	IIIA1i	Lymph node metastasis not more than 10 mm in greatest dimension
N1b	IIIA1ii	Lymph node metastasis more than 10 mm in greatest dimension
T3a any N	IIIA2	Microscopic extrapelvic (above the pelvic brim) peritoneal involvement with or without retroperitoneal lymph node, including bowel involvement

(Continued)

Table 52-2		International Federation of Gynecology and Obstetrics (FIGO) Staging System for Carcinoma of the Ovary, Fallopian Tube, and Primary Peritoneal Cancer[a] *(Continued)*
TNM Categories	**FIGO Stages**	**Definition**
T3b any N	IIIB	Macroscopic peritoneal metastasis beyond pelvic brim, 2 cm or less in greatest dimension, including bowel involvement outside the pelvis with or without retroperitoneal nodes
T3c any N	IIIC	Peritoneal metastasis beyond pelvic brim more than 2 cm in greatest dimension and/or retroperitoneal lymph node metastasis (includes extension of tumor to capsule of liver and spleen without parenchymal involvement of either organ)
M1	IV	Distant metastasis (excludes peritoneal metastasis)
M1a	IVA	Pleural effusion with positive cytology
M1b[c]	IVB	Parenchymal metastasis and metastasis to extra-abdominal organs (including inguinal lymph nodes and lymph nodes outside the abdominal cavity)

[a]From Tokunaga H, Shimada M, Ishikawa M, Yaegashi N. TNM classification of gynaecological malignant tumours, eighth edition: changes between the seventh and eighth editions. *Jpn J Clin Oncol.* 2019;49(4):318. Reproduced by permission of Oxford University Press.
[b]Liver capsule metastasis is T3/stage III.
[c]Liver parenchymal metastasis is M1/stage IV.

The standard surgical approach involves a vertical midline incision to allow for adequate exposure, although more recent advances in laparoscopic surgery have made minimally invasive options available (Table 52-3).

- Ovarian cancer can spread by direct extension, by exfoliation of cells into the peritoneal cavity (transcoelomic spread), via the bloodstream, or via the lymphatic system. The most common pathway of spread is transcoelomic. Cells from the tumor are shed into the peritoneal cavity and circulate following the clockwise path of the peritoneal fluid. All peritoneal surfaces are at risk. Lymphatic spread to the pelvic and para-aortic lymph nodes can occur. Hematogenous spread to the liver or lungs can occur in advanced disease.

Prognostic Factors

- The most important prognostic factors are stage, grade, histology of the tumor, the amount of residual disease remaining after initial debulking surgery, and the age of the patient.
- The 5-year survival rate of patients with epithelial ovarian cancer correlates directly with **tumor stage** (Table 52-4).

Table 52-3	Surgical Staging Procedures for Ovarian Cancer

Obtain ascites for cytologic evaluation.
Washings from the pelvis, gutters, and diaphragm
Systematic exploration of all organs and surfaces
Hysterectomy[a]
Bilateral salpingo-oophorectomy[a]
Infracolic omentectomy
Sampling pelvic and para-aortic lymph nodes
Multiple biopsy specimens from peritoneal sites
   Pelvic side walls
   Surfaces of the rectum and bladder
   Cul-de-sac
   Lateral abdominal gutters
   Diaphragm

[a]May be preserved in select patients, particularly if future fertility is desired.

- Within each **histologic subtype**, tumors may be described as benign, of LMP, or malignant.
  - **Serous.** The serous subtype is the most common, accounting for over 50% of all malignant ovarian tumors. Approximately one-third are malignant, half are benign, and one-sixth are LMP. Serous carcinoma of the ovary closely resembles fallopian tube and peritoneal cancer in histology as well as in clinical behavior, and thus they are often referred to as one entity. The mean age of patients at diagnosis is 57 years. Psammoma bodies are present in 25% of serous tumors.
  - **Mucinous** tumors are lined by cells that resemble endocervical glands or intestinal epithelium. Primary ovarian mucinous tumors account for 3% to 4% of epithelial tumors. Sixty percent of mucinous tumors are stage I, and most are

Table 52-4	Stage Distribution and 5-Year Survival for Ovarian Cancer (2009-2015)[a]

Stage at Diagnosis	Stage Distribution (%)	5-y Relative Survival (%)
Localized	15	92.4
Regional	21	75.2
Distant	59	29.2
Unknown	6	24.3

[a]From National Cancer Institute/Surveillance, Epidemiology, and End Results Program. Cancer stat facts: ovarian cancer. Surveillance, Epidemiology, and End Results Program Web site. https://seer.cancer.gov/statfacts/html/ovary.html. Accessed July 2, 2019.

unilateral. They are typically large, often filling the abdominal cavity, cystic, and multiloculated. The mean age of patients diagnosed with malignant mucinous tumors is 54 years. The CA-125 levels may not be markedly elevated.

- ○ Pseudomyxoma peritonei is a condition associated with mucinous neoplasms, usually of gastrointestinal origin, and is characterized by gelatinous mucus or ascites in the abdomen.
- ○ Primary ovarian mucinous tumors may be difficult to differentiate from metastatic neoplasms of the gastrointestinal tract (colon, appendix, pancreas). Prior studies have shown that, in general, primary ovarian mucinous tumors are unilateral and measure ≥10 cm, whereas metastatic tumors are bilateral and measure <10 cm in diameter. Using these criteria, approximately 84% of all mucinous tumors are correctly classified, including 100% of primary ovarian tumors.

- **Endometrioid** tumors resemble the histology of the endometrium and account for 6% of epithelial tumors. Most are malignant; 20% may be tumors of LMP. The mean age of patients diagnosed with malignant tumors is 56 years. About 14% of women will also have endometrial cancer, and 15% to 20% or more will have endometriosis. Endometrioid tumors appear to have a better prognosis than serous tumors, most likely because of their early stage at diagnosis.

- **Clear cell** carcinomas account for 3% of epithelial ovarian cancers. These are the most chemoresistant type of ovarian cancer and overall are associated with a poor prognosis among subtypes. Endometriotic implants are present in 30% to 35% of cases, and although an uncommon occurrence, clear cell carcinomas may be associated with paraneoplastic syndromes such as hypercalcemia. About 50% of patients present with stage I disease. Tumors are large, with a mean diameter of 15 cm. Histologically, **hobnail-shaped cells** are characteristic of these tumors. The mean age at diagnosis is 57 years.

- **Transitional cell** tumors histologically resemble the bladder. The two types of malignant transitional cell tumors are Brenner tumors and transitional cell carcinomas. Approximately 10% to 20% of advanced stage ovarian carcinomas contain a transitional cell carcinoma component. The mean age for malignant Brenner tumors is 63 years.

- **Grade** is an important independent prognostic factor, particularly in patients with early-stage disease.
  - Grade is based on a combination of architecture (glandular, papillary, or solid), degree of nuclear atypia, and mitotic index.
  - Grade 1 is well differentiated, grade 2 is moderately differentiated, and grade 3 is poorly differentiated.
  - More recently, a two-tiered grading system has been proposed. Low-grade tumors exhibit a low degree of atypia with infrequent mitotic figures and are thought to develop from adenofibromas or borderline tumors in a slow, step-wise process. High-grade tumors demonstrate atypical nuclei and numerous mitotic figures. These tumors are thought to develop rapidly de novo.

- **Debulking**, also called **cytoreduction**, is defined as removal of as much tumor as possible during surgical exploration. Optimal cytoreduction implies that any remaining tumor nodules are less than 1 cm in diameter. Cytoreduction of all visible disease is associated with the greatest survival advantage, reinforcing the importance of a gynecologic oncologist's involvement in cytoreductive surgery for ovarian cancer.

Management of Epithelial Ovarian Cancer

- Treatment of epithelial ovarian cancer depends on the stage and grade of the disease, type of disease (ie, primary or recurrent), previous treatment, and the patient's performance status.

Tumors of Low Malignant Potential

- These tumors show a different pattern of behavior than does malignant ovarian disease. Approximately 15% of all epithelial ovarian tumors are classified as LMP, and they are often found in younger patients. They are most commonly of serous histology (85%), followed by mucinous.
- Serous LMP tumors with invasive implants tend to behave as low-grade carcinomas with a mortality rate of 34%.
- Mucinous LMP tumors confined to the ovary have a survival rate approaching 100%, whereas those with advanced-stage disease have a survival rate of 40% to 50%. They may be associated with a concurrent appendiceal primary tumor, and affected patients should also undergo appendectomy. Mucinous LMPs that display aggressive behavior are associated with pseudomyxoma peritonei, which is indicative of appendiceal origin.
- Surgical staging of LMPs is advocated because of the possibility of identifying an invasive cancer on final pathology. Surgical staging for LMPs incorporates a total abdominal hysterectomy, bilateral salpingo-oophorectomy, and resection of any visible residual disease. Unlike standard ovarian cancer staging, lymphadenectomy has not been shown to increase survival and is not required for such cases. If invasive peritoneal implants are not identified, then the patient may be observed. Patients with invasive implants have not been shown to benefit from adjuvant chemotherapy but are at higher risk for recurrence. If disease recurs, it does so an average of 10 years after initial diagnosis, and resection can be performed again at the time of recurrence. Most patients die *with* disease rather than *from* disease.
- In addition, early-stage disease in women who desire future fertility may be treated with unilateral salpingo-oophorectomy, or even with unilateral cystectomy, with good outcomes.

Early Invasive Disease (Stage I or II)

- **Initial surgical resection** is necessary for establishing a histologic diagnosis and appropriate staging. Options exist for young patients who wish to preserve fertility. If intraoperative findings are consistent with stage I disease and the contralateral ovary is normal in appearance, unilateral salpingo-oophorectomy with thorough surgical staging may be performed. The uterus and normal-appearing contralateral ovary may remain in situ. The patient should be counseled about the potential for a second primary in the preserved ovary, and a total hysterectomy with removal of the remaining tube and ovary should be considered after childbearing is completed.
- **Chemotherapy.** For patients with stage IA, grade 1 or 2 disease, chemotherapy is not required. For patients with early-stage disease with prognostic factors placing them at higher risk for recurrence (stage IC or II, grade 3 disease, or clear cell histology of any stage), postoperative platinum-based chemotherapy is recommended (see chapter 56).
- **Radiation.** With relatively effective chemotherapeutic options available as well as frequency of widespread metastasis, radiation therapy is used infrequently in the treatment of ovarian cancer.

Advanced Invasive Disease

- **Advanced disease** requires surgical staging, debulking, and a course of platinum-based chemotherapy.
- **Primary cytoreductive surgery**, or debulking, is central in the treatment of advanced disease because optimal cytoreduction is one of the most powerful predictors of survival in patients with advanced ovarian cancer.
  - The determination of residual disease on completion of the procedure does not include the total volume of tumor cells left behind but rather the diameter of the largest single residual nodule. For example, a patient with one unresected nodule measuring 2.5 cm has not undergone optimal debulking, whereas debulking is considered to be optimal in a patient with residual miliary studding of the entire peritoneal cavity.
  - More recent studies have demonstrated that primary cytoreductive surgery no longer needs to include systemic lymphadenectomy in the setting of clinically negative lymph nodes given lack of effect of progression-free or overall survival.
- **Neoadjuvant therapy.** Randomized trial data have demonstrated that neoadjuvant chemotherapy followed by surgical debulking is not inferior to primary debulking surgery in patients with advanced stage disease. However, complete resection of all macroscopic disease remained the main predictor of overall survival—more so at the time of interval cytoreduction than at primary cytoreduction. At this time, neoadjuvant chemotherapy is primarily used in patients whose performance status prohibits surgery or who have unresectable disease.
- **Combination chemotherapy** is most often used as postoperative (adjuvant) treatment for advanced epithelial ovarian cancer. Combination chemotherapy with six cycles of carboplatin plus paclitaxel is the treatment of choice for patients with advanced disease. The optimal method of chemotherapy administration has recently become less clear due to publication of several large randomized trials. As such, the superiority of recently developed regimens including intraperitoneal chemotherapy and/or weekly paclitaxel are less clear than previously appreciated.
- **Consolidation treatment.** Eighty percent of patients who complete optimal tumor debulking followed by six cycles of carboplatin and paclitaxel will achieve a clinical remission. Consolidation treatment strategies to lengthen time to recurrence are currently being investigated. Prior studies using platinum and taxane agents for maintenance chemotherapy have not shown significant improvements in overall survival. Recent studies have demonstrated an improvement in progression-free survival when bevacizumab was administered along with intravenous carboplatin and paclitaxel and continued as a single agent for 10 months, although there was no significant improvement in overall survival. Consideration of its use must reflect on its significantly increased cost without an improvement in overall survival. In patients with estrogen-positive primary tumors, hormonal therapies such as tamoxifen or aromatase inhibitors can also be considered.

Posttreatment Surveillance

Asymptomatic Patients

- Appropriate follow-up for asymptomatic patients after primary surgery and chemotherapy should include a physical examination with rectovaginal examination. The utility of CA-125 testing and imaging are unproven but frequently employed to detect recurrent disease prior to the development of symptoms. Patients should be seen every 3 to 4 months for the first 2 years and then every 4 to 6 months for the next 3 years.

- In patients whose CA-125 level was elevated preoperatively, CA-125 is a reliable marker of disease recurrence with a sensitivity of 62% to 94% and specificity of 91% to 100%. Levels are often elevated 2 to 5 months prior to clinical detection of recurrence. A recent prospective randomized trial showed no survival advantage for patients who were treated for recurrent ovarian cancer based on CA-125 level alone versus waiting for the development of symptomatic disease.
- The CT scans have a sensitivity and specificity of 40% to 93% and 50% to 98%, respectively, for recurrent disease. One limitation is the poor sensitivity of detecting small-volume disease. In a retrospective study, asymptomatic patients with recurrence detected by CT scan had a higher rate of optimal secondary cytoreductive surgery and improved overall survival compared to patients with symptomatic recurrence.
- Combined positron emission tomography imaging and CT (PET-CT) may have clinical use in detecting disease recurrence in select patients and is often recommended prior to secondary cytoreduction.
- **Second-look surgery** by laparotomy or laparoscopy can be performed on patients with advanced epithelial ovarian cancer who have no clinical evidence of disease after undergoing primary debulking and adjuvant chemotherapy. The use of second-look surgery remains controversial and should be performed only in the setting of a clinical trial or on an individualized basis because there are no data demonstrating improved survival with this approach. Patients need to be counseled that the procedure is not therapeutic but may provide prognostic information.

Recurrent or Persistent Disease

- **Secondary cytoreductive surgery.** Patients with recurrent or persistent disease may be candidates for further surgical therapy or secondary cytoreduction. Surgery should be reserved for patients in whom additional therapy has a good chance of prolonging life or palliating symptoms. The best candidates for secondary cytoreduction are those with longer disease-free intervals (at least 6-12 mo) and fewer sites of recurrence.
- **Second-line chemotherapy.** Response rates for second-line chemotherapy are in the range of 20% to 40%. A host of chemotherapy options are available for recurrent ovarian cancer.
- **Targeted therapy.** A more novel approach to the treatment of ovarian cancer is the use of poly(adenosine diphosphate ribose) polymerase inhibitors. Studies have demonstrated a substantial clinical benefit in the treatment of *BRCA* mutation patients. More recent studies have also demonstrated its efficacy in the general population of platinum-sensitive relapsed ovarian cancer patients regardless of the presence of BRCA or homologous recombination deficiency. Ultimately, the greatest use of this therapy is as maintenance therapy for those with recurrent disease. Bevacizumab, a monoclonal antibody inhibitor of vascular endothelial growth factor 1, has been shown to benefit patients in a variety of settings, including maintenance therapy and salvage therapy alone or in combination with chemotherapy in patients with recurrent disease.

- **Hormone therapy** has been used as salvage treatment. Both megestrol acetate (Megace) and tamoxifen have been used to treat recurrent disease. Response rates are low.
- **Radiation therapy** is generally not used except for palliation of distant metastases.
- **Experimental studies.** Many investigators are currently studying the underlying molecular biology of epithelial ovarian cancer. Microarray analysis and proteomics provide insight into the differential expression of mRNA and proteins, respectively. Translational studies to further characterize these molecular changes, as they relate to the clinical disease state, provide an opportunity for novel therapeutic agents. Clinical trials are also currently investigating immunotherapy agents such as checkpoint inhibitors.

Complications of Advanced Ovarian Cancer

- **Intestinal obstruction.** Many women with ovarian cancer develop intestinal obstruction, either at initial diagnosis or with recurrent disease. Obstruction may be related to mechanical blockage or carcinomatous ileus. Correction of intestinal obstruction at initial treatment is usually possible; obstruction associated with recurrent disease, however, is a more complex problem. Some of these obstructions may be treated conservatively with intravenous hydration, total parenteral nutrition, and gastric decompression. The decision to proceed with palliative surgery must be based on the physical condition of the patient and her expected survival. If patients are unable to undergo surgery or are judged to be poor operative candidates, placement of a percutaneous gastric tube may offer some symptomatic relief. In cases of large bowel obstruction, the use of colorectal stents may be an option in order to avoid the significant morbidity and mortality associated with surgical management.
- **Ascites.** Ascites is often present at diagnosis in patients with advanced ovarian cancer and almost always resolves following debulking surgery and adjuvant chemotherapy. Persistent ascites at the completion of primary therapy can be difficult to manage and is a poor prognostic sign. For many years, the only treatment option was serial paracentesis; however, newer data support the use of bevacizumab to reduce the production of malignant ascites in patients with recurrent disease.

Survival

- **Age.** The 5-year overall survival rate in women younger than 65 years of age is nearly twice that of women over age 65 years (57% and 28%, respectively).
- **Stage.** Patients with local (stage I) disease have about 92% 5-year survival rate. In contrast, overall survival for women with distant disease on presentation (majority of the cases) is 29% (see Table 52-4).
- **Performance status.** The Karnofsky Performance Scale Index classifies patients according to their functional impairment and can be used to assess prognosis in individual patients. Lower scores are associated with inferior survival regardless of stage.
  - Able to carry on with normal activities of daily living (ADL) with no special care needed
    - KPS 100%: no evidence or symptoms of disease, no complaints
    - KPS 90%: minor signs or symptoms of disease, still able to carry on with ADL
    - KPS 80%: some signs or symptoms of diease, can carry on independentaly with ADL with effort

- Able to live at home, but requires assistance for ADL and is unable to work
  - KPS 70%: unable to carry on with usual ADL or work, but can still care for self
  - KPS 60%: unable to carry on with usual ADL, but, with occasional assistance, can care for most personal needs
  - KPS 50%: requires considerable assistance and significant medical care
- Requires institutional or hospital care, unable to care for self, disease may be rapidly progressing
  - KPS 40%: requires specialized assistance as patient is disabled
  - KPS 30%: although death is not imminent, hospitalization is indicated as patient is severely disabled
  - KPS 20%: patient is very sick and hospitalization is necessary for active supportive treatment and care
  - KPS 10%: rapidly progressing toward death
  - KPS 0%: patient is dead

Peritoneal Carcinoma

- Primary malignant transformation of the peritoneum is termed **primary peritoneal carcinoma**, which clinically and pathologically resembles serous epithelial ovarian cancer. Primary peritoneal carcinoma presents with similar symptoms as ovarian cancer but can occur in women with a history of oophorectomy or with pathologically normal-appearing or minimally involved ovaries. Extensive upper abdominal disease is common, and clinical course, management, and prognosis are similar to those for epithelial ovarian cancer.

GERM CELL OVARIAN TUMORS

Epidemiology

- Approximately 20% of all ovarian tumors are of germ cell origin, with only 2% to 3% of these being malignant. Types include the following: dysgerminoma, endodermal sinus tumor, embryonal carcinoma, polyembryoma, choriocarcinoma, and teratoma.
- Roughly 70% to 80% of all germ cell tumors occur before age 20 years, and approximately one-third of these are malignant. The median age of women diagnosed with a malignant germ cell tumor is 16-20 years. About 50% to 75% of patients with malignant germ cell tumors present with stage I disease. Overall survival rates, including those with advanced disease, are 60% to 80%.
- The most common germ cell tumor is a benign cystic teratoma (dermoid), and the most common malignant tumor is the dysgerminoma.

Pathology

- Germ cell tumors are derived from the primordial germ cells of the ovary; however, they are a heterogeneous group of tumors. They gradually differentiate to mimic tissues of embryonic origin (ectoderm, mesoderm, endoderm) and extraembryonic origin (trophoblast, yolk sac). They are aggressive tumors, frequently unilateral, and usually curable if treated early.

| Table 52-5 | Serum Markers for Germ Cell and Sex Cord–Stromal Ovarian Tumors | | | | | | | |

Tumor	LDH	AFP	hCG	E_2	Inhibin	Testosterone	Androgen	DHEA
Dysgerminoma	±	−	±	−	−	−	−	−
Embryonal	−	±	+	−	−	−	−	−
Endodermal sinus tumor	−	+	−	−	−	−	−	−
Polyembryoma	−	±	+	−	−	−	−	−
Choriocarcinoma	−	−	+	−	−	−	−	−
Immature teratoma	−	±	−	±	−	−	−	±
Granulosa cell	−	−	−	±	+	−	−	−
Thecoma-fibroma	−	−	−	−	−	−	−	−
Sertoli-Leydig cell	−	−	−	−	±	+	+	−
Gonadoblastoma	−	−	−	±	±	±	±	±

Abbreviations: AFP, α-fetoprotein; DHEA, dehydroepiandrosterone; E_2, estradiol; hCG, human chorionic gonadotropin; LDH, lactate dehydrogenase.

Diagnosis

- Clinically, germ cell malignancies grow quickly and are often characterized by acute pelvic pain. The pain can be caused by distention of the ovarian capsule, hemorrhage, necrosis, or torsion. A palpable pelvic mass is a common finding on presentation. Abdominal distention and abnormal vaginal bleeding may also be the presenting complaint. The tumors are often large at presentation, with a median diameter of 16 cm.
- Ovarian masses that are 2 cm or larger in premenarchal girls or >8 to 10 cm in premenopausal patients generally require exploratory surgery.
- **Preoperative workup.** Measurement of serum tumor markers may assist in the diagnosis of germ cell malignancies (Table 52-5). Workup should include measurement of serum human chorionic gonadotropin (hCG), α-fetoprotein (AFP) titers, lactate dehydrogenase levels, a complete blood count, and liver function tests. A chest radiograph is important to rule out pulmonary metastases. A preoperative CT scan should be considered to assess for the presence or absence of liver metastases and retroperitoneal lymphadenopathy.

Germ Cell Tumor Types

- **Dysgerminomas** are the most common malignant germ cell tumor, comprising up to 50% of all cases. All dysgerminomas are malignant; however, not all are aggressive. Seventy-five percent of dysgerminomas occur in the second or third decades of life. They are the only germ cell tumor that occur bilaterally (10%-15% of cases). The 5-year survival rate for stage IA disease is 95% and for all stages is 85%.

- **Endodermal sinus tumors** (yolk sac tumors) are derived from cells of the primitive yolk sac and are the second most common malignant germ cell tumor, accounting for 20% of cases. Histologically, they are characterized by **Schiller-Duval bodies**. These tumors tend to grow rapidly and secrete AFP. The disease-free survival for all stages is >80%.
- **Embryonal carcinoma.** These tumors are extremely rare and occur in children and young adults. They may secrete both hCG and AFP. Patients may present with sexual precocity and vaginal bleeding.
- **Polyembryoma.** These tumors are exceedingly rare and highly malignant. They resemble early embryos and may secrete AFP or hCG.
- **Nongestational choriocarcinoma.** Pure, nongestational choriocarcinoma involving the ovary is very rare and is histologically similar to gestational choriocarcinoma (see chapter 55). Almost all patients are premenarchal. This tumor often produces remarkably high levels of hCG, which may in turn increase thyroid function. Precocious puberty is seen occasionally, and patients may present with vaginal bleeding. Historically, choriocarcinomas have had a poor prognosis but tend to respond to combination chemotherapy.
- **Immature malignant teratomas** contain tissues resembling those in an embryo. They account for 20% of malignant germ cell tumors and 1% of ovarian malignancies. Half of immature teratomas occur in patients between ages 10 and 20 years. These tumors may secrete AFP. The most important prognostic factor is tumor grade. The 5-year survival rate is 95% for stage I disease and 75% for advanced disease.
- **Mixed germ cell tumors** account for 10% of malignant germ cell tumors and contain elements of two or more of the germ cell tumors discussed previously.

Management of Germ Cell Tumors

- **Surgical.** Primary treatment for all germ cell tumors is surgical and should include proper surgical staging to rule out the presence of extraovarian microscopic disease. Because most patients are of reproductive age, preservation of fertility is important.
  - Unilateral oophorectomy is performed along with unilateral pelvic and para-aortic lymphadenectomy. A frozen section should be obtained. Bilateral involvement is rare in germ cell tumors, with the exception of dysgerminomas (10%-15% bilaterality). The contralateral ovary should be inspected, and a biopsy may be performed if there is suspicion of involvement. The ovary should only be removed in a young patient if disease is present, with the exception of dysgerminomas, in which case even a grossly positive ovary can be retained due to high response rates to chemotherapy. The remaining pelvic organs may be left in situ to preserve fertility.
  - For patients who have completed childbearing, a total abdominal hysterectomy with bilateral salpingo-oophorectomy is reasonable. If metastatic disease is present on initial surgery, cytoreductive surgery is recommended, although data are limited.
  - Surgical therapy alone is recommended for stage IA dysgerminomas and stage IA, grade I immature teratomas. These patients have a 5-year survival of >90%. Approximately 15% to 25% will recur but can be treated successfully

at the time of presentation. For endodermal sinus tumors, staging is not always recommended because chemotherapy should be given regardless.

- **Adjuvant therapy.** The decision to administer adjuvant therapy depends on the histologic type of germ cell tumor. Except those with stage IA, grade I immature teratoma and stage IA dysgerminoma that have undergone surgical staging including lymphadenectomy, all patients require postoperative chemotherapy. Dysgerminomas are very sensitive to radiation therapy; however, fertility is lost as a consequence of irradiation. Therefore, chemotherapy is the first-line treatment. Combination therapy with three agents (bleomycin, etoposide, and cisplatin, or BEP) is recommended. In some cases, bleomycin may be omitted due to the risk of pulmonary toxicity, although analogous studies performed in patients with testicular cancer suggest inferior outcomes in patients with high-risk disease in whom bleomycin was omitted. Prognosis has significantly improved with platinum-based chemotherapy.
- Ninety percent of patients with germ cell tumors who experience a **recurrence** will do so in the first 2 years after therapy. If initially treated with surgery alone, BEP chemotherapy can be used. Patients who initially received chemotherapy can be treated with alternative platinum-based regimens.

SEX CORD–STROMAL OVARIAN TUMORS

Sex cord–stromal tumors are derived from the sex cords and mesenchyme of the embryonic gonad and account for 5% to 8% of all ovarian neoplasms. Most of these tumors are hormonally active (see Table 52-5). Types include the following: granulosa-stromal cell, Sertoli-Leydig, sex cord tumor, and gynandroblastoma.

Granulosa Cell Tumor

- **Incidence.** The granulosa cell tumor is the most common malignant sex cord–stromal tumor, accounting for 70% of cases. Adult granulosa cell tumors occur primarily in the perimenopausal years, with a mean age of 52 years at presentation. Two forms exist: an adult form (95%) and a much rarer juvenile form (5%). The tumor is bilateral in <10% of cases.
- **Diagnosis and presentation.** In the majority of cases, tumors secrete estrogen and inhibin. Histologically, **Call-Exner bodies** are seen. Patients may present with abnormal vaginal bleeding, abdominal distention, pain, or a mass, usually >10 cm in diameter. Granulosa cell tumors are characteristically hemorrhagic and can present with a hemoperitoneum.
  - The incidence of concurrent endometrial hyperplasia is at least 30%. The incidence of concurrent endometrial adenocarcinoma ranges from 3% to 27%, demonstrating the importance of endometrial biopsy when the diagnosis of granulosa cell tumor is made. The majority (90%) of affected patients present with stage I disease, mainly because the hormonal effects of the tumor cause symptoms early in the disease. In the juvenile type, patients present with pseudo-precocious puberty and have elevated serum estradiol.
- **Treatment.** Surgery alone is usually sufficient treatment for stage IA or IB disease. For all other stages, platinum-based chemotherapy is recommended. Carboplatin and paclitaxel have been increasingly used; however, regimens used for germ cell tumors (BEP) can also be considered. Radiation and/or chemotherapy can be used

to treat recurrent disease. If the patient desires to maintain fertility, a unilateral salpingo-oophorectomy is adequate for treating stage IA tumors, and surgical staging should also be performed. With completion of childbearing, a total abdominal hysterectomy and bilateral salpingo-oophorectomy should be performed. If the uterus is left in situ, the patient should undergo dilation and curettage to rule out endometrial hyperplasia or adenocarcinoma. Chemotherapy after surgery has not been shown to reduce the recurrence risk.

- **Prognosis and survival.** Granulosa cell tumors have a propensity for late recurrence, which has been reported as long as 30 years after treatment of the primary tumor. The 10-year and 20-year survival rates are 90% and 75%, respectively.

Sertoli-Leydig Cell Tumor

- **Incidence.** Sertoli-Leydig cell tumors account for only 0.2% of ovarian neoplasms. The average age at diagnosis is 25 years, but they can occur at any age. These tumors are most frequently low-grade malignancies, and nearly all patients (97%) present with stage I disease.
- **Diagnosis and presentation.** Sertoli-Leydig cell tumors often produce androgens. Patients present with virilization (30%-50%), menstrual disorders, and symptoms related to an abdominal mass. The average size of these tumors is about 16 cm. They may produce testosterone, androstenedione, or AFP.
- **Treatment.** In young patients, unilateral salpingo-oophorectomy with staging may be performed to preserve fertility. In older patients, a total abdominal hysterectomy and bilateral salpingo-oophorectomy should be performed as well. Treatment of those with higher stage and/or grade typically includes chemotherapy.
- **Prognosis and survival.** Prognosis is related to stage and histologic grade. The 5-year survival rate is 70% to 90%.

SPECIAL CONSIDERATIONS IN OVARIAN CANCER

- **Metastatic tumors** account for 5% to 20% of ovarian malignancies and are often, but not always, bilateral.
  - **Gastrointestinal tract tumors** are the most likely to metastasize to the ovary. **Krukenberg** tumors of the stomach are usually bilateral and account for 30% to 40% of metastatic tumors to the ovary. These tumors are characterized histologically by signet-ring cells, in which the nucleus is flattened against the cell wall by the accumulation of cytoplasmic mucin. In postmenopausal women who undergo evaluation for an adnexal mass, metastatic colon cancer should be ruled out, using colonoscopy if possible.
  - **Breast cancer** is the second most likely cancer to metastasize to the ovary.
  - **Lymphomas** can also metastasize to the ovary. Burkitt lymphoma may affect children or young adults. Rarely, ovarian lesions are the primary manifestation of disease in lymphoma patients.
  - **Metastatic gynecologic tumors** may involve the ovaries. Fallopian tube cancer is the most common malignancy to metastasize to the ovaries and occurs by direct extension. Cervical cancer very rarely spreads to the ovaries without other sites of metastasis. Endometrial cancer may metastasize to the ovaries; however, synchronous endometrioid adenocarcinoma, primary to both the ovary and the endometrium, can also occur.

- Ovarian carcinosarcomas, also known as **malignant mixed-mesodermal tumors of the ovary**, are extremely rare. These lesions are very aggressive, and treatment consists of surgical resection followed by combination chemotherapy. They are associated with a low response to treatment and overall poor outcome.
- **Ovarian tumors during pregnancy** are very rare. The incidence of an adnexal mass during pregnancy is approximately 1 in 800. The majority of adnexal masses discovered during the first trimester resolve by the second trimester. However, approximately 1% to 6% of these masses are malignant.
  - Germ cell tumors (primarily dysgerminoma) account for approximately 45% of ovarian malignancies diagnosed in pregnancy.
  - Masses are usually diagnosed during routine ultrasonography or at the time of cesarean delivery. The majority of patients (74%) are diagnosed with stage I disease.
  - Early-stage disease can be treated with conservative surgery in the second trimester of pregnancy, usually with good maternal and fetal outcomes. Late-stage and high-grade disease should be treated aggressively after appropriate counseling of the patient.

SUGGESTED READINGS

American College of Obstetricians and Gynecologists Committee on Gynecologic Practice. ACOG Committee Opinion No. 774: opportunistic salpingectomy as a strategy for epithelial ovarian cancer prevention. *Obstet Gynecol.* 2019;133:e279-e284.

American College of Obstetricians and Gynecologists Committee on Practice Bulletins—Gynecology. ACOG Practice Bulletin No. 174: evaluation and management of adnexal masses. *Obstet Gynecol.* 2016;128:e210-e226.

American College of Obstetricians and Gynecologists Committee on Practice Bulletins—Gynecology, Committee on Genetics, Society of Gynecologic Oncology. ACOG Practice Bulletin No. 182: hereditary breast and ovarian cancer syndrome. *Obstet Gynecol.* 2017;130:e110-e126.

Armstrong DK, Bundy B, Wenzel L, et al; for Gynecologic Oncology Group. Intraperitoneal cisplatin and paclitaxel in ovarian cancer. *N Engl J Med.* 2006;354:34-43.

Burger RA, Brady MF, Bookman MA, et al; for Gynecologic Oncology Group. Incorporation of bevacizumab in the primary treatment of ovarian cancer. *N Engl J Med.* 2011;365:2473-2483.

Chi DS, Berchuck A, Dizon DS, Yashar C, eds. *Principles and Practice of Gynecologic Oncology.* 7th ed. Philadelphia, PA: Wolters Kluwer Heath; 2017.

Kurman RJ, Shih I-M. The origin and pathogenesis of epithelial ovarian cancer: a proposed unifying theory. *Am J Surg Pathol.* 2010;34(3):433-443.

Hereditary Cancer Syndromes

Anja Frost and Deborah K. Armstrong

- It is essential that providers identify patients who may harbor a genetic predisposition to cancer. Recognition of certain familial patterns and appropriate referral is critical for the diagnosis and management of potential hereditary cancer syndromes. **Family history** should be reviewed and updated during annual gynecologic visits. Family cancer history is fluid and changes with time, as do research and discovery of new gene mutations.

- Historically, hereditary cancer syndromes in women have focused predominantly on hereditary breast and ovarian cancer syndromes (HBOC). There are now known to be many more relevant genes and syndromes outside of *BRCA1/BRCA2* mutations. These include Lynch syndrome; Cowden syndrome; Peutz-Jeghers syndrome; and mutations in *ATM*, *PALB2*, and other genes.

- Primary prevention of cancer should be a goal for any health care provider. Given the high rates of cancer development in those with an identified hereditary/familial cancer syndrome, these patients will have unique needs for screening and prevention.

  - Accessibility to genetic testing has increased, and the cost of testing has decreased since the June 2013 Supreme Court ruling that "a naturally occurring DNA segment" (ie, a gene) cannot be patented, removing the preexisting patent on the *BRCA1/BRCA2* genes.

  - Identification of germline mutations will allow application of comprehensive, targeted screening and management recommendations.

IDENTIFICATION OF HIGH-RISK WOMEN AND REFERRAL STRATEGIES

- Two distinct populations will present for consideration of genetic testing: (1) individuals with a cancer diagnosis and (2) unaffected individuals with a strong family history of cancer or with an identified mutation in a blood relative.

- Data show that only a quarter of women diagnosed with ovarian cancer receive genetic testing despite the National Comprehensive Care Network Clinical Practice Guidelines in Oncology (NCCN Guidelines®) for Genetic/Familial High-Risk Assessment: Breast, Ovarian, and Pancreatic recommending genetic counseling and testing for all women with ovarian cancer.

  - Patient barriers include a lack of perceived importance (ie, already affected, no offspring); concerns about cost; fear, anxiety, and misinformation about genetic issues including insurability; and resistance to the need of seeing a counselor.

  - Provider barriers include a lack of understanding of genetic syndromes, unfamiliarity with testing procedures, and insufficient time for comprehensive genetic counseling.

- Identification of individuals at high genetic risk for cancer has the potential to have a significant impact on mortality given the availability of well-defined and proven risk-reducing strategies. Even among cancer-affected individuals, genetic testing

Table 53-1	Features Suggestive of Hereditary Cancer

- Early age of cancer onset
- Multiple primary cancers in a single individual
- Bilateral cancer in paired organs or multifocal disease (eg, bilateral breast cancer)
- Clustering of the same type of cancer in close relatives
- Rare tumors that are part of defined genetic syndromes (eg, retinoblastoma, adrenocortical carcinoma, pheochromocytoma/paraganglioma, ocular melanoma, medullar thyroid cancer)
- Occurrence of epithelial ovarian, fallopian tube, or primary peritoneal cancer
- Geographic or ethnic populations known to be at high risk for hereditary cancers (eg, Ashkenazi Jewish ancestry)

has implications for targeted therapy in affected mutation carriers, and knowledge of mutation status can guide therapy and impact disease outcomes.

- Suspicion for hereditary cancer syndromes is increased with multiple affected family members, early age of onset, and the presence of multiple primary and/or bilateral primary cancers. Criteria for genetic evaluation have been largely agreed on by entities including the American College of Medical Genetics and Genomics, the National Society of Genetic Counselors, NCCN®, and the Society of Gynecologic Oncology (SGO). Table 53-1 details the features suggestive of hereditary cancer. Although these tables encompass general recommendations for genetic evaluation, there are instances in which there should be a lower threshold, including the following:
  - Gender imbalance in families or generations of the family
  - Hysterectomy/oophorectomy at a young age in multiple family members (predisposition to hereditary cancers may be masked)
  - Adoption or estrangement from parental lineage(s)
  - Deaths of family members at an early age, before cancer onset
- Evaluation of a patient's predisposition to gynecologic cancer syndromes allows physicians to provide individualized assessments of risk as well as tailored screening and prevention strategies including surveillance, chemoprevention, and prophylactic surgery to reduce overall morbidity and mortality.
  - **Pretest counseling** should provide the patient with the information needed to make a decision about genetic testing. This should include the rationale for genetic testing and the potential implications of genetic test results. Table 53-2 outlines the recommended components for pretest counseling.
  - Whereas these services have traditionally been provided by genetic counselors, the growing demand for genetic testing has surpassed the capacity of these specialists. The traditional referral model for genetic testing is also known to suffer from poor patient compliance, and thus, pretest genetic counseling and initiation of genetic testing is increasingly being provided by primary care providers, including obstetrician-gynecologists. Many will provide this service under

Table 53-2	Recommended Components of Pretest Cancer Genetic Evaluation

- Review the individual's personal medical history.
- Thoroughly review family history.
  - Document at least three generations of the family history of cancer.
- Provide information on role of genes in causing cancer.
- Provide a targeted discussion of possible syndromes that could explain the family history.
- Provide a general estimate of the individual's risk of having a cancer genetic syndrome.
  - Include cancer risks associated with the syndrome(s).
- Identify the benefits, risks, and limitations of proposed testing.
- Address cost of testing.
- Address genetic discrimination and impact of the genetic testing results on insurability.
- Agree on method of disclosure of test results.
- Address in advance possible results.
  - Briefly address screening, prevention, and risk reduction.
- Discuss implications of test results for family members.

guidance from a cancer genetics service. Fortunately, there are a number of online and Web-based services to aid the patient and the provider in pretest counseling.

- When considering genetic testing of an individual due to a family history of cancer, it is always **preferable to test a cancer-affected family member first**. Unfortunately, this is not always possible. When possible, testing of unaffected family members closest to the affected individual(s) can help inform genetic evaluation in the family. Although selection of gene(s) for testing can be based on particular familial patterns as well as ethnicity, in most cases, a broad and comprehensive panel of cancer-related genes will be tested.
  - Genetic testing of an unaffected individual for an identified deleterious gene mutation in a blood relative is referred to as "**cascade testing**." Before testing proceeds, the provider should obtain documentation of the positive test result so that the specific mutation (variant) can be identified. In most cases, testing can be "single site testing" for the identified mutation alone. However, there should be careful review of the family history to ensure that testing for other genes should not be included. For example, a woman with a maternal first cousin with ovarian cancer and an identified *BRCA1* germline mutation should undergo testing for that mutation. However, if her paternal cancer family history is suspicious, testing may be broadened to include other genes. The Centers for Disease Control and Prevention has highlighted HBOC syndrome and Lynch syndrome as high priority for cascade testing to identify more at-risk and/or affected individuals to ultimately prevent progression to any relevant cancers related to the known gene mutation.

- An often overlooked element in genetic services is **posttest counseling**, particularly for cancer-free individuals who test negative. Unless there is a known gene mutation in the family, a negative test cannot be reassuring and does not remove the risk associated with the cancer family history. It is important for patients and providers to not be falsely reassured by this "**uninformative negative**" test if a mutation has not been identified in the family.
  - In most cases, a positive test is an indication for a formal referral to a genetics service to comprehensively address the implications of test results. In addition, the identification of a "variant of undetermined significance," for which cancer risk is unknown, may also prompt referral.

SPECIFIC HEREDITARY GYNECOLOGIC CANCER SYNDROMES

Hereditary Breast and Ovarian Cancer

Testing of women with advanced ovarian cancer reveal that about 15% will have a mutation in *BRCA1* or *BRCA2*, whereas 5% will have a mutation in one of a number of other cancer-associated genes.

BRCA1 and BRCA2

- *BRCA1* and *BRCA2* are tumor suppressor genes. *BRCA* mutations are inherited in an autosomal dominant fashion.
- *BRCA1* and *BRCA2* mutations account for most cases of HBOC and are associated with an increased lifetime risk of multiple other cancers, including pancreatic cancer, melanoma, and prostate cancer. A summary of cancer risks associated with *BRCA1* and *BRCA2* mutations are shown in Table 53-3.
- *BRCA1* mutation carriers have a particularly early onset of disease, with both breast and ovarian cancers developing in some before age 40 years. *BRCA2*-associated breast and ovarian cancers generally develop one decade prior to the general population.

Table 53-3	*BRCA1* and *BRCA2* Penetrance: Cumulative Lifetime Cancer Risk[a]		
	General Population	*BRCA1*	*BRCA2*
Breast cancer	13%	50%-72%	40%-69%
Ovarian cancer	1%-2%	35%-60%	10%-27%
Prostate cancer	11%	15%-25%	
Pancreatic cancer	1%-2%	2-fold increase	2- to 5-fold increase

[a]From Chen S, Parmigiani G. Meta-analysis of *BRCA1* and *BRCA2* penetrance. *J Clin Oncol.* 2007;25(11):1329-1333.

- **Genetic testing** is recommended when a detailed risk assessment suggests a high risk for HBOC: number of affected relatives, degree of relativity between patient and affected family member(s), younger age at diagnosis, personal history of two breast cancer primaries, male breast cancer, diagnosis of triple negative breast cancer. Additionally, SGO and the NCCN Guidelines® for Genetic/Familial High-Risk Assessment: Breast, Ovarian, and Pancreatic recommend genetic testing, which may include *BRCA1* and *BRCA2*, in all newly diagnosed epithelial ovarian, tubal, and primary peritoneal cancers.
- **Surveillance to reduce breast and ovarian cancer**
  - **Breast cancer surveillance.** Women with *BRCA* mutations are recommended to have a clinical breast exam and breast imaging as shown in Table 53-4.
  - **Ovarian cancer surveillance.** Although screening for ovarian cancer has not been shown to clearly impact mortality, women at increased risk are recommended to consider annual transvaginal ultrasound and cancer antigen 125 levels. See Table 53-4.
- **Risk-reducing strategies** (See Table 53-4.)
  - Risk-reducing strategies for breast cancer:
    - Medications: Hormonal prevention with **tamoxifen**, a selective estrogen receptor modulator, has shown a significant breast cancer risk reduction in women with *BRCA2* mutations. The same benefits have not been seen in *BRCA1* carriers, likely because these carriers generally present with estrogen receptor–negative breast cancers. **Raloxifene** has also been studied in women at high risk for breast cancer, and the Study of Tamoxifen and Raloxifene trial showed that both agents significantly decreased the lifetime risk of breast cancer, although a greater benefit with tamoxifen with the caveat of increased risk of thromboembolic events and cataracts, and a nonstatistically significant increase in the number of uterine cancer diagnoses with tamoxifen. Aromatase inhibitors have also been documented to reduce risk of breast cancer and are the preferred hormonal chemoprevention agent in postmenopausal women. None of these hormonal chemoprevention approaches impacts the risk of ovarian cancer.
    - Surgery: Women with *BRCA* mutations should be offered risk-reducing **bilateral mastectomy**, which reduces the risk of breast cancer by over 90% in this patient population. Bilateral **risk-reducing salpingo-oophorectomy** for ovarian cancer prevention also decreases breast cancer risk in *BRCA* carriers.
  - Risk-reducing strategies for ovarian cancer:
    - Medications: The use of **oral contraceptives (OCPs)** for 5 or more years has been shown to decrease ovarian cancer in the general population and in women with *BRCA* mutations. However, there is a concern about OCP-associated breast cancer risk for these women, particularly with use of OCPs past age 35 years.
    - Surgery: The most effective risk-reducing strategy for women with *BRCA1* or *BRCA2* mutations is **bilateral risk reducing salpingo-oophorectomy (RRSO)** and is recommended once childbearing is complete. For women with a *BRCA1* mutation, this is considered by ages 35 to 40 years and ages 40 to 45 years for *BRCA2* mutation carriers. Given that a significant portion of serous ovarian cancers likely originate in the distal fallopian tube, one can consider bilateral salpingectomy with delayed bilateral oophorectomy, depending on the patient's age and desire for fertility, although the standard of care remains RRSO. There is ongoing research with clinical trials to see if bilateral salpingectomy alone will be able to replace RRSO.

Table 53-4	Surveillance and Risk-Reduction Considerations for Known Mutation Carriers		
Gene	Genetic Syndrome	Surveillance and Age to Initiate	Risk Reduction and Age to Consider
BRCA1	HBOC	Every 6 mo/annual TVUS and CA-125 (ages 30-35 y) Breast awareness (age 18 y) Clinical breast exam every 6-12 mo (age 25 y) Annual breast MRI (ages 25-29 y) Annual mammogram (age 30 y, alternating every 6 mo with annual MRI)	RRSO (ages 35-40 y) Offer RR mastectomy Consider RR medical therapy (OCPs, tamoxifen, raloxifene, aromatase inhibitors)
BRCA2	HBOC	Same as BRCA1	RRSO (ages 40-45 y) Offer RR mastectomy Consider RR medical therapy
BRIP1, RAD51C, RAD51D		No recommendations	Consider RRSO (ages 45-50 y)
MLH1, MSH2, MSH6, PMS2	LS	Colonoscopy beginning ages 20-25 y EMB every 1-2 y (ages 30-35 y) Consider annual TVUS. Consider annual CA-125.	RRSO when childbearing complete (start discussion by 40s) RR hysterectomy when childbearing complete Consider RR medications (OCPs, progestins, aspirin)
POLD1	PPAP	No recommendations	No recommendations
PTEN	Cowden syndrome	Consider annual TVUS + EMB (ages 30-35 y). Breast awareness (age 18 y) Clinical breast exam every 6-12 mo (age 25 y) Annual breast MRI (ages 30-35 y) Annual mammogram (ages 30-35 y)	Discuss RR hysterectomy when childbearing complete Discuss RR mastectomy

Table 53-4	Surveillance and Risk-Reduction Considerations for Known Mutation Carriers *(Continued)*		
Gene	Genetic Syndrome	Surveillance and Age to Initiate	Risk Reduction and Age to Consider
STK11	PJS	Annual pelvic exam + pap smear (ages 18-20 y) Consider annual TVUS. Clinical breast exam every 6 mo (age 25 y) Annual breast MRI (age 25 y) Annual mammogram (age 25 y)	Discuss RR mastectomy
TP53	LF	Breast awareness (age 18 y) Clinical breast exam every 6-12 mo (ages 20-25 y) Annual breast MRI (ages 20-25 y) Annual mammogram (ages 20-25 y)	Discuss RR mastectomy

Abbreviations: CA-125, cancer antigen 125; EMB, endometrial biopsy; HBOC, hereditary breast and ovarian cancer syndrome; LF, Li-Fraumeni syndrome; LS, Lynch syndrome; MRI, magnetic resonance imaging; OCPs, oral contraceptives; PJS, Peutz-Jeghers syndrome; PPAP, polymerase proofreading–associated polyposis; RR, risk-reducing; RRSO, risk-reducing salpingo-oophorectomy; TVUS, transvaginal ultrasound.

Other Ovarian Cancer–Associated Gene Mutations

- There are other gene mutations associated with development of hereditary ovarian cancer that function in the same homologous recombination pathway responsible for DNA double-strand repair as *BRCA*. These genes include *PALB2*, *ATM*, *RAD51C*, *RAD51D*, *BRIP1*, and others. Most of these are low- or moderate-penetrance genes, increasing lifetime risk up to 10%, a 2- to 6-fold increase over the general population.
- Risk-reducing strategies: The recommendation for RRSO holds true for additional high-risk mutations including *BRIP1*, *RAD51C*, and *RAD51D* by the age of 45 to 50 years old. The OCPs can also be considered, although ovarian cancer risk reduction with OCPs has not been validated in these populations. Percentage of risk reduction with regard to both of these options has not yet been well evaluated prospectively. See Table 53-4.

		Gene		
Cancer	General Population	MLH1 or MSH2[b]	MSH6	PMS2
Colon cancer	4.5%	52%-82%	10%-22%	15%-20%
Endometrial cancer	2.7%	25%-60%	16%-26%	15%
Prostate cancer	11.6%	~30%	~30%	NR
Ovarian cancer	1.3%	11%-24%	NR	[c]
Stomach cancer	<1%	6%-13%	≤3%	[c]
Sebaceous neoplasms	<1%	1%-9%	NR	NR

Table 53-5 Lynch Syndrome Lifetime Cancer Risks Up to Age 70 y[a]

Abbreviation: NR, not reported.

[a]Adapted with permission from the NCCN Clinical Practice Guidelines in Oncology (NCCN Guidelines®) for Genetic/Familial High Risk Assessment: Colorectal V.1.2018. © 2018 National Comprehensive Cancer Network, Inc. All rights reserved. The NCCN Guidelines® and illustrations herein may not be reproduced in any form for any purpose without the express written permission of NCCN. To view the most recent and complete version of the NCCN Guidelines, go online to NCCN.org. The NCCN Guidelines are a work in progress that may be refined as often as new significant data becomes available. NCCN makes no warranties of any kind whatsoever regarding their content, use or application and disclaims any responsibility for their application or use in any way.

[b]MLH1 or MSH2 mutations: The individual risks of urinary tract, hepatobiliary, small bowel, brain/central nervous system, and pancreatic cancers range between 1% and 7%.

[c]PMS2 mutation: The combined risk for renal, stomach, ovary, small bowel, ureter, and brain is 6%.

Lynch Syndrome

- Lynch syndrome, previously known as hereditary nonpolyposis colorectal cancer, is inherited in an autosomal dominant fashion and increases the lifetime risk of multiple cancers, including cancers of the gastrointestinal tract, endometrium, the genitourinary tract, and others. **Colorectal and endometrial cancers** are the most common. See Table 53-5.

- The most common gynecologic cancer associated with Lynch syndrome is **endometrial cancer**, and approximately 2% to 6% of endometrial cancers are in individuals affected by Lynch syndrome. Furthermore, disease onset will be earlier in women with Lynch syndrome (mean age 47-49 years). Endometrial cancer can be the presenting cancer in 40% to 50% of Lynch syndrome–affected women.

- There are three approaches to guide which patients should undergo testing for Lynch syndrome (Table 53-6): (1) when a detailed risk assessment suggests a high risk for Lynch Syndrome, (2) when a patient is diagnosed with endometrial or colorectal cancer before age 60 years, or (3) when a patient is diagnosed with endometrial or colorectal cancer at any age. Approach should be determined by local pathology and genetic resources, availability of genetic counseling, and cost.

Table 53-6	Three Approaches to Guide Who Should Receive Genetic Screening for Lynch Syndrome

Approach 1
- Diagnosis of endometrial or colorectal cancer before age 50 y
- Patient with endometrial or ovarian cancer with a synchronous colon or other Lynch syndrome–associated tumor
- Patients with endometrial or colorectal cancer and
  - A first-degree relative affected with a Lynch syndrome–associated tumor diagnosed before age 50 y OR
  - Two or more first- or second-degree relatives with Lynch syndrome–associated tumors OR
  - Tumor displaying microsatellite instability or loss of expression of a DNA mismatch repair protein (MLH1, MSH2, MSH6, PMS2) expression
- Patients with a first- or second-degree relative or other close family member with a known mutation in a DNA mismatch repair gene

Approach 2
- Diagnosis of endometrial or colorectal cancer before age 60 y

Approach 3
- Diagnosis of endometrial or colorectal cancer at any age

Data from American College of Obstetricians and Gynecologists Committee on Practice Bulletins—Gynecology, Society of Gynecologic Oncology. ACOG Practice Bulletin No. 147: Lynch syndrome. *Obstet Gynecol.* 2014;124:1042-1054. (Reaffirmed 2019); and Lancaster JM, Powell CB, Kauff ND, et al. Society of Gynecologic Oncologists Education Committee statement on risk assessment for inherited gynecologic cancer predispositions. *Gynecol Oncol.* 2007;107(2):159-162.

- There are two approaches for testing for Lynch syndrome: (1) direct germline DNA testing and (2) testing of the tumor using immunohistochemistry (IHC) or microsatellite instability testing. Whenever possible, testing the tumor directly is the preferred initial approach.
  - The most common germline mutations are those in the mismatch repair proteins, which include MLH1, MSH2, MSH6, and PMS2 as well as in EpCAM, a regulator of MSH2.
  - An IHC for expression of the DNA mismatch repair protein expression from MLH1, MSH2, MSH6, and PMS2 and/or polymerase chain reaction–based microsatellite instability analysis can be performed on tumors to aid in identifying Lynch syndrome and can help inform recommendations for germline testing.
  - Two additional genes, *POLD1* and *POLE*, have an increased risk of malignancy, most commonly colonic polyps and colon cancers; however, *POLD1* germline mutations carry a risk of endometrial cancer as well. These conditions have been named **polymerase proofreading–associated polyposis** and often mimic Lynch syndrome–associated cancers histologically and can have loss of expression of Lynch proteins on IHC and microsatellite instability.

- Surveillance for women with Lynch syndrome:
  - Endometrial biopsy every 1 to 2 years (start age 30-35 years)
  - Colonoscopy every 1 to 2 years (start age 20-25 or 2-5 y before earliest cancer diagnosis in a family member, whichever is earlier)
  - Although of limited benefit, NCCN Guidelines® for Genetic/Familial High-Risk Assessment: Colorectal recommend consideration of transvaginal ultrasound and cancer antigen 125 for management of patients with Lynch syndrome as surveillance/prevention strategies for endometrial and ovarian cancers.
- Risk-reducing strategies:
  - Medications: The OCPs and progestin therapy alone can reduce endometrial cancer risk. It is not clear whether OCP use has an impact on Lynch syndrome–associated ovarian cancer risk. Taking daily aspirin (600 mg) for more than 2 years reduces colorectal cancer risk, although data on long-term adverse effects is lacking.
  - Surgery: risk-reducing hysterectomy and bilateral salpingo-oophorectomy at the completion of childbearing. The SGO and American College of Obstetricians and Gynecologists recommend this discussion by the early to mid-40s.

Cowden Syndrome

- Cowden syndrome is caused by a germline mutation in the *PTEN* gene and is inherited in the autosomal dominant fashion.
- Cowden syndrome is associated with multiple cancers, most commonly **breast cancer** and **endometrial cancer** with a 25% to 50% and 28% lifetime risk, respectively. Other associated cancers include thyroid (most commonly follicular, 3%-10% risk), colon, and renal cancers.
- Individuals affected with Cowden syndrome often have associated physical characteristics including macrocephaly, multinodular goiters, trichilemmomas, gastrointestinal hamartomas, and Lhermitte-Duclos disease (hamartomatous outgrowths of the cerebellum).
- Risk-reducing strategies for women include hysterectomy at the completion of childbearing and mastectomy on an individualized basis. See Table 53-4 for screening and risk-reducing strategies.

Peutz-Jeghers Syndrome

- Mutations in the *STK11/LKB1* gene, which are inherited in an autosomal dominant fashion, increase the risk of **cervical (adenoma malignum)**, **ovarian (sex cord stromal tumors)**, and **breast cancers** by approximately 10%, 20%, and 50% lifetime risk, respectively.
- Peutz-Jeghers syndrome is also associated with many clinical characteristics such as benign hamartomatous polyps of the gastrointestinal tract, mucocutaneous pigmented macules, and an increased risk of gastrointestinal tumors (colon, gastric, pancreatic) as well as nongastrointestinal tumors mentioned above.
- Recommendations for risk reduction are individualized. Risk-reducing mastectomy can be considered for women with Peutz-Jeghers syndrome. See Table 53-4 for screening and risk-reducing strategies.

Li-Fraumeni Syndrome

- Li-Fraumeni syndrome is defined by inherited mutations in the *TP53* gene, a critical tumor-suppressor gene regulating repair of DNA damage.
- Individuals with these mutations are at an increased risk for multiple cancers, frequently in childhood, with the highest risk being that of **breast cancer** with up to a 60% lifetime risk, and presenting often in the third decade of life.

- Given the large number of cancers associated with Li-Fraumeni syndrome, screening recommendations are very complex. There is also a general recommendation to minimize radiation exposure complicating screening in these individuals. There are, to date, no recommendations for risk-reducing hysterectomy or salpingo-oophorectomy, and patients should be individually evaluated following a detailed family history. Risk-reducing mastectomy is considered for women with Li-Fraumeni syndrome. See Table 53-4.

Newly Defined Nonsyndrome Mutations

- With the advancement in hereditary panel testing and increasing research, additional mutations have been discovered that are associated with an increased risk of ovarian cancer. Germline mutations in *DICER1* and *SMARCA4* genes have been associated with Sertoli-Leydig tumors and ovarian small cell carcinoma, respectively.
- As increased single gene and panel testing is performed, it is expected that mutation-associated cancers will be better defined and penetrance will be clarified. It is also expected that the list of cancer-associated genes will continue to expand.

TARGETED THERAPY FOR MUTATION CARRIERS

- Determination of a patient's gene mutation status is important not only for screening and primary prevention but also for new and emerging targeted therapies. For example, poly(adenosine diphosphate ribose) polymerase inhibitors have shown benefit for BRCA-associated ovarian cancer in multiple settings, including maintenance therapy after initial chemotherapy, primary treatment of recurrent disease, and maintenance therapy after successful treatment of recurrent platinum-sensitive serous ovarian cancer. It is unclear whether ovarian cancers associated with other homologous recombination pathway gene mutations, such as *PALB2*, *ATM*, and others, might have similar benefits from poly(adenosine diphosphate ribose) polymerase inhibitor therapy.

SUGGESTED READINGS

American College of Obstetricians and Gynecologists Committee on Gynecologic Practice. ACOG Committee Opinion No. 727: cascade testing: testing women for known hereditary genetic mutations associated with cancer. *Obstet Gynecol*. 2018;131:e31-e34.

American College of Obstetricians and Gynecologists Committee on Practice Bulletins—Gynecology. ACOG Practice Bulletin No. 182: hereditary breast and ovarian cancer syndrome. *Obstet Gynecol*. 2017;130:e110-e126.

American College of Obstetricians and Gynecologists Committee on Practice Bulletins—Gynecology, Society of Gynecologic Oncology. ACOG Practice Bulletin No. 147: Lynch syndrome. *Obstet Gynecol*. 2014;124:1042-1054. (Reaffirmed 2019)

Frost AS, Toaff M, Biagi T, Stark E, McHenry A, Kaltman R. Effects of cancer genetic panel testing on at-risk individuals. *Obstet Gynecol*. 2018;131(6):1103-1110.

Lancaster JM, Powell CB, Chen L, Richardson DL. Society of Gynecologic Oncology statement on risk assessment for inherited gynecologic cancer predispositions. *Gynecologic Oncology*. 2015;136:3-7.

Shaw J, Bulsara C, Cohen PA, et al. Investigating barriers to genetic counseling and germline mutation testing in women with suspected hereditary breast and ovarian cancer syndrome and Lynch syndrome. *Patient Educ Couns*. 2018;101(5):938-944.

Premalignant and Malignant Disease of the Vulva and Vagina

Megan E. Gornet and Rebecca Stone

PREMALIGNANT NEOPLASTIC DISEASES OF THE VULVA AND VAGINA

Vulvar Intraepithelial Neoplasia

- Vulvar intraepithelial neoplasia (VIN) is the putative precursor lesion to vulvar squamous cell carcinoma (VSCC).
- Histologic criteria for VIN include disordered maturation and nuclear abnormalities, loss of polarity, pleomorphism, mitotic figures, cytologic atypia, and coarsened nuclear chromatin. Historically, the degree of maturation present in the surface epithelium defined the grade of dysplasia.
  - VIN 1 (mild dysplasia) demonstrates loss of squamous maturation in the lower one-third of the epithelium.
  - VIN 2 (moderate dysplasia) shows loss of maturation in the lower two-thirds of the epithelium. Surface maturation is present.
  - VIN 3 (severe dysplasia, carcinoma in situ) presents with full-thickness loss of squamous maturation. Cytologic atypia may be severe, but there is no stromal invasion.
- In 2004, the International Society for the Study of Vulvovaginal Disease proposed that the term *VIN* refers more specifically to VIN 2 and VIN 3. New histologic subtypes were also introduced: usual VIN (uVIN) for human papillomavirus (HPV)-related lesions and differentiated VIN (dVIN) for lesions not associated with HPV but rather with vulvar dermatoses such as lichen sclerosis.
- The most recent 2015 International Society for the Study of Vulvovaginal Disease revised classification includes three types of VIN, each with distinct underlying etiologies and malignant potential:
  - Low-grade squamous intraepithelial lesion of the vulva, equivalent to uVIN 1: benign manifestations of the skin's reaction to HPV infection, low-risk HPV types 6 and 11 account for over 90%, should not be considered neoplastic
  - High-grade squamous intraepithelial lesion of the vulva, equivalent to uVIN 2 and 3: driven by the oncogenic types of HPV (particularly oncotypes 16, 18, 33) and risk factors for HPV persistence, such as cigarette smoking; seen in younger women; tends to be multifocal with synchronous or metachronous squamous neoplasia of other lower genital tract sites; accounts for 20% of VSCC; 5% to 6% progress to invasive cancer (9% in untreated and 3% in treated cases)
  - The dVIN: not typically associated with HPV and generally seen in older women, associated with atrophy and inflammatory dermatoses (eg, lichen sclerosis, lichen simplex chronicus), often unifocal, accounts for 80% of VSSC, aggressive with one-third progressing to invasive cancer, has a worse prognosis even when adjusting for age/stage
- One-third of VIN cases will recur, regardless of how they are treated.

Vaginal Intraepithelial Neoplasia

- This rare condition affects approximately 0.2 per 100 000 US women.
- Vaginal intraepithelial neoplasia (VAIN) is the putative precursor lesion to vaginal squamous cell carcinoma.
- A VAIN is a preinvasive lesion defined by the presence of squamous cell atypia without invasion. Lesions are classified according to the depth of epithelial involvement.
  - VAIN 1: Cytologic atypia is present throughout the lower one-third of the epithelium.
  - VAIN 2: Cytologic atypia is present throughout the lower two-thirds of epithelium.
  - VAIN 3: Cytologic atypia involves more than two-thirds of the epithelium.
- A VAIN is usually asymptomatic, although patients can present with postcoital spotting or vaginal discharge. It is diagnosed by persistently abnormal Pap smears with no evidence of cervical neoplasia. After VAIN is diagnosed, invasive disease must be excluded by colposcopy and biopsy, especially before undertaking nonexcisional therapy. A VAIN progresses to invasive cancer in 3% to 7% of patients.
- The majority of lesions are located in the upper one-third of the vagina.
- Common risk factors include HPV infection (HPV 16 is most common), smoking, current or prior lower genital preinvasive or invasive lesions, immunosuppression, and history of radiation exposure.
- The risk of VAIN or vaginal cancer is extremely low (0.12%) in women who have undergone total hysterectomy for benign disease (excluding grades 2-3 cervical intraepithelial neoplasia); screening guidelines recommend discontinuation of vaginal cytology posthysterectomy for benign disease other than grades 2 and 3 cervical intraepithelial neoplasia.
- Forty percent to 50% of VAIN cases will recur, regardless of how they are treated.

Treatment of Vulvar Intraepithelial Neoplasia and Vaginal Intraepithelial Neoplasia

- Among low-grade VAIN and uVIN lesions, there appears to be a high rate of spontaneous regression. Thus, low-grade VAIN and VIN can be expectantly managed.
- Surgical excision is the mainstay of treatment for uVIN 2/3, dVIN, and VAIN 2/3 and should be performed if invasion cannot be excluded. Biopsies to exclude invasive disease are mandatory prior to pursuing medical or ablative therapies.
  - Wide local excision: 1-cm margin, ideal for small, unifocal lesions
  - Simple vulvectomy: often needed for large or multifocal lesions
  - Simple vaginectomy
- Ablative techniques (carbon dioxide laser vaporization, argon beam ablation, ultrasonic surgical aspiration): must rule out invasion with pretreatment biopsies, useful with multifocal disease, minimal scarring and sexual dysfunction. The VIN lesions should be ablated to 3 mm in hair-bearing areas and 1 mm on nonhairy surfaces.
- Topical agents (5% imiquimod and 5-fluorouracil cream): useful for persistent low-grade, multifocal lesions or women who are poor surgical candidates
- Intracavitary radiation therapy is effective for VAIN but is associated with morbidity and should be reserved for women who are poor surgical candidates, have extensive disease burden with concern for invasion, and/or have failed other more conservative treatment approaches.
- There is prospective evidence that earlier detection and proactive management of lichen sclerosis with long-term topical corticosteroid treatment may lead to reduced risk of dVIN and development of VSCC.

- Six months is a reasonable surveillance interval for detection of recurrent/progressive VIN/VAIN; patients with persistent VAIN following treatment have an approximately 10% risk of progression to invasive vaginal cancer.

MALIGNANT NEOPLASTIC DISEASES OF THE VULVA

- Vulvar cancer is relatively rare, accounting for 0.71% of all cancers in women and for 5% to 6% of all primary malignancies of the female genital tract. There were an estimated 6020 new cases and 1150 deaths from vulvar cancer in the United States in 2017. Importantly, incidence has risen 0.6% over last 10 years, with now over 20% of new cases occurring in women younger than 50 years old. This is in stark contrast to several decades ago, when the incidence of vulvar cancer in women under 50 years old was only 2%. Although there is an increasing proportion of younger women diagnosed with vulvar cancer, death rates have been increasing an average of 0.7% per year, and 5-year disease-free specific survival has dropped from 75% to 68% since 2004.
- Squamous cell carcinoma is the most common, followed by melanoma, basal cell carcinoma (BCC), sarcoma, and other more rare histologies.
- Vulvar cancer most commonly presents as pruritus, bleeding, or vulvodynia and are often misdiagnosed by health care providers. Many advanced vulvar cancers are a result of delayed diagnosis and treatment due to patient/provider factors.

Vulvar Squamous Cell Carcinoma

- Squamous cell lesions account for 80% or more of vulvar malignancies.
- The VIN is the precursor lesion to VSCC (see Vulvar Intraepithelial Neoplasia).
- Invasive VSCC is present at the time of excision in 10% to 22% of women with high-grade VIN on initial biopsy.
- **Patient evaluation:** Diagnosis of vulvar cancer requires biopsy. Definitive excisional biopsy to obtain gross surgical margins of at least 1 cm circumferentially can often be used to address small lesions (typically ≤2 cm). For larger lesions, wedge biopsy at the tumor-skin interface should be performed.
- **Staging:** Revised in 2009, the International Federation of Gynecology and Obstetrics (FIGO) staging system defines stage based, in part, on information derived from surgical assessment of the groin nodes (Table 54-1).
- Nodal status has the most prognostic significance and directs treatment for VSCC.
- National Comprehensive Cancer Network guidelines should direct treatment. These are available online free-of-charge at www.NCCN.org.
- **Primary treatment**
  - In general, treatment options include radical vulvectomy as primary surgery, pelvic exenteration (ultraradical surgery), radiotherapy (primary or neoadjuvant), chemoradiation (primary or neoadjuvant), and neoadjuvant chemotherapy followed by surgery.
  - The initial management decision for vulvar cancer is based on clinical features including the extent of the primary lesion and the presence or absence of detectable node metastases as well as age, comorbidities, and patient preference.
  - Wide local excision alone (simple/skinning excision with 1-cm circumferential margins) is considered adequate for stage IA lesions. Except when surgery would compromise functionally important midline structures (eg, clitoris, urethra, anus), radical local excision (1- to 2-cm circumferential margins and deep

Table 54-1 International Federation of Gynecology and Obstetrics Staging for Carcinoma of the Vulva (2009) and 5-Year Survival[a]

Stage	Description	5-y Survival[b]
0	Carcinoma in situ, intraepithelial neoplasia	
I	Tumor confined to vulva or perineum	98%
IA	Tumor confined to vulva or perineum; lesion ≤2 cm with stromal invasion ≤1 mm, no nodal metastasis	
IB	Tumor confined to vulva or perineum; lesion >2 cm or stromal invasion >1 mm, with negative nodes	
II	Tumor of any size with extension to adjacent perineal structures (lower one-third urethra, lower one-third vagina, anus) with negative nodes	85%
III	Tumor of any size with or without extension to adjacent perineal structures with positive inguinofemoral lymph nodes	74%
IIIA	1. With one lymph node metastasis (≥5 mm) or 2. One to two lymph node metastasis(es) (<5 mm)	
IIIB	1. With two or more lymph node metastases (≥5 mm) or 2. Three or more lymph node metastases (<5 mm)	
IIIC	Positive nodes with extracapsular spread	
IV	Tumor invading other regional (upper two-thirds urethra, upper two-thirds vagina) or distant structures	31%
IVA	Tumor invading any of the following: 1. Upper urethra and/or vaginal mucosa, bladder mucosa, rectal mucosa, or fixed to pelvic bone 2. Fixed or ulcerated inguinofemoral lymph nodes	
IVB	Distant metastasis to any site including pelvic lymph nodes	

[a]Adapted from Pecorelli S. FIGO Committee on Gynecologic Oncology. Revised FIGO staging for carcinoma of the vulva, cervix, and endometrium. *Int J Gynaecol Obstet.* 2009;105(2):103-104. Copyright © 2009 International Federation of Gynecology and Obstetrics. Reprinted by permission of John Wiley & Sons, Inc.
[b]Five-year survival data according to previous International Federation of Gynecology and Obstetrics staging system.

margin at the perineal membrane) with groin node assessment is the preferred initial approach to stage IB lesions and some cases of early stage II disease.

- **Neoadjuvant therapy:** largely considered when adequate surgical margins (1- to 2-cm clinical margins, ≥8 mm in fixed tissue) may be difficult to obtain. Advantages may include reduced tumor volume increasing operability, allowance for more effective radiotherapy, and treatment of micrometastatic disease.

- **Primary surgical treatment**
  - A radical excisional procedure (total radical vulvectomy, partial radical vulvectomy, radical local excision) obtains 1- to 2-cm clinical margins and dissects down to the perineal membrane.
  - In the setting of close (<8 mm) or positive surgical margin, re-resection versus adjuvant therapy should be considered.
  - Groin node assessment is accomplished by surgical exploration of the groin nodes. The most widely accepted surgical practice is to obtain histologic examination of ipsilateral inguinofemoral lymph nodes for well-lateralized lesions of the vulva (lesions located >2 cm from midline) and of bilateral nodes for lesions within 2 cm of midline.
- **Groin evaluation:** Sentinel lymph node biopsy (SLNB) has been accepted as the standard of care for groin node assessment in early-stage VSCC. A SLNB is preferable to inguinofemoral lymphadenectomy due to the decreased risk of lymphedema and wound complications.
  - A negative sentinel node excludes metastasis beyond it with a negative predictive value of >95%. Candidates for SLNB should have clinically negative lymph nodes, tumor size <4 cm, and unifocal disease.
  - Pathologic ultrastaging of sentinel lymph nodes increases sensitivity for detection of micrometastatic disease.
  - The Groningen International Sentinel Node for Vulvar Cancer trial showed an overall survival of 97% and a 3% relapse rate 2 years after excision with a negative SLNB in women with vulvar cancers <4 cm.
  - An SLNB is more successful with combined use of radiocolloid (technetium-99) and blue dye (isosulfan) for identification of the sentinel node.
  - Inguinofemoral lymphadenectomy: Boundaries of dissection are the adductor longus muscle, the sartorius muscle, and the inguinal ligament; should be performed when SLNB is not feasible or sentinel lymph node is not identified
- **Primary nonsurgical treatment.** Chemoradiation is the preferred treatment strategy for cases that would require exenterative procedures or other significantly deforming surgical interventions.
- **Adjuvant treatment.** Indications for adjuvant radiotherapy following upfront surgical resection include patients with negative groin nodes but with adverse primary tumor risk factors and patients with groin node involvement.
  - In node-negative cases, adjuvant radiation may be administered based on primary tumor risk factors including involved or close surgical margins (<8 mm), deep invasion (>5 mm), pattern of invasion, and/or the presence of lymphvascular invasion.
  - Adjuvant therapy for sentinel lymph node–positive disease: radiation with or without concurrent chemotherapy for patients with micrometastasis (nodal met ≤2 mm) with no additional dissection, or completion of inguinofemoral lymphadenectomy in cases of macrometastases (nodal met >2 mm), followed by radiation with or without concurrent chemotherapy
  - Unilateral or bilateral radiation to the groin and low pelvic lymph nodes is recommended following surgical resection of positive inguinofemoral nodes, particularly when there are ≥2 positive nodes or a metastatic focus with extracapsular extension.
  - Metastatic disease: Chemotherapeutic agents active against squamous cancer are often offered, but response is generally poor.
  - Recurrence: Outcome highly dependent on site of relapse and prior treatment history. Several reports have suggested that up to 75% of patients with a local

vulvar recurrence may be cured with surgical reexcision. Groin node recurrence, particularly in a radiated field, is typically fatal.

- Five-year survival rates range from 86% for localized disease (stage I/II), 57% for regional or locally advanced disease (stage III/IVA), and to 17% for patients with distant metastasis (stage IVB).

Verrucous Carcinoma

- **Verrucous carcinoma** is a variant of squamous carcinoma that occurs in postmenopausal women. These tumors are large, fungating masses that may be mistakenly diagnosed as condyloma acuminata recalcitrant to treatment. Because the histologic appearance of verrucous carcinoma closely resembles normal squamous epithelium, a sufficiently deep biopsy must be obtained for diagnosis. Although lymph node metastasis is exceedingly rare, local destruction and tumor recurrence are common.
- **Treatment** consists of radical local excision. Radiation therapy is contraindicated because it may actually be tumor promoting.

Basal Cell Carcinoma

- In contrast to other cutaneous sites where BCC is the most common skin cancer, this malignancy accounts for only 2% to 3% of all vulvar carcinomas. The BCCs occur most commonly in postmenopausal white women. In contrast to other cutaneous sites, ultraviolet light exposure plays no role in the etiology of vulvar BCC.
- Grossly, these lesions appear as flesh/white-colored nodules or plaques; ulceration can be present. The prognosis is good, despite a 20% local recurrence risk. Groin metastasis is rare.
- **Treatment:** wide, local excision

Melanoma

- **Melanomas** constitute the second most common primary malignancy of the vulva, comprising 5% to 10% of vulvar neoplasms. Anogenital lesions account for 3% of all melanomas. Vulvar melanoma most commonly occurs in the sixth to seventh decades of life.
- *BRAF* and *c-KIT* gene mutations may be present and provide opportunity for targeted therapy.
- Melanomas are typically raised lesions, with irregular pigmentation and borders. They are found with equal frequency on the labia majora and mucosal surfaces. Prognosis depends primarily on tumor thickness and on the presence or absence of lymph node involvement.
- They may be staged via the American Joint Committee on Cancer, FIGO, Clark, Breslow, or Chung system.
- **Treatment.** Wide, local excision of the primary tumor with clinically negative circumferential margins should be attempted. The acceptable clinical margins for melanoma in situ, melanomas with Breslow thickness (depth of deepest invasive cells) ≤2 mm, and thickness >2 mm are 0.5, 1, and 2 cm, respectively.
- Although nodal status has prognostic significance, the therapeutic role of regional lymphadenectomy is not well defined. Thus, groin assessment is typically limited to SLNB.
- As a rough approximation, prognosis of melanoma of the vulva parallels prognosis by stage of cutaneous melanomas, but overall prognosis is worse because of characteristically advanced stage at the time of diagnosis.

- High recurrence rate, higher than that seen in other cutaneous/mucosal melanomas. Nearly 60% of vulvar melanomas will recur.
- There are limited therapeutic agents for advanced, metastatic, and/or recurrent melanomas not amenable to surgery. At present, radiation therapy has no established role in the routine management of vulvar melanomas.
- Although 5-year overall survival as high as 50% has been reported, most series report 5-year overall survival of 15% to 30% except for patients with stage I disease.

Paget Disease of the Vulva

- Paget disease of the vulva is rare. Most affected patients are in their seventh or eighth decade of life and experience local irritation, pruritus, and bleeding.
- Paget lesions typically have slightly raised edges and are erythematous, with islands of white epithelium. Lesions are multifocal and are sharply demarcated and often have foci of excoriation and induration. The lesions are characterized histologically by large, vacuolated pathognomonic Paget cells with bluish cytoplasm located in the basal layer of the vulvar epithelium.
- Adenocarcinoma of the underlying apocrine glands is found in 10% to 15% of patients who have intraepithelial Paget disease. Ten percent of patients with vulvar Paget disease are found to have associated breast, colon, or genitourinary cancer; thus, the workup should include colonoscopy, cystoscopy, mammogram, and colposcopy. If the disease is limited to the epithelium, its clinical course is usually prolonged and indolent.
- **Treatment:** Although radical surgery was formerly the mainstay of therapy, newer evidence suggests that local excision with 2- to 3-cm borders of all involved tissue carries similar prognosis. Negative surgical margins are difficult to obtain because "pagetoid" changes may extend microscopically in the epidermis well beyond the margins of what can be appreciated on clinical examination. Negative surgical margins have only limited correlation with freedom from local relapse.

Bartholin Gland Carcinoma

- Squamous carcinoma (arising in ductal epithelium) constitutes approximately 50% of cases of Bartholin complex carcinomas; adenocarcinoma is slightly less common.
- Bartholin gland malignancies typically occur in the sixth decade of life, and resection of Bartholin cysts/abscesses is recommended in women aged 40 years and older (as opposed to just drainage/marsupialization).
- **Treatment.** Because of anatomic proximity of the complex to both the inferior ischial ramus and the anorectum, adequate surgical margins are rarely obtained, and management frequently entails combinations of conservative surgery and radiation therapy or primary therapy with chemoradiation therapy. Because these are medial and deep vulvar tumors, staging should include assessment of the nodes bilaterally.

Vulvar Sarcoma

- Sarcomas of the vulva are rare and account for 1% to 2% of vulvar malignancies. The age range is broader than for VSCC. Lymphatic metastasis is uncommon.
- **Treatment.** Wide, local excision is recommended, followed by adjuvant radiation, chemotherapy, or both. Other than the special problems associated with treating tumors in proximity to multiple functionally important structures, there is nothing that distinguishes treatment of vulvar sarcomas from the treatment of soft tissue sarcomas at other sites.

MALIGNANT NEOPLASTIC DISEASES OF THE VAGINA

Most malignancies identified in the vagina are secondary (ie, recurrent or metastatic cervical cancer). Primary vaginal cancer is very rare and accounted for approximately 4810 new cancer cases and 1240 cancer deaths in the United States in 2017. Vaginal cancers comprise approximately 0.56% of all cancers in women and 4.5% of gynecologic malignancies. Squamous cell carcinoma is the most common histopathology (80%), followed by melanoma (3%), sarcoma (3%), adenocarcinoma, and other more rare histologies.

Squamous Cell Vaginal Cancer

- Patients may present with painless vaginal bleeding and discharge or an abnormal Pap smear.
- Most are associated with HPV infection and the precursor lesion, VAIN.
- Visual inspection of the vagina as the speculum is being inserted or removed may reveal a gross lesion. Alternatively, vaginal tumors can be detected incidentally as a result of cytologic screening for cervical cancer. The posterior wall of the upper one-third of the vagina is the most commonly affected site. Colposcopy is helpful for visualization. Definitive diagnosis is accomplished by biopsy.
- Staging is performed clinically, based on findings from physical and pelvic examination, cystourethroscopy, proctosigmoidoscopy, and chest radiography. Careful examination of the cervix and vulva is required because involvement would allocate to primary cervical or vulvar cancer, respectively. The prognosis of squamous cell carcinoma of the vagina depends on FIGO staging (Table 54-2).

Table 54-2	International Federation of Gynecology and Obstetrics Staging Classification of Vaginal Cancer and 5-Year Survival[a]	
Stage	Description	5-y Survival
0	Carcinoma in situ, intraepithelial neoplasia	
I	The carcinoma is confined to the vaginal wall.	95%
II	The carcinoma involves subvaginal tissue but has not extended to the pelvic sidewall.	67%
III	The carcinoma extends to the pelvic sidewall.	32%
IV	The carcinoma extends beyond the true pelvis or involves the bladder or rectum; bullous edema as such does not permit a case to be allotted to stage IV.	
IVA·	Tumor invades bladder or rectal mucosa or there is direct extension beyond the true pelvis.	18%
IVB	Spread to distant organs.	Closest to 0%

[a]Adapted from FIGO Committee on Gynecologic Oncology. Current FIGO staging for cancer of the vagina, fallopian tube, ovary, and gestational trophoblastic neoplasia. *Int J Gynaecol Obstet.* 2009;105(1):3-4. Copyright © 2009 International Federation of Gynecology and Obstetrics. Reprinted by permission of John Wiley & Sons, Inc.

Lymphatic dissemination from lesions in the upper third of the vagina spreads to pelvic and para-aortic lymph nodes, whereas tumors in the distal third of the vagina spread to inguinofemoral and then pelvic nodes.

- **Treatment.** Treatment depends on the location, size, and clinical stage of the tumor. Invasive disease can be treated with surgery and/or radiation. Irradiation is treatment of choice for most patients.
  - Surgery is preferred if negative surgical margins can be achieved. Disease limited to the vaginal fornix can be treated with radical hysterectomy and/or partial vaginectomy with parametrectomy and pelvic lymphadenectomy. If the distal third of the vagina is involved, dissection of groin nodes should be performed. Lymph nodes are not accounted for in the FIGO staging system, but identification of nodal disease is important for treatment planning and prognostication. An SLNB is still experimental.
  - Radiotherapy can be delivered by brachytherapy with or without external beam radiation therapy and/or interstitial implants. Proximity of the bladder, urethra, and rectum to the vagina makes radiation treatment planning challenging. Cisplatin is often used for chemosensitization in the setting of radiation therapy.
  - Vaginal brachytherapy includes multiple techniques, with choice based on various factors such as tumor location, disease extent, and response to external beam radiation therapy, with the goal of delivering adequate dose to the target while limiting dose to critical organs.
  - Stage I disease is defined as cancer that is limited to the vaginal mucosa. Primary surgical excision with adjuvant radiation may be appropriate for small primary tumors that do not encroach on important midline structures. Otherwise, treatment of choice most commonly is definitive brachytherapy.
  - Stage II disease is defined as tumor invading submucosal tissues, without positive lymph nodes. Stage II disease is treated with brachytherapy with or without external beam radiation and/or chemotherapy. A primary surgical approach may be selectively applied.
  - Stage III disease is treated with irradiation; an extenterative surgical approach may be selectively applied.
  - Stage IV disease
    - If pelvic nodes are involved, treatment is external beam radiation with or without brachytherapy and/or chemotherapy.
    - Stage IVA disease is defined as tumor invading the bladder or rectum. Consider pelvic exenteration versus external beam radiation.
    - Stage IVB disease: Patients with distant metastases should receive supportive care with palliative intent chemotherapy and/or radiation.
  - Recurrent disease may require pelvic exenteration or other diverting surgeries.

Adenocarcinoma of the Vagina

- Vaginal adenocarcinoma is very rare because the normal vagina does not contain glandular cells. Vaginal adenocarcinomas account for <10% of vaginal cancers. Adenocarcinomas are commonly metastatic from other primary sites (uterus, colon, ovary, kidney, breast) with the exception of primary clear cell cancers. Clear cell adenocarcinoma may arise from areas of adenosis in women exposed to diethylstilbestrol in utero. Diethylstilbestrol was used from 1948 to the early 1970s to support high-risk pregnancies and prevent threatened spontaneous abortion. Screening in these patients should begin at menarche or 14 years of age. Possibly because of early occurrence of abnormal bleeding, the majority of cases are stage I or stage II at diagnosis.

- **Treatment.** In general, adenocarcinoma is treated similarly to squamous cell carcinoma, with both surgery and radiation/chemoradiation as primary treatment options.

Melanoma

- Primary malignant melanoma of the vagina is rare. Bleeding or protrusion of a mass from the vagina is the most common presentation. Importantly, they are often nonpigmented. Staging should be based on tumor thickness (Breslow or American Joint Committee on Cancer, not FIGO or other melanoma staging systems).
- Primary treatment includes radical surgery, radiation, or combinations of radiation and surgery. Modality of treatment does not appreciably affect survival. Groin SLNB may be reasonable for prognostic reasons in women with distal vaginal lesions.
- The majority of relapses are local or regional, often with distant metastases. The lung and liver are the most common remote organs affected. The rate of survival is much lower than that for cutaneous melanomas but is consistent with survival at other mucosal sites. The 5-year survival rate for vaginal melanomas is usually <20%.

Sarcoma

- These rare vaginal malignancies often follow a history of pelvic radiation therapy.
- Treatment is preferably surgery.

Embryonal Rhabdomyosarcoma (Sarcoma Botryoides)

- **Sarcoma botryoides** is a highly malignant tumor that occurs during infancy and early childhood. It usually presents as soft nodules that resembles a bunch of grapes. The polypoid mass may fill or protrude from the vagina (see also chapter 38).
- **Treatment.** Treated with multimodality chemotherapy with vincristine, dactinomycin, and cyclophosphamide and limited surgery in order to preserve reproductive function.

SUGGESTED READINGS

American College of Obstetricians and Gynecologists Committee on Gynecologic Practice, American Society for Colposcopy and Cervical Pathology. ACOG Committee Opinion No. 675: management of vulvar intraepithelial neoplasia. *Obstet Gynecol.* 2016;128:e178-e182. (Reaffirmed 2019)

Apgar B, Cox JT. Differentiating normal and abnormal findings of the vulva. *Am Fam Physician.* 1996;53:1171-1180.

Dellinger TH, Hakim AA, Lee SJ, Wakabayashi MT, Morgan RJ, Han ES. Surgical management of vulvar cancer. *J Natl Compr Canc Netw.* 2017;15(1):121-128.

Duong TH, Flowers LC. Vulvo-vaginal cancers: risks, evaluation, prevention, and early detection. *Obstet Gynecol Clin N Am.* 2007;34:783-802.

Hiniker SM, Roux A, Murphy JD, et al. Primary squamous cell carcinoma of the vagina: prognostic factors, treatment patterns, and outcomes. *Gynecol Oncol.* 2013;131(2):380-385.

Homesley HD, Bundy BN, Sedlis A, et al. Prognostic factors for groin node metastasis in squamous cell carcinoma of the vulva (a Gynecologic Oncology Group study). *Gynecol Oncol.* 1993;49(3):279-283.

Koh WJ, Greer BE, Abu-Rustum NR, et al. Vulvar Cancer, Version 1.2017, NCCN clinical practice guidelines in oncology. *J Natl Compr Canc Netw.* 2017;15(1):92-120.

Leitao MM Jr, Cheng X, Hamilton AL, et al. Gynecologic Cancer InterGroup (GCIG) consensus review for vulvovaginal melanomas. *Int J Gynecol Cancer.* 2014;24(9 suppl 3):S117-S122.

Shrivastava SB, Agrawal G, Mittal M, Mishra P. Management of vaginal cancer. *Rev Recent Clin Trials.* 2015;10(4):289-297.

Te Grootenhuis NC, van der Zee AG, van Doorn HC, et al. Sentinel nodes in vulvar cancer: long-term follow-up of the GROningen INternational Study on Sentinel nodes in Vulvar cancer (GROINSS-V) I. *Gynecol Oncol.* 2016;140(1):8-14.

Van der Zee AG, Oonk MH, De Hullu JA, et al. Sentinel node dissection is safe in the treatment of early-stage vulvar cancer. *J Clin Oncol.* 2008;26:884-889.

Gestational Trophoblastic Disease

Danielle B. Chau and Kimberly Levinson

Gestational trophoblastic disease (GTD) is a heterogeneous group of interrelated but distinct neoplasms derived from the trophoblastic cells of the placenta. Lesions may be benign entities such as placental site tumors; premalignant complete and partial hydatidiform moles; or malignant invasive mole, choriocarcinoma, placental site trophoblastic tumor (PSTT), and epithelioid trophoblastic tumor (ETT). Most women with GTD can be cured with their fertility preserved.

TYPES OF TROPHOBLASTIC CELLS

- Trophoblasts are specialized cells of the early blastocyst that play a role in implantation of the embryo and eventually form the placenta.
- There are three types of placental trophoblastic cells: cytotrophoblast, syncytiotrophoblast, and intermediate trophoblast.
  - **Cytotrophoblasts** comprise the inner layer of the trophoblast. They are primitive trophoblastic cells that are polygonal to oval in shape. They exhibit a single nucleus and clearly defined borders. Mitotic activity is evident because these cells behave like stem cells. Implantation of the embryo is dependent on functioning cytotrophoblasts. Cytotrophoblasts do not produce either β-human chorionic gonadotropin (β-hCG) or human placental lactogen (hPL).
  - **Syncytiotrophoblasts** comprise the outer layer of the trophoblast. They are well-differentiated cells that interface with the maternal circulation and produce most of the placental hormones. No mitotic activity is evident. Syncytiotrophoblasts demonstrate β-hCG production at 12 days of gestation. Secretion rapidly increases and peaks by 8 to 10 weeks, with a decline thereafter. By 40 weeks, β-hCG is present only focally in syncytiotrophoblasts. At 12 days, hPL is also present in syncytiotrophoblasts. Production continues to rise throughout pregnancy.

- **Intermediate trophoblasts** show infiltrative growth into decidua, myometrium, and blood vessels, and in a normal pregnancy, they anchor the placenta to maternal tissue. Intermediate trophoblasts characteristically invade the wall of large vascular channels until the wall is completely replaced. As early as 12 days after conception, β-hCG and hPL are present focally in intermediate trophoblasts. However, at 6 weeks, β-hCG production disappears, whereas secretion of hPL peaks at 11 to 15 weeks gestation.

CLASSIFICATION OF GESTATIONAL TROPHOBLASTIC DISEASE: ETIOLOGY, PATHOLOGY, AND CLINICAL PRESENTATION

GTD is unique among human neoplastic disorders because each type is genetically related to fetal tissues. The molecular pathogenesis of these tumors is an area of active research interest. Classification can be divided into nonneoplastic trophoblastic lesions, molar pregnancy, and gestational trophoblastic neoplasia (GTN).

Nonneoplastic Trophoblastic Lesions: Exaggerated Placental Sites and Placental Site Nodules

Exaggerated Placental Sites

- **Etiology:** Exaggerated placental sites (EPSs) can occur after any pregnancy; however, they more frequently occur with molar pregnancies. They likely represent excessive production of placental tissue rather than a separate pathologic process.
- **Pathology:** EPSs are characterized by extensive infiltration of the endometrium and myometrium by intermediate trophoblastic cells that often have irregularly shaped nuclei without evidence of mitotic activity. Chorionic villi are present, given that EPSs occur with a concurrent pregnancy. These lesions will show strong staining for hPL and focal staining for placental alkaline phosphatase (PLAP).
- **Clinical presentation:** These are most often incidental findings.

Placental Site Nodules

- **Etiology:** Placental site nodules (PSNs) are lesions most commonly found in the endometrium of reproductive aged women. Occasionally, extrauterine PSNs can be found in the fallopian tubes (4%), likely as a result of a tubal ectopic pregnancy, or in the endocervix (up to 40% in one case series).
- **Pathology:** Gross findings include well-circumscribed yellow-tan nodules and, less frequently, multiple nodules or plaques. PSNs contain intermediate trophoblasts separated by an abundant fibrinous extracellular matrix. These lesions show strong staining for PLAP and focal staining for hPL.
- **Clinical presentation:** These are most often incidental findings.

Molar Pregnancy: Complete and Incomplete Mole

Hydatidiform moles, or molar pregnancies, have an excess of paternal genetic material compared to maternal genetic material. See Table 55-1 for comparison of complete versus incomplete (partial) molar pregnancy.

Complete Mole

- **Etiology:** In most cases of complete moles, all of the chromosomal complements are paternally derived. The more common 46,XX genotype typically results from

Table 55-1	Comparison of Complete Versus Partial Hydatidiform Mole[a]	
	Complete	**Partial**
Karyotype	Most commonly 46,XX or 46,XY	Most commonly 69,XXX or 69,XXY
Uterine size		
Large for gestational age	33%	10%
Small for gestational age	33%	65%
Diagnosis by ultrasonography	Common	Rare
Theca lutein cysts	25%-35%	Rare
β-hCG (mIU/mL)	>50 000	<50 000
Malignant potential	15%-25%	<5%
Metastatic disease	<5%	<1%

[a]Adapted with permission from Soper JT. Gestational trophoblastic disease. *Obstet Gynecol.* 2006; 108(1):176-187. Copyright © 2006 by The American College of Obstetricians and Gynecologists.

duplication of a haploid sperm pronucleus in an empty ovum. Three percent to 13% of complete moles have a 46,XY chromosome complement, presumably as a result of dispermy, in which an empty ovum is fertilized by two sperm pronuclei.

- **Pathology:** Gross findings include massively enlarged, edematous villi that give the classic grape-like appearance to the placenta and lack embryonic tissue. Microscopic examination shows hydropic swelling in the majority of villi, accompanied by a variable degree of trophoblastic proliferation. Complete moles have widespread, diffuse immunostaining for β-hCG; moderately diffuse staining for hPL; and focal staining for PLAP.

- **Clinical presentation:** Vaginal bleeding is the most common presenting symptom, occurring in 97% of cases. Uterine size may be greater than expected for gestational age; however, in approximately one-third of patients, the uterus is small for gestational age. Ovarian enlargement caused by theca lutein cysts occurs in 25% to 35% of cases. Serum β-hCG levels are generally above 50,000 mIU/mL.

- Complications may occur and include severe hyperemesis and pregnancy-induced hypertension, which can develop in up to 25% of women, with hyperthyroidism in 7% of cases.

Incomplete Mole

- **Etiology:** Karyotyping of incomplete moles most frequently shows triploidy with two paternal and one maternal chromosome. The chromosomal complement is 69,XXY in 70% of cases, 69,XXX in 27% of cases, and 69,XYY in 3% of cases. The abnormal conceptus in these cases arises from the fertilization of an egg with a haploid set of chromosomes either by two sperm, each with a set of haploid chromosomes, or by a single sperm with a diploid 46,XY complement.

- **Pathology:** Gross findings reveal fetal tissue in nearly all instances, although its discovery may require careful examination because early fetal death often takes place (ie, 8-9 wk gestational age). Microscopic examination finds two populations of chorionic villi: one of normal size and the other grossly hydropic. Partial moles show focal to moderate immunostaining for β-hCG and diffuse staining for hPL and PLAP.

- **Clinical presentation:** A clinical diagnosis of a missed or spontaneous abortion is made in 91% of women with incomplete molar pregnancy, and patients report abnormal uterine bleeding in about 75% of cases. Uterine size is generally small for gestational dates, and excessive uterine size is observed in less than 10% of patients. Serum β-hCG levels are in the normal or low range for gestational age. Preeclampsia occurs with a lower incidence (2.5%) and presents much later with partial mole than with a complete mole but can be equally severe.

Gestational Trophoblastic Neoplasia: Invasive Mole, Choriocarcinoma, and Placenta Site and Epithelioid Trophoblastic Tumor

Invasive Mole

- **Etiology:** Invasive mole is an important complication of hydatidiform mole, representing 70% to 90% of cases of persistent GTD.
- **Pathology:** Histologically, hydropic chorionic villi migrate into the myometrium, vascular spaces, or outside of the pelvis in 20% of cases to the vagina, perineum, or lungs. Grossly, invasive moles present as erosive, hemorrhagic lesions extending from the uterine cavity into the myometrium. Metastasis can range from superficial penetration to extension through the uterine wall, with subsequent perforation and life-threatening hemorrhage. Molar vesicles are often apparent. Microscopically, the diagnostic feature of invasive mole is the presence of molar villi and trophoblast within the myometrium or at an extrauterine site. Lesions at distant sites are usually composed of molar villi confined within blood vessels, without invasion into adjacent tissue.
- **Clinical presentation:** A plateau or rise in β-hCG titers is typically the first indication of an invasive mole. Patients may also present with recurrent vaginal bleeding after dilation and curettage (D&C).

Choriocarcinoma

- **Etiology:** Gestational choriocarcinoma is a highly malignant epithelial tumor that can be associated with any type of gestational event, most often a complete hydatidiform mole. In the United States, choriocarcinoma occurs in 1 in 20,000 to 40,000 pregnancies. Approximately 25% of gestational choriocarcinomas develop after term pregnancies, 50% after molar gestations, and 25% after abortion or ectopic pregnancies. Early systemic hematogenous metastasis often takes place.
- **Pathology:** On gross examination, these tumors appear as dark red, hemorrhagic masses with shaggy, irregular surfaces. Metastatic lesions outside the uterus are well circumscribed. On microscopic examination, sheets of syncytiotrophoblasts and cytotrophoblasts are seen without chorionic villi, invading surrounding tissue or permeating vascular spaces.
- **Clinical presentation:** A plateau or rise in β-hCG titers is typically the first indication of choriocarcinoma. Other presenting signs and symptoms are related to the anatomic sites involved with metastatic disease: chest pain, hemoptysis, or persistent cough with pulmonary involvement; bleeding from vaginal extensions; and focal neurologic deficits from cerebral hemorrhage. Eighty percent of patients with extrauterine disease show pulmonary metastases, whereas approximately 30% demonstrate extension to the vagina. Ten percent of women also exhibit liver and CNS involvement.

Placental Site and Epithelioid Trophoblastic Tumor

- **Etiology:** PSTT and ETT are rare gestational trophoblastic neoplasms, accounting for 1% of persistent GTD. Both can develop long after prior gestational events. Most cases of PSTT and ETT are confined to the uterus, but 15% to 25% of cases present with local invasion or distant spread.
- **Pathology:** In contrast to the normal implantation site, where invasion of the extravillous subtype of intermediate trophoblast is tightly regulated and confined to the inner third of the myometrium, tumor cells of PSTT and ETT are invasive and infiltrate deeply into the myometrium. Although PSTT and ETT share similar clinical features, careful examination of tumor histology and gene-expression patterns show that PSTT and ETT are composed of different extravillous trophoblastic cells. Gross lesions may be barely visible or may result in diffuse nodular enlargement of the myometrium. Most tumors are well circumscribed. Microscopically, invasion may extend to the uterine serosa and, in rare instances, extends to adnexal structures.
- **Clinical presentation:** PSTTs and ETTs usually remain confined to the uterus and metastasize late. In some cases, recurrent or metastatic PSTT/ETTs can occur in patients long after initial treatment. These tumors typically produce only small amounts of β-hCG, despite a large tumor burden. Serum hPL, produced by the intermediate trophoblasts that predominate, serves as a better marker for disease progression or recurrence. Approximately 15% of lesions metastasize to extrauterine sites (eg, lungs, liver, abdominal cavity, and brain).

DIAGNOSIS AND MANAGEMENT

Nonneoplastic Trophoblastic Lesions

- EPSs and PSNs are benign forms of GTD that are often incidental findings on a biopsy or hysterectomy specimen.

Molar Pregnancy

- Incidence of molar pregnancy varies widely throughout the world, with the highest rates reported in Asia, Africa, and Latin America. In the United States, hydatidiform moles are observed in 1 in 600 therapeutic abortions and 1 in 1000 to 1200 pregnancies.
- Approximately 20% of patients require treatment for malignant sequelae after evacuation of hydatidiform mole.

Risk Factors

- **Extremes of reproductive age.** Women over age 40 years have a 5.2-fold increased risk, whereas women younger than age 20 years have a 1.5-fold increased risk. Persistent GTD occurs more frequently in older patients.
- **History of previous hydatidiform mole.** The risk of a subsequent hydatidiform mole rises by 10- to 20-fold. With two previous molar pregnancies, the risk increases by 40-fold. Conversely, term pregnancies and live births produce a protective effect.
- **History of spontaneous abortions** doubles the risk of molar gestation.
- **Race.** Asian and Latin American women demonstrate a higher risk of being diagnosed with GTD, whereas North American and European women have lower risk.

- **Low socioeconomic status** and **dietary factors** (such as vitamin A deficiency and low carotene intake) as well as **cigarette smoking** and **oral contraceptive use** may be associated. However, these associations are weak and not demonstrated consistently across all studies.

Imaging and Lab Evaluation

The following imaging should be performed for evaluation:
- **Pelvic ultrasound.** Ultrasound usually establishes the diagnosis, identifying a mixed echogenic pattern (villi and blood clots replace normal placental tissue). Ultrasonography often, but not always, shows a classic "snowstorm" appearance for complete hydatidiform moles and fetal parts/tissue for incomplete hydatidiform moles.
- **Chest radiograph.** If the chest x-ray is positive for metastases, it should be managed as GTN (see below) after initial uterine evacuation.

The following imaging should be obtained preoperatively:
- Quantitative serum β-hCG level
- Complete blood count
- Complete chemistry profile including liver and renal function tests
- Thyroid function tests
- Blood type and screen (Rh-negative patients must be given $Rh_O[D]$ immune globulin.)

Pathologic Diagnosis

- The **pathologic diagnosis** of hydatidiform mole is typically made following D&C performed for an incomplete abortion or because of suspicion of hydatidiform mole based on clinical findings (see above for pathologic features).

Management

Despite the cytogenetic, pathologic, and clinical differences between a complete and incomplete (partial) mole, the management is similar. The **primary treatment** for hydatidiform mole is suction D&C, preferably under ultrasound guidance.
- **Preoperative considerations**
  - Stabilization of medical complications
  - Full operating room support in a hospital setting
  - Large-bore intravenous access
  - Induction of regional or general anesthesia
- **Intraoperative considerations**
  - Uterine evacuation should be accomplished with the largest cannula that can be safely introduced through the cervix. Uterotonic drugs should be initiated at the time of uterine evacuation, keeping in mind that oxytocin receptors may not be present. Therefore, alternatives to Pitocin should be available.
  - Hysterectomy may be considered as initial treatment for hydatidiform mole in patients who are older or do not wish to preserve fertility.
  - Prophylactic chemotherapy with methotrexate (MTX) or dactinomycin may be considered at the time of evacuation of a hydatidiform mole in patients at high risk for postmolar GTN (age >40 y, β-hCG >100 000 mIU/mL, excessive uterine enlargement, theca lutein cysts >6 cm) or if β-hCG follow-up is unavailable or unreliable.

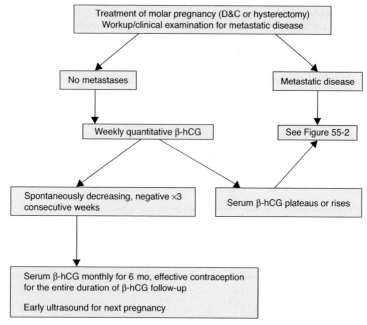

Figure 55-1. Follow-up of molar pregnancy. Abbreviations: β-hCG, β-human chorionic gonadotropin; D&C, dilation and curettage. Data from Berkowitz RS, Horowitz NS, Goldstein DP. Gestational trophoblastic disease. In: Berek JS, ed. *Berek & Novak's Gynecology.* 16th ed. Philadelphia, PA: Wolters Kluwer; 2020:1170-1185.

- **Postoperative considerations**
  - **Medical complications** occur in approximately 25% of patients and are more prominent in those with uterine enlargement >14 to 16 weeks' gestational size. Complications include anemia, infection, hyperthyroidism, pregnancy-induced hypertension or preeclampsia, and theca lutein cysts.
  - **Postevacuation follow-up** should include the following:
    - ○ Effective contraception for the entire interval of β-hCG follow-up testing. Preventing pregnancy is important, as a rising β-hCG titer due to a normal pregnancy cannot be distinguished from persistent GTD.
    - ○ Pelvic examination 1 month after initial treatment to monitor for involution of pelvic organs and for detection of metastasis
    - ○ β-hCG level 48 hours after evacuation, then weekly β-hCG levels until three consecutive negative results, and then monthly until results are negative for 6 consecutive months (Figure 55-1).

Considerations for Future Pregnancies

- Patients with a history of molar pregnancy should be counseled that there is no difference in reproductive outcomes such as stillbirth and miscarriage compared to the general population. However, because of the increased risk (1%-2%) of a second mole in subsequent pregnancies, all future pregnancies should be evaluated by ultrasonography early in their course.

Persistent Gestational Trophoblastic Disease/Gestational Trophoblastic Neoplasia

- Persistent GTD or GTN includes invasive mole, choriocarcinoma, PSTT, and ETT. Persistent disease occurs in approximately 20% of cases of complete mole; approximately 15% develop invasive GTD and <5% develop metastatic GTD. The risk of persistent GTD is considerably lower for partial moles (1%-5%). Gestational choriocarcinoma, by comparison, occurs in about 1 in 20,000 to 40,000 pregnancies.
- Although much less common than hydatidiform mole or choriocarcinoma, PSTT and ETT can develop after any type of pregnancy. Over 95% of malignant sequelae occur within 6 months after surgical evacuation.
- If β-hCG levels plateau or rise, immediate evaluation is required, and treatment for persistent GTD may be indicated.

Risk Factors

- Risk factors for persistent GTD include large-for-dates uterus, ovarian enlargement due to theca lutein cysts, recurrent molar pregnancy, uterine subinvolution, advanced maternal age, significantly elevated β-hCG level, and acute pulmonary compromise.

Imaging and Lab Evaluation

A plateau or rise in β-hCG titers is typically the first indication of persistent GTD. PSTTs and ETTs typically demonstrate low β-hCG levels; however, serum hPL level is often elevated and may be a more useful serologic marker.

- All patients suspected of having persistent GTD should undergo the following workup to evaluate the extent of disease (Figure 55-2):
  - Pelvic ultrasound
  - Chest radiograph
  - Computed tomography of pelvis, abdomen, chest, and brain (only if chest radiograph shows metastases)
  - Serum β-hCG level, possibly serum hPL level
  - Complete blood count
  - Complete chemistry profile including liver and renal function tests
  - Thyroid function tests

Diagnostic Criteria

- **Criteria** for persistent GTD include the following:
  - β-hCG level plateau of four measurements ± 10% recorded over a 3-week duration
  - β-hCG level increase of >10% for three measurements over a 2-week duration
  - Detectable β-hCG for >6 months after molar evacuation
  - Presence of metastatic disease
  - Histologic diagnosis of choriocarcinoma. Rarely, the diagnosis of persistent GTD is made via histologic evidence or pathologic diagnosis; however, obtaining a tissue diagnosis is not necessary and may be associated with significant hemorrhage.

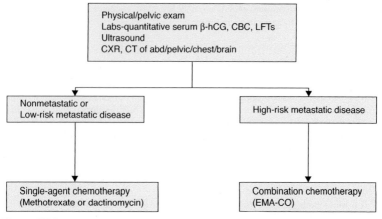

Figure 55-2. Management of persistent gestational trophoblastic disease. Abbreviations: abd, abdomen; β-hCG, β-human chorionic gonadotropin; CBC, complete blood count; CT, computed tomography; CXR, chest radiograph; EMA-CO, etoposide, methotrexate, dactinomycin, cyclophosphamide, and vincristine; LFTs, liver function tests. Data from Berkowitz RS, Goldstein DP. Gestational trophoblastic disease. In: Berek JS, Hacker NF, eds. *Berek & Hacker's Gynecologic Oncology.* 6th ed. Philadelphia, PA: Wolters Kluwer; 2015:625-648.

Staging and Management of Gestational Trophoblastic Neoplasia

- **Staging.** International Federation of Gynecology and Obstetrics (FIGO) staging describes stage I disease as GTN confined to the uterus with varying levels of metastases for stages II to IV (Table 55-2).
- **Treatment** depends on the stage of disease and risk assessment based on the World Health Organization (WHO) prognostic scoring system. Factors include age, antecedent pregnancy, time since antecedent pregnancy, initial β-hCG levels, largest tumor size, site and number of metastases, and prior failed chemotherapy (Table 55-3).

Table 55-2	International Federation of Gynecology and Obstetrics Staging System for Gestational Trophoblastic Neoplasia[a,b]
Stage	Description
I	Strictly confined to uterus
II	Extension outside uterus but limited to pelvic structures
III	Extension to lungs
IV	All other metastatic sites

[a]Each stage is divided into high or low risk using the World Health Organization Prognostic Scoring Index.

[b]From FIGO Committee on Gynecologic Oncology. Current FIGO staging for cancer of the vagina, fallopian tube, ovary, and gestational trophoblastic neoplasia. *Int J Gynecol Obstet.* 2009;105(1):3-4. Copyright © 2009 International Federation of Gynecology and Obstetrics. Reprinted by permission of John Wiley & Sons, Inc.

Table 55-3	International Federation of Gynecology and Obstetrics/ World Health Organization Prognostic Scoring Index for Gestational Trophoblastic Neoplasia[a,b]			
Score	0	1	2	4
Age	<40 y	≥40 y		
Antecedent pregnancy	Mole	Abortion	Term	
Time since pregnancy	<4 mo	4-6 mo	7-12 mo	>12 mo
Initial β-hCG levels (mIU/mL)	<1000	1000-9999	10 000-99 999	≥100 000
Largest tumor size (in cm, including uterus)	<3	3-4	5 or more	
Site of metastases	Lung, vagina	Spleen, kidney	Gastrointestinal tract	Brain, liver
Number of metastases	0	1-4	5-8	>8
Prior failed chemotherapy	None		Single drug	≥2 drugs

Abbreviation: β-hCG, β-human chorionic gonadotropin.
[a]The total score is obtained by adding the scores for individual prognostic factors. Scores from 0 to 6 are categorized as low risk, whereas a score of 7 or higher is high risk.
[b]Adapted from Kohorn EI. The new FIGO 2000 staging and risk factor scoring system for gestational trophoblastic disease: description and clinical assessment. *Int J Gynecol Cancer.* 2001;11:73-77.

- Note that the prognostic scoring system does not apply to intermediate trophoblastic tumors, and their treatment is discussed separately.

Management of Nonmetastatic Disease and Low-Risk Metastatic Disease

- **Low-risk disease** is GTN with a calculated WHO prognostic score ≤6.
- **Primary treatment** is most commonly single-agent chemotherapy with either Methotrexate (MTX) or dactinomycin.
  - The MTX is alternated with folinic acid in most institutions for a total 8-day course and administered every 2 weeks; however, MTX can also be given daily for 5 days without folinic acid and repeated every 2 weeks, most commonly for disease with a WHO score <5. Although some evidence suggests that dactinomycin may provide slightly higher remission rates than MTX, MTX is typically considered first-line therapy for low-risk GTN, given the high toxicity profile of dactinomycin. Pulsed dactinomycin (higher dose administered every 2 wk) generally is used more frequently than the biweekly 5-day regimen.
- **Duration of course.** During chemotherapy, β-hCG levels are monitored every 2 weeks at the start of each cycle. Systemic treatments are administered until two to

three full cycles past normalization of β-hCG levels. Chemotherapy cycles should be held if white blood cell count $<3.0 \times 10^3/\mu L$ and absolute neutrophil count $<1.5 \times 10^3/\mu L$, or in the presence of persistent mucositis.

- **Surgical considerations.** Repeat D&C may also be considered and may decrease the number of patients requiring chemotherapy. Hysterectomy with salpingectomy may also be considered for disease confined to the uterus in patients who do not desire future fertility. Ovaries should be left in situ, regardless of the presence of theca lutein cysts.
  - For disease treated with surgical intervention alone, further monitoring is with serial lab values similar to GTD (β-hCG every 2 wk until 3 consecutive normal assays, followed by monthly β-hCG for 6 mo). Treatment failure require chemotherapy.

Management of Treatment Failure for Low-Risk Disease

- If a patient has a good response to initial therapy followed by plateau of β-hCG levels (<10% decrease in β-hCG over two treatment cycles), the patient is considered **resistant** to that particular chemotherapeutic agent, and the alternative single-agent chemotherapy may be instituted. *Note:* Pulsed dactinomycin cannot be used as secondary therapy and instead should be given daily for 5 days and repeated every 14 days. If no response is seen after both single agents, then a repeat workup for metastasis should be performed, and combination chemotherapy with EMA-CO is required.
- If β-hCG titers have a rapid rise (>10% from last value) after the first treatment cycle or titers plateau (<10% decrease over two treatment cycles) with the first two treatment cycles, the patient is considered to have a **poor response to initial therapy** and single-agent therapy should be discontinued and replaced by EMA-CO (see "Management of High-Risk or Metastatic Disease").

Prognosis for Low-Risk Disease

- Following completion of chemotherapy, patients are followed with monthly β-hCG levels for 12 months. Oral contraceptive pills are the preferred method of birth control during surveillance because they suppress luteinizing hormone/follicle-stimulating hormone, which may interfere with β-hCG at low levels.
- Overall, 85% to 95% of patients can be cured with single-agent chemotherapy without hysterectomy. The cure rate for patients with low-risk disease approaches 100% with recurrence rates <5%.

Management of High-Risk or Metastatic Disease

- **High-risk disease** is GTN with a calculated WHO prognostic score ≥7.
- **Primary treatment** for patients with high-risk disease is combination chemotherapy with etoposide, MTX, dactinomycin, cyclophosphamide, and vincristine (EMA-CO).
- **Induction chemotherapy.** Low-dose etoposide and cisplatin given weekly on days 1 and 2 for one to three courses can be considered prior to starting EMA-CO therapy in patients with WHO prognostic scores >12, who are at significant risk for pulmonary, intraperitoneal, or intracranial hemorrhage.
- **Duration of course.** EMA-CO is administered every 2 weeks until remission or until intolerable side effects occur. During chemotherapy, β-hCG levels are monitored every 2 weeks at the start of each cycle. After the normalization of β-hCG levels, an additional three courses should be given as consolidation therapy.
- **Prophylaxis considerations.** Granulocyte-colony stimulating factor can be administered on days 9 through 14 of each EMA-CO cycle for secondary prophylaxis of neutropenic fever.

Management of Treatment Failure for High-Risk Disease

- If the patient has a **poor response to initial EMA-CO therapy**, salvage therapy often consists of platinum etoposide combinations like EMA-EP (etoposide, MTX, dactinomycin, etoposide, cisplatin). Bleomycin and ifosfamide regimens (VIP, ICE) have also been used. Experimental protocols may also be investigated in these patients. Additionally, if feasible, consideration should be given to surgical resection of chemotherapy-resistant disease.
- If patients have a good response to initial therapy, followed by plateau of β-hCG levels (<10% decrease in β-hCG over two treatment cycles), the patient is considered **resistant to EMA-CO therapy**, and platinum/etoposide combination chemotherapy should be initiated. Similarly, if a patient has return of positive β-hCG after treatment, she is considered to have a **relapse from remission** and would require platinum/etoposide combination therapy.

Specific Considerations for Management of Metastatic Disease Sites

For patients with **complications** of metastatic disease specific to the organ involved, the following interventions can be instituted:

- **Vaginal involvement.** These lesions can bleed profusely, and biopsy should therefore be avoided. Bleeding can be controlled with packing for 24 hours. Prompt radiation to the affected region may provide further hemostasis. Embolization of the pelvic vessels may also be implemented in women with life-threatening or recurrent hemorrhage.
- **Pulmonary metastases.** These lesions usually respond to chemotherapy. Occasionally, thoracotomy is required to remove a persistent viable tumor nodule. Favorable outcomes from resection include absence of other metastatic sites, presence of a solitary nodule, no uterine involvement, and β-hCG <1500 mIU/mL. Not all chest lesions clear radiographically due to scarring and fibrosis from the injury and healing process.
- **Hepatic lesions.** If these lesions fail to respond to systemic chemotherapy, other options include hepatic arterial infusion of chemotherapy or partial hepatic resection to remove resistant tumor. These lesions are usually hypervascular and prone to hemorrhage if biopsied.
- **Cerebral metastases.** The MTX and folinic acid doses in EMA-CO therapy are increased in the setting of brain metastases. Whole-brain irradiation (typically 30 Gy in 15 fractions) may also be considered. Radiation and chemotherapy reduce the risk of spontaneous cerebral hemorrhage. However, concurrent whole brain radiation and chemotherapy increase treatment-related toxicity, especially leukoencephalopathy (radiographic diffuse white matter changes with symptoms of lethargy, seizures, and dysarthria, and rarely ataxia, dementia, memory loss, and death). Alternatively, cerebral metastases can be treated with stereotactic brain radiotherapy with or without intrathecal MTX. Craniotomy can be considered for peripheral isolated drug-resistant lesions.
- **Extensive uterine disease.** Hysterectomy can be considered in cases with large intrauterine tumor burden, infection, or hemorrhage. Concurrent removal of the ovaries is not indicated given that ovarian metastases are rare.

Prognosis for High-Risk Disease

- Following completion of chemotherapy, patients are followed with monthly β-hCG levels for 12 months. The importance of birth control during this surveillance period should be emphasized with the patients, as previously stated.
- Following EMA-CO, the overall remission rate is 80% to 90%. Approximately 25% of high-risk patients demonstrate incomplete responses to first-line therapy and relapse. When brain metastases are present, the overall remission rate drops to

50% to 60%. Higher failure rates are also seen with stage IV disease, greater than eight metastatic lesions, and a history of previous chemotherapy.

Considerations for Future Pregnancies

- Although some studies have demonstrated that patients who have received chemotherapy for treatment of GTN have a slightly increased risk of stillbirth in subsequent pregnancies, patients should be counseled that overall, they can expect similar pregnancy outcomes compared to the general population.
- Surveillance in subsequent pregnancies can include pathologic analysis of the placenta for evidence of GTD and a β-hCG level at 6 weeks' postpartum.

Management of Intermediate Trophoblastic Tumors: Placental Site Trophoblastic Tumor and Epithelioid Trophoblastic Tumor

- **Primary treatment.** For intermediate trophoblastic tumors, treatment decisions are based on FIGO stage of disease. In contrast to other trophoblastic tumors, these tumors are relatively insensitive to chemotherapy, and surgical excision is usually the best treatment modality.
- For patients with **stage I PSTT**, or disease confined to the uterus, the primary treatment is hysterectomy with or without pelvic lymph node biopsy (given estimated incidence of positive nodes in 5%-15% of clinical stage I tumors). Patients with poor prognostic factors (high mitotic rates [5/10 HPFs], deep myometrial invasion, extensive coagulative necrosis, lymphovascular space invasion [LVSI], and interval since last pregnancy >2 years) should be considered for systemic therapy.
- For patients with **metastatic intermediate trophoblastic disease**, treatment is with hysterectomy, possible excision of metastatic disease (if feasible), and initiation of a platinum/etoposide-containing regimen such as EMA-EP.
- **Prophylaxis considerations.** Granulocyte-colony stimulating factor can be administered on days 9 through 14 of each EMA-CO cycle for secondary prophylaxis of neutropenic fever.

Prognosis for Intermediate Trophoblastic Tumors

- Poor prognostic factors in PSTT are high mitotic rates (5/10 HPFs), deep myometrial invasion, extensive coagulative necrosis, LVSI, and interval since last pregnancy >2 years.
- The β-hCG is often not a reliable marker for patients with intermediate trophoblastic disease. Serum hPL can serve as a better marker for disease progression or recurrence. If no reliable serum marker is available, surveillance can be performed with imaging. Consider PET/CT for follow-up at the completion of chemotherapy and then every 6 to 12 months for 2 to 3 years.

SUGGESTED READINGS

Lurain JR. Gestational trophoblastic disease I: epidemiology, pathology, clinical presentation and diagnosis of gestational trophoblastic disease, and management of hydatidiform mole. *Am J Obstet Gynecol.* 2010;203(6):531-539.

Lurain JR. Gestational trophoblastic disease II: classification and management of gestational trophoblastic neoplasia. *Am J Obstet Gynecol.* 2011;204(1):11-18.

56 Chemotherapy, Antineoplastic Therapy, and Radiation Therapy

Tiffany Nicole Jones and Stéphanie Gaillard

- Treatment of gynecologic cancer typically requires a multidisciplinary and multi-treatment approach, often involving a combination of surgery, **chemotherapy**, and **antineoplastic and radiation therapy**. These modalities can be administered sequentially or in combination, as with chemoradiation or intraoperative radiation therapy.
- **Primary** treatment refers to initial therapy, including two special cases: (1) **adjuvant** therapy, which is treatment administered for micrometastatic disease after surgical management, and (2) **neoadjuvant** therapy, consisting of induction chemotherapy, radiation therapy, targeted therapy, or combination therapy administered before definitive surgical management. In the recurrent setting, therapies are often referred to by their sequence after primary treatment (second line, third line, etc).
- Methods used to treat gynecologic cancer are potentially damaging to normal tissue. Thus, the governing principle of all antineoplastic therapies is to maximize the therapeutic cytotoxic effect on cancer cells while minimizing toxicity to normal tissues. Unfortunately, obtaining a therapeutic effect without temporarily or permanently altering function of healthy cells, tissues, or organs is not always possible. The **therapeutic index** is the ratio of a toxic dose to the effective dose. An optimal treatment goal is to use chemotherapy agents and radiation doses that have a high therapeutic index.

CELL CYCLE

- The cell cycle is a sequence of events that results in the division of a cell into two identical daughter cells (Figure 56-1). Within the cell cycle are two main phases: interphase and mitosis. Interphase is composed of **G1 phase** (the period of cell growth before the DNA is duplicated), **S phase** (the period when chromosomal DNA is duplicated), and **G2 phase** (the period when DNA duplication is complete and the cell prepares for division). **Mitosis** refers to the division of the parent cell into two daughter cells. Tumor cells grow as a result of deregulation between proliferation and growth suppression or cellular death. Our understanding of cancer cell kinetics and the classical cell cycle has led to the development of drugs that disrupt cell cycle progression or induce cellular death.
- Chemotherapies are chemical compounds found to have general cytotoxic properties. Chemotherapeutic agents may be characterized by their effect on the cell cycle.
  - **Cell cycle–specific** chemotherapeutic agents depend on the proliferative capacity of the cell and the phase of the cell cycle for their mechanism of action. They are effective against tumors with relatively long S phases and rapid proliferation rates.
  - **Cell cycle–nonspecific** chemotherapeutic agents kill cells in all phases of the cell cycle; their effectiveness is not dependent on proliferative capacity. Radiation therapy is considered cell cycle nonspecific.

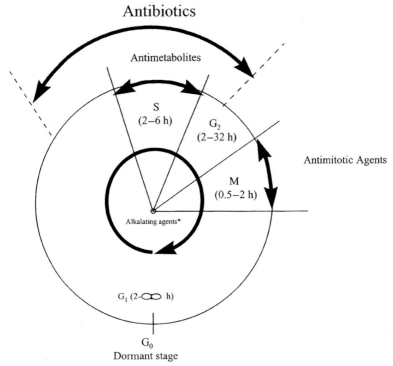

Figure 56-1. Phases of the cell cycle, relative time intervals, and sites of action of the various classes of antineoplastic agents. Reprinted with permission from Trimble EL, Trimble CL. *Cancer Obstetrics and Gynecology.* Philadelphia, PA: Lippincott Williams & Wilkins; 1999:60.

CHEMOTHERAPY, TARGETED THERAPY, AND HORMONAL AGENTS

Chemotherapy

Chemotherapeutic agents commonly used for the treatment of gynecologic cancer may be grouped into the following categories (Table 56-1):

- **Alkylating agents** are **cell cycle nonspecific** (eg, cyclophosphamide, ifosfamide, cisplatin, carboplatin). They contain an alkyl group that forms a covalent bond with the DNA helix, preventing DNA duplication. They also function by attaching to free guanine bases of DNA, thereby prohibiting their action as templates for new DNA formation.

- **Antimetabolites** are **cell cycle specific** (eg, 5-fluorouracil [5-FU], methotrexate, gemcitabine) and are similar in chemical structure to compounds required by normal and tumor cells for cell division. These antimetabolites may be incorporated into new nuclear material or combined with enzymes to inhibit cell division.

Table 56-1	Chemotherapeutic Agents Commonly Used in Gynecologic Cancers and Their Most Common Toxicities

Chemotherapeutic Agent	Toxicity
Alkylating agents	
Cyclophosphamide (Cytoxan)	• Myelosuppression (WBCs > Plt), hemorrhagic cystitis, bladder fibrosis, alopecia, hepatitis, amenorrhea
Ifosfamide	• Myelosuppression, hemorrhagic cystitis, CNS dysfunction, renal toxicity, vomiting
Alkylating-like agents	
Cis-dichloro-diamino-platinum (Cisplatin)	• Nephrotoxicity, vomiting, tinnitus and hearing loss, myelosuppression, peripheral neuropathy characterized by paresthesia of the extremities
	• Renal insufficiency is the major dose-limiting toxic effect causing elevations in BUN, serum creatinine, and serum uric acid levels within 2 wk of treatment. Can lead to irreversible damage. Prevention with IV hydration; diuretics is important during treatment. Obtain 24-h creatinine clearance to establish baseline renal function prior to treatment.
	• Tinnitus or high-frequency hearing loss may be cumulative and possibly irreversible. Audiograms may be obtained prior to and during treatment to assess hearing loss.
Carboplatin	• Less neuropathy, ototoxicity, and nephrotoxicity but more myelosuppression (Plt > WBC) than cisplatin
Antitumor antibiotics	
Actinomycin D (Dactinomycin)	• Nausea and vomiting, skin necrosis, mucosal ulceration, myelosuppression, alopecia
Bleomycin sulfate	• Pulmonary toxicity, fever, anaphylactic reactions, dermatologic reactions, mucositis, alopecia
	• May cause significant pulmonary fibrosis. Generally, both dose and age related but can be idiopathic. Pulmonary function tests are performed to assess baseline pulmonary capacity before the first dose is administered.
	• Can cause anaphylaxis, skin reactions, fever, and chills. Because of the high incidence of allergic reactions, patients are given a test dose of 2-4 U intramuscularly prior to first dose of drug.

(Continued)

Table 56-1	Chemotherapeutic Agents Commonly Used in Gynecologic Cancers and Their Most Common Toxicities *(Continued)*
Chemotherapeutic Agent	**Toxicity**
Doxorubicin hydrochloride (Adriamycin)	• Myelosuppression, cardiac toxicity, alopecia, mucosal ulcerations, vomiting, cholestasis, hyperpigmentation
	• Irreversible cardiomyopathies involve progressive congestive heart failure, pleural effusions, heart dilation, and venous congestion. These are generally cumulative; therefore, dosages are kept under the maximum. The MUGA scans are commonly obtained prior to treatment to obtain a baseline ejection fraction and may be repeated as necessary.
Liposomal doxorubicin (Doxil)	• Myelosuppression, skin and mucosal toxicity, hand-foot syndrome, significantly reduced risk of cardiomyopathy compared to doxorubicin
Antimetabolites	
5-Fluorouracil (5-FU)	• Myelosuppression, vomiting, anorexia, alopecia, hyperpigmentation, mucosal ulceration, cardiotoxicities (MI, angina, arrhythmia)
Methotrexate sodium (MTX)	• Myelosuppression, mucosal ulceration (stomatitis and mucositis), hepatotoxicity, acute pulmonary infiltrates that respond to steroid therapy, vomiting, alopecia, peripheral neuropathy
Gemcitabine hydrochloride (Gemzar)	• Mild myelosuppression, flu-like syndrome, vomiting
Plant alkaloids	
Vincristine sulfate (Oncovin)	• Neurotoxicity (peripheral, central, and visceral neuropathies that are cumulative), alopecia, myelosuppression, cranial nerve palsies
Epipodophyllotoxin (etoposide, VP-16)	• Myelosuppression, alopecia, hypotension, allergic reaction, vomiting
Paclitaxel (Taxol)	• Myelosuppression (WBC > platelets), alopecia, allergic reactions, cardiac arrhythmias, peripheral neuropathies, vomiting
	• Asymptomatic and transient bradycardia (40-60 beats/min), ventricular tachycardia, and atypical chest pain during infusion. These symptoms resolve with slowing of infusion.
	• Hypersensitivity reactions with characteristic bradycardia, diaphoresis, hypotension, cutaneous flushing, and abdominal pain. Premedication of diphenhydramine hydrochloride, dexamethasone, and ranitidine are given prophylactically.

Table 56-1	Chemotherapeutic Agents Commonly Used in Gynecologic Cancers and Their Most Common Toxicities *(Continued)*

Chemotherapeutic Agent	Toxicity
Docetaxel (Taxotere)	• Myelosuppression (neutropenia), hypersensitivity; cutaneous reactions, alopecia, mucosal ulcerations, paresthesia
Biologics	
Bevacizumab (Avastin): monoclonal antibody, anti-VEGF	• Hypertension, proteinuria, small risk of bowel perforation
Erlotinib, gefitinib: anti-EGFR	• Skin rash, diarrhea
Rapamycin: anti-mTOR	• Mucositis, rash, nausea, vomiting, weakness, fatigue
Immune checkpoint inhibitors	
Pembrolizumab, nivolumab: anti-PD-1 Ipilimumab, tremelimumab: anti-CD4	• Skin rash, diarrhea, hypothyroidism, hepatitis, and other immune-related toxicities
Poly(ADP-ribose) polymerase (PARP) inhibitors	
Olaparib, rucaparib, niraparib	• Nausea and vomiting, myelosuppression, skin rash
Miscellaneous	
Topotecan hydrochloride (Hycamtin): topoisomerase I inhibitor	• Myelosuppression (WBC > Plt), mucosal ulcerations, vomiting, paresthesia

Abbreviations: ADP, adenosine diphosphate; BUN, blood urea nitrogen; CNS, central nervous system; EGFR, epidermal growth factor receptor; IV, intravenous; MI, myocardial infarction; mTOR, mammalian target of rapamycin; MUGA, multiple-gated acquisition; PD-1, programmed cell death protein 1; Plt, platelet; VEGF, vascular endothelial growth factor; WBC, white blood cell.

- **Plant alkaloids** are **cell cycle specific** (eg, paclitaxel, docetaxel, etoposide, vincristine) and are derived from various plants and trees, including the periwinkle plant (*Vinca rosea*), the May apple (*Podophyllum peltatum*), and the Pacific yew (*Taxus brevifolia*). They bind to tubules, blocking microtubule formation and interfering with spindle formation. This leads to the arrest of metaphase and inhibits mitosis.
- **Antitumor antibiotics** are **cell cycle specific** (eg, actinomycin D, bleomycin, doxorubicin) and have multiple modes of action, including increasing cell membrane permeability, inhibiting DNA and RNA synthesis, and preventing DNA replication.

- **Camptothecin analogs** (eg, topotecan, irinotecan) are topoisomerase inhibitors, preventing DNA religation during replication and ultimately causing cell death.

Targeted Therapy

Targeted therapies are developed to interact with a specific molecular entity to alter signal transduction pathways essential to cancer cell proliferation and survival. They may be used alone or in combination with chemotherapy or radiation. Common classes of targeted agents, along with specific examples and their targets (in parentheses) are listed below.

- **Monoclonal antibodies** frequently target cell surface growth factor receptors or their growth factor ligand.
  - Bevacizumab (vascular endothelial growth factor [VEGF]), trastuzumab (human epidermal growth factor receptor 2/neu), cetuximab (epidermal growth factor receptor)
- **Immune checkpoint inhibitors** are a form of **immunotherapy** and target key regulators of the immune system to eradicate malignant cells. **Cytotoxic T lymphocyte–associated protein 4 (CTLA-4)** and **programmed cell death protein 1 (PD-1)** are receptors present on T cells; they act to downregulate T-cell function. Some cancer cells are able to downregulate T-cell function, and these antibodies assist in restoring T-cell function.
  - Nivolumab, pembrolizumab (PD-1 antibodies)
  - Avelumab, durvalumab, atezolizumab (programed cell death ligand 1 antibodies)
  - Ipilimumab, tremelimumab (CTLA-4 antibodies)
- **Poly(adenosine diphosphate ribose) polymerase (PARP) inhibitors** target proteins that repair single-strand DNA breaks. Inhibition leads to eventual cell death. Tumors with homologous recombination deficiencies or BRCA1 or BRCA2 mutations lack double-stranded repair mechanisms of their cells and are more sensitive to treatment with PARP inhibitors due to the synthetic lethality.
  - Olaparib, rucaparib, niraparib, talazoparib, veliparib
- Small molecule tyrosine kinase inhibitors disrupt signaling through pathways dependent on phosphorylation of tyrosine.
  - Cediranib (vascular endothelial growth factor receptor [VEGFR]), gefitinib, erlotinib (epidermal growth factor receptor), imatinib (Bcr-Abl, c-kit), pazopanib (VEGFR, platelet-derived growth factor receptor, c-kit), sorafenib (Raf/Mek/Erk, VEGFR), sunitinib (VEGFR, platelet-derived growth factor receptor)

Hormonal Therapy

Hormonal agents take advantage of the fact that well-differentiated neoplastic gynecologic tissues generally express and may be dependent on both estrogen and progesterone receptors for growth. These receptors are commonly lost as tumors become less well differentiated.

- Antiestrogens (also known as selective estrogen receptor modulators or selective estrogen receptor disruptors): tamoxifen, fulvestrant
- Progestins: medroxyprogesterone acetate, megestrol acetate
- Aromatase inhibitors: anastrozole, letrozole, exemestane
- Gonadotropin-releasing hormone agonists/antagonists: leuprolide

COMMON SIDE EFFECTS OF CHEMOTHERAPY, TARGETED THERAPY, AND HORMONAL AGENTS

- **Hematologic toxicity** and myelosuppression are dangerous effects of chemotherapy that vary in severity, depending on the drug administered. A nadir in white cell, red cell, or platelet count is usually observed 7 to 14 days after drug administration. Most agents are readministered every 3 to 4 weeks if the patient has recovered from pancytopenia.
  - **Neutropenia** is defined as an absolute neutrophil count less than 1500/mL. Neutropenia is expected with most chemotherapy and mild neutropenia (absolute neutrophil count >1000/mL) is commonly tolerated without need for dose or schedule adjustment. However, if severe or prolonged neutropenia is expected, recombinant human granulocyte colony-stimulating factor (G-CSF), such as filgrastim (Neupogen) or pegylated filgrastim (Neulasta), is administered as primary prophylaxis. The G-CSF is generally not administered during neutropenic fever because it has not been shown to meaningfully shorten the duration or reduce complications. The G-CSF is contraindicated during the actual administration of chemotherapy.
    - **Neutropenic fever is a medical emergency** because these patients can quickly become septic. Common causes of infection include enteric gram-negative bacteria, gram-positive bacteria, viruses (herpes simplex and herpes zoster), and fungi (*Candida* and *Aspergillus* species), although often an offending agent is not identified.
  - **Anemia** can be treated acutely with blood transfusions and/or managed long-term with ferrous sulfate and erythropoietin stimulating agents (eg, epoetin α: Epogen, Procrit). No specific hemoglobin target is set, and therapy should be considered if a patient is symptomatic. All of these interventions have potentially significant risks that must be considered against their benefits prior to their use. In particular, worse survival outcomes have been associated with erythropoietin-stimulating agents in cancer patients. These agents should be used with caution and only with extensive patient counseling.
  - **Thrombocytopenia** is treated with platelet transfusion when the platelet count drops below 20 000/mL or if signs of spontaneous bleeding are evident. In patients who develop significant thrombocytopenia, changes to the chemotherapy dose or schedule may be necessary. Rarely, thrombopoietic growth factors (eg, oprelvekin, romiplostim) may also be given.
- Gastrointestinal side effects are common after chemotherapy.
  - **Nausea and vomiting** are the most common side effects of chemotherapy due to decreased intestinal motility. The severity and incidence of these symptoms vary greatly, but the inability to effectively control them can result in the patient refusal to carry out potentially curative treatment. Nausea and vomiting can be
    - Acute, occurring during or immediately after chemotherapy administration
    - Delayed, occurring several days after chemotherapy administration
    - Anticipatory, occurring before the administration of chemotherapy
  - The incidence and severity are related to the emetogenic potential of the drug, the dose, the route and time of day of administration, patient characteristics, and the combination of drugs used. Gastrointestinal obstruction must be considered if abdominal distention or obstipation is present.

- Antiemetic regimens, including a combination of serotonin 5-HT3 receptor–blocking agents (eg, ondansetron, granisetron), NK_1 receptor antagonists (eg, aprepitant, fosaprepitant), and dexamethasone have been shown to be particularly effective in reducing acute and delayed emesis.
- **Diarrhea** may occur in association with chemotherapy and is typically not infectious; however, necrotizing enterocolitis must always be considered if diarrhea is watery, bloody, and associated with abdominal pain and fever.
- **Stomatitis and mucositis** occur most commonly following therapy with antimetabolites because these cells are naturally rapidly proliferating. Treatment is with either Larry solution (three equal parts diphenhydramine hydrochloride elixir [Benadryl], magnesium and aluminum oral suspension [Maalox], and viscous lidocaine) or nystatin swish and swallow. Severe cases may require hospitalization for nutrition supplementation, intravenous hydration, and pain management.
- **Dehydration** may occur in the setting of emesis and diarrhea. Patients are encouraged to increase their fluid intake to prevent postchemotherapy dehydration, which increases the risk of nephrotoxicity or electrolyte disturbances.
- **Hepatic toxicity**, including transient elevations in transaminase and alkaline phosphatase levels, may occur with chemotherapy. Cholangitis, hepatic necrosis, and hepatic veno-occlusive disease, although rare, must be considered.
- Common dermatologic toxicities are **alopecia** and **photosensitivity**. Extravasation of chemotherapeutic agents can additionally cause skin necrosis. Once identified, the infusion should be immediately stopped and the patient given topical steroids and hyaluronidase or sodium thiosulfate.
- Acute allergic or infusion reactions may occur with the use of chemotherapeutic agents. For agents that cause **hypersensitivity**, such as paclitaxel, premedication with diphenhydramine hydrochloride, dexamethasone, and ranitidine are given. For agents that may cause **anaphylaxis**, such as bleomycin, a test dose should be performed prior to administration. *Platinum agents* commonly cause hypersensitivity reactions after several doses have been administered, and prompt recognition of anaphylaxis is key.
- Neurologic side effects of chemotherapy include damage to peripheral nerves as well as subtle changes in cognitive function. **Peripheral nerve damage** may range from paresthesia (ie, "pins and needles" sensation) to chronic loss of sensitivity and fine motor control. Changes in **cognitive function** are generally perceived as difficulties with concentration and short-term memory. To date, there are no interventions proven to prevent or ameliorate this neurologic damage.
- **Fatigue** is commonly reported. The mechanisms causing fatigue are not well understood; however, correction of anemia, good sleep hygiene, and regular exercise can help reduce symptoms.
- **Cardiac toxicity** is rare with chemotherapy because myocytes do not readily divide. However, *doxorubicin* is classically associated with cardiomyopathy. Additionally, use of bevacizumab (Avastin) has been associated with the development of hypertension, venous thromboembolism, and rarely, arterial thromboembolism. Anti-VEGF agents have also been associated with left ventricular hypertrophy and subsequent reduced left ventricular ejection fraction.
- **Pulmonary toxicity** in the form of interstitial pneumonitis with pulmonary fibrosis is classically seen with *bleomycin*. Once diagnosed, the medication should be stopped and steroids started.

- **Genitourinary toxicity** is typically seen in the form of renal tubular toxicity with platinum agents, especially cisplatin. A variety of antineoplastic agents is associated with renal toxicity in the form of proteinuria, secondary to glomerulonephritis, interstitial nephritis, and acute tubular necrosis. Additionally, **hemorrhagic cystitis** can occur with the alkylating agents ifosfamide and cyclophosphamide. Preventative measures include hydration and administration of diuretics. Treatment includes dosage reduction or discontinuation of the drug. Mesna, a uroprotector, is administered simultaneously to protect against bladder toxicity. Mesna acts to detoxify *acrolein*, the common metabolite of both cyclophosphamide and ifosfamide.

RADIATION THERAPY

- X-rays or γ rays destroy tumor and normal cells by creating oxygen-free radicals and a multitude of other reactions, which ultimately results in DNA and cell membrane injury. Radiation therapy is cell cycle nonspecific.
- The absorption of energy by tissue is measured in rads. One gray is 100 rad, and 1 cGy is 1 rad. The **inverse square law** states that the dose of radiation at a given point is inversely proportional to the square of the distance from the source of radiation.

Clinical Radiation Sources

- **Teletherapy** is external beam radiation. During external beam radiation, the patient may be in the prone or supine position. The usual total dose to the pelvis ranges from 4000 to 5000 cGy given in daily fractions of 180 to 200 cGy in 5 weeks.
- **Brachytherapy** involves placement of a radiation device either within or close to the target tumor volume (ie, interstitial and intracavitary irradiation); the radiation dose to the tissue is determined largely by the inverse square law. The radiation applicators are called **intrauterine tandems** and **ovoids/colpostats**. Intrauterine tandems are placed in the uterine cavity while the patient is under anesthesia and position is confirmed with radiographic studies. Vaginal ovoids are designed for placement in the vaginal vault and support the position of the tandem, but they may also be loaded with radioactive sources themselves.
  - Vaginal, endometrial, and cervical cancers may be treated with either high- or low-dose rate intracavitary implants. Replacing low-dose rate (usually cesium) with high-dose rate intracavitary brachytherapy treatments (usually iridium 192) is increasingly common in the United States and Europe. High-dose rate applications do not require anesthesia or operating room time and radiation exposure is 10 to 20 minutes for each outpatient visit (usually four to six visits are required), whereas use of low-dose rate cesium implants requires hospitalization for 48 to 72 hours.
  - **Interstitial implants** are another form of brachytherapy configured as radioactive wires or seeds and placed directly within tissues. Hollow guide needles are inserted in a geometric pattern to deliver a relatively uniform dose of radiation to a target tumor volume. After the position of the guide needle is confirmed, they can be threaded with the radioactive sources and the hollow guides removed. Interstitial implants are sometimes used in the treatment of locally advanced cervical cancer or for women with pelvic recurrences of endometrial or cervical cancer.

Common Side Effects of Radiation Therapy

- **Hematologic toxicity** is dependent on the volume of marrow irradiated and the total radiation dose. In adults, 40% of active marrow is in the pelvis, 25% is in the vertebral column, and 20% is in the ribs and skull. Extensive radiation to these sites may result in need for blood product transfusions or administration of erythropoietin to support patient's hematologic function during therapy.
- **Gastrointestinal toxicity** may be acute or chronic.
  - Acutely, nausea, vomiting, and diarrhea commonly occur 2 to 6 hours after abdominal or pelvic irradiation. Supportive therapy with hydration and administration of antiemetics and antidiarrheals are used for first-line therapy. In patients with severe diarrhea, opiates, such as opium tincture, paregoric elixir, or codeine may be used to decrease peristalsis, whereas octreotide acetate may be given to reduce the volume of persistent, high-output diarrhea.
  - Chronic diarrhea, obstruction caused by bowel adhesions, and fistula formation are serious complications of irradiation that occur in less than 1% of cases. Small bowel and rectovaginal fistulas can be caused by radiation effects or by recurrent disease. Once recurrence is ruled out as an etiology, the patient may require temporary or permanent colostomy to allow healing of the affected bowel.
- **Dermatologic toxicity**, such as an acute skin reaction, typically becomes evident by the third week of therapy. The reaction is characterized by erythema, desquamation, and pruritus and should be completely resolved within 3 weeks of the end of treatment.
  - Symptoms are treated with topical corticosteroids or moisturizing creams. If the reaction worsens, treatment is discontinued and zinc oxide or silver sulfadiazine is applied to affected area.
  - The perineum is at greater risk for skin breakdown because of its increased warmth, moisture, and lack of ventilation; therefore, patients should be instructed to keep the perineal area clean and dry.
  - Late subcutaneous fibrosis can develop, especially with doses >6500 cGy.
- Genitourinary toxicity typically presents as cystitis (dysuria, urgency, hematuria, and urinary frequency). The bladder is relatively tolerant of radiation, but with doses higher than 6000 to 7000 cGy over a 6- to 7-week period, cystitis can develop.
  - The diagnosis of **radiation cystitis** may be made after normal urine culture is obtained. Hydration, frequent sitz baths, and possibly use of antibiotics and antispasmodic agents may be necessary for treatment.
  - **Hemorrhagic cystitis** may lead to symptomatic anemia that requires blood transfusions and hospitalization. Clot evacuation of the bladder with continuous bladder irrigation is often necessary. Bladder irrigation with 1% alum or 1% silver nitrate can alleviate bleeding. Significant bleeding from the bladder may require immediate cystoscopy to localize and control the bleeding.
- **Vesicovaginal fistulas** and ureteral strictures are long-term complications that can occur due to radiation therapy. Nephrostomy placement, insertion of ureteral stents, and, less commonly, surgical intervention, may be necessary.
- **Vulvovaginitis** occurs secondary to erythema, inflammation, mucosal atrophy, inelasticity, and ulceration of the vaginal tissue. Adhesions and vaginal stenosis are common, resulting in pain during pelvic examination and intercourse. Vaginal dilators may be needed for treatment. Additionally, use of estrogen cream may also be helpful in promoting epithelial regeneration. Infections, including candidiasis, trichomoniasis, and bacterial vaginosis may be related to radiation-induced vaginitis.

- The most common neurologic side effect is fatigue. This may continue for several months after completion of therapy. As with chemotherapy-induced fatigue, correction of anemia, good sleep hygiene, and regular exercise can help decrease radiation-induced fatigue.

PRIMARY TREATMENT MODALITIES ACCORDING TO CANCER SITE

Epithelial Ovarian Cancer

- Women with epithelial ovarian cancer (EOC) need surgical staging to confirm the diagnosis and guide treatment planning (see chapter 52 for detailed description of surgical staging of EOC). Of note, carcinoma of the fallopian tube and primary peritoneal carcinoma should be managed the same way as EOC.
- Chemotherapy is recommended based on stage and grade of EOC:
  - Patients with stages IA and IB, grades 1 to 2, EOC do not benefit from adjuvant chemotherapy.
  - Patients with stages IA to IB, grade 3 disease, and those with stage IC, all grades, should receive three to six cycles of intravenous platinum-based adjuvant chemotherapy.
  - Patients with stage II EOC should receive platinum-based adjuvant chemotherapy.
  - Patients with stages III and IV EOC require optimal surgical cytoreduction (residual tumor implants less than 1 cm in diameter) either at the time of initial surgery or after three to four cycles of neoadjuvant chemotherapy. Neoadjuvant chemotherapy is considered for patients unfit for surgery at the time of presentation due to extent of disease, comorbidities, or poor performance status.
- The EOCs that persist or progress despite surgery and primary platinum-based chemotherapy are termed *platinum refractory*. The EOCs that recur within 6 months of the last platinum-based treatment are termed *platinum resistant*, and neoplasms that recur more than 6 months later than the last platinum treatment are considered *platinum sensitive*. Drugs commonly used for the treatment of women with platinum-resistant disease include topotecan, liposomal doxorubicin, docetaxel, gemcitabine, weekly paclitaxel, and bevacizumab. Patients with platinum-sensitive disease are generally treated with a combination of platinum and another active agent.

Nonepithelial Ovarian Cancers

- **Ovarian germ cell cancers.** As with EOC, comprehensive surgical staging is critical for patients with ovarian germ-cell cancers. Most women who are diagnosed at an early stage have excellent prognosis (see chapter 52).
  - Stage IA pure dysgerminoma and stage IA (grade 1) immature teratoma are treated with surgery alone. No adjuvant chemotherapy is recommended.
  - Those with stages IB to IV dysgerminoma or stages IA (grade 2 or 3) to IV immature teratoma undergo adjuvant chemotherapy with three to four courses of bleomycin, etoposide, and cisplatin after primary surgery.
  - Postoperative radiation is also an option for patients with dysgerminoma, although use is limited for those who desire to maintain fertility.
- **Ovarian sex cord–stromal cancer.** Most ovarian sex cord–stromal cancers are diagnosed at an early stage, and surgery is the primary treatment followed by adjuvant chemotherapy with platinum-based chemotherapy.

Cervical Cancer

- Surgery, chemotherapy, and radiation therapy all play a role in the management of women with cervical cancer limited to the pelvis (stages IA to IVA). Early-stage cervical cancer is most often treated surgically. However, later stage cervical cancer usually requires chemotherapy and/or radiation therapy (see chapter 50).
- Radiation sensitization with concomitant cisplatin improves both progression-free and overall survival for women with cervical cancer. It is important to note, however, that patients who undergo both surgery and radiation (or chemoradiation) for the treatment of their cervical cancer will experience more short- and long-term toxicity than those who are treated with one modality alone.
- Treatment for women with stage IVB disease should focus on symptom control because the disease is not curable. Radiation may be used for palliation of central disease and/or distant metastases. Typical initial therapy for stage IVB disease involves cisplatin, paclitaxel, and bevacizumab based on the results of the Gynecologic Oncology Group (GOG) 240 study showing an overall survival benefit with the addition of bevacizumab to chemotherapy.

Vulvar Cancer

- The goals for treatment of vulvar cancer include efforts to decrease the extent of surgery and preserve normal urinary, rectal, and sexual functions while providing curative therapy. Early vulvar cancer is often treated surgically (see chapter 54).
- Locally advanced disease may be treated with neoadjuvant chemoradiation, including cisplatin, 5-FU/cisplatin, and 5-FU/mitomycin-C, and radical vulvectomy and lymph node dissection. Recurrent or persistent local disease may be treated with pelvic exenteration.
- Current treatment options for patients with distant metastatic vulvar cancer is limited; these include radiation and/or chemotherapy with the single-agents, cisplatin, carboplatin, paclitaxel, and erlotinib, or with the two-drug combinations, cisplatin-vinorelbine, cisplatin-paclitaxel, and carboplatin-paclitaxel.

Vaginal Cancer

- Early vaginal cancer may be treated with either surgery or radiation (intracavitary with or without interstitial radiation). More advanced disease (stages II to IV) is generally treated with radiation alone. Platinum-based chemoradiation is also commonly used (see chapter 54).

Uterine Cancers

Endometrioid Endometrial Carcinoma

- Endometrioid endometrial carcinomas are thought to arise in the hormonal milieu of estrogen excess relative to progesterone. Prolonged progesterone therapy has been shown to induce histologic regression of cancer in about 50% to 78% of women with well-differentiated endometrioid endometrial carcinoma confined to the endometrium. Hormonal therapy, therefore, is a treatment option among young women who wish to preserve fertility as well as among patients with multiple comorbidities for whom the operative risks outweigh the benefits (see chapter 51).

- The choice of radiation, chemotherapy, or combination therapy for the adjuvant therapy of endometrial cancer is based on histologic subtype, grade, and the presence of negative prognostic factors.
- Patients found to have endometrial cancer recurring in the pelvis may benefit from surgical resection and radiation. Those with distant metastatic disease should receive platinum-based chemotherapy, if not recently received as part of adjuvant therapy. The small subset of women with recurrent grade I disease may benefit from hormonal therapy.

Uterine Leiomyosarcomas

- The primary treatment for leiomyosarcomas remains total abdominal hysterectomy and bilateral salpingo-oophorectomy. The use of adjuvant chemotherapy for uterus-limited high-grade leiomyosarcomas has not been shown to improve outcomes. Similarly, adjuvant pelvic radiation does not appear to be beneficial. The most active agents for women with recurrent or metastatic disease include the combination of gemcitabine and docetaxel or doxorubicin-based regimens.

Uterine Carcinosarcomas

- The primary treatment for uterine carcinosarcomas is total abdominal hysterectomy, bilateral salpingo-oophorectomy, omentectomy or omental biopsy, and lymphadenectomy with resection of grossly visible disease. Adjuvant therapy is recommended in all stages of disease, due to the high likelihood of recurrence. Adjuvant chemotherapy is recommended given improved progression free and overall survival. Carboplatin and paclitaxel are recommended over ifosfamide combinations for initial treatment based on results of GOG261. Adjuvant pelvic radiation is often offered in addition due to decreased risk of local recurrence, although overall survival is not impacted.

Gestational Trophoblastic Tumors

- Hydatidiform mole is treated with dilation and curettage, although hysterectomy is advised if childbearing is completed. When postmolar gestational trophoblastic neoplasia is suspected (serum human chorionic gonadotropin levels that rise or plateau), women with low-risk disease (an International Federation of Gynecology and Obstetrics score of 0-6) are treated with either methotrexate with leucovorin or single-agent dactinomycin. Those with an International Federation of Gynecology and Obstetrics score ≥7 or recurrent gestational trophoblastic tumors after primary chemotherapy are treated with EMA-CO, a five-drug combination of etoposide, methotrexate, actinomycin-D, cyclophosphamide, and vincristine (Oncovin) (see chapter 55).

SUGGESTED READINGS

American College of Obstetricians and Gynecologists Committee on Practice Bulletins—Gynecology. ACOG Practice Bulletin No. 149: endometrial cancer. *Obstet Gynecol*. 2015;125(4):1006-1026. (Reaffirmed 2017)

Colombo N, Preti E, Landoni F, et al. Endometrial cancer: ESMO clinical practice guidelines for diagnosis, treatment and follow-up. *Ann Oncol*. 2013;24(suppl 6):vi33-vi38.

DiSaia PJ, Creasman WT, Mannel RT, McMeekin DS, Mutch DG, eds. *Clinical Gynecologic Oncology*. 9th ed. Philadelphia, PA: Elsevier; 2018.

El-Khalfaoui K, du Bois A, Heitz F, Kurzeder C, Sehouli J, Harter P. Current and future options in the management and treatment of uterine sarcoma. *Ther Adv Med Oncol.* 2014;6(1):21-28.

Gaillard SL, Secord AA, Monk B. The role of immune checkpoint inhibition in the treatment of ovarian cancer. *Gynecol Oncol Res Pract.* 2016;3:11.

Koh W, Greer BE, Abu-Rustum NR, et al. NCCN vulvar cancer, Version 1.2017: clinical practice guidelines in oncology. *J Nar Compr Canc Netw.* 2017;15(1):92-102.

Machado KK, Gaillard SL. Emerging therapies in the management of high-grade serous ovarian carcinoma: a focus on PARP inhibitors. *Curr Obstet Gynecol Rep.* 2017;6(3):207-218.

Marth C, Landoni F, Mahner S, McCormack M, Gonzalez-Martin A, Colombo N. Cervical cancer: ESMO clinical practice guidelines for diagnosis, treatment and follow-up. *Ann Oncol.* 2017;28(suppl 4):iv72-iv83.

Menczer J. Review of recommended treatment of uterine carcinosarcoma. *Curr Treat Options Oncol.* 2015;16(11):53.

Pakish JB, Zhang Q, Chen Z, et al. Immune microenvironment in microsatellite-instable endometrial cancers: hereditary or sporadic origin matters. *Clin Cancer Res.* 2017;23(15): 4473-4481.

Ray-Coquard I, Morice P, Lorusso D, et al. Non-epithelial ovarian cancer: ESMO clinical practice guidelines for diagnosis, treatment and follow-up. *Ann Oncol.* 2018;29(suppl 4): iv1-iv18.

Reichardt P. The treatment of uterine sarcomas. *Ann Oncol.* 2012;23(suppl 10):x151-x157.

Seckl MJ, Sebire NJ, Fisher RA, et al. Gestational trophoblastic disease: ESMO clinical practice guidelines for diagnosis, treatment and follow-up. *Ann Oncol.* 2013;24(suppl 6): vi39-vi50.

Palliative and End-of-Life Care

Melissa H. Lippitt and Stephanie L. Wethington

DEFINITIONS

Palliative Care

- Palliative care, as defined by the National Consensus Project, means patient- and family-centered care that optimizes quality of life by anticipating, preventing, and treating suffering. Palliative care throughout the continuum of illness involves addressing physical, intellectual, emotional, social, and spiritual needs and facilitating patient autonomy, access to information, and choice.
- Essential components of palliative care:
  - Rapport and relationship building with patients and family caregivers
  - Symptom, distress, and functional status management
  - Exploration of understanding and education about illness and prognosis
  - Clarification of treatment goals
  - Assessment and support of coping needs

- Assistance with medical decision making
- Coordination with other care providers
- Provision of referrals to other care providers as indicated
- Palliative care uses an interdisciplinary team that may include primary physicians, specialists (eg, oncologist), board-certified palliative care physicians, advance practice nurses, physician assistants, social workers, chaplains, and pharmacists.
- Primary palliative care is care led by the patient's primary physician. Subspecialty palliative care is care led by a board-certified palliative care physician.
- Palliative care may be delivered in the inpatient setting (by the admitting service, a consult service, or an inpatient palliative care unit), in an outpatient clinic, or at home.
- All cancer patients should be screened for palliative care needs at their initial visit, at appropriate intervals, and as clinically indicated.
- According to the American Society of Clinical Oncology, patients with advanced cancer should be referred to interdisciplinary palliative care teams that provide inpatient and outpatient care early in the course of disease, alongside active treatment of their cancer.
- Clinical trials have demonstrated that palliative care for patients with cancer improves symptom management and quality of life and may even increase overall survival when introduced early in the course of disease.

Hospice Care

- Hospice care delivers palliative care to patients with a terminal condition whose life expectancy is 6 months or less if the disease continues to run its usual course.
- Hospice aims to maintain or improve quality of life for someone whose illness, disease, or condition is not curable and provides medical, psychological, and spiritual support to the patient and their family. Additionally, the primary focus is to assist the dying individual in achieving peace, comfort, and dignity during the process.
- Hospice care is provided by an interdisciplinary team, including nurses, physicians, volunteers, therapists, social workers, spiritual counselors, home health aides, and bereavement counselors.
- Hospice services are provided at a patient's place of residence (eg, private residence, nursing home, residential facility), a hospice inpatient facility, or an acute care hospital.
- It is covered under Medicare, Medicaid, and most private insurance plans. In the United States, the Medicare Hospice Benefit (MHB) pays for 80% of all hospice care.
- Eligibility for the MHB:
  - Two physicians (hospice medical director and referring physician) determine the patient has a prognosis of 6 months or less to live if the patient's disease runs its natural course.
  - Eligibility is reassessed at regular intervals, but there is no limit to the amount of time a patient can spend under hospice care.
  - A "Do Not Resuscitate" status cannot be used as a requirement for admission.
  - The patient must be entitled to Medicare Part A (hospital payments) and once the patient decides to enter hospice care, they sign off Part A and elect for the MHB. This process is reversible, and patients may elect to return to Medicare Part A.

- The following interventions are not routinely covered during hospice care but may be covered for specific indications: parenteral fluids, enteral feeding, total parenteral nutrition, radiation therapy, blood transfusions, platelet transfusions, chemotherapy, antibiotics, and laboratory/diagnostic services.

SYMPTOM MANAGEMENT

Pain

- Pain is one of the most common symptoms for chronically and terminally ill patients.
- Patient surveys have shown that pain associated with advanced illness is often undertreated and that approximately 40% of cancer pain is undertreated.
- Pain should be treated with multimodal therapy, and selection of the pain regimen should be based on the pain etiology.
  - About 30% of cancer patients will have inadequate pain control despite large doses of opiates or will have intolerable side effects at opiate doses that do control pain.
- If a patient has refractory pain, a referral to a pain specialist may be indicated.
- Pharmacologic treatment options:
  - Nonsteroidal anti-inflammatory drugs (NSAIDs)
    - Can act synergistically with opioids.
    - No NSAID has greater efficacy than another.
    - Should be given around the clock if pain is constant—twice daily options can aid in compliance.
    - Side effects include platelet inhibition (some nonsteroidals, such as trilisate, do not inhibit platelets), gastrointestinal effects, and nephrotoxicity. These can be especially pronounced in older and/or frail patients.
    - Often contraindicated in clinical trials or while receiving chemotherapy.
    - Gastrointestinal prophylaxis usually indicated for long-term palliative use.
    - Acetaminophen is often just as effective and may be safer in some situations.
  - Opiates
    - Both short- and long-acting formulations are available.
    - When pain is constant, escalate to around-the-clock dosing or longer acting narcotics with rescue doses as needed.
    - There are multiple formulations and routes of administration (there is variation in response to these formulations and none is universally preferred over another).
    - Refer to dosing guidelines (see equianalgesic table, Table 57-1). Because intravenous (IV) opioids are more potent than oral doses, direct conversion risks overadministration, side effects, and overdose. Hydromorphone and fentanyl are much more potent than other opiates.
    - Side effects
      - To alleviate side effects, decrease the dose, change to a different narcotic, change the route, or treat the symptoms.
      - See section "Nausea/Vomiting" for treatment of nausea and vomiting.
      - Constipation is frequently a problem for patients on an around-the-clock opioid. A bowel regimen should be prescribed when opioids are initiated.

Table 57-1 Opioid Analgesics: Equivalent Dosing for Various Narcotic Formulations[a]

Drug	Oral (mg)	IM (mg)	Half-Life (h)	Peak Effect (h)	Duration (h)	Comment[b]
Morphine	20-30[c]	10	2-3	0.5-1.0	3-6	Standard for comparison
Morphine CR	20-30	10	2-3	3-4	8-12	Various formulations are not bioequivalent.
Morphine SR	20-30	10	2-3	2-3	12-24	
Codeine	200	130	2-3	1.5-2.0	3-6	Combined with aspirin or acetaminophen; usually for moderate pain; also available without coanalgesic
Hydromorphone	7.5	1.5	2-3	0.5-1.0	2-4	Potency may be greater: ie, hydromorphone: morphine = 3:1 rather than 6.7:1 during prolonged use
Oxycodone	20	n/a	2-3	1	3-4	Combined with aspirin or acetaminophen, for moderate pain; available orally without coanalgesic and useful for severe pain
Oxycodone CR	20	n/a	2-3	2-3	8-12	
Oxymorphone CR	20 (oral)	n/a	2-3	1.5-3.0	2-4	

(Continued)

Table 57-1 Opioid Analgesics: Equivalent Dosing for Various Narcotic Formulations[a] *(Continued)*

Drug	Oral (mg)	IM (mg)	Half-Life (h)	Peak Effect (h)	Duration (h)	Comment[b]
Methadone	20	10	12-190	0.5-1.5	4-12	Although 1:1 ratio with morphine was in single-dose study, there is a change with chronic dosing and large dose reduction (75%-90%) is needed when switching to methadone; risk of delayed toxicity
Levorphanol	4	2	12-15	0.5-1	4-6	Usage limited because only 2-mg tablets are available
Fentanyl	n/a	n/a	7-12	0.08-0.16	2-4	Can be administered as a continuous IV infusion or SC infusion; based on clinical experience, 100 µg/h is roughly equianalgesic to morphine 4 mg/h
Fentanyl TTS	n/a	n/a	16-24	12-24	48-72	Based on clinical experience, 100 µg is roughly equianalgesic to morphine 4 mg.
Meperidine	300	75	2-3	0.5-1.0	3-4	Not preferred for cancer patients owing to potential toxicity
Tapentadol	50	n/a	4-5	1	4-6	

Abbreviations: CR, controlled release; IM, intramuscular; IV, intravenous; SC, subcutaneous; SR, sustained release.
[a]Adapted with permission from Barakat RR. *Principles and Practice of Gynecologic Oncology.* Philadelphia, PA: Wolters Kluwer Health/Lippincott Williams & Wilkins; 2013:1014. Table 31.6.
[b]All opioids may produce various common side effects (eg, constipation, nausea, sedation). Respiratory depression is rare in cancer patients.
[c]Extensive survey data suggest that the relative potency of IM to oral morphine of 1:16 changes to 1:23 with chronic dosing.

- ○ Sedation is common, although tolerance often develops.
- ○ Treat pruritus with diphenhydramine or low-dose nalbuphine or naloxone.
- Specialist pain procedures
  - ○ Myofascial injections may work for pain from localized muscle contractions. Relief lasts from days to weeks.
  - ○ Neurostimulation (implanted device) has an unclear mechanism of action.
    - ○ Stimulation can be given to the spinal cord or thalamic nuclei.
    - ○ Spinal cord stimulators are electrodes placed in the epidural space. They are very expensive and require patient involvement, which may not be ideal for end of life.
  - ○ Epidural or spinal patient-controlled analgesia can decrease narcotic doses and reduce side effects.
  - ○ A somatic nerve block works for pain localized to a single nerve, plexus, or dermatome.
    - ○ The block can disrupt motor, sensory, or autonomic pathways.
    - ○ Sympathetic blocks can relieve visceral pain.
- Severe pain crisis
  - Treat with a rapid taper of a fast-acting IV narcotic, or with IV patient-controlled analgesia.
  - Once acute pain is controlled, calculate the dose and convert to a long-acting form.
- Management strategies for specific cancer pain syndromes
  - Associated with inflammation
    - ○ Recommend a trial of NSAIDs or corticosteroids.
  - Bone pain without oncologic emergency
    - ○ Recommend NSAIDs, acetaminophen, steroids.
    - ○ Consider bone-modifying agents (bisphosphonates, denosumab).
    - ○ For local bone pain, consider radiation, nerve block (eg, rib pain), vertebral augmentation, or radiofrequency ablation.
    - ○ Consider physical medicine evaluation.
  - Bowel obstruction (see section "Malignant Bowel Obstruction")
  - Nerve pain
    - ○ If thought to be secondary to nerve compression or inflammation, consider corticosteroids.
    - ○ For neuropathic pain, may opt for a trial of antidepressant (eg, amitriptyline), anticonvulsant (eg, gabapentin or pregabalin), or topical agent.
    - ○ Somatic nerve blocks work for pain localized to a single nerve, plexus, or dermatome.
    - ○ Superior hypogastric plexus blocks relieve pain from the pelvic viscera.
- Severe refractory pain in an imminently dying patient may be treated with palliative sedation.

Dyspnea

- Dyspnea is the sensation of uncomfortable breathing or shortness of breath.
- Differential diagnosis includes pulmonary embolus, pleural effusion, anemia, lung metastasis, pneumonia, anxiety, and fatigue/weakness.
- Treatment of the underlying cause (eg, with antibiotics, anticoagulation, blood transfusion, thoracentesis) can provide relief.

- Symptom relief may be achieved using one or more of the following:
  - Oxygen for symptomatic hypoxia
  - Nonpharmacologic therapies including fans, cooler temperature, stress management, relaxation therapy, and physical comfort measures
  - Medications including morphine, benzodiazepines, corticosteroids, and bronchodilators
  - Noninvasive positive-pressure ventilation support if clinically indicated for severe reversible condition
- For dyspnea at the end of life, the focus should be on comfort.
  - Symptom relief may be achieved with fans and oxygen.
  - If fluid overload is a possibility, may opt to decrease or discontinue enteral or parental fluid; consider low-dose diuretic.
  - Consider morphine if opioid naïve or benzodiazepines.
  - Reduce excessive secretions with antisecretory agents.

Anorexia/Cachexia

- Usually a symptom of functional decline and not the cause; may be a symptom of the dying process
- **Anorexia** refers to decreased appetite.
- **Cachexia** implies wasting; seen in cancer patients at the end of life.
- Assessment and management includes the following:
  - Treat reversible causes: oral-pharyngeal candidiasis, depression, symptoms that interfere with intake, early satiety, nausea/vomiting, dyspnea, constipation, and fatigue.
  - Evaluate for endocrine abnormalities (hypogonadism, thyroid dysfunction, metabolic abnormalities).
  - Consider an exercise program.
  - Assess social and economic factors.
  - Consider nutrition consult and nutrition support as appropriate.
  - Consider appetite stimulant such as dexamethasone, Megace, or dronabinol.
    - Appetite stimulants can restore appetite briefly but are not associated with improved survival.
    - Use when appetite is a significant quality-of-life issue and potential benefits outweigh side effects.
- At end of life
  - Absence of hunger and thirst is normal in the dying patient.
  - Nutritional support may not be metabolized in patients with advanced cancer.
  - There are risks associated with artificial nutrition and hydration, including fluid overload, infection, and hastened death.
  - Symptoms like dry mouth should be treated with local measures (eg, mouth care, small amounts of liquids).
  - Withholding or withdrawing nutrition is ethically permissible and may improve some symptoms. Forced feeding has not been shown to improve survival.

Nausea/Vomiting

- Determining the cause of the nausea and/or vomiting will help to determine the appropriate treatment strategy.

- Causes of nausea/vomiting in cancer patients include chemotherapy, radiation, severe constipation/fecal impaction, gastroparesis, bowel obstruction, gastric outlet obstruction, gastritis/gastroesophageal reflux disease, medication, a psychogenic disorder, hypercalcemia, uremia, dehydration, and nonspecific causes, including anxiety, a vertiginous component, or nonpharmacologic therapies.
- Nausea and vomiting due to chemotherapy can often be prevented (or mitigated) by selecting an appropriate acute and delayed emesis prevention plan depending on the emetic risk of the IV chemotherapy regimen.
- Around-the-clock dosing with rescue and escalation regimens using drugs from different categories is often successful:
  - Corticosteroids (dexamethasone)
  - 5-Hydroxytryptamine type 3 receptor antagonists (ondansetron)
  - Antipsychotic (haloperidol)
  - Anticholinergic (eg, scopolamine patch)
  - Antihistamine (eg, diphenhydramine and promethazine)
  - Antidepressant (mirtazapine)
  - Anxiolytic (lorazepam)
  - Oral cannabinoid (dronabinol)
  - Dopamine receptor antagonists (prochlorperazine)
  - Neurokinin receptor antagonist (aprepitant)
- Acupuncture may be of benefit.

Ascites

- A frequent problem in late-stage ovarian cancer
- Treatment options are limited. High-dose spironolactone has shown some benefit in small trials.
- Therapeutic paracentesis can be performed for acute relief.
  - Mean duration of relief is only 10 days.
  - Large volume drainage leads to hypovolemia.
  - Repetitive taps increase the risk of infection.
- Permanent tunneled catheters are available and may reduce infection risk and allow patients to drain their ascites at home.

Malignant Bowel Obstruction

- Initial assessment
  - Screening for and treating underlying reversible causes: adhesions, radiation-induced strictures, or internal hernias
  - Evaluating for malignant causes that may be secondary to tumor mass or carcinomatosis
  - Assessing goals of treatment of the patient to help guide intervention (eg, decrease nausea/vomiting, allow patient to eat, decrease pain, or allow patient to go home/to hospice)
- Small bowel obstruction (SBO)
  - Usually managed conservatively with bowel rest and decompression (ie, nasogastric tube) unless bowel ischemia or closed loop is present
  - Operative intervention may be considered, but perioperative morbidity and mortality are high, and repeat obstruction is common.

- Risk factors for poor surgical outcome include ascites, carcinomatosis, palpable intra-abdominal masses, recurrent or multiple sites of obstructions, previous abdominal radiation, advanced disease for which no further treatment options exist, and poor performance status.
- A percutaneous gastrostomy tube can be placed for venting.
- Hyoscyamine or octreotide decreases gastric secretion and slows intestinal motility, thereby decreasing the nausea/vomiting associated with SBO. This is supported by several randomized trials.
- Large bowel obstruction
  - Less frequent than SBO.
  - Surgical correction is indicated.
  - Endoscopic stents may work in select circumstances.

Constipation

- Common for women with gynecologic malignancies secondary to disease burden and due to chronic opioid use
- Preventative measures include fluids, dietary fiber, exercise if appropriate, prophylactic medications (stimulant $\pm$ stool softener, increase dose of laxative $\pm$ stool softener with goal of 1 nonforced bowel movement every 1-2 d).
- Assessment and treatment of constipation
  - Assess for cause and severity and discontinue any nonessential constipating medications.
  - Rule out impaction, especially if diarrhea accompanies constipation because there may be overflow around impaction.
  - Rule out obstruction.
  - Treat other causes, including hypercalcemia, hypokalemia, hypothyroidism, diabetes, and medication-induced constipation.
  - Add and titrate Bisacodyl (stimulant to increase bowel motility) with a goal of 1 nonforced bowel movement every 1 to 2 days. Stool softeners (eg, docusate sodium) are usually ineffective when used alone.
  - If impacted
    - Administer glycerin suppository $\pm$ mineral oil retention enema.
    - Perform manual disimpaction following premedication with analgesic $\pm$ anxiolytic.
  - If constipation persists
    - Reassess for cause and severity.
    - Recheck for impaction or obstruction.
    - Consider adding other laxatives or, if severe, consider colonic cleanout with a bowel preparation regimen.
    - Consider peripherally acting μ-opioid receptor antagonist for opioid-induced constipation, except for postoperative ileus and mechanical bowel obstruction.
    - Administer tap water enema until clear.
    - Consider use of a prokinetic agent.

Sleep/Wake Disturbances

- Sleep/wake disturbances are common in women with cancer.
- Contributing factors may include pain, depression, anxiety, delirium, nausea, medication side effects, and primary sleep disorders.

- Insomnia may be alleviated by treating the underlying contributing factors.
- Sleep hygiene is often helpful.
- Options for pharmacologic therapy include antipsychotics, sedatives/hypnotics, benzodiazepines, and antidepressants. In an actively dying patient consider chlorpromazine.

Fatigue

- The pathophysiology of fatigue from cancer is unclear.
- Fatigue can significantly decrease quality of life.
- Differential diagnosis includes underlying disease, anemia, chronic stress reaction, inflammation/immune reaction, disrupted circadian rhythm or sleep disturbance, hormonal changes, depression, and direct central nervous system toxicity.
- Treatment of reversible causes should promptly be initiated and can include fatigue-causing medication adjustment, transfusion, electrolyte repletion, pain management, or antidepressants.
- At the end of life, reassurance for the family may be the most appropriate step.
- Psychostimulant use is not well supported.

Delirium

- Mental status changes can be very distressing for families and can complicate home care.
- Screening and treating underlying reversible causes is critical. The following mnemonic can be helpful in identifying causes:
  - **D:** drugs (eg, anticholinergics, ranitidine, lorazepam, opiates)
  - **E:** electrolytes, emotions (eg, hyponatremia, hypophosphatemia, hyperammonemia)
  - **L:** low oxygen, lack of drugs (eg, pneumonia, pulmonary embolus, withdrawal)
  - **I:** ictal (eg, stroke, brain metastases, seizure disorder)
  - **R:** retention (eg, of carbon dioxide, urine, or stool)
  - **I:** ischemia, infection (eg, transient ischemic attack, stroke, meningitis, urosepsis, pneumonia)
  - **U:** uremia (eg, renal failure)
  - **M:** myocardial (eg, infarction, arrhythmia, heart failure)
- Management
  - Nonpharmacologic modalities including reorientation, cognitive stimulation, and sleep hygiene
  - Reducing and eliminating unnecessary medications
  - Pharmacologic therapy with haloperidol or other antipsychotic medication; may also consider addition of a benzodiazepine

Mood Disorders

- Depression
  - Adjustment reaction to a terminal diagnosis is expected; however, depression should be formally evaluated and treated when diagnosed.
  - Counseling and cognitive-behavioral therapy are useful adjuncts.
  - All antidepressants have side effects, which should be considered in the choice of treatment.
    - Tricyclic antidepressants are sedating and have anticholinergic effects (eg, dry mouth, constipation, urinary retention).

- Selective serotonin reuptake inhibitors are less sedating and less anticholinergic than tricyclics.
- Bupropion can lower seizure threshold.
- Anxiety
  - Benzodiazepines are the mainstay of acute treatment.
    - Short-acting options include alprazolam and lorazepam.
    - Longer acting options include clonazepam and diazepam.
  - Many antidepressants, especially selective serotonin reuptake inhibitors, also have anxiolytic effects.
  - Neuroleptics such as thioridazine or haloperidol may be used if benzodiazepines are ineffective.
  - Other options include methotrimeprazine and chlorpromazine. Although these are more sedating, they are also analgesic.
  - Atypical antipsychotics (eg, olanzapine and risperidone) may be useful in frail, older patients.
  - Buspirone may be used for chronic anxiety, although it takes 5 to 10 days to see any effect.

COMMUNICATION

- Communication and shared decision making is one of the key domains of palliative care.
- Oncologists often are faced with the task of breaking bad news. One framework for effectively communicating bad news is SPIKES:
  - **Setting:** setting up the interview
  - **Perception:** assessing the patient's perception
  - **Invitation:** obtaining the patient's permission to discuss the news
  - **Knowledge:** giving knowledge and information to the patient
  - **Emotion:** addressing the patient's emotion with empathic responses
  - **Strategy and summary:** summarizing the discussion and making a plan for next steps

ADVANCE CARE PLANNING

- Advance care planning is about determining the type of health care a patient would want if they were too sick to tell the doctor themselves.
- Advance care planning includes the following:
  - Assessing decision-making capacity and need for surrogate decision makers
  - Preparation of a living will, an advanced directive that communicates a patient's wishes concerning medical treatment at the end of life when they are otherwise unable to communicate wishes
  - Selecting a medical power of attorney (or health care proxy) allows a patient to appoint a trusted person to act as her health care agent or surrogate decision maker.
  - Exploring goals of care and patient values to establish recommendations regarding future treatment
  - Discussions regarding code status
    - Code status discussion should take place in the context of the larger goals of care discussion.

○ It is important to know the outcomes of cardiopulmonary resuscitation. And meta-analysis suggests less than 10% of cancer patients will survive cardiopulmonary resuscitation to discharge.
○ Patient preferences should be documented in the medical record, including Medical Orders for Life-Sustaining Treatment or Physician Orders for Life-Sustaining Treatment.

END-OF-LIFE CARE ISSUES

- Caring for the imminently dying patient includes focusing on physical, psychosocial, and practical interventions.
  - **Physical**
    ○ Hospice evaluation if not already enrolled in hospice.
    ○ Intensify comfort measures.
    ○ Discontinue unnecessary diagnostic tests and interventions.
    ○ Replace vital sign checks with symptom assessments.
    ○ Treat terminal secretions, dyspnea, restlessness, and agitation.
    ○ Be prepared to discuss request for organ donation and autopsy.
  - **Psychosocial**
    ○ Support the patient and family in the process of discontinuing interventions that will not add to the patient's comfort.
    ○ Consider social work and chaplain consults, if not already complete.
    ○ Educate the family about signs and symptoms of imminent death and offer support.
    ○ Offer anticipatory bereavement support.
    ○ Support culturally meaningful rituals.
    ○ Ensure caregivers understand and will honor advance directives.
    ○ Promote healthy grieving.
  - **Practical**
    ○ Ensure patient's advance directives are documented and implemented.
    ○ Discuss and document patient/family wishes for resuscitation.
    ○ Provide the patient/family/caregiver with respectful space and uninterrupted time together.
    ○ Provide information on funeral planning.
    ○ Assist with estate and financial planning.
- Palliative sedation may be used when a patient has refractory symptoms and is imminently dying.
- Strive for a "peaceful death" that is
  - Free from avoidable distress and suffering for the patient, family, and caregiver(s).
  - In general accord with the patient's and family's wishes.
  - Consistent with clinical, cultural, and ethical standards.

CAREGIVER SUPPORT

- Family and/or friends providing care may also experience distress.
- Providing appropriate referrals to palliative care or social work may help to relieve caregiver burden.

SUGGESTED READINGS

Dahlin C. *Clinical Practice Guidelines for Quality Palliative Care*. 3rd ed. Pittsburgh, PA: National Consensus Project for Quality Palliative Care; 2013. https://www.hpna.org/multimedia/NCP_Clinical_Practice_Guidelines_3rd_Edition.pdf. Accessed March 7, 2018.

Ferrell BR, Temel JS, Temin S, et al. Integration of palliative care into standard oncology care: American Society of Clinical Oncology clinical practice guideline update. *J Clin Oncol*. 2017;35(1):96-112.

Lefkowits C, Solomon C. Palliative care in obstetrics and gynecology. *Obstet Gynecol*. 2016; 128(6):1403-1420.

VI

Surgery in Obstetrics and Gynecology

58 Anatomy of the Female Pelvis

Katherine F. Chaves and Jean R. Anderson

ABDOMINAL WALL

The **anterior abdominal wall** lies ventrally and is outlined superiorly by the lower edge of the rib cage and inferiorly by the iliac crests, inguinal ligaments, and pubic bone.

Layers of the Anterior Abdominal Wall

- **Skin**
- **Subcutaneous layer.** This consists of fat globules in a meshwork of fibrous septa. **Camper fascia** is the more superficial aspect of the subcutaneous layer. **Scarpa fascia** is the deeper portion and has a more organized consistency than Camper fascia secondary to more fibrous tissue.
- **Musculoaponeurotic layer.** Located immediately below the subcutaneous layer, the musculoaponeurotic layer consists of layers of fibrous tissue and muscles that hold the abdominal viscera in place.
  - **Rectus sheath.** The aponeuroses of the external oblique, internal oblique, and transversus abdominis muscles comprise the rectus sheath.
  - The anterior rectus sheath is anatomically different above and below the **arcuate line**. The arcuate line (linea semicircularis, semilunar fold of Douglas) is located midway between the umbilicus and symphysis pubis. It marks the lower edge of the posterior rectus sheath.
    - **Above the arcuate line**, the anterior rectus sheath is composed of the aponeuroses of the external oblique and ventral half of the internal oblique muscles. The posterior rectus sheath is composed of the aponeuroses of the dorsal half of the internal oblique and transversus abdominis muscles (Figure 58-1).

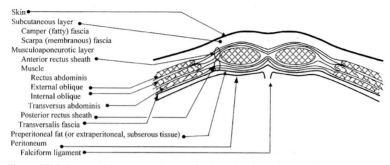

Skin
Subcutaneous layer
  Camper (fatty) fascia
  Scarpa (membranous) fascia
Musculoaponeurotic layer
  Anterior rectus sheath
  Muscle
    Rectus abdominis
    External oblique
    Internal oblique
    Transversus abdominis
  Posterior rectus sheath
  Transversalis fascia
Preperitoneal fat (or extraperitoneal, subserous tissue)
Peritoneum
  Falciform ligament

Figure 58-1. Layers of the anterior abdominal wall cephalad to the arcuate line.

- o **Below the arcuate line**, the anterior rectus sheath is composed of the aponeuroses of all the muscles previously mentioned (Figure 58-2).
- o The **linea alba** is the midline between the rectus abdominis muscles. Above the arcuate line, the linea alba marks the fusion of the anterior and posterior rectus sheaths.
- **Abdominal wall muscles**
  - **Oblique flank muscles** lie lateral to the rectus abdominis muscles.
    - o The **external oblique muscle** originates from the lower eight ribs and iliac crest and runs obliquely anteriorly and inferiorly.
    - o The **internal oblique muscle** originates from the anterior two-thirds of the iliac crest, the lateral part of the inguinal ligament, and the thoracolumbar fascia in the lower posterior flank. It runs obliquely, anteriorly, and superiorly.
    - o The **transversus abdominis muscle** runs transversely, originating from the lower six costal cartilages, the thoracolumbar fascia, the anterior three-fourths of the iliac crest, and the lateral inguinal ligament. The nerves and vasculature of the flank are found between the internal oblique and transversus abdominis muscles and, therefore, are susceptible to injury in transverse incisions.
  - **Longitudinal muscles**
    - o The **rectus abdominis muscle** is a paired muscle, found on either side of the midline, originating from the sternum and cartilage of ribs 5 through 7 and inserting into the anterior surface of the pubic bone.

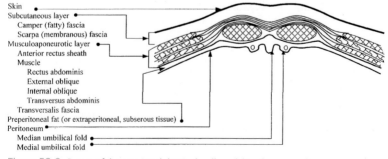

Skin
Subcutaneous layer
  Camper (fatty) fascia
  Scarpa (membranous) fascia
Musculoaponeurotic layer
  Anterior rectus sheath
  Muscle
    Rectus abdominis
    External oblique
    Internal oblique
    Transversus abdominis
  Transversalis fascia
Preperitoneal fat (or extraperitoneal, subserous tissue)
Peritoneum
  Median umbilical fold
  Medial umbilical fold

Figure 58-2. Layers of the anterior abdominal wall caudal to the arcuate line.

- o The **pyramidalis muscle** is a vestigial muscle with a variable presence among individuals. It arises from the pubic bone and inserts into the linea alba several centimeters cephalad to the symphysis and ventral to the rectus abdominis muscle.
- The **transversalis fascia** is a layer of fibrous tissue, located underneath the abdominal wall muscles and outside the peritoneum. The transversalis is separated from the peritoneum by a variable layer of adipose tissue.
- **Peritoneum.** A single layer of serosa lines the posterior aspect of the anterior abdominal wall. Five vertical folds converge toward the umbilicus.
  - The **median umbilical fold** is a single fold created by the **median umbilical ligament** or **obliterated urachus**.
    - o The apex of the bladder blends into the median umbilical ligament and is highest in the midline. This relationship should be considered when entering the peritoneal cavity.
  - The **medial umbilical folds** are paired folds lateral to the median umbilical fold, remnants of the obliterated umbilical arteries; they converge at the umbilicus.
  - The **lateral umbilical folds** are paired folds caused by the inferior epigastric vessels.

Vasculature of the Abdominal Wall

- **Subcutaneous vascular supply** (Figure 58-3)
- The **superficial epigastric artery** branches from the femoral artery after it descends through the femoral canal. It runs superomedially approximately 5 cm lateral to the midline.
- The **superficial circumflex iliac artery** branches from the femoral artery and runs laterally toward the flank.
- **Musculofascial blood supply** parallels the subcutaneous supply (see Figure 58-3).
  - The **inferior epigastric artery** branches from the external iliac artery, proximal to the inguinal ligament. It runs cephalad, deep to the transversalis fascia and lateral to the rectus muscle. Midway between the pubis and umbilicus, the vessels intersect the lateral border of the rectus muscle and course between the dorsal aspect of the rectus and the posterior rectus sheath. These vessels run between 4 and 8 cm lateral to the midline. After entering the posterior rectus sheath, numerous branches supply all layers of the abdominal wall and anastomose with the superior epigastric vessels.
  - The **superior epigastric artery** branches from the internal thoracic artery and runs caudally to form anastomoses with the inferior epigastric artery.
  - The **deep circumflex iliac artery** also branches from the external iliac artery and runs laterally between the internal oblique and transverses abdominis muscles.

PELVIC VISCERA

Vagina

- The **vagina** is shaped like a flattened tube, starting at the distal hymenal ring and ending at the fornices surrounding the proximal cervix. Its average length is 8 cm; this varies greatly with age, parity, and surgical history.
- The vaginal epithelium is nonkeratinized, stratified squamous epithelium lacking mucous glands and hair follicles.

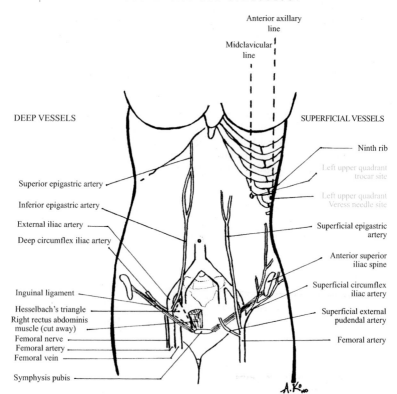

Figure 58-3. Vasculature and laparoscopic landmarks of the anterior abdominal wall. Original drawing by Alice W. Ko, from *The Johns Hopkins Manual of Gynecology and Obstetrics.* 2nd ed. Philadelphia, PA: Lippincott Williams & Wilkins; 2002.

- Deep to the epithelium is the vaginal muscularis or endopelvic fascia. The term *fascia* is misleading because this is actually fibromuscular tissue that includes fibroblasts, smooth muscle cells, elastin, and a collagen network, all loosely arrayed to create an elastic supportive layer. At the vaginal apex, this fibromuscular layer coalesces to create the **cardinal** and **uterosacral** ligaments. The fan-shaped cardinal ligament creates a sheath that envelops the uterine artery and vein, fusing medially with the paracervical ring. The uterosacral portion inserts into the posterior and lateral aspect of the paracervical ring and then curves laterally along the pelvic sidewall to attach to the presacral fascia that overlies the second, third, and fourth sacral vertebrae. Together, the cardinal and uterosacral ligaments pull the vagina proximally toward the sacrum, suspending it over the muscular levator plate.
- The endopelvic fascia of the anterior and posterior vaginal wall are known as the **pubocervical fascia** and **rectovaginal fascia**, respectively. Again, these layers are not true fasciae but are composed of fibromuscular sheets. Superiorly, the pubocervical fascia attaches to the cervix and the cardinal/uterosacral support of the vaginal apex. Laterally, it coalesces with the fascia of the obturator internus muscle to create

Figure 58-4. Illustration of attachment of rectovaginal fascia (RVF) and arcus tendineus fascia pelvis (ATFP) to the pelvic sidewall. The RVF represents the ideal line of suture placement during lateral defect repair. Abbreviations: ATFRV, arcus tendineus fascia rectovaginalis; IS, ischial spine; PCF, pubocervical fascia. Reprinted from Leffler KS, Thompson JR, Cundiff GW, et al. Attachment of the rectovaginal septum to the pelvic sidewall. *Am J Obstet Gynecol.* 2001;185(1):41-43. Copyright © 2001 Elsevier. With permission.

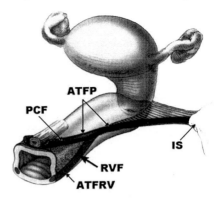

the **arcus tendineus fascia pelvis (ATFP)** or "white line." Inferiorly, it attaches to the pubic symphysis. The rectovaginal fascia in the upper vagina coalesces with the lateral support of the anterior vaginal wall and fuses with the ATFP. The lower half of the rectovaginal fascia fuses with the aponeurosis of the levator ani muscles along a line referred to as the **arcus tendineus fascia rectovaginalis**. At its most inferior point, the rectovaginal septum fuses with the perineal body (Figure 58-4).

Uterus

- The **uterus** is a fibromuscular organ composed of the corpus and the cervix.
- **Corpus.** The **endometrium** is the innermost lining of the uterus made up of columnar epithelium and specialized stroma. The superficial layer of the endometrium contains hormonally sensitive spiral arterioles, which shed with each cycle. The **myometrium** contains interlacing smooth muscle fibers, and the **serosal** surface of the uterus is formed by peritoneal mesothelium. The **fundus** is the portion of the uterus cephalad to the endometrial cavity. The **cornua** are located where the fallopian tubes insert into the uterine cavity, lateral to the fundus.
- **Cervix.** The cervix is generally 2 to 4 cm in length and has two parts: the **portio vaginalis** (protruding into the vagina) and the **portio supravaginalis** (lying above the vagina). The cervix is made up of dense fibrous connective tissue and is surrounded in a circular fashion by a small amount of smooth muscle into which the cardinal and uterosacral ligaments and pubocervical and rectovaginal fascia insert. The cervix contains a central longitudinal canal connecting the endometrial cavity with the vagina, called the **endocervical canal.** The **internal os** of the cervix is at the junction of the endocervical canal and the endometrial cavity. The **external os** is the distal opening of the cervical canal to the vagina. The **squamocolumnar junction** is located at the external os. It marks the transition from the squamous epithelium of the ectocervix to the columnar epithelium of the endocervical canal at the external os. The position of this junction varies in response to hormonal influences. The **transformation zone** is the area of squamous metaplasia surrounding the squamocolumnar junction. The transformation zone is sampled with Pap smears and is a common site for cervical dysplasia and cancer. The **ectocervix** is the outer portion of the cervix.

Ligaments of the Uterus

- These ligaments are formed by thickening of the endopelvic fascia or folds of peritoneum.
- The **round ligament** courses from the anterolateral aspect of the uterine corpus through the inguinal canal to insert into the labia majora. It has a fibromuscular element and can give rise to leiomyomas. It contains the **artery of Sampson**. This ligament provides no support for the uterus.
- The **utero-ovarian ligament** contains the anastomotic vasculature of the uterine and ovarian vessels and connects the uterus and ovaries.
- The **cardinal ligaments (Mackenrodt ligaments)** extend from the lateral pelvic walls and insert into the lateral portion of the vagina, uterine cervix, and isthmus. These contain both the uterine artery and vein and play an important role in support of the pelvic organs.
- The **infundibulopelvic ligament (IP ligament, suspensory ligament of the ovary)** contains the ovarian vessels. The ovarian arteries branch directly off the aorta. The right ovarian vein feeds into the inferior vena cava, whereas the left vein drains into the left renal vein.
- The **uterosacral ligaments** extend from the sacral fascia and insert into the posterior portion of the uterine isthmus and endopelvic fascia. Together, the cardinal and uterosacral ligaments form the parametrium and play an important role in pelvic organ support.
- The **broad ligament** is the peritoneum that covers the uterus and fallopian tubes. It is divided into the mesometrium that surrounds the uterus, the mesosalpinx that surrounds the fallopian tube, and the mesovarium that surrounds the utero-ovarian ligament.

Adnexae

- The **fallopian tubes** are bilateral tubular structures that connect the endometrial cavity to the peritoneal cavity. They are, on average, 10 cm in length. Distally, the tubes have a fimbriated end that receives each ovum after ovulation. The lumen is lined by ciliated columnar epithelium. The fallopian tube has four regions (from proximal to distal): interstitial, isthmic, ampullary, and infundibular.
- The **ovaries** are bilateral, white, flattened oval structures that store ova. The ovary is suspended laterally from the pelvic sidewall by the IP ligament and medially from the uterus by the utero-ovarian ligament. Each ovary rests in the ovarian fossa, which is bordered dorsomedially by the hypogastric artery and ventrolaterally by the external iliac artery. The ureter runs at the base of this fossa. The ovary has a fibromuscular and vascular medulla and an outer cortex that contains specialized stroma with follicles, corpora lutea, and corpora albicantia. The ovary is covered by cuboidal epithelium.

Ureter

- The **ureter** courses from the kidneys retroperitoneally, crosses the pelvic brim at the level of the bifurcation of the common iliac artery, and continues in the medial leaf of the broad ligament. It enters the tunnel of Wertheim as it passes under the uterine artery 1.5 cm lateral to the cervix at the level of the internal cervical os and enters the trigone of the bladder. The three most common areas of ureteral injury during gynecologic surgery are at the pelvic brim during clamping of the

IP ligaments, during clamping of the uterine artery at time of hysterectomy, and during the colpotomy incision.

SURGICAL SPACES OF THE PELVIS

The reproductive, urinary, and gastrointestinal organs found in the pelvis have the ability to change their size and shape independently of each other, which is made possible by their loose attachments via connective tissue planes composed of fat and areolar tissue. These planes are potential spaces that can be entered with surgical dissection. The neurolymphovascular supply to the organs remains in the connective tissue septae, permitting blunt and bloodless dissection of the surgical spaces. Eight avascular spaces are described: prevesical, vesicovaginal, paravesical (2), pararectal (2), rectovaginal, and retrorectal (Figure 58-5).

- The **prevesical space**, also known as the **space of Retzius** or **retropubic space**, is separated ventrally from the rectus abdominis by the transversalis fascia. Laterally, the muscles of the pelvic wall, cardinal ligament, and attachment of the pubocervical fascia to the ATFP border the prevesical space. Important structures within the space of Retzius include the dorsal clitoral vessels, obturator nerves and vessels, nerves of the lower urinary tract, iliopectineal line, ATFP, and the arcus tendineus levator ani. Burch urethropexies are performed in this space.

- The **vesicovaginal spaces (also called vesicocervical)** are separated by a thin supravaginal septum. The spaces are bound caudally by the fusion of the junction of the proximal one-third and distal two-thirds of the urethra with the vagina, ventrally by the urethra and bladder, cephalad by the peritoneum, forming the vesicocervical reflection. This is the space entered when developing a "bladder flap" during cesarean delivery or hysterectomy.

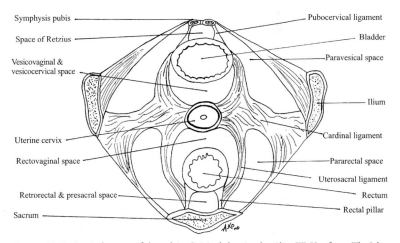

Figure 58-5. Surgical spaces of the pelvis. Original drawing by Alice W. Ko, from *The Johns Hopkins Manual of Gynecology and Obstetrics*. 2nd ed. Philadelphia, PA: Lippincott Williams & Wilkins; 2002.

- The **paravesical spaces** are paired spaces adjacent to the bladder. They are bordered medially by the bladder and obliterated umbilical artery, laterally by the obturator internus, dorsally by the cardinal ligament, ventrally by the pubic symphysis, and caudally by the levator ani. The ureter can be found in the tissue between the paravesical and vesicovaginal spaces. Parametrial tissue obtained in a radical hysterectomy is located between the paravesical and pararectal spaces.

- The **pararectal spaces** are paired spaces adjacent to the rectum. The space is bordered medially by the ureter, uterosacral ligament, and rectum; laterally by the hypogastric vessels and pelvic wall; ventrolaterally by the cardinal ligament; and dorsally by the sacrum. The coccygeus forms the floor of this space. Bleeding can be encountered from the lateral sacral and hemorrhoidal vessels if dissection is carried to the pelvic floor. These spaces allow access to the sacrospinous ligaments as well as identification of the ureter for ureterolysis when indicated.

- The **rectovaginal space** is bordered caudally by the apex of the perineal body; laterally by the uterosacral ligament, ureter, and rectal pillars; ventrally by the vagina; and dorsally by the rectum. The **pouch of Douglas** or **posterior cul-de-sac** is the space between the uterus and rectum bounded inferiorly by the peritoneum. The rectovaginal space is below this peritoneum and cul-de-sac and is developed by incising the peritoneal fold between the uterus and rectum.

- The **retrorectal space** is caudal to the presacral space and bordered ventrally by the rectum, posteriorly by the sacrum, and laterally by the uterosacral ligaments. The **presacral space** is bordered laterally by the internal iliac arteries, cephalad by the bifurcation of the aorta, dorsally by the sacrum, and ventrally by the colon. It contains the presacral nerve (superior hypogastric plexus), the middle sacral artery and vein (originating from the dorsal aspect of the aorta and vena cava), and the lateral sacral vessels. This space is entered for sacrocolpopexy for pelvic organ prolapse, presacral neurectomy for pelvic pain, and para-aortic lymph node dissection.

VASCULATURE OF THE ABDOMEN AND PELVIS

- **Aorta.** From cephalad to caudad, the arteries that stem from the aorta below the diaphragm are inferior phrenic, celiac trunk, suprarenal, superior mesenteric, renal, lumbar, ovarian, inferior mesenteric, and median sacral. The aorta then bifurcates into the common iliac arteries at the level of the fourth lumbar vertebra.

- **Celiac trunk.** The celiac trunk has three main branches: the **left gastric**, the **splenic**, and the **common hepatic** arteries. The **left gastric artery** divides into the esophageal branches and branches that supply the lesser curvature of the stomach. The **splenic artery** divides into pancreatic branches, **short gastric arteries**, which supply the fundus of the stomach, and the **left gastroepiploic artery**, which supplies the greater omentum and the greater curvature of the stomach. The left gastroepiploic artery anastomoses with the right gastroepiploic, which is a terminal branch of the common hepatic. The **common hepatic artery** has two main divisions: the **proper hepatic artery** and the **gastroduodenal artery**. The proper hepatic artery divides into the **right gastric artery** and enters the lesser omentum to anastomose with the **left gastric artery** and terminates into the **right and left hepatic arteries**. The **cystic artery** often branches from the right hepatic artery and supplies the gallbladder. The **gastroduodenal artery** branches into the **supraduodenal artery**, the **right gastroepiploic artery**, and the **superior pancreatoduodenal artery**. The **right gastroepiploic artery** enters the greater omentum and anastomoses with the left gastroepiploic artery along the greater curvature of the stomach. The **superior pancreatoduodenal artery** supplies the second part of the duodenum and the head of the pancreas.

- The **superior mesenteric artery** branches into the **jejunal** and **ileal artery** branches, the **ileocolic artery**, the **right colic artery**, and the **middle colic artery**.
- The **inferior mesenteric artery** branches into the **left colic artery**, the **sigmoid branches**, and the **superior rectal artery**.
- **Ovarian vessels.** The ovarian arteries originate from the anterior aspect of the aorta and course toward the pelvis, crossing laterally over the **ureters** at the level of the pelvic brim, and passing branches to the ureters and fallopian tubes. They then cross medially over the proximal external iliac vessels and run medially in the IP ligaments. The left ovarian vein drains into the left renal vein, whereas the right ovarian vein drains directly into the inferior vena cava.
- The aorta bifurcates into the **common iliac arteries** at the level of the fourth lumbar vertebra. The common iliac then bifurcates into the **external and internal** (hypogastric) **arteries**. The hypogastric artery divides into an anterior and posterior division 3 to 4 cm after the branching off of the common iliac artery. The **ureter** courses anteriorly to the division of the hypogastric and external iliac arteries.
  - **Anterior division of the hypogastric artery.** Some variance exists in the branching pattern. The branches include the obturator, uterine, vaginal, inferior and superior vesical, middle rectal, internal pudendal, and inferior gluteal arteries. The **ureter** passes laterally under the **uterine artery** at the level of the internal cervical os. During hypogastric artery ligation, the anterior division of the hypogastric artery should be doubly ligated with 1-0 silk (do not divide) 2.5 to 3.0 cm distal to the bifurcation of the common iliac. The dissection is done laterally to medially to avoid damaging the hypogastric vein.
  - **Posterior division of the hypogastric artery.** The branches include the iliolumbar, lateral sacral, and superior gluteal arteries, all of which have anastomosing channels in the pelvis.
- **External iliac artery.** The deep epigastric and deep circumflex iliac arteries branch from the external iliac artery before it travels under the inguinal ligament and into the femoral canal, where it becomes the femoral artery.
- **Anastomoses.** The **superior rectal artery** branches off the inferior mesenteric artery, the **middle rectal artery** branches off the anterior division of the hypogastric artery, and the **inferior rectal artery branches** off the pudendal artery (a branch of the hypogastric). This allows for redundant blood flow to the pelvis.

VULVA AND PERINEUM

External Anatomy

- The bony pelvic outlet is bordered anteriorly by the ischiopubic rami and posteriorly by the coccyx and sacrotuberous ligaments. The outlet can be divided into anterior and posterior triangles sharing a common base along a line between the ischial tuberosities.
- **Skin and subcutaneous layer.** The subcutaneous tissue has two nondiscrete layers: Camper fascia and Colles fascia.
  - **Camper fascia** includes the continuation of this layer from the anterior abdominal wall.
  - **Colles fascia** is similar to Scarpa fascia of the anterior abdominal wall. It fuses posteriorly with the perineal membrane and laterally with the ischiopubic rami.

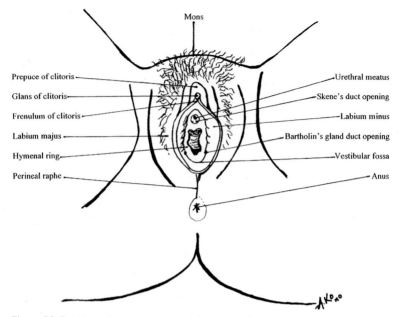

Figure 58-6. Vulva and perineum. Original drawing by Alice W. Ko, from *The Johns Hopkins Manual of Gynecology and Obstetrics*. 2nd ed. Philadelphia, PA: Lippincott Williams & Wilkins; 2002.

- The **mons (mons pubis, mons veneris)** is hair-bearing skin overlying adipose tissue that lies on the pubic bones (Figure 58-6).
- The **labia majora** extend posteriorly from the mons and contain similar hair-bearing skin. The labia majora contain the insertion of the round ligaments.
- The **labia minora** are hairless skin folds that split anteriorly to form the prepuce and frenulum of the clitoris. They overlie loosely organized connective tissue rather than adipose tissue.
- **Gland duct openings**
  - The **greater vestibular (Bartholin) gland** duct opening is seen on the posterolateral aspect of the vestibule 3 to 4 mm lateral to the hymenal ring.
  - The **minor vestibular gland** duct opening is seen in a line above the greater vestibular gland duct opening toward the urethra.
  - The **Skene ducts** are located inferolateral to the urethral meatus at approximately 5 and 7 o'clock.
- **Specialized glands**
  - **Holocrine sebaceous glands** are located in the labia majora and are associated with hair shafts.
  - **Apocrine sweat glands** are located lateral to the introitus and anus. **Hidradenitis suppurativa** can occur if these glands become chronically infected. **Hidradenomas** are neoplastic enlargements of these glands.
  - **Eccrine sweat glands** are also located laterally to the introitus and anus. They can enlarge and form a **syringoma**.

Superficial Compartment of the Vulva

- This compartment lies between the subcutaneous layer and the perineal membrane (Figure 58-7).
- The **clitoris** consists of the glans, a shaft that is attached to the pubis by a subcutaneous suspensory ligament, and paired crura that stem from the shaft and attach to the inferior aspect of the pubic rami.
- **Ischiocavernosus muscles** overlie the crura of the clitoris. They originate at the ischial tuberosities and free surfaces of the crura and insert into the upper crura and clitoral shaft.
- **Bulbospongiosus muscles** originate in the perineal body and insert into the clitoral shaft. They overlie the centrolateral aspects of the vestibular bulbs and Bartholin gland.
- **Superficial transverse perineal muscles** originate from the ischial tuberosities and insert into the perineal body.
- The **perineal body (central tendon of the perineum)** is connected anterolaterally with the bulbospongiosus muscle and anteriorly with the perineal membrane, which attaches the perineal body to the inferior pubic rami. The perineal body is attached laterally to the superficial transverse perineal muscles, posteriorly to the external anal sphincter, and superiorly to the distal rectovaginal fascia.
- The **vestibular bulbs** are paired erectile tissues that lie immediately under the skin of the vestibule and under the bulbocavernosus muscles.

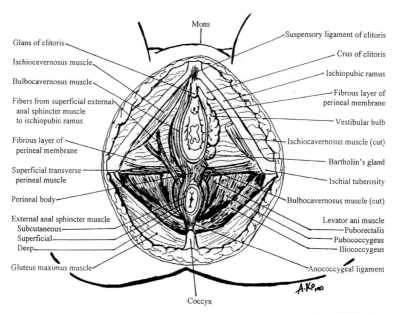

Figure 58-7. Superficial compartment of the vulva. Original drawing by Alice W. Ko, from *The Johns Hopkins Manual of Gynecology and Obstetrics.* 2nd ed. Philadelphia, PA: Lippincott Williams & Wilkins; 2002.

- **Bartholin glands** lie between the bulbocavernosus muscles and the perineal membrane at the tail end of the vestibular bulb. Their ducts empty into the vestibular mucosa.

Pelvic Floor

- The **pelvic floor** comprises the perineal membrane and the muscles of the pelvic diaphragm. It helps support the pelvic contents above the pelvic outlet.
- The **perineal membrane** is a triangular sheet of dense fibromuscular tissue that spans the anterior triangle. It provides support by attaching the urethra, vagina, and perineal body to the ischiopubic rami. The perineal membrane contains the dorsal and deep nerves and vessels to the clitoris.
- The **muscles of the pelvic diaphragm** comprise the levator ani and coccygeal muscles. These are covered by the superior and inferior fascias (Figure 58-8).
  - **Levator ani muscles**
  - The **puborectalis** arises from the inner surface of the pubic bones and inserts into the rectum. Some fibers form a sling around the posterior aspect of the rectum.
  - The **pubococcygeus** arises from the pubic bones and inserts into the anococcygeal raphe and superior aspect of the coccyx.

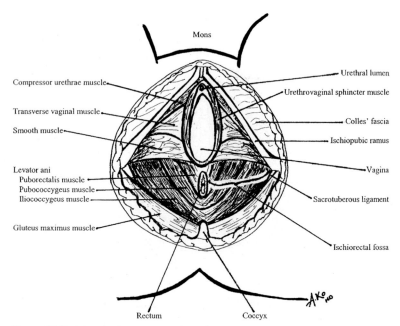

Figure 58-8. Pelvic diaphragm. Original drawing by Alice W. Ko, from *The Johns Hopkins Manual of Gynecology and Obstetrics.* 2nd ed. Philadelphia, PA: Lippincott Williams & Wilkins; 2002.

- The **iliococcygeus** arises from the **arcus tendineus levator ani** and inserts into the anococcygeal raphe and coccyx.
- The **coccygeus muscle** arises from the ischial spine and inserts into the coccyx and lowest area of the sacrum. It lies cephalad to the sacrospinous ligament.

Posterior Triangle

- This area is bounded bilaterally by the ischial tuberosities and posteriorly by the coccyx.
- **External anal sphincter**
  - The superficial portion is attached anteriorly to the perineal body and posteriorly to the coccyx.
  - The deep portion encircles the rectum and blends in with the puborectalis muscle.
- **Internal anal sphincter.** This sphincter is a smooth muscle that is separated from the external sphincter by the intersphincteric groove as well as fibers from the longitudinal layer of the bowel.
- The **ischioanal fossa** contains the pudendal neurovascular trunk; it is bordered medially by the levator ani muscles and laterally by the obturator internus muscles. It has an anterior recess that lies above the perineal membrane and a posterior portion that lies above the gluteus maximus. This space allows for physiologic expansion of the rectum.

NERVES OF THE PELVIS AND PERINEUM

Pelvic Diaphragm

- The **pudendal nerve** supplies the external anal sphincter and the urethral sphincter.
- The **anterior branch of the ventral ramus of S3 and S4** innervates the levator ani and coccygeal muscles.

Perineum

- The **pudendal nerve** is the sensory and motor nerve of the perineum.
  - The pudendal nerve originates from the sacral plexus (S2-S4), exits the pelvis through the greater sciatic notch, hooks around the ischial spine and sacrospinous ligament, and enters the pudendal canal (**canal of Alcock**) in the lesser sciatic notch. The pudendal nerve has several terminal branches:
    - The **clitoral nerve** runs along the superficial aspect of the perineal membrane to supply the clitoris.
    - The **perineal nerve** runs along the deep aspect of the perineal membrane. Its branches supply the muscles of the superficial compartment, subcutaneum, and skin of the vestibule, labia minora, and medial aspect of the labia majora.
    - The **inferior hemorrhoidal nerve (inferior rectal)** innervates the external anal sphincter and the perianal skin.
- A pudendal block is performed by injecting anesthetic just inferior to the ischial spine; this provides local analgesia for vaginal deliveries. This block may also be performed in cases of nerve injury or compression and resulting pudendal neuralgia.
- Nerve injuries can be encountered during gynecologic surgery from positioning, incisions, use of retractors, and hematoma formation (see chapter 60).

LYMPHATIC DRAINAGE OF THE PELVIS

* The vulva and lower vagina drain to the **inguinofemoral lymph nodes** and then to the **external iliac nodes**.
* The cervix drains through the cardinal ligaments to the **pelvic nodes (hypogastric, obturator, and external iliac)** and then to the **common iliac and para-aortic lymph nodes**.
* The **uterus** drains through the broad ligament and intraperitoneal ligament to the **pelvic and para-aortic lymph nodes**.
* The **ovaries** drain to the **pelvic and para-aortic lymph nodes**.

SUGGESTED READINGS

Ashton-Miller JA, DeLancey JO. Functional anatomy of the female pelvic floor. *Ann N Y Acad Sci.* 2007;1101:266-296.

DeLancey JO. Surgical anatomy of the female pelvis. In: Jones HW, Rock JA, eds. *Te Linde's Operative Gynecology.* 11th ed. Philadelphia, PA: Wolters Kluwer; 2015:93-122.

Law YM, Fielding JR. MRI of pelvic floor dysfunction: review. *AJR Am J Roentgenol.* 2008;191:S45-S53.

Weber AM, Walters MD. Anterior vaginal prolapse: review of anatomy and techniques of surgical repair. *Obstet Gynecol.* 1997;89:311-318.

Surgical Approaches in Gynecologic Surgery

MaryAnn Wilbur and Kristin Patzkowsky

Choosing the most appropriate route of surgery for a patient and her pathology is a critical step to ensure good operative outcomes. Gynecologic surgery is unique in that more than one approach, including vaginal, hysteroscopic, laparoscopic, robotic, or abdominal, may be reasonable for similar surgical procedures.

* **Minimally invasive surgery (MIS)** approaches include vaginal, hysteroscopic, laparoscopic, or robotic-assisted laparoscopic surgery.
* MIS can be safely used in most gynecologic conditions (both benign and malignant).
* Whenever appropriate for the particular clinical situation and safely feasible, MIS should be prioritized over open procedures based on their advantages over laparotomy.
* For hysterectomies, an MIS approach should be performed over abdominal hysterectomy whenever clinically appropriate. Additionally, a transvaginal approach is preferred over laparoscopy for many clinical situations.
* Both standard laparoscopy and robotic-assisted laparoscopy can be performed using multiple port sites or with a single site. When a single incision is used for such approaches, it is termed *single-site surgery, laparoendoscopic single-site surgery,* or *single-site incision laparoscopic surgery.*

MINIMALLY INVASIVE SURGERY IN GYNECOLOGY

Benefits of Minimally Invasive Surgery

- Although most patients will heal well from either an MIS or an open approach, MIS is associated with decreased blood loss, need for transfusion, postoperative pain and narcotic requirement, wound infection, length of hospital stay, and need for readmission.
- Patients with obesity and diabetes particularly benefit from the decreased risk of wound infection and readmission; therefore, an MIS approach should be strongly considered for these patients whenever feasible.

Laparoscopy

- Laparoscopic surgery is an operation performed through a number of small abdominal incisions with the abdominal cavity insufflated with carbon dioxide (CO_2) gas for visualization.
- The number of incisions varies depending on the procedure to be performed, the size of the pathology, and the complexity of the case.
- A trocar, or port, is placed through each incision through which instruments can be passed into and out of the abdomen without loss of intra-abdominal gas. Trocars vary in size, 3 to 15 mm, depending on what instruments will be used and the size of the specimen to be removed from the abdomen.
- For laparoscopic surgery, especially for complex cases, surgeons may have a long learning curve because one has to learn how to operate in 2-dimensional space with its resultant loss of depth perception and challenging hand-eye coordination.

Robot-Assisted Laparoscopic Surgery

- The da Vinci system was US Food and Drug Administration approved for use in gynecology in 2005 as a tool to improve surgeon experience of laparoscopy and to increase the number of patients that can be offered a minimally invasive approach.
- What a robotic-assisted procedure offers above and beyond standard laparoscopy includes (1) wristed instruments, (2) 3-dimensional vision from the dual eye technology, and (3) opportunity for a third arm that can be used for retraction. It also improves the ergonomic experience of the surgeon.
- Robot-assisted laparoscopy removes the surgeon from the patient bedside and removes the ability for tactile feedback.
- The decision to perform a procedure via conventional laparoscopy or robotically is surgeon dependent. Reasons often cited for choosing a robotic approach over a conventional laparoscopic approach are (1) anticipation of a difficult dissection (adhesions, extensive surgical history, stage IV endometriosis), (2) complex myomectomy, (3) morbid obesity, (4) surgeon preference, and (5) an extremely large uterus.

Laparoendoscopic Single Site/Single-Site Incision Laparoscopic Surgery

- Single incision surgery typically uses a single, larger (approximately 2-3 cm) port at the umbilicus with three trocars that triangulate. Pros of such a procedure include improved cosmesis and an independent surgeon who requires an assistant to hold the camera. Cons include a slightly increased risk of hernia and a steep learning curve to master the mechanics of triangulated ports where the right and left hand control the opposite instrument in the surgical field.

- A robotic single-site platform is available that uses curved instruments that allow for greater ease of manipulating the instruments.
- Although any number of gynecologic procedures can be performed by a minimally invasive method, two of the commonly performed procedures are hysterectomy and myomectomy.

Minimally Invasive Hysterectomy

Transvaginal Hysterectomy

- Despite the frequent discussions about laparoscopy and robotics in operative gynecology, the 2017 American College of Obstetrics and Gynecologists Committee Opinion continues to affirm that, when feasible, a **total vaginal hysterectomy (TVH)** remains the preferred method for removal of the uterus and cervix.
- A TVH is the most cost-effective and least invasive hysterectomy approach.
- Uterine size, mobility, accessibility, and absence of adnexal pathology or suspected adhesions are all factors that should be considered when determining the appropriateness for offering TVH.

Laparoscopically Assisted Vaginal Hysterectomy

- A **laparoscopically assisted vaginal hysterectomy** uses a laparoscope to visualize the peritoneal cavity and assess the pelvis. Many surgeons will use this approach to take down adhesions and ligate the ovarian vessels laparoscopically before performing what is otherwise a vaginal hysterectomy. Other surgeons will continue laparoscopically and ligate the uterine vessels prior to completing the colpotomy and hysterectomy vaginally.

Laparoscopic Hysterectomy (Including Robotic Assisted)

- A **total laparoscopic hysterectomy** is performed laparoscopically up to and including the colpotomy. Depending on surgeon training/preference, the colpotomy can be closed by sewing the vaginal cuff vaginally or laparoscopically, and evidence is conflicting regarding superiority of closure route.
  - Vaginal cuff dehiscence is an uncommon complication ($<1\%$) after hysterectomy, although it occurs more frequently after robotic and laparoscopic approaches compared to abdominal and vaginal approaches. There are no clear risk factors. Factors likely contributing to the increased risk after laparoscopic and robotic hysterectomy are the use of electrosurgery for colpotomy, magnified view leading to inadequate bites for closure, and inadequate integrity of laparoscopically tied knots (by knot pusher or other device).
- **Supracervical hysterectomy (SCH)** is commonly performed at sacrocolpopexy to provide a site for mesh fixation, thus reducing the risk of vaginal mesh erosion. Outside of this indication, SCH is less commonly performed because of the 20% risk of ongoing cyclic bleeding, continued need for cervical cancer surveillance and no difference in sexual satisfaction, bladder/bowel function, or pelvic organ prolapse. After SCH, the woman can resume sexual intercourse sooner because there is no risk of vaginal cuff dehiscence.

Minimally Invasive Myomectomy

- When feasible, myomectomy should be performed via an MIS approach, including hysteroscopic (for type 0 and 1 submucosal fibroids <5 cm and select type 2 fibroids) or laparoscopic/robotic approach (see chapter 33). To date, evidence suggests no difference in surgical outcomes between laparoscopic and robotic myomectomies.

- Although surgical approach is based on surgeon preference, the main reason cited for choosing a robotic approach for myomectomy is the need for excessive suturing and the inherent benefit of wristed instruments for this task. This is particularly beneficial for the closure of posterior uterine defects, which pose a distinct technical challenge.
- Preoperative magnetic resonance imaging is critical to myomectomy planning because it does the following:
  - Precisely details fibroid burden to help the surgeon map out the excision
  - Helps to guide counseling regarding potential fibroid impact on fertility
  - Allows for evaluation for concurrent adenomyosis or adenomyoma

Laparoscopic Entry Techniques

- There are several entry techniques available, and none are without risks. The appropriate choice will depend on patient anatomy, surgical history, and a surgeon's preference.
  - **Open or Hassan technique** allows for entering the abdominal cavity under direct visualization. This approach can be used to enter the abdomen in any quadrant but is most commonly used at the umbilicus. A 10- to 120-mm skin incision is made at the umbilicus and dissected down so that the fascia and peritoneum can be entered directly. Once entry is visualized and noted to be free of adhesions, the fascia is typically tagged with suture(s) and a blunt trocar placed directly into the peritoneal cavity, which allows CO_2 gas insufflation and placement of a laparoscopic camera.
  - For the **closed or Veress needle** approach, the base of the umbilicus is everted, a skin incision made (5-10 mm to accommodate planned trocar) with a scalpel and the Veress needle is placed into the peritoneal cavity. Classically, two "pops" are heard/felt, representing passage of the Veress through the fascia and peritoneum. Once the Veress needle is intraperitoneal, the abdomen is insufflated with CO_2 gas, the Veress is removed, and a trocar is placed blindly or by direct visualization through an optical trocar. Several tests can be used to assess if the Veress is in the correct position:
    - Water drop test: A saline filled syringe (without the plunger) is attached to the Veress. If tip of the Veress is within the peritoneal cavity, saline will pass easily into this space, whereas if it is preperitoneal, saline will pass slowly.
    - Drawing back on a syringe: Attach a syringe to the Veress and draw back. Blood or bowel contents would indicate incorrect placement.
    - Opening pressure: Attach CO_2 tubing to the Veress needle and initiate gas flow. The pressure on opening the valve should be <5 mm Hg if within the peritoneal cavity.
  - **Direct visualization technique** using an optical trocar. A zero-degree laparoscope is backloaded into an optical (clear-tipped) trocar, and the layers of the abdominal wall are visually passed until the peritoneal cavity is entered. Once peritoneal entry is suspected, CO_2 insufflation is initiated and correct placement is confirmed by direct visualization.
- Although there are risks associated with all entry techniques and entry sites, the risk of vascular and bowel injuries is very small, far less than 1%. A Cochrane review from 2015 indicates there is no difference in vascular or bowel injury for

open- versus closed-entry techniques. The closed-/Veress needle–entry technique is associated with an increased risk of failed entry (ie, preperitoneal placement) as compared to the open technique. There is no superior entry option, and the surgeon must gauge risks for each patient.

Laparoscopic Entry Sites

- Any of the entry techniques can be used at the different **entry sites**.
- The most common site of entry is at the **umbilicus** due to its central location and the anatomic phenomenon that all layers essentially become one at the level of the umbilical stalk. Alternative sites are considered in the presence of previous abdominal or pelvic surgeries, umbilical hernia, or concern for adhesions or in the setting of very large pathology.
- **Left upper quadrant or Palmer's point.** For left upper quadrant entry, an incision is made in the left midclavicular line, generally 1 to 2 fingerbreadths beneath the inferior costal margin. Layers traversed are skin, subcutaneous fat, external oblique aponeurosis, internal oblique aponeurosis, transversalis muscle fibers, extraperitoneal fat, and peritoneum. To avoid injury to the stomach, decompress the stomach with orogastric or nasogastric tube before entry.
- **Right upper quadrant.** Right upper quadrant entry can be helpful in a patient with previous gastric surgery. Entry is made with great care to avoid injury to the liver. This entry site may not be ideal in someone with prior cholecystectomy or Fitz-Hugh–Curtis syndrome.
- **Supraumbilical.** In the setting of large pathology, a **supraumbilical entry** point can be used.

Port Placement

- Although there are many variations, for standard **pelvic laparoscopy**, the most common approach is one umbilical entry trocar followed by placement of two additional trocars, in the bilateral lower quadrants, under direct laparoscopic visualization.
  - Care should be made to **avoid the inferior epigastric artery** when placing additional trocars. The inferior epigastric artery, which arises from the external iliac artery above the inguinal ligament, can be identified just medial to the insertion of the round ligament into the inguinal canal. This trajectory can be followed cephalad, and trocars should be placed lateral to this line. If the vessels cannot be seen, a safe location to place a lower quadrant trocar is typically 5 to 8 cm superior to the pubic symphysis and 8 cm lateral from the midline.
  - Subsequent ports are placed depending on type of surgery and anatomic findings (including size of uterus or adnexa, spread of disease, presence of adhesions, need for lymph node dissection). More complicated surgeries may require up to five ports, and these locations should be adjusted according to surgical needs, anatomy, and disease process.
- Robotic procedures use three to four robotic ports and a laparoscopic accessory port. The robotic camera port is typically placed above or around the umbilicus. Two to three robotic ports are placed laterally for the operating arms. The laparoscopic accessory port can be various sizes and locations depending on the planned procedure and the suture/instruments/specimens intended to be passed into and out of the abdomen. Consideration should be made for distance between robotic arms to minimize external collisions.

Removal of Large Specimens

- Safe specimen removal, particularly with larger specimens, should be carefully considered with all MIS procedures. The surgeon will need to choose one of the following options for specimen removal:
  - Vaginally: through the vagina at time of hysterectomy
  - Colpotomy: creating an incision in the posterior vaginal fornix
  - Port site: If needed, any port site can be extended for specimen removal. The umbilicus is often extended because this is the thinnest point of the abdominal wall and the larger incision can be hidden in the folds of the umbilicus.
  - Minilaparotomy: typically well tolerated because manipulation of this incision is far less than when it is used for a cesarean delivery or other open procedure
- Previously, power morcellation was routinely used for specimen removal. Power morcellation is not contained, allowing for macroscopic and microscopic fragments of tissue to spread in the abdomen at the time of specimen removal. Subsequent complications can include the growth/spread of fibroids, adenomyomas, and endometriosis in various sites (bowel mesentery, pelvic side wall, abdominal wall) or the iatrogenic spread of cancer in the event of undiagnosed malignancy.
  - For these reasons, the US Food and Drug Administration issued a warning in 2014 and power morcellation is now used sparingly, if at all. Whenever feasible, morcellation should now be "contained," meaning that a sterile bag is placed into the peritoneal cavity and the intact specimen placed within the bag before morcellation so that no fragments spread into the abdomen. In-bag morcellation can be performed with a scalpel (with the bag brought up the abdominal wall or the vaginal opening for access), power morcellator, or a modified technique.
  - Contained morcellation obviates the need for a full laparotomy and provides the postoperative benefits of MIS to many patients with larger specimens.
  - The histopathologic issues of a fragmented specimen, however, remain. Thus, the surgeon must consider when the importance of an intact histopathologic inspection supersedes the benefits of an MIS approach. If there is high level of concern for malignancy, morcellation is not appropriate. However, there is always a risk of occult malignancy and patients should be carefully counseled to this fact when being offered MIS hysterectomy. For example, literature suggests the risk of leiomyosarcoma may approach 1 in 350.

Port Closure and Trocar Site Complications

- Due to the very low risk of hernia, the general consensus is that ports that are ≤8 mm do not require fascial closure (hernia risk of <0.25%).
- Fascial defects ≥10 mm require closure. Risk factors for hernia include trocar size ≥10 mm, umbilical site, and increased manipulation. Two closure techniques:
  - Direct closure using a curved needle
  - Use of an endoscopic closure instrument, such as a Carter-Thomason
- Hernia is not the only iatrogenic trocar site complication that has been reported. Deposits of endometriosis and/or metastatic disease can occur. The incidence of such port site deposits is approximately 2% to 3% and is correlated with the amount of peritoneal disease present as well as volume of ascites and the concentration of cancer cells in the ascitic fluid.

Uterine Manipulation During Minimally Invasive Surgery Procedures

- For many MIS procedures, adequate uterine manipulation is critical. There are many devices available for manipulation.
- Key components of uterine manipulators:
  - Different tip lengths to correspond to the size of the uterus (allows for improved ability to manipulate a large uterus)
  - Colpotomy ring/cup. The colpotomy ring/cup sits around the cervix at the cervicovaginal junction. It provides a physical structure on which to perform a colpotomy and a visual guide point for uterine artery insertion at the level of the internal os. The appropriate size ring/cup is selected based on the diameter of the cervix.
  - Vaginal pneumo-occluder. Many manipulators come with this built-in device, an additional ring or a balloon, to maintain pneumoperitoneum once colpotomy is performed.

Minimally Invasive Surgery in the Obese Patient

- Obese patients create a particular technical challenge for MIS. However, this population often benefits the most from this less invasive approach. Therefore, the extra time, effort, and considerations should be made to offer MIS to obese patients.
- Positioning considerations: There are many different options for stabilizing the patient on the bed including specialized foam pads, gel pads, and vacuum pads that will mold around the patient to help keep her from shifting once in Trendelenburg. The extra weight of the thighs can cause the knees and hips to slowly abduct during the procedure, putting extra pressure on lateral knee against the yellow fins. Consider adding extra padding between the lateral knee and the yellow fin in an effort to avoid injury to the peroneal nerve. If needed, place bed extenders on one or both sides of the table to support the arms and decrease the risk of injury to the ulnar nerve.
- Ventilation can pose a challenge in obese patients during minimally invasive procedures. Increased adiposity leads to increased airway pressures, particularly in Trendelenburg position, which is a requisite for pelvic surgery. Pneumoperitoneum further increases these pressures. There are several strategies that can improve airway pressures and subsequent ability to tolerate Trendelenburg.
  - Reduce intra-abdominal pressure: Reducing insufflation pressure from standard 15 mm Hg to 10 to 12 mm Hg can improve anesthesia's ability to ventilate with little negative effect on surgeon visualization intraoperative.
  - Limit the degree of Trendelenburg to only what is absolutely necessary to safely complete the procedure.
  - Retraction: Laparoscopic paddles or fans are designed to help retract bowel or fat away from the surgical field, thus requiring less Trendelenburg. Passing a temporary stitch through bowel epiploica or bladder and passing extracorporeally can be used for retraction.

LAPAROTOMY IN OPERATIVE GYNECOLOGY

- Despite the many benefits of MIS, there will be patients who are not candidates for MIS and require an open procedure. The following is a nonexhaustive list of indications for laparotomy (which may also be variable dependent on surgeon experience/preferences):
  - Medical comorbidities precluding pneumoperitoneum
  - Large uterine size (Size cutoff will depend on patient anatomy and surgeon experience.)

- Desire for myomectomy with innumerable fibroids or massive uterine size
- Uterine size that would preclude intact removal but is not appropriate for contained morcellation
- Spread of disease malignant disease

Abdominal Wall Incisions

- **Midline vertical incision** provides optimal exposure to the abdomen. It allows extension up toward the xiphoid process and down to the pubic symphysis and provides (1) greatest exposure, (2) flexibility in length of incision, and (3) minimal blood loss. However, a midline vertical incision can be associated with increased pain, risk of hernia, and poorer cosmesis.
  - The anterior rectus sheath is incised longitudinally in the midline. If the incision extends above the arcuate line, the posterior sheath is then identified and incised longitudinally. The peritoneum is then identified and entered, taking care to avoid underlying structures including the superior aspect of the bladder and bowel. Once entry to the peritoneal cavity is confirmed, a visual and tactile inspection is performed to assure that no adhesions are present and that no visceral organs were harmed during entry.
- **Transverse incisions**
  - **Pfannenstiel incision** is one of the most common incisions in obstetrics and gynecology. A transverse skin incision is made approximately 2 fingerbreadths (3-4 cm) above the pubic symphysis; the fascia is transversely incised and the rectus muscles are separated from the anterior rectus sheath, thus disturbing many of the small perforating vessels that supply the rectus muscles. Then, the rectus muscles are separated in the midline to gain entry to the peritoneum.
    - The greatest limitation of a Pfannenstiel incision is limited exposure, both laterally and vertically.
    - Lateral extension of the skin incision runs a risk of injury to the ilioinguinal and iliohypogastric nerves either by direct incision or more often by entrapment during fascial closure.
  - **Maylard incision** uses a transverse skin incision, typically made at the level of the anterior superior iliac spine but can be made anywhere along the abdominal wall. The key difference between a Pfannenstiel and Maylard incision is that the rectus muscles are not separated from the fascia. Rather, they are left attached to the rectus sheath, and the muscles are transected after the inferior epigastric vessels are identified and ligated. The rectus muscles do not have to be reapproximated at the completion of the surgery.
    - This incision provides excellent lateral exposure and improved cosmesis and less pain as compared to midline vertical.
    - When comparing Maylard to Pfannenstiel incisions, Maylard offers better exposure, and no difference was noted in postoperative pain at 1 and 3 months and no difference in abdominal muscle strength at 3 months.
  - **Cherney incision** provides better exposure to the pelvis than the Pfannenstiel incision. This incision provides excellent lateral exposure and access to the space of Retzius. After the rectus muscle is dissected off the fascia, as in a Pfannenstiel, the tendinous insertion of the rectus muscle is cut approximately 0.5 cm above the insertion site at the posterior aspect of the pubic bones. The rectus bellies are then moved cephalad, providing excellent exposure to the pelvis. Note the importance of leaving enough tendon on the pubic bone so that the caudal aspect of the rectus

muscles can be reapproximated to the tendon with a delayed absorbable suture in a horizontal mattress fashion during closure. Because of the risk of osteomyelitis, the rectus muscles should NOT be sutured to the periosteum of the symphysis pubis.

- If a Pfannenstiel incision is found to offer inadequate exposure, it can be converted to a Cherney incision. A conversion to a Maylard incision should not be performed because of (1) the risk of rectus muscle necrosis that can occur after taking both the inferior epigastric arteries and the perforating fascial vessels that provide blood supply to the rectus abdominis and (2) the risk that the rectus muscles will not reapproximate because the muscle edges have likely retracted with separation of the rectus from the anterior rectus sheath.

Closure Techniques

- Proper closure techniques are an important part of every successful laparotomy procedure.
- For most patients, surgeons generally favor **primary fascia closure** without a peritoneal closure and with minimal involvement of the rectus muscles.
  - Although some surgeons opt to close the peritoneum prior to fascial closure in hopes of reducing postoperative adhesions, this adds operative time and a recent Cochrane review suggests that there is no clinical benefit to closing the peritoneum.
  - Fascial closure:
    - Use delayed absorbable or nonabsorbable suture to reduce hernia risk.
    - Postoperative outcomes (including infection, hernia, pain) were improved with continuous closure when compared to interrupted suture closure.
- For patients at high risk for fascial dehiscence, some surgeons prefer a **mass closure** (involving the peritoneum, muscles, and fascia together).
- There may be times when the patient is not a candidate for primary closure and will need to return to the operating room for closure at a later time. These situations usually involve massive hemorrhage or infection but can also occur due to extensive fluid resuscitation and a prolonged open abdomen (often during cytoreduction for malignancy) leading to bowel edema and inability to close the abdomen without risking abdominal compartment syndrome. These patients should have advanced surgeons and anesthesia closely involved in their care whenever possible.

SUGGESTED READINGS

Ahmad G, Gent D, Henderson D, O'Flynn H, Phillips K, Watson A. Laparoscopic entry techniques. *Cochrane Database Syst Rev*. 2015;(8):CD006583.

American College of Obstetricians and Gynecologists Committee on Gynecologic Practice. Committee Opinion No. 701: choosing the route of hysterectomy for benign disease. *Obstet Gynecol*. 2017;129:e155-e159.

Conrad LB, Ramirez PT, Burke W, et al. Role of minimally invasive surgery in gynecologic oncology: an updated survey of members of the Society of Gynecologic Oncology. *Int J Gynecol Cancer*. 2015;25(6):1121-1127.

Jernigan AM, Auer M, Fader AN, Escobar PF. Minimally invasive surgery in gynecologic oncology: a review of modalities and the literature. *Womens Health (Lond)*. 2012;8(3):239-250.

Uccella S, Malzoni M, Cromi A, et al. Laparoscopic vs transvaginal cuff closure after total laparoscopic hysterectomy: a randomized trial by the Italian Society of Gynecologic Endoscopy. *Am J Obstet Gynecol*. 2018;218(5):500.e1-500.e13.

Perioperative Care and Complications of Gynecologic Surgery

Katelyn A. Uribe and Karen C. Wang

PREOPERATIVE CARE

The main objectives of the **preoperative assessment** are
- completion of a thorough history and physical examination
- selection of the ideal surgery, considering both procedure and route
- identification of potential limitations
- optimization of the patient's medical condition

The goal is to decrease perioperative morbidity and complications and to optimize outcomes.

Informed Consent

- **Informed consent** should include the rationale and explanation of the procedure as well as alternatives such as expectant management, nonsurgical interventions, and other surgical options. An interactive dialogue should occur between physician and patient. When more than one option is available, the surgeon should provide education and guidance without coercion. Ultimately, the patient must determine which of the options is appropriate.
- Risk discussion should address the specific procedure as well as general surgical risks and should be accompanied by a discussion of interventions intended to minimize those risks. These risks may include, but are not limited to; pain; bleeding; and possible blood transfusion, infection, organ injury (bladder, ureter, bowel, vessel, or nerve), unanticipated organ removal, need for additional surgery, myocardial infarction, congestive heart failure, thromboembolic complications, stroke, unexpected malignancy, and perioperative death. Injury and failure rates should be cited based on personal data and current literature when available. Discussion of interventions such as perioperative antibiotics, deep vein thrombosis (DVT) prophylaxis, and postoperative incentive spirometry should be included. Possible changes in plans due to intraoperative surgical findings should be included in the consent document as well as the possibility of a change in mode of access (eg, laparoscopic to open procedure, vaginal to abdominal procedure). Documentation of the preoperative discussions and the patient's response and acceptance of risk, including informed refusal, is crucial.
- Postoperative expectations should be reviewed as well, including expected symptoms, postoperative management, expected length of stay, restrictions, and anticipated follow-up.

Medical Evaluation and Optimization

Preoperative Evaluation

- **Preoperative evaluation.** History and physical examination are essential for evaluating surgical eligibility and the need for further testing or consultation. Identifying occult disease and optimizing preexisting conditions are of utmost importance.

Abnormal findings and comorbid conditions need to be evaluated appropriately. Routine health maintenance evaluation and screening should be considered especially in the absence of regular medical care. It may be beneficial for patients with complex preexisting conditions to be comanaged with a medical specialist. Preoperative consultation with an anesthesiologist is advised for the medically complicated patient, those with known difficult airways, and those with a history of anesthesia complications.

- **Preoperative testing and imaging.** Preoperative testing should be based on risk factors for abnormal physiology, including comorbid conditions, tobacco use, exercise intolerance, and irregular examination findings. Mild and even asymptomatic conditions that may be exacerbated by medical and surgical interventions should be anticipated. Guidelines are available from the American Society of Anesthesiologists and American Heart Association/American College of Cardiology.
  - Gynecologic patients are strongly advised to have current Pap smear and mammography results (as appropriate). Red blood cell type and screen should be performed on most patients, with exceptions made for very minor outpatient procedures. **A pregnancy test will be required on all reproductive age women (<50 years), and endometrial biopsy is recommended by American College of Obstetricians and Gynecologists for women with abnormal uterine bleeding over the age of 45 or <45 years of age if risk factors are present or unresponsive to medical therapy.** Imaging should be individualized, but pelvic ultrasound, computed tomography (CT), or magnetic resonance imaging may be helpful for illustrating anatomy and extent of disease, thereby optimizing surgical planning.

- **Preoperative cardiac evaluation.** The preoperative cardiac evaluation should be directed toward the detection of symptoms using directed questioning looking for conditions such as angina, heart failure, and arrhythmias. The 2014 American College of Cardiology/American Heart Association guidelines recommend electrocardiogram (ECG) for patients with known coronary artery disease, significant arrhythmia, peripheral arterial disease, cerebrovascular disease, structural heart disease, and obesity with one risk factor for coronary heart disease. The ECGs are not needed for low-risk procedures. A baseline ECG may be helpful for women age >50 years in major gynecologic procedures. Additional cardiac workup depends on the planned surgery and the patient's functional status.
  - In low-risk procedures (minimally invasive, minimal blood loss, and fluid shifts), no additional workup or treatment is needed, and most patients can proceed directly to surgery.
  - Major intraperitoneal surgery is considered intermediate risk with a reported cardiac risk of 1% to 5%. These patients should be assessed by their functional status. Functional status is based on a patient's ability to perform 4 metabolic equivalents (METs) of activity or greater without chest pain, dyspnea, or fatigue.
    - An MET is a unit equal to the MET of oxygen uptake while quietly seated. Activities that use 4 METs include walking on a flat surface or climbing a flight of stairs. If the patient can perform 4 METs of activity without dyspnea or fatigue, she is considered to have a normal functional status and may proceed to intermediate risk surgery without further cardiac testing. If her functional status is <4 METs, additional evaluation may be indicated

based on clinical risk factors that include history of ischemic heart disease, history of compensated or prior heart failure, history of cerebrovascular disease (stroke), diabetes mellitus, and chronic kidney disease (defined as a creatinine >2 mg/dL).

- For gynecologic surgeries that are considered high risk (prolonged surgeries that involve large fluid shifts), patients with a functional capability <4 METs and one to three risk factors may warrant further cardiac testing, such a cardiac stress test or echocardiogram.

Preoperative Management

- **Thromboembolic prophylaxis.** The approximate risk of DVT in hospitalized patients after major gynecology procedures is 10% to 40%. It is the standard of care to offer DVT prophylaxis (Table 60-1).
- **Reducing surgical site infection (SSI).** Measures should be taken to reduce the risk of SSI.
  - Do not shave the incision site. Use only electric clippers if hair removal is necessary.
  - Implement perioperative glycemic control with a goal serum glucose level of <200 mg/dL to reduce the risk of SSI.
  - Recommend preoperative bath or shower with a soap or an antiseptic agent for those scheduled to undergo an abdominal procedure.
  - Unless contraindicated, an alcohol-based agent (ie, chlorhexidine) should be used for the preoperative surgical site skin preparation.
- **Antibiotic prophylaxis.** See Table 60-2 for preoperative antibiotic prophylaxis. Single-dose prophylaxis appears to be as effective as multiple doses, with less risk of adverse events and microbial resistance. To reduce SSI, cephalosporins are preferred for most patients. A combination of clindamycin or metronidazole *plus* gentamicin is recommended for those with severe penicillin allergy or anaphylaxis.
  - Antibiotics should be administered within 1 hour prior to incision. Antibiotics should be redosed according to half-life and blood loss (eg, cefazolin is redosed every 4 h or if >1500 mL of blood loss).
  - Postoperative antibiotic prophylaxis has not been shown to be effective.
  - Preoperative treatment of bacterial vaginosis is recommended. Bacterial vaginosis is a known risk factor for SSI, and treatment with metronidazole 4 days prior to surgery has been demonstrated to decrease the risk of cuff cellulitis.
- **Antibiotic prophylaxis for subacute bacterial endocarditis.** The American Heart Association no longer recommends routine prophylaxis for bacterial endocarditis for routine genitourinary or gastrointestinal (GI) tract procedures. One exception is in patients undergoing a genitourinary or GI procedure in the setting of active infection.
  - For patients with a prosthetic cardiac valve, previous history of endocarditis, unrepaired cyanotic congenital heart defect including palliative shunts and conduits, completely repaired congenital heart defect with prosthetic material or device during the first 6 months after the procedure, repaired congenital heart defect with residual defect at the site or adjacent to the site of a prosthetic patch or device, cardiac transplant, or cardiac valvulopathy, it may be reasonable to use an antibiotic regimen that covers organisms known to cause endocarditis, particularly *enterococci*. Preferred agents include penicillin, ampicillin, piperacillin, or vancomycin.

Table 60-1	Thromboprophylaxis for Gynecologic Procedures[a]	
Level of Risk	Definition	Successful Prevention Strategies
Low	• Surgery <30 min in patients younger than 40 y with no additional risk factors	No specific prophylaxis; early and "aggressive" mobilization
Moderate	• Surgery >30 min in patients with additional risk factors • Surgery <30 min in patients aged 40-60 y with no additional risk factors • Major surgery in patients <40 y with no additional risk factors	Low-dose unfractionated heparin (5000 units every 12 h), low-molecular-weight heparin (2500 units dalteparin or 40 mg enoxaparin daily), graduated compression stockings, or intermittent pneumatic compression device
High	• Surgery <30 min in patients >60 y or with additional risk factors • Major surgery in patients >40 y or with additional risk factors	Low-dose unfractionated heparin (5000 units every 8 h), low-molecular-weight heparin (5000 units dalteparin or 40 mg enoxaparin daily), or intermittent pneumatic compression device
Highest	• Major surgery patients >60 y plus prior venous thromboembolism, cancer, or molecular hypercoagulable state	Low-dose unfractionated heparin (5000 units every 8 h), low-molecular-weight heparin (5000 units dalteparin or 40 mg enoxaparin daily), or intermittent pneumatic compression device/ graduated compression stockings + low-dose unfractionated heparin or low-molecular-weight heparin Consider continuing prophylaxis for 2-4 wk after discharge.

[a]Modified from Geerts WH, Pineo GF, Heit JA, et al. Prevention of venous thromboembolism: the Seventh ACCP Conference on Antithrombotic and Thrombolytic Therapy. *Chest.* 2004;126(3 suppl):338S-400S. Copyright © 2004 The American College of Chest Physicians. With permission.

- **Bowel preparation.** Mechanical bowel preparation has not been shown to improve visualization or outcomes. A clear liquid diet for 24 hours on the day before surgery is a safe alternative to a mechanical bowel preparation that can cause electrolyte abnormalities and dehydration.
- **Medications.** Antihypertensive, cardiac, reflux, psychiatric, asthma, and antiseizure medications should be taken on the morning of surgery, with a sip of water.
  - Diabetic patients should take one-third of the long-acting insulin, and those with an insulin pump should be on their basal rate. Oral hypoglycemics should

Table 60-2 Indications for Antibiotic Prophylaxis[a]

Antibiotic	Indication	Dose
Cefazolin	Hysterectomy (supracervical, vaginal, abdominal, laparoscopic, robotic) Colporrhaphy Vaginal sling placement Consider for laparotomy without entry into bowel or vagina.	2 g, 3 g IV for patients weighing >120 kg Redose at 4 h or if EBL >1500 mL. If PCN allergic (anaphylaxis, urticaria, bronchospasm), use metronidazole or clindamycin + gentamicin or aztreonam.
Doxycycline	Uterine evacuation (suction D&C, D&E)	200 mg
None	Cervical tissue excision procedures (LEEP, biopsy, endocervical curettage) Cystoscopy Endometrial biopsy Laparoscopy without entry into bowel or vagina Hysterosalpingogram (HSG)[b] (chromotubation, saline-infused sonohysterogram) Hysteroscopy (operative, diagnostic) Intrauterine device insertion Oocyte retrieval Nonobstetrical D&C Urodynamics	

Abbreviations: D&C, dilation and curettage; D&E, dilation and evacuation; EBL, estimated blood loss; IV, intravenous; LEEP, loop electrosurgical excision procedure; PCN, penicillin.

[a]Data from American College of Obstetricians and Gynecologists Committee on Practice Bulletins—Gynecology. ACOG Practice Bulletin No. 195: prevention of infection after gynecologic procedures. *Obstet Gynecol.* 2018;131:e172-e189.

[b]To prevent the incidence of postprocedural pelvic inflammatory disease (PID), Doxycycline 100 mg twice a day for 5 days is recommended for women undergoing HSG or chromotubation with a history of PID or evidence of dilated fallopian tubes.

not be taken on the day of surgery. Metformin should be stopped 2 days before surgery and not restarted for at least 48 hours after surgery due to the risk of lactic acidosis.

- Aspirin and Plavix should be discontinued ideally 7 days before surgery; other nonsteroidal anti-inflammatory drugs should be stopped 3 days before surgery. Patients on an anticoagulant will require a detailed plan of management. Coumadin therapy should be discontinued 4 to 5 days prior to surgery and converted to subcutaneous low-molecular-weight heparin (LMWH). On the day of surgery, the morning dose of heparin is held and coagulation studies are drawn immediately before surgery to avoid operating with a hypocoagulable state.

- Patients who were treated with steroids within the last year on a long-term basis (eg, prednisone >5 mg/d for >3 wk) should receive intraoperative stress doses of steroids. Two options are hydrocortisone 50 or 100 mg intravenous or methylprednisolone 100 mg intravenous at the time of surgery. The steroids are continued for 24 hours postsurgery.

- Herbal supplements are discontinued 1 to 2 weeks prior to surgery because many have anticoagulant or coagulopathic effects.

- These medication adjustments should be arranged in coordination with the patient's primary care physician. Postoperative instructions should address resumption of any discontinued medications.

- Perioperative β-blockade should be continued for patients who are already on them, to prevent cardiac events associated with surgery.

Hemorrhage Prevention Optimization

- For procedures at high risk for severe blood loss, preoperative optimization with uterine artery embolization may be prudent. Usually performed 1 day prior to surgery with admission overnight, this intervention has been shown to significantly reduce intraoperative blood loss.

- Patients who do not accept blood products for religious or personal reasons require particular preoperative counseling that includes a thorough review of what products a patient is or is not willing to accept in the event of a hemorrhage. These patients must be counseled of the potential consequences should they refuse blood products in the setting of extreme blood loss. If acceptable to the patient, the use of cell salvage systems can be of great value and consideration to these systems can also be given to any high blood loss procedure.

- The use of medications intraoperatively can also assist in reduction of blood loss. At the time of myomectomy or cervical procedures, injection of vasopressin (off-label use) can be used to decrease blood flow to the site of operation and by default, blood loss. The maximum recommended dose is 20 units, which can be diluted to meet the needs of the surgeon. The medication has a relatively short half-life, and repeat administration may be necessary, with care taken to avoid intravascular injection due to the associated reflex cardiac changes.

- Prior to myomectomy, the placement of 800 μg of rectal Cytotec (off-label use) can also be considered to decrease blood loss.

- In the setting of acute bleeding intraoperatively, intravenous tranexamic acid can also be administered at dosage of 10 mg/kg.

INTRAOPERATIVE COMPLICATIONS

Hemorrhage

- Incidence of pelvic hemorrhage in major gynecologic surgery is reported as 1% to 2% in abdominal hysterectomy, 0.6% to 1.2% in laparoscopic hysterectomy, and 0.7% to 2.5% for vaginal hysterectomy. Other procedures associated with higher rates of hemorrhage are Burch colposuspension, abdominal sacrocolpopexy, and lymph node dissection. Previous surgery, large malignant or benign masses, history of pelvic inflammatory disease, and endometriosis can cause anatomic distortion predisposing a patient to injury and pelvic hemorrhage.
  - Control of pelvic bleeding starts with **preventive measures**, such as proper patient positioning, choosing an appropriate incision to ensure adequate exposure, meticulous surgical technique, and limited blunt dissection. Once hemorrhage is encountered, communication with anesthesia and operating room staff is essential.
  - Hemorrhage management is centered on four basic actions: (1) assess vital signs, (2) obtain adequate intravenous access, (3) resuscitate with judicious use of fluid or blood components, and (4) achieve hemostasis.
    - **Direct pressure** should be applied to sites of bleeding, allowing time for proper identification and control with electrocautery, ligation, or surgical clips. Bleeding in the presacral area can also be managed with **bone wax** or **sterile tacks**.
    - **Hypogastric artery ligation** may be used for uncontrolled venous bleeding because it lowers pulse pressure.
    - Topical hemostatic agents, such as fibrin glue, Gelfoam, and Surgicel, can be applied to small venous bleeding sites.
    - **Pelvic packing**, using moist laparotomy pads, may be used temporarily for continued hemorrhage or left intra-abdominally with postoperative intensive care unit monitoring. The patient is usually returned to the operating room in 48 to 72 hours to remove the packs, irrigate, and close the abdomen.
  - If a patient can be stabilized, consideration for intraoperative uterine artery embolization can also be given. However, this option is not always readily available and requires coordination between both the surgical team, anesthesia, and interventional radiology.
  - Tranexamic acid can be considered in the case of a hemorrhage where estimated blood loss exceeds 1.5 L.
- **Postoperative bleeding** may be detected through changes in vital signs consistent with hypovolemia, patient restlessness, disproportionate pain relative to surgery or analgesics, abdominal ecchymosis, and abdominal distention. A larger than anticipated reduction in postoperative hematocrit should raise suspicion. These findings should prompt further evaluation to determine whether active bleeding is present. Orthostatic blood pressures, serial blood counts, and imaging studies (ie, ultrasound or CT) should be performed as indicated. A stable hematoma can often be managed conservatively. Active bleeding requires blood replacement, and reexploration is often necessary. With the availability of interventional radiology, **pelvic artery embolization** has clinical success rates of 90% for postsurgical hemorrhage and avoids the additional morbidity of reoperation.

Ureteral Injury

- **Ureteral injury** rates have been reported from 1% to 2% during benign pelvic surgery, and only one-third are recognized intraoperatively. A recent study sites an average ureteral rate injury of 1.7%, which does not vary across route of hysterectomy; however, other studies have found that ureteral injury may be higher in laparoscopic hysterectomies than abdominal or vaginal hysterectomies.
- **Prevention and detection.** Steps taken to avoid ureteral injury during hysterectomy include development of the vesicouterine space, skeletonization of the uterine arteries, and cephalad traction on the uterus, all of which deflect the ureters laterally and downward. These measures are equally important in laparoscopic and abdominal surgery. The ureter can be visualized in the pararectal space on the medial leaf of the broad ligament, and ureterolysis in the case of adhesions or altered anatomy can be prudent. The pelvic ureter approaches within 1 cm of the infundibulopelvic ligament, lies approximately 1.5 cm lateral to the internal cervical os, and approaches within 0.9 cm of the upper third of the vagina. These distances are important during dissection, clamp placement, and in the consideration of thermal injury with the use of electrosurgery. Preoperative intravenous pyelograms and ureteral stenting have a questionable role in decreasing ureter injury risk.
- **Intraoperative cystoscopy** is an excellent test for assessing ureteral integrity and allows immediate corrective surgery to be undertaken if injury is detected. This technique is recommended for urogynecologic surgery and laparoscopic hysterectomies to identify and prevent sequelae of intraoperative urinary tract injury as well as decrease liability from an undetected injury.
- **Management.** In cases of crush injury without transection, stenting the ureter for an extended period and placing a drain at the site of injury may be sufficient therapy. Complete transection above the pelvic brim or partial transection is repaired by suturing the defect end-to-end (**ureteroureterostomy**). Reimplantation into the bladder (**ureteroneocystostomy**) is performed if the injury is within 6 cm of the ureterovesical junction. Mobilization of the bladder along the external iliac vessels with attachment to the psoas tendon (**psoas hitch**) can be used to bridge the gap and decrease tension at the anastomotic site when necessary. In cases of insufficient residual ureteral length, a Boari flap or ileal interposition can be performed. **Transureteroureterostomy** for injuries high in the pelvis is no longer recommended. Drains should be placed near the anastomosis to prevent urinoma formation and detect leakage. Delayed diagnosis of a ureteral injury may require retrograde pyelography with cystoscopy and stent placement or percutaneous nephrostomy with antegrade stent placement. The recovery potential of the kidney depends on the duration of the obstruction, the degree of obstruction, the degree of backflow, the presence or absence of infection, and the extent to which each kidney was functional before the injury.

Bladder Injury

- The rate of **bladder injury** in benign gynecologic surgery is 0.5% to 1%. Major lacerations may require mobilization of the bladder for tension-free repair. Multiple cystotomies may be joined into one defect. A two-layer closure with 2-0 or 3-0 synthetic absorbable suture is recommended, and the seal is assessed by placing sterile milk or methylene blue retrograde into the bladder. A Foley or suprapubic catheter is left in place for 7 to 14 days. A small cystotomy that occurs with a trocar during placement of a midurethral sling requires catheterized bladder decompression; some surgeons recommend drainage for only 24 to 72 hours.

- A missed bladder or ureteral injury usually results in postoperative urinary ascites or urinoma, abdominal or flank pain, and distention with fever, chills, oliguria, nausea, and vomiting. These patients may have elevated blood urea nitrogen and creatinine levels and may respond to aggressive hydration and bladder rest. Unrecognized surgical injuries are the most common cause of genitourinary fistulas in the developed world.

Bowel Injury

- Inadvertent **bowel injury** occurs most often in gynecologic surgeries from an abdominal approach and is reported in 0.1% to 1% of abdominal hysterectomies, 0.3% to 0.4% of laparoscopic hysterectomies, and 0.1% to 0.8% of vaginal hysterectomies.
- A systematic evaluation of the bowel should be performed at the end of procedures where extensive lysis of adhesions is performed. Serosal injuries can be closed with permanent or delayed absorbable 3-0 suture. Lacerations to the stomach, small bowel, and large bowel may be closed in two layers, using a continuous mucosal repair with 2-0 absorbable suture and an imbricating seromuscular interrupted 2-0 permanent suture.
  - Suture lines should be perpendicular to the longitudinal axis of the lumen to avoid luminal constriction. In cases of multiple enterotomies, the bowel may need to be resected and anastomosed. A nasogastric tube can be used for decompression in stomach and small bowel injuries. Distal colonic injury does not warrant colostomy except in cases of previous radiation or infection.

Nerve Injury

- Malpositioning or retractor placement is the usual cause of **nerve injury** in gynecologic surgery. However, hematoma formation, a foreign body, or transection can also be complicating factors (Table 60-3).
- Most compression and stretch injuries resolve completely over several weeks to months. Physical therapy is required in cases with motor deficits. The key to treatment is prevention: proper patient positioning, periodic reassessment during long surgeries, proper retractor placement, and careful dissection.

Complications Specific to Laparoscopy

- **Port placement**
  - Intra-abdominal access can be gained using Veress entry, open entry, or direct visual entry. Selection of the entry method and location should be made by surgeon comfort and preference based on the planned procedure and patient history (see chapter 59).
  - The majority of injuries during laparoscopy occur during access. During primary port placement, the small bowel, iliac artery, and colon are the most commonly injured structures. With secondary ports, abdominal wall vessels, iliac arteries, and the aorta are at most risk for injury. A systematic review of the field should be performed in every case after gaining primary access prior to

Table 60-3 Nerve Injuries During Gynecologic Surgery

Nerve	Injury	Motor Loss	Sensory Paresthesia/Pain
Femoral L2-L4	Deep retraction on psoas muscle, excessive hip flexion	Hip flexion, knee extension, knee DTR, leg adduction	Anteromedial thigh, anteromedial leg and foot
Lateral femoral cutaneous L2-L3	Deep retraction on psoas muscle, excess hip flexion	None	Anterolateral thigh
Genitofemoral branch L1-L2	Pelvic sidewall dissection	None	Mons, labia majora, anterior superior thigh
Obturator L2-L4	Retroperitoneal dissection, paravaginal defect repair, trocar placement (TOT)	Leg adduction	Anteromedial thigh
Sciatic L3-L4	Extensive endopelvic resection, excessive external hip rotation	Hip extension, knee flexion, foot dorsiflexion (foot drop)	Lateral calf, dorsomedial foot
Common peroneal L4-S2	Compression from stirrups on lateral epicondyle	Foot dorsiflexion (foot drop)	Lateral calf, dorsomedial foot
Iliohypogastric T12	Transverse abdominal incision or trocar placement	None	Mons, labia, inner thigh
Ilioinguinal L1	Transverse abdominal incision or trocar placement	None	Groin, symphysis pubis

Abbreviations: DTR, deep tendon reflexes; TOT, transobturator tape.

Trendelenburg positioning. All secondary ports should be inserted under direct visualization.

- **Extraperitoneal insufflation of carbon dioxide.** Misplacement of a Veress needle in the preperitoneal space causes this complication and can impair visualization due to peritoneal tenting. In most cases, carbon dioxide can be allowed to escape and needle placement attempted again. If this is not successful, open entry is performed. Mediastinal emphysema is an uncommon complication that requires observation for respiratory compromise and, in severe cases, may require ventilation.

- **Vessel injury.** The Veress needle or trocar may traumatize omental, mesenteric, major abdominal, or pelvic vessels. Trendelenburg position should never be obtained prior to initial trocar placement; the table should be flat. The sacral promontory should be palpated as a landmark of the aortic bifurcation. In thin patients, the Veress needle is directed at 45 degrees and in obese patients at 90 degrees to avoid tracking. The most accurate confirmation of peritoneal access is an opening pressure of <10 mm Hg.

  - The *superficial epigastric* vessels may be identified by transillumination, especially in thinner patients; however, the deeper *inferior epigastric* vessels should be identified intra-abdominally prior to accessory trocar placement (see chapter 59).

  - Management of inferior epigastric vessel injury includes balloon tamponade with a Foley or suture ligature using a Carter-Thomason or Endo Close device. Consider enlarging the incision at the trocar site or proceeding to laparotomy to improve visualization. Damage to major retroperitoneal vessels generally requires emergent laparotomy, packing, and consultation with a vascular surgeon.

- **Bowel injury.** Intestinal injuries have been reported at a rate of <0.5%. Approximately half of these injuries occur on entry, and half occur as a result of electrocautery. Most bowel injuries are not recognized at the time of surgery. If bowel perforation with the Veress needle is suspected, the needle should be withdrawn and insufflation attempted at another site. Generally, puncture sites from the Veress needle can be managed conservatively. If the laparoscope enters the bowel lumen, it should be left in place to limit contamination and to facilitate identification of the injured site. Repair may be accomplished by routine laparoscopic or open techniques. A thermal injury is often treated by resection or oversewing of the bowel in cases of smaller injury. Monopolar energy has been shown to have a thermal spread up to several centimeters away; therefore, extreme caution should be used when using electrosurgery on strands of tissues attached to bowel. Symptoms of bowel injury can range from increased pain at the trocar site to abdominal distention and diarrhea to sepsis. The CT scan is the best imaging study to confirm the diagnosis. Access injuries or traumatic injuries often present early, in the first hours or days postoperatively. Thermal injury may present late (3-7 d after surgery) due to delayed necrosis at the site of injury and subsequent bowel perforation. Unrecognized bowel injury is one of the most common causes of postoperative death from laparoscopy.

- **Bladder injury.** Prevention is best achieved by decompression of the bladder with a Foley catheter, avoiding low suprapubic ports, and with direct visualization during trocar placement. Bladder injury is not restricted to port placement and also occurs during dissection of the vesicouterine space. Low anterior fibroids and history of prior cesarean delivery increase that risk. Injury may be detected by the presence of air or blood in the drainage bag of an indwelling Foley catheter or loss of pneumoperitoneum in the case of a large cystotomy. The size of the injury dictates treatment. Needle perforations can be managed expectantly. Lacerations <10 mm long will heal spontaneously if the bladder is drained continuously with a Foley catheter for 3 to 4 postoperative days. Larger injuries require suturing, as described earlier. This can be performed laparoscopically by surgeons experienced in laparoscopic suturing technique.

- **Ureteral injury.** Laparoscopic-assisted vaginal hysterectomy is the leading gynecologic procedure in which ureteral injury occurs. Cautery can cause inadvertent thermal injury that may be missed at the time of the procedure. Careful exposure and identification of anatomy is the best way to reduce risk of injury to the ureter. If ureteral injury is suspected, intravenous indigo carmine, methylene blue, or fluorescein should be administered and cystoscopy performed intraoperatively.
- **Dehiscence and hernia.** The overall incidence of incisional dehiscence and hernia is approximately 0.02% and is greater with trocar-cannula systems >10 mm in diameter. Richter hernias, which typically have a delayed diagnosis, contain a portion of the intestinal wall in a peritoneal defect. General recommendations for fascial closure are to close all defects >10 mm and defects >5 mm that are lateral to the rectus sheath after significant tissue extraction or peritoneal stretch.

Complications Specific to Hysteroscopy

- **Fluid overload.** Fluids can be delivered into the uterine cavity with sufficiently high pressure to allow intravasation of the distention media into the vascular system. Serious complications can occur if intravasation is excessive. The risks and allowable fluid deficits vary according to type of distention media used. Absorption is increased as a function of increasing flow pressure, uterine size, and operative time. Automated fluid-monitoring systems have made the exact measurements of input and output of the distending medium much easier. The surgeon should be aware of the deficit at all times and should be updated frequently by operating room staff (Table 60-4).
  - Electrolyte-containing media (normal saline and lactated ringer) are relatively safe, but fluid overload is still possible. These media can be used with bipolar instruments.

Table 60-4	Guidelines for Fluid Management During Operative Hysteroscopy[a]		
Fluid Type	Examples	When to Consider Stopping Procedure	Maximum Fluid Deficit
Hypotonic Low viscosity Electrolyte-poor solution	1.5% glycine 3% sorbitol 5% mannitol	1000 mL	1500 mL
Isotonic Electrolyte-rich solution	Normal saline Lactated Ringer	2000 mL	2500 mL
High viscosity	Hyskon/dextran[b]	300 mL	500 mL

[a]Data from American College of Obstetrics and Gynecologists. ACOG Technology Assessment No. 13: hysteroscopy. *Obstet Gynecol.* 2018;131(5):e151-e156.
[b]Dextran rarely used due to crystallization of fluid, anaphylaxis, and disseminated intravascular coagulation.

- Alternative fluid media carry increased risk of overload and electrolyte abnormalities.
  - Three percent sorbitol and 1.5% glycine are low-viscosity, hypotonic, electrolyte-poor solutions, which allow the use of monopolar instruments. When absorbed into the bloodstream in high volumes, they cause hyponatremia, arrhythmias, cerebral edema, coma, and death.
  - Mannitol 5% is an iso-osmolar medium that can also cause hyponatremia.
- **Uterine perforation** may be managed conservatively, particularly when caused by a blunt instrument, with close monitoring or overnight hospitalization. In cases of active bleeding or perforation with electrosurgical instruments, conversion to laparoscopy or laparotomy is required.

POSTOPERATIVE COMPLICATIONS

Postoperative Fever

- A commonly accepted diagnosis of fever requires a temperature at or above 38°C (100.4°F) on two occasions at least 4 hours apart. Febrile morbidity within the first 48 hours of laparotomy has been estimated to occur in up to 30% of gynecologic surgery patients. Atelectasis, an often-cited reason for low-grade febrile illnesses, has not been shown to be causal for fever during this period in the literature, and the majority is attributed to cytokine flares. Noninfectious etiologies, such as medications, malignant hyperthermia, thrombotic or embolic events, ureteral injuries, cardiovascular events, endocrine abnormalities, and transfusion reactions, should be included in the differential diagnosis and workup for postoperative fever.
- **Evaluation.** Evaluation should include a review of the patient's history and a thorough examination, with specific attention to sites as follows: pulmonary examination; palpation of the suprapubic region and costovertebral angles; evaluation of incisions; catheter and line sites; extremities; and pelvic examination to evaluate the vaginal cuff for cellulitis, hematoma, or abscess.
- **Testing.** Initial laboratory and radiologic assessment should be tailored to the individual patient. Complete blood count with differential, urinalysis, and urine culture should be performed. Urinalysis will be of limited value in patients with bladder catheters. Blood cultures seldom yield positive results except in patients with high fever or risk factors for endocarditis and are most sensitive when drawn at the time of the fever. Imaging studies may include chest and abdominal radiographs, intravenous pyelograms, ultrasonography of the pelvis and kidneys, contrast bowel studies, and CT scan. Chest CT or ventilation perfusion (V/Q) scan should also be considered to rule out pulmonary embolism (PE).

Postoperative Infection

- **Urinary tract infection.** The bladder is a common site of infection in surgical patients, largely due to contamination with indwelling Foley catheters. Pyelonephritis is a rare complication. The treatment is hydration and antibiotic therapy tailored to the pathogen.
- **Respiratory infection.** Preventive measures are early ambulation and intensive respiratory therapy (ie, incentive spirometry, chest physical therapy) for reversal of hypoventilation and atelectasis. Patients at risk for postoperative pneumonia

include those with an American Society of Anesthesiologists status of 3 or higher, preoperative hospital stay of 2 days or longer, surgery lasting 3 hours or longer, surgery in the upper abdomen or thorax, nasogastric suction, postoperative intubation, or a history of smoking or obstructive lung disease. Smoking cessation should be encouraged preoperatively not only for respiratory complications but also for wound healing.

Wound Infection

- **Risk factors** for SSI include age, nutritional status, diabetes, smoking, obesity, coexistent infections at a remote body site, colonization with microorganisms, altered immune response, and length of preoperative stay.
- **Prevention.** Hair removal should only be performed with surgical clippers rather than a razor. Appropriate prophylactic antibiotic for the specific procedure should be given within 1 hour of starting the procedure.
- **Surgical closure.** Studies in cesarean delivery patients have shown closure of the subcutaneous fat compared with nonclosure reduces wound complications (defined as hematoma, seroma, wound infection, wound separation). In women with fat thickness >2 cm, suture closure of subcutaneous fat decreases the risk of wound disruption. Further trials are justified to investigate suturing materials and techniques. Whether these findings can be extrapolated to gynecologic surgery is unclear. Recent meta-analyses have failed to show that the routine use of closed suction drains prevents surgical infections.
- **Wound care.** Wound care has recently shifted away from an aggressive cleaning approach to one that emphasizes a clean but moist environment and minimizes the mechanical irritation caused by frequent dressing changes. Hydrogel applications play an important role, and vacuum systems in high-risk patients can aid in wound drainage and facilitation of blood flow to the wound, resulting in a seemingly more rapid closure.

Incisional or Vaginal Cuff Cellulitis

- Fever, leukocytosis, and pain localizing to the pelvis may accompany a severe cellulitis in which adjacent pelvic tissues are involved. Broad-spectrum antibiotic therapy should be initiated. If an abscess is suspected at the cuff or incision, drainage is indicated. Radiologic confirmation with ultrasonography or CT scan is usually needed for diagnosis.
- Treatment involves parenteral antibiotics, with possible drainage in cases of large collections or failure to improve on antibiotics alone. In many circumstances, sonographic or CT-guided drain placement has obviated the need for surgical exploration, which is associated with high morbidity.

Necrotizing Fasciitis

- **Risk factors** include diabetes, obesity, age >50 years, malnutrition, chronic disease, immunosuppression.
- *Group A Streptococcus* can cause a progressive, inflammatory infection of the deep fascia, with necrosis of the subcutaneous tissues. Surgeons must be acutely aware of this potentially life-threatening complication in any patient with a wound infection. Clinically, the infection results in extensive soft-tissue destruction, including

necrosis of skin, subcutaneous tissue, and muscle. Erythema and induration around the wound should be marked and followed closely. Extensive and aggressive surgical debridement and broad-spectrum antibiotic therapy are warranted at first suspicion. Treatment delay and obesity increase an already high mortality rate.

Venous Thromboembolism

- **Risk factors** include age >40 years, obesity, prolonged surgery, prior venous thromboembolism, malignancy, immobility, thrombophilia condition, diabetes, and heart failure.
- **Deep vein thrombosis** can cause unilateral lower extremity swelling, pain, and erythema. A palpable cord may be detected. Duplex Doppler ultrasonographic imaging has replaced venography as the gold standard for diagnosing DVT.
- **Pulmonary embolism.** The signs and symptoms of PE include anxiety, shortness of breath, tachypnea, chest pain, hypoxia, tachycardia, and mental status changes. Symptoms should prompt a thorough evaluation; chest radiograph, ECG, and arterial blood gas assessment are the first-line tests. The chest radiograph helps distinguish between pneumonia and embolism. The ECG findings are usually nonspecific except for sinus tachycardia, but they help rule out an ischemic cardiac event. Laboratory evaluation with arterial blood gas test may show hypoxemia, hypocapnia, respiratory alkalosis, and an increased arterial-alveolar gradient.

Imaging

- Radionucleotide imaging ($\dot{V}/\dot{Q}$ scan) and contrast-enhanced CT arteriography (CTA) are the current studies available for the evaluation of a suspected PE. The $\dot{V}/\dot{Q}$ scans have a high sensitivity but a low specificity. A CTA is rapid, easily accessible in most large hospitals, and less prone to interference from other underlying pulmonary disease. Its sensitivity is greatest for detecting emboli in the main, lobar, or segmental pulmonary arteries. In most institutions, the CTA has replaced the $\dot{V}/\dot{Q}$ scan as the first-line diagnostic imaging study (see chapter 20).

Therapy

- Intravenous unfractionated heparin (UFH) has been the traditional treatment for DVT and PE. Recent studies have established that LMWH and the pentasaccharide fondaparinux are equivalent to UFH. The half-life of LMWH is longer, the dose response is more predictable, and less bleeding may occur while producing an equivalent antithrombotic effect. When using UFH, oral therapy with Coumadin is started as early as possible, and the patient can discontinue UFH when a therapeutic international normalized ratio value is reached. Vena caval filter may be needed in patients with acute thromboembolism and active bleeding or a high risk of bleeding, patients on medical therapy with a history of multiple venous thrombi, and patients with a history of heparin-induced thrombocytopenia. Bleeding that occurs after the use of heparin-related compounds can be reversed with protamine sulfate; Coumadin-related bleeding can be reversed with vitamin K or with plasma or factor IX concentrates.

Ileus and Bowel Obstruction

- **Diagnosis.** Infection, peritonitis, electrolyte disturbances, extensive manipulation of the GI tract, and prolonged procedures may cause postoperative ileus.

Postoperative adhesions occur in about 25% but can be up to 90% in patients who undergo major gynecologic surgery and represent one of the most common causes of intestinal obstruction. The prevalence of ileus or small bowel obstruction following hysterectomy is 0.2% to 2.2%. Nausea, vomiting, and distention may be present with both. Absent and hypoactive bowel sounds are more likely to occur with ileus, whereas borborygmi, rushes, and high-pitched tinkles are more characteristic of postoperative obstruction. Abdominal radiographs show distended loops of large and small bowel, with gas present in the rectum in the setting of ileus. Single or multiple loops of distended bowel with air-fluid levels are seen in postoperative obstruction. These findings may be difficult to distinguish in the early postoperative period. In prolonged cases, it may be helpful to obtain a study with oral contrast to identify a transition point.

- **Treatment.** Ileus is treated with bowel rest, intravenous fluids, electrolyte repletion, and nasogastric suction in cases of persistent vomiting. Most cases of partial obstruction will respond to conservative management with bowel rest and nasogastric decompression. Increasing abdominal pain, progressive distention, fever, leukocytosis, or acidosis should increase the suspicion for complete bowel obstruction, which may require reexploration. In cases with delayed improvement, a CT scan may help identify bowel perforation or abscess. Parenteral nutrition should also be considered in patients with prolonged GI compromise.

Diarrhea

- **Diarrhea** is not uncommon after abdominal and pelvic surgery. Prolonged or multiple episodes, however, may represent a pathologic process, such as impending small bowel obstruction, colonic obstruction, or pseudomembranous colitis. *Clostridium difficile*–associated colitis may result from exposure to any antibiotics; stool testing can confirm clinical suspicions. Extended oral metronidazole therapy and hydration are needed for adequate treatment, and oral vancomycin may be necessary in refractory cases.

Genitourinary Fistulae

- In the United States, most **genitourinary fistulae** are the result of pelvic surgery, usually after an abdominal hysterectomy for benign conditions. In the developing world, most fistulas are due to obstetric trauma secondary to absent or poor obstetric care. Patients may present with persistent vaginal discharge or recurrent urinary tract infections.
- The simplest initial test for a genitourinary fistula is the tampon test. A tampon is inserted into the vagina. The bladder is then filled with methylene blue or indigo carmine through a Foley catheter. The patient is given an oral dose of Pyridium. The appearance of blue dye on the tampon suggests a vesicovaginal fistula. An orange tampon is suggestive of a ureteral-vaginal fistula. Fluid pooling in the vagina can also be sent for a creatinine level. Further workup may include intravenous pyelograms, cystoscopy, voiding cystourethrogram, retrograde ureteral studies, and magnetic resonance imaging. Simple fistulas often resolve with drainage by either Foley catheter or percutaneous nephrostomy tube placement. Surgical repair is necessary if this is unsuccessful.

ENHANCED RECOVERY AFTER SURGERY

Enhanced recovery after surgery (ERAS), an evidence-based care improvement process for surgical patients, is a multidisciplinary approach to the care of postoperative patients, focusing on improvements in clinical outcomes and cost saving. General principles including laxity of nothing-by-mouth restrictions prior to surgery, intraoperative fluid management, focus on minimally invasive approach, early ambulation, and early enteral feeding.

Preadmission/Preoperatively

- Efforts should be made to optimize patient status prior to surgical intervention, including nutritional support (if needed), encouragement of smoking cessation, and control of alcohol intake. In conjunction with anesthesia and medical consultations, optimize any significant medical conditions prior to surgery, particularly major procedures. A detailed informational session with nursing or surgeons should occur prior to surgery with instructions for preoperative diet, bowel preparation (if indicated), and surgical skin preparation.
- Bowel regimens should only be implemented if absolutely necessary. It can cause significant dehydration and has no clear evidence of improved outcomes. There are few gynecologic procedures that warrant such a preparation.
- Nothing-by-mouth status can deviate from the traditional teaching of nothing by mouth after midnight and, depending on institution, will often allow patients to consume clear liquids up to 2 hours before arriving to the preoperative area.
- Many institutions have begun to premedicate patients with a combination of antiemetics to prevent postoperative nausea or vomiting with a combination of analgesics to reduce intraoperative and postoperative pain requirements. Although regimens vary by institution, medications such as acetaminophen, gabapentin, and cyclooxygenase 2 inhibitors are commonly included.

Intraoperatively

- Management of the patient intraoperatively requires coordination of care between the surgeon and anesthesiologist. Development of protocols for intraoperative management can streamline care and reduce costs.
- As is possible and appropriate, the surgeon should prioritize the use of minimally invasive procedures, shorten operative time, and minimize the placement of drains and tubes remaining in place following completion of a procedure.
- Anesthesia protocols in ERAS focus on the use of regional anesthesia such as epidural anesthesia or local anesthesia blocks to reduce both intraoperative and postoperative narcotic use. Opioid-sparing anesthesia is preferred. Maintaining temperature control in the operating room using devices such as warming blankets or Bair Hugger systems are recommended. In addition, balanced fluid infusion and the use of colloid over crystalloid when clinically appropriate has been emphasized in numerous protocols to prevent postoperative fluid overload and third space extravasation while also maintaining delivery of oxygen and nutrients to vital organs.

Postoperatively

- Early enteral feeding remains a tenant of ERAS protocol when clinically appropriate. Early nutrition helps to promote bowel motility preventing postoperative ileus, provides important nutritional support in a catabolic state, and allows for early discontinuation of intravenous fluid support.
- Removal of drains and catheters as soon as is clinically appropriate helps to encourage mobilization and reduce infection risk. If at all possible, urinary catheters should be discontinued intraoperatively or on the first postoperative day.
- Early ambulation should be encouraged because it helps to regain strength and reduce the rate of postoperative ileus. If clinically appropriate, a patient should be encouraged to be out of bed on the day of surgery or first postoperative day.
- Pain control should be multimodal in the postoperative period in an attempt to reduce the use of opiates. The use of a transverse abdominis plane block or epidural is frequently used for laparotomy procedures. In addition, local anesthesia should be used at incision sites. Routine use of nonsteroidal anti-inflammatory drugs, acetaminophen, and other nonnarcotics is encouraged and should be prioritized for pain management over narcotics.

Outcomes

- The ERAS protocol has been shown to significantly reduce length of stay, complication rates, and readmission. In addition, the number of patients requiring reoperation or admission to the intensive care unit has decreased significantly. As such, implementation of an ERAS protocol should be considered when feasible.

SUGGESTED READINGS

AAGL. AAGL practice report: practice guidelines for intraoperative cystoscopy in laparoscopic hysterectomy. *J Minim Invasive Gynecol*. 2012;19:407-411.

American College of Obstetricians and Gynecologists Committee on Practice Bulletins—Gynecology. ACOG Practice Bulletin No. 84: prevention of deep vein thrombosis and pulmonary embolism. *Obstet Gynecol*. 2007;110:429-440. (Reaffirmed 2018)

American College of Obstetricians and Gynecologists Committee on Practice Bulletins—Gynecology. ACOG Practice Bulletin No. 195: prevention of infection after gynecologic procedures. *Obstet Gynecol*. 2018;131:e172-e189.

American College of Obstetricians and Gynecologists. ACOG Technology Assessment No. 13: hysteroscopy. *Obstet Gynecol*. 2018;131:e151-e156.

Kuroki LM, Mutch DG. Control of pelvic hemorrhage. In: Jones HW, Rock JA, eds. *Te Linde's Operative Gynecology*. 11th ed. Philadelphia, PA: Wolters Kluwer; 2015:336-358.

Wilson W, Taubert KA, Gewitz M, et al. Prevention of infective endocarditis: guidelines from the American Heart Association. *Circulation*. 2007;116(15):1736-1754.

Critical Care

Lauren Thomaier and Arthur Jason Vaught

Intensive care unit (ICU) admission is indicated for patients requiring intensive monitoring and physiologic support for organ failure. Indications for intensive care include hemodynamic instability, single or multisystem organ failure, active or potential requirement for ventilator support or vasoactive medications, severe medical illness, and postoperative care after major surgery.

CARDIOVASCULAR CRITICAL CARE

* **Cardiovascular function** in critical care can be assessed with **invasive hemodynamic monitoring** that provides information on the cardiac performance, fluid status, tissue perfusion, and arterial pressure.
* **Arterial catheterization**, most commonly performed in the radial or femoral artery, is preferred for direct blood pressure (BP) measurement and is used to facilitate blood gas analysis in the critically ill.
* A **pulmonary artery catheter (PAC, Swan-Ganz catheter)** can be used to measure or calculate hemodynamic parameters. It is placed via the subclavian or internal jugular vein (preferred) and has two lumens. The proximal lumen is positioned in the superior vena cava or right atrium, whereas the other opens at the tip of the catheter and contains a balloon that can be "floated" through the right atrium and ventricle into the pulmonary artery.
    * **Indications** include distinguishing cardiogenic from other noncardiogenic causes of pulmonary edema; diagnosis of pulmonary hypertension; guiding fluid resuscitation and pharmacologic therapy in patients with shock, renal failure, or unexplained acidosis; and guiding ventilator management. Of note, there is no confirmed medical benefit from PACs in critically ill patients.
    * The **hemodynamic parameters** that can be measured directly and indirectly with a PAC are central venous pressure (CVP), pulmonary capillary wedge/occlusion pressure, right ventricular and atrial pressures, pulmonary arterial pressure, cardiac output, mixed venous oxygen saturation, right and left ventricular stroke work index, cardiac index (CI), stroke volume index, systemic and pulmonary vascular resistance, arterial oxygen delivery (DO_2), and mixed venous oxygen saturation.
* **Central venous pressure** is recorded from the proximal lumen of the PAC and reflects **right atrial pressure**. A normal value is 1 to 6 mm Hg. When there is no obstruction between the right atrium and ventricle, CVP = right atrial pressure = right ventricular end-diastolic pressure. It exhibits a complex waveform that can be affected by various pathologic processes and is most often interpreted as a proxy for fluid status and therefore used to guide fluid management. However, CVP can be misleading and vary based on patient position, changes in thoracic pressure (from respiration or ventilation settings), and cardiac disease.
* **Pulmonary capillary wedge pressure (PCWP)** is recorded with the PAC balloon inflated and wedged in a branch of the pulmonary artery. A normal value is 6 to

12 mm Hg. When there is no obstruction between the left atrium and ventricle, PCWP = left atrial pressure = left ventricular end-diastolic pressure. As with CVP, PCWP values can be misleading. Left ventricular end-diastolic pressure reflects left ventricular preload only with normal ventricular compliance, which often is not the case in critically ill patients.

- Recently, use of CVP and PAC has fallen out of favor when used in critical care medicine to guide fluid resuscitation. A CVP has been shown to be unreliable when assessing fluid responsiveness in studies, and in a large meta-analysis, PAC did not change all-cause mortality.
- **Cardiac index** is cardiac output (stroke volume × heart rate) / body surface area. A normal value is 2.4 to 4 L/m^2. Cardiac output is measured with a PAC using a thermodilution technique. A thermistor located near the end of the PAC tip detects the flow of a cold fluid injected via the proximal port to calculate blood flow rate (equivalent to cardiac output).
- **Mixed venous oxygen saturation** can help assess tissue oxygen delivery and can be used to determine whether a patient's cardiac output is high enough to provide adequate oxygen delivery. A decrease in this variable (normal value 65%-75%) implies increased oxygen utilization by the tissue.

Heart Failure

Heart failure is categorized by right sided versus left sided, acute versus chronic, and reduced left ventricular ejection fraction versus preserved left ventricular ejection fraction. **Systolic heart failure** occurs due to impaired ventricular contraction. **Diastolic heart failure or heart failure with preserved ejection fraction** is a disorder of ventricular relaxation and therefore inadequate filling. The two can be distinguished by the end-diastolic volume, which increases in systolic heart failure, and decreases in diastolic heart failure. Although ejection fraction is decreased in systolic heart failure, it is often maintained in diastolic heart failure.

- Common **etiologies** of heart failure include cardiac ischemia, hypertensive heart disease, cardiac arrhythmias, pulmonary embolism (PE), and cardiomyopathy.
- In **acute decompensated heart failure**, patients most commonly exhibit dyspnea, orthopnea, tachypnea, tachycardia, and anxiety. Decreased peripheral perfusion, pulmonary crackles, wheezing, elevated jugular venous pressure, and peripheral edema may be noted on physical exam.
- The **workup** for heart failure includes an electrocardiogram (ECG), arterial blood gas and cardiac enzymes, echocardiography, and chest radiography. Although there is no consensus on the role of brain natriuretic peptide and diagnosing and monitoring heart failure in the ICU setting, it can be useful because of its high negative predictive value. In severe cases, invasive hemodynamic monitoring may be used to manage treatment.
- In addition to correcting any precipitating factors such as hypertension, myocardial ischemia, or cardiac arrhythmias, **treatment** should be aimed at improving symptoms, optimizing volume status, and restoring oxygenation. After the patient recovers from the acute phase, chronic heart failure therapy should be optimized.
  - **Therapy for acute heart failure:** In the presence of hypoxia, patients should receive **supplemental oxygen** and be positioned upright. Noninvasive positive pressure ventilation should be considered in patients with severe dyspnea and pulmonary edema.

- If there is evidence of fluid overload, **loop diuretics** should be administered while monitoring daily weights, strict intake and output, and electrolytes.
- Afterload reduction with intravenous (IV) **vasodilators** such as nitroglycerin, nitroprusside, or nesiritide can be considered in patients with left-sided **systolic heart failure** without hypotension. If these patients exhibit hypotension, **inotropes and vasopressors** such as milrinone or dobutamine and norepinephrine are more appropriate.

Acute Coronary Syndrome

Acute coronary syndrome is composed of **unstable angina** and myocardial infarction (MI) with and without associated ST-segment elevation (**non-ST segment elevation myocardial infarction** and **ST segment elevation myocardial infarction [STEMI]**). Factors that cause coronary artery obstruction including thrombus formation or vasospasm lead to myocardial ischemia, hypoxia, and acidosis. Diagnosis is based on patient symptoms, ECG findings, and cardiac biomarker values.

- Myocardial ischemia can be divided into different categories:
  - Type 1 MI: spontaneous MI related to ischemia due to a primary coronary event such as plaque erosion and/or rupture, fissuring, dissection
  - Type 2 MI: secondary to ischemia due to either increased oxygen demand or decreased supply
  - Type 3 MI: sudden unexpected cardiac death often with symptoms suggestive of myocardial ischemia
  - Type 4 MI: ischemia associated with a percutaneous intervention (4a) or stent thrombosis (4b)
  - Type 5 MI: ischemia associated with cardiac surgery
- The type of MI should be elucidated in the setting of critical illness because the treatment can differ substantially. Type 1 MI typically requires percutaneous intervention, where type 2 MI (demand ischemia) usually requires the treatment of underlying oxygen demand (ie, sepsis) with volume resuscitation and vasopressor support with or without blood transfusion if indicated.
- Patients with suspected myocardial ischemia should be treated with oxygen, sublingual nitroglycerin, and chewable aspirin (162-325 mg) as soon as possible. Opiates should be administered for pain and to reduce anxiety, which in turn may help reduce myocardial demand.
- Patients with **STEMI** symptom onset within the last 12 hours should receive immediate reperfusion therapy.
  - Depending on risk factors and eligibility criteria, primary percutaneous coronary intervention, rather than fibrinolytic therapy, is recommended.
  - Patients undergoing reperfusion therapy should receive a loading dose of a thienopyridine such as clopidogrel as early as possible. Anticoagulation, with unfractionated heparin or other agents depending on the type of reperfusion therapy to be performed, should also be administered. Expert consultation should be sought.
  - *Depending on the situation*, other medications such as β-blockers and angiotensin-converting enzyme inhibitors should be administered within 24 hours of a STEMI.
- In the absence of contraindications, patients with **unstable angina** and **non-ST segment elevation myocardial infarction** should be treated with aspirin, a second antiplatelet agent such as clopidogrel, β-blockade, anticoagulant therapy, and a glycoprotein IIb/IIIa inhibitor until a revascularization decision is made.

- If a patient experiences **cardiac arrest**, code team activation, early and proficient provision of cardiopulmonary resuscitation, and early defibrillation for ventricular fibrillation (VF) or pulseless ventricular tachycardia (VT) should occur immediately.

Cardiac Arrhythmias

- **Tachycardia** is defined as a heart rate >100 beats per minute. In pregnancy, a higher threshold, typically 120 beats per minute, is used. Tachycardias can be classified by the site of origin and regularity of rhythm. Typically, tachycardias that originate above the atrioventricular (AV) node are narrow complex, whereas those that originate below the AV node are wide complex. Patients with rate-related cardiovascular compromise should proceed to immediate synchronized cardioversion per advanced cardiac life support protocol; adenosine can be considered in patients with narrow complex regular tachycardia with monomorphic QRS complexes.
  - **Narrow complex, regular rhythm** tachycardias include sinus tachycardia, atrial flutter and AV nodal reentry tachycardia. The atrial rate with **atrial flutter** is typically 250 to 350 beats per minute most often with a 2:1 ventricular conduction ratio. Treatment is similar to that in atrial fibrillation, as described below. Acute episodes of **AV nodal reentry tachycardia** can be terminated with vagal maneuvers, adenosine, or calcium channel blockers.
  - **Narrow complex, irregular rhythm** tachycardias include atrial fibrillation, multifocal atrial tachycardia, and atrial flutter with variable AV block. Medical management for **atrial fibrillation** involves rate control and prevention of thromboembolic events. Rhythm control with chemical or electrical cardioversion is generally a second-line treatment. In patients with atrial fibrillation with rapid ventricular response, IV β-blockers, amiodarone, and nondihydropyridine calcium channel blockers (eg, diltiazem) can be used.
  - **Wide complex, regular rhythm** tachycardias include monomorphic VT or supra-VT with aberrancy. Preferred treatment for stable patients with likely VT is elective cardioversion or antiarrhythmics.
  - **Wide complex, irregular rhythm** tachycardias include VF, polymorphic VT, and atrial fibrillation with aberrancy.
- **Bradycardia** is defined as a heart rate <60 beats per minute. Common causes include electrolyte abnormalities, increased vagal tone, myocardial ischemia, myocarditis, cardiomyopathy, and medications. Initial therapy for persistent bradyarrhythmia in an unstable patient is atropine. If this fails, transcutaneous pacing, transvenous pacing, dopamine, or epinephrine can be attempted.

Hypotension and Shock

Shock is a clinical syndrome in which decreased perfusion causes cellular injury due to inadequate delivery of oxygen. This triggers an inflammatory cascade that leads to symptoms of vital organ dysfunction, including tachycardia, hypotension, oliguria, and altered mentation. In patients with gynecologic malignancy, common postoperative causes include hemorrhage, PE, MI, and sepsis.

- No absolute criteria for hypotension define shock, but systolic BP <90 mm Hg or a decrease of >40 mm Hg from baseline deserves further evaluation.
- The Weil-Shubin classification scheme defines four categories of shock: **hypovolemic**, **cardiogenic**, **obstructive**, and **distributive**. See Table 61-1 for a comparison

Table 61-1	Hemodynamic Profiles for Critical Care Diagnosis			
	PCWP or CVP	CO	SVR	SvO₂
Hypovolemic	↓	↓	↑	↓
Cardiogenic	↑	↓	↑	↓
Obstructive				
Tamponade	↑	↓	↑	↓
Pulmonary embolus	nl or ↓	↓	↑	↓
Distributive				
Early septic shock	↓	↑	↓	↑
Late septic shock	↓	↑↓	↓	↑↓
Neurogenic shock	↓	↓	↓	↓

Abbreviations: CO, cardiac output; CVP, central venous pressure; nl, normal; PCWP, pulmonary capillary wedge pressure; SvO₂, mixed venous oxygen saturation; SVR, systemic vascular resistance; ↑, increased; ↓, decreased; ↑↓, either decreased or increased.

of hemodynamic parameters in various shock states. Because a patient may exhibit multiple types of shock, strict classification can be difficult.

- Management starts with determining and correcting the etiology of the underlying disease process. Ensuring sufficient perfusion and adequate oxygenation is the primary goal.

- **Hypovolemic shock** is due to intravascular fluid loss (eg, bleeding, nasogastric suction, diarrhea). **Hemorrhagic shock** is a type of hypovolemic shock classified by the volume of blood loss and physiologic response (Table 61-2). Expedient volume resuscitation is required when blood loss exceeds 30% to 40%. The mainstay of treatment in hypovolemic shock is volume replacement.

  • It is important to **replace blood products** in patients with significant bleeding or severe anemia (hemoglobin <7 g/dL). Patient core temperature should be closely monitored during massive transfusion. Hematologic critical care is further addressed later in this chapter.

  • The IV fluids should be considered as drugs, and as such, their pharmacokinetic and pharmacodynamics properties should be taken into account prior to administration. **Indications for IV fluids** include replacement of extracellular fluid volume losses, correction of electrolyte or acid-base disorders, providing a source of glucose, and maintenance of fluid and electrolyte balance.

    ◦ **Crystalloid** (normal saline, lactated Ringer or Ringer lactate) is typically available on any unit, is inexpensive, and carries less risk than colloid administration, making it a common first choice for volume resuscitation. Ringer lactate is less acidic than normal saline and can ameliorate the hyperchloremic metabolic acidosis that results from large-volume saline infusion, although there is no important physiologic difference in the degree of resuscitation provided by Ringer lactate versus normal saline.

    ◦ **Colloid** therapy (albumin, dextrans, hydroxyethyl starches, gelatins) is more costly but may provide better short-term volume expansion, although it has not been shown to confer a survival benefit. **Albumin 5%** is generally considered

		Updated Advanced Trauma Life Support Classification for Hemorrhagic Shock		
Table 61-2				
Parameter	Class I	Class II (Mild)	Class III (Moderate)	Class IV (Severe)
Approximate blood loss	<15%	15–30%	31–40%	>40%
Heart rate	↔	↔/↑	↑	↑/↑↑
Blood pressure	↔	↔	↔/↓	↓
Pulse pressure	↔	↓	↓	↓
Respiratory rate	↔	↔	↔/↑	↑
Urine output	↔	↔	↓	↓↓
Glasgow Coma Scale score	↔	↔	↓	↓
Base deficit[a]	0 to −2 mEq/L	−2 to −6 mEq/L	−6 to −10 mEq/L	−10 mEq/L or less
Need for blood products	Monitor	Possible	Yes	Massive Transfusion Protocol

[a]Base excess is the quantity of base (HCO_3^-, in mEq/L) that is above or below the normal range in the body. A negative number is called a base deficit and indicates metabolic acidosis.
Reprinted from American College of Surgeons. *Advanced Trauma Life Support.* 10th ed. Chicago, IL: American College of Surgeons, Committee on Trauma; 2018.

safe in ICU patients; however, **hetastarch** has been shown to increase the risk of renal failure and death in ICU patients and should therefore be avoided.

- **Vasoactive pharmacotherapy** may be required along with fluid resuscitation. Intensive care and possibly invasive monitoring are required. Norepinephrine is often employed in the treatment of severe hypotensive shock (Table 61-3).
- **Cardiogenic shock** occurs with decreased myocardial contractility and function. Common etiologies include MI, congestive heart failure, cardiac arrhythmias, and valvular disease.
  - Treatment is targeted at improving myocardial function. For example, inotropes may be used to improve contractility, and vasopressor agents may be used to increase aortic diastolic pressure in order to improve myocardial perfusion. Where these fail, a mechanical assist device such as an intra-aortic balloon pump should be considered.
  - Fluid administration in patients with cardiogenic shock should be approached with caution.
- **Obstructive shock** occurs secondary to mechanical obstruction of blood flow (eg, cardiac tamponade, tension pneumothorax, massive PE, prosthetic valve thrombosis) rather than primary cardiac disease.
- **Distributive shock** results from loss of peripheral vascular tone, which in turn results in relative hypovolemia. It encompasses a wide range of conditions including

Table 61-3	Selected Vasoactive Agents in Critical Care				
Drug	Main Effects	Dose	Mechanism	Use	Warnings
Dobutamine	Increased inotropy and systemic vasodilation	3-15 µg/kg/min	Potent β_1 agonist, weak β_2 agonist	Primarily for decompensated heart failure	Adverse effects include tachycardia and ventricular ectopy. Contraindicated with hypertrophic cardiomyopathy
Dopamine	Low dose: renal and splanchnic vasodilation and natriuresis; medium dose: increased inotropy and systemic vasodilation; high dose: systemic vasoconstriction	1-3 µg/kg/min; 3-10 µg/kg/min; >10 µg/kg/min	Dose-dependent agonist for dopamine receptors (low), β-adrenergic receptors (medium), and peripheral α-adrenergic receptors (high)	May be useful for cardiogenic or hypotensive shock where both cardiac stimulation and peripheral vasoconstriction are needed	Low-dose dopamine is not appropriate for acute renal failure. Adverse effects include tachyarrhythmia, ischemic limb necrosis, increased intraocular pressure, and delayed gastric emptying.
Epinephrine	Dose-dependent increase in cardiac output, increased systemic vascular resistance, relaxation of bronchial smooth muscle	0.3-0.5 µg IM; 2-8 µg/min infusion	β-adrenergic receptor agonist (low dose) and α agonist (high dose)	Drug of choice for anaphylaxis. Used in ACLS protocols for cardiac arrest. Nebulized racemic epimer used for laryngospasm and severe asthma exacerbation	Contraindicated with narrow-angle glaucoma, ischemic cardiac disease. Local infiltration can cause tissue necrosis.

(Continued)

Table 61-3 Selected Vasoactive Agents in Critical Care *(Continued)*

Drug	Main Effects	Dose	Mechanism	Use	Warnings
Norepinephrine	Dose-dependent increase in systemic vascular resistance	0.2-5 µg/kg/min	α-Adrenergic receptor agonist and cardiac β agonist	Preferred vasopressor for septic shock or refractory hypotension	Extreme vasoconstriction can exacerbate end-organ damage. Extravasation can produce local tissue necrosis.
Nitroglycerin	Low dose: venodilation; high dose: arteriodilation	1-50 µg/min; >50 mg/min	Metabolized in endothelial cells to produce NO that stimulates cGMP production causing smooth muscle relaxation. Dose-dependent vasodilator	Used for unstable angina and to augment cardiac output in decompensated heart failure	Rapid onset and metabolism. Tolerance develops quickly. Contraindicated for patients taking phosphodiesterase inhibitors
Nitroprusside	Systemic vasodilation	0.3-2 µg/kg/min	Releases NO in bloodstream; similar mechanism to nitroglycerin	Used for rapid control of severe hypertension and for decompensated heart failure	Risk for accumulation of cyanide metabolite

Abbreviations: ACLS, advanced cardiac life support; cGMP, cyclic guanosine monophosphate; IM, intramuscularly; NO, nitric oxide.

septic shock, other systemic inflammatory response syndrome (SIRS) responses (eg, trauma, surgery, pancreatitis, hepatic failure), anaphylaxis, neurogenic shock (eg, spinal cord injury), acute adrenal insufficiency, and toxic shock syndrome.
- The initial approach to treatment is similar to in hypovolemic shock. The goal is to restore and maintain adequate intravascular volume and add vasoactive agents as needed.
- In addition, adjunctive agents should be added depending on etiology. Epinephrine should be administered in anaphylaxis. Corticosteroids should be provided in acute adrenal insufficiency. Underlying conditions should be addressed.
- Sepsis and toxic shock syndrome are discussed later in this chapter.

RESPIRATORY CRITICAL CARE

Respiratory support is frequently required for critical care patients.
- **Hypoxic respiratory failure** is characterized by decreased arterial partial pressure of oxygen (PaO_2) <60 mm Hg and/or arterial oxygen saturation (SaO_2) <90% and is typically associated with tachypnea and hypocapnia. Initially, the SaO_2 may be normal or elevated from baseline.
  - The differential diagnosis includes drug-induced hypoventilation, acute neuromuscular dysfunction, PE, heart failure, congestive obstructive pulmonary disease, pulmonary edema, pneumonia, atelectasis, and acute respiratory distress syndrome (ARDS).
- **Hypercapnic respiratory failure** is characterized by increased arterial partial pressure of carbon dioxide ($PaCO_2$) >46 mm Hg and pH <7.35 and is associated with hypoventilation. The SaO_2 may be normal.
  - The differential diagnosis includes infection, seizures, overfeeding, shock, chronic neuromuscular disorder, electrolyte abnormalities, cardiac surgery, obesity, and drug-induced respiratory depression. Consider hypercapnia as a cause of hypertension in somnolent, tachycardic postoperative patients who may be overmedicated, and avoid administering additional narcotics.
- A stepwise **evaluation of respiratory failure** (ie, hypoxemia or hypercapnia) begins with an arterial blood gas and calculation of the alveolar-arteriolar (A-a) oxygen gradient.
  - The **A-a gradient** = FIO_2 ($P_{atmosphere} - P_{H2O}$) − $PaCO_2$ / RQ − PaO_2. It is the difference in the PaO_2 between the alveolus and the arterial blood. The FIO_2 is the fraction of inspired oxygen, and RQ is the respiratory quotient. A patient at sea level breathing room air (FIO_2 = 21%) would therefore have an A-a gradient of 148 − 1.2 ($PaCO_2$) − PaO_2. The **expected A-a gradient** can be estimated using the formula Age / 4 + 4. Supplemental oxygen increases the normal gradient by 5 to 7 mm Hg for every 10% increase in FIO_2.
    - **If the A-a gradient is normal/unchanged**, the culprit is hypoventilation. To distinguish central hypoventilation from a neuromuscular disorder, maximum inspiratory effort (PI_{max}) is evaluated. The PI_{max} is measured by having the patient inspire maximally against a closed valve. For most adults, PI_{max} should be >80 cm H_2O but varies with age and sex.
      - If the PI_{max} is normal, drug-induced central hypoventilation should be considered.
      - If the PI_{max} is low, neuromuscular cause of hypoventilation should be considered.

- If the A-a gradient is increased with hypoxemia, measure the mixed venous oxygen pressure (P_{VO_2}) to assess for ventilation-perfusion ($\dot{V}/\dot{Q}$) abnormalities. The P_{VO_2} is ideally measured from pulmonary arterial blood using a PAC, but superior vena caval blood can be used. Normal values from the pulmonary artery are 35 to 45 mm Hg.
  - If the P_{VO_2} is normal, consider a $\dot{V}/\dot{Q}$ abnormality.
  - $\dot{V}/\dot{Q} > 1$ indicates increased dead space ventilation and occurs with PE, CHF, emphysema, and alveolar overdistension from positive pressure ventilation.
  - $\dot{V}/\dot{Q} < 1$ indicates intrapulmonary shunt and occurs with asthma, bronchitis, pulmonary edema, pneumonia, and atelectasis. The portion of cardiac output in an intrapulmonary shunt is called the shunt fraction and is normally $<10\%$. Shunt fractions $>50\%$ will not improve with oxygen supplementation.
  - If the P_{VO_2} is low, consider an imbalance in oxygen delivery/uptake (DO_2/VO_2) such as anemia, low cardiac output, or hypermetabolism.
- If the A-a gradient is increased with hypercapnia, measure the rate of CO_2 production ($\dot{V}_{CO_2}$) to assess metabolic versus other disorders. The $\dot{V}_{CO_2}$ is evaluated by a metabolic cart using infrared light to measure CO_2 in expired gas. Normal $\dot{V}_{CO_2}$ is 90 to 130 mL/min/m^2.
  - If the $\dot{V}_{CO_2}$ is increased, consider overfeeding (especially with carbohydrate load), fever, sepsis, and seizures.
  - If the $\dot{V}_{CO_2}$ is normal, consider increased dead space ventilation (see above) and hypoventilation from respiratory weakness (eg, shock, multisystem organ failure, prolonged neuromuscular blockade, electrolyte imbalances, cardiac surgery) or central hypoventilation (eg, opiate or benzodiazepine depression, obesity).

Acute Respiratory Distress Syndrome

- The ARDS is a leading cause of acute respiratory failure, resulting from inflammatory lung injury. The pathophysiology involves activation of diffuse pulmonary inflammation and endothelial damage producing inflammatory alveolar exudates, microvascular thrombosis, pulmonary fibrosis, and high mortality rates exceeding 50% to 60%. Predisposing conditions include sepsis, blood product transfusion, aspiration or chemical pneumonitis, pneumonia, pancreatitis, multiple or long bone fractures, intracranial hypertension, cardiopulmonary bypass, amniotic fluid embolism, and pyelonephritis in pregnancy. Clinically, ARDS is characterized by severe early hypoxemia, normal pulmonary capillary hydrostatic pressures, and diffuse pulmonary infiltrates.
- **Diagnosis** is by clinical criteria: acute onset, bilateral infiltrates on chest radiograph, PaO_2/FiO_2 ratio <300, and PCWP <18 mm Hg or no clinical evidence of left atrial hypertension. By the Berlin criteria, ARDS can be further subdivided into mild (PaO_2/FiO_2 ratio <300 mm Hg with positive end-expiratory pressure [PEEP] >5 cm H_2O), moderate (PaO_2/FiO_2 ratio <200 mmHg with PEEP >5 cm H_2O), and severe (PaO_2/FiO_2 ratio <100 mm Hg with PEEP >5 cm H_2O). The ARDS can have different causes, such as pneumonia, intra-abdominal sepsis, preeclampsia, transfusion-related lung injury, pancreatitis, and amniotic fluid embolism.
- **Management** of ARDS is essentially supportive. The underlying disorder should be corrected while respiratory support is provided. Multiple clinical trials have demonstrated the value of low tidal volume (TV) "lung protective" ventilation (<6 mL/kg

ideal body weight) with low-level PEEP, permissive hypercapnia, and limitation of plateau pressure ($<$30 mm Hg) to avoid the destructive proinflammatory effects of ventilator-induced barotrauma. Lower SaO_2 ($>$88%) and PaO_2 ($>$55 mm Hg) can be tolerated. Additional supportive measures that are sometimes used include prone positioning, conservative fluid management, and steroid treatment.

Oxygen Therapy

- **Oxygen therapy** can be used in many patients to improve oxygenation of peripheral tissues but should be applied judiciously. Oxygen can contribute directly to cellular injury and pathophysiology: it increases toxic-free radical metabolites; stimulates peripheral vasoconstriction, which decreases systemic blood flow; directly injures pulmonary tissues at high concentrations; and has a negative cardiac inotropic effect, which reduces cardiac output. An FiO_2 of $>$60% for longer than 48 hours is generally considered toxic. In critically ill patients, even an FiO_2 of $>$21% may be toxic. Therefore, oxygen supplementation should only be used when there is evidence or risk of inadequate tissue oxygenation such as PaO_2 $<$60 mm Hg, venous oxygen saturation $<$50%, serum lactate $>$4 mmol/L, or CI $<$2 L/min/m². Respiratory treatments should be assessed and optimized frequently.
- **Oxygen delivery systems** are classified as low flow (eg, nasal cannula, face mask with and without bags) and high flow.
  - **Nasal cannulas** use the patient's oronasopharynx as an oxygen reservoir (about 50 mL capacity). A patient with normal ventilation (ie, TV, 500 mL; respiratory rate, 20 breaths per minute; inspiratory/expiratory ratio, 1:2) increases their FiO_2 by 3% to 4% for each additional volume (L/min) of oxygen flow. The increase in FiO_2 is significantly reduced with hyperventilation when minute ventilation exceeds the system flow rate, and as the oxygen reservoir is drained, the patient inspires only room air. Above the maximum flow rate of 6 L/min, there is no increase in FiO_2 (approximately 45%).
  - **Face masks without bags** have an oxygen reservoir of 100 to 200 mL. In order to clear exhaled gases, a minimum flow rate of 5 L/min is required. The maximum flow rate of 10 L/min provides an FiO_2 of 60%.
  - **Face masks with bags** have an oxygen reservoir of 600 to 1000 mL. There are two types of reservoir mask devices:
    ○ A **partial rebreather** has a maximum FiO_2 of 70% to 80%. It "captures" initial exhaled air containing a higher proportion of oxygen from the upper airway (anatomic dead space) in the reservoir bag and releases the terminal exhaled air containing more CO_2. The reservoir bag maintains a high oxygen content.
    ○ A **nonrebreather** has a maximum FiO_2 of 100%. It requires a tight seal during use and can be used to administer nebulizer treatments but does not allow easy oral feeding. The reservoir bag maintains 100% oxygen content.
  - **High-flow oxygen masks** deliver a constant FiO_2 at a flow rate that exceeds the peak inspiratory rate, preventing the variability seen with low flow systems. They may be useful in patients with chronic hypercapnia who require a constant FiO_2 to avoid increased CO_2 retention. The maximum FiO_2 is 50%.
  - **Noninvasive positive pressure ventilation** can be a useful alternative to invasive (ie, endotracheal or tracheostomy) intubation in suitable patient populations. It has been used to successfully manage obstructive sleep apnea in general medical patients but is also appropriate for critical care patients with moderate respiratory compromise due to mild neuromuscular weakness, congestive heart

failure/cardiogenic pulmonary edema, and decompensated congestive obstructive pulmonary disease.

- o A cooperative patient with no risk for emergent intubation and moderate dyspnea, tachypnea, increased work of breathing, hypercapnia, or hypoxemia can be considered for noninvasive ventilation (NIV).
- o Contraindications include cardiac or respiratory arrest or severe cardiopulmonary compromise, coma, status epilepticus, potential airway obstruction, patient inability to protect her airway, and emergent conditions.
- o The NIV can be supplied via mouthpiece, nasal pillows, face mask, or helmet; the device must fit properly to avoid air leaks. The FiO_2 is titrated to the necessary minimum and the backup rate, pressure support, and PEEP are adjusted to maintain an appropriate TV (5-7 mL/kg/breath).
- o Complications with NIV include facial or nasal pressure sores, gastric distension, aspiration, and inspissated uncleared secretions.

- **Mechanical ventilation** should be instituted for patients who cannot be adequately managed with the systems above, are in respiratory distress, or are at risk for cardiopulmonary collapse. Indicators for endotracheal intubation include tachypnea >35 breaths per minute; PaO_2 <60 mm Hg; $PaCO_2$ >46 mm Hg with pH <7.35; and absent gag reflex. Standard positive pressure ventilation is delivered with a preset volume-cycled device; additional modes of ventilation such as high-frequency and proportional-assist ventilation are not discussed here. Selection of ventilation modes is tailored to the patient and is largely selected by provider preference.
  - o In **assist-control ventilation**, the patient initiates breaths and the ventilator delivers a set TV. If the patient fails to initiate, the ventilator "assists" at a preset "controlled" rate and TV. Tachypnea is not well tolerated in this mode and can lead to overventilation, respiratory alkalosis, and hyperinflation. Patients with respiratory muscle weakness are appropriately ventilated with assist-control ventilation.
  - o In **intermittent mandatory ventilation (IMV)**, a breath is delivered at a preset rate and volume, but the patient can breathe spontaneously between machine breaths without assistance. In **synchronized IMV**, machine breaths are coordinated with spontaneous respirations to avoid respiratory alkalosis and "stacking" breaths. Asynchronous IMV is not ideal because it can deliver a breath at any time during the patient's spontaneous breaths (ie, during expiration).
- In **pressure-controlled ventilation (PCV)**, regardless of how or when breaths are delivered, a constant pressure is provided by regulating the inspiratory flow rate throughout each breath. This may result in variable inflation volumes, especially as lung compliance changes. The PCV is well suited to patients with neuromuscular disease with stable lung mechanics.
  - o In **inverse-ratio ventilation (IRV)**, PCV is delivered with a prolonged inspiratory phase. A normal inspiratory:expiratory ratio is 1:2 to 1:4. In IRV, the ratio is reversed to 2:1, which prevents alveolar collapse and provides auto-PEEP but may lead to reduced cardiac output. The main use of IRV is for ARDS with hypoxemia or hypercapnia that is refractory to conventional ventilation modes.
  - o In **pressure support ventilation**, the patient breathes spontaneously and the machine adds extra support to maintain inspiratory pressures. It is a common weaning mode of ventilation.

- **Ventilator management** is a continuous and dynamic process, ideally leading to weaning from mechanical ventilation and extubation. The following basic parameters can be adjusted: mode, FIO_2, TV, PEEP, and pressure support.
  - The FIO_2 is initially set to 100% and then titrated to the minimum needed to maintain PaO_2 above 60 mm Hg or SaO_2 above 90%. Although oxygen can be toxic, in acute respiratory distress, treatment of hypoxemia takes precedence.
  - Normal **minute ventilation** (respiratory rate × TV) is 6 to 8 L/min. Infection, inflammation, and acid-base disorders can effect large variation in the required ventilation.
  - The PEEP is the positive airway pressure at the end of respiration (ie, alveolar pressure higher than atmospheric pressure) that prevents alveolar collapse.
    - **Extrinsic PEEP** is created by a device that stops exhalation at a preselected pressure. The PEEP reduces the risk of oxygen toxicity by improving gas exchange, increasing lung compliance, and increasing the PaO_2, which allows reduced FIO_2.
    - **Intrinsic PEEP** (auto-PEEP) is created by increasing minute ventilation or shortening the expiratory phase. It is common in patients with prolonged expiration such as during an asthma exacerbation.
    - The PEEP can progress to the point of sudden cardiovascular collapse; elevated auto-PEEP requires immediate disconnection from the ventilator to allow the patient to fully exhale. This may take 30 to 60 seconds, but it is lifesaving.
- **Weaning from mechanical ventilation** is the gradual process of reducing ventilation to minimum settings (ie, FIO_2 <50%, IMV, with PEEP and pressure support <5 cm H_2O each) or T-piece ventilation, followed by extubation. Duration of mechanical ventilation is directly related to complications, so extubation should be performed as soon as feasible. A daily sedation break and spontaneous breathing trial should be performed on all eligible patients. Criteria for extubation include progressive clinical recovery from illness; intact neurologic status (ie, alert, oriented) with ability to follow commands; patent airway without concern for occlusion (see cuff test below); and normal arterial blood gas on minimal supplemental oxygen.
  - Assessment of airway patency and **respiration mechanics** helps assess whether a patient is ready for extubation. Patients who cannot meet minimum criteria or are neurologically impaired and unable to cooperate with the evaluation may not be ready for unassisted respiration.
    - The "**cuff test**" can be used to assess the airway. The endotracheal tube cuff is deflated, and the patient is asked to breathe while the tube is occluded. A positive cuff leak demonstrates tracheal edema is not to the point that the endotracheal tube is required, and extubation can be considered.
    - **Forced vital capacity** should be at least 10 mL/kg and is typically at least 1000 mL.
    - **Negative inspiratory force (NIF)** should be −25 to −30 cm H_2O. When performed as an "occlusion NIF," the test is not effort dependent. A normal person can generate NIF of −80 cm H_2O.
    - **Rapid shallow breathing index (RSBI or Tobin index)** should be <80 and predicts the patient's ability to remain extubated for 24 hours. It is measured by switching from any ventilator mode to continuous positive airway pressure and assessing the patient's respiratory rate (f) and TV over 1 minute. The RSBI = f/TV.
      - Patients with RSBI <80 are 8- to 9-fold more likely to remain extubated.
      - Patients with RSBI >100 are 8- to 9-fold more likely to require reintubation.
      - Patients with RSBI between 80 and 100 require clinical judgment regarding suitable timing for extubation.

○ After extubation, **secretions** should be cleared and humidified oxygen should be supplied by face mask. The patient should be encouraged to cough and breathe deeply at regular intervals. If reintubation is necessary, perform a complete assessment of the reasons for failure and attempt extubation again within 24 to 72 hours.

FLUIDS AND ELECTROLYTES

Fluid and electrolyte disorders are common for critically ill patients and for women with obstetric morbidity or undergoing major gynecologic surgery. Some of the most common issues are addressed here.

Hyponatremia

• **Hyponatremia** is defined as serum sodium <136 mEq/L. It can be classified on the basis of volume status and further diagnosed with urine sodium and osmolality (Figure 61-1). Management includes treating the underlying condition and replacing the sodium deficit if present.

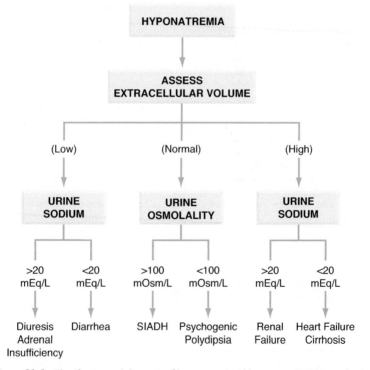

Figure 61-1. Classification and diagnosis of hyponatremia. Abbreviation: SIADH, syndrome of inappropriate antidiuretic hormone secretion. Reprinted with permission from Marino PL, ed. *The ICU Book*. 3rd ed. Philadelphia, PA: Wolters Kluwer Health/Lippincott Williams & Wilkins; 2012:606.

- Rapid **correction of chronic or severe hyponatremia** can cause cerebral edema and increased intracranial pressure leading to a demyelinating encephalopathy or central pontine myelinolysis. Hyponatremia can be corrected as follows:
  - **Step 1:** Calculate the sodium deficit. Sodium deficit = Total body water (TBW) × (desired sodium − actual sodium). In women, **TBW** in liters = 50% of lean body weight in kilograms.
  - **Step 2:** Calculate the volume of crystalloid needed to correct the deficit. This volume is the (sodium deficit) / (mEq of sodium found in replacement fluid in sodium per liter). For reference, 3% sodium chloride contains 513 mEq sodium per liter.
  - **Step 3:** Calculate the infusion rate to correct the sodium at no more than 0.5 mEq/L/h. Use serial serum sodium measurements to assess response.
    - ○ For example, a 60-kg woman with a sodium level of 120 mEq/L with a goal sodium of 130 mEq/L has a calculated sodium deficit of 300 mEq that should be corrected by total infusion of 585 mL of 3% sodium chloride over 20 hours at a rate of 29 mL/h.

Hypernatremia

- **Hypernatremia** is defined as serum sodium >145 mEq/L. It reflects a relative deficiency of free water as occurs with vomiting, diarrhea, overdiuresis, diabetes mellitus with nonketotic hyperglycemia, and diabetes insipidus. Iatrogenic hypernatremia from hypertonic saline or sodium bicarbonate (HCO_3) infusion is also possible. Clinical findings can vary from tachycardia and decreased urine output to encephalopathy, seizures, and coma.
- **Management** is generally directed toward volume replacement with crystalloid or colloid and maintenance of cardiac output. It is based on accurate assessment of extracellular volume by invasive monitoring or clinical evaluation.
  - **Hypovolemic hypernatremia** should be corrected by replacing the free water deficit over 24 to 72 hours. The serum sodium should be lowered at a rate less than 0.5 mEq/L/h, in order to avoid cerebral edema. The free water deficit is TBW × (serum sodium − 140) / 140.
  - **Euvolemic hypernatremia** is treated with isotonic saline to slowly replace the water deficit.
  - **Hypervolemic hypernatremia** will be corrected by the kidneys via renal sodium excretion. In some cases, diuresis may be helpful, but care must be taken to avoid hypovolemia and exacerbating the problem.

Hypokalemia

- **Hypokalemia** is defined as serum potassium <3.5 mEq/L. It can be caused by artifactual dilution (ie, drawn near an IV infusion site), decreased potassium intake, insufficient replacement of nasogastric tube output, diuretic therapy, diarrhea, and laxative abuse.
- **Clinical findings** of severe hypokalemia include muscle weakness and mental status changes. The ECG changes can be seen, such as flattened T waves, prolonged QT intervals, and U waves. Chronic hypokalemia can result in renal tubular disorders with concentrating abnormalities, phosphaturia, and azotemia.
- **Management** includes correcting the underlying cause (eg, alkalosis) and replacing the potassium deficit to a level of 4 mEq/L. Typically, potassium repletion is not an

emergency, except in the most severe cases with active arrhythmias or in patients who are on digoxin therapy.

- For each 10 mEq oral or IV potassium chloride, the serum potassium rises by about 1 mEq/L.
- Rapid increases in serum potassium can predispose to cardiac arrest, so the maximum rate of IV potassium chloride infusion is 20 mEq/L via central catheter or 10 mEq/L via peripheral IV.
- Hypomagnesemia can cause refractory hypokalemia and should be replaced along with potassium. Serum magnesium levels are not generally helpful unless the patient is receiving magnesium infusion (eg, for preeclampsia) or the patient has impaired renal function.
- Patients with significant kidney disease (ie, glomerular filtration rate [GFR] <25 mL/min) should have potassium therapy titrated using serial serum potassium levels. Patients taking potassium-sparing diuretics may also require close monitoring.

Hyperkalemia

- **Hyperkalemia** is defined as serum potassium >5.0 mEq/L. It is not as well tolerated and can be life-threatening. It can be caused by laboratory artifact (ie, hemolyzed specimen), cellular redistribution associated with acidosis (eg, diabetic ketoacidosis, sepsis), renal insufficiency, adrenal insufficiency, and tissue injury (eg, hemolysis, rhabdomyolysis, crush injury, burns).
- **Clinical findings** in the majority of patients are unimpressive. The ECG changes are seen when serum potassium approaches 6 mEq/L; the earliest findings include peaked T waves, especially in precordial leads, flattened P waves, and prolonged PR intervals. This progresses to absent P waves, wide QRS complexes, and ultimately VF and asystole.
- **Management** in an asymptomatic patient with unexpected hyperkalemia starts with repeating the measurement and discontinuing any potassium supplementation. If the abnormal value is confirmed, acute management as described below is guided by serum potassium and ECG findings, if any.
  - **Calcium gluconate** stabilizes the myocardium, but response lasts only 20-30 minutes.
  - **Insulin/glucose** facilitates movement of potassium into cellular compartment and can reduce serum concentrations by 1 mEq/L for 1 to 2 hour.
  - **Kayexalate** is a cation exchange resin that facilitates removing potassium from the body but may require time and multiple doses to take effect.
  - **Loop diuretics** enhance urinary potassium secretion but should be avoided in renal failure and hemodynamically unstable patients.
  - **Urgent hemodialysis** is necessary in cases of life-threatening hyperkalemia.

Hypocalcemia

- **Hypocalcemia** is defined as total serum calcium <8.5 mg/dL or ionized serum calcium <1.1 mmol/L. A "normal" plasma calcium is lower in patients with hypoalbuminemia, due to decreased protein binding. Causes of hypocalcemia include hypoparathyroidism, hypomagnesemia, alkalosis, blood transfusion, chronic renal failure, pancreatitis, some drugs (eg, aminoglycosides, heparin), and sepsis.

- **Clinical findings** include hyperreflexia, paresthesias, tetany, seizures, hypotension, cardiac arrhythmias, heart block, and VT.
- **Management** is directed toward diagnosis and correction of the underlying condition. Symptomatic hypocalcemia or ionized calcium <0.65 mmol/L should be immediately corrected with calcium chloride or calcium gluconate IV, preferably through a central vein.

Hypercalcemia

- **Hypercalcemia** is defined as total serum calcium >10.5 mg/dL or ionized serum calcium >1.3 mmol/L. In 90% of cases, the underlying cause is hyperparathyroidism or malignancy; severe hypercalcemia (ie, total calcium >14 mg/dL or ionized calcium >3.5 mmol/L) is associated with neoplasm. Other causes include thyrotoxicosis, thiazide diuretics, and lithium treatment. The most common mechanism of hypercalcemia in gynecologic oncology patients is increased osteoclastic bone resorption without direct bone metastases.
- **Clinical findings** are nonspecific but can include gastrointestinal (eg, nausea, constipation, ileus, abdominal pain, pancreatitis), cardiovascular (eg, hypovolemia, hypotension, hypertension, shortened QT interval), renal (eg, polyuria, nephrolithiasis), and neurologic (eg, lethargy, confusion, coma) abnormalities. Symptoms are usually present when total serum calcium exceeds 12 mg/dL.
- **Acute management** aims to increase excretion and storage of calcium.
  - Hydration with **isotonic saline** promotes renal natriuresis and thereby increases calcium excretion.
  - Diuresis with **furosemide** (40-80 mg IV every 2 h) with a goal of 100 to 200 mL urine output per hour further promotes urinary calcium excretion. Urine output, stimulated by hydration or pharmacologic diuresis, should be replaced with isotonic saline to prevent hypovolemia.
  - **Calcitonin** (salmon calcitonin 4 U/kg subcutaneously or intramuscularly every 12 h) rapidly inhibits bone resorption and may decrease serum calcium levels, although the effect is not profound.
  - **Hydrocortisone** (200 mg IV daily divided into 3 doses) inhibits some lymphoid neoplastic growth, decreasing bone calcium release.
  - **Pamidronate disodium** (90 mg IV over 2 h) or zoledronate are effective for severe hypercalcemia, with peak effect in 2 to 4 days.
  - **Dialysis** is appropriate for patients with severe renal failure.

Acid-Base Disorders

Evaluation of acid-base disorders requires arterial blood gas interpretation. A stepwise approach for basic analysis is outlined here.
- **Step 1. Determine the primary disorder.** Assess the pH and $PaCO_2$. If either the pH or $PaCO_2$ is abnormal, a disorder is present.
  - If the pH is <7.36, the patient is acidemic. A **respiratory acidosis** is present if the $PaCO_2$ >44, and a **metabolic acidosis** is present if the HCO_3 <22.
  - If the pH is >7.44, the patient is alkalemic. A **respiratory alkalosis** is present if the $PaCO_2$ <36, and a **metabolic alkalosis** is present if HCO_3 >26.
  - A mixed disorder is present if either the pH or the $PaCO_2$ is normal. Compensatory responses never completely correct the primary acid-base disturbance, so equal and opposite processes are occurring.

Table 61-4	Normal Values and Expected Changes in Various Acid-Base Disorders[a]

Primary Disorder	Expected Result
Metabolic acidosis	Expected $Paco_2$ = $(1.5 \times HCO_3) + (8 \pm 2)$
Metabolic alkalosis	Expected $Paco_2$ = $(0.7 \times HCO_3) + (21 \pm 2)$
Acute respiratory acidosis	$DpH = 0.008 \times DPaco_2$
	Expected pH = $7.40 - [0.008 \times (Paco_2 - 40)]$
Acute respiratory alkalosis	$DpH = 0.008 \times DPaco_2$
	Expected pH = $7.40 + [0.008 \times (40 - Paco_2)]$
Chronic respiratory acidosis	$DpH = 0.003 \times DPaco_2$
	Expected pH = $7.40 - [0.003 \times (Paco_2 - 40)]$
Chronic respiratory alkalosis	$DpH = 0.003 \times DPaco_2$
	Expected pH = $7.40 - [0.003 \times (40 - Paco_2)]$

Normal values: pH = 7.36-7.44; Pco_2 = 36-44 mm Hg; HCO_3 = 22-26 mEq/L

Normal in pregnancy: pH = 7.40-7.45; Pco_2 = 27-32 mm Hg; HCO_3 = 19-25 mEq/L

Abbreviations: $DPaco_2$, change in arterial CO_2; DpH, change in arterial pH; HCO_3, serum bicarbonate.
[a]Adapted with permission from Marino PL, ed. *The ICU Book*. 3rd ed. Philadelphia, PA: Wolters Kluwer Health/Lippincott Williams & Wilkins; 2012:535.

- **Step 2: Determine the expected compensatory response:** See Table 61-4.
  - In metabolic disorders, if the measured $Paco_2$ is higher than expected, there is a **superimposed respiratory acidosis**. If the measured $Paco_2$ is lower than expected, there is a **superimposed respiratory alkalosis**.
  - In respiratory disorders, if the change in pH is more than 0.008 times the change in Pco_2, then a superimposed metabolic disorder is present.
- **Step 3: Calculate the anion gap.** The anion gap = $Na^+ - (Cl^- + HCO_3^-)$. For every 1 g/dL reduction of **albumin** from 4 g/dL, add another 2.5 to the anion gap. The normal range is 10 to 14 mEq/L. If an anion gap is present, the patient has an anion gap metabolic acidosis, regardless of what other disturbances are present.
  - **Causes of normal anion gap acidosis** (mnemonic **USEDCAR**) include **U**rinary diversion (ureterosigmoidostomy), **S**aline administration (in the face of renal dysfunction), **E**ndocrine disorder (Addison disease, primary hyperparathyroidism), **D**iarrhea/**D**rugs (spironolactone, triamterene, amiloride, amphotericin), **C**arbonic anhydrase inhibitors (acetazolamide, methazolamide, topiramate), **A**mmonium chloride/hyper**A**limentation, and **R**enal tubular acidosis.
  - **Causes of increased anion gap acidosis** (mnemonic **MUDPILES**) include **M**ethanol, **U**remia, **D**iabetes (ketoacidosis)/**D**rugs (metformin), **P**araldehyde, **I**soniazid/ **I**nfection/**I**schemia, **L**actic acidosis, **E**thylene glycol, **S**alicylates/**S**tarvation.
- **Step 4: If there is an anion gap, calculate the delta gap:** The delta gap = $(25 - HCO_3)$ − (anion gap − 12). If this is >5, there is a coexisting nonanion gap metabolic acidosis.

- **Step 5: Calculate the osmolar gap in patients with unexplained anion gap metabolic acidosis**: Osmolar gap = measured OsM − calculated OsM. Calculated OsM = 2 × sodium + glucose / 18 + blood urea nitrogen (BUN) / 2.8.
  - Increased osmolar gap is seen in ingestion of ethylene glycol, alcohol, methanol, isopropyl alcohol, mannitol, sorbitol, and paraldehyde.
- **Treatment** is based on the severity and diagnosis. Typically, it is only necessary to treat the underlying cause(s). In patients with profound disturbances (ie, pH <7.2 or bicarbonate levels <10 mEq/L), bicarbonate infusion may be warranted.

RENAL FAILURE

- **Acute kidney injury** (AKI) is characterized by an abrupt decrease in the GFR and resulting disruption in fluid and electrolyte homeostasis. Severity is classified by the RIFLE criteria (risk, injury, failure, loss, end-stage kidney disease), which correlates well with overall mortality.
- The **differential diagnosis** of AKI is classified by anatomic location of the problem.
  - A **prerenal disorder** causing decreased kidney perfusion is the etiology in approximately 40% of AKI cases.
    - In obstetrics and gynecology, the most common causes are intravascular volume depletion from hemorrhage, third-spacing of fluids (eg, with preeclampsia), or inadequate fluid resuscitation. Other common causes include hypotension, heart failure, renal vasoconstriction (eg, from nonsteroidal anti-inflammatory drugs), and reduced glomerular filtration pressure (eg, from angiotensin-converting enzyme inhibitors).
    - A prerenal disorder is suggested by elevated urine specific gravity, decreased fractional excretion of sodium (FE_{Na}) of <1%, BUN:creatinine ratio >20, and urine sodium <20 mEq/L.
  - An **intrinsic renal disorder** from direct injury to the kidney is the etiology in up to 50% of AKI cases in ICU patients. Causes include ischemia/hypoperfusion injury, inflammation, sepsis, radiocontrast dye, myoglobinuria, and other drugs/toxins. These can result in three types of renal pathology: acute tubular necrosis (ATN), acute glomerulonephritis, and acute interstitial nephritis (AIN).
    - The **ATN** is the most common cause of intrinsic renal dysfunction and is typically the result of any process that leads to renal hypoperfusion. The renal tubules and parenchyma are damaged but glomeruli are usually intact. Injured tubular epithelial cells are shed, blocking the proximal tubular lumen and reducing net GFR. The ATN is suggested by FE_{Na} >2%, fractional excretion of urea (FE_{urea}) >50%, urine sodium >40 mmol/L, urine osmolarity <350 mOsm/L, and granular casts on microscopy.
    - The **AIN** is the result of inflammatory injury to the renal interstitium and can often present as AKI without oliguria. It is classically precipitated by antibiotics such as penicillins, aminoglycosides, and vancomycin. The AIN is suggested by eosinophils and leukocyte casts on urine microscopy.
  - A **postrenal disorder** results from obstruction of the urinary tract distal to the kidney and rarely leads to oliguria unless there is a single kidney or the condition is bilateral (eg, advanced cervical cancer).
    - The obstruction may occur in the collecting system (eg, papillary necrosis), ureters (eg, compression, calculus, tumor, papillary sloughing, clot/hematoma), bladder (eg, calculus, neurogenic bladder, carcinoma, clot/hematoma), and urethra (eg, calculus, stricture, clot/hematoma).

- o Assessment includes bladder catheterization, urinary tract ultrasound/imaging, and laboratory evaluation for prenatal and intrarenal diseases.
- o Early treatment can prevent permanent kidney damage. Significant postobstructive diuresis occurs with resolution of bilateral obstruction, leading to electrolyte abnormalities and volume contraction. Decompression of an overly distended bladder can reveal capillary bleeding with hematuria or even frank hemorrhage.

- **Clinical assessment** should include review of strict intake and output and medications administered; identifying problems with urinary drainage such as an obstructed catheter; and evaluating for signs and symptoms of hypovolemia, cardiac dysfunction, and infection.
- **Laboratory assessment** includes the following:
  - The **urine specific gravity** (range: 1.003-1.030) is elevated in the setting of dehydration. False elevations can occur with mannitol, glucose, and radiocontrast dye.
  - **Urine microscopy** helps distinguish intrinsic disorders; it is not useful for prerenal diagnoses. Tubular epithelial cells and granular casts are pathognomonic for ATN. Leukocyte casts suggest interstitial nephritis (pyelonephritis). Red cell casts suggest glomerulonephritis. Pigmented casts suggest myoglobinuria. Sloughed papillae from papillary necrosis may be seen in postrenal disorders involving the renal collecting system.
  - The **urine sodium level (urine$_{Na}$)** is best assessed with a 24-hour urine specimen, but a random 10-mL specimen may also be used. Urine$_{Na}$ <20 mEq/L suggests a prerenal disorder; renal hypoperfusion leads to increased sodium reabsorption and decreased excretion. Urine$_{Na}$ >40 mEq/L suggests impaired sodium reabsorption from an intrinsic renal disorder, although it does not rule out coexisting prerenal disorders and may not be useful if diuretics have been administered or in elderly patients with obligatory urinary sodium loss.
  - **Fractional excretion of sodium** is the fraction of sodium filtered at the glomerulus that is ultimately excreted in the urine. An FE$_{Na}$ <1% suggests a prerenal disorder, and an FE$_{Na}$ >2% suggests an intrinsic renal disorder. It is not a useful test for nonoliguric renal dysfunction. Calculation of this value in the setting of oliguria is one of the most reliable tests for distinguishing prerenal causes from intrarenal causes of AKI. The FE$_{Na}$ is calculated by the formula

$$[(Urine_{Na} / Plasma_{Na}) / (Urine_{Cr} / Plasma_{Cr})] \times 100$$

  - **Fractional excretion of urea** may be useful in patients on diuretics. A value <35% indicates prerenal disorders, whereas FE$_{urea}$ >50% suggests an intrarenal cause. It is calculated by the formula

$$[(Urine_{urea} \times Plasma_{creatinine}) / (Urine_{creatinine} \times Plasma_{urea})] \times 100$$

  - **Creatinine clearance (Cl$_{Cr}$)** is best assessed with a 24-hour urine collection. Normal Cl$_{Cr}$ for women is 72 to 110 mL/min at our institution. Renal impairment is considered at a Cl$_{Cr}$ level of 50 to 70 mL/min, renal insufficiency at a level of 20 to 50 mL/min, and renal failure at a level of 4 to 20 mL/min. Note that serum creatinine level of 1.2 mg/dL in a pregnant patient indicates >50% reduction in GFR. The Cl$_{Cr}$ is calculated by the formula

$$Cl_{Cr} \text{ (mL/min)} = [Cr_{urine} \text{ (mg/dL)} \times \text{Volume of urine (mL)}] / [Cr_{serum} \text{ (mg/dL)} \times \text{Time (min)}]$$

- **Management** of acute oliguria should optimize central hemodynamics and increase glomerulotubular flow. Precipitating factors should be identified and corrected. Nephrotoxic agents should be minimized and all medications renally dosed. Electrolytes should be monitored and repleted.
  - If there is evidence for volume depletion, a fluid challenge should first be administered and volume infused until cardiac output is restored. In patients with invasive hemodynamic monitoring, base the management on cardiac filling pressures (CVP and PCWP), cardiac output (using CI), and BP.
  - There is no evidence that low "renal dose" dopamine or furosemide treatments are beneficial. Dopamine may increase risk for bowel ischemia.
  - Low-dose dopamine (5 mg/kg/min) has traditionally been used to improve inotropy in oliguric renal failure. However, recent studies have shown that dopamine has little benefit in these situations and may increase risk for bowel ischemia.
  - Similarly, loop diuretics are often used to treat oliguric renal failure, but multiple studies have suggested that not only is there no benefit but also their use may harm critically ill patients. If loop diuretics are used, it should be as a continuous infusion. Rarely, a "Lasix-dependent" patient is encountered who requires diuretic to maintain adequate urine output. This is very uncommon, however, and most postoperative patients with oliguria are simply hypovolemic. Volume status and cardiac output should be optimized before proceeding with pharmacologic management.
  - Special attention should be given to urine output in postoperative gynecologic oncology patients who have had malignant ascites removed. The fluid tends to reaccumulate in the abdominal cavity quickly after drainage and may require massive ongoing fluid replacement.
  - Patients who fail conservative management of AKI may require **renal replacement therapy**. Indications include volume overload, uremia, hyperkalemia, severe acidosis, and rapidly increasing serum creatinine.

HEMATOLOGIC CRITICAL CARE

Anemia

- Hemoglobin levels of 7 g/dL, or even lower, are typically well tolerated in patients without cardiovascular disease.
- The decision to transfuse depends on the clinical situation and should balance the potential risks of a blood transfusion with patient symptoms, comorbidities, and risk of further bleeding. A landmark study that compared a conservative transfusion threshold (<7 g/dL) with a liberal threshold (<10 g/dL) demonstrated a lower complication rate and 28-day mortality in the conservative group.
- However, higher hemoglobin levels may be desired in preoperative patients in whom blood loss is anticipated; patients with cardiac ischemia who need better oxygen delivery; and in patients undergoing radiation therapy, where availability of oxygen to form free radicals may contribute to better treatment outcomes.
- Adverse effects include hypocalcemia due to citrate anticoagulant in banked blood, hyperkalemia in patients with circulatory shock, hemolytic reactions, transmission of infectious diseases, and transfusion-related acute lung injury.
- Due to the risk of developing coagulopathy during **massive hemorrhage**, resuscitation should include transfusing a combination of red blood cells (RBCs),

fresh frozen plasma (FFP), and platelets. There does not yet exist consensus regarding the optimal ratio, but some institutions have proposed a 1:1:1 ratio of RBC:FFP:platelets.

Thrombocytopenia

- **Thrombocytopenia** is defined as a platelet count of less than 140 000/μL. Bleeding complications typically do not occur until levels fall below 50 000 /μL.
- Drugs that may cause thrombocytopenia include trimethoprim-sulfamethoxazole, penicillins, thiazide diuretics, chemotherapeutic agents, and heparin. **Heparin-induced thrombocytopenia** is an antibody-mediated reaction that most often occurs 4 to 10 days after initiating heparin treatment. The diagnosis should be considered in patients receiving heparin in whom platelet count drops >50%. After heparin-induced thrombocytopenia is diagnosed, heparin should immediately be discontinued and an alternative anticoagulant such as lepirudin, bivalirudin, and argatroban should be initiated.

Disseminated Intravascular Coagulation

- **Disseminated intravascular coagulation** is a disorder of hemostasis in which intravascular activation of both clotting and fibrinolytic systems leads to consumption of coagulation factors and platelets. Widespread endothelial damage causes release of **tissue factor** that activates these systems. Clinically, a patient will experience systemic hemorrhage concurrent with widespread microvascular thrombosis.
- **Lab abnormalities** include increased prothrombin time, partial thromboplastin time, and fibrin split products (D-dimer). Platelet counts and fibrinogen are decreased. Peripheral blood smears show fragmented RBCs (ie, schistocytes) and thrombocytopenia with large platelets.
- Risk factors include **sepsis**, **trauma**, **obstetric complications**, **malignancy**, **liver failure**, and **renal failure**.
- **Treatment** is supportive and difficult. Any inciting factors should be addressed. **Transfusion therapy** with platelets, FFP, and/or cryoprecipitate may be provided. However, this rarely helps and may feed the consumption of platelets and coagulation factors, leading to further microvascular thrombosis.

INFECTIOUS DISEASES

Sepsis

- **Sepsis** is defined as life-threatening organ dysfunction caused by a dysregulated host response to infection. It is characterized by a host inflammatory response to infection including vasodilation, complement activation, loss of hemostatic balance, and increased microvascular permeability. This results in widespread microvascular and cellular injury, which causes further inflammation, multiorgan dysfunction, and ultimately organ failure. Table 61-5 lists definitions for the SIRS, sepsis, septic shock, and sequential organ failure assessment (SOFA) scoring.
  - The SIRS was initially a harbinger of sepsis diagnosis. However, SIRS focuses on inflammation, which does not take into account endogenous factors such as bacterial versus fungal infection, resistance pattern, and the ability to obtain

Table 61-5	Criteria for Sepsis and Related Disorders
SIRS[a]	At least two of the following: Temperature >38°C or <36°C Heart rate >90 beats/min Respiratory rate >20 breaths/min or $Paco_2$ <32 mm Hg WBC >12 000 cells/mm^3 or <4000 cells/mm^3 or >10% bands
Sepsis	SIRS that is the result of an infection
Septic shock	Severe sepsis with hypotension refractory to volume resuscitation adequate volume resuscitation
qSOFA	A "positive" qSOFA score (≥2) suggests high risk of poor outcome in patients with suspected infection. These patients should be more thoroughly assessed for evidence of organ dysfunction. Altered mental status (GCS <15) = 1 point Respiratory rate greater than or equal to 22 breaths/min = 1 point Systolic BP less than or equal to 100 mm Hg = 1 point

Abbreviations: BP, blood pressure; GSC, Glasgow Coma Scale; qSOFA, quick sequential organ failure assessment; SIRS, systemic inflammatory response syndrome; WBC, white blood cell.
[a]No longer used to diagnose (rule in or rule out) sepsis alone.

source control. The SIRS also diagnosed hospitalized patients without infections and did not account for hypotension, oliguria, or other forms of end-organ dysfunction. For this reason, SIRS alone is not adequate to diagnose (rule in or rule out) sepsis.

- Sepsis is a spectrum of disease; SOFA scoring has been used to assess severity. Quick SOFA (qSOFA) is an easier assessment that does not require labs.
- Early septic shock is **distributive**, whereas later stages of septic shock *can* produce **cardiogenic** shock when hypotension, acidosis, and ischemia suppress myocardial function or when there is demand ischemia. Additionally, infection, tissue trauma, or obstetric accidents can activate the intrinsic coagulation pathway with subsequent intravascular thrombosis and fibrinolysis, causing disseminated intravascular coagulation and massive bleeding.
- Successful management of sepsis includes early recognition, aggressive but appropriate fluid replacement, broad-spectrum antibiotics, source identification and control, and ongoing supportive care. Table 61-6 contains the sepsis management guidelines proposed by the Surviving Sepsis Campaign. This and guidelines for managing sepsis can be found at http://www.survivingsepsis.org.
  - Goals for **initial resuscitation** during the first 6 hours in patients with sepsis-induced hypotension (hypotension despite initial fluid challenge or a lactate >4 mmol/L) include CVP 8 to 12 mm Hg, mean arterial pressure ≥65 mm Hg, urine output 0.5 mL/kg/h, central venous or mixed oxygen saturation of 70% or 65%, respectively, and normalizing lactate.
  - Crystalloids are the initial fluids of choice. Albumin can be considered if significant amounts of fluids are required. Current evidence argues against the use of hydroxyethyl starches.

Table 61-6	Surviving Sepsis Campaign Recommendations[a,b]

1. Measure lactate levels.
2. Obtain cultures (aerobic and anaerobic) prior to antibiotic administration.
3. Administer broad-spectrum antibiotics (within 1 h).
4. Within the first 3 h, administer at least 30 mL/kg crystalloid for hypotension or lactate >4 mmol/L.
5. For hypotension that does not respond to initial fluid resuscitation, administer vasopressors (norepinephrine is first line) to maintain a mean arterial pressure ≥65 mm Hg.
6. Remeasure lactate if initial lactate was elevated. Guide resuscitation to normalize lactate levels.
7. Identify a specific anatomic source of infection as rapidly as possible and implement any source control intervention as soon as safely possible.
8. Narrow antimicrobial therapy once pathogen identification and sensitivities are established and/or adequate clinical improvement is noted.

---

[a]Sepsis and septic shock are medical emergencies for which treatment and resuscitation should begin immediately.
[b]Adapted with permission from Rhodes A, Evans LE, Alhazzani W, et al. Surviving sepsis campaign: international guidelines for management of sepsis and septic shock: 2016. *Crit Care Med.* 2017;45(3):486-552. Copyright © 2016 by the Society of Critical Care Medicine and Wolters Kluwer Health, Inc.

- If vasopressors are required, norepinephrine is generally used first line. Epinephrine is the adjunctive agent of choice.
- If none of these measures successfully restores hemodynamic stability, IV hydrocortisone 200 mg/d can be considered.
- **Diagnosis** should include obtaining cultures as long as collection does not delay antimicrobial therapy >60 minutes and imaging studies if this will help confirm the source of infection.
- Broad-spectrum antibiotics should be initiated within 1 hour of recognizing sepsis or septic shock. Regimens should be assessed daily, and empiric therapy should not be continued beyond 3 to 5 days. Early source control should be pursued aggressively and should involve removal of nonessential intravascular devices.
- **Toxic shock syndrome** occurs in <5 per 100 000 reproductive age women. Staphylococcal toxic shock syndrome (STSS) results from toxin 1 produced by *Staphylococcus aureus*. Toxic shock–like syndrome (TSLS) results from pyrogenic exotoxin produced by group A *Streptococcus* (GAS). Both can cause dramatic and rapid critical illness, including fever, hypotension, malaise, mucosal hyperemia, erythroderma and desquamation, and diarrhea. There is an association with extended or superabsorbent tampon use, surgical wounds, skin infection, and abscesses. An STSS can occur in otherwise healthy individuals, whereas a TSLS typically presents with a prior infection. Blood cultures can be negative.
- The **diagnostic criteria** for STSS are the following: fever >39.9°C; diffuse blanching erythroderma progressing to desquamation at 10 to 14 days, especially on the palms and soles; hypotension with systolic BP <90 mm Hg or orthostasis; and involvement of three or more organ systems such as gastrointestinal

(diarrhea, vomiting), musculoskeletal (severe myalgia, creatine kinase > twice upper limit of normal), mucous membrane hyperemia (oropharynx, conjunctiva, vagina), renal dysfunction (BUN or creatinine > twice upper limit), liver dysfunction (bilirubin, aspartate aminotransferase, or alanine transaminase > twice the upper limit), hematologic abnormalities (platelets <100 000/mL), or mental status changes without focal findings. Diagnostic criteria for TSLS are similar but require isolation of GAS and dysfunction in at least two organ systems.

- The **differential diagnosis** includes Rocky Mountain spotted fever, Stevens-Johnson syndrome, scarlet fever, viral exanthems, drug reaction, meningococcemia, leptospirosis, and heat stroke.
- **Treatment** includes early recognition, elimination/debridement of infectious source if identified, antibiotics, and ICU supportive care with fluids, oxygen, and vasopressors if needed. Mortality ranges from 5% to 60% depending on the bacterial strain and severity of illness.
    - β-Lactam agents, including penicillin G are effective against GAS, whereas STSS requires vancomycin, nafcillin, or oxacillin.
    - Clindamycin is given for its inhibitory action on protein synthesis including toxin suppression.
    - In patients who do not show rapid clinical response, immunoglobulins may be administered to neutralize superantigens and potentially shorten the disease course.

SPECIAL OBSTETRIC CONSIDERATIONS IN CRITICAL CARE

Hypertension, hemorrhage, sepsis, and cardiopulmonary conditions account for the majority of intensive care admissions in the antepartum and postpartum period. Physiologic alterations in pregnancy can continue into the postpartum period and are important to account for when interpreting critical care data.

- Profound **hemodynamic alterations** occur during pregnancy, including a 40% to 50% increase in blood volume, 30% to 50% increase in cardiac output, decrease in systemic vascular resistance, and increase in heart rate. Little data exists to determine the utility of invasive hemodynamic monitoring in obstetric patients.
- Although the need for **cardiopulmonary resuscitation** is rare, left lateral uterine displacement is essential to maximizing cardiac output generated during chest compressions.
- In addition to etiologies typically seen outside of pregnancy, chorioamnionitis, pyelonephritis, tocolytic therapy, and preeclampsia should be considered when an obstetric patient presents with **ARDS**. In this condition, pregnancy-induced respiratory alkalosis may be exacerbated by hyperventilation. Otherwise, management with supportive care and lung protective ventilation is similar to that for nonobstetric patients.
- Colloid osmotic pressure is decreased by up to 20% in pregnancy thereby increasing the risk of developing cardiogenic and noncardiogenic pulmonary edema, especially in women with underlying cardiac conditions. Careful fluid management in these patients is paramount.
- In critically ill obstetric patients, the decision to move toward delivery should be evaluated as a patient's clinical course evolves. If a condition is exacerbated by pregnancy and is refractory to all conservative interventions, delivery can be considered.

The risks of prematurity should be carefully balanced with the risks to the mother of maintaining her pregnancy.

- Cardiac arrest in pregnancy: If return to spontaneous circulation does not occur within the first few minutes of maternal resuscitation (including cardiopulmonary resuscitation), resuscitative hysterotomy and delivery of the fetus via a perimortem cesarean delivery is recommended if the uterine size is at or above the umbilicus (about 20 wk size).

SUGGESTED READINGS

Carson JL, Guyatt G, Heddle NM, et al. Clinical practice guidelines from the AABB: red blood cell transfusion thresholds and storage. *JAMA*. 2016;316(19):2025-2035.

Finfer S, Bellomo R, Boyce N, et al; for Safe Study Investigators. A comparison of albumin and saline for fluid resuscitation in the intensive care unit. *N Engl J Med*. 2004;350:2247-2256.

Guntupalli KK, Hall N, Karnad DR, Bandi V, Belfort M. Critical illness in pregnancy: part I: an approach to a pregnant patient in the ICU and common obstetric disorders. *Chest*. 2015;148(4):1093-1104.

Guntupalli KK, Karnad DR, Bandi V, Hall N, Belfort M. Critical illness in pregnancy: part II: common medical conditions complicating pregnancy and puerperium. *Chest*. 2015;148(5):1333-1345.

Marino P. *Marino's the ICU Book*. 4th ed. Philadelphia, PA: Lippincott Williams & Wilkins; 2014.

Rhodes A, Evans LE, Alhazzani W, et al. Surviving sepsis campaign: international guidelines for management of sepsis and septic shock: 2016. *Crit Care Med*. 2017;45(3):486-552.

Ricci Z, Cruz D, Ronco C. The RIFLE criteria and mortality in acute kidney injury: a systematic review. *Kidney Int*. 2008;73(5):538-546.

Yancy CW, Jessup M, Bozkurt B, et al. 2017 ACC/AHA/HFSA focused update of the 2013 ACCF/AHA guideline for management of heart failure: a report of the American College of Cardiology/American Heart Association Task Force on Clinical Practice Guidelines and the Heart Failure Society of America. *J Am Coll Cardiol*. 2017;70(6):776-803.

Quality, Safety, and Value in Women's Health

Anna Jo Smith and Judy M. Lee

According to the Merriam-Webster dictionary, *quality* can be defined as a "degree of excellence." Within the health care setting, achieving a high degree of excellence in patient care starts with responsive leadership and a culture of safety. Traditional models of care and quality assurance focused on individuals and individual events. Today, the focus has shifted to an educational model, where structure, process, and outcomes are the basis for continuous quality assessment and improvement. By being responsive to changes needed to reduce risk, and promote a culture of safety, health care organizations can inspire, cultivate, and innovate delivery of the highest quality of care for its patients.

BACKGROUND

- The United States has the highest maternal and infant mortality rates of any high-income country. African American women are more than 3 times as likely to die during pregnancy and postpartum than white women and twice as likely to die of cervical cancer than white women. Although some differences may be related to underlying health status (eg, hypertension, obesity, smoking), there is substantial variance between hospitals in rates of cesarean deliveries, postpartum hemorrhage, and infection that contributes to health disparities. Improving the quality and safety of women's health care nationwide can help address these disparities.
- In 2001, the Institute of Medicine Committee on Quality of Health Care in United States published their vision to improve health care quality. Their aim is for health care to be (1) safe, (2) effective, (3) timely, (4) patient centered, (5) equitable, and (6) efficient. Three major components or strategies of a quality program that can be considered in building this Institute of Medicine vision of a health care system are quality assurance, continuous improvement, and clinical innovation.

QUALITY ASSURANCE

- Quality assurance eliminates or prevents substandard practices.
- External examples of quality assurance can include oversight or recognition through organizations or processes such as the following:
  - Accreditation Council for Graduate Medical Education: among other standards, includes procedure minimums for resident surgical training
  - Specialty-specific board exams, certification, and maintenance of certification requirements
  - Hospital accreditation by organizations, such as The Joint Commission
  - Recognition for nursing excellence and high-quality patient care by the American Nurses' Credentialing Center in awarding a hospital Magnet status
- Internal examples of quality assurance can be at the department or hospital level such as the following:
  - A credentialing and privileging process that verifies, evaluates, and oversees practitioners in their practice, judgment, and technical skills
  - Chart review process or chart audit for major events, such as shoulder dystocias
  - A period of focused professional practice evaluation if needed and as defined by The Joint Commission, such as when concern is raised over a particular competency or behavior
  - A peer review process
  - The "**Checklist**" movement in medicine takes complex processes, such as preparing a patient for the operating room and breaks these processes down into simple standardized steps. Such checklists have identified safety hazards, such as missed antibiotics or venous thromboembolism prophylaxis, and helped decrease surgical complications. Others have resulted in decreasing catheter-associated urinary tract infections and central line–associated bloodstream infections. Institutions can optimize the use of checklists in at-risk clinical situations and measuring compliance.

CONTINUOUS IMPROVEMENT

- Whereas there is a spectrum of care within which organizations operate, by ensuring there is a process for identifying areas for improvement, organizations can make effective, consistent progress over time.
- Continuous improvement, or quality improvement, projects are best designed with specific, measurable, attainable, relevant, and time-bound goals.
- The Alliance for Innovation on Maternal Health, an initiative of the American College of Obstetricians and Gynecologists and 30 other organizations, is one such model currently being rolled out nationwide. The Alliance for Innovation on Maternal Health provides hospitals and providers with **patient safety "bundles,"** such as strategies to reduce postpartum hemorrhage, tools to identify women at high risk for adverse obstetrical outcomes, data to benchmark individual practices against national trends, and patient education resources. These tools are available free online.
- Examples of quality improvement projects are the following:
  - **Enhanced recovery after surgery** programs have reduced lengths of stay, decreased complications, and/or increased patient satisfaction (see chapter 60).
  - **Emergency drills** allow providers, including interdisciplinary (nurses, midwives, anesthesia) team members, to practice the skills and team-based coordination needed for an emergency.
  - **Simulation** exercises can be designed and employed for technically complicated and/or uncommon procedures such as minimally invasive techniques, including robotic surgery, repair of fourth-degree lacerations, and neonatal resuscitation. Two common scenarios for team-based simulation include shoulder dystocia and postpartum hemorrhage.
  - Regular unit-based meetings or huddles about patient safety introduce a systematic way through which staff can communicate to improve patient care, patient safety, and teamwork; they can also result in a cultural shift in attitude toward communication and patient safety.
- The plan-do-study-act or plan-do-check-act cycle is a frequently used tool to test interventions, observe outcomes, and adapt to lessons learned. Through an iterative process, ideas are refined to achieve desired outcomes.
- **Root cause analysis (RCA)** is a retrospective process aimed at analyzing adverse events or sentinel events. The goal is not only to identify solutions for what went wrong but also to prevent or mitigate such an event occurring in the future. It is important to perform team-based debriefing and reviews after safety events or near misses where findings from an RCA can be communicated back to the team. The goal of the RCA is to identify fixable problems without placing blame and to build a culture of safety on the unit.
- **Clinical audits** are commonly employed to ensure compliance with certain clinical guidelines or practices. These measure a set of outcomes or processes and compare the results against desired standards, benchmarks, or evidence-based medicine; the aim of which is to identify changes to improve quality of care. Ensuring compliance can also be seen in the form of a clinical pathway or order sets that default to important settings that require indicators or quality metrics fundamental to the performance of a hospital, department, or service.
- **Quality metrics or clinical indicators** involve evaluating a process (eg, time to patient appointment, rate of cesarean delivery among nulliparous women) or an outcome (eg, surgical site infection, venous thromboembolism, unplanned hospital

readmission, term admission to the neonatal intensive care unit, unplanned return to the operating room, mortality).

- A metric can have a goal of increasing or decreasing use of an intervention, such as vaccination administration or cesarean deliveries. Involving patients and/or their families and local communities in developing metrics can help identify unexpected ways to improve patient centeredness and equity of obstetrician-gynecologist services.
- Quality metrics may also be a way to improve efficiency of health care, especially by reducing overused services. For example, the "**Choosing Wisely**" campaign, an international initiative to decrease low-value care in partnership with physician groups, has identified hundreds of small changes to decrease health care costs. There are "Choosing Wisely" recommendations from American College of Obstetricians and Gynecologists, Society for Maternal-Fetal Medicine, American Society for Colposcopy and Cervical Pathology, American Society for Reproductive Medicine, and the Society for Gynecologic Oncology.

CLINICAL INNOVATION

- Clinical innovation is aimed at moving health care practice and delivery forward into new areas through innovation and research.
- Innovation in health care can include anything from new surgical techniques to drug delivery systems, genomics, and diagnosis methods. It can include innovative processes in streamlining access to care, such as providing home-based telehealth to patients with chronic diseases, providing wearable biosensors, and improving patient education through intelligent app-based care modules. Often, clinical innovation is hospital or clinic specific; therefore, awareness of what is happening in your clinical area can lead to a small but highly effective projects.
- One survey of leaders across the health care industry noted the following top 10 health care innovations: next generation sequencing, 3-dimensional printed devices, immunotherapy, artificial intelligence, point-of-care diagnostics, virtual reality, leveraging social media to improve patient experience, biosensors and trackers, convenient care, and telehealth.
- With the shift toward value-based care and the exponential growth in innovation and technology, hospitals and providers will have to innovate to stay competitive while providing safe, quality care and reducing costs.

SUGGESTED READINGS

ABIM Foundation. Choosing Wisely recommendations. Choosing Wisely Web site. http://www.choosingwisely.org/getting-started/lists/. Accessed November 5, 2018.

American College of Obstetricians and Gynecologists, Women's Health Care Physicians. *Quality and Safety in Women's Health Care*. 2nd ed. Washington, DC: American College of Obstetricians and Gynecologists; 2010.

Council on Patient Safety in Women's Health Care. Alliance for Innovation on Maternal Health. Council on Patient Safety in Women's Health Care Web site. https://safehealthcareforeverywoman.org/aim-program/. Accessed November 5, 2018.

Institute of Medicine Committee on Quality of Health Care in America. *Crossing the Quality Chasm: A New Health System for the 21st Century*. Washington, DC: National Academies Press; 2001.

Pellegrini JE, Toledo P, Soper DE, et al. Consensus bundle on prevention of surgical site infections after major gynecologic surgery. *Obstet Gynecol*. 2017;129(1):50-61.

Pettker CM, Grobman WA. Obstetric safety and quality. *Obstet Gynecol*. 2015;126(1):196-206.

Index

Page numbers followed by *f* indicate a figure; page numbers followed by *t* indicate a table.